W.-B. Schill · F. H. Comhaire · T. B. Hargreave (Eds.)
Andrology for the Clinician

W.-B. Schill · F. H. Comhaire ·
T. B. Hargreave (Eds.)

Andrology for the Clinician

With 225 Figures in 300 Parts and 120 Tables

Springer

Prof. em. Dr. Dr. Wolf-Bernhard Schill
Center of Dermatology and Andrology, Justus Liebig University Giessen
Gaffystraße 14
35385 Giessen, Germany

Prof. em. Dr. Frank Comhaire
Center for Medical and Urological Andrology and Reproductive
Endocrinology, University Hospital Ghent 6K12IE
De Pintelaan 185
9000 Ghent, Belgium

Prof. Dr. Timothy B. Hargreave
Department of Oncology, University of Edinburgh
Human Genetics Building, Western General Hospital
Edinburgh EH4 2XU
Scotland UK

ISBN 3-540-23171-4 Springer-Verlag Berlin Heidelberg New York

Library of Congress Control Number: 2005935881

Springer is a part of Springer Science+Business Media
http://www.springer.com

Editor: Marion Philipp
Desk Editor: Ellen Blasig
Production Editor: Joachim W. Schmidt

Cover design: eStudio Calamar, Spain

Typesetting: FotoSatz Pfeifer GmbH, D-82166 Gräfelfing
Printed on acid-free paper - 24/3151 - 5 4 3 2 1 0

Foreword

Andrology in its widest sense is a fast growing medical discipline with special emphasis on the disturbances of male reproductive function including erectile dysfunction and problems of the ageing male. There is a great need to educate both the specialists who practise as andrologists, such as endocrinologists, urologists and dermatologists, as well as the general practitioner, who is often involved in the management of these patients. Three international scientists from different medical disciplines (dermatology, endocrinology and urology) have created an alternative to a classical textbook by providing a new format in this book to facilitate the review of information in the field provided by a large number of international experts.

This textbook is written in two parts. Part I provides easily accessible, brief, problem-oriented information about modern andrology including male factor infertility, male contraception, male genital tract infection and tumours. The book is intended to be of use to the busy clinician and to provide quick access to didactic information about current practice. Part II is subject-oriented and provides the background scientific information for the recommendations in Part I. The three editors are recognized experts in the field and have invited key international scientists to write various sections of this book but, by their extensive sub-editing, have created a homogeneous concept. The key features of this book are the clear recommendations about current practice and easy access to the underlying science. I have no doubt that this textbook will be an asset to the clinical andrologist by facilitating information on to the rapidly increasing scientific data in the fast growing field of andrology.

It is the aim of this textbook to reach doctors working in the field of andrology all over the world but should be of particular value in European countries. The book will be valuable for urologists, andrologists, dermatologists, endocrinologists, gynaecologists, reproductive biologists, general practitioners, gerontologists, psychologists, psychiatrists, paediatricians and paramedicals including all professions allied to medicine as well as pharmaceutical companies working in the field of andrology. I am sure that the book will be a great success and will be of great value to its readers.

David de Kretser
Monash Institute of Medical Research
Monash University, Melbourne

Preface

Andrology is the medical practice of disorders that afflict men. These include congenital and acquired abnormalities of the male reproductive system as well as disorders of the male endocrine system. As these may be treated by different disciplines including endocrinology, dermatology, urological surgery, plastic surgery, oncology, venereology, and sexual medicine, it is difficult for doctors in these various specialties to have a holistic view of andrology. We hope that this book will be a source of reference to the broad spectrum of andrological conditions and that it will promote a holistic view of andrology and catalyse interdisciplinary co-operation in the management of andrological disorders.

The book is written in two parts: Part I presents current clinical practice, whereas PartII provides the reader with more detail on the theoretical background. The reader will find chapters on the diagnosis and treatment of disorders of male fertility, disorders of male sexual function, sexually transmitted infections, disorders of androgen status, including ageing changes, and chapters on benign and malignant growths of the male reproductive organs. In addition, we have included chapters on phytotherapeutics and aesthetic dermatology and medical cosmetics because in practice many men seek these treatments and the competent andrologist needs to understand alternative as well as traditional approaches.

Our contributors are from many different countries and each is an acknowledged expert. Wherever possible, reference has been made to the results of randomized clinical trials and it has been our intention that the information in this book should be evidence-based. All contributors were asked to present a comprehensive review of their field as well as their own work.

In previous years, andrological problems have been relatively ignored but this is changing because of the development of effective treatments such as phosphodiesterase inhibitors for erectile dysfunction and 5-α-reductase inhibitors for prostatic enlargement, and as a result, greater media coverage of andrological disorders. Therefore, more men seek treatment and increasingly men expect their clinician to be well informed about all aspects of andrology. We hope that this book will help advance towards that objective.

Wolf-Bernhard Schill, Frank Comhaire, Timothy Hargreave
Giessen – Ghent – Edinburgh, February 2006

Contents

List of Contributors

Wolf-Bernhard Schill, Co-ordinating Editor
Centre of Dermatology and Andrology, Justus Liebig University Giessen, Gaffystr. 14, 35385 Giessen, Germany (e-mail: wb@prof_schill.de/www.prof-schill.de)

Tevita F. 'Aho
Addenbrooke's NHS Foundation Trust, Department of Urology, Box 43, Hills Rd, Cambridge CB2 2QQ, UK (e-mail: tevita.aho@addenbrookes.nhs.uk

William Derval Aiken
Department of Surgery, University of the West Indies Mona, Kingston 7, Jamaica (e-mail: uroplum23@yahoo.com)

Omer Baldo
Pyrah Department of Urology, St. James University Hospital, Beckett Street, Leeds LS9 7TF, UK

Arnold M. Belker
University of Louisville School of Medicine, Department of Urology, Louisville, Kentucky 40292, USA, 250 E. Liberty St., Suite 602, Louisville, KY 40202 USA (e-mail: abelker@aol.com)

Martin Bergmann
Institute of Veterinary Anatomy, Histology and Embryology, Justus Liebig University, Frankfurterstr. 98, 35392 Giessen, Germany (e-mail: martin. bergmann@vetmed.uni-giessen.de)

Manfred Beutel
Clinic and Policlinic for Psychosomatic Medicine and Psychotherapy, Johannes Gutenberg University, Untere Zahlbacher Str. 8, 55131 Mainz, Germany (e-mail: beutel@psychosomatik.klinik.uni-mainz.de)

M.C. Bishop
Department of Urology, Nottingham City Hospital NHS Trust, Nottingham, NG5 1 PB, UK (e-mail: tguyler@ncht.trent.nhs.uk)

N. Bliesener
Institute for Clinical Biochemistry, Endocrinology, University of Bonn, Sigmund-Freud-Str. 25, 53105 Bonn, Germany

Jens Peter Bonde
Department of Occupational Medicine, Århus University Hospital, Nørrebrogade 44, Building 2 C, 8000 Århus C, Denmark (e-mail: jpbon@akh.aaa.dk)

Riana Bornman
Department of Urology, Faculty of Health Sciences, University of Pretoria, PO Box 169 Pretoria 0001, South Africa (e-mail: mbornman@medic.up.ac.za)

Marc E. Bracke
Laboratory of Experimental Cancerology, Department of Radiotherapy and Nuclear Medicine, University Hospital, De Pintelaan 185, 9000 Ghent, Belgium, Laboratory Nuytinck, Reibroekstraat 13, 9940 Evergem, Belgium (e-mail: brackemarc@hotmail.com)

Burkhard Brosig
Centre of Psychosomatic Medicine, Clinic for Psychosomatics and Psychotherapy, Ludwigstr. 76, 35392 Giessen, Germany (e-mail: Burkhard.Brosig@psycho.med.uni-giessen.de)

Giovanni M. Colpi
Unità di Andrologia, Ospedale San Paolo, Polo Universitario, Milano, Italy (e-mail: gmcolpi@yahoo.com)

Frank Comhaire
Centre for Medical and Urological Andrology and Reproductive Endocrinology, University Hospital Ghent 6K12IE, De Pintelaan 185, 9000 Ghent, Belgium (e-mail: Frank.Comhaire@Ugent.be)

K. Dawson
Monash Immunology and Stem Cell Laboratories, Monash University, Wellington Road, Clayton, Victoria, 3800, Australia

Christophe Depuydt
Laboratory for Clinical Pathology, Amerikalei 62–64, 2000 Antwerp, Belgium (e-mail: Christophe.Depuydt@riatol.be)

J. Michael Dixon
Edinburgh Breast Unit, Western General Hospital, Crewe Road South, Edinburgh EH4 2XU, UK (e-mail: mike.dixon@ed.ac.uk)

Gert R. Dohle
Department of Urology, Erasmus Medisch Centrum Rotterdam, P.O. Box 2040, 3000 CA Rotterdam, The Netherlands (e-mail: G.R.Dohle@erasmusmc.nl)

Ian Eardley
Pyrah Department of Urology, St. James University Hospital, Beckett Street, Leeds LS9 7TF, UK (e-mail: ian.eardley@btinternet.com)

Jakob Eberhard
Department of Oncology, Lund University Hospital, Lund, Sweden (e-mail: jakob.eberhard@kir.mas.lu.se)

David J. Elliott
Institute of Human Genetics, International Centre for Life, University of Newcastle-upon-Tyne, Central Parkway, Newcastle NE1 3BZ, UK (e-mail: David.Elliott@ncl.ac.uk)

Christine Mary Evans
Smithy Cottage, Llanarmon-yn-ial, Mold, CH74QXN, Wales, UK (e-mail: christinemaryevans@hotmail.com)

K. Everaert
Department of Urology, Ghent University Hospital, De Pintelaan 185, 9000 Ghent, Belgium (e-mail: karel.everaert@UGent.be, Tel.: + 32-92-402276)

Harry Fisch
Clinical Urology Department of Urology, Columbia University, Columbia University Medical Center of New York, Presbyterian Hospital, 944 Park Avenue, New York, NY, USA (e-mail: harryfisch@aol.com)

Yigal Gat
Andrology Unit, Department of Obstetrics and Gynecology, Rabin Medical Center, Beilinson Campus, Petah Tiqva and Sackler Faculty of Medicine, Tel Aviv University, Tel Aviv, Israel (e-mail: yigalgat@yahoo.com)

Aleksander Giwercman
Fertility Centre, Malmö University Hospital, 20502 Malmö, Sweden (e-mail: aleksander.giwercman@kir.mas.lu.se)

Louis J.G. Gooren
Department of Endocrinology, Andrology section, Vrije Universiteit Medical Centre, P.O. Box 7057, 1007 MB Amsterdam, The Netherlands (e-mail: ljg.gooren@vumc.nl)

Michael Gornish
Department of Radiology and the Interventional and Vascular Unit, Rabin Medical Center, Beilinson Campus, Petah Tiqva and Sackler Faculty of Medicine, Tel Aviv University, Tel Aviv, Israel

Alexander von Graevenitz
Department of Medical Microbiology, University of Zürich, Gloriastrasse 32, 8028 Zürich, Switzerland (e-mail: avg@immv.unizh.ch)

Gerhard Haidl
Department of Dermatology/Andrology Unit, University of Bonn, Sigmund-Freud-Str. 25, 53105 Bonn, Germany (e-mail: gerhard.haidl@ukb.uni-bonn.de)

David J. Handelsman
ANZAC, Research Institute & Department of Andrology, Concord Hospital, University of Sydney, Sydney NSW 2139, Australia (e-mail: djh@anzac.edu.au)

Timothy B. Hargreave
Department of Oncology, Edinburgh University, Human Genetics Building, Western General Hospital, Edinburgh EH4 2XU, UK (e-mail: tbhargreave@btinternet.com)

Christiaan Frederik Heyns
Department of Urology, Faculty of Health Sciences, University of Stellenbosch and Tygerberg Hospital, PO Box 19063, Tygerberg 7505, South Africa (e-mail: Cfh2@sun.ac.za)

Emmanuele A. Jannini
Course of Medical Sexology and Endocrinology, Dept. of Experimental Medicine, University of L'Aquila Coppito, Bldg. 2, Room A2/54. Via Vetoio, 67100 L'Aquila, Italy (e-mail: eaj@iol.it)

Andreas Jung
Justus Liebig University Giessen, Gaffkystr. 14, 35385 Giessen, Germany (e-mail: Andreas.Jung@derma-med.uni-giessen.de)

Jean M. Kaufman
Department of Endocrinology, Laboratory of Hormonology and Unit for Osteoporosis and Metabolic Bone Diseases, Ghent University Hospital, De Pintelaan 185, 9000 Ghent, Belgium (e-mail: Jean.Kaufman@ugent.be)

David Kirk
Urology Department, Gartnavel General Hospital, 1053 Great Western Road, Glasgow G12 0YN, UK (e-mail: Dkirk70683@aol.com)

Dietrich Klingmüller
Institute for Clinical Biochemistry, Endocrinology, University of Bonn, Sigmund-Freud-Str. 25, 53105 Bonn, Germany (e-mail: d.Klingmueller@uni-bonn.de)

Frank-Michael Köhn
Department of Dermatology and Allergology, Technical University, Biedersteiner Str. 29, 80802 Munich, Germany (e-mail: Frank.Koehn@lrz.tu-muenchen.de)

Kenjiro Kohri
Department of Nephro-urology, Nagoya City University Graduate School of Medical Sciences, 1 Kawasumi, Mizuho-cho, Mizuho-ku, Nagoya 467-8601, Japan (e-mail: kohri@med.nagoya-cu.ac.jp)

Yoshiyuki Kojima
Department of Nephro-urology, Nagoya City University Graduate School of Medical Sciences, 1 Kawasumi, Mizuho-cho, Mizuho-ku, Nagoya 467-8601, Japan (e-mail: ykojima@med.nagoya-cu.ac.jp)

Gabor Thomas Kovacs
Monash University, Department of Obstetrics and Gynaecology, Box Hill Hospital, Victoria, Australia (e-mail: gab.kovacs@boxhill.org.au)

Walter Krause
Department of Andrology and Venerology, University Hospital, Philipp University, 35033 Marburg, Germany (e-mail: Krause@mailer.uni-marburg.de)

John N. Krieger
Department of Urology, University of Washington School of Medicine, Box 356510, Seattle, WA 98195, USA (e-mail: jkrieger@u.washington.edu)

Pardeep Kumar
The St Peter's Andrology Centre and Institute of Urology, 48 Riding House St, London W1P 7PN, UK (e-mail: pardeepkumar@hotmail.com)

Jan Kunnen
Department of Radiology and Medical Imaging, ZNA Middelheim Hospital, Lindendreef 1, 2020 Antwerp, Belgium (e-mail: Jan.Kunnen@zna.be)

Marc Kunnen
Department of Radiology and Medical Imaging, University Hospital Ghent, De Pintelaan 185, 9000 Ghent, Belgium

Andrea Lenzi
Chair of Clinical Pathology, Department of Medical Physiopathology, University of Rome „La Sapienza“ Policlinico Umberto I, 00161 Rome, Italy (e-mail: andrea.lenzi@uniroma1.it)

Steve Ken Wing Leung
Prostate Research Group, School of Molecular and Clinical Medicine, The University of Edinburgh, Western General Hospital, Crewe Road South, Edinburgh EH4 2XU, UK (e-mail: Steem21@hotmail.com)

Yvonne Lundberg Giwercman
Department of Urology, Wallenberg Laboratory, Malmö University Hospital, 20502 Malmö, Sweden (e-mail: Yvonne.Giwercman@kir.mas.lu.se)

Ahmed Mahmoud
Center for Medical and Urological Andrology and Reproductive Endocrinology, University Hospital Ghent 6K12IE, De Pintelaan 185, 9000 Ghent, Belgium (e-mail: ahmed.mahmoud@ugent.be)

Mario Mancini
Unità di Andrologia, Ospedale San Paolo, Polo Universitario, Milano, Italy

S. Alan McNeill
Department of Urology, Western General Hospital, Crewe Road, Edinburgh, EH4 2XU, UK (e-mail: alan.mcneill@luht.scot.nhs.uk)

Andreas Meinhardt
Department of Anatomy and Cell Biology, Justus-Liebig University Giessen, Aulweg 123, 35385 Giessen, Germany (e-mail: Andreas.Meinhardt@anatomie.med.uni-giessen.de)

E.J.H. Meuleman
Free University of Amsterdam, Medical Centre Department of Urology, de Boelelaan 1117, 1081 HV Amsterdam, The Netherlands

Ian David Cumming Mitchell
Department of Urology, Queen Margaret Hospital, Whitefield Road Dunfermline, Fife KY12 0SU, UK (e-mail: iandcmitchell@btinternet.com)

Christina Müller
Centre of Dermatology and Andrology, Justus Liebig University, Gaffkystr. 14, 35385, Giessen, Germany (e-mail: Christina.mueller@derma.med.uni- giessen.de)

David Edgar Neal
Department of Urology, Addenbrooke's NHS Foundation Trust, Department of Oncology, Oncology Centre, Box 193, Addenbrooke's Site, Hills Road, Cambridge CB2 2QQ, UK (e-mail: Den22@cam.ac.uk)

Els L.F. Nijs
Department of Radiology, University Hospitals Gasthuisberg, Katholieke Universiteit Leuven, Herestraat 49, 3000 Leuven, Belgium (e-mail: Els.Nijs@uz.kuleuven.ac.be)

Agneta Nordenskjöld
Department of Molecular Medicine, CMM 02, Karolinska Hospital, 17176 Stockholm, Sweden (e-mail: Agneta.Nordenskjold@cmm.ki.se)

F.R. Ochsendorf
Centre of Dermatology and Venerology, J.W. Goethe University, Theodor-Stern-Kai 7, 60590-Frankfurt/M, Germany (e-mail: ochsendorf@em.uni-frankfurt.de)

Willem Ombelet
Genk Institute for Fertility Technology, Schiepse Bos 6, 3600 Genk, Belgium (e-mail: willem.ombelet@pandora.be)

Raymond H. Oyen
Department of Radiology, University Hospitals Gasthuisberg, Katholieke Universiteit Leuven, Herestraat 49, 3000 Leuven, Belgium (e-mail: Raymond.Oyen@uz.kuleuven.ac.be)

Guido Piediferro
Unità di Andrologia, Ospedale San Paolo, Polo Universitario, Milano, Italy

Roberto Ponchietti
University of Siena, Cattedra di Urologia, Policlinico S., Maria alle Scotte, Viale Bracci 13, 53110 Siena, Italy (e-mail: ponchietti@unisi.it)

David J. Ralph
The St Peter's Andrology Centre and Institute of Urology, 48 Riding House St, London W1P 7PN, UK (e-mail: dralph@andrology.co.uk)

Shoichi Sasaki
Department of Nephro-urology, Nagoya City University Graduate School of Medical Sciences, 1 Kawasumi, Mizuho-cho, Mizuho-ku, Nagoya 467–8601, Japan (e-mail: ssk@med.nagoya-cu.ac.jp)

Hans Gerd Schiefer
Department of Medical Microbiology, Justus Liebig University Giessen, Schubertstr. 1, 35392 Giessen, Germany (e-mail: agnes.kroener@mikrobio.med.uni-giessen.de)

Frank Schoonjans
Centre for Medical and Urological Andrology and Reproductive Endocrinology, University Hospital Ghent, 6K12IE, De Pintelaan 185, 9000 Ghent, Belgium (e-mail: Frank.Schoonjans@ugent.be)

Hans-Christian Schuppe
Centre of Dermatology and Andrology, Justus Liebig University, Gaffkystr. 14, 35385 Giessen, Germany (e-mail: Hans-Christian.Schuppe@derma.med.uni-giessen.de)

Fabrizio I. Scroppo
Unità di Andrologia, Ospedale San Paolo, Polo Universitario, Milano, Italy

Jay B. Shah
Squier Urological Clinic, Columbia University Medical Center, 161 Fort Washington Avenue, New York, NY 10032, USA (e-mail: jbs58@columbia.edu)

P.S.H. Soon
Edinburgh Breast Unit, Western General Hospital, Crewe Road South, Edinburgh EH4 2XU, UK

Olof Ståhl
Department of Oncology, Lund University Hospital, Lund, Sweden (e-mail: olof.stahl@kir.mas.lu.se)

Oleg Tatarov
Urology Department, Gartnavel General Hospital, 1053 Great Western Road, Glasgow G12 0YN, UK (e-mail: olegtatarov@hotmail.com)

Herman J. Tournaye
Centre for Reproductive Medicine, Dutch-speaking Brussels Free University Hospital, 101, Laarbeeklaan, 1090 Brussels, Belgium (e-mail: tournaye@az.vub.ac.be)

Alan Trounson
Monash Immunology and Stem Cell Laboratories, Monash University, Wellington Road, Clayton, Victoria, 3800, Australia (e-mail: jill.mcfadyean@med.monash.edu.au)

Guy G.R. T'Sjoen
Department of Endocrinology, University Hospital, Belgium 9K12IE, De Pintelaan 185, 9000 Ghent, Belgium (e-mail: guy.tsjoen@ugent.be)

Kevin James Turner
Department of Urology, Western General Hospital, Edinburgh, EH4 2XU, UK (e-mail: kevin@kkturner.freeserve.co.uk)

Lynne Turner-Stokes
Regional Rehabilitation Unit, Northwick Park Hospital, Watford Road Harrow, Middlesex HA1 3UJ, UK

Justin Alastair Vale
Consultant Urological Surgeon, St Mary's Hospital, Praed Street, London W2 1NY, UK (e-mail: j.vale@imperial.ac.uk)

Dirk Vanderschueren
Laboratory for Experimental Medicine and Endocrinology, Katholieke Universiteit Leuven, Campus Gasthuisberg, Onderwijs & Navorsing, Herestraat 49, 3000 Leuven, Belgium (e-mail: Dirk.Vanderschueren@uz.kuleuven.ac.be)

A.J. Visser
Garden City Hospital, Johannesburg, South Africa

Gorm Wagner
Dept. Medical Physiology, University of Copenhagen, Blegdamsvej 3, 2200 Copenhagen N, Denmark (e-mail: gorm@mfi.ku.dk)

Geoffrey Malcolm Hasting Waites (deceased)
ANZAC, Research Institute & Department of Andrology, Concord Hospital, University of Sydney, Sydney NSW 2139, Australia

R.F.A. Weber
Department of Andrology Erasmus MC, Dr. Molewaterplein, 40 3015 GD Rotterdam, The Netherlands (e-mail: r.f.a.weber@erasmusmc.nl)

Peter F. Wieacker
Institute for Human Genetics, Otto-von-Guericke University of Magdeburg, Leipziger Strasse 44, 39120 Magdeburg, Germany
(e-mail: Peter.Wieacker@medizin.uni-magdeburg.de)

Stefan A. Wudy
Centre of Child and Adolescent Medicine, Justus Liebig University, Feulgenstr. 12, 35392 Giessen, Germany
(e-mail: Stefan.wudy@paediat.med.uni-giessen.de)

Introduction

Andrology: Definition, Clinical Issues and Prevalence

W.-B. Schill, F. Comhaire, T.B. Hargreave

Andrology is a young interdisciplinary medical specialty derived linguistically from the Greek word "andros", which deals with the male with special emphasis of the physiology and pathophysiology of male reproductive functions. Therefore, primarily, its clinical focus is the diagnosis and therapy of male fertility disturbances. Thus, andrology is the male equivalent of gynaecology and deals with the disorders of the male reproductive organs. In some parts of the world, andrology is closely connected or even an integral part of in vitro fertilization centres. According to the definition of the World Health Organization (WHO), andrology is engaged in all aspects of male reproductive health.

In addition, andrology is concerned with problems of erectile dysfunction. Approximately 10% to 15% of andrology patients consult for disturbed sexual dysfunctions. The diagnosis and management of penis problems includes lack of firmness of penis erection or bending and deformity of the erect penis (Peyronie's disease). Recently, treating the ageing male has become another important issue. Because of dramatic changes in the demographic development of the age pyramid, there will be a tremendous change of the ratio old to young men within the next 20 years. Therefore, consultations on the part of older men will greatly increase, particularly in terms of health prevention and hormone dysfunction.

Further areas of andrological activities are the diagnosis and management of testicle problems and prostate disorders, for example prostate enlargement, inflammation or cancer (the latter being mostly a genuine problem of urology) prevention and rehabilitation, primary and secondary hypogonadism, delayed puberty, adverse drug side effects and environmental pollutants with regard to fertility, cryopreservation of semen and testicular tissue, forensic paternity problems, family planning, male contraception and basic andrological research. All these issues are of increasing importance for the further development of clinical andrology.

In summary, the following subjects are within the field of responsibility of andrology:

1. Male fertility and infertility
2. Erectile dysfunction and sexual disturbances
3. Ageing male and hormone replacement therapy
4. Male reproductive tract inflammation and infection
5. Testicle problems (testicular tumours)
6. Prostate disorders (BPH, carcinoma)
7. Primary and secondary hypogonadism
8. Delayed puberty
9. Prevention and rehabilitation
10. Adverse drug side effects
11. Environmental pollutants
12. Cryopreservation of semen and testicular tissue
13. Forensic paternity problems
14. Family planning
15. Male contraception
16. Basic andrological research

Historically, the term "andrology" was introduced in Germany in 1951 by the gynaecologist Harald Siebke from the university of Bonn, who considered andrology as a counterpart to gynaecology (Schirren 1985). Thereafter, andrology developed within the field of dermatovenereology (as in Egypt), where it was associated with names such as Döpfmer, Heinke, Adam, Meyhöfer, and Schirren (Adam 1986; Schirren 1989). The importance of andrology was acknowledged in 1958 when the newly established German Society for the Study of Fertility and Sterility considered andrology as a main part of its activities. In 1970, the Comité International de Andrología (CIDA) was founded in Barcelona, followed in 1973 by the Nordic Association of Andrology, in 1974 by the American Association of Andrology, and in 1975 by the German Society of Andrology. In 1976, the American Society of Andrology was established, followed in 1981 by the formation of the International Society of Andrology (www.andrology.org), which in 2005 was made up of 41 national member societies with more than 10,000 members. In 1992, the European Academy of Andrology was founded with the formation of andrology training centres on a European level (European Academy of Andrology, 2001). Today more than 16 training centres in Europe (Belgium, Denmark, Germany, Italy, the Netherlands, Poland, and Spain) have been appointed after a stringent international reviewing process by the European Academy of Andrology. Andrological activities have also been strengthened by ESHRE and other international societies involved in reproductive medicine. Dramatic changes have occurred after the availability of in vitro fertilization in the years after 1978, followed by intracytoplasmic sperm injection in the early 1990s. It is particularly remarkable that apart from infertility treatment, the spectrum of diseases treated is expanding via erection and ejaculation disorders to problems of the ageing male as well as to urological issues concerning inflammatory and neoplastic diseases of the testes, epididymides, and the prostate.

The international development of andrology shows that the field is mainly represented by clinicians from urology, endocrinology, dermatology, and gynaecology, depending on history and scientific activities. Thus the rapid development of andrology over the past 25 years (Prins and Bremner 2004) is reflected by the fact that in addition to several national andrological journals there are presently five international andrological periodicals available (*Andrologia* as the first international journal founded by Carl Schirren in 1969, *Journal of Andrology, International Journal of Andrology, Asian Journal of Andrology, Archives of Andrology*) and at least ten journals that are exclusively concerned with scientific questions of reproductive medicine and reproductive biology.

Curiously, the term "andrology" was first anecdotally used as early as 1891, when *JAMA* published an editorial entitled "Andrology as a speciality" (Niemi 1987). This editorial was soon forgotten but contained passages that are still valid today, after more than 110 years, and can therefore be considered a milestone of reproductive medicine. Later, in 1902, the first surgeon to treat the problem of obstructive azoospermia successfully was Edward Martin (1859–1938), who as a clinician already pointed out the need for accurate diagnosis in the treatment of male infertility and thus was recently considered as the founding father of modern clinical andrology (Jequier 1991).

Remarkably, from the historical point of view, one of the first books on human semen came from Joel (1953), Thaddeus Mann (1964, 1981) and Rune Eliasson (1971), the two latter particularly on seminal plasma biochemistry. In 1960, two German books were published on the subject of andrology: *Male Fertility Disturbances*, with more than 880 pages edited by the dermatologists Schuermann and Döpfmer, and *The Male Gonad* by the anatomist Tonutti in collaboration with colleagues from internal medicine and dermatology. Thus today most of the German university clinics of dermatology have training facilities and departments in andrology. In addition, during the last 50 years andrology was substantially influenced by urology (Macleod 1951; Macleod and Gold 1951a–c; Macleod et al. 1964; Tulloch 1953; Amelar et al. 1977; Kelami 1980; Whitfield et al. 1998) endocrinology (Hellinga 1950, 1957, 1976; Rosemberg and Paulsen 1970; Steinberger 1970, 1971; Comhaire 1996; Nieschlag and Behre 2000), immunology (Rümke and Hellinga 1959; Rümke 1965, 1970), and gynaecology (Schoysman 1961, 1964, 1968; Insler and Lunenfeld 1986). For example, andrology has been firmly integrated into the graduation rules for urologists, where important surgical procedures to overcome a severe male factor had been established. Historically, the term "andrology" as a medical subspecialty officially has been used in Italy since 1989, in France since 1993, in Poland since 1995, and in the Netherlands since 2003. Also, the European Dermatology Forum (EDF) is using the term "andrology". Therefore, the activities of the European Academy of Andrology (EAA) are of particular importance for the proclamation of andrology to receive more attention and awareness by the European health politicians. The most recent progress is the acceptance of andrology as a medical specialty by the medical associations of Indonesia (2002), and Germany (2003). In the latter, the acquisition of an additional skill in andrology may be acquired by dermatologists, endocrinologists, and urologists, but not by gynaecologists. A medical qualification officially certified by the medical association allows the identification of the specialist by the patient, guarantees quality control and efficiency assurance, and attracts more medical professionals to the field.

The diagnosis and treatment of childless couples require a particularly close cooperation between andrology and gynaecology, which has been conducted to the formation of centres of reproductive medicine in many places throughout the world. The causes of barren marriage stem equally from the female and the male, but in some cases may be compensated by the high fertility of the other partner. If there is coincidentally a sterility factor in both partners, a compensation is no longer possible, leading to a severe infertility problem. The definition of infertility commonly used is that more than 12 months are required to conceive. However, infertility shows considerable geographic variation. In general, the male factor contributes one-third to one-half of all factors that contribute to a couple's problem with conception (Hull et al. 1985). The prevalence of primary and secondary infertility is estimated to be 15% or more of all couples in their reproductive age (Bruckert 1991). Thus, the percentage of couples seeking medical advice and treatment for infertility is in the range of 5% to 17%. Lastly, 3% to 4% of all couples remain involuntarily childless at the end of their reproductive life phase (Templeton 1992).

Concerning the prevalence of male factor infertility, it is estimated to be in the range of 7 % of all men, under the assumption that a male factor is responsible in about half of the involuntarily childless couples. This incidence is above the prevalence of diabetes mellitus (Nieschlag and Behre 2000). In contrast to earlier reports that the male's age does not influence the couple's fertility, new data suggest that in addition to the female age factor, the age of the male should not be neglected (Dunson et al. 2004).

Besides a careful medical history, physical examination, and at least two spermiograms, andrological diagnosis comprises the enlarged semen analysis, including biochemical parameters and sperm function tests, hormonal diagnosis, immunological and microbiological examinations, cytogenetic analysis and, if necessary, testicular biopsies. Further diagnostic and therapeutic procedures may be required in interdisciplinary cooperation with urology, gynaecology, endocrinology, radiotherapy, sexology, psychosomatic medicine, neurology, psychiatry, and cytogenetics.

Both history taking and clinical examination of the male patient are essential for the andrological workup and the diagnosis of a male factor in the case of infertility. Often only the clinical examination of the patient allows the correct interpretation of the semen parameters, leading to an aetiopathologically orientated therapy. Therefore, to improve the management of andrological problems, formal training and training courses in clinical andrology are urgently required (Jequier 2004). This is underscored by the fact that presently only a few textbooks and WHO guidelines on the subject of andrology are available (Rowe et al. 1993, 2000; WHO 1999; Nieschlag and Behre 2000), together with some international congress proceedings (Waites et al. 1997; Robaire et al. 2001). In conclusion, further training and education in all aspects of clinical andrology is urgently needed.

References

Adam W (1986) Where stands andrology today? Retrospection and perspectives (in German) Hautarzt 37:472 – 475

Amelar RD, Dubin L, Walsh PC (1977) Male infertility. Saunders, Philadelphia, Pa.

Bruckert E (1991) How frequent is unintentional childlessness in Germany? Andrologia 23:245 – 250

Comhaire FH (1996) Male infertility. Clinical investigations, cause evaluation and treatment. Chapman and Hall Medical, London

Dunson DB, Baird DD, Colombo B (2004) Increased infertility with age in men and women. Obstet Gynecol 103:51 – 56

Eliasson R (1971) Standards for investigation of human semen. Andrologie 3:49 – 64

European Academy of Andrology (2001) Membership list 2001, statutes, andrology centres. Int J Androl 24, Suppl 1

Hellinga G (1957) Classification of male hypogonadism. Acta Endocrinol 31:148

Hellinga G (1959) Analysis of the seminal picture in the etiologic diagnosis of seminal pathology (Dutch). Ned Tijdschr Verloskd Gynaecol 50:267 – 284

Hellinga G (1976) Clinical andrology. William Heinemann Medical, London

Hull MG, Glazener CM, Kelly NJ, Conway DI, Foster PA, Hinton RA, Coulson C, Lambert PA, Watt EM, Desai KM (1985) Population study of causes, treatment and outcome of infertility. Br Med J 291:1693 – 1697

Insler V, Lunenfeld B (1986) Infertility: male and female. Churchill Livingstone, Edinburgh

Jequier AM(1991) Edward Martin (1859 – 1938).The founding father of modern clinical andrology. Int J Androl 14:1 – 10

Jequier AM (2004) Clinical andrology- still a major problem in the treatment of infertility. Hum Reprod 19:1245 – 1249

Joel CA (1953) Studies an human semen (in German). Schwabe, Bale

Kelami A (1980) Atlas of operative andrology. Selected operations on male genitalia and their accessory glands. Walter de Gruyter, Berlin

Macleod J (1951) Semen quality in 1000 men of known fertility and in 800 cases of infertile marriage. Fertil Steril 2:115 – 139

Macleod J, Gold RZ (1951a) The male factor in fertility and infertility. II. Spermatozoon counts in 1000 men of known fertility and in 1000 cases of infertile marriage. J Urol 66:436 – 449

Macleod J, Gold RZ (1951b) The male factor in fertility and infertility. III. An analysis of motile activity in the spermatozoa of 1000 fertile men and 1000 men in infertile marriage. Fertil Steril 2:187 – 207

Macleod J, Gold RZ (1951c) The male factor in fertility and infertility. VI. Sperm morphology in fertile and infertile marriage. Fertil Steril 2:394 – 414

Macleod J, Pazianos A, Ray BS (1964) Restoration of human spermatogenesis by menopausal gonadotrophins. Lancet 1:1196

Mann T (1964) The biochemistry of semen and of the male reproductive tract. Methuen, London

Mann T, Lutwak-Mann C (1981) Male reproductive function and semen. Springer, Berlin Heidelberg New York

Niemi M (1987) Andrology as a speciality – its origin. J Androl 8:201 – 202

Nieschlag E, Behre HM (2000) Andrology. Male reproductive health and dysfunction 2nd edn. Springer, Berlin Heidelberg New York

Prins GS, Bremner W (2004) The 25th volume: President's message: Andrology in the 20th century: a commentary on our progress during the past 25 years. J Androl 25:435 – 440

Robaire B, Chemes H, Morales CR (2001) Andrology in the 21st century. Proceedings of the VIIth International Congress of Andrology, Montreal, Canada. Medimond, Englewood, N.J.

Rosemberg E, Paulsen CA (1970) The human testis. Plenum, New York

Rowe PJ, Comhaire FH, Hargreave TB, Mellows HJ (1993, 2000) WHO manual for the standardized investigation and diagnosis of the infertile couple. Cambridge University Press, Cambridge

Rümke P (1965) Autospermagglutinins: a cause of infertility in men. Ann N Y Acad Sci 1234:696 – 701

Rümke P (1970) Sperm antibodies and their action upon human spermatozoa. Ann Inst Pasteur (Paris) 118:525 – 528

Rümke P, Hellinga G (1959) Autoantibodies against spermatozoa in sterile men. Am J Clin Pathol 32:357 – 363

Schirren C (1985) Andrology: origin and development of a special discipline in medicine. Andrologia 17:117 – 125

Schirren C (1989) History of andrology within dermatology (in German). Andrologia 21 [Suppl 1]

Schoysman R (1961) Exploration and physiological treatment of a case of male infertility (in French). Bull Soc R Belge Gynecol Obstet 31:445 – 450

Schoysman R (1964) Preliminary studies of the treatment of average oligospermia by human gonadotropins extracted from the urine of menopausal women (H.M.G.) (in French). Bull Soc R Belge Gynecol Obstet 34:399–407

Schoysman R (1968) Creation of an artificial spermatocele in agenesis of the deferent duct (in French). Bull Soc R Belge Gynecol Obstet 38:307–317

Schuermann H, Doepfmer R (1960) Fertility disturbances in man (in German) In: Jadassohn J (ed) Handbook of skin and venereal diseases. Supplementum VI/3. Springer, Berlin Heidelberg New York

Steinberger A, Steinberger E (1970) In vitro growth and development of mammalian testes. In: Johnson AD, Gomes WR, Vandemark NL (eds) The testis, vol II. Academic, New York, pp 363–391

Steinberger E (1971) Hormonal control of mammalian spermatogenesis. Physiol Rev 51:1

Templeton AA (1992) The epidemiology of infertility. In: Templeton AA, Drife JO (eds) Infertility. Springer, Berlin Heidelberg New York, pp 23–32

Tonutti E, Weller O, Schuchardt E, Heinke E (1960) The male gonad-structure, function, clinic – main features of andrology (in German). Georg Thieme, Stuttgart

Tulloch WS (1953) Testicular biopsy: indications and technique. Proc R Soc Med 46:838–839

Waites GMH, Frick J Baker GWH (1997) Current advances in andrology. Proceedings of the VI International Congress of Andrology, Salzburg, Austria. Monduzzi Editore, Bologna, Italy

Whitfield HN, Hendry WF, Kirby RS, Duckett JW (1998) Textbook of genitourinary surgery, 2nd edn, vol 1, 2. Blackwell, Oxford

World Health Organization (1999) WHO laboratory manual for the examination of human semen and sperm-cervical mucus interaction, 4th edn. Cambridge University Press, Cambridge

Layout and How to Use the Book

F. Comhaire

In everyday practice, the clinician is faced with patients consulting for different problems related to the broader field of andrology.

The first concern will be to rapidly gain information that is immediately applicable for the management of the patient.

The first part of the present book aims at providing this "express" information in a condensed manner and using a systematic sequence. Under the heading "Problem: . . .," the following items are addressed in sequence:

1. Definition of the disease
2. Aetiology and pathogenesis
3. History taking, physical examination, technical and laboratory findings
4. Differential diagnosis (when applicable)
5. Treatment
6. Expected treatment results
7. Prognosis
8. Prevention (when applicable)
9. Complementary considerations

The second part of the book includes more extended and detailed information giving the rationale, scientific background, and literature references and is organized into four major sections:

1. Understanding normal anatomy and function
2. Mechanisms of dysfunction and pathogenesis
3. Diagnostic tools
4. Therapeutic options

Whenever required or desired, the clinician can cross-reference from Part I to Part II in order to discover or ascertain the consensus-based and current knowledge supporting the guidelines that are summarized in Part I.

Although this book can perfectly serve as a teaching instrument, this is not its primary purpose. The editors have instead aimed at creating a working instrument for the everyday practice of the busy clinician. Neither the choice of the topics nor the contents of the book focus on completeness or considerations which are mostly irrelevant for clinical practice.

General Considerations

Evidence-Based Medicine in Reproductive Medicine and Andrology

F. Comhaire, A. Mahmoud

In modern, rational and scientific medicine, the pressure of society on practitioners is continuously increasing. Good health is considered a right, rather than a privilege, and the population expects diseases to be overcome promptly and efficiently. This applies to all diseases, including infertility.

More than before, it is emphasized that diagnosis and treatment must be based on the current best evidence that is acquired by high-standard scientific research and is applied judiciously and conscientiously.

Good clinicians have always relied on their personal experience and judgment to decide on the treatment strategy for individual patients, which may sometimes differ from current evidence (Kirk-Smith and Stretch 2001). The approach based on personal experience is sometimes questioned and even rejected as "authority-based" and, therefore, unscientific. The seeming difference between experience and evidence may result in conflicting views on, for example, the treatment of the infertile male with far-reaching ethical and economic consequences. The problem is complicated by the fact that different therapeutic strategies affect not only the consulting couple, but also the health and happiness of the future child.

First of all, there may be problems in defining the outcomes of treatment, e.g. of infertility. In the heterosexual couple, it is not just the dichotomy between whether or not there is a successful delivery, but several nuances must be considered. The time needed to reach the desired pregnancy, the physical and emotional invasiveness of treatment and its economic impact on society and the couple, possible adverse effects of the treatment for the mother, and the health of the offspring must be included in the decision-making process.

Men can only prove their fertility through the intermediate of their female partner (Steinberger et al. 1981), and the potential fertility of the latter is suboptimal in approximately half of the couples consulting for male infertility (WHO 1987). Therefore, some trials rely on an intermediate end-point to estimate the effect of treatment, namely sperm quality. However, the relation between semen characteristics and men's fertility is complicated, and techniques of sperm analysis are often poorly reproducible. So far, there is no single test on semen that can confidently predict the fertilizing potential. Treatment by means of in vitro fertilization (IVF) with or without ICSI hold an increased risk for congenital malformations (In't Veld et al. 1995; Sutcliffe et al. 1999; Koudstaal et al. 2000; Wennerholm et al. 2000; Hansen et al. 2002) or impaired development of the offspring (Strömberg et al. 2002), and must be used with extreme restraint. Such techniques should be reserved as an ultimate option when other solutions are excluded or have turned out to be ineffective (Mitchell 2002). Otherwise "children may become the nameless, faceless, voiceless victims of reproductive technology, because they do not have standing to oppose the use of those new technologies" (Berry 2002).

In the second place, the quality of current best evidence must be questioned and put through serious scrutiny. Evidence-based medicine attaches the highest value to evidence gained from double-blind randomized prospective trials (Ellis and Adams 1997). The crossover method should, however, be avoided in trials of reproductive medicine (Khan et al. 1996). Meta-analysis of selected trials is also considered highly valuable; whereas prospective (open label) cohort trials score much lower as to their scientific reliability. The lowest level is awarded to retrospective cohort studies and case studies. The reliability of meta-analysis is, however, highly questionable (Editorial 1997). It has indeed been documented that the correspondence between the conclusions of meta-analysis as compared to those of (subsequent) large-scale randomized trials is only 67% (LeLorier et al. 1997), so hardly better than by chance (50%). Hence, selecting treatment based on the evidence of meta-analyses may be incorrect in as many as one-third of patients! We should not bestow too much confidence to the conclusions of meta-analyses, particularly if these contradict medical experience or results of either prospective or retrospective cohort studies. This is particularly true if the trials on which the meta-analysis is based yield highly divergent outcomes (Comhaire and Mahmoud 2004; Evers and Collins 2004).

In addition, concern has risen about the reliability of the published randomized trials. Many of these are co-ordinated and financed ("sponsored") by companies (Miller and Shorr 2002) that have direct interest in a favourable outcome of the trial (Smith 1998; Stelfox et al. 1998), whereas the results of trials not generating the expected positive outcome may never be published, disclosed or cited (Kjaergard and Gluud 2002). Similarly, centres that dispose of particular techniques have a commercial interest in claiming high success rates (Teris 1998; Van Steirteghem 1998; Wilson 2002), and it may take years or even decades before the statistical manipulations are unveiled. For example, recent publications report the "real" effective success rate of assisted reproductive techniques such as IVF and ICSI to be more than 40 % lower than those claimed or extrapolated from theoretical models (Schroder et al. 2004).

There are many pitfalls that are inherent to the proper methodology of randomized trials (Cleophas 1996; Schulz and Grimes 2002). In correctly performed trials, the "blind" assignment to patients to groups is done by an external and independent body (Kiene 1996a, b; Fergusson et al. 2004), and not by the clinician or the centre directly involved in patient care. Furthermore, inevitably an unintentional bias in selecting cases will take place as soon as patients must consent to participate in a placebo-controlled trial, since a particular type of person may refuse to do so, or indeed accept recruitment because of perceived opportunistic self-interest.

It is usually accepted as self-evident that results obtained in randomized trials may confidently be extrapolated to the general population. However, participants of such trials are recruited on the basis of well-defined inclusion and exclusion criteria, and the selected "cases" may not be representative of the real-life patient population seen by clinicians. In the case of infertility treatment, many different factors can coincide in each particular couple and the implementation of recommendations gained from another (trial) population to individual couples may be unwarranted (Ellis and Adams 1997). Examples of confusing factors that are usually not considered are lifestyle (tobacco, alcohol, sedentary lifestyle, stress), educational and social status, exposure to environmental or professional agents, ethnic background, genetic constitution, etc.

Too often, no (statistical) evidence of effect is interpreted as evidence of no effect. Whereas the latter may be true, there are many reasons why it may in fact not be correct. Evidencing the effect of a particular treatment that results in relatively minor improvement (e.g. from 15 % to 25 % success) requires a large number of cases in the treated and the control groups in order to reach a reasonable power of confidence. Any trial not reaching this number of participants will suffer from a type 2 or beta error, and the conclusions are invalid. Large trials commonly require a multi-centre effort, which introduces additional confounders such as the diagnostic adequacy (Kassirer and Kopelman 1989) and the therapeutic (surgical) expertise of the clinicians (Nilsson et al. 1979; Olive 1996), the quality of the laboratory (Clements et al. 1995; Neuwinger et al. 1990), etc.

Finally, randomized trials are subjected to ethical concerns when the implementation of a reasonably validated treatment comes into conflict with the requirements of trial protocol (Hope 1995). From the philosophical point of view, evidence suggests that something is scientifically proven, and therefore the observations are in agreement with the "truth" (Kaptchuk 2001). Whether the truth always corresponds to the "good" is another question (Hope 1995).

Progress in medicine depends on high-quality scientific research and on the evidence gained from this. But the outcome of trials and meta-analyses must be confronted with the knowledge on, for example, pathogenesis and epidemiology, as well as the experience from individual and cohort observations, which may all contribute valuable indirect evidence. Furthermore, the quality of current practice must continuously be controlled by means of auditing. The judicious amalgamation of the so-called hard direct evidence with more soft indirect evidence, well-balanced and validated by a group of experts, will produce the best possible evidence by consensus. It is this consensus-based evidence that is implemented in the present book.

References

Berry JJ (2002) Congenital anomalies after IVF/ICSI. Tulane Law Review 72:248–256

Clements S, Cooke ID, Barratt CL (1995) Implementing comprehensive quality control in the andrology laboratory. Hum Reprod 10:2096–2106

Cleophas TJ (1996) Clinical trials: design flaws associated with use of a placebo. Am J Ther 3:529–534

Comhaire FH, Mahmoud AM (2004) Editorial commentary. J Androl 25:771–772

Editorial (1997) Meta-analysis under scrutiny. Lancet 350:675

Ellis SJ, Adams RF (1997) The cult of the double-blind placebo-controlled trial. Br J Clin Pract 51:36–39

Evers J, Collins J (2004) Surgery or embolisation for varicocele in subfertile men. Cochrane Database Syst Rev 3:CD000479

Fergusson D, Glass KC, Waring D, Shapiro S (2004) Turning a blind eye: the success of blinding reported in a random sample of randomised, placebo controlled trials. BMJ 328:432

Hansen M, Kurinczuk JJ, Bower C, Webb S (2002) The risk of major birth defects after intracytoplasmic sperm injection and in vitro fertilization. N Engl J Med 346:725–730

Hope T (1995) Evidence based medicine and ethics. J Med Ethics 21:259 - 260
In't Veld P, Brandenburg H, Verhoeff A, Dhont M, Los F (1995) Sex chromosomal abnormalities and intracytoplasmic sperm injection. Lancet 346:773
Kaptchuk TJ (2001) The double-blind, randomized, placebo-controlled trial: gold standard or golden calf? J Clin Epidemiol 54:541 - 549
Kassirer JP, Kopelman RI (1989) Cognitive errors in diagnosis: instantiation, classification, and consequences. Am J Med 86:433 - 441
Khan KS, Daya S, Collins JA, Walter SD (1996) Empirical evidence of bias in infertility research: overestimation of treatment effect in crossover trials using pregnancy as the outcome measure. Fertil Steril 65:939 - 945
Kiene H (1996a) A critique of the double-blind clinical trial. Part 1. Altern Ther Health Med 2:74 - 80
Kiene H (1996b) A critique of the double-blind clinical trial. Part 2. Altern Ther Health Med 2:59 - 64
Kirk-Smith MD, Stretch DD (2001) Evidence-based medicine and randomized double-blind clinical trials: a study of flawed implementation. J Eval Clin Pract 7:119 - 123
Kjaergard LL, Gluud C (2002) Citation bias of hepato-biliary randomized clinical trials. J Clin Epidemiol 55:407 - 410
Koudstaal J, Bruinse HW, Helmerhorst FM, Vermeiden JP, Willemsen WN, Visser GH (2000) Obstetric outcome of twin pregnancies after in-vitro fertilization: a matched control study in four Dutch University hospitals. Hum Reprod 15: 935 - 940
LeLorier J, Gregoire G, Benhaddad A, Lapierre J, Derderian F (1997) Discrepancies between meta-analyses and subsequent large randomized, controlled trials. N Engl J Med 337:536 - 542
Miller FG, Shorr AF (2002) Ethical assessment of industry-sponsored clinical trials: a case analysis. Chest 121:1337 -1342
Mitchell AA (2002) Infertility treatment-more risks and challenges. N Engl J Med 346:769 - 770
Neuwinger J, Behre HM, Nieschlag E (1990) External quality control in the andrology laboratory: an experimental multicenter trial. Fertil Steril 54:308 - 314
Nilsson S, Edvinsson A, Nilsson B (1979) Improvement of semen and pregnancy rate after ligation and division of the internal spermatic vein: fact or fiction? Br J Urol 51:591 - 596
Olive DL (1996) Evidence based medicine and the surgical procedure. Course on evidence based medicine: contemporary mode of practice. Am Soc Reprod Med 1 - 65
Schroder AK, Katalinic A, Diedrich K, Ludwig M (2004) Cumulative pregnancy rates and drop-out rates in a German IVF programme: 4102 cycles in 2130 patients. Reprod Biomed Online 8:600 - 606
Schulz KF, Grimes DA (2002) Blinding in randomised trials: hiding who got what. Lancet 359:696 - 700
Smith R (1998) Beyond conflict of interest. Transparency is the key. BMJ 317:291 - 292
Steinberger E, Rodriguez-Rigau LJ, Smith KD (1981) The interaction between the fertility potentials of the two members of an infertile couple. In: Frajese G, Hafez ES, Conti C, Fabbrini A (eds) Oligozoospermia: recent progress in andrology. Raven, New York, pp 9 - 19
Stelfox HT, Chua G, O'Rourke K, Detsky AS (1998) Conflict of interest in the debate over calcium-channel antagonists. N Engl J Med 338:101 - 106
Strömberg B, Dahlquist G, Ericson A, Finnstrom O, Koster M, Stjernqvist K (2002) Neurological sequelae in children born after in-vitro fertilisation: a population-based study. Lancet 359:461 - 465
Sutcliffe AG, Taylor B, Li J, Thornton S, Grudzinskas JG, Lieberman BA (1999) Children born after intracytoplasmic sperm injection: population control study. Br Med J 318:704 - 705
Teris B.(ed) (1998) Recombinant FSH: a collection of previously published papers. Fertil Steril 69 (Suppl 2)
Van Steirteghem A (1998) Outcome of assisted reproductive technology. N Engl J Med 338:194 - 195
Wennerholm U, Bergh C, Hamberger L, Lundin K, Nilsson L, Wikland M, Kallen B (2000) Incidence of congenital malformations in children born after ICSI. Hum Reprod 15: 944 - 948
WHO (1987) Towards more objectivity in diagnosis and management of male infertility. Int J Androl Suppl 7
Wilson AM (2002) Press communication. The Independent, 22 October 2002

Economic Cost and Cost-Effectiveness

F. Comhaire, A. Mahmoud

Optimal health care is a universal human right. Alas, this right can be claimed by only a fraction of the world's population, and many persons in large areas are deprived of this right. On the other hand, the financial cost to implement this right in both poor and wealthier parts of the world is enormous. In addition, providing adequate health care to the population seems to be a rather low priority in certain countries where greater financial means are being invested in other projects (e.g. waging wars). In so-called developed and wealthier countries, the care for an increasing proportion of ageing persons, the enhanced prevalence of certain diseases related to the modern lifestyle, unsuitable nutrition and environmental contamination, for example, and the availability of new but commonly expensive modalities of treatment make the cost of medical care for the entire population hardly bearable.

Therefore it is mandatory and, in fact, part of the deontological obligation of all clinicians to make the best possible use of financial means, both public and private money, by selecting the most cost-effective modalities for diagnosing and treating the patient. Also, the cost-effectiveness of methods for the prevention and/or early detection of diseases, or of impaired health and function must be assessed.

For the majority of problems in the field of clinical andrology, there are several possible options with regard to investigation and management. Aside from the fact that internal and external auditing is required to assess the good quality of the care delivered, medical strategies must continuously be evaluated as to their cost-effectiveness and the optimal approach.

In the field of surgery, the endoscopic approach may sometimes be as effective but less expensive compared to open surgery, by shortening the duration of hospital stay and the time needed to recover and to resume economically rewarding work, for example.

Also, in vasectomized patients surgical reversal is more cost-effective than IVF with ICSI (Pavlovich and Schlegel 1997).

Another example relates to the systematic and periodic measurement of prostate-specific antigen (PSA) in the blood of men over a certain age, in view of the early detection and more effective treatment of cancer of the prostate.

With respect to the management of reproductive disorders, the World Health Organization and the United Nations Population Fund have set the goal to universal access to reproductive health care no later than 2015, including the prevention and appropriate treatment of infertility (WHO 2003). Considering the enormity of this task and its massive financial consequences (Collins et al. 1997), methods for the diagnosis and management of the infertile male in particular should be scrupulously evaluated for their cost-effectiveness (Comhaire 1995). Cost not only refers to expenses carried by the public healthcare systems and insurance, but also by the patients involved (Collins 2002; Pratt 2004). In doing so, it is the cost per delivery of a healthy singleton that must be the end-point, but the effective cumulative pregnancy rate and the time needed to attain the desired pregnancy are also important (Comhaire et al. 1996).

Calculation of the direct cost per delivery is rather simple and can be done by dividing the cost per treatment by the rate of success in terms of the probability of a healthy singleton will result from that particular treatment. A clear-cut example of this calculation is the cost per delivery after in vitro fertilization in case of couple infertility due to oligozoospermia (Neumann et al. 1994). The net cost per treatment cycle, including medication for ovarian hyperstimulation, cycle monitoring, pick-up and laboratory expenses amounts to a minimum of 2,500 €. The take-baby-home rate per treatment cycle is approximately 20 %, so the direct cost per delivery is between at least 12,500 €. Other estimations result in a cost per successful outcome in the first treatment cycle of US $60,000 (Griffin and Panak 1998). This cost increases with the increasing number of treatment cycles (Trad et al. 1995), reaching approximately US $114,000 in the 6th cycle (Neumann et al. 1994). Estimations do not include indirect costs and economic factors, such as time away from work, cost for postnatal care of the newborn which is approximately five times higher than after natural conception (Callahan et al. 1994; Wolner-Hanssen and Rydhstroem 1998), and complementary expenses for the treatment of congenital defects or problems during development.

Using this approach, it is possible to estimate the cost per successful delivery for different modes of treatment of the infertile male (Fig. 1; Comhaire 1995). The best

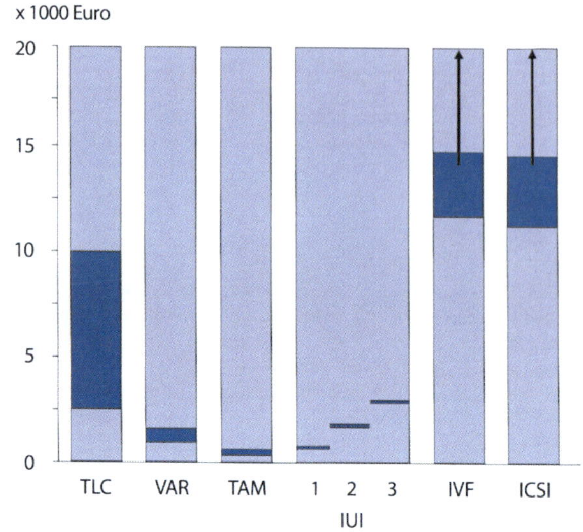

Fig. 1. Cost per delivery in euros. [*1* First cycle, *2* second cycle, *3* third cycle, *ICSI* in vitro fertilization plus intracytoplasmic sperm injection (first cycle), *IUI* intrauterine insemination, *IVF* in vitro fertilization (first cycle), *TAM* treatment with tamoxifen, *TLC* tender loving care, or treatment-independent pregnancies, *VAR* varicocele treatment]

cost-effectiveness is, in order: tamoxifen treatment, one or two cycles of IUI (Goverde et al. 2000; Philips et al. 2000), and varicocele treatment (Schlegel 1997; Penson et al. 2002). Since the spontaneous pregnancy rate during counselling (also referred to as treatment-independent pregnancy rate or tender loving care) is relatively low, the cost-effectiveness of this approach is poor, particularly in couples with longer duration of infertility (Mol et al. 2000). Also, the cost per delivery of IUI is high in the 3rd and 4th cycles of IUI, because of the decreasing conception rates. There is preliminary evidence that complementing established treatment modalities by food supplementation may decrease the time to pregnancy, reducing the cost per delivery. The cost per delivery of IVF for male subfertility is highest, even more when used in older women (Legro et al. 1997), while ICSI may be slightly better from this point of view because of the higher immediate success rate. It is a matter of debate whether or not insemination with donor semen should also be included in the comparison of cost-effectiveness (Granberg et al. 1996).

Knowing the frequency of particular aetiological andrological diagnoses in the patient population visiting infertility clinics, the effective cumulative pregnancy rates and cost per successful outcome of various treatment modalities, it is estimated that no more than 80 deliveries can be obtained with an investment of 1 million € when IVF is used as primary treatment, as compared to approximately 300 deliveries when treating the subfertile men in agreement with the WHO guidelines (Comhaire 1995). Therefore, the latter approach must be taken as part of good medical practice (Collins 1994; Karande et al. 1999).

References

Callahan TL, Hall JE, Ettner SL, Christiansen CL, Greene MF, Crowley WF Jr (1994) The economic impact of multiple-gestation pregnancies and the contribution of assisted-reproduction techniques to their incidence. N Engl J Med 331:244–249

Collins J (2002) An international survey of the health economics of IVF and ICSI. Hum Reprod Update 8:265–277

Collins JA (1994) Reproductive technology – the price of progress. N Engl J Med 331:270–271

Collins JA, Feeny D, Gunby J (1997) The cost of infertility diagnosis and treatment in Canada in 1995. Hum Reprod 12: 951–958

Comhaire F (1995) Economic strategies in modern male subfertility treatment. Hum Reprod 10 [Suppl 1]:103–106

Comhaire F, Zalata A, Mahmoud A (1996) Critical evaluation of the effectiveness of different modes of treatment of male infertility. Andrologia 28 [Suppl 1]:31–35

Goverde AJ, McDonnell J, Vermeiden JP, Schats R, Rutten FF, Schoemaker J (2000) Intrauterine insemination or in-vitro fertilisation in idiopathic subfertility and male subfertility: a randomised trial and cost-effectiveness analysis. Lancet 355:13–18

Granberg M, Wikland M, Hamberger L (1996) Cost-effectiveness of intracytoplasmic sperm injection in comparison with donor insemination. Acta Obstet Gynecol Scand 75: 734–737

Griffin M, Panak WF (1998) The economic cost of infertility-related services: an examination of the Massachusetts infertility insurance mandate. Fertil Steril 70:22–29

Karande VC, Korn A, Morris R, Rao R, Balin M, Rinehart J, Dohn K, Gleicher N (1999) Prospective randomized trial comparing the outcome and cost of in vitro fertilization with that of a traditional treatment algorithm as first-line therapy for couples with infertility. Fertil Steril 71:468–475

Legro RS, Shackleford DP, Moessner JM, Gnatuk CL, Dodson WC (1997) ART in women 40 and over. Is the cost worth it? J Reprod Med 42:76–82

Mol BW, Bonsel GJ, Collins JA, Wiegerinck MA, van d, V, Bossuyt PM (2000) Cost-effectiveness of in vitro fertilization and embryo transfer. Fertil Steril 73:748–745

Neumann PJ, Gharib SD, Weinstein MC (1994) The cost of a successful delivery with in vitro fertilization. N Engl J Med 331:239–243

Pavlovich CP, Schlegel PN (1997) Fertility options after vasectomy: a cost-effectiveness analysis. Fertil Steril 67:133–141

Penson DF, Paltiel AD, Krumholz HM, Palter S (2002) The cost-effectiveness of treatment for varicocele related infertility. J Urol 168:2490–2494

Philips Z, Barraza-Llorens M, Posnett J (2000) Evaluation of the relative cost-effectiveness of treatments for infertility in the UK. Hum Reprod 15:95–106

Pratt KT (2004) Inconceivable? Deducting the costs of fertility treatment. Cornell Law Rev 89:1121–1200

Schlegel PN (1997) Is assisted reproduction the optimal treatment for varicocele-associated male infertility? A cost-effectiveness analysis. Urology 49:83–90

Trad FS, Hornstein MD, Barbieri RL (1995) In vitro fertilization: a cost-effective alternative for infertile couples? J Assist Reprod Genet 12:418–421

WHO (2003) Measuring Access to reproductive health services, Summary Report of WHO/UNFPA Technical Consultation, 2–3 December 2003

Wolner-Hanssen P, Rydhstroem H (1998) Cost-effectiveness analysis of in-vitro fertilization: estimated costs per successful pregnancy after transfer of one or two embryos. Hum Reprod 13:88–94

Ethics of Reproductive Research and Treatment

T.B. Hargreave

Key Messages

- Three ethical principles underpinning all medical ethics are respect for autonomy, beneficence and justice.
- Consideration of these principles has to be balanced between the individual, the couple, the future child, the family and society as a whole.
- In general, consideration of the interests of the future child takes precedence over consideration of other parties.
- Consent is a process of giving the individual all the information necessary for that individual to make a free choice.
- Consent is not just signing a piece of paper.
- Reproductive advances such as intracytoplasmic sperm injection (ICSI), sex selection, cloning and germ-line genetic repair pose particular ethical problems.

Introduction

Any clinician involved in clinical practice or clinical research will face ethical problems; this is particularly relevant for those engaged in fertility clinic work. Each clinician, both individually and in the context of guidance from regional and national ethical committees, must formulate his or her own ideas. No one person has the competence to pronounce on ethical issues because these depend on culture, religion and national and international law. There are different perspectives in different countries. The purpose of the following text is to help the clinician think about the ethical issues.

Basic Principles Underlying Ethical Considerations

Three principles underlying ethical considerations have been stated namely autonomy, beneficence and justice (Beauchamp and Childress 1983).

Respect for Autonomy

Individuals should be able to choose freely what they will do, unless or until their actions cause (serious) harm to others or (seriously) limit others' liberty.

Beneficence

There are two aspects of beneficence:

- Promoting the welfare of others
- Doing no harm to others.

Justice

Justice concerns the distribution of liberties, benefits and harms. The subject is controversial because there is no agreed answer to the question "What is due to various individuals and on what basis is it due?" Possible answers include:

- To everyone according to his or her merit
- To everyone according to his or her need
- To everyone an equal share
- To everyone what he or she has acquired by proper means.

Dignity

The principle of respect for human dignity is separated by some authorities from the principle of autonomy, especially when a narrow definition of autonomy is used. For some, human dignity begins at the moment of conception although the degree of autonomy of an early embryo is very limited.

Proportionality

Proportionality means using the appropriate and least risky means to an end.

The Precautionary Principle

Where risks are unquantifiable, certain lines of research or treatment may not be appropriate until more is known.

It is also helpful to list the interested parties:

- Society as a whole
- The couple (a man and a woman trying to have a child; in certain circumstances this may be a woman alone)
- Any third party (gamete donor, surrogate mother, laboratory animal)
- The products of conception (pre-embryo, embryo, foetus, child and ultimately another person).

Consent

In almost all circumstances, people should be given the opportunity to consent before any medical intervention. Special situations include the very young and those who are unconscious or have mental incapacity. Proper consent has nothing to do with signing documents but is all about giving the patient all relevant information in a way that the patient can understand, including all appropriate information about risks and benefits of receiving or not receiving the medical intervention. Patients expect and trust their doctor to give impartial advice and if there is any reason why advice might be biased, then the patient should be made aware of this; for example, if the doctor is receiving a personal payment for recruiting the patient into a clinical trial.

It is usual to document the consent process with a consent form. In general, the consent form should be a simple document where the patient is able to sign consent to a specific treatment. Unfortunately many consent forms are taken as a substitute for giving proper information and often institutional authorities add wording that has nothing to do with consent but is all about protecting the institution. "I understand" statements on consent forms are in general bad practice, as it is for the clinician to communicate the necessary information in a comprehensible fashion and to ensure that, as far as possible, the patient has understood. A very simple guideline for the consent process is to give your patient the information that you would wish to be given yourself or would give to your brother, sister, mother or father. It is always a good idea to document the information that you have given, and a helpful way to do this is to include the information in the form of a letter and send this to your patient after the consultation and before the medical intervention starts. Further information about consent is included in the extension to this chapter, including consent for blood and tissue for research is given in the second part of this chapter. Except in emergency, people should be given sufficient time to consider information before giving consent. Thus in andrology, a young man with a testicular torsion may be asked to sign a consent form for treatment almost as soon as he has been seen by a doctor, but in almost all other situations patients can be given a minimum of 24 h before giving consent to an invasive procedure.

Applying the Principles to Reproductive Medicine

Thus when considering ethics of reproduction and reproduction-related research, the above principles should be implemented in relation to each of the interested parties. When this is done, there are often conflicts of interest. As a general rule, the interests of a future child take precedence over the interests of the parents. The following is a brief survey of some common reproduction-related ethical problems. Extensive reference has been made to three major inquiries, namely the Warnock Committee (Warnock 1984), the Ethics Committee of the American Fertility Society (American Fertility Society 1986) and Adoption of an Opinion on Ethical Aspects of Human Stem Cell Research and Use of the European Commission (Anonymous 2000).

The Right to Procreate

There are a number of issues to be addressed:

- Does the couple have a right to procreate?
- Should this right be curtailed by the needs of society, e.g. overpopulation?
- Is it ethical to provide care for couples with an infertility problem in those countries which have insufficient resources for general medical care?

The Universal Declaration of Human Rights speaks of the "right of men and women of suitable age to marry and found a family" (UN 1978). In the USA, the right not to procreate has been legally ratified but the right to have children is not clearly indicated in the American constitution or legally tested. In the People's Republic of China, there is a State policy of only one child per couple. It is relevant to note that this stricture is applied to the vast majority of couples in the interests of the State because of overpopulation. In the UK, the point was made that it is very difficult to balance the needs of society against the desires of an individual. A further point was made that the number of children born as a result of treatments of infertility will always be insignificant in comparison with the naturally increasing world population. In summary, it seems that there is a right to reproduce but the extent of reproduction may be censored by the overwhelming needs of society, provided this censorship is applied equally to all couples.

Artificial Insemination with Husband's Semen

Artificial insemination with husband's semen (AIH) is generally acceptable. The point was made that the results of AIH are uncertain when it is used for indications such as oligozoospermia and in that context it must be regarded as a clinical trial.

Sex Selection

Sex selection is possible by separating X- and Y-bearing sperm, by embryo biopsy and selective sex replacement during in vitro fertilization (IVF), by amniocentesis and sex determination and selective termination, and by infanticide. In Asian societies where there is strong cultural preference for a son and heir, and particularly in the People's Republic of China and in India (Kusum 1993) these techniques are being used extensively, with the result that by 1990 it was estimated that there are 100 million missing women in Asia and South East Asia (Benagiano and Bianchi 1999). The use of embryo biopsy and selective replacement has been called "Girl Interrupted" by Ms Puri (Times of India 2001). Many people feel that sex selection for social reasons is not acceptable, but the European experience indicates that families choose more girls than boys and that the technique does not threaten population sex ratios as is the case in parts of China and India. Most people accept that sex selection is justified for prevention of sex-linked disease, but concerns remain on sex selection for nonmedical reasons. These concerns centre on the threat to population ratios, the charge of sexism, the danger of reinforcing gender stereotypical behaviour in sex-selected children, and the fear of the slippery slope towards designer babies (Dahle 2003).

The use of sex selection for family balancing would seem to overcome many concerns because the intention is to provide a child of the missing or underrepresented sex in the family and there is evidence that a second, third or subsequent child who does not have the sex desired by the parents would receive less affection and attention than if the child is of the desired sex. Sex selection based on sperm separation is to be preferred over any other technique because the intervention is before conception and is less risky.

There is also the question of whether a technique can be unethical on one continent if it is acceptable somewhere else in the world.

Insemination of Donor Semen

Insemination of donor semen (DI) is much more controversial. The majority view in both the USA and UK reports was that artificial insemination by donor semen is acceptable because there is no evidence of substantial risk to the couple concerned or the resulting child. Also, the benefit of a child that is at least genetically the mother's is deemed to outweigh any concerns. There is no evidence that giving sperm is harmful to the donor either physically or psychologically.

However, there was a lack of uniformity of opinion amongst the expert committees drawing up the reports and, although reports concluded that the procedure was ethical, a formal note of dissent was recorded in the

USA report. The main worry is that DI introduces a third party in the (marriage) relationship and there is a body of opinion that this is never acceptable. This view also applies to surrogacy and ovum donation. DI and indeed all "artificial methods" are considered unacceptable by the Roman Catholic Church, but acceptable – albeit under particular circumstances – by the Protestant and Jewish religions.

There is ongoing controversy about the anonymity of the donor, in relation to the alleged "universal" right of children to know their biological parents. In this respect, legal constraints are different in different countries.

Egg Donation

The major ethical considerations of egg donation are the same as for sperm donation, namely concerns about third-party intrusion, legal considerations, particularly who is the parent, and possible genetic risks. This practice was considered acceptable for certain indications in both the USA and UK reports. The extra dimension compared with sperm donation is because there may be additional risk to the donor associated with obtaining the eggs. In situations where eggs are being obtained anyway, for example if the donor herself is undergoing IVF attempts and there are spare eggs, there will not be any additional risk. In this situation, the ethical considerations will be analogous to those relevant to donation of sperm.

In many countries, egg donation is considered ethically acceptable under certain conditions, but the problem of anonymity remains a matter of debate in view of the perceived right of all children to know their biological parents.

Surrogacy

There is divided opinion about surrogacy. In the USA, surrogate motherhood was acceptable only as an experiment until such time as adequate data were assembled to assess risk and benefits. The US committee recognized surrogacy as one of the most problematical areas of the new reproductive technologies. In the UK, surrogacy was generally considered unacceptable, although it was recognized that it is impossible to legislate against private noncommercial arrangements. It was emphasized that should this happen the child from such an arrangement must not be stigmatized.

The main arguments centre on:

1. The degree of involvement of the third party.
   - The involvement of the third party is much greater than with egg or sperm donation.
   - The effects of bonding between the surrogate and the foetus in utero.
2. Whether the surrogate mother will exercise due care during pregnancy.
3. The fate of the child, should it prove to have a nonlethal abnormality or handicap.
4. The surrogate mother will run risks associated with pregnancy without benefit.
5. In the case of close relatives, there may be a degree of coercion.
6. Adults should be free to take decisions, even if these involve risk. A rather similar situation is seen when a person gives a kidney to a relative (living related kidney donation).
7. Commercialization of surrogacy.

In the UK, the committee recommended that all surrogacy agreements should be regarded as illegal contracts, and therefore unenforceable in courts of law. The second recommendation was that it should be regarded as a criminal offence for professionals or others to assist in surrogacy arrangements. In several other countries, surrogacy is either not regulated by law, or it is considered acceptable under strict conditions. Commercial surrogacy is always formally rejected.

IVF and ICSI

IVF and ICSI are considered acceptable practice in both the USA and UK and in almost all other countries in the world. The objections to IVF have much in common with the objections to any of the new reproductive technologies:

- Separation of procreation from sexual union; it is held by some that children should be conceived in the act of sexual love-making.
- The procedure may result in foetal abnormality. There are ongoing concerns about the level of risk to babies born of ICSI.
- IVF is the start of a slippery slope to unacceptable forms of manipulation.
- Infertility is not life-threatening, and it is inappropriate to devote expensive healthcare resources to this form of help. IVF involves the use of expertise and resources to produce offspring in an already overpopulated world.
- IVF will produce more embryos than can be transferred, and it is morally unacceptable to create embryos and then to allow them to die.
- In both the USA and UK reports, much emphasis was placed on the need for quality control of IVF and indeed all the reproductive technologies.

Research on Embryos

This is one of the most difficult areas because of the fear that by allowing work on human material this is the "thin end of the wedge" or what others have called the "slippery slope" to unacceptable forms of experimenta-

Characteristics of the products of conception

	Human	Alive	Brain life	Potential to develop into more than one individual	Longer term viability
Gametes	yes	yes	no	no	no
Fertilised egg (Zygote)	yes	yes	no	yes	no
Pre-embryo (8 cells)	yes	yes	no	yes	no
Embryo	yes	yes	no	no	no
Foetus < 24 weeks	yes	yes	yes	no	perhaps
Foetus > 24 weeks	yes	yes	yes	no	yes
New born baby	yes	yes	yes	no	yes
Organ for transplant e.g. Kidney	yes	yes	no	no	no
Hamster egg – human sperm	Half	yes	no	no	no
Organ culture from stem cells	yes	yes	no	no	no

tion. The table may be helpful for thinking about experimentation on human products of conception. The concept of "brain life" has been used to help thinking about the early stages of human life. In transplantation practice, it is now acceptable in a number of countries to remove organs for transplantation when there is evidence that the brain stem is dead, "brain death". What has been proposed is the exact opposite, i.e. "brain life". Clearly a certain degree of organization of tissues is necessary before there is any form of brain life, and by restricting research on embryos to a time before the central nervous system develops, there can be no possibility of "brain life". In various reports (the Waller Commission in Australia 1983, the Ethics Committee of the American Fertility Society 1986 and the Warnock Enquiry UK 1984), an arbitrary limit has been set at 14 days.

Manipulation of Embryos

Various forms of manipulation are possible and there are two main areas of concern. In those situations where embryos are to be used for experiments or as a source of stem cells, the debate is about the value and dignity of human life in the early embryo and whether such techniques can ever be legitimate. In those situations where there is manipulation to the embryo prior to embryo replacement, the debate is about risks to the future baby. These areas of concern have to be considered in relation to the following techniques:

- Embryonic biopsy to determine genetic details prior to IVF transfer
- Nucleus substitution (nuclear cloning)
- Cloning by dividing the embryo before the eight-cell stage.
- Parthenogenesis (manipulation of the unfertilized egg to induce development). For example, it might be possible to fuse two eggs to create a diploid cell that will develop into an embryo.

Some of these are speculative. There are two approaches to dealing with future new reproductive technology. One approach is to issue guidelines including moratoria on particular techniques; another is to have national ethical review bodies or, as in the UK, a statutory body (Human Fertilization and Embryo Authority, HFEA) to license new technologies. In ethical guidelines issued by the Council of Europe, the following procedures have been censored:

- Implantation of human embryos into another species
- Cross-species fertilization
- Creation of embryos with sperm of different individuals
- The creation of chimaeric individuals
- The bringing to term of an embryo outside the female uterus
- The creation of an individual from parents of the same sex
- The choice of sex of offspring except for therapeutic reasons
- The creation of identical twins
- The creation of embryos specifically as a source of tissue or for research.

  There is varying opinion about the use of embryos left over after IVF.

However, such lists of rules reflect public prejudice at the time and are constantly challenged by technology. For example, is it really wrong to take a cell from an early embryo and use this to culture replacement tissue such as bone marrow cells?

Conclusion

In this chapter, few answers are given but instead there is a framework for thought about ethical matters. Andrologists must be equipped to join the debate about what is right and what is wrong, or more importantly – to keep an open mind and to see the pros and cons of new developments. It is particularly important for those who have an understanding of andrological medicine and biology to be able to contribute to public debate on ethical questions in andrological practice.

References

American Fertility Society (1986) Ethical considerations of the new reproductive technologies. The Ethics Committee of the American Fertility Society. Fertil Steril [Suppl 1]46

Anonymous (2000) Adoption of an Opinion on Ethical Aspects of Human Stem Cell Research and Use, The European Group on Ethics in Science and New Technologies to the European Commission, Paris 14th November 2000, revised edn. January 2001

Beauchamp TL, Childress JF (1983) The principles of biomedical ethics, 2nd edn. Oxford University Press, New York

Benagiano G, Bianchi P (1999) Sex preselection: an aid to couples or a threat to humanity? Hum Reprod 14:870–872

Dahle E (2003) Procreative liberty: the case for preconception sex selection. Reproductive Biomedicine online: www.rbmonline.com/article/1105 18 Sept 2003 7:380–384

Kusum (1993) The use of prenatal diagnostic techniques for sex selection: the Indian scene. Bioethics 7:149–165

Times of India (2001) Interview with Ms Nina Puri, Chairperson of the South Asia IPPF, 15 May 2001

Warnock (1984) Report of the Committee of Enquiry into Human Fertilisation and Embryology – The Warnock Report. Department of Health and Social Security, HMSO, London

Human Tissue for Research

T. Hargreave

Until recent years much molecular cancer research has been concerned with single gene defects and using limited numbers of tissue samples. However, now that the human chromosome has been sequenced there is a need to apply techniques to investigate the interaction of multiple genes. New molecular techniques have been developed that enable the analysis of many hundreds of genes, and in order to further this work large banks of normal and abnormal tissue for research will be needed. Ideally, all abnormal tissue that is in excess of diagnostic requirements should be available for research. However, obtaining consent for tissue for research is complicated because the most valuable research is when the tissue can be linked to the individual, but if the identity link is preserved then the research could have consequences for the individual and his or her family.

When samples are to be obtained for research in the context of a planned therapeutic surgical procedure, the patient/subject should be told that refusal to consent to provide specimens for research will not prejudice their medical or surgical care.

In order that the potential research subject can make a fully informed decision about whether or not to agree to her/his samples being used for research, the subject should be given detailed information verbally and in an information sheet. This information should also be detailed in the research protocol submitted to the research ethics committee.

Whenever possible, researchers should consider obtaining consent for use of the samples in future studies. However, individuals must be free to consent for the use of their samples in the immediate specified research only, or for the use of these samples in the immediate specified research and also in future research, either of a specified or unspecified nature.

The major consequence and major research benefit of giving human samples for research depend on whether the research results can be relayed back to the donor or not. All research subjects should be given information about whether the research results can be linked to them and about the measures taken to ensure protection of medical confidentiality. The identifying link between the research subject and the sample or research result may be kept or removed (Table 1). Because all samples are originally linked to personal clinical information, researchers should ensure appropriate

Table 1. Categories of identification of human tissue research samples

Unidentified The identity is removed so that nobody knows from whom the sample came, and there is no possibility of tracing the donor. Removal of identity may be at the time of sample collection (samples collected in this way are known as anonymous samples) or a researcher may remove the identity or unlink the code from samples after conclusion of the research for which they were obtained (samples handled in this way are known as anonymized samples). Research subjects should be given the information that it will not be possible to provide them with any personal results from the study, since it will not be possible to identify their samples
Coded The sample is labelled with a code known only to certain researchers, rather than with personal identifying information. Coding of samples may be done by the person collecting the samples, which are then given to the researcher, or the researcher may arrange with a third party to code samples. It is not possible for the researcher using the sample to link the biological information from the sample without breaking the code. Research subjects should be given information about who has access to the code and the circumstances in which the code will be broken
Identified The sample is labelled with the name of the donor or other personal identifying information. Any researcher using these samples would be able to link the biological information from the sample directly to the individual from whom the sample was obtained. Research subjects should be given information about who will have access to the samples and how personal information will be made secure against invasions of privacy and breaches of medical confidentiality

measures are in place to provide appropriate protection of medical confidentiality and privacy.

Acknowledgements. Tim Hargreave has developed this brief summary from a longer guideline prepared by himself, Dr David Griffin, and Professor Ruth Maklin for the Reproductive Health Research Programme, World Health Organization, Geneva

Appendix

Summary of Information About Research Samples that Should Be Given to Research Subjects

What the Sample is and how the Sample will be Obtained

- Degree of invasiveness
- In case of invasive procedures, any additional risks
- Arrangements for treating complications that may arise during or after invasive procedure to collect specimens
- Consequences of any variation in normal histopathological examination caused by specimen collection
- In the case of vaginal examination or other intimate examination, how privacy will be protected

What Consent Is Being Asked?

- Consent for the specific research project only (fully restricted)
- Partially restricted consent
- Unrestricted consent to use sample for any type of research

Whether Identity Will Be Retained or Not

- Unidentified (anonymous or anonymized)
- Coded (linked or identifiable)
- Identified

How Will Confidentiality Be Ensured

- How confidentiality and privacy of personal information will be protected
- Where samples and any clinical information will be kept
- Who will have access to the samples and the research results
- Whether the results of the research will be relayed back to the research subject
- How long samples will be kept
- The final disposition of the samples and information

Additional Information

In addition, it may be appropriate to give information about:

- Arrangements for disposal of the samples at the end of the research project
- If the proposed studies will involve genetic research
- The possibility of revealing nonpaternity
- Detection of infectious disease
- Whether the results may affect insurability
- Whether the research involves "fertilization"
- Whether the research involves alteration to germ lines or embryos
- That the research subject will not receive any money from commercial applications of the research
- Who is funding the research
- Whether the researcher will receive per subject payments
- What treatment will be provided in the case of research-related injury in obtaining the sample, and whether monetary compensation will be available for any such injuries

Diagnosing and Solving Clinical Problems

Problem: Gender Dysphoria and Disorders of Sexual Differentiation

I.1

I.1.1 Gender Dysphoria

G.G.R. T'Sjoen

Key Messages

- Transsexualism is a condition in which a person with apparently normal somatic sexual differentiation is convinced that he or she is actually a member of the opposite sex.
- The aetiology of transsexualism remains uncertain.
- Clinical examination, like measurement of sex hormone levels and karyotyping, is unlikely to yield anything more than confirmation of biological sex.
- Hormonal reassignment aims at reducing the hormonally induced secondary sex characteristics of the original sex and at inducing the secondary sex characteristics of the new sex.
- The quality of surgical construction of the genitalia is crucial for all transsexuals.
- Transsexual individuals require long-term assistance to optimize cross-sex hormone treatment.
- Few transsexuals regret undergoing treatment.

I.1.1.1 Definition

Transsexualism is a condition in which a person with apparently normal somatic sexual differentiation is convinced that he or she is actually a member of the opposite sex. It is associated with an irresistible urge to be hormonally and surgically adapted to that sex.

Gender dysphoria is a self-diagnosis with no supporting tests other than persistence of dysphoria for at least 2 years, alleviated by cross-gender identification psychosocially, anatomically, and hormonally. Self-diagnosis is confirmed by psychological assessment, which includes a trial period, "the real life test". This period when hormonal treatment starts and subjects are required to live socially the life of the desired sex is necessary before irreversible surgical reassignment is considered.

Gender identity disorder has three criteria according to DSM-IV:

1. The desire to live and be accepted as a member of the opposite sex, usually accompanied by the wish to make his or her body as congruent as possible with the preferred sex through surgery and hormone treatment.
2. The transsexual identity has been present persistently.
3. The disorder is not a symptom of another mental disorder or a chromosomal abnormality.

I.1.1.2 Aetiology and Pathogenesis

The aetiology of transsexualism remains uncertain (Gooren 1990; Zhou et al. 1995). The most recent prevalence information from the Netherlands is 1 in 11,900 males and 1 in 30,400 females (van Kesteren et al. 1996).

I.1.1.3 Clinical Findings

Before any physical intervention is considered, extensive exploration of psychological, family and social issues should be undertaken. A clear explanation of the irreversible effects of hormone therapy on body habitus is necessary. The physician should counsel the patient about realistic expectations from treatment and discuss the treatment options, both hormonal and surgical.

Biologic males, especially those who have not already reproduced, should be informed about sperm preservation options, and they can consider banking sperm prior to hormonal therapy (De Sutter 2001). Biologic females do not presently have readily available options for gamete preservation, other than cryopreservation of fertilized embryos.

Physical assessment, to be approached with care, should include a full examination of secondary sexual characteristics. Clinical examination, like measurement of sex hormone levels and karyotyping, baseline cholesterol, urea and electrolytes, glucose and liver function tests, is unlikely to yield anything more than confirmation of biological sex, aside from potentially disclosing evidence of self-treatment (Levy et al. 2003). Basic medical monitoring should include serial physical examinations relevant to treatment effects and side effects, vital sign measurements before and during treatment, weight measurements, and laboratory assessment.

For those receiving oestrogens, the minimum laboratory assessment should consist of a pretreatment (free) testosterone level, fasting glucose, liver function tests, and complete blood count with reassessment at 6 and 12 months and annually thereafter. A pretreatment prolactin level should be obtained and repeated on a yearly basis. Biologic males undergoing oestrogen treatment should be monitored for breast cancer and encouraged to engage in routine self-examination. As they age, they should be monitored for prostatic cancer (van Haarst et al. 1998).

For those receiving androgens, the minimum laboratory assessment should consist of pretreatment liver function tests and haematocrit/complete blood count with reassessment at 6 months, 12 months, and yearly thereafter.

I.1.1.4 Treatment

I.1.1.4.1 Standards of Care

The international organization involved with professional help to transsexuals, the Harry Benjamin International Gender Dysphoria Association, has drafted standards of care. The major purpose of the standards of care is to articulate this organization's professional consensus about the psychological, medical, and surgical management of gender identity disorders. These standards provide guidance to professionals practising in this area.

I.1.1.4.2 Physical Interventions

A staged process is recommended to keep options open through the reversible stage. Moving from one state to another should not occur until there has been adequate time for the person and his or her family to assimilate fully the effects of earlier interventions. Arguments include psychosocial reasons and, furthermore, a more gradual adaptation of the body to a changing hormonal milieu. It is our belief that a slow transition phase of usually 2 years, rather than a quick one, may be more advisable (T'Sjoen et al. 2004).

Reversible Interventions

These interventions involve the use of luteinizing hormone releasing hormone (LHRH) agonists, cyproterone acetate or medroxyprogesterone to suppress oestrogen or testosterone production in order to reduce the hormonally induced secondary sex characteristics of the original sex as much as possible.

Irreversible Interventions

These include hormonal interventions that masculinize or feminize the body, such as administration of testosterone to biologic females and oestrogen to biologic males, and the surgical procedures.

I.1.1.4.3 Hormonal Sex Reassignment

Hormonal treatment, when medically tolerated, should precede any genital surgical interventions. Satisfaction with the hormone's effects consolidates the person's identity as a member of the preferred sex and gender and further adds to the conviction to proceed. Dissatisfaction with hormonal effects may signal ambivalence about proceeding to surgical interventions. Some individuals who receive hormonal treatment will not desire genital or other surgical interventions (Table I.1.1).

Table I.1.1. Recommended hormonal treatment regimens and follow-up for transsexuals

	Male to female	Female to male
Treatment		
Psychological assessment		
Hormonal treatment		
Reversible phase	Antiandrogen	Progestin
Irreversible phase	Antiandrogen + oestrogens	Testosterone
Follow-up		
Initial visit	Karyotype Measurement of sex hormone levels Weight Lipid profile Liver function tests	Karyotype Measurement of sex hormone levels Weight Lipid profile Liver function tests
Every 4 months preoperative	Testosterone levels Weight Lipid profile Liver function tests Serum prolactin	Testosterone levels Weight Lipid profile Liver function tests Complete blood count
Every 6 months to 1 year postoperative	Same parameters, include Dexa scan. Over 50 years: PSA Encourage breast exams	Same parameters, include Dexa scan.

Hormonal reassignment has two aims (Asscheman and Gooren 1992):

1. To reduce the hormonally induced secondary sex characteristics of the original sex as much as possible, but complete elimination is rare. For example, in male-to-female transsexuals, the previous effects of androgens on the skeleton, such as the greater height of men than women, the size and shape of hands, feet, jaws and pelvis, cannot be reversed. Conversely, the relatively lower height and the broader hip configuration of female-to-male transsexuals compared to men will not change with androgen treatment.
2. To induce the secondary sex characteristics of the new sex.

Biologic Males

- Antiandrogens
  Several agents are available to inhibit androgen secretion or action. In Europe, the most widely used drug is cyproterone acetate (usually 50 mg daily), a progestational compound with antiandrogenic properties. If it is not available, medroxyprogesterone acetate, 5–10 mg/day, is an alternative, although less effective. Nonsteroidal antiandrogens, such as flutamide and nilutamide, are also used, but they increase gonadotrophin secretion, causing increased secretion of testosterone and oestradiol; the latter is a desirable effect in this context. Spironolactone (100 mg twice daily), a diuretic with antiandrogenic properties, has similar effects. Long-acting gonadotrophin-releasing hormone (GnRH) agonists, used as monthly injections, also inhibit gonadotrophin secretion. Finasteride (1–5 mg/day), a 5α-reductase inhibitor, might also be considered.
- Oestrogens
  Oestrogen treatment can realistically be expected to result in breast growth, some redistribution of body fat to approximate a female body habitus, decreased upper body strength, softening of skin, decrease in body hair, slowing or stopping the loss of scalp hair, decreased fertility and testicular size and less firm erections. Breast formation starts almost immediately after initiation of oestrogen administration. Androgens have an inhibitory effect on breast formation and, therefore, oestrogens will be most effective in a milieu devoid of androgen action. After 2 years of oestrogen administration, no further development can be expected. It is estimated to be quantitatively satisfactory in 40% to 50% of subjects. The attained size is often disproportional to the male dimension of the chest and height of the subject, so the subject may desire surgical breast augmentation. Adult male beard growth is very resistant to inhibition by combined hormonal intervention, and in Caucasian subjects additional measures to eliminate facial hair are necessary. Sexual hair growth on other parts of the body responds more favourably (Giltay and Gooren 2000). Antiandrogens and oestrogens have no effect on the properties of the voice, so male-to-female transsexuals may wish to consult a specialized phoniatric centre for speech therapy (Van Borsel et al. 2001).

There is a wide range of oestrogens from which to choose. The use of transdermal oestrogen patches should be considered for males over 40 years of age or those with clotting abnormalities or a history of venous thrombosis (Moore et al. 2003). Attempts to mimic the menstrual cycle by prescribing interrupted oestrogen therapy or substituting progesterone for oestrogen during part of the month are not necessary to achieve feminization.

Biologic Females

The goal of treatment in female-to-male transsexuals is to induce virilization, including a male pattern of sexual hair and male physical contours, and to stop menses.

- Progestins, e.g. medroxyprogesterone acetate 5–10 mg/day, to stop menstrual bleeding
- Testosterone

Androgen administration induces the following permanent changes: a deepening of the voice after 6–10 weeks, clitoral enlargement, mild breast atrophy, increased facial and body hair and male pattern baldness. Other changes include increased upper body strength, weight gain, increased social and sexual interest and arousability, and decreased hip fat. Viable options of androgen treatment include oral, injectable, and transdermal delivery systems. Treatment principles are equal to those for treatment of the hypogonadal male patient.

Potential Negative Medical Side Effects

In a review of 816 male-to-female transsexuals and 293 female-to-male transsexuals (total exposure 10,152 patient years), mortality was no higher than in a comparison group (Van Kesteren et al. 1997). However, cross-sex hormone administration may be associated with the side effects listed below.

Increased propensity in biologic males treated with oestrogens and antiandrogens to blood clotting (venous thrombosis with a risk of fatal pulmonary embolism), development of benign pituitary prolactinomas, infertility, weight gain, emotional lability, liver disease, somnolence, hypertension, and diabetes mellitus.

Side effects in biologic females treated with testosterone may include infertility, acne, emotional lability, increases in sexual desire, and shift of lipid profiles to male patterns which increase the risk of cardiovascular disease. Ovaries of female-to-male transsexuals taking androgens show similarities with polycystic ovaries, which are also more likely to develop malignancies. Therefore, it seems reasonable to remove the ovaries of androgen-treated female-to-male transsexuals after a successful transition to the male role.

Contraindications against the use of high doses of either sex steroid are cardiovascular disease, cerebrovascular disease, thromboembolic disease, marked obesity, poorly controlled diabetes mellitus, and active liver disease. Risk-benefit ratios should be considered collaboratively by the patient and prescribing physician (Michel et al. 2001).

Post-transition Follow-up

Postoperative patients may also sometimes exclude themselves from follow-up with the physician prescribing hormones, not recognizing that these physicians are best able to prevent, diagnose and treat possible long-term medical conditions that are unique to hormonally and surgically treated patients. Postoperative patients should undergo regular medical screening according to recommended guidelines for their age.

Close monitoring and yearly reevaluation of treatment are also important to minimize the adverse effects while maximizing the benefits. After reassignment surgery, including orchiectomy, hormone therapy must be continued. Continuous oestrogen therapy is required to avoid symptoms of hormone deprivation and, most importantly, to prevent osteoporosis. After bilateral oophorectomy, androgen therapy must be continued to maintain virilization and prevent osteoporosis (Van Kesteren 1998).

I.1.1.4.4 Surgical Sex Reassignment

The procedures differ depending upon the direction of the sex change (Monstrey et al. 2001).

Male-to-female: A neovagina is surgically constructed, usually using the penile skin for vaginal lining and scrotal skin for the labia. If breast development is judged to be insufficient, the breasts may be surgically augmented. Because immobilization is also a risk factor for venous thromboembolic events, oral oestrogen administration should be discontinued 3–4 weeks before elective surgical interventions. Once subjects are fully mobilized again, oral oestrogen therapy may be resumed.

Female-to-male: The breasts, uterus and ovaries are surgically removed. In rare cases, the hypertrophied clitoris may serve as a phallus. In other cases a so-called metaidoioplasty may be performed. Free flaps removed from arms or legs can be used to construct a neophallus. These surgical interventions allow the person to urinate standing. From the labia majora, a scrotum can be constructed in which testicular prostheses can be implanted. An erection prosthesis may be optional. The quality of surgical construction of the genitalia is crucial for all transsexuals to permit them to adopt credibly the role of a member of the new sex.

I.1.1.5 Prognosis

Although more evidence would be welcome, adequately treated gender dysphoria is likely to be safer than the untreated condition, which is associated with an enhanced risk of depression and suicide. Reassuringly, few transsexuals regret undergoing treatment (Pfäfflin 1992).

A team of professionals with an interest in the gender identity disorders can provide optimal care. Doubts about the authenticity of gender dysphoria as a diagnosis, lack of approbation from peers and perhaps personal phobias may lead some members of the medical profession to withhold treatment. Transsexual individuals require long-term assistance to optimize cross-sex hormone treatment and should not be subject to discrimination when they seek health care.

References

Asscheman H, Gooren LJ (1992) Hormone treatment in transsexuals. J Psychol Hum Sex 5:39

De Sutter P (2001) Gender reassignment and assisted reproduction: present and future reproductive options for transsexual people. Hum Reprod 16:612–614

Futterweit W (1998) Endocrine therapy of transsexualism and potential complications of long-term treatment. Arch Sex Behav 27:209

Giltay EJ, Gooren LJ (2000) Effects of sex steroid deprivation/administration on hair growth and sebum production in transsexual males and females. J Clin Endocrinol Metab 85:2913

Gooren L (1990) The endocrinology of transsexualism: a review and commentary. Psychoneuroendocrinology 15:3

Levy A, Crown A, Reid R (2003) Endocrine intervention for transsexuals. Clin Endocrinol (Oxf) 59:409–418

Michel A, Mormont C, Legros JJ (2001) A psycho-endocrinological overview of transsexualism. Eur J Endocrinol 145:365–376

Monstrey S, Hoebeke P, Dhont M, De Cuypere G, Rubens R, Moerman M, Hamdi M, Van Landuyt K, Blondeel P (2001) Surgical therapy in transsexual patients: a multi-disciplinary approach. Acta Chir Belg 101:200–209

Moore E, Wisniewski A, Dobs A (2003) Endocrine treatment of transsexual people: a review of treatment regimens, outcomes, and adverse effects. J Clin Endocrinol Metab 88:3467

Pfäfflin F (1992) Regrets after sex reassignment surgery. J Psychol Hum Sex 5:69

Standards of care for gender identity disorders. The Harry Benjamin International Gender Dysphoria Association. (http://www.hbigda.org)
T'Sjoen G, Rubens R, De Sutter P, Gooren L (2004) Author's response: the endocrine care of transsexual people. J Clin Endocrinol Metab 89:1014–1015
Van Borsel J, De Cuypere G, Van den Berghe H (2001) Physical appearance and voice in male-to-female transsexuals. J Voice 15:570–575
van Haarst EP, Newling DW, Gooren LJ et al (1998) Metastatic prostatic carcinoma in a male-to-female transsexual. Br J Urol 81:776
Van Kesteren PJ, Gooren LJ, Megens JA (1996) An epidemiological and demographic study of transsexuals in The Netherlands. Arch Sex Behav 25:589
Van Kesteren PJ, Megens JA, Asscheman H, Gooren LJ (1997) Side effects of cross-sex hormone administration in transsexuals. Clin Endocrinol 47: 337
Van Kesteren P, Lips P, Gooren LJ et al (1998) Long term follow-up of bone mineral density in transsexuals treated with cross-sex hormones. Clin Endocrinol 48:347
Zhou JN, Hofman MA, Gooren LJ, Swaab DF (1995) A sex difference in the human brain and its relation to transsexuality. Nature 378:68

I.1.2 Disorders of Sexual Differentiation

G.G.R. T'Sjoen

Key Messages

- Individuals who have a genital appearance that does not permit gender declaration are said to have ambiguous genitalia.
- Intersex is not confined to infants at birth.
- The commonest cause of newborn intersex is congenital adrenal hyperplasia (CAH) due to 21-hydroxylase deficiency.
- The commonest cause of the under-masculinized male is the group of androgen insensitivity syndromes.
- Gonadal histology is needed to confirm a diagnosis of hermaphroditism.
- The urgent medical issue is the possibility of adrenal crisis (a life-threatening emergency) in infants with the salt-wasting form of CAH.
- The birth of an infant with ambiguous genitalia is a psychosocial emergency for the family.

I.1.2.1 Definition

Individuals who have a genital appearance that does not permit gender declaration are said to have ambiguous genitalia. This includes infants with perineal hypospadias with bifid scrotum, bilateral cryptorchidism, clitoromegaly, posterior labial fusion, phenotypic female appearance with palpable gonad, and infants with discordant genitalia and sex chromosomes. XY infants with palpable gonads and simple hypospadias or microphallus, although under-virilized, do not have truly ambiguous genitalia and are discussed separately in other chapters. Intersex is not confined to infants at birth. Nonisosexual development can occur at puberty. Examples include 17β-hydroxydehydrogenase deficiency and 5α-reductase enzyme deficiencies, late-onset congenital adrenal hyperplasia (CAH) and partial androgen insensitivity syndrome (PAIS).

I.1.2.2 Aetiology and Pathogenesis

The investigation and management of disorders of sexual differentiation is dependent on an understanding of the embryology, genetics and hormonal control of normal foetal sex development (see Sects. 2.1.2 and 2.2.2 in Chap. 2). Knowledge of postnatal psychosexual development and an appreciation of the sociocultural influences on gender is very important. History taking should include the following information: family tree with females who are childless or have amenorrhea, history of consanguinity, prenatal exposure to androgens (e.g. danazol, testosterone) or teratogens or endocrine disruptors (phenytoin, aminoglutethimide) (Dessens et al. 2001), and a history of unexplained infant deaths (CAH).

I.1.2.3 Classification of Intersex

We have traditionally used prefixes to the word, hermaphroditism, to classify intersex: female pseudohermaphroditism (e.g. congenital adrenal hyperplasia) and male pseudohermaphroditism (androgen insensitivity syndrome) (Table I.1.2).

This terminology is confusing for medical staff and patients. A simpler format, as has been suggested by ex-

Table I.1.2. Phenotypic characteristics possibly reflecting disordered sexual differentiation

Female phenotype	Ambiguous phenotype	Male phenotype
Isolated clitoromegaly	Ambiguous genitalia	Male with nonpalpable testes
Isolated labial fusion		Micropenis, bifid scrotum
Palpable gonads, inguinal herniae	Syndromal genital anomalies	Severe hypospadias ± undescended testes

perts in this field, is: "the masculinized female" and "the under-masculinized male", and reserve the word "hermaphroditism" to describe its precise meaning: the presence of both testicular and ovarian tissues in the same individual.

I.1.2.4 Clinical Findings

I.1.2.4.1 Which Newborns to Investigate?

The examiner should note phallus size, position of the urethral orifice, fusion of the labia, bifid scrotum and descent, and size of the gonads (Diamond 2001).

I.1.2.4.2 Technical Investigations

The following is not an exhaustive list of all the possible investigations in a case of newborn intersex. The clinical assessment will influence the approach (Table I.1.3).

- Genetics
  - Peripheral blood karyotype
  - DNA, identification of genetic mutations
  - Fluorescence in situ hybridization (FISH) using SRY (sex-determining region on the Y chromosome) -specific probes (useful in clarifying the results of the karyotype)
- Endocrine
  - 17-Hydroxyprogesterone, 11-deoxycortisol, 17-hydroxypregnenolone, dehydroepiandrosterone (DHEA), electrolytes, renin, aldosterone, adrenocorticotrophic hormone (ACTH), urine steroids
  - Testosterone (T), dihydrotestosterone (DHT)
  - Androstenedione
  - Luteinizing hormone (LH), follicle-stimulating hormone (FSH), AMH (anti-Müllerian hormone)
  - hCG test (human chorionic gonadotrophin)
- Imaging
  - Pelvic ultrasound
  - MRI
  - Cystourethroscopy
- Surgical
  - Exploratory laparoscopy
  - Biopsy of gonads

Table I.1.3. Simple classification of intersex

Type/cause	Result
Masculinized female	
Female androgens	CAH, placental aromatase deficiency, adrenal tumours, ovarian tumours
Maternal androgens	
Under-masculinized male	
Abnormal testis determination	Gonadal dysgenesis, XO/XY mosaicism
Defects in androgen biosynthesis and metabolism	17α-OH-dehydrogenase deficiency, 5α-reductase deficiency
Resistance to androgens	Partial AIS
True hermaphroditism	
Presence of both testicular and ovarian (with follicles) tissue	XX, XY, XX/XY

The commonest cause of newborn intersex is CAH due to 21-hydroxylase deficiency characterized by a 46, XX karyotype, increased 17-hydroxyprogesterone levels and the presence of a uterus (Speizer 2001) (Fig. I.1.1). The commonest cause of the under-masculinized male is the group of androgen insensitivity syndromes (Wisniewski et al. 2000) (Fig. I.1.2). The diagnostic process in under-virilized XY infants is more difficult because of the phenotypic variability and the large number of potential causes (Ahmed and Hughes 2002).

XY intersex is a diagnostic challenge (Migeon et al. 2002b). The hCG stimulation test is a key investigation, although consistent protocols and defined normal responses have not been established for the neonatal period and infancy (Forest 1979). Serum AMH is a simple and useful marker of testis development and probably function (Lee et al. 1997; Rey et al. 1999; Misra et al. 2002). Gonadal histology is needed to confirm a diagnosis of hermaphroditism (Krob et al. 1994). The genetic cause of gonadal dysgenesis is unknown in most cases.

I.1.2.5 Management

The urgent medical issue is the possibility of adrenal crisis (a life-threatening emergency) in infants with the salt-wasting form of CAH. Symptoms of salt-wasting include vomiting, diarrhoea, hypovolaemia, hyponatraemia with hyperkalaemia, hypoglycaemia and cardiovascular collapse (Speiser 2001). To prevent potentially life-threatening manifestations of adrenal crisis, stress doses of glucocorticoids should be initiated in all infants in whom CAH is a consideration (25–50 mg hydrocortisone i.v., i.m. or p.o. per day), and particularly so if the infants are medically stressed. Once diagnosis of salt-wasting is confirmed, infants should begin to receive glucocorticoid and mineralocorticoid replacement therapy (25–30 mg/m^2 per day divided into three doses administered three times per day).

The birth of an infant with ambiguous genitalia is a psychosocial emergency for the family. Careful and complete evaluation by an experienced team of endo-

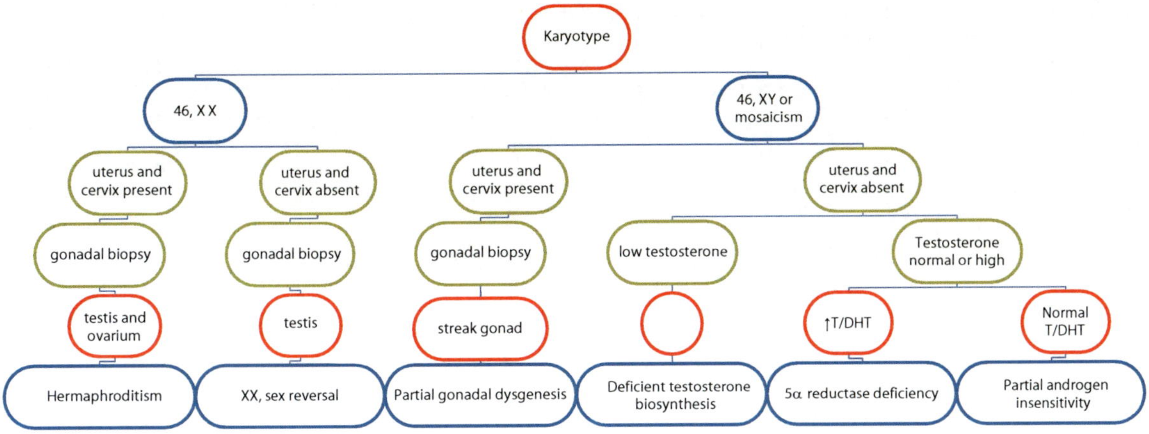

Fig. I.1.1. Ambiguous genitalia, palpable gonads

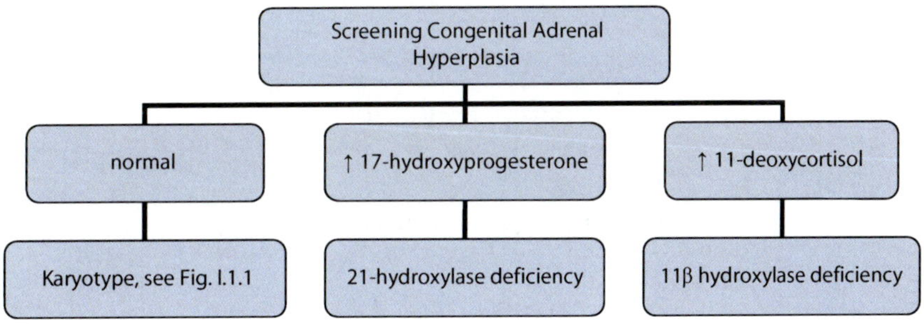

Fig. I.1.2. Ambiguous genitalia, nonpalpable gonads

crinologist, geneticists and surgeons, and psychologists is necessary before an appropriate therapeutic plan can be developed. The management of infants with ambiguous genitalia is critical and often controversial in the absence of well-defined outcome-based guidelines. Many experts have begun to question the wisdom of previous management paradigms that promoted early genital surgery and gender assignment based on potential for reproduction and traditional sexual function (Money 1955; Gourlay et al. 1994; Slijper et al. 1998; Migeon et al. 2002a; Berenbaum et al. 2003). The issue of timing and approach to genital reconstruction is controversial and evolving.

I.1.2.6 Prevention

Prenatal diagnosis is possible in pregnant women with a family history of 21-hydroxylase deficiency. Dexamethasone (20 μg/kg per day) is administered starting in the 5th week of pregnancy. This treatment is continued throughout the pregnancy when the female foetus is diagnosed with the condition. If the foetus is male or the female foetus is not affected, dexamethasone is stopped (New et al. 2001).

References

Ahmed SF, Hughes IA (2002) The genetics of male undermasculinization. Clin Endocrinol (Oxf) 56:1–18

Ahmed SF, Cheng A, Dovey L, Hawkins JR, Martin H, Rowland J, Shimura N, Tait AD, Hughes IA (2000) Phenotypic features, androgen receptor binding, and mutational analysis in 278 clinical cases reported as androgen insensitivity syndrome. J Clin Endocrinol Metab 85:658–665

Berenbaum SA, Bailey JM (2003) Effects on gender identity of prenatal androgens and genital appearance: evidence from girls with congenital adrenal hyperplasia. J Clin Endocrinol Metab 88:1102–1105

Burgner DP, Kinmond S, Wallace AM et al (1996) Male pseudohermaphroditism secondary to panhypopituitarism. Arch Dis Child 75:153–155

Cara JF, Moshang T Jr, Bongiovanni AM, Marx BS (1985) Elevated 17-hydroxyprogesterone and testosterone in a newborn with 3-beta-hydroxysteroid dehydrogenase deficiency. N Engl J Med 313:618–621

Consensus statement on 21-hydroxylase deficiency from the Lawson Wilkins Pediatric Endocrine Society and the European Society for Paediatric Endocrinology. J Clin Endocrinol Metab 87:4048–4053

Dessens AB, Cohen-Kettenis PT, Mellenbergh GJ et al (2001) Association of prenatal phenobarbital and phenytoin exposure with genital anomalies and menstrual disorders. Teratology 64:181–188

Diamond M, Sigmundson HK (1997) Management of intersexuality. Guidelines for dealing with persons with ambiguous genitalia. Arch Pediatr Adolesc Med 151:1046–1050

Faisal Ahmed S, Iqbal A, Hughes IA (2000) The testosterone:androstenedione ratio in male undermasculinization. Clin Endocrinol (Oxf) 53:697–702

Forest MG (1979) Pattern of the response of testosterone and its precursors to human chorionic gonadotropin stimulation in relation to age in infants and children. J Clin Endocrinol Metab 49:132–137

Gourlay WA, Johnson HW, Pantzar et al (1994) Gonadal tumors in disorders of sexual differentiation. Urology 43:537–540

Imperato-McGinley J, Gautier T, Pichardo M, Shackleton C (1986) The diagnosis of 5-alpha-reductase deficiency in infancy. J Clin Endocrinol Metab 63:1313–1318

Krob G, Braun A, Kuhnle U (1994) True hermaphroditism: geographical distribution, clinical findings, chromosomes and gonadal histology. Eur J Pediatr 153:2–10

Lee M, Donahoe P, Silverman B et al (1997) Measurement of serum mullerian inhibiting substance in the evaluation of children with nonpalpable gonads. N Engl J Med 336:1480–1486

Mendonca BB, Inacio M, Arnhold IJ, Costa EM (2000) Male pseudohermaphroditism due to 17 beta-hydroxysteroid dehydrogenase 3 deficiency. Diagnosis, psychological evaluation, and management. Medicine (Baltimore) 79:299–309

Migeon CJ, Wisniewski AB, Gearhart JP et al (2002a) Ambiguous genitalia with perineoscrotal hypospadias in 46,XY individuals: long-term medical, surgical, and psychosexual outcome. Pediatrics 110:e31

Migeon CJ, Wisniewski AB, Brown TR et al (2002b) 46,XY intersex individuals: phenotypic and etiologic classification, knowledge of condition, and satisfaction with knowledge in adulthood. Pediatrics 110:e32

Minto CL, Liao LM, Woodhouse CR et al (2003) The effect of clitoral surgery on sexual outcome in individuals who have intersex conditions with ambiguous genitalia: a cross-sectional study. Lancet 361:1252–1257

Misra M, MacLaughlin DT, Donahoe PK, Lee MM (2002) Measurement of Mullerian inhibiting substance facilitates management of boys with microphallus and cryptorchidism. J Clin Endocrinol Metab 87:3598–3602

Money J, Hampson JG, Hampson JL (1955) Hermaphroditism: recommendations concerning assignment of sex, change of sex, and psychologic management. Bull Johns Hopkins Hosp 97:284–300

New MI, Carlson A, Obeid J, Marshall I, Cabrera MS, Goseco A, Lin-Su K, Putnam AS, Wei JQ, Wilson RC (2001) Prenatal diagnosis for congenital adrenal hyperplasia in 532 pregnancies. J Clin Endocrinol Metab 86:5651–5657

Rey RA, Belville C, Nihoul-Fekete C et al (1999) Evaluation of gonadal function in 107 intersex patients by means of serum antimullerian hormone measurement. J Clin Endocrinol Metab 84:627–631

Schnitzer JJ, Donahoe PK (2001) Surgical treatment of congenital adrenal hyperplasia. Endocrinol Metab Clin North Am 30:137–154

Slijper F, Drop S, Molenaar J, de Muinck Keizer-Schrama S (1998) Long-term psychological evaluation of intersex children. Arch Sex Behav 27:125–144

Speiser PW (2001) Congenital adrenal hyperplasia owing to 21-hydroxylase deficiency. Endocrinol Metab Clin North Am 30:31–59

Verp MS, Simpson JL (1987) Abnormal sexual differentiation and neoplasia. Cancer Genet Cytogenet 25:191–218

Wisniewski AB, Migeon CJ, Meyer-Bahlburg, HF et al (2000) Complete androgen insensitivity syndrome: long-term medical, surgical, and psychosexual outcome. J Clin Endocrinol Metab 85:2664–2669

Problem: Abnormal Pubertal Development I.2

S.A. Wudy

Key Message

- Puberty is a landmark of development. It begins with increased and nocturnal pulsatile secretion of gonadotrophin-releasing hormone (GnRH). The primary guidelines for management of precocious as well as of delayed puberty are to rule out an organic disorder that requires treatment in and of itself.

I.2.1 Physiology

During puberty – the period of transition between childhood and adulthood – full sexual maturation, the adolescent growth spurt and fertility (production of mature gametes) are attained. Puberty starts with an increase in pulsatile secretion of the hypothalamic hormone gonadotrophin-releasing hormone (GnRH, LHRH). Consequently, the pituitary gonadotrophins (LH, luteinizing hormone; FSH, follicle-stimulating hormone) are stimulated and their release consecutively leads to an increase in gonadal steroids (predominantly testosterone in males).

In boys, the first sign of pubertal development is an increase in testicular volume (4 ml), which occurs at a mean age of 12 years (Marshall and Tanner 1970). To characterize the physical changes in individuals and in populations, Tanner developed standards for assessing sexual maturation (Table I.2.1).

Table I.2.1. Tanner stages of pubertal development in boys

A. Genital development
Stage 1: Preadolescent. Testes, scrotum, and penis are about the same size and proportion as in early childhood.
Stage 2: The scrotum and testes have enlarged; the scrotal skin shows a change in texture and also some reddening.
Stage 3: Growth of the penis has occurred, at first mainly in length but with some increase in breadth; there is further growth of the testes and scrotum.
Stage 4: The penis is further enlarged in length and breadth with development of the glans. The testes and scrotum are further enlarged. The scrotal skin has further darkened.
Stage 5: Genitalia are adult in size and shape. No further enlargement takes place after stage 5 is reached.
B. Pubic hair development
Stage 1: Preadolescent. The vellus over the pubes is not further developed than that over the abdominal wall; i.e. there is no pubic hair.
Stage 2: Sparse growth of long, slightly pigmented, downy hair, straight or slightly curled, appearing chiefly at the base of the penis.
Stage 3: Hair is considerably darker, coarser, and curlier and spreads sparsely over the junction of the pubes.
Stage 4: Hair is now adult in type, but the area it covers is still considerably smaller than in most adults. There is no spread to the medial surface of the thighs.
Stage 5: Hair is adult in quantity and type, distributed as an inverse triangle. The spread is to the medial surface of the thighs but not up the linea alba or elsewhere above the base of the inverse triangle. Most men will have further spread of the pubic hair

I.2.2 Precocious Puberty

In boys, puberty is considered precocious if typical secondary sex characteristics occur prior to 9 years of age. Because of the premature closing of the epiphyses, subjects who have undergone precocious puberty are generally shorter than normal.

It is important to separate *true* (i.e. *central*) precocious puberty – which is due to the premature activation of the hypothalamic-pituitary-gonadal axis – from *pseudoprecocious* puberty – which is generally due to a secreting tumour, inducing only the development of the secondary sex characteristics (Partsch et al. 2002).

In gonadotrophin-dependent true precocious puberty, the premature activation of the hypothalamic GnRH pulse generator induces an increase in amplitude and frequency of episodic secretion of pituitary LH and FSH. This form of precocious puberty can be classified into two types: one with identifiable neurological lesions (e.g. intracranial tumours, congenital malformations, traumatic causes, postinfectious causes, etc.); in the absence of such a lesion, the precocious puberty is said to be idiopathic (sporadic, familial forms).

True precocious puberty must be distinguished from the gonadotrophin-independent form of sexual precocity. Its differential diagnosis comprises gonadotrophin-secreting tumours (inside or outside the central nervous system), increased androgen secretion by the adrenals (congenital adrenal hyperplasia, adrenal neoplasms) or by the testes (Leydig cell adenoma or testotoxicosis).

In case an underlying cause resulting in early puberty can be identified, therapy should be directed to treating this cause if possible. Such a treatment could consist in surgery, radiation, or chemotherapy for cerebral, ectopic gonadotrophin-producing, gonadal, or adrenal tumours. Congenital adrenal hyperplasia warrants adrenal suppression. In gonadotrophin-independent precocity, testolactone or ketoconazole have been used. Among patients with central puberty – idiopathic or otherwise – the current treatment of choice consists in stopping gonadotrophin production with gonadotrophin-releasing hormone (GnRH) analogues. Adequacy of treatment should be monitored by clinical indices and hormonal testing.

I.2.3 Delayed Puberty

In boys, puberty is considered delayed when secondary sex characteristics (testicular volume <4 ml) do not occur prior to 14 years of age.

There is a multitude of causes for delayed puberty (Pozo and Argente 2003). Constitutional delay of growth and puberty is the most frequent cause of delayed puberty in boys. Usually there is a family component of late maturation. Furthermore, functional hypogonadotrophic hypogonadism can be due to chronic pathology such as chronic illnesses, nutritional disorders, isolated growth hormone deficiency, other hormonal disturbances or stress. The spectrum of permanent hypogonadotrophic conditions comprises entities such as Kallmann's syndrome, isolated gonadotrophin deficiency, fertile eunuch syndrome, or multiple pituitary hormone deficiencies. Chromosomal anomalies, anomalies of hormone biosynthesis and receptivity, malformation syndromes, agenesis of the gonads, gonadal hypoplasia and acquired primary gonadal failure lead to hypergonadotrophic hypogonadism.

Full replacement of androgen to attain and maintain an adult male state physically and sexually requires parenteral administration of testosterone. The dosage of initial therapy depends on age and maturational status of the patient and the rapidity of pubertal development desired. Traditionally, testosterone is given as a depot injection. Transdermal application via patches or gels may become a substitute for this mode of therapy; data in children are still scarce. Although observation is the main recommendation in individuals with constitutional delay of growth and puberty, short-term administration of testosterone can be beneficial in some situations.

References

Marshall WA, Tanner JM (1970) Variations in the pattern of pubertal changes in boys. Arch Dis Child 45:13–23

Partsch CJ, Heger S, Sippell WG (2002) Management and outcome of central precocious puberty. Clin Endocrinol 56:129–148

Pozo J, Argente J (2003) Ascertainment and treatment of delayed puberty. Horm Res 60 [Suppl 3]:35–48

Male Factor Fertility Problems

I.3

I.3.1 The Consensus-Based Approach to Standardized Diagnosis and Management of the Infertile Male

F. Comhaire, A. Mahmoud

In the past, several workshops and meetings have been convened trying to reach consensus on different aspects of andrology. These have addressed, among other items, the following questions: the usefulness of advanced diagnostic techniques of semen analysis (ESHRE 1996; Comhaire 1997; Fraser et al. 1997), management of testicular germ cell tumours (Krege et al. 2001), couples' perception of contraception (Neal and Groat 1976), the role of counselling of the infertile couple (Monach 2003), vasectomy reversal (Chawla et al. 2004) and managed care (Hull 1996). In trying to overcome confusion on terminology in the unregulated field of infertility (Easton 1998), several working definitions have been introduced by WHO (Rowe et al. 1993).

The term "infertility" is used to describe the situation where a couple does not succeed in achieving a spontaneous pregnancy in spite of the exposure to the risk of pregnancy during a given period of time. A time limit of 12 months is commonly accepted (Rowe et al. 2000). Although arbitrary, the time period corresponds with the fact that the majority (approximately 85 %) of couples who have achieved spontaneous pregnancy did so within 12 months.

This does not imply, however, that investigation for infertility must be postponed until the period of 12 months has elapsed, particularly if the couple has events in the history to suspect infertility in either partner, or the age of the female partner is relatively high, approaching 35 years or older.

The term "primary male infertility" is used when a man has never impregnated a woman. Impregnation means that conception was attained, independent of the outcome of pregnancy.

"Secondary male infertility" is when the man has impregnated a woman, irrespective of whether she is the present partner and irrespective of the outcome of pregnancy. Certain diagnoses are less likely to be found in these men, such as congenital disorders, or severe impairment of sperm quality with azoospermia or extreme oligozoospermia, whereas varicocele and male accessory gland infection are more common.

The duration of involuntary infertility is defined as the number of months during which the couple has been having sexual intercourse without the use of any contraceptive method. This gives prognostic information about the couple's future probability of spontaneous conception (Fig. I.3.1).

The investigation of the infertile couple must always include the investigation of both partners. In general, a male factor is detected in half of the couples with demonstrable abnormalities. In approximately half of these, there is a female factor as well (Steinberger et al. 1981; WHO 1987). Treatment should always aim at cre-

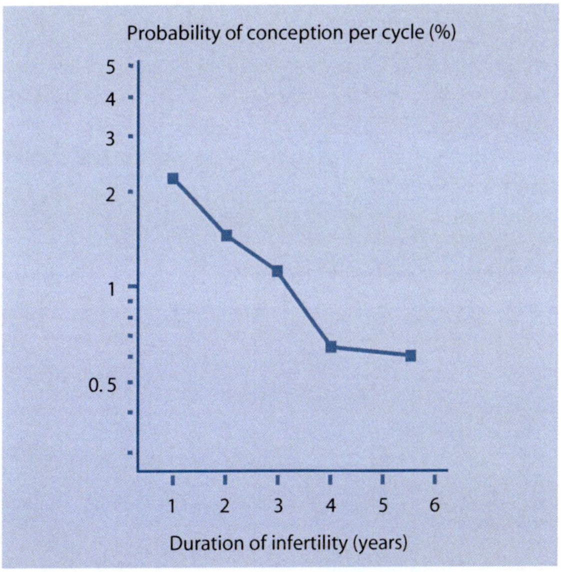

Fig. I.3.1. The probability of conception per cycle of exposure (P/C) is shown in relation to the duration of infertility. Note that P/C values are plotted on a logarithmic scale

ating optimal conditions for impregnation, including the correction of all causal factors in both partners. Clearly, improving the fertility potential of the female partner will increase the probability of the couple, in which the male partner is subfertile, in attaining conception (Rodriguez-Rigau et al. 1978; Silber 1989). There is some evidence to suggest that a male factor may also be involved in certain cases of unexplained recurrent spontaneous abortion (Bernardini et al. 2004). It is speculated that, in such cases, the DNA quality is not optimal, e.g. because of a high level of oxidative damage, whereas sperm–oocyte fusion can occur.

WHO has performed a comprehensive trial including a very large number of couples consulting for infertility who where investigated using a fixed protocol and standardized methodology, complemented by external quality control by an independent expert group (WHO 1987). After thorough analysis of all the data, a simplified system for the standardized investigation, diagnosis and management was created (Rowe et al. 2000) and implemented in an expert computer programme. Every item included in the system was validated as to its contribution to diagnosis and management.

A working group of ten clinical experts, with longstanding experience in the field of andrology, carefully reviewed the evidence gained from the WHO study, from retrospective and prospective cohort studies and from published randomized trials and meta-analyses. Also, the results of prospective trials conducted by WHO were taken into account. In case of contradictory conclusions from different trial designs, for example, regarding the effect of treatment with tamoxifen or of varicocele, the expert group also considered evidence from physiopathology, anatomy and epidemiology to formulate recommendations. In doing so, several levels of quality of evidence were taken into account, and this was reflected in the choice of phrasing.

In the present chapter covering male factor fertility problems, the consensus-based viewpoints expressed in the WHO manual are updated by recently published findings, both regarding the clinical approach and assisted reproductive technologies.

References

Bernardini LM, Costa M, Bottazzi C, Gianaroli L, Magli C, Venturini PL, Francioso R, Conte N, Ragni N (2004) Sperm aneuploidy and recurrent pregnancy loss. Reprod Biomed Online 9:312–320

Chawla A, O'Brien J, Lisi M, Zini A, Jarvi K (2004) Should all urologists performing vasectomy reversals be able to perform vasoepididymostomies if required? J Urol 172:1048–1050

Comhaire F (1997) Consensus workshop on advanced diagnostic andrology techniques [letter]. Hum Reprod 12:872–872

Easton M (1998) Infertility treatment: lack of consensus plagues an unregulated field. CMAJ 158:1345–1348

ESHRE (1996) Consensus workshop on advanced diagnostic andrology techniques. ESHRE (European Society of Human Reproduction and Embryology) Andrology Special Interest Group. Hum Reprod 11:1463–1479

Fraser L, Barratt CL, Canale D, Cooper T, DeJonge C, Irvine S, Mortimer D, Oehninger S, Tesarik J (1997) Consensus workshop on advanced diagnostic andrology techniques. ESHRE Andrology Special Interest Group. Hum Reprod 12:873

Hull MG (1996) Managed care of infertility. Curr Opin Obstet Gynecol 8:305–313

Krege S, Souchon R, Schmoll HJ (2001) Interdisciplinary consensus on diagnosis and treatment of testicular germ cell tumors: result of an update conference on evidence-based medicine (EBM). Eur Urol 40:372–391

Monach J (2003) Counselling – its role in the infertility team. Hum Fertil (Camb) 6:S17–S21

Neal AG, Groat HT (1976) Consensus in the marital dyad: couples' perceptions of contraception, communication, and family life. Sociol Focus 9:317–329

Rodriguez-Rigau LJ, Smith KD, Steinberger E (1978) Relationship of varicocele to sperm output and fertility of male partners in infertile couples. J Urol 120:691–694

Rowe PJ, Comhaire FH, Hargreave TB, Mellows HJ (1993) WHO manual for the standardized investigation and diagnosis of infertile couple. Cambridge University Press, Cambridge

Rowe PJ, Comhaire FH, Hargreave TB, Mahmoud AMA (2000) WHO manual for the standardized investigation, diagnosis and management of the infertile male. Cambridge University Press, Cambridge

Silber SJ (1989) The relationship of abnormal semen parameters to male fertility. Hum Reprod 4:947–953

Steinberger E, Rodriguez-Rigau LJ, Smith KD (1981) The interaction between the fertility potentials of the two members of an infertile couple. In: Frajese G, Hafez ES, Conti C, Fabbrini A (eds) Oligozoospermia: recent progress in andrology. Raven, New York, pp 9–19

WHO (1987) Towards more objectivity in diagnosis and management of male infertility. Int J Androl Suppl 7

I.3.2 The WHO Recommended Diagnostic Flow Chart

F. Comhaire, A. Mahmoud

It is still common practice in many countries for the female partner of an infertile couple to be investigated, and possibly treated, before the male partner is evaluated. In other cases, the clinician (usually the gynaecologist, sometimes the general practitioner) has ordered semen analysis to be performed from the very beginning of the couple's investigation.

In order to assess the diagnosis of the infertile male, a systematic approach must be adopted, and it is recommended to accurately complete the questionnaire and record of physical findings. This will help to avoid overlooking details that may be of crucial importance and may completely change the management and prognosis in particular couples (e.g. effect of hot baths or alcohol abuse).

Once all the information has been put together, the clinician will introduce these into the flow chart (Fig. I.3.2), which is meant to help with the diagnostic process, and will lead to one or more applicable diagnoses, in agreement with objective criteria for the diagnostic categories.

Clearly, a man may encounter problems with erection and/or intromission, or he may be unable to deposit his semen into the vagina at the appropriate period of the cycle. There are several reasons for sexual and/or ejaculatory inadequacy, which must be explored and treated whenever possible. In such cases, the diagnosis of sexual and ejaculatory dysfunction is applicable and treatment should be applied independent of the quality of the spermatozoa. Nonetheless, semen analysis should be performed, if semen can be obtained, since the outcome of this analysis will influence the infertility management. Also, sexual or ejaculatory dysfunction may not have been detected during history taking, and may be revealed by a repeatedly negative postcoital test with no spermatozoa being present, in spite of spermatozoa being found upon semen analysis.

If sexual and ejaculatory function are normal and intercourse occurs with adequate frequency and is timely, semen analysis is of pivotal importance.

Independent of the characteristics of the spermatozoa (concentration, motility and morphology), the presence of antisperm antibodies (ASAs) on motile spermatozoa will induce the diagnosis of immunological cause. In these cases, the management will depend on several factors, including the type of antibodies and other characteristics of the spermatozoa.

If sexual and ejaculatory functions are normal and no antisperm antibodies are detected, the diagnosis and management will entirely depend on the result of the semen analysis. If the characteristics of spermatozoa are better than the reference limits, possible abnormalities of seminal plasma may be involved, such as increased viscosity, abnormal liquefaction or abnormal ejaculate volume. In these cases, the diagnostic category of isolated seminal plasma abnormalities is applicable, and it is recommended to have a postcoital test performed. If this test reveals a normal number of motile sperm, the isolated seminal plasma abnormality is not considered the cause of the couple's infertility. If the test is abnormal, there are reasons to accept that the seminal plasma abnormality does contribute to the infertility problem, which will result in appropriate treatment.

The finding of abnormal characteristics of the spermatozoa *must* induce a systematic and state-of-the art search for causal factors. Information from history taking often is of primordial importance for the diagnosis of iatrogenic factors, systemic and congenital causes, and acquired testicular damage. The diagnoses of varicocele, male accessory gland infection and endocrine causes are mostly based on clinical examination and complementary investigations.

In cases with normal sexual and ejaculatory function and abnormal spermatozoa, but with no demonstrable causal factor, the classification idiopathic is applied. It should be stressed that the latter classification requires the formal exclusion of all possible or probable causes.

If spermatozoa are present in the ejaculate, the diagnostic classification will be either idiopathic oligozoospermia, idiopathic asthenozoospermia, or idiopathic teratozoospermia, or any combination of these. This classification is relevant for the prediction of the probability of spontaneous conception, and for the choice of treatment. The term "cryptozoospermia" is used for the situation where no spermatozoa are seen in the fresh preparation, but some spermatozoa are detected in the sediment after centrifugation. The approach of patients belonging to this group is the same as for cases classified as idiopathic oligozoospermia.

Men in whom no spermatozoa are detected, neither in the fresh preparation nor after centrifugation, are classified as suffering from azoospermia. Provided there is no demonstrable cause for the absence of spermatozoa, the classification as idiopathic is accepted. Further investigations are needed to differentiate between obstructive or primary testicular azoospermia.

The diagnoses of idiopathic abnormal sperm quality (oligospermia and/or asthenospermia and/or teratozoospermia or azoospermia) can never be combined with any causal diagnosis, but several causal diagnoses

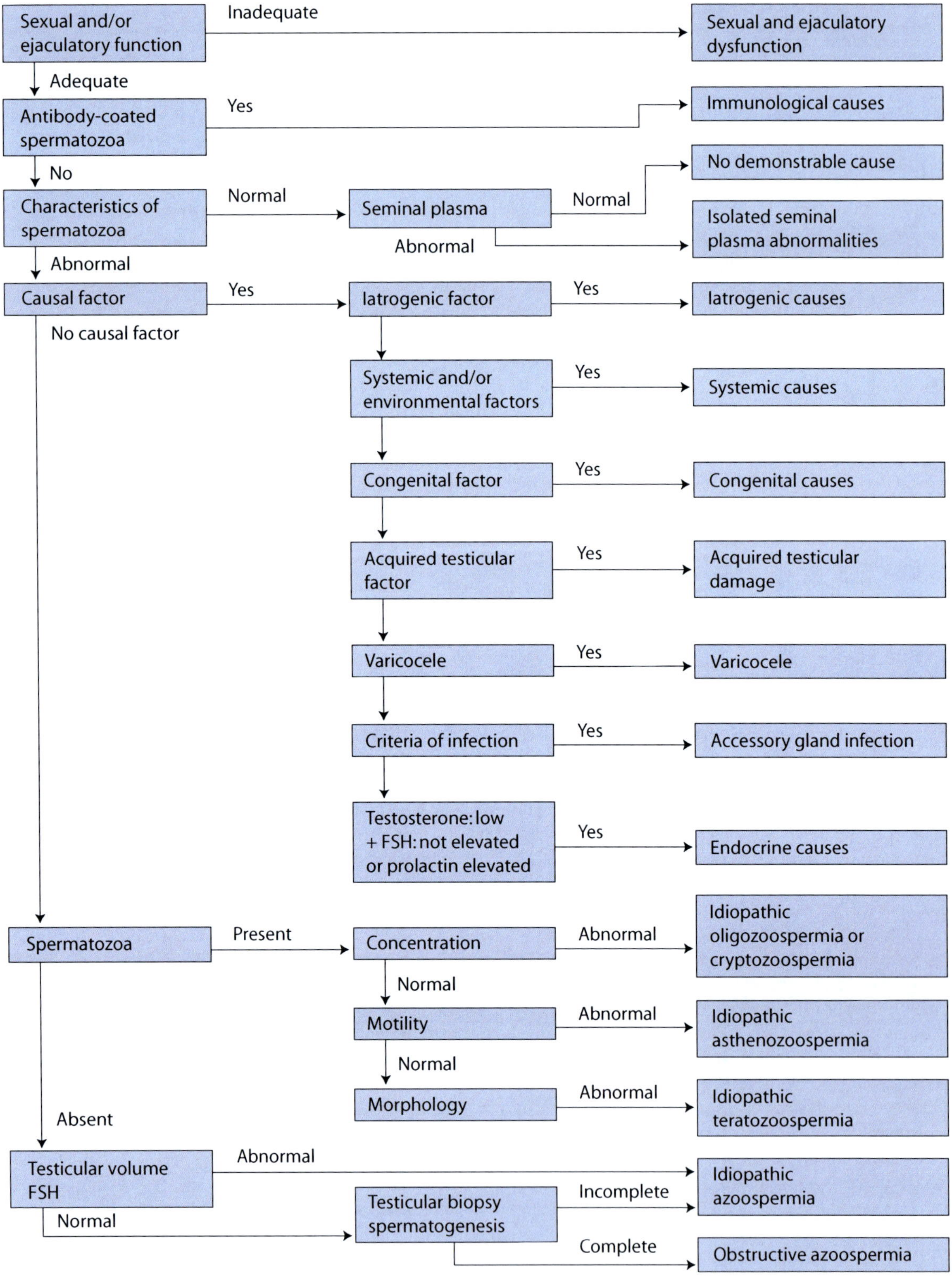

Fig. I.3.2. The WHO recommended diagnostic flow chart

may be combined, where, for example, the patient may suffer from both an immunological factor and male accessory gland infection (MAGI), or varicocele and systemic causes.

It is recommended to use the flow chart to assist the clinician in making the diagnosis for each individual patient. Also, the diagnostic flow chart has been implemented in a computer programme that will automatically generate all applicable diagnoses and suggest the optimal treatment.

I.3.3 Implications of Multifactorial Aetiology in the Diagnosis and Management of Male Infertility

F. Comhaire, A. Mahmoud

Similar to many other diseases, the aetiology of male infertility is commonly multifactorial. Aside from the typical andrological diseases, as listed in the following chapters and summarized in the diagnostic flow chart, there are three complementary groups of factors that may exert an unfavourable influence on men's reproductive potential (Fig. I.3.3).

Genetic factors include the well-known abnormalities in the number of chromosomes and structural defects such as translocations. These and the alterations found in patients with congenital bilateral agenesis of the vasa deferentia and seminal vesicles associated with mutant cystic fibrosis transmembrane conductance regulator (CFTR), and the microdeletions of the DAZ region of the Y-chromosome, are to be classified as congenital abnormalities.

However, other minor genetic defects may play a role in the pathogenesis of sperm deficiency, and may possibly come to expression if the DNA repair mechanisms (McMurray and Kortun 2003; Karagiannis and El Osta 2004; Rockett et al. 2004) of spermatogenic cells are unable to correct the defect(s). The latter could well result from oxidative overload, which itself may be due to a number of factors at the testicular level (e.g. varicocele), the genital tract (e.g. infection or inflammation) (Depuydt et al. 1996), or from external origin (Aitken 2003; Schrader and Cooke 2003).

Lifestyle factors include nutritional state and intake of certain subgroups of essential fatty acids, obesity and overweight, abuse of alcohol (more than 6 units per day) or tobacco (more than ten cigarettes per day) (Mahmoud et al. 1998), the regular use of hot baths, tight clothing, and severe stress. These may directly suppress spermatogenesis and/or are associated with the generation of excessive amounts of reactive oxygen species.

Another group of factors with adverse effects are the exposure to toxic substances such as heavy metals (Bonde et al. 2002), carbon disulphide (Vanhoorne et al. 1994), or benzenes at the workplace. Also, exposure to high ambient temperature may suppress spermatogenesis. In addition, internal exposure to environmental agents that disrupt the hormonal balance, including xeno-oestrogens or antiandrogens, seem to play an important role.

Finally, several causal diagnoses may be given in the same patient, reinforcing each other's impact because of (negative) synergy.

Evaluating the population of men consulting because of infertility by means of the sperm production

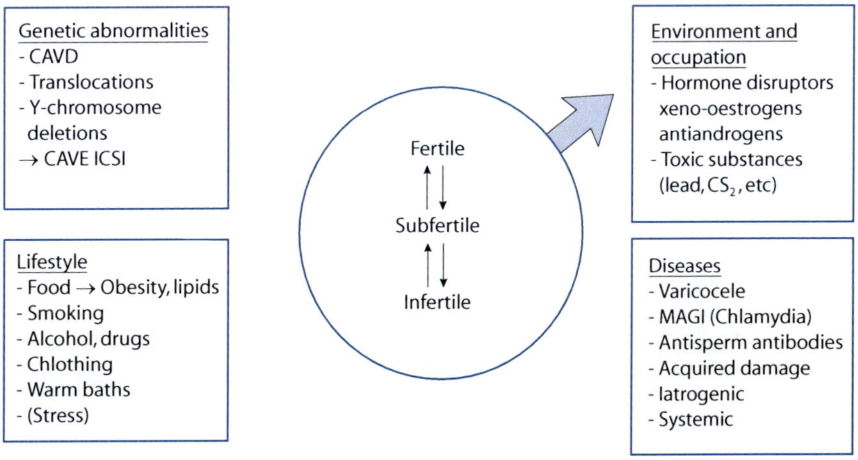

Fig. I.3.3. Subfertility/infertility: a multifactorial disease. *CAVD* congenital agenesis of the vasa deferentia, *CAVE ICSI* beware of transmission by intracytoplasmic sperm injection, *MAGI* Male accessory gland infection

index demonstrates a cumulative distribution (Fig. I.3.4). The sperm production index is calculated by dividing the sperm output per ejaculate (sperm concentration multiplied by ejaculate volume) by the total testicular volume. In normal men, the sperm production index is estimated at 4.9 or more million spermatozoa per millilitre of testicular volume per ejaculate. The distribution observed in Fig. I.3.4 suggests a multifactorial causality in a large proportion of infertile men (Everaert et al. 2003). For instance, smoking and varicocele have an additive effect in decreasing the sperm production index (Fig. I.3.5). This index is decreased in men with more than 2 million peroxidase-positive white blood cells who present no other abnormalities of the genital organs. In contrast, a decrease in the index is already observed when 0.3 million white blood cells are found in the ejaculate of men with varicocele, again suggesting a synergy between these two factors.

The body mass index of men consulting for infertility was higher than that of the average male population of the same region (Fig. I.3.6), with more patients being classified as overweight or obese. Furthermore, the intake of essential fatty acids belonging to the omega-3 group was lower in infertile men than in fertile controls, and there was a positive correlation between the nutritional intake of alpha-linolenic acid (18:3 ω3) and both sperm concentration and progressive motility (Christophe et al. 1998).

In view of these and many other findings, it is mandatory to take into account that fertility in a particular man may result from the synergistic interaction between several factors, namely the genetic constitution, the patient's lifestyle, the amount of toxic agents he is exposed to in his workplace and local environment,

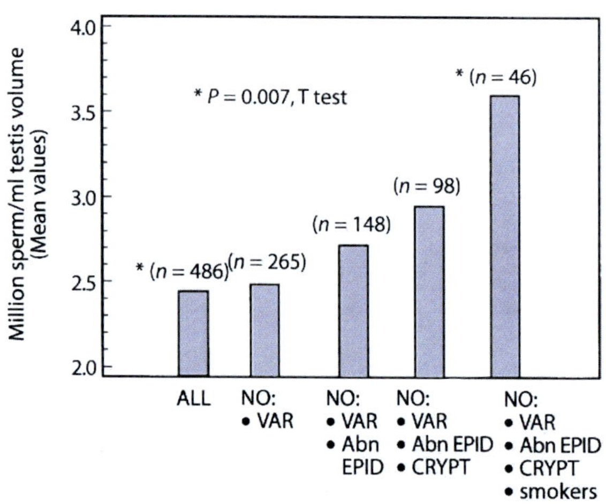

Fig. I.3.4. Cumulative effect of different factors on sperm production (non-azoospermic subfertile men). *VAR* varicocele, *AbnEPID* abnormal epididymis, *CRYPT* cryptorchidism

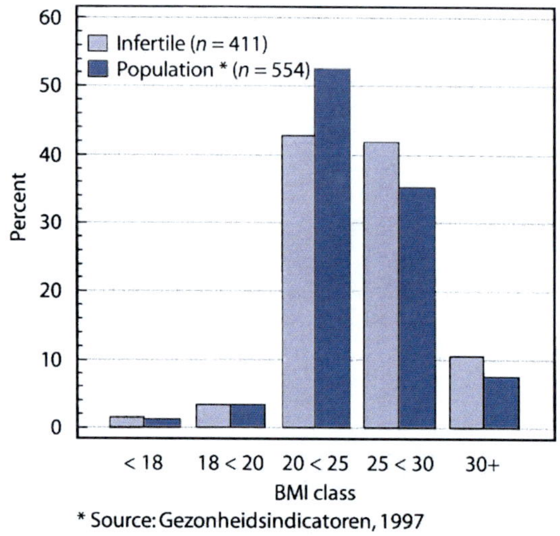

Fig. I.3.6. Body mass index in subfertile men compared to a matched normal population

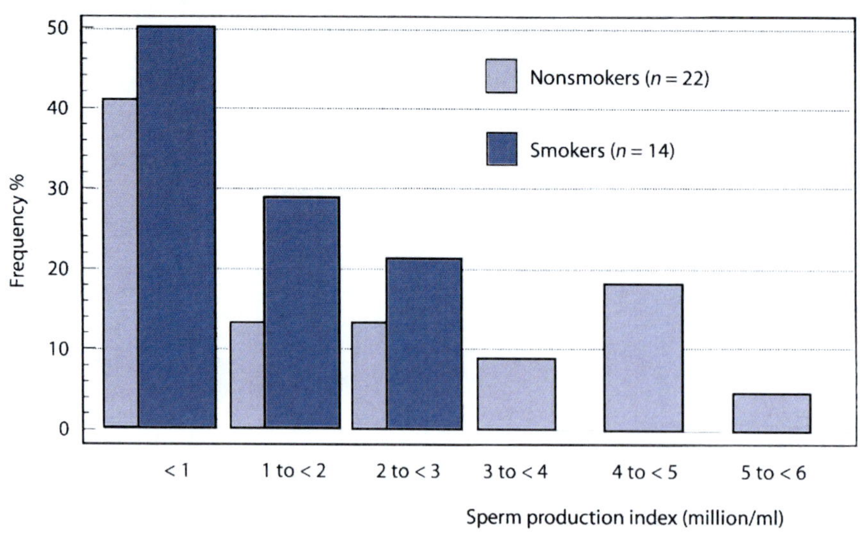

Fig. I.3.5. Effect of smoking on sperm production in subfertile men with varicocele (azoospermia, cryptorchidism, abnormal epididymis excluded)

and the possible presence of disease(s) of the urogenital region. Hence, management may not be limited to treating the latter, but it must also improve the circumstantial factors as part of a holistic approach.

References

Aitken J (2003) Oxidative stress in the male germinal cell line and its role in the aetiology of male infertility and genetic disease. Reprod Biomed Online 7:65–70

Bonde JP, Joffe M, Apostoli P, Dale A, Kiss P, Spano M, Caruso F, Giwercman A, Bisanti L, Porru S, Vanhoorne M, Comhaire F, Zschiesche W (2002) Sperm count and chromatin structure in men exposed to inorganic lead: lowest adverse effect levels. Occup Environ Med 59:234–242

Christophe A, Zalata A, Mahmoud A, Comhaire F (1998) Fatty acid composition of sperm phospholipids and its nutritional implications. Middle East Fertil Soc J 3:46–53

Depuydt CE, Bosmans E, Zalata A, Schoonjans F, Comhaire FH (1996) The relation between reactive oxygen species and cytokines in andrological patients with or without male accessory gland infection. J Androl 17:699–707

Everaert K, Mahmoud A, Depuydt C, Maeyaert M, Comhaire F (2003) Chronic prostatitis and male accessory gland infection–is there an impact on male infertility (diagnosis and therapy)? Andrologia 35:325–330

Karagiannis TC, El Osta A (2004) DNA damage repair and transcription double-strand breaks: signaling pathways and repair mechanisms. Cell Mol Life Sci 61:2137–2147

Mahmoud AM, Schoonjans F, Zalata AA, Comhaire FH (1998) The effect of male smoking on semen quality, reducing capacity, reactive oxygen species, and spontaneous and assisted conception rates. Andrology in the nineties. Genk, Belgium, 22–25 April

McMurray CT, Kortun IV (2003) Repair in haploid male germ cells occurs late in differentiation as chromatin is condensing. Chromosoma 111:505–508

Rockett JC, Patrizio P, Schmid JE, Hecht NB, Dix DJ (2004) Gene expression patterns associated with infertility in humans and rodent models. Mutat Res 549:225–240

Schrader TJ, Cooke GM (2003) Effects of Aroclors and individual PCB congeners on activation of the human androgen receptor in vitro. Reprod Toxicol 17:15–23

Vanhoorne M, Comhaire F, De Bacquer D (1994) Epidemiological study of the effects of carbon disulfide on male sexuality and reproduction. Arch Environ Health 49:273–278

I.3

I.3.4 Sexual Dysfunction and Male Fertility

T.B. Hargreave

Key Messages

- Sexual dysfunction is the primary cause in approximately 1 % of cases of infertility.
- Male sexual dysfunction as a consequence of infertility is common and this should be considered in the overall management of the couple.
- Assessment of the man should include a complete clinical examination including examination of the penis, and the foreskin should be retracted to ensure the diagnosis of minor anatomical problems such as phimosis or tight frenulum.
- Performance anxiety is often a problem following surgical procedures such as circumcision or correction of congenital penile deformity, and in such cases postsurgical treatment with type-5 phosphodiesterase (PDE5) inhibitors may prevent subsequent sexual dysfunction.

I.3.4.1 Definition of the Disease

Sexual dysfunction as a cause of male infertility can be defined as those physical or psychological problems causing inadequate erection and or inadequate frequency of sexual intercourse, sufficient to prevent deposition of semen in the vagina. Ejaculatory problems include anejaculation, retrograde ejaculation or psychological or physical problems resulting in ejaculation outside the vagina, for example epispadias. Erectile problems include failure of development of the penis, insufficient rigidity of erections or deformity of erection sufficient to penetration. Sexual dysfunction as a primary cause of male infertility accounts for approximately 1 % of cases (Fertility Problems Clinic, Western General Hospital, Edinburgh, unpublished data). Sexual dysfunction as a consequence of male infertility is more common.

I.3.4.2 Aetiology and Pathogenesis

Anatomical problems sufficient to interfere with erections include congenital abnormalities such as micropenis, hypospadias and epispadias and acquired abnormalities such as phimosis, scarring of the frenulum, and trauma including paraplegia. Although primary psychological problems account for a proportion of cases, failure of erection secondary to infertility problems is much more common, although not the cause of the infertility per se. Anejaculation is rare but may occur in association with spinal cord disease. Premature ejaculation is common in young men with a new sexual partner, but more recently it has been shown that there are a proportion of men with lifelong premature ejaculation. Retrograde ejaculation is another

Table I.3.1. Causes of retrograde ejaculation

Neurogenic	Spinal cord + cauda equina lesion	Injury Tumour Stenosis Tethered spinal cord (Shibahara et al. 2000) After anterior interbody lumbar fusion (Tiusanen et al. 1995)
	Neuropathies	Multiple sclerosis Diabetes
	Surgical injury to nerves	Retroperitoneal lymph node dissection (men with testicular cancer) Sympathectomy Abdominoperineal resection
Bladder neck incompetence	Congenital defects	Exstrophy Hemitrigone
	Congenital dysfunction Bladder neck resection	
	Prostatectomy	Effect more pronounced after open prostatectomy compared with TURP or TUIP (De Paula et al. 1997)
Obstruction	Congenital	Ectopic ureterocele Urethral valves
	Acquired	Urethral stricture

common ejaculatory problem. This may be congenital or acquired (see Table I.3.1). In acquired cases, there may be history of pelvic fracture or urological surgery in childhood or infancy such as treatment of urethral valves.

I.3.4.2.1 Sexual Dysfunction as a Consequence of Infertility

A typical problem is a man who has erectile dysfunction because he and his wife understand that sexual intercourse for procreation has to occur on day 14 of the cycle and her drive for pregnancy becomes so consuming that eroticism is lacking and sexual intercourse becomes stressful. This problem can be aggravated by lack of proper organization in the fertility clinic and can often be prevented by ensuring that couples are given proper information about tests and treatments and are not subject to long trials of unproven treatments. Occasionally, one may see a couple where secondary psychosexual problems have caused major disharmony and in such cases referral for counselling or psychotherapy should be in parallel to any fertility treatment.

I.3.4.3 Clinical Findings: History, Physical Examination, Technical Investigations, Laboratory Findings

Erectile deficiency as a cause of male infertility can be difficult to diagnose because the man with psychological problems may hide the problem, which only becomes apparent to the clinician after talking to both partners and once both partners have gained confidence in the treating physician. This process may take more than one consultation and the time required can be difficult to find in the context of a busy fertility clinic. Indicators of a possible sexual problem are the inability of the man to provide semen samples and or an unexpectedly poor postcoital test. If the man says he is unable to produce a semen sample by masturbation, then many clinics encourage the couple to collect a semen sample using a silicon condom; however, if the man is still unable to comply the clinician should take the time to question the couple about sexual intercourse, including finding out whether the man and his partner have a basic understanding of penetrative intercourse and female anatomy. It can help to take a history about sexual technique at the same time as genital and vaginal examination, posing the question about whether penetration is successful or not. If it is established that the man is unable to try to have penetrative intercourse and after penile anatomical abnormalities have been excluded, further management is with professional psychosexual assessment (see Chap. II.4.8).

Anatomical penile problems such as phimosis can be detected during clinical examination by retraction of the foreskin or by asking the man to do this. It may be necessary to examine the penis when erect (see Chap. I.4), especially if the man complains of erectile deformity and there is no significant abnormality on examination of the flaccid penis.

Diagnosis of retrograde ejaculation may be suspected if the man gives the history of no external ejaculation or if he is unable or only produces a very small volume of ejaculate and particularly if he describes passing cloudy material in his urine after orgasm. The diagnosis may be confirmed by asking the man to produce a postorgasm urine sample and the finding of a large numbers of sperm in the centrifuged deposit.

I.3.4.4 Differential Diagnosis

The main differential diagnosis when considering penile erection problems and fertility is between organic and psychological causes. In general in younger men and in the absence of any clear indication on physical examination, psychological problems are more likely but can be difficult to diagnose.

The main differential diagnosis when there is a lack of external ejaculation is between retrograde ejaculation and ejaculatory duct obstruction and congenital absence of the seminal vesicles. This latter condition is usually associated with congenital bilateral absence of the vas deferens and thus the distinction is usually by means of clinical examination and the finding of absent vasa. Retrograde ejaculation can be distinguished from the various obstructive disorders by the finding of sperm in the postorgasm urine.

I.3.4.5 Treatment

Treatment depends on the cause of the problem. Usually severe congenital problems such as epispadias, exstrophy and micropenis are evident from infancy and treatment of the fertility problem is in the context of a series of treatments from infancy onwards to restore anatomical integrity and urinary and sexual function. In this situation, it is often best to use treatments to enable fertility such as microscopic epididymal sperm aspiration and intracytoplasmic sperm injection (MESA, ICSI) separately from treatments to restore sexual function such as penile reconstructive surgery. Minor anatomical problems may need surgical correction, e.g. circumcision for a tight phimosis. In addition to the anatomical problem, there is nearly always considerable performance anxiety, and following any surgical treatment, it is usually helpful to offer adjunctive treatment in the postoperative period with PDE inhibitors such as sildenafil. For men with primary psychopathology, treatment should be undertaken by a psychiatrist with special expertise in sexual problems. In this situation, the couple may be helped towards fertility with artificial insemination techniques but this should only be offered in the context of psychotherapy and with the agreement of the treating psychiatrist.

Treatment to restore antegrade ejaculation is relatively unsuccessful, whereas treatment of the fertility problem can be done by obtaining sperm and using artificial insemination or IVF techniques. The various types of treatment that can be used are shown in the Table I.3.2.

I.3.4.5.1 Achieving Fertility for Men with Paraplegia

The andrologist may be concerned with helping men with paraplegia in two respects – firstly to achieve fertility and secondly to enable sexual intercourse. In general, treatment to improve these functions is separate. Various treatments to obtain sperm are shown in Table I.3.3. Treatments to help the man achieve sexual intercourse are described in Chap. I.4

Men with paraplegia have on average lower sperm concentration and motility than intact men. This is because of nondrainage, genitourinary infection and raised testicular temperature when sitting in a wheel chair. Semen quality can be improved by regular ejaculation. This is easily achieved if the man has a hypogastric plexus stimulator or if he is able to achieve ejaculation with a vibrator. Although improvement has been reported with repeated electro-ejaculation this is much more difficult to organize (Chen et al. 1999). Genital tract infection is reduced by good management of the bladder as well as regular ejaculation. Testicular temperature when in a wheelchair can be reduced by propping the legs apart and attention to clothing.

I.3.4.6 Results of Treatment

When there is a sexual problem, the results of treatment may be assessed in terms of the couple achieving fertility and the couple achieving penetrative sexual intercourse. Ideally, conception occurs as a result of natural intercourse but in some of the above problems this will not be so. As a general rule, spermatogenesis is normal and sperm are of normal quality; therefore it is nearly always possible to obtain sperm and the results of fertility treatments are the same as the results of intracytoplasmic sperm injection (ICSI). Sexual dysfunction in the context of severe psychopathology can be very resistant to treatment and difficult to manage. When there is a simple problem such as phimosis, the results of treatment are excellent, especially if adjuvant PDE inhibitor treatment is offered.

I.3.4.7 Prevention

Young men with erectile or ejaculatory problems often have secondary performance anxiety and if unrecognized this can be the cause of failure of treatment. The problem can be prevented by proper organization of the fertility problems clinic and by offering adjunctive PDE5 therapy after surgical correction. Proper organi-

Table I.3.2. Treatment of retrograde ejaculation

Treatment	Description of treatment	Comment about success and risks
Treatment to restore antegrade ejaculation		
Drugs which stimulate alpha receptors in the bladder neck (Sandler 1979)	Ephedrine taken 1 h before intercourse. Desipramine 50 mg alternate days	These are often used as a first-line treatment but do not work in the majority of cases
Pyridazines (new antihypertensive)	Amezinium 10 mg once a day (Ichiyanagi et al. 2003)	
	Imipramine 25–50 mg for 7 days	Reported after node dissection (Ochsenkuhn et al. 1999)
Intercourse with a full bladder	The man has intercourse with an uncomfortably full bladder. In this situation, the bladder neck tends to close more firmly and sometimes antegrade ejaculation results (see Shibahara et al. 2000)	Simple inexpensive treatment that most couples can try but more often than not does not work. The discomfort from the overfull bladder is not very sexy
Bladder neck surgery (Pryor 1988)	In theory it is possible to tighten the bladder neck by surgery or injection of bulking agents	However, the risks include urinary tract obstruction and as the consequence of this could be very damaging; most clinicians would not recommend surgical treatment
Treatment to achieve fertility		
Extraction of sperm from urine and artificial insemination	Acidic urine is harmful to sperm (Crich and Jequier 1978). The man is taught how to test the pH of his urine and is then instructed to take sufficient sodium bicarbonate (baking powder) to alkalinize the urine. After 24–48 h when the urine PH is alkaline he masturbates to orgasm and then immediately voids urine into a container with a buffer solution. This solution is centrifuged and the sperm are resuspended in tissue culture medium. Depending on sperm number, the sperm are used for artificial insemination or IVF	The whole process is quite laborious and requires that the man is able to understand what needs to be done and can comply with the instructions. When artificial insemination is used, this methodology avoids the need for any invasive procedure to obtain sperm and avoids IVF
Catheterization shortly after orgasm. Hotchkiss procedure (Ranieri et al. 1995; Silva et al. 2000). Introduction of modified Hams F10 solution into the bladder (Saito et al. 1998)	The man alkalinizes his urine as above. Immediately before orgasm he empties his bladder. Immediately after orgasm a silicon catheter is passed and the bladder is washed out with a buffer solution	This treatment requires a lot of cooperation from the man but when successful may avoid the need for IVF, as sometimes large numbers of sperm are obtained
Electro-ejaculation	Except for men with paraplegia, the procedure is painful and general anaesthesia is required. The bladder is washed out with buffer solution and then electro-ejaculation is performed and the bladder washed out again to obtain sperm	This treatment requires a general anaesthetic and is therefore more difficult to organize and more expensive. Also the equipment and expertise for electro-ejaculation are not universally available
ICSI with sperm extracted from the urine	Sperm are extracted from the urine (Nikolettos et al. 1999)	Only small numbers of sperm can be obtained and IVF or IVF ICSI is required
ICSI with sperm from MESA	This technology is widely available in IVF units and MESA is more and more frequently offered for men with retrograde ejaculation because of the lack of andrological expertise in any of the above techniques in many IVF clinics (Ranieri 1998)	

zation of the fertility problems clinic includes allowing the time to take a full medical history and complete physical examination, giving the couple a realistic prognosis and not recommending time-consuming unproven treatments. Also, wherever possible, the couple should see the same clinician at successive consultations.

Table I.3.3. Obtaining sperm from men with paraplegia

Reflex ejaculation in coitus or by masturbation (with or without drugs – see below)	This is achieved by 5% of men with complete cervical, upper thoracic and midthoracic lesions (Brindley 1994)	
Vibrator 60–100 Hz with amplitude of 3 mm peak to peak when the vibrator knob is held against the glans penis (Brindley 1994). Many vibrators available from sex shops do not fulfil these criteria with an amplitude of only 1 mm	Does not work unless T11–S4 segments are intact. Whether these segments are intact can be determined by checking that hip flexion occurs in response to scratching the sole of the foot	Vibrators Ling 201 (Ling dynamic systems of Royston Herts. UK) Ferticare (Multicept ApS, 95 Gentofte gade 2820 Gentofte, Denmark Wahl 2 speed massager Wahl clipper corporation, 2902 Locust St, Sterling, IL 61081 Vibrion, 15 Rue Charles de Gaulle, 42000 Saint Etienne, France Whirlimixer Fisons scientific instruments
Drugs to facilitate reflex ejaculation	Physostigmine (Chapelle 1984) Alpha-2 adrenoreceptor blockers Dopamine receptor stimulants	Side effect of vomiting Idazoxan Yohimbine Bromocriptine Apomorphine
Electro-ejaculation	Seager rigid electrode probe and sinusoidal stimulation of 50–60 Hz. Equipment modified from veterinary practice. Most widely used technique	Small risk of rectal injury. Rectal probes are fitted with temperature sensor and cut out device
Hypogastric plexus stimulators (Brindley et al. 1989)	The stimulator is implanted surgically and once implanted has a long life with function up to 10 years postimplantation	Allows the couple to obtain sperm at home and practice home insemination. Disadvantage of the need for a surgical procedure and limited availability of the necessary expertise
Sperm reservoirs (Brindley et al. 1986) and vas cannula	These reservoirs are no longer used because of limited success and the nowadays widespread availability of MESA	
MESA	The widespread availability of MESA is such that the technique has superseded most of the above techniques with perhaps the exception of electro-ejaculation	Lack of andrology expertise in some IVF units results in MESA being offered as the first-line treatment when some of the above treatments may be more appropriate

I.3

References

Brindley GS (1994) Neurophysiology of ejaculation and treatment of infertility in men with spinal cord injuries. In: Hargreave TB (ed) Male infertility. Springer, Berlin Heidelberg New York, pp 312

Brindley GS, Scott GI, Hendry WH (1986) Vas cannulation with implanted reservoirs for obstructive azoospermia or ejaculatory failure. Br J Urol 58:721–723

Brindley GS, Sauerwein D, Hendry WF (1989) Hypogastric plexus stimulators for obtaining semen from paraplegic men. Br J Urol 64:72–77

Chapelle PA (1984) Traitment de l'anéjaculation du paraplégique complet par association métoclopramide-eserine. In: Buvat J (ed) L'éjaculation et ses perturbations. Simep, Lyon

Chen D, Hartwig DM, Roth EJ (1999) Comparison of sperm quantity and quality in antegrade V retrograde ejaculates obtained by vibratory penile stimulation in males with spinal cord injury. Am J Phys Med Rehabil 78:46–51

Crich JP, Jequier AM (1978) Infertility in men with retrograde ejaculation: the action of urine on sperm motility and a simple method for achieving antegrade ejaculation. Fertil Steril 30:572–576

De Paula F, Donadio D, Lauretti S, Brisciani A, Florio A (1997) Transurethral incision of prostate (TUIP) and retrograde ejaculation. Arch Ital Urol Androl 69:163–166

Ichiyanagi O, Sasagawa I, Suzuki Y, Matsuki S, Itoh K, Miura M, Tomita Y (2003) Successful treatment of retrograde ejaculation with amezinium. Arch Androl 49:215–217

Nikolettos N, Al-Hasani S, Baukloh V, Schopper B, Demirel LC, Baban N, Sturm R, Rudolf K, Tomalak K, Tinneberg HR, Diedrich K (1999) The outcome of intracytoplasmic sperm injection in patients with retrograde ejaculation. Hum Reprod 14:2293–2296

Ochsenkuhn R, Kamischke A, Nieschlag E (1999) Imipramine for successful treatment of retrograde ejaculation caused by retroperitoneal surgery. Int J Androl 22:173–177

Pryor JP (1988) Reconstruction of the bladder neck for retrograde ejaculation. In Gingell C, Abrahms P (eds) Controversies and innovations in urological surgery. Springer, Berlin Heidelberg New York, pp 433–437

Ranieri DM (1998) Is IVF/ICSI always the first step to treat couples with infertility due to retrograde ejaculation? [letter] Fertil Steril 69:1160–1161

Ranieri DM, Simonetti S, Vicino M, Cormio L, Selvaggi L (1995) Successful establishment of pregnancy by superovu-

lation and intrauterine insemination with sperm recovered by a modified Hotchkiss procedure from a patient with retrograde ejaculation. Fertil Steril 64:1039–1042
Saito K, Kinoshita Y, Yumura Y, Iwasaki A, Hosaka M (1998) Successful pregnancy with sperm retrieved from the bladder after the introduction of a low-electrolyte solution for retrograde ejaculation. Fertil Steril 69:1149–1151
Sandler B (1979) Idiopathic retrograde ejaculation. Fertil Steril 32:474–475
Shibahara H, Toji H, Shigeta M, Yoshimoto T, Shima H, Koyama K (2000) Successful pregnancies in a case of retrograde ejaculation associated with tethered spinal cord syndrome. J Assist Reprod Genet 17:233–237
Silva PD, Larson KM, Van Every MJ, Silva DE (2000) Successful treatment of retrograde ejaculation with sperm recovered from bladder washings. A report of two cases. J Reprod Med 45:957–960
Tiusanen H, Seitsalo S, Osterman K, Soini J (1995) Retrograde ejaculation after anterior interbody lumbar fusion. Eur Spine J 4:339–342

I.3.5 Reference Values of Semen Variables and Their Interpretation

F. Comhaire, A. Mahmoud

Key Messages

- Approximately half of the couples consulting for an infertility problem present a "male factor".
- Commonly, the male partner is subfertile rather than infertile.
- The level of relative fertility can be expressed as probability of treatment-independent, naturally attained conception per menstrual cycle (or month) of exposure to the risk of pregnancy.
- The relative fertility potential depends on the degree of impairment of semen quality.
- Interpretation of the result of semen analysis must take into account the variability of fertilizing potential.

The majority of couples coming to consultation because they fail to initiate the desired pregnancy are subfertile rather than infertile or sterile (Comhaire et al. 1988). Fertility should be considered as a spectrum varying from as good as normal to completely sterile. The relative probability of each couple depends on several factors and is rather constant (Majumdar and Sheps 1970; Leridon 1980). Changes in the relative fertility can be brought about by many factors, either decreasing the probability of spontaneous conception (such as intercurrent disease) or improving it thanks to treatment (Wood et al. 1984; Comhaire and Kunnen 1985).

It has been demonstrated that the probability of treatment-independent conception in subfertile couples decreases with the duration of infertility (Schwartz et al. 1981; Hargreave and Nillson 1984). Other factors that can influence the treatment-independent conception rate include the type and severity of the causal pathology in the male, the age and possible pathology of the female partner, and whether or not the couple has previously achieved a pregnancy (Collins et al. 1983; Eimers et al. 1994).

Based on empirical observations, a model has been developed estimating the treatment-independent or spontaneous pregnancy rate for each individual couple (Comhaire et al. 1987) (Table I.3.4).

The relative fertility of a couple can be expressed as probability of conception per cycle of exposure (also called fecundability), which may vary from 0 in sterile couples to 30% or more in couples with high fertility. For practical reasons, fecundability is generally expressed as the probability of successful conception per month (P/M). The application of this concept is exemplified in two hypothetical model populations with fecundability of 15% and 5%. The cumulative probability of conception was calculated after different durations of exposure up to 12 months (Fig. I.3.7). In model A, a theoretic population of 100 couples is considered all having an identical fecundability of 15% per month. If all these couples try to achieve pregnancy starting at time 0, 15 (15% of 100) will be successful in the first cycle. Of the remaining 85 couples, 13 (15% of 85) will achieve pregnancy in the second cycle, 11 (15% of 72) in the third cycle, etc. (Fig. I.3.7). After 12 cycles of exposure, the cumulative conception rate is 86, whereas the remaining 14 couples will be considered "infertile" in agreement with the working definition. Model B consists of a population of 100 couples with reduced fertility and fecundability of 5% per month. When calculations are performed as above, 54% of couples will remain infertile after 12 cycles. It is important to realize that a couple can be categorized as infertile with highly variable degrees of fertility in terms of probability of conception per month.

Sperm quality is a major determinant of the probability of spontaneous conception. Not only the severity

Table I.3.4. A model for the calculation of the expected probability of spontaneous conception per month (P/M) in couples consulting for infertility

Formula I

Proportion of infertile and fertile couples (in %) related to the conception rate per cycle (P/C) and duration of exposure (n = number of months of trial to conceive).

Ia infertile couples = (1 – P/M)n × 100

Ib fertile couples = [1 – (1 – P/M)n] × 100

Formula II

IIa Probability of conception per cycle (P/M in %) related to the duration of infertility (n in months) in couples consulting for infertility of 12–48 months duration.

P/M = 4 × 0.97n

IIb Probability of spontaneous conception per cycle in couples consulting for infertility of more than 4 years duration (X is the number of years of unsuccessful exposure).

P/M = 1.3 – 0.1 X

Formula III

Probability of conception per cycle (P/M in %) related to duration of infertility (n in months), type of infertility (a), severity of male (bm) and female factor (bf).

P/M = 4 × 0.97n × (a) × (bm) × (bf)

Estimated coefficients expressing the relative influence of different factors affecting the spontaneous conception rate of infertile couples:

IIIa Primary infertility = 0.9

Secondary infertility = 1.35

bm: Male factors

No antisperm-antibodies present

Sperm concentration > 20 million/ml = 1.25

Sperm concentration 1.9 – 19.9 million/ml = 0.8

Sperm concentration 0.1 – 1.9 million/ml = 0.4

Idiopathic azoospermia = 0.08

Significant presence of antisperm antibodies on spermatozoa

Sperm concentration > 20 million/ml = 0.4

Sperm concentration 1.9 – 19.9 million/ml = 0.25

Sperm concentration 0.1 – 1.9 million/ml = 0.15

bf: Female factors

No demonstrable abnormality or minimal endometriosis (AFS I)

Age 20 – 30 years = 1.25

Age 30 – 40 years = 0.75

Age > 40 years = 0.50

Demonstrable pathology present

Functional ovulatory disturbances = 1.2

Cervical factor or mild endometriosis (AFS II) = 0.8

Minor tubal pathology or moderate endometriosis (AFS III) = 0.6

Bilateral tubal occlusion on hysterosalpingography or severe endometriosis (AFS IV) = 0.3

of impairment of sperm quality, but also the presence or absence of any demonstrable causal factor affects the conception rate (Comhaire et al. 1992). In general, the probability of conception in cases with sperm concentration exceeding 20 million/ml depends to a lesser extent on sperm motility and morphology (Zaini et al. 1985). The rather poor prognostic significance of the latter sperm characteristics contrasts with the fact that their power is relatively high to discriminate between semen of fertile as compared to subfertile men (Comhaire et al. 1987).

Men with sperm concentration over 20 million/ml, but abnormal motility or morphology of unknown origin (idiopathic astheno- and/or teratozoospermia) have a 40% higher probability of achieving spontaneous conception than men in whom the sperm abnormalities are related to a demonstrable cause such as varicocele, accessory gland infection, or congenital causes. Also, the fecundability of semen with sperm concentration over 20 million/ml but presence of antisperm antibodies is decreased (Table I.3.4).

Moderate oligozoospermia with sperm concentration between 3 and 19.9 million/ml results in a roughly 40% reduction of fecundability, while severe oligozoospermia between 0.1 and 2.9 million/ml reduces the probability of conception to almost zero (Collins et al. 1983).

It should be clear that answering the question "what is a normal semen analysis result?" is complex (Rogers et al. 1983) and hotly debated. In order to find a scientifically founded response, two approaches can be taken. The first one assesses the sperm characteristics of normally *fertile men* (who have attained successful

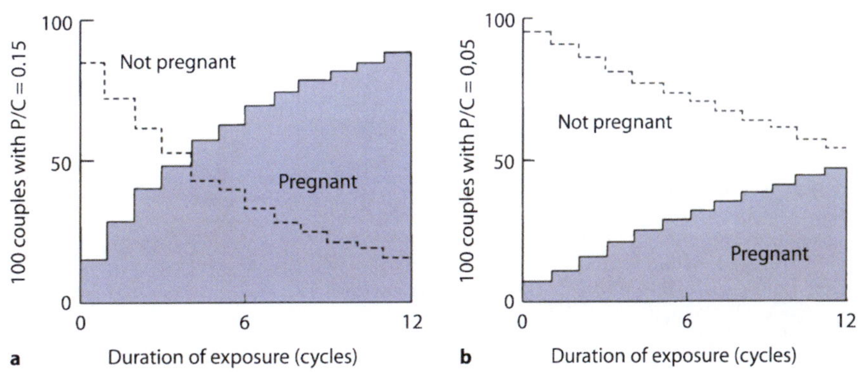

Fig. I.3.7a, b. The hatched area indicates the calculated cumulative conception rate related to the number of cycles of exposure in a model population of 100 couples with probability of conception of 15% per cycle (**a**) or 5% per cycle (**b**). The *broken line* shows the number of couples at risk

pregnancy within 12 months of exposure) and compare these with the characteristics of the spermatozoa of men who either did attain pregnancy but needed longer than 12 months to do so (*subfertile* group), and *sterile* men who completely failed in attaining spontaneous pregnancy in spite of the absence of demonstrable abnormalities in the female partner (Wang et al. 1988). Statistical methods such as the receiver-operating characteristic curves (ROC) (Schoonjans et al. 1996; Ombelet et al. 1997) are used to determine the accuracy of the different sperm characteristics in discriminating between the three groups (Fig. I.3.8). The 5th percentile of characteristics of the fertile and subfertile groups are used as lower reference values, and the 95th percentile as higher reference value, when applicable (Comhaire et al. 1987; Menkveld et al. 2001).

Another approach consists of performing semen analysis in first-pregnancy planners, and to relate the result of this analysis with the subsequent occurrence of pregnancy and time to pregnancy (Bonde et al. 1998) (Fig. I.3.9).

Comparison of the results of these approaches is feasible for those measurements where the same or comparable techniques of semen analysis have been used, e.g. ejaculate volume, sperm concentration, and percentage of progressive motility. The power of discrimination may also be better when objective methods for the assessment of, for example, sperm motility are implemented (Hinting et al. 1988). For other variables, comparison is impossible because different criteria are applied, for example in assessing sperm morphology (Panidis et al. 2003).

It should also be remembered that the discriminating power between fertile, subfertile and sterile is different for the different variables. Therefore, the finding of a concentration of type (a) motile sperm below the reference value gives a higher level of probability than a particular sample that belongs to, for example, subfertile man rather than a fertile man (accuracy of correct classification 87%), than if only the sperm concentration is lower than the reference value (accuracy of correct classification 66%) (Marmar et al. 1979; Homonnai et al. 1980).

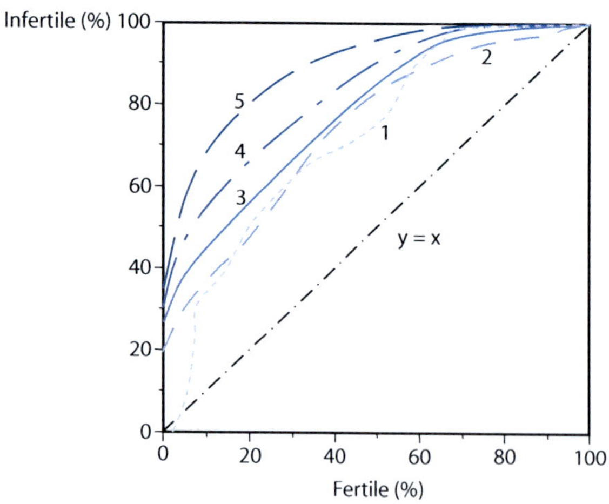

Fig. I.3.8. Receiver operating characteristics curves of the characteristics of spermatozoa in fertile compared to subfertile men (Comhaire et al. 1987). [*1* Peroxidase-negative cells per 100 spermatozoa, *2* sperm count, *3* sperm concentration, *4* grade (a) and (b) motile sperm concentration, *5* grade (a) motile sperm concentration]

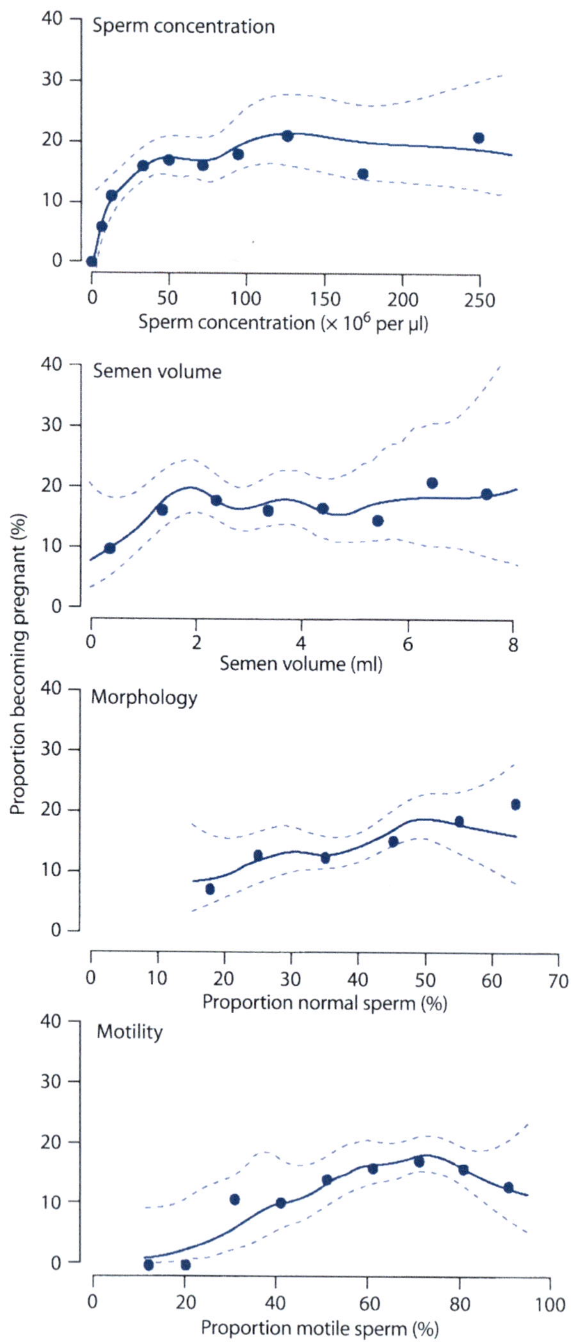

Fig. I.3.9. Relation between sperm characteristics and the fecundability in first pregnancy planners (Bonde et al. 1998)

Table I.3.5. Reference values and areas

	Sterile		Subfertile		Fertile
Concentration (million/ml)		3–4		35–40	
Grade (a) motility (%)		3		25–28	
Grade (a) + (b) motility (%)		14		48–50	
Grade (a) motile sperm concentration (million/ml)		0.3		8–10	
Grade (a) + (b) motile sperm concentration (million/ml)		0.6		20	
Morphology (% ideal)		4		14–15	
White blood cells		< 1.0 million/ml			
Ejaculate volume		1.5–6 ml			
pH		7.2–7.9			
Direct IgG MAR test		Suspect 10%–40% Positive > 40%			

Table I.3.5 lists reference values for the basic characteristics of semen and spermatozoa. The reference values divide the spectrum of semen data into three groups. If all the characteristics of the semen sample are better than the higher reference values, it is 95% probable that the semen originates from a man who is potentially fertile (green area). If the results are lower than the lower reference values, the semen originates from a man whose probability to (ever) attain pregnancy by natural conception is less than 5% and, therefore, he will be considered sterile (red area) (Ducot et al. 1988). If the results are situated between the two limits, and so are lower than the highest reference values but higher than the lowest reference values (orange area), the man is subfertile. This means that the probability that he will attain spontaneous conception with his partner is decreased. He may still attain conception, but the time needed may be longer than "normal" (Bostofte et al. 1990). Clearly, the closer the sperm results are to the higher reference values, the less severe is the degree of subfertility, and vice versa. With regard to sperm concentration, it has become usual to assign the term "oligozoospermia" to semen samples with less than 20 million spermatozoa per millilitre (Small et al. 1987)

The reference values given in Table I.3.5 may only be applied if semen analysis is performed following the methods described in Chap. II.3.2. It must again be stressed that the values are no more than indicative, and that their power to differentiate between fertile and subfertile semen is higher than to differentiate between subfertile and infertile semen. Also, the values refer to the occurrence of spontaneous conception, and may not be extrapolated for the selection of cases for intrauterine insemination or in vitro fertilization. Finally, semen characteristics may present a relatively high variability in the same person, so that classification may differ between semen samples produced at a different moment in time (Schaefer et al. 1991; Cooper et al. 1993).

References

Bonde JP, Ernst E, Jensen TK, Hjollund NH, Kolstad H, Henriksen TB, Scheike T, Giwercman A, Olsen J, Skakkebaek NE (1998) Relation between semen quality and fertility: a population-based study of 430 first-pregnancy planners. Lancet 352:1172–1177

Bostofte E, Bagger P, Michael A, Stakemann G (1990) Fertility prognosis for infertile men: results of follow-up study of semen analysis in infertile men from two different populations evaluated by the Cox regression model. Fertil Steril 54: 1100–1106

Collins JA, Wrixon W, Janes LB, Wilson EH (1983) Treatment-independent pregnancy among infertile couples. N Engl J Med 309:1201–1206

Comhaire FH, Kunnen M (1985) Factors affecting the probability of conception after treatment of subfertile men with varicocele by transcatheter embolization with Bucrylate. Fertil Steril 43:781–786

Comhaire FH, Vermeulen L, Schoonjans F (1987) Reassessment of the accuracy of traditional sperm characteristics and adenosine triphosphate (ATP) in estimating the fertilizing potential of human semen in vivo. Int J Androl 10:653–662

Comhaire FH, Rowe PJ, Farley TM (1988) How should we evaluate infertility in men and in women. Acta Clin Belg 43:78–85

Comhaire FH, Farley TMM, Rowe PJ (1992) Adenosine triphosphate (ATP) in semen and other sperm characteristics: their relevance for fertility prediction in men with normal sperm concentration. Fertil Steril 6:877–881

Cooper TG, Keck C, Oberdieck U, Nieschlag E (1993) Effects of multiple ejaculations after extended periods of sexual abstinence on total, motile and normal sperm numbers, as well as accessory gland secretions, from healthy normal and oligozoospermic men. Hum Reprod 8:1251–1258

Ducot B, Spira A, Feneux D, Jouannet P (1988) Male factors and the likelihood of pregnancy in infertile couples. II. Study of clinical characteristics-practical consequences. Int J Androl 11:395–404

Eimers JM, te Velde ER, Gerritse R, Vogelzang ET, Looman CW, Habbema JD (1994) The prediction of the chance to conceive in subfertile couples. Fertil Steril 61:44–52

Hargreave TB, Nillson S (1984) Seminology. In: Hargreave TB (eds) Male infertility. Springer, Berlin Heidelberg New York, pp 56–74

Hinting A, Comhaire F, Schoonjans F (1988) Capacity of objectively assessed sperm motility characteristics in differentiating between semen of fertile and subfertile men. Fertil Steril 50:635–639

Homonnai ZT, Paz GF, Weiss JN, David MP (1980) Relation between semen quality and fate of pregnancy: retrospective study on 534 pregnancies. Int J Androl 3:574–584

Leridon H (1980) The efficacy of natural insemination : a comparative standard for AID. In: David G, Price WS (eds) Human artificial insemination and semen preservation, Plenum Press, New York, pp 191–196
Majumdar H, Sheps M (1970) Estimation of a type I geometric distribution from observations on conception types. Demography 7:349–360
Marmar JL, Praiss DE, DeBenedictis TJ (1979) An estimate of the fertility potential of the fractions of the split ejaculate in terms of the motile sperm count. Fertil Steril 32:202–205
Menkveld R, Wong WY, Lombard CJ, Wetzels AM, Thomas CM, Merkus HM, Steegers-Theunissen RP (2001) Semen parameters, including WHO and strict criteria morphology, in a fertile and subfertile population: an effort towards standardization of in-vivo thresholds. Hum Reprod 16:1165–1171
Ombelet W, Bosmans E, Janssen M, Cox A, Vlasselaer J, Gyselaers W, Vandeput H, Gielen J, Pollet H, Maes M, Steeno O, Kruger T (1997) Semen parameters in a fertile versus subfertile population: a need for change in the interpretation of semen testing. Hum Reprod 12:987–993
Panidis DK, Rousso DH, Kourtis AI, Mavromatidis GA, Makedos GA, Kalahanis JA (2003) Prognostic value of evaluation of total number of morphological anomalies in 100 sperm in semen of infertile men. Arch Androl 49:351–354
Rogers BJ, Bentwood BJ, Van Campen H, Helmbrecht G, Soderdahl D, Hale RW (1983) Sperm morphology assessment as an indicator of human fertilizing capacity. J Androl 4:119–125
Schaefer F, Seidel C, Mitchell R, Scharer K, Robertson WR (1991) Pulsatile immunoreactive and bioactive luteinizing hormone secretion in adolescents with chronic renal failure. The Cooperative Study Group on Pubertal Development in Chronic Renal Failure (CSPCRF). Pediatr Nephrol 5:566–571
Schoonjans F, Depuydt C, Comhaire F (1996) Presentation of receiver-operating characteristics (ROC) plots [letter]. Clin Chem 42:986–987
Schwartz D, Mayaux MJ, Spira A, Moscato ML, Jouannet P, Czyglik F, David G (1981) Study of a group of 484 fertile men. Part II: relation between age (20–59) and semen characteristics. Int J Androl 4:450–465
Small DR, Collins JA, Wilson EH, Wrixon W (1987) Interpretation of semen analysis among infertile couples. CMAJ 136:829–833
Wang C, Chan SY, Ng M, So WW, Tsoi WL, Lo T, Leung A (1988) Diagnostic value of sperm function tests and routine semen analyses in fertile and infertile men. J Androl 9:384–389
Wood C, BG, Trounson A (1984) Current status and future prospects. In: Wood C, Trounson A (eds) Clinical in vitro fertilization, Springer Verlag, Berlin Heidelberg New York, pp 11–26
Zaini A, Jennings MG, Baker HW (1985) Are conventional sperm morphology and motility assessments of predictive value in subfertile men? Int J Androl 8:427–435

I.3.6 Normal Spermatozoa and Isolated Abnormalities of Seminal Plasma

F. Comhaire, A. Mahmoud

Key Messages

- Men producing ejaculates with normal concentration, motility and morphology of spermatozoa, but abnormal seminal plasma, may not be optimally fertile.
- Isolated abnormalities of seminal plasma may result from multiple causes affecting the function of the accessory sex glands, which usually is irreversible.
- If the postcoital test is abnormal, intrauterine insemination of spermatozoa prepared in vitro yields excellent success rates.

I.3.6.1 Definition

The diagnostic classification of normal spermatozoa and isolated seminal plasma abnormalities is given when sperm concentration, sperm motility and sperm morphology are better than the reference values for fertile men, but there are abnormalities in the physical, biochemical or bacteriological composition of the seminal plasma, an increased number of white blood cells, or agglutination with a negative test for antisperm antibodies. These patients do not fulfil the criteria for the diagnosis of male accessory gland infection or any other pathology. The significance of isolated abnormalities of seminal plasma for the couple's infertility has to be assessed by means of complementary tests (Rowe et al. 2000).

I.3.6.2 Aetiology and Pathogenesis

Seminal plasma is composed of the secretion products of the accessory sex glands: mainly the epididymides, the seminal vesicles and the prostate (Mann and Lutwak-Mann 1951; Eliasson 1968). During normal ejaculation, the fluids from the prostate and epididymides are expelled first (Bjorndahl and Kvist 2003). This first fraction of the ejaculate has a volume of 0.5–1.0 ml, is liquid, and has an acidic pH (6.0–6.5). The second fraction contains the secretions of the seminal vesicles. It is coagulated (Robert and Gagnon 1999), has an alkaline pH and the normal volume varies between 1.0 and 5.0 ml. In vitro, the coagulum is liquefied after approximately 30 min thanks to the enzymatic activity of the prostate-specific antigen (PSA) (Robert et al. 1997). Inadequate secretion by the accessory sex glands, in quantity and/or in quality, will result in abnormal ejaculate volume (less than 1.5–2 ml or more than 6 ml), and/or abnormal seminal pH, and/or poor or absent liquefaction. Normal seminal plasma is relatively clear. It may become cloudy due to the presence of mucous streaks or an increased number of white blood cells. Poor liquefaction occurs in case of decreased secretion of PSA by the prostate (Elzanaty et al. 2002, 2004). These abnormalities may impair the transition of spermatozoa, which are normal in number, motility and morphology, from the semen into the cervical mucus, decreasing the probability of conception.

Also, the osmolarity of the seminal plasma may be abnormal, decreasing the longevity of the spermatozoa and inducing curling of the sperm tails.

There is some evidence suggesting that abnormal seminal plasma may impair sperm function (Carpino et al. 1994; Lin et al. 2000) and chromatin stability (Gonzales and Sanchez 1994; Elzanaty et al. 2002) because of the inadequate amount of substances such as zinc (Malm et al. 2000) or calcium. Also, the secretions of the epididymides and the prostate are the major source of antioxidants in semen. Impaired epididymal function may be associated with decreased antioxidant capacity of the seminal plasma, causing an imbalance between oxidative stress and antioxidant protection (Gavella et al. 1996; Koca et al. 2003). This then will damage both the sperm membrane and the DNA composition.

Isolated seminal plasma abnormalities may be found after successful eradication of male accessory gland infection, or in cases with inflammation but no current infection. It may be associated with varicocele or hypoandrogenism, but in these cases the characteristics of the spermatozoa are commonly abnormal, excluding the diagnosis of isolated seminal plasma abnormalities.

I.3.6.3 Clinical and Laboratory Findings

History taking may reveal an episode of infection of the urinary tract that has disappeared either spontaneously or after treatment. Some patients report decreased orgasmic feeling or may have observed either a decreased volume or abnormal appearance of the ejaculate.

The epididymides may be enlarged or nodular upon palpation, or painful in case of current inflammation. Usually testicular volume and consistency are normal.

Echography of the pelvic organs may reveal signs of past infection of the prostate, or abnormal appearance of the seminal vesicles.

Analysis of blood, including tests for infection and hormone measurements, are normal. There should be no antisperm antibodies in serum. The test for antibodies against *Chlamydia trachomatis* may be positive. Urine analysis may reveal signs of inflammation of the urinary tract, and the urine obtained after massage of the prostate may contain an increased number of white blood cells.

Upon semen analysis, the concentration, motility and morphology of spermatozoa must be better than the reference values. Obviously and by definition, the seminal plasma must be abnormal from the physical, biochemical or bacteriological point of view, or contain an increased number of white blood cells, or spermatozoa may present agglutination. A test for the detection of antibodies attached to the spermatozoa must be performed, and should be negative.

In order to assess the importance of the isolated seminal plasma abnormality as a cause of the couple's infertility, an in vivo test of semen-cervical mucus interaction is recommended, namely the postcoital test (also called the Sims-Huhner test) (see WHO 1999). If the result of this test is normal, the isolated seminal plasma abnormalities are considered not to be the cause of the infertility. Nonetheless, the functional capacity of the spermatozoa may be impaired due to oxidative stress, and treatment with food supplements is suggested to counteract this. If, by contrast, the postcoital test is abnormal (poor or negative after repeated performance), the isolated abnormality of the seminal plasma may be relevant for the infertility problem, and treatment by means of intrauterine insemination may be indicated.

I.3.6.4 Differential Diagnosis

Abnormal seminal plasma may occur in combination with abnormal spermatozoa in diseases such as male accessory gland infection, varicocele, or endocrine cause. The diagnosis of isolated seminal plasma abnormalities is not applicable in these cases, since this requires spermatozoa to be normal. Also, immunological infertility must be excluded by means of a test detecting the presence of antisperm antibodies on the spermatozoa.

I.3.6.5 Treatment

It is generally not possible to correct an abnormality of the seminal plasma, since it is commonly related to a permanently inadequate function and secretion of the accessory sex glands. This implies that the secretory cells have been damaged beyond repair. Since the spermatozoa are normal, and in case the postcoital test is abnormal, insemination should be recommended. For optimal results, artificial insemination is performed within 5–6 h after ovulation, which requires careful monitoring of the cycle, possibly associated with induction of ovulation by means of human chorionic gonadotrophin. The semen is ejaculated directly into a receptacle containing culture medium with 3% human serum albumin, in an amount equal to the volume of semen. Alternatively, a small amount of bromelain or alpha-chymotrypsin can be added to the semen after ejaculation in order to liquefy it in cases of hyperviscosity of the seminal plasma. It is suggested to immediately prepare the semen for insemination using a density gradient column. Intrauterine insemination may be preferable, but intracervical insemination can be considered as well. There is no advantage to inducing hyperovulation, since this will increase the risk of multiple pregnancies, without increasing the clinical pregnancy rate (Guzick et al. 1999).

Giving the male patient a combination of antioxidants in the form of a food supplement will reduce the oxidative damage to the spermatozoa. This improves their functional capacity, increases the induced acrosome reaction, improves the rate of sperm–oocyte fusion, and increases the probability of successful pregnancy.

In vitro fertilization with or without intracytoplasmic sperm injection is rarely indicated.

I.3.6.6 Results of Treatment

Provided there is no demonstrable abnormality in the female partner or a possible abnormality has been corrected, the result of the treatment described above is excellent. In cases with abnormal postcoital test, more than 75% of couples attain normal pregnancy upon the first insemination cycle. Up to 90% of couples are successful within three cycles of insemination. Some cases with normal postcoital test may also benefit from insemination and food supplementation of the male partner.

If correctly performed insemination remains unsuccessful, in vitro fertilization with ICSI may be indicated, and will have the success rate that is typical for this treatment.

I.3.6.7 Prognosis

Isolated seminal plasma abnormalities usually remain present, but they may sometimes disappear spontaneously after some time. The number of white blood cells may decrease spontaneously with time, and this is accelerated by the intake of an antioxidant food supplement.

I.3.6.8 Prevention

The early diagnosis and correct treatment of every infectious or inflammatory condition of the urogenital tract can prevent inadequate functioning of the accessory sex glands and abnormalities of the seminal plasma.

I.3.6.9 Other

In summary, the finding of isolated seminal plasma abnormalities in the male partner of infertile couples needs careful evaluation. The condition may be permanent, but the negative effects on sperm function may be reversible. Insemination, if performed under optimal circumstances, will result in a high probability of successful pregnancy, and in vitro fertilization is rarely indicated.

References

Bjorndahl L, Kvist U (2003) Sequence of ejaculation affects the spermatozoon as a carrier and its message. Reprod Biomed Online 7:440–448

Carpino A, Sisci D, Aquila S, Salerno M, Siciliano L, Sessa M, Ando S (1994) Adnexal gland secretion markers in unexplained asthenozoospermia. Arch Androl 32:37–43

Eliasson R (1968) Biochemical analyses of human semen in the study of the physiology and pathophysiology of the male accessory genital glands. Fertil Steril 19:344–350

Elzanaty S, Richthoff J, Malm J, Giwercman A (2002) The impact of epididymal and accessory sex gland function on sperm motility. Hum Reprod 17:2904–2911

Elzanaty S, Malm J, Giwercman A (2004) Visco-elasticity of seminal fluid in relation to the epididymal and accessory sex gland function and its impact on sperm motility. Int J Androl 27:94–100

Gavella M, Lipovac V, Vucic M, Rocic B (1996) Superoxide anion scavenging capacity of human seminal plasma. Int J Androl 19:82–90

Gonzales GF, Sanchez A (1994) High sperm chromatin stability in semen with high viscosity. Arch Androl 32:31–35

Guzick DS, Carson SA, Coutifaris C, Overstreet JW, Factor-Litvak P, Steinkampf MP, Hill JA, Mastroianni L, Buster JE, Nakajima ST, Vogel DL, Canfield RE (1999) Efficacy of superovulation and intrauterine insemination in the treatment of infertility. National Cooperative Reproductive Medicine Network. N Engl J Med 340:177–183

Koca Y, Ozdal OL, Celik M, Unal S, Balaban N (2003) Antioxidant activity of seminal plasma in fertile and infertile men. Arch Androl 49:355–359

Lin YC, Chang TC, Tseng YJ, Lin YL, Huang FJ, Kung FT, Chang SY (2000) Seminal plasma zinc levels and sperm motion characteristics in infertile samples. Changgeng Yi Xue Za Zhi 23:260–266

Malm J, Hellman J, Hogg P, Lilja H (2000) Enzymatic action of prostate-specific antigen (PSA or hK3): substrate specificity and regulation by Zn(2+), a tight-binding inhibitor. Prostate 45:132–139

Mann T, Lutwak-Mann C (1951) Secretory function of male accessory organs of reproduction in mammals. Physiol Rev 31:27–55

Robert M, Gagnon C (1999) Semenogelin I: a coagulum forming, multifunctional seminal vesicle protein. Cell Mol Life Sci 55:944–960
Robert M, Gibbs BF, Jacobson E, Gagnon C (1997) Characterization of prostate-specific antigen proteolytic activity on its major physiological substrate, the sperm motility inhibitor precursor/semenogelin I. Biochemistry 36:3811–3819
Rowe PJ, Comhaire FH, Hargreave TB, Mahmoud AMA (2000) WHO manual for the standardized investigation, diagnosis and management of the infertile male. Cambridge University Press, Cambridge
WHO (1999) WHO laboratory manual of the examination of human semen and sperm-cervical mucus interaction. Cambridge University Press, Cambridge

I.3.7 Immunological Causes

A. Mahmoud, F. Comhaire

I.3

Key Messages

- Antisperm antibodies (ASAs) in the male are a cause of subfertility and low spontaneous pregnancy rates.
- ASA formation may follow infection/inflammation, surgery, trauma and obstruction of the (uro)genital tract.
- Test every subfertile patient for ASA using direct mixed antiglobulin reaction (MAR) or the immunobead test.
- If positive (>50%), evaluate the biological significance of ASAs (e.g. sperm–cervical mucus interaction).
- Treat the accompanying pathology if feasible.
- If treatment of the cause is not successful try intrauterine insemination (IUI) or in more severe cases in vitro fertilization/intracytoplasmic sperm injection (IVF/ICSI).
- When most spermatozoa are ASA-coated (>80%), ICSI is usually recommended, although some success was reported using chymotrypsin-treated spermatozoa for IUI.
- In patients with azoospermia, ASAs >40% in serum may indicate a better chance of sperm retrieval during testicular sperm extraction (TESE).

I.3.7.1 Introduction

Rümke (1954) and Wilson (1954) demonstrated half a decade ago that the occurrence of antisperm antibodies (ASAs) in man was associated with infertility. Since that time, many studies have shown that immune infertility may result from immunological response against spermatozoa, both cellular and humoral. Several reports have indicated that immunological causes may be present in 3%–36% of infertile couples (WHO 1987; Naz 2004). Although ASAs were considered to cause a relative reduction in fertility, but not to absolutely prevent conception, it is now clear that the presence of ASAs on the surface of spermatozoa can impair the sperm fertilizing capacity at different levels, including diminished sperm vitality, motility and mucous penetration, and impaired sperm-egg interaction (Mahmoud et al. 1996; Lombardo et al. 2001; Marin-Briggiler et al. 2003). Antisperm antibodies are associated with excessive generation of reactive oxygen species, which may adversely affect sperm quality via oxidation of the sperm plasma membranes, axonemal proteins and DNA (Zalata et al. 1995).

I.3.7.2 Mechanisms of Male Immunity to Spermatozoa

Spermatozoa are not present at the time when, during embryological development, the immune system establishes tolerance to self antigens (Billingham et al. 1953). Furthermore, spermatozoa have a different chromosomal make-up than the somatic cells. As a consequence, sperm-specific antigens are viewed as foreign antigens by the immune system. As soon as the spermatozoa appear during puberty, these foreign cells must be completely isolated from the immune system. Within the testis, this isolation is achieved relatively completely by the blood–testis barrier formed by tight junctional complexes between the tubular cells of Sertoli (Dym and Fawcett 1970). In other regions of the male genital tract, the epithelial lining, probably supplemented by a local immunosuppressive barrier, are responsible for this isolation (el Demiry et al. 1985). Alternatively, the immunosuppression theory (Tung 1980) postulates that small amounts of spermatozoal antigens continuously leak from the genital tract, leading to the activation of suppressor T lymphocytes, which inhibit immune responsiveness.

The pathogenesis of the formation of antisperm antibodies is still a matter of discussion. Antisperm immune responses occur probably as a result of the disruption of the epithelial or blood–testis barrier (Mengel and Zimmermann 1982; Haas 1987), an immunosuppression defect (Witkin 1988), or as a result of an insult to the genital tract that would provide an excess of spermatozoal antigens that could override the mechanism of immunosuppression (Haas 1991). Vasectomy is a major cause of antigen leakage causing ASA formation (Hendry 1989; Meinertz et al. 1990; Wen et al. 1994). Other conditions may also stimulate ASA formation such as vas obstruction (Hendry 1989), testicular trauma, torsion, malignancy, infection of the genital tract, semen deposition at nongenital tract sites, and perhaps, varicocele (WHO 1987; Knudson et al. 1994; Mahmoud et al. 1996) and intolerance to heavy metals (Podzimek et al. 2003).

I.3.7.3 Detection of Antisperm Antibodies

Four major types of tests are used in practice to detect and quantify antisperm antibodies, namely agglutination tests, complement-dependent tests, immunoglobulin binding, and ELISA tests.

I.3.7.3.1 Agglutination Tests

Agglutination tests detect the presence of antibodies to the surface antigens on spermatozoa by their ability to cause agglutination of normal spermatozoa. This agglutination may be observed macroscopically (Kibrick et al. 1952) or microscopically (for details, see Andreou et al. 1995). A drawback of these tests is that agglutination can also occur in the absence of specific antibodies as a result of the presence of bacteria, fungi, or amorphous material in seminal plasma, or under the influence of sex steroids or nonimmunoglobulin proteins in serum (Beer and Neaves 1978; Jones 1980; Bronson et al. 1984). The reference test commonly used is the tray agglutination test (TAT), introduced by Friberg (1974, 1980). The titre, type, and degree of agglutination can adequately be determined with TAT. Nonimmunological agglutination may, however, occur in TAT, particularly when female sera are tested, and at low serum dilutions (Ingerslev 1981).

I.3.7.3.2 Complement-Dependent Tests

Complement-dependent tests detect the presence of antibodies reacting with antigens of the sperm membrane by the induction of a cytotoxic effect which occurs in the presence of complement. Cytotoxicity results in the loss of sperm motility, which is used as a marker in the sperm immobilization test (SIT) (Isojima et al. 1968) or in membrane damage. The latter is revealed by the fact that the cell membrane allows specific dyes to enter the head portion of the spermatozoa (Eliasson 1977) or by leakage of adenosine triphosphate (ATP) out of the cell. The results of the ATP release cytotoxicity test (ARCT) present an excellent correlation with those of the sperm immobilization test (Linnet and Suominen 1982). We have simplified the method by testing only one serum dilution (1/4) and calculating the sperm toxicity index. The latter is closely correlated with the sperm cytotoxic titre. Our study confirms that sperm cytotoxic antibodies belong mainly to the IgG class. The simplified ARCT appears to be useful as an objective and specific method to detect and quantify cytotoxic ASAs in serum (Hinting et al. 1988a). In general, complement-dependent tests are considered to be specific and reproducible, but they have the disadvantage of not detecting IgA class antibodies (Clarke et al. 1985b).

I.3.7.3.3 Immunoglobulin Binding Tests

The presence of antibodies on spermatozoa can be detected by means of antibodies directed against human immunoglobulin. These antiglobulins can either be labelled or bound to indicator cells or particles. The antiglobulin labels commonly used are a fluorescence molecule in the immunofluorescence technique (Cross and Moore 1990), a radioactive isotope in the radiolabelled antiglobulin assay (Haas et al. 1980), or an enzyme in the enzyme-linked immunosorbent assay (Ackerman et al. 1981). Antiglobulin indicators are either red blood cells, as in the original mixed antiglobulin reaction, or latex particles as in the Latex-MAR test (Jager et al. 1978), or polyacrylamide beads, as in the immunobead binding technique (Clarke et al. 1985a).

Mixed Antiglobulin Reaction and Immunobead Tests

In 1978, Jager and co-workers described the direct mixed antiglobulin reaction (MAR) test for the detection of ASAs bound to spermatozoa in fresh semen (Jager et al. 1978). In this test, the presence of immunoglobulins bound to spermatozoa is revealed by the occurrence of a mixed agglutination of red blood cells coated with immunoglobulins with motile spermatozoa in the presence of an antiglobulin. By selecting the class of the immunoglobulins on the indicator cells and the type of antiglobulin, it is possible to identify the class of immunoglobulins bound on the spermatozoa. Initially, only IgG class antibodies could be detected, but this technique has recently been adapted to allow for the detection of IgA class antibodies. The test can also be performed indirectly to detect ASAs in serum or in seminal plasma (Vermeulen and Comhaire 1983).

In order to make the test more practical and sensitive, the coated red blood cells have been replaced by coated latex particles (Vermeulen and Comhaire 1983). The MAR test with latex particles is simple to carry out since it is performed in untreated semen. Moreover, the test provides information on the presence, the localization, and the Ig class of ASAs.

In the immunobead test (Clarke et al. 1985a), polyacrylamide beads are coated with polyclonal antibodies against human IgG, IgA, or IgM. This test requires washing the spermatozoa through repeated centrifugation-resuspension, in order to remove the bulk of immunoglobulins present in seminal plasma. The adequate diagnostic performance of the SpermMAR test has been established in many laboratories (Ackerman et al. 1988; Kay and Boettcher 1992; Eggert-Kruse et al. 1993). The presence of 50 % or more adherence of particles to the motile spermatozoa is strong evidence for an immunological cause of infertility. If the result of the test was doubtful or the test was not feasible due to low sperm motility, detection may be performed on the serum sample. In general, the performance of the immunobead test was found to be less adequate, with both lower specificity and sensitivity than the SpermMAR test (Khoo et al. 1991; Kay and Boettcher 1992; Andreou et al. 1995). Neither test can be performed if the number of motile spermatozoa in the ejaculate is too low but the number of motile spermatozoa needed for the MAR test is smaller.

We have developed a simple procedure for the detection of ASAs of the IgG class in human serum using the indirect MAR test. The test uses only one dilution of serum (1/16) and no washing procedures (Hinting et al. 1988b).

Our data indicate that the direct MAR test result for IgG correlated better with the indirect MAR result for IgG in seminal plasma and serum than did the direct immunobead test result for IgG (Andreou et al. 1995). The latter could be expected since the bulk of IgG in semen is probably derived from serum, and enters the ejaculate via the prostate (Rumke 1974; Tauber et al. 1975). Furthermore, the results of indirect MAR IgG test on serum correlate better than the immunobead test with the results of TAT and ARCT on serum. Using the cut-off value of 40 %, motile spermatozoa attached to coated latex particles as the lower limit of significant activity, the indirect MAR test has a sensitivity of 96 % and specificity of 87 % (Andreou et al. 1995) in comparison with the TAT test as a reference. Few studies have evaluated the clinical relevance of antisperm antibodies in the male serum. The presence of IgG in serum in cases with azoospermia is probably a marker of both seminal tract obstruction and the presence of some degree of spermatogenesis. The majority of our vasectomized men develop high percentages of IgG antibodies at follow-up. A recent study also indicated that, in men with azoospermia, the presence of IgG antibodies in serum is predictive of sperm recovery from the testis in testicular sperm extraction (TESE). In the majority of patients with a serum IgG over 10 % and in all with a serum IgG greater than 40 %, at least one sperm could be retrieved during TESE (Kazemeyni 2003).

I.3.7.3.4 Enzyme Linked Immunosorbant Assays

Antibody-enzyme-immunoglobulin complexes are detected by addition of a specific enzyme substrate, usually resulting in a colour change. The advantage of this method is that it is both specific and quantitative. The major disadvantage of the enzyme linked immunosorbant assay (ELISA) is that samples are generally subjected to fixation, disrupting the plasma membrane of spermatozoa, which may result in the detection of internal antigens. Binding to nonspecific antigens, the time and cost involved, poor sensitivity, and inability to determine ASA location and isotype are the main disadvantages (Mazumdar and Levine 1998). Recently, an ELISA test based on the detection of antiprostasome antibodies was able to identify most TAT-positive sera (Carlsson et al. 2004).

I.3.7.3.5 Other Tests

Other techniques are continuously emerging, such as the panning procedure for ASA detection on spermatozoa (Hancock and Faruki 1984), polyacrylamide gel electrophoresis and immunoblotting for detailed analysis of both spermatozoal antibodies and antigens (Snow and Ball 1992; Bohring and Krause 2001), and flow cytometry (for a review, see Mazumdar and Levine 1998). In this regard, the immunoblotting technique provides more information on the molecular nature of the antigen that elicits ASAs. These techniques are mostly applied for research purposes and sometimes do not seem to give reliable results. They also offer little advantage over the less costly and user-friendly immunoglobulin binding tests (Eggert-Kruse et al. 1993; Mazumdar and Levine 1998).

I.3.7.4 Antisperm Antibodies in Male Infertility

Routine testing for antisperm antibodies is an essential step in the diagnosis and management of male infertility (Bronson 1999a; WHO 1999; Rowe et al. 2000). Several techniques are available for ASA detection in serum as well as in genital secretions. Important questions are whether the assay actually measures antibodies against spermatozoa, and whether the antibodies that are detected do interfere with fertility. It seems that no single test is capable of detecting ASA with 100 % accuracy, for all classes of immunoglobulins and against all antibody activities. Hence, the evaluation of male immune infertility should employ several tests, starting with the most sensitive one for screening, and confirming with the most specific one.

The presence of antibodies coating the spermatozoa reduces the sperm fertilizing ability independently of other sperm characteristics (Mahmoud et al. 1996; Lombardo et al. 2001; Marin-Briggiler et al. 2003). Therefore, the detection of IgG-coated spermatozoa by means of the MAR or immunobead tests has been included as a standard procedure in the World Health Organization's recommended methodology of routine semen analysis (WHO 1999). Although the effect of antisperm antibodies on fertility is regarded as a continuum (Bronson 1999b), results from our studies using the MAR test indicated that the finding of 40% or more adherence of particles to motile spermatozoa must be considered strong evidence for an immunological cause of infertility (Comhaire et al. 1988). The limit of 40% reaction is close to that recommended by the World Health Organization, which suggests 50% motile spermatozoa coated by IgG as the critical limit (WHO 1999).

The direct tests for IgG seem to be ideal screening procedures for ASA detection since they are simple and sensitive. In positive cases, however, one should perform more specific tests such as complement-dependent tests. Further, in order to ascertain that fertility prognosis is adequately assessed, ASA class must also be detected. ASAs of the IgA class appear to be more important than ASA of the IgG class in impairing sperm migration through the female reproductive tract (Steen et al. 1994; Yeh et al. 1995). Since the bulk, if not all, of IgA is produced locally, these must be detected on spermatozoa rather than in serum. It should be stressed that ASAs of the IgA class rarely occur without ASAs of the IgG class (Andreou et al. 1995). Hence, IgA testing is not considered necessary as a routine diagnostic screening procedure.

Several biological tests are available to assess the functional impact of ASAs. These include the sperm-cervical mucuscontact test (Jager et al. 1979) in which fresh sperm is mixed with cervical mucus. In case ASAs are present on the spermatozoa, a shaking phenomenon of the motile spermatozoa is observed. Other functional aspects of ASAs can be evaluated in the human zona-binding assay (Burkman et al. 1988), the acrosome reaction test (Talbot and Chacon 1981), and the zona-free hamster oocyte test (Yanagimachi et al. 1976). Antisperm antibodies are associated with excessive generation of reactive oxygen species, which may adversely affect sperm quality via oxidation of the sperm plasma membranes, axonemal proteins and DNA (Zalata et al. 1995).

I.3.7.5 Clinical Aspects of Men with Antisperm Antibodies

Clinical evaluation can give relevant information in men with ASAs. Medical history of urogenital tract infection, sexually transmitted diseases, varicocele, autoimmune disease and surgery of the urogenital tract or in the groin are very common (Sinisi et al. 1993; Hinting et al. 1996; Mahmoud et al. 1996). A high frequency of epididymal thickness is also found on physical examination (Mahmoud et al. 1996). It seems that the pathogenesis of male immune infertility may originate from inflammation of the genital tract, vas lesion and/or partial obstruction (Hinting et al. 1996).

Treatments to overcome immunological infertility at present are still controversial. Pathology suspected as aetiological should be initially treated, such as appropriate antibiotics in cases of actual infection, and nonsteroidal anti-inflammatory medication in patients with signs of inflammation but no actual infection (Rowe et al. 2000). In some clinics, surgical treatment has been performed for partial obstruction (Hendry 1989) but is rarely done nowadays due to the availability of ICSI.

In cases where no infective or obstructive cause can be found, empirical immunosuppressive treatment has been attempted (Shulman and Shulman 1982; Hendry 1989). Recent studies clearly indicated that high-dose corticosteroid therapy was ineffective, and it carries a serious risk of side effects (Bals-Pratsch et al. 1992). Another approach has been the use of assisted reproductive technology with special sperm treatment. In assisted reproduction, the sperm preparation may reduce the agglutinating and cytotoxic effects of antibody bound to spermatozoa (Hinting et al. 1989). It is suggested that three to six cycles of intrauterine insemination (IUI) of motile sperm concentration was reasonable. This results in a pregnancy rate of about 9% per cycle (Grigoriou et al. 1996; Mahmoud et al. 1996). In a comparative crossover study, IUI has been found to result in higher pregnancy rates compared to low-dose cyclic corticosteroid therapy of the male with immunological factor (Lahteenmaki et al. 1995).

In severe cases with lower motile sperm concentration or after failing IUI, IVF or ICSI should be attempted. When most of the spermatozoa (>80%) are antibody-coated, ICSI is usually recommended, although a recent retrospective study indicated that in vitro treatment of these spermatozoa with chymotrypsin prior to IUI with semen samples where all spermatozoa were antibody-coated results in a pregnancy rate per cycle of 11% (Check et al. 2004).

I.3.7.6 Perspectives

Several antibody-binding proteins have been described in human seminal plasma. These proteins potentially have the ability to reduce the actions of antisperm antibodies (for a review, see Chiu and Chamley 2003). However, knowledge of their physiological role is limited. The immunological characterization of sperm proteins as cognate antigens has identified many antibodies that affect sperm functions. This line of research may lead to a better delineation of antibodies that are relevant for fertilization and the development of immunological contraceptives (for a review, see Bohring and Krause 2003).

References

Ackerman SB, Wortham JW, Swanson RJ (1981) An indirect enzyme-linked immunosorbent assay (ELISA) for the detection and quantitation of antisperm antibodies. Am J Reprod Immunol 1:199–205

Ackerman S, McGuire G, Fulgham DL, Alexander NJ (1988) An evaluation of a commercially available assay for the detection of antisperm antibodies. Fertil Steril 49:732–734

Andreou E, Mahmoud A, Vermeulen L, Schoonjans F, Comhaire F (1995) Comparison of different methods for the investigation of antisperm antibodies on spermatozoa, in seminal plasma and in serum. Hum Reprod 10:125–131

Bals-Pratsch M, Doren M, Karbowski B, Schneider HP, Nieschlag E (1992) Cyclic corticosteroid immunosuppression is unsuccessful in the treatment of sperm antibody-related male infertility: a controlled study. Hum Reprod 7:99–104

Beer AE, Neaves WB (1978) Antigenic status of semen from the viewpoints of the female and male. Fertil Steril 29:3–22

Billingham RE, Brent L, Medawar PB (1953) Activity acquired tolerance of foreign cells. Nature 172:603–606

Bohring C, Krause W (2001) Differences in the antigen pattern recognized by antisperm antibodies in patients with infertility and vasectomy. J Urol 166:1178–1180

Bohring C, Krause W (2003) Immune infertility: towards a better understanding of sperm (auto)-immunity: the value of proteomic analysis. Hum Reprod 18:915–924

Bronson R (1999a) Detection of antisperm antibodies: an argument against therapeutic nihilism. Hum Reprod 14: 1671–1673

Bronson RA (1999b) Antisperm antibodies: a critical evaluation and clinical guidelines. J Reprod Immunol 45:159–183

Bronson R, Cooper G, Rosenfeld D (1984) Sperm antibodies: their role in infertility. Fertil Steril 42:171–183

Burkman LJ, Coddington CC, Franken DR, Krugen TF, Rosenwaks Z, Hogen GD (1988) The hemizona assay (HZA): development of a diagnostic test for the binding of human spermatozoa to the human hemizona pellucida to predict fertilization potential. Fertil Steril 49:688–697

Carlsson L, Nilsson BO, Ronquist G, Lundquist M, Larsson A (2004) A new test for immunological infertility: an ELISA based on prostasomes. Int J Androl 27:130–133

Check JH, Hourani W, Check ML, Graziano V, Levin E (2004) Effect of treating antibody-coated sperm with chymotrypsin on pregnancy rates following IUI as compared to outcome of IVF/ICSI. Arch Androl 50:93–95

Chiu WW, Chamley LW (2003) Human seminal plasma antibody-binding proteins. Am J Reprod Immunol 50:196–201

Clarke GN, Elliott PJ, Smaila C (1985a) Detection of sperm antibodies in semen using the immunobead test: a survey of 813 consecutive patients. Am J Reprod Immunol Microbiol 7:118–123

Clarke GN, Stojanoff A, Cauchi MN, Johnston WI (1985b) The immunoglobulin class of antispermatozoal antibodies in serum. Am J Reprod Immunol Microbiol 7:143–147

Comhaire FH, Hinting A, Vermeulen L, Schoonjans F, Goethals I (1988) Evaluation of the direct and indirect mixed antiglobulin reaction with latex particles for the diagnosis of immunological infertility. Int J Androl 11:37–44

Cross NL, Moore S (1990) Regional binding of human antisperm antibodies assessed by indirect immunofluorescence. Hum Reprod 5:47–51

Dym M, Fawcett DW (1970) The blood-testis barrier in the rat and the physiological compartmentation of the seminiferous epithelium. Biol Reprod 3:308–326

Eggert-Kruse W, Bockem-Hellwig S, Doll A, Rohr G, Tilgen W, Runnebaum B (1993) Antisperm antibodies in cervical mucus in an unselected subfertile population. Hum Reprod 8:1025–1031

El Demiry MI, Hargreave TB, Busuttil A, James K, Ritchie AW, Chisholm GD (1985) Lymphocyte sub-populations in the male genital tract. Br J Urol 57:769–774

Eliasson R (1977) Supravital staining of human spermatozoa. Fertil Steril 28:1257

Friberg J (1974) A simple and sensitive micro-method for demonstration of sperm-agglutinating activity in serum from infertile men and women. Acta Obstet Gynecol Scand Suppl 21–29

Friberg J (1980) Immunoglobulin concentration in serum and seminal fluid from men with and without sperm-agglutinating antibodies. Am J Obstet Gynecol 136:671–675

Grigoriou O, Konidaris S, Antonaki V, Papadias C, Antoniou G, Gargaropoulos A (1996) Corticosteroid treatment does not improve the results of intrauterine insemination in male subfertility caused by antisperm antibodies. Eur J Obstet Gynecol Reprod Biol 65:227–230

Haas GG Jr (1987) Antibody-mediated causes of male infertility. Urol Clin North Am 14:539–550

Haas GG Jr (1991) Male fertility and immunity. In: Lipshultz LI, Howards SS (eds) Infertility in the male, Mosby-Year Book, St.Louis, pp 277–296

Haas GG Jr, Cines DB, Schreiber AD (1980) Immunologic infertility: identification of patients with antisperm antibody. N Engl J Med 303:722–727

Hancock RJ, Faruki S (1984) Detection of antibody-coated sperm by 'panning' procedures. J Immunol Methods 66: 149–159

Hendry WF (1989) Detection and treatment of antispermatozoal antibodies in men. Reprod Fertil Dev 1:205–220

Hinting A, Vermeulen L, Comhaire F (1988a) Evaluation of a simplified adenosine triphosphate release cytotoxicity test for the detection of sperm antibodies in human serum. J Reprod Immunol 13:123–131

Hinting A, Vermeulen L, Comhaire F (1988b) The indirect mixed antiglobulin reaction test using a commercially available kit for the detection of antisperm antibodies in serum. Fertil Steril 49:1039–1044

Hinting A, Vermeulen L, Goethals I, Dhont M, Comhaire F (1989) Effect of different procedures of semen preparation on antibody-coated spermatozoa and immunological infertility. Fertil Steril 52:1022–1026

Hinting A, Soebadi DM, Santoso RI (1996) Evaluation of the immunological cause of male infertility. Andrologia 28: 123–126

Ingerslev HJ (1981) Antibodies against spermatozoal surface-membrane antigens in female infertility. Acta Obstet Gynecol Scand Suppl 100:1–52

Isojima S, Li TS, Ashitaka Y (1968) Immunological analysis of sperm-immobilizing factor found in sera of women with unexplained sterility. Am J Obstet Gynecol 101:677–683

Jager S, Kremer J, van Slochteren-Draaisma T (1978) A simple method of screening for antisperm antibodies in the human male. Detection of spermatozoal surface IgG with the direct mixed antiglobulin reaction carried out on untreated fresh human semen. Int J Fertil 23:12–21

Jager S, Kremer J, van Slochteren-Draaisma T (1979) Presence of sperm agglutinating antibodies in infertile men and inhi-

bition of in vitro sperm penetration into cervical mucus. Int J Androl 2:117–130
Jones WR (1980) Immunologic infertility-fact or fiction? Fertil Steril 33:577–586
Kay DJ, Boettcher B (1992) Comparison of the SpermMar test with currently accepted procedures for detecting human sperm antibodies. Reprod Fertil Dev 4:175–181
Kazemeyni SM (2003) Correlation between antisperm antibodies and successful testicular sperm extraction in azoospermic men. Reprod Biomed Online 7 [Suppl 1]:30–40
Khoo D, Feigenbaum SL, McClure RD (1991) Screening assays for immunologic infertility: a comparison study. Am J Reprod Immunol 26:11–16
Kibrick S, Belding DL, Merrill B (1952) Methods for the detection of antibodies against mammalian spermatozoa. II. A gelatin agglutination test. Fertil Steril 3:430–438
Knudson G, Ross L, Stuhldreher D, Houlihan D, Bruns E, Prins G (1994) Prevalence of sperm bound antibodies in infertile men with varicocele: the effect of varicocele ligation on antibody levels and semen response. J Urol 151:1260–1262
Lahteenmaki A, Veilahti J, Hovatta O (1995) Intra-uterine insemination versus cyclic, low-dose prednisolone in couples with male antisperm antibodies. Hum Reprod 10:142–147
Linnet L, Suominen JJ (1982) A comparison of eight techniques for the evaluation of the auto-immune response to spermatozoa after vasectomy. J Reprod Immunol 4:133–144
Lombardo F, Gandini L, Dondero F, Lenzi A (2001) Antisperm immunity in natural and assisted reproduction. Hum Reprod Update 7:450–456
Mahmoud AM, Tuyttens CL, Comhaire FH (1996) Clinical and biological aspects of male immune infertility: a case-controlled study of 86 cases. Andrologia 28:191–196
Marin-Briggiler CI, Vazquez-Levin MH, Gonzalez-Echeverria F, Blaquier JA, Miranda PV, Tezon JG (2003) Effect of antisperm antibodies present in human follicular fluid upon the acrosome reaction and sperm-zona pellucida interaction. Am J Reprod Immunol 50:209–219
Mazumdar S, Levine AS (1998) Antisperm antibodies: etiology, pathogenesis, diagnosis, and treatment. Fertil Steril 70:799–810
Meinertz H, Linnet L, Fogh-Andersen P, Hjort T (1990) Antisperm antibodies and fertility after vasovasostomy: a follow- up study of 216 men. Fertil Steril 54:315–321
Mengel W, Zimmermann FA (1982) Immunologic aspects of cryptorchidism. Urol Clin North Am 9:349–352
Naz RK (2004) Modalities for treatment of antisperm antibody mediated infertility: novel perspectives. Am J Reprod Immunol 51:390–397
Podzimek S, Prochazkova J, Pribylova L, Bartova J, Ulcova-Gallova Z, Mrklas L, Stejskal VD (2003) [Effect of heavy metals on immune reactions in patients with infertility]. Cas Lek Cesk 142:285–288
Rowe PJ, Comhaire FH, Hargreave TB, Mahmoud AMA (2000) WHO manual for the standardized investigation, diagnosis and management of the infertile male. Cambridge University Press, Cambridge
Rumke P (1954) The presence of sperm antibodies in serum of two patients with oligozoospermia. Vox Sang 4:135–140
Rumke P (1974) The origin of immunoglobulins in semen. Clin Exp Immunol 17:287–297
Shulman JF, Shulman S (1982) Methylprednisolone treatment of immunologic infertility in male. Fertil Steril 38:591–599
Sinisi AA, Di Finizio B, Pasquali D, Scurini C, D'Apuzzo A, Bellastella A (1993) Prevalence of antisperm antibodies by SpermMARtest in subjects undergoing a routine sperm analysis for infertility. Int J Androl 16:311–314
Snow K, Ball GD (1992) Characterization of human sperm antigens and antisperm antibodies in infertile patients. Fertil Steril 58:1011–1019
Steen Y, Forssman L, Lonnerstedt E, Jonasson K, Wassen AC, Lycke E (1994) Anti-sperm IgA antibodies against the equatorial segment of the human spermatozoon are associated with impaired sperm penetration and subfertility. Int J Fertil Menopausal Stud 39:52–56
Talbot P, Chacon RS (1981) A triple-stain technique for evaluating normal acrosome reactions of human sperm. J Exp Zool 215:201–208
Tauber PF, Zaneveld LJ, Propping D, Schumacher GF (1975) Components of human split ejaculates. I. Spermatozoa, fructose, immunoglobulins, albumin, lactoferrin, transferrin and other plasma proteins. J Reprod Fertil 43:249–267
Tung KSK (1980) Autoimmunity of the testis. In: Dhindsa DS, Schumacher GFB (eds) Immunological aspects of infertility and fertility regulation, Elsevier-North Holland, New York, pp 33–91
Vermeulen A, Comhaire F (1983) Le test "MAR" aux particules de Latex, et le test spermatoxique selon Suominen: simplification et nouveauté dans l'arsenal du diagnostic immunologique. Contraception, Fertilité, Sexualité 11:381–384
Wen RQ, Li SQ, Wang CX, Wang QH, Li QK, Feng HM, Jiang YJ, Huang JC (1994) Analysis of spermatozoa from the proximal vas deferens of vasectomized men. Int J Androl 17:181–185
WHO (1987) Towards more objectivity in diagnosis and management of male infertility. Int J Androl Suppl 7
WHO (1999) WHO laboratory manual of the examination of human semen and sperm-cervical mucus interaction. Cambridge University Press, Cambridge
Wilson L (1954) Sperm agglutinins in human semen and blood. Proc Soc Exp Biol Med 85:652–655
Witkin SS (1988) Mechanisms of active suppression of the immune response to spermatozoa. Am J Reprod Immunol Microbiol 17:61–64
Yanagimachi R, Yanagimachi H, Rogers BJ (1976) The use of zona-free animal ova as a test-system for the assessment of the fertilizing capacity of human spermatozoa. Biol Reprod 15:471–476
Yeh WR, Acosta AA, Seltman HJ, Doncel G (1995) Impact of immunoglobulin isotype and sperm surface location of antisperm antibodies on fertilization in vitro in the human. Fertil Steril 63:1287–1292
Zalata A, Hafez T, Comhaire F (1995) Evaluation of the role of reactive oxygen species in male infertility. Hum Reprod 10:1444–1451

I.3.8 Iatrogenic Causes of Abnormal Spermatozoa

G. Haidl

Key Messages

- Many drugs, in particular cytostatic and hormonally active agents, can exert deleterious effects on male fertility.
- Vasectomy and vasectomy reversal can result in formation of antisperm antibodies; therefore patients should be counselled accordingly.
- Inguinal hernia repair may be complicated by obstruction of the vas deferens.
- Lumbar sympathectomy can result in ejaculatory disorders.
- Cryobanking of spermatozoa for patients undergoing unavoidable drug treatment affecting male fertility or irradiation is strongly recommended.

I.3.8.1 Definition

Iatrogenic causes of male fertility disturbances are coded when the abnormal spermatozoa are considered to stem from medical or surgical causes. This diagnosis requires the following to be true:

- History of medical treatment with possible adverse effect on fertility
- And/or history of surgery with possible adverse effect on fertility

I.3.8.2 Aetiology and Pathogenesis

I.3.8.2.1 Medical Treatments

Therapeutic drugs may cause a temporary or permanent disturbance of male fertility by impairment of the following functions: spermatogenesis, epididymal sperm maturation, sperm transport, sperm metabolism, motility, capacitation and egg penetration.

I.3.8.2.2 Gonadotoxic Interventions

Testicular cancer, Hodgkin's disease, non-Hodgkin lymphomas and leukaemia may affect young people, and the disease or its treatment may have deleterious effects on fertility. Impairment of spermatogenesis substances with direct antiproliferating effects on the germinal epithelium is caused by alkylating substances such as cyclophosphamide and chlorambucil and after cytostatic treatment with cisplatin and adriamycin as well as methotrexate and vincristine or bleomycin.

I.3.8.2.3 Further Drugs with Possible Negative Influence on Fertility

Apart from cytostatic agents, direct inhibition of proliferation of the spermatogenesis can be caused by neuroleptics and tricyclic antidepressives (Neumann 1984), by antiemetics and antiepileptics, as well as by antibiotics and chemotherapeutics at higher dosages and long-term treatment (nitrofurantoin, co-trimoxazole, gentamicin and niridazole). Salazosulphapyridine leads to a direct inhibition of spermatogenesis by absorption of toxic metabolites (sulphapyridine). More agents with potentially blocking effects on spermatogenesis belong to the groups of analgesics and immunosuppressants. However, reliable studies are not available for most of these frequently used drugs.

I.3.8.2.4 Hormones and Hormone Antagonists

Hormonal active drugs influence spermatogenesis indirectly by inhibition of the gonadotrophic functions of the pituitary. Impairment of spermatogenesis is possible by oestrogens, gestagens, androgens, anabolics, antiandrogens, luteinizing hormone releasing hormone (LHRH), gonadotrophin releasing hormone (GnRH) (super)agonists or antagonists and glucocorticoids. Drugs may interfere with androgen production by different mechanisms, for example, a decrease in LH production by opiates, blockage of enzymes for steroid production by aminoglutethimide and ketoconazole, an increase in testosterone metabolism by barbiturates, anticonvulsives and further liver enzyme-inducing agents, blockage of the effects of testosterone by androgen receptor antagonists such as cimetidine, spironolactone, cyproteronacetate, an influence such as the physiologic antagonist of androgen effects by digoxin with oestrogenic mode of action and drugs causing hyperprolactinaemia.

Reduction in sperm count, motility and percentage of normally formed sperm is reversible after discontinuation of administration of androgenic hormones. In bodybuilders who have taken anabolic steroids at doses exceeding those generally applied for clinical purposes by up to 40-fold, recovery of sperm numbers into the normal range may vary considerably after stopping the steroids. Time intervals between 4 and 12 months are reported (Knuth et al. 1989; Gazvani et al. 1997). In another case, the patient remained azoospermic even after 12 months of abstinence from the steroid and subsequent treatment with gonadotrophins was initiated (Menon 2003).

I.3.8.2.5
Drugs Affecting Sperm Function

Despite the major clinical significance of therapeutic drugs which may have an influence on gamete functions, there is only scarce knowledge on this subject because of the lack of epidemiological studies. There are reports on certain drugs demonstrating influences on sperm functions or sperm–egg interaction by in vitro tests or by application to small groups of patients. For example, treatment with the calcium-channel blocker nifedipine was shown to block sperm–egg interaction, obviously by alteration of the lipid composition of the cell membranes (Benoff et al. 1994). More relevant substances may be verapamil (alteration of sperm membranes, decline of sperm motility), antiepileptics (damage of sperm membranes, decline of motility), sulphasalazine (decrease in sperm count and motility), tetracyclines (in vitro direct toxic effect), macrolides at high concentrations (in vitro decrease in sperm motility), and amantadine and colchicine (impairment of sperm–egg interaction).

Finally, sperm motility can be impaired by damage of sperm membrane-bound functions. Drugs with motility-disturbing effects in vitro are nitrofurantoin, 2,6-diamino-3-phenazopyridine, tetracyclines, gentamicin, metoclopramide, imipramine, chlorpromazine, nortriptyline, lithium, trifluoperazine, levamisole, propranolol, phentolamine, dibenamine, stropine and bentropinmesylate (Table I.3.6).

Table I.3.6. Drugs with possible influence on male fertility

Suppression of spermatogenesis
Cytostatic agents
Hormones and hormonally active drugs: androgens, antiandrogens, oestrogens, progestagens, glucocorticoids, anabolics, cimetidine, spironolactone, digoxin, ketoconazole
Psychotropic drugs, antiepileptics, antiemetics, analgesics, certain antibiotics and chemotherapeutics, anthelmintics such as niridazole, salazosulphapyridine
Impairment of sperm function
Calcium channel blockers (sperm motility and sperm-egg binding)
Antiepileptics (sperm motility)
Sulphasalazine (sperm count and motility)
Antibiotics (sperm motility)
Amantadine and colchicine (Sperm–egg interaction)
Psychotropic drugs, alpha- and beta-blockers (sperm motility)
Inhibition of sperm transport
Antihypertensive drugs
Psychotropic drugs

I.3.8.2.6
Inhibition of Sperm Transport

α-Adrenolytic acting substances influence sperm transport by inhibition of the emission phase (chemical sympathectomy) of the ejaculatory reflex: antihypertensive drugs (guanethidine, reserpine, methyldopa), psychotropic drugs (thioridazine, chlorprothixene, tricyclic antidepressives, chlordiazepoxide), ganglion blockers (hexamethonium, mecamylamine) as well as alpha receptor blockers (phentolamine, phenoxybenzamine) (Forman et al. 1996; Rowe et al. 2000) (Table I.3.6).

I.3.8.2.7
Surgery

There may be temporary depression of fertility, which may last for 3–6 months after any surgical procedure, particularly after general anaesthesia has been administered.

Testicular biopsy may result in a temporary suppression of spermatogenesis. Unsuccessful operations such as herniotomies or corrections of testicular maldescent may result in damage to the vas deferens and testis, respectively, with subsequent loss of testicular function. Iatrogenic obstructions may have been provoked by herniotomies (particularly during infancy) or surgical procedures at the ejaculatory ducts or vasographs of the ductus deferentes using irritating contrast media. Incidentally performed epididymal incisions or biopsies during testicular biopsies usually result in obstructions as well. Hernia repair may additionally result in an immunological reaction with production of antisperm antibodies. This may also occur after hydrocelectomy or any other genital or inguinal surgery. Vasectomy is the most common cause of surgical obstruction and also results in production of antisperm antibodies.

Aspermia may be caused by disturbances of the function of the bladder neck after transurethral prostatectomy, treatment of urethral valves in infancy, bladder neck incision for outflow obstruction, lumbar sympathectomy, retroperitoneal lymphadenectomy as well as abdominoperineal surgery.

Urinary catheterization may be complicated by urinary tract infection or by urethral stricture. Urethral stricture repair may result in pooling of ejaculate material in a flaccid segment of the urethra and its contamination with urine. There may be ejaculatory disturbance after reconstructive surgery for hypospadias, epispadias and vesicular exstrophy.

Operations for varicocele, testicular torsion or testicular maldescent are recorded separately. Other operations should be noted if the investigator suspects relevance to infertility (Rowe et al. 2000).

I.3.8.2.8
Irradiation

Irradiation in the genital region will most probably cause irreversible arrest of spermatogenesis with subsequent sterility. An organ dosage of 3 Gy, which usually is achieved by irradiation of the inguinal region or the contralateral testicle, is lethal for spermatogenesis or leads at least temporarily to extensive suppression of spermatogenesis (Rowley et al. 1974).

I.3.8.3
Clinical and Laboratory Findings

History taking should reveal medical or surgical treatment with possible negative influences on fertility.

In patients with a history of gonadotoxic chemotherapy for reasons other than testicular cancer, testicular volume and consistency usually are normal; in patients with testicular cancer in their history, the testicle being left after operation may either be normal or may reveal a smaller volume in cases with a history of cryptorchidism. In patients treated with hormonally active compounds, testicular atrophy, gynaecomastia or skin alterations such as acne may be observed. In patients presenting with a history of vasectomy, the epididymis may be enlarged; further physical signs depend on the procedure done.

There may be a large variability of semen parameters ranging from azoospermia after chemotherapy with alkylating substances or after irradiation to severe oligoasthenoteratozoospermia and only minor aberrations in patients, for example after treatment with drugs affecting only sperm motility. In cases of sperm transport disturbances with complete retrograde ejaculation, aspermia will be observed with spermatozoa present only in the postejaculatory urine.

The biochemical marker substance α-glucosidase will be markedly decreased after procedures causing obstruction (vasectomy or failed hernia repair).

After operations for testicular torsions and refertilization after vasectomy, frequently antisperm antibodies, as reflected by a positive MAR test, and agglutinations of spermatozoa in combination with low sperm motility and vitality are observed.

Elevated levels of FSH and decreased concentrations of inhibin-B may occur after orchidectomy due to testicular cancer and after chemotherapy as well as after irradiation.

In patients with epilepsy, frequently low testosterone levels are observed, which is deteriorated by antiepileptic drugs; these also may lead to impaired sperm motility and morphology (Isojärvi et al. 2004). Low testosterone concentrations can also be caused by other drugs interfering with the testosterone metabolism.

In patients with a history of vasectomy, antisperm antibodies are also detected in the serum.

I.3.8.4
Differential Diagnosis

Further factors contributing to the fertility disturbance such as varicoceles, inflammations of the genital tract, genetic causes or anatomical aberrations have to be excluded before establishing the diagnosis of iatrogenic fertility disorder.

I.3.8.5
Treatment

Toxic medication should be replaced with an alternative treatment whenever possible. In vasectomized patients, a microsurgical reversal is recommended (Schroeder-Printzen and Weidner 2003). If vasectomy reversal fails, treatment as idiopathic azoospermia or oligoasthenozoospermia is indicated, but genetic evaluation may be omitted. If toxic medication cannot be replaced or if there is no restoration of normal fertility, treatment as idiopathic abnormality according to semen quality should be given.

I.3.8.6
Results of Treatment

Microsurgical vasovasostomy is the most frequently performed procedure for refertilization. Usually patency rates of about 90% are achieved, the pregnancy rates are partly dependent on the interval between vasectomy and vasovasostomy, pregnancy rates of 49% are reported after an obstruction interval of 15–19 years, and spouses of men with obstruction for 20–25 years had pregnancy rates of 33% (Fuchs and Burt 2002). Refertilization after childhood herniorrhaphy achieves patency rates of 44% and pregnancy rates of 36% (Matsuda 2000). Some authors suggest that a second trial of refertilization after failure of vasovasostomy may be worthwhile since they found it to be more cost effective than ICSI with epididymal spermatozoa (Donovan et al. 1998).

I.3.8.7
Prognosis

Impairment of spermatogenesis finally resulting in azoospermia by substances with direct antiproliferating effects on the germinal epithelium is caused by alkylating substances such as cyclophosphamide and chlorambucil, which lead to mostly irreversible azoospermia.

Recovery of spermatogenesis has been observed after cytostatic treatment with cisplatin and adriamycin as well as after treatment with methotrexate and vincristine or bleomycin (Forman et al. 1996).

Vasectomy is the most common cause of surgical obstruction and also results in production of antisperm antibodies. These antibodies persist after the repair operation and may hinder natural conception, even if obstruction has been relieved correctly. Therefore, methods of assisted fertilization may be necessary in a considerable percentage of couples after successful refertilization surgery (Rowe et al. 2000).

Irradiation in the genital region will most probably cause irreversible arrest of spermatogenesis with subsequent sterility. Recoveries have been observed after a time interval up to 5 years (Rowley et al. 1974).

Prognosis of medical therapy in patients finally classified as idiopathic depends on the degree of the disturbance provoked by the causative agent.

I.3.8.8 Prevention

Prior to chemotherapy or radiotherapy, sperm banking should be offered to all patients.

Any drug treatment with possible influence on fertility should be carefully deliberated in younger men whose family planning is not completed.

I.3.8.9 Other

Iatrogenic causes of male infertility cannot simply be avoided. Therefore, extensive counselling of patients undergoing vasectomy with regard to the problems arising from a potential reversal is necessary. Cryopreservation of sperm must be offered to cancer patients before chemo- or radiotherapy, and this could also be an option for patients receiving drug treatment with possible adverse effects on fertility.

References

Benoff S, Cooper GW, Hurley I et al (1994) The effect of calcium channel blockers on sperm fertilizing potential. Fertil Steril 62:606–617

Donovan DF, DiBaise M, Sparks AET, Kessler J, Sandlow JI (1998) Comparison of microscopic epididymal sperm aspiration and intracytoplasmic sperm injection/in-vitro fertilization with repeat microscopic reconstruction following vasectomy: is second attempt at reversal worth the effort? Hum Reprod 13:387–393

Forman R, Gilmour-White S, Forman N (1996) Drug-induced infertility and sexual dysfunction. Cambridge University Press, Cambridge, pp 168

Fuchs EF, Burt RA (2002) Vasectomy reversal performed 15 years or more after vasectomy: correlation of pregnancy outcome with partner age and with pregnancy results of in vitro fertilization with intracytoplasmic sperm injection. Fertil Steril 77:516–519

Gazvani MR, Buckett W, Luckas MJM, Aird IA, Hipkin LJ, Lewis-Jones DI (1997) Conservative management of azoospermia following steroid abuse. Hum Reprod 12:1706–1708

Isojärvi JIT, Löfgren E, Juntunen KST, Pakarinen AJ, Päivänsalo M, Rautakorpi I, Tuomivaara L (2004) Effect of epilepsy and antiepileptic drugs on male reproductive health. Neurology 62:247–253

Knuth UA, Maniera H, Nieschlag E (1989) Anabolic steroids and semen parameters in bodybuilders. Fertil Steril 52:1041–1047

Matsuda T (2000) Diagnosis and treatment of post-herniorrhaphy vas deferens obstruction. Int J Urol 7:35–38

Menon DK (2003) Successful treatment of anabolic steroid-induced azoospermia with human chorionic gonadotropin and human menopausal gonadotropin. Fertil Steril 79 [Suppl 3]:1659–1661

Neumann F (1984) Effects of drugs and chemicals on spermatogenesis. Arch Toxicol 7 [Suppl]:109–117

Rowe PJ, Comhaire FH, Hargreave TB, Mahmoud AMA (2000) WHO Manual for the standardized investigation, diagnosis and management of the infertile male. Cambridge University Press, pp 10–11

Rowley MJ, Leach DR, Warner GA, Heller CG (1974) Effect of graded doses of ionizing radiation on the human testis. Radiat Res 59:665 – 678

Schroeder-Printzen I, Weidner W (2003) Limits of microsurgical refertilization under urological aspects. Andrologia 35:178 – 179

WHO (1999) WHO laboratory manual of the examination of human semen and sperm-cervical mucus interaction. Cambridge University Press, Cambridge

I.3.9 Systemic Causes of Male Infertility

A. Mahmoud, F. Comhaire

Key Messages

- Many systemic diseases can negatively affect male fertility and sperm quality, but only in a small percentage of infertile men.
- A good general physical examination and selective screening tests are essential.
- In addition to genetic and endocrine causes, organ failure, infectious diseases, obesity, and exposure to toxins, drugs and medications can cause male infertility.
- If possible, treatment of the underlying cause(s) of infertility is advisable before resorting to assisted reproductive techniques.

I.3.9.1 Introduction

Although the majority of infertile men are otherwise asymptomatic and healthy, many systemic diseases can negatively affect male fertility and sperm quality. Therefore a good general physical examination and selective screening tests are essential (Rowe et al. 2000). Systemic diseases may cause the so-called dual defect, i.e. a combination of both primary (hypergonadotrophic) and secondary (hypogonadotrophic) testicular failure. Transient secondary hypogonadism is predominant in acute illnesses, while in chronic illnesses primary hypogonadism prevails. Genetic factors are responsible for the diverse responses in men with the same illness (for a review, see Baker 1998).

I.3.9.2 Systemic Causes

I.3.9.2.1 Fever

A fever exceeding 38.5°C may suppress spermatogenesis for a period of up to 6 months (WHO 1987).

Carlsen et al. (2003) found that sperm concentration, morphology and motility parameters were adversely affected by a febrile episode during the postmeiotic period of human spermatogenesis (spermiogenesis). Their study indicated that sperm concentration was also adversely affected by fever during the period of meiosis, whereas fever at other time points during spermatogenesis did not seem to significantly affect these sperm parameters. The adverse effect seemed to be dependent upon the number of days with fever. Fever may also be associated with sperm DNA damage (Evenson et al. 2000).

Details should be recorded of the disease or condition causing the hyperthermia, its duration and treatment. It is not known, for example, whether the deleterious influence of an attack of influenza may be less than that following a severe malarial episode.

I.3.9.2.2 Excessive Heat

Excessively hot environments may depress spermatogenesis (Thonneau et al. 1996, 1998) and some studies suggest that exposure of the testis to elevated temperature may temporarily have the same effect. Examples include hot bathing, prolonged car driving and lap top computer use in a laptop position (Mieusset and Bujan 1995; Bujan et al. 2000; Sheynkin et al. 2005).

I.3.9.2.3 Mumps and Other Viral Diseases

Orchitis

The classical orchitis is associated with infectious parotitis (mumps), but orchitis is seen with other viral infections such as coxsackie or herpes. Following an attack of mumps orchitis, the recovery of fertility is variable; some men remain sterile and in other cases the time to recovery of sperm production may take as long as 2 years. Mumps occurring before puberty and mumps not accompanied by orchitis do not interfere with fertility. Orchitis associated with infectious parotitis (mumps) is actually a possible cause of acquired testicular damage rather than a systemic disease.

Human Immunodeficiency Virus Infection

In patients with HIV infection, the impairment of spermatogenesis is related to the severity of the disease (Politch et al. 1994; Muller et al. 1998). The mechanisms of HIV-associated infertility include primary and later secondary hypogonadism, leucocytospermia, cytokine release, direct involvement of the testes or epididymides by HIV, opportunistic infections, malignancy (for a review, see Baker 1998; Umapathy et al. 2001), and the popular use of anabolic steroids (Pena et al. 2003).

Using sperm processing accompanied by antiretroviral therapy, assisted reproductive techniques are offered by some centres to HIV-serodiscordant couples where the man is seropositive to achieve pregnancy while minimizing the risk of HIV transmission (Sauer 2005).

I.3.9.2.4 Chronic Renal Failure

Reduced sexual activity and libido as well as diminished fertility have consistently been reported in the dialysis population. These factors may reduce the well-being and quality of life of these patients. The reasons for these disturbances are complex. Recent developments, however, improved therapeutic possibilities.

Mechanism of Male Infertility

Azoospermia, severe oligozoospermia, and decreased sperm viability are common in patients with chronic renal failure. Especially when FSH is elevated, sperm deficiency is usually severe (Mastrogiacomo et al. 1984; Prem et al. 1996). Studies in rats suggest chronic renal failure also has adverse effects on the overall sperm fertilizing capacity (Yamamoto et al. 1997). Spermatogenesis is impaired and testicular histology frequently shows hypospermatogenesis, maturation arrest or germ cell aplasia (Mastrogiacomo et al. 1984; Prem et al. 1996; Schmidt and Holley 1998; Kheradmand and Javadneia 2003). Also, the rete testis may present cystic transformation (Nistal et al. 1989).

Many investigators believe that these defects represent primary gonadal damage by uremic toxins (Mahajan et al. 1984; Lim 1987), probably via impairing the activity of the enzyme 17-beta-hydroxysteroid-dehydrogenase. A derangement of the peripheral conversion of steroids cannot, however, be excluded. Increased oestradiol secretion by patients with renal failure has been described, and this may interfere with steroid biosynthesis. The coexistence of central neuroendocrine disorders in the regulation of gonadotrophin secretion has been proposed (Lim 1987). Other changes in reproductive hormones include suboptimal serum testosterone with elevated LH, FSH, and prolactin levels (Kheradmand and Javadneia 2003).

Treatment of Renal Failure and Male Infertility

Earlier studies came to the contradictory conclusions that maintenance haemodialysis either had no effect or exerted a deleterious influence on sperm concentration (Holdsworth et al. 1978; Tourkantonis et al. 1981; Mastrogiacomo et al. 1984). A more recent study, however, reported improvements of sperm motility during haemodialysis (Kheradmand and Javadneia 2003).

After successful renal transplantation, semen quality and testicular histology may show a striking improvement, sometimes reaching complete recovery of spermatogenesis (Mastrogiacomo et al. 1984; Prem et al. 1996) with reversal of azoospermia (Kheradmand and Javadneia 2003) and restoration of fertility (Phadke et al. 1970; Holdsworth et al. 1978; Prem et al. 1996). Abnormalities in reproductive hormones are frequently corrected following transplantation (Kheradmand and Javadneia 2003). Nevertheless, a high prevalence of abnormalities of the hypothalamic–pituitary–testicular axis was demonstrated in renal transplant recipients with well-functioning allografts. Alterations of the hypothalamic–pituitary–testicular axis are probably multifactorial, being influenced prevalently by immunosuppressive treatments with further influence by allograft function and time elapsed from transplant (Tauchmanova et al. 2004).

Immunosuppressive therapy with cyclosporine A does not seem to adversely affect fertility in renal transplant patients (Haberman et al. 1991), although another study reported negative correlations between the levels of this medication in whole blood and both sperm concentration and motility parameters (Eid et al. 1996). Corticosteroids apart, little is known about the effect of other immunosuppressants used in renal transplant patients on sperm quality.

In patients with symptomatic secondary hyperparathyroidism, a marked improvement in sperm motility has been reported following total parathyroidectomy combined with partial autotransplantation of 60–90 mg of parathyroid tissue subcutaneously (Chou et al. 2003).

Studies on zinc therapy give contradictory results, which may (Mahajan et al. 1982) or may not cause significant improvement in sperm characteristics (Rodger et al. 1989).

Stimulation of Leydig cell function by human chorionic gonadotrophin (hCG) for 4 months did not improve fertility (Bundschu et al. 1976); neither were there any significant changes in sperm counts after pergolide administration (Rodger et al. 1989).

The effect of clomiphene citrate on spermatogenesis in dialysis patients is inconclusive, as either improvement or deterioration may occur (Lim and Fang 1976). This is similar to observations in men with idiopathic oligozoospermia, and may be related to the combined anti-oestrogenic and slightly oestrogenic activity of this drug. So far, there are no data on the use of the pure anti-oestrogen tamoxifen in the treatment of male infertility associated with renal failure.

Present-day assisted reproductive technology, especially in vitro fertilization (IVF) with intracytoplasmic sperm injection (ICSI), offers new hope for subfertile men with otherwise untreatable severely impaired semen quality.

I.3.9.2.5 Alcoholism

Excessive alcohol consumption causes systemic disease in multiple organs, including the liver and probably indirectly the testis. Chronic excessive alcohol consumption may interfere with spermatogenesis and also reduce sexual function through inhibition of testosterone biosynthesis. These effects are prominent if alcohol abuse occurs on an almost daily basis and exceeds approximately 6 units per day.

I.3.9.2.6
Liver Cirrhosis

Hypogonadism and feminization are common features of liver cirrhosis and are related to the severity of cirrhosis. Serum oestradiol, sex hormone-binding globulin and gonadotrophins are elevated, while testosterone levels are low (for a review, see Kaymakoglu et al. 1995; Baker 1998). Loss of libido, erectile dysfunction, infertility, reduced secondary sex hair, testicular atrophy, and gynaecomastia are frequent. The pathogenesis of hypogonadism in liver cirrhosis is not well understood. This has been attributed to oestrogen excess, primary testicular failure, or a dual defect (see introduction) (for a review, see Baker 1998). Animal experiments, however, indicate the blood-testis barrier is altered from an early stage of cirrhosis and that insulin-like growth factor 1 deficiency might play a pathogenetic role in hypogonadism of cirrhosis. The administration of this growth factor for a short period of time reverted the testicular atrophy associated with advanced experimental cirrhosis in rats (Castilla-Cortazar et al. 2004).

In the majority of men with chronic liver failure, the hypothalamic-pituitary-testicular hormone axis and gonadal tissue resume normal function after liver transplantation (Madersbacher et al. 1994).

I.3.9.2.7
Cancer

Testicular cancer, Hodgkin's disease, non-Hodgkin lymphomas and leukaemia may affect young people and the disease or its treatment may have deleterious effects on fertility (Bahadur et al. 2005). As a result of the increasing incidence of many cancers and improvements in cancer therapy, an increasing proportion of boys and young men with cancer will survive their disease and desire fertility. Unfortunately, cancer treatment may have a negative and in many cases permanent impact on the individual's fertility potential (see Chap. II.2.7). This effect is highly dependent on the type and dose of therapy as well as the age at which it was given (Giwercman and Petersen 2000). Irradiation in the genital region will most probably cause irreversible arrest of spermatogenesis with subsequent sterility. Among cancer chemotherapy, the alkylating agents usually cause irreversible damage. Cisplatin-based regimens for testis neoplasm induce temporary azoospermia but permanent damage can occur with high doses (400 – 600 mg/m^2) (Colpi et al. 2004). Recovery, if it occurs, is expected up to roughly 5 years after cancer treatment (Bahadur et al. 2005). Another aspect of the relationship between cancer and infertility is the possibility that men with testicular dysfunction may have an increased risk of testicular cancer. Screening for early testicular malignancy may therefore be advisable in some groups of men with poor semen quality (Giwercman and Petersen 2000). Additional risk factors for testicular cancer include cryptorchidism, low testicular volume, gonadal dysgenesis, testicular (micro)lithiasis and most importantly, carcinoma in situ testis (Otite et al. 2001; Dieckmann and Pichlmeier 2004) (Chap. II.2.8). All these abnormalities occur with an increased frequency in subfertile men.

Management

Because cancer treatment may be associated with sperm DNA damage (Morris 2002; Deane et al. 2004), semen cryopreservation should be offered prior to treatment and not during treatment in all cases where fertility is desired (Meistrich 1993). Multiple samples should be frozen, especially when the sperm quality is impaired. In cases with ejaculatory problems, the use of a vibrator or medical induction of an erection may be attempted. Many children and young adolescents, however, are unable to ejaculate, although the testis may contain spermatozoa or their precursors. Freezing of testicular tissue may be considered in these cases, although the fertilizing potential of the spermatozoa is unknown. It is hoped that the recent advances in the fields of in vitro sperm culture and maturation techniques (Tesarik and Mendoza 2003) and autotransplantation of germ cells (McLaren 1998) will help to achieve successful fertilization using frozen testicular cells from this young population. Proper protection of the gonads is essential during radiotherapy in the proximity of the gonads; precautions to protect the bowel and bladder must also be taken when a radioactive substance is administered parenterally, e.g. radioactive iodine for thyroid cancer.

I.3.9.2.8
Respiratory Tract Diseases

Chronic respiratory tract disease includes chronic sinusitis, chronic bronchitis, and bronchiectasis. These conditions are sometimes associated with disorders of the sperm flagellum such as in the immotile cilia syndrome, or with secretory disturbance in the epididymis with obstructive azoospermia. The latter problem may also occur in men with cystic fibrosis; these men have an increased incidence of dysgenesis or absence of the vas deferens based on the same genetic defect (Chap. I.3.7).

I.3.9.2.9
Body Composition

Several syndromes are typically associated with childhood obesity and hypogonadism (see Chap. I.3.11). Obesity is associated with relatively low androgen/oestrogen ratio due to increased peripheral conversion of androgens to oestrogens by the enzyme aromatase in adipose tissue. Disturbed testicular thermoregulation has also been proposed as a mechanism for impaired testicular function in obese men (for a review, see Baker 1998). In addition to their possible role as a cause of male infertility, the chemical calorie theory suggests that endocrine disruptors (see Chap. I.3.11) are, at least in part, responsible for the pandemic of obesity in the last few decades (Baillie-Hamilton 2002). Our data indicates that subfertile men have a significantly higher body mass index (BMI) than the general population (see Fig. I.3.10). An abnormal BMI of less than 19 or over 30 kg/m^2 has been associated with reduced testicular volume (WHO 1987) and reduced semen quality, suggesting impairment of spermatogenesis (Jensen et al. 2004).

I.3.9.2.10
Medication

Certain medical treatments may cause temporary or permanent damage to spermatogenesis (see Chap. I.3.5).

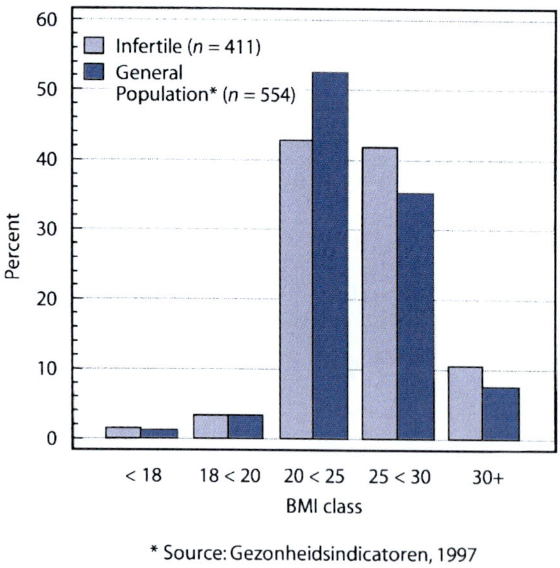

Fig. I.3.10. Frequency distribution of body mass index in infertile men and an age-matched general population

I.3.9.2.11
Environmental Factors

Chronic exposure to heavy metals, e.g. lead, cadmium and mercury or other substances, e.g. pesticides, herbicides, carbon disulphide may also reduce fertility (see Chap. I.3.11).

I.3.9.2.12
Smoking and Recreational Drugs

Recent literature meta-analyses indicate tobacco smoking is associated with modest reductions in semen quality, increased oxidative damage to the sperm DNA, and alterations in serum hormone levels. It has been reported that excessive tobacco smoking can enhance the deleterious effects of genital diseases (e.g. varicocele) (Klaiber et al. 1987; Mahmoud et al. 1998) or other environmental factors on spermatogenesis. In addition, men who smoke have a higher number of white blood cells in semen (Close et al. 1990), an increased risk of urethritis (Martin-Boyce et al. 1977) and impaired secretory functions of male accessory sex glands (Pakrashi and Chatterjee 1995). Male smoking is associated with lower spontaneous pregnancy rates and lower success rates following intrauterine insemination (Mahmoud et al. 1998), in vitro fertilization and ICSI (Zitzmann et al. 2003).

There have been reports that marihuana smoking is associated with reduction in fertility. Men who become addicted to opiate drugs often have multiple episodes of septicaemia and poor general health, and it is difficult to know if any damage to fertility is a direct result of the drug or rather self-neglect.

I.3.9.2.13
Others

Tuberculosis may cause epididymitis and prostatitis associated with impairment of sperm transport. Diabetes mellitus and neurological disease may cause erectile impotence and disorders of ejaculation. In addition, both conditions may damage spermatogenesis and the function of the accessory sex glands (Colpi et al. 1987; Padron et al. 1997; Sexton and Jarow 1997). Other nongenital diseases may be associated with infertility (see Table I.3.7).

Table I.3.7. Diseases associated with male infertility (adapted from Hargreave 1994)

Disease	Mechanism
Congenital disorders	
Genetic disorders	
Kartagener's syndrome	Immotile sperm
Cystic fibrosis	Associated with agenesis of vas deferens and also with secretory disturbance in epididymis
Androgen receptor deficiency	Lack of development of genitalia
Prune Belly syndrome	Testicular maldescent
Coeliac disease	Testicular damage
Testicular maldescent	Testicular damage
Von-Hippel-Lindau syndrome	Cystadenoma of epididymis
Acquired disorders	
Infections	
Infectious parotitis (mumps)	Orchitis
HIV infection	See text
Tuberculosis	Obstruction and orchitis
Bilharziasis	Obstruction
Gonorrhoea	Obstruction (and orchitis)
Chlamydial epididymitis	Obstruction
Filariasis	Obstruction
Typhoid	Orchitis
Influenza	Orchitis
Undulant fever (Brucellosis)	Orchitis
Syphilis	Orchitis
Pemphigus foliaceus in South America	Azoospermia (? obstruction)
Endocrine disease	
Thyrotoxicosis	Hormonal abnormality
Diabetes mellitus	Testicular failure and ejaculatory disturbance
Hepatic failure	Hormonal abnormality
Renal failure	Testicular failure and loss of libido
Secondary testicular failure	Pituitary failure; usually there will also be androgen deficiency
Chromophobe adenoma	
Astrocytoma	
Hamartoma	
Teratoma	
Sarcoidosis	
Neurological disease	Erectile impotence and disorders of ejaculation; damage to spermatogenesis; damage to accessory sex glands
Paraplegia	
Chronic respiratory tract disease	
Bronchiectasis	May be associated with abnormal sperm cilia in the immotile cilia syndrome, situs inversus or secretory disturbance in the epididymis such as in Young's syndrome
Chronic sinusitis	
Chronic bronchitis	

References

Bahadur G, Ozturk O, Muneer A, Wafa R, Ashraf A, Jaman N, Patel S, Oyede AW, Ralph DJ (2005) Semen quality before and after gonadotoxic treatment. Hum Reprod 20:774–781

Baillie-Hamilton PF (2002) Chemical toxins: a hypothesis to explain the global obesity epidemic. J Altern Complement Med 8:185–192

Baker HW (1998) Reproductive effects of nontesticular illness. Endocrinol Metab Clin North Am 27:831–850

Bujan L, Daudin M, Charlet JP, Thonneau P, Mieusset R (2000) Increase in scrotal temperature in car drivers. Hum Reprod 15:1355–1357

Bundschu HD, Rager K, Heller S, Hayduk K, Pfeiffer EH, Luders G, Liebau G (1976) Effects of long-term HCG administration on testicular function in hemodialysis patients. Klin Wochenschr 54:1039–1046

Carlsen E, Andersson AM, Petersen JH, Skakkebaek NE (2003) History of febrile illness and variation in semen quality. Hum Reprod 18:2089–2092

Castilla-Cortazar I, Diez N, Garcia-Fernandez M, Puche JE, Diez-Caballero F, Quiroga J, Diaz-Sanchez M, Castilla A, Casares AD, Varela-Nieto I, Prieto J, Gonzalez-Baron S (2004) Hematotesticular barrier is altered from early stages of liver cirrhosis: effect of insulin-like growth factor 1. World J Gastroenterol 10:2529–2534

Chou FF, Lee CH, Lee CT, Huang FJ, Hsu KL (2003) Spermatogenesis after parathyroidectomy in patients with symptomatic secondary hyperparathyroidism. J Am Coll Surg 196: 854–858

Colpi GM, Casella F, Zanollo A, Ballerini G, Balerna M, Campana A, Lange A (1987) Functional voiding disturbances of the ampullo-vesicular seminal tract: a cause of male infertility. Acta Eur Fertil 18:165–179

Colpi GM, Contalbi GF, Nerva F, Sagone P, Piediferro G (2004) Testicular function following chemo-radiotherapy. Eur J Obstet Gynecol Reprod Biol 113 [Suppl 1]:S2–S6

Deane L, Sharir S, Jarvi K, Zini A (2004) High levels of sperm DNA denaturation as the sole semen abnormality in a patient after chemotherapy for testis cancer. J Androl 25: 23–24

Dieckmann KP, Pichlmeier U (2004) Clinical epidemiology of testicular germ cell tumors. World J Urol 22:2–14

Eid MM, Abdel-Hamid IA, Sobh MA, el-Saied MA (1996) Assessment of sperm motion characteristics in infertile renal transplant recipients using computerized analysis. Int J Androl 19:338–344

Evenson DP, Jost LK, Corzett M, Balhorn R (2000) Characteristics of human sperm chromatin structure following an episode of influenza and high fever: a case study. J Androl 21: 739–746

Giwercman A, Petersen PM (2000) Cancer and male infertility. Baillieres Best Pract Res Clin Endocrinol Metab 14: 453–471

Haberman J, Karwa G, Greenstein SM, Soberman R, Glicklich D, Tellis V, Melman A (1991) Male fertility in cyclosporine-treated renal transplant patients. J Urol 145:294–296

Hargreave TB (1994) History and examination. In: Hargreave TB (ed) Male infertility. Springer, Berlin Heidelberg New York, pp 17–36

Holdsworth SR, de Kretser DM, Atkins RC (1978) A comparison of hemodialysis and transplantation in reversing the uremic disturbance of male reproductive function. Clin Nephrol 10:146–150

Jensen TK, Andersson AM, Jorgensen N, Andersen AG, Carlsen E, Petersen JO, Skakkebaek NE (2004) Body mass index in relation to semen quality and reproductive hormones among 1,558 Danish men. Fertil Steril 82:863–870

Kaymakoglu S, Okten A, Cakaloglu Y, Boztas G, Besisik F, Tascioglu C, Yalcin S (1995) Hypogonadism is not related to the etiology of liver cirrhosis. J Gastroenterol 30:745–750

Kheradmand AR, Javadneia AH (2003) Efficacy of hemodialysis and renal transplantation on reproductive function in men with end stage renal disease. Transplant Proc 35:2718–2719

Klaiber EL, Broverman DM, Pokoly TB, Albert AJ, Howard PJJ, Sherer JFJ (1987) Interrelationships of cigarette smoking, testicular varicoceles, and seminal fluid indexes. Fertil Steril 47:481–486

Lim VS (1987) Reproductive function in patients with renal insufficiency. Am J Kidney Dis 9:363–367

Lim VS, Fang VS (1976) Restoration of plasma testosterone levels in uremic men with clomiphene citrate. J Clin Endocrinol Metab 43:1370–1377

Madersbacher S, Grunberger T, Maier U (1994) Andrological status before and after liver transplantation. J Urol 151: 1251–1254

Mahajan SK, Abbasi AA, Prasad AS, Rabbani P, Briggs WA, McDonald FD (1982) Effect of oral zinc therapy on gonadal function in hemodialysis patients. A double-blind study. Ann Intern Med 97:357–361

Mahajan SK, Prasad AS, McDonald FD (1984) Sexual dysfunction in uremic male: improvement following oral zinc supplementation. Contrib Nephrol 38:103–111

Mahmoud AM, Schoonjans F, Zalata AA, Comhaire FH (1998) The effect of male smoking on semen quality, reducing capacity, reactive oxygen species, and spontaneous and assisted conception rates. Andrology in the Nineties, Genk, Belgium, 22–25 April

Martin-Boyce A, David G, Schwartz D (1977) Genitourinary infection, smoking and alcohol in the male. Rev Epidemiol Santé Publique 25:209–216

Mastrogiacomo I, De Besi L, Zucchetta P, Serafini E, Gasparotto ML, Marchini P, Pisani E, Dean P, Chini M (1984) Effect of hyperprolactinemia and age on the hypogonadism of uremic men on hemodialysis. Arch Androl 12:235–242

McLaren A (1998) Germ cells and germ cell transplantation. Int J Dev Biol 42:855–860

Mieusset R, Bujan L (1995) Testicular heating and its possible contributions to male infertility: a review. Int J Androl 18: 169–184

Morris ID (2002) Sperm DNA damage and cancer treatment. Int J Androl 25:255–261

Muller CH, Coombs RW, Krieger JN (1998) Effects of clinical stage and immunological status on semen analysis results in human immunodeficiency virus type 1-seropositive men. Andrologia 30 [Suppl 1]:15–22

Nistal M, Santamaria L, Paniagua R (1989) Acquired cystic transformation of the rete testis secondary to renal failure. Hum Pathol 20:1065–1070

Otite U, Webb JA, Oliver RT, Badenoch DF, Nargund VH (2001) Testicular microlithiasis: is it a benign condition with malignant potential? Eur Urol 40:538–542

Padron OF, Brackett NL, Sharma RK, Lynne CM, Thomas AJ Jr, Agarwal A (1997) Seminal reactive oxygen species and sperm motility and morphology in men with spinal cord injury. Fertil Steril 67:1115–1120

Pakrashi A, Chatterjee S (1995) Effect of tobacco consumption on the function of male accessory sex glands. Int J Androl 18:232–236

Pena JE, Thornton MH Jr, Sauer MV (2003) Reversible azoospermia: anabolic steroids may profoundly affect human immunodeficiency virus-seropositive men undergoing assisted reproduction. Obstet Gynecol 101:1073–1075

Phadke AG, MacKinnon KJ, Dossetor JB (1970) Male fertility in uremia: restoration by renal allografts. Can Med Assoc J 102:607–608

Politch JA, Mayer KH, Abbott AF, Anderson DJ (1994) The effects of disease progression and zidovudine therapy on semen quality in human immunodeficiency virus type 1 seropositive men. Fertil Steril 61:922–928

Prem AR, Punekar SV, Kalpana M, Kelkar AR, Acharya VN (1996) Male reproductive function in uraemia: efficacy of haemodialysis and renal transplantation. Br J Urol 78: 635–638

Rodger RS, Sheldon WL, Watson MJ, Dewar JH, Wilkinson R, Ward MK, Kerr DN (1989) Zinc deficiency and hyperprolactinaemia are not reversible causes of sexual dysfunction in uraemia. Nephrol Dial Transplant 4:888–892

Rowe PJ, Comhaire FH, Hargreave TB, Mahmoud AMA (2000) WHO manual for the standardized investigation, diagnosis and management of the infertile male. Cambridge University Press, Cambridge

Sauer MV (2005) Sperm washing techniques address the fertility needs of HIV-seropositive men: a clinical review. Reprod Biomed Online 10:135–140

Schmidt RJ, Holley JL (1998) Fertility and contraception in end-stage renal disease. Adv Ren Replace Ther 5:38–44

Sexton WJ, Jarow JP (1997) Effect of diabetes mellitus upon male reproductive function. Urology 49:508–513

Sheynkin Y, Jung M, Yoo P, Schulsinger D, Komaroff E (2005) Increase in scrotal temperature in laptop computer users. Hum Reprod 20:452–455

Tauchmanova L, Carrano R, Sabbatini M, De Rosa M, Orio F, Palomba S, Cascella T, Lombardi G, Federico S, Colao A (2004) Hypothalamic-pituitary-gonadal axis function after successful kidney transplantation in men and women. Hum Reprod 19:867–873

Tesarik J, Mendoza C (2003) Using the male gamete for assisted reproduction: past, present, and future. J Androl 24: 317–328

Thonneau P, Ducot B, Bujan L, Mieusset R, Spira A (1996) Heat exposure as a hazard to male fertility. Lancet 347:204–205

Thonneau P, Bujan L, Multigner L, Mieusset R (1998) Occupational heat exposure and male fertility: a review. Hum Reprod 13:2122–2125

Tourkantonis A, Spiliopoulos A, Pharmakiotis A, Settas L (1981) Haemodialysis and hypothalamo-pituitary-testicular axis. Nephron 27:271–272

Umapathy E, Simbini T, Chipata T, Mbizvo M (2001) Sperm characteristics and accessory sex gland functions in HIV-infected men. Arch Androl 46:153–158

WHO (1987) Towards more objectivity in diagnosis and management of male infertility. Int J Androl Suppl 7

Yamamoto Y, Sofikitis N, Miyagawa I (1997) Effects of chronic renal failure on the sperm fertilizing capacity. Urol Int 58:105–107

Zitzmann M, Rolf C, Nordhoff V, Schrader G, Rickert-Fohring M, Gassner P, Behre HM, Greb RR, Kiesel L, Nieschlag E (2003) Male smokers have a decreased success rate for in vitro fertilization and intracytoplasmic sperm injection. Fertil Steril 79 [Suppl 3]:1550–1554

I.3.10 Congenital Disorders and Male Infertility

T. Hargreave

Key Messages

- Newborn male babies should be examined to check that both testicles are in the scrotum. Babies with suspected testicular maldescent should be re-examined at 1 year of age.
- There is a need for long-term studies of the fertility of men who had orchiopexy for testicular maldescent in infancy but such studies are very difficult to undertake. At present, treatment recommendation is for orchiopexy as soon as it is safe and ideally before the age of 2–3 years.
- Klinefelter syndrome is probably under-diagnosed and should be considered in all men with azoospermia or very low sperm counts who also have small testicles.
- Long-term follow-up of androgen status and if necessary androgen replacement should probably be offered to all men with Klinefelter syndrome and especially to those men who have had extensive testicular biopsy to recover sperm.

I.3.10.1 Definition of the Disease

Included in this category are karyotype disorders, genetic disorders, and congenital phenotypic disorders where the genetic basis is complex or unknown such as testicular maldescent. Chromosomal and genetic disorders are more fully described in Chap. II.3.10. Congenital anatomical disorders of the penis sufficient to prevent sexual intercourse are included in the chapter on sexual dysfunction (Chap. I.4). Most of the conditions discussed in this chapter are more fully described elsewhere in this book, and for underlying references the reader is referred to the numerous cross-references to the appropriate chapters.

I.3.10.2 Aetiology and Pathogenesis

Karyotype and genetic disorders may be inherited from parents. Karyotype abnormalities may also occur during meiosis. Testicular maldescent may occur in association with defined chromosome abnormality but may also occur because of environmental and endocrine factors during foetal development. The cause of penile abnormalities such as unilateral agenesis of the corpus cavernosa is unknown but may relate to fusion abnormalities of the two genital tubercles and this in turn may relate to unknown genetic factors, or mechanical or environmental factors, at this stage in foetal development.

I.3.10.3 Clinical Findings: History, Physical Examination, Technical Investigations, Laboratory Findings

The history and clinical findings depend on the nature of the problem. Clinical examination is important and careful note should be made of any abnormality that may be congenital.

Chromosomal abnormalities are more common in infertile than fertile men. Standard karyotype analysis should be offered to all men with damaged spermatogenesis who are seeking fertility treatment by in vitro fertilization (IVF) or intracytoplasmic sperm injection (ICSI). Fluorescent in situ hybridization (FISH) analysis of spermatozoa is a research investigation.

The commonest chromosomal abnormality is Klinefelter syndrome 47XXY: the clinical findings may be subtle and easily overlooked. The leg length is disproportionately long to the trunk length and the testicles are small and firm but virilization is often normal. The diagnosis is confirmed by karyotype analysis using a peripheral blood sample. Klinefelter's mosaicism is present in about 15% to 20% of cases. Low levels of mosaicism may be missed by some laboratories but should be identified if possible because the prospects for sperm recovery are much better than with nonmosaic Klinefelter's syndrome. At least three ejaculates should be tested in the laboratory with examination of the centrifuged deposit for sperm. If sperm are seen, then it is usually possible to find sperm in testicular tissue but extensive biopsy may be needed. A later consequence of extensive biopsy is androgen deficiency because of damage to the testicle. Probably all men with Klinefelter's should be offered long-term follow-up of androgen status, particularly if they have had sperm recovery by biopsy. Also, there is a risk that sperm recovered are 47 XXY aneuploid spermatozoa. Before proceeding with IVF ICSI, the couple should be informed of the risk of having children with Klinefelter syndrome. Counselling can be very difficult because the potential father may have a poor understanding because low intelligence is sometimes a feature of Klinefelter syndrome. Full genetic counselling should include discussion about preimplantation diagnosis and amniocentesis.

Men with congenital absence of the vas deferens account for approximately 2% of men with azoospermia in European populations. This is associated with mutations in the coding and noncoding regions of the cystic fibrosis transmembrane conductance regulator gene (CFTR). These men may also have mild stigmata of cystic fibrosis such as increased tendency to chest infections or if they smoke a pronounced smoker's cough. The condition is often missed on hurried clinical examination and may be first suspected because semen analysis shows azoospermia with an ejaculate volume of less than 1 ml and acidic Ph.

Testicular maldescent is categorized according to the position of the testicle. Impalpable testes may be intra-abdominal or atrophic and within the inguinal canal. Intra-abdominal testes are usually sited within the pelvic cavity, with blood vessels arising from the lower half of the abdominal aorta. Incompletely descended testes may lie within the inguinal canal. Often there is an associated hernia sac and the testicle may flip in and out of the internal inguinal ring into the abdominal cavity. In this situation, the man may give the history of an intermittent inguinal lump.

Ectopic testes are defined as those testes that have left the abdominal cavity but deviated from the normal pathway of descent through the inguinal canal. The most common site for ectopic testis is in the superficial inguinal pouch; in this situation the testis descends through the inguinal canal and lies above the external inguinal ring. The cord including the testicular blood vessels thus run inferiorly from the testicle before entering the superficial inguinal ring to run superiorly into the abdominal cavity. Surgeons need to understand this anatomical relationship to avoid damaging blood vessels during corrective surgery. Very rarely the ectopic descent is through the femoral canal. Retraction of the testes into the external inguinal ring is normal in boys from the age of 1.5 years until the testicles enlarge at puberty. The best time to differentiate testis maldescent from retractile testes is by clinical examination before 1 year of age, which is before the cremasteric reflex has developed. A reasonable screening strategy is to examine all male babies at birth and to re-examine at 1 year those babies with potential testicular maldescent. It is more difficult to distinguish retractile testes from maldescended testes at the time of school medical examination when boys are 8–9 years old boys because at this age the cremasteric reflex is very marked.

Imaging investigations to locate impalpable testes include inguinal canal ultrasound and magnetic resonance imaging of the abdominal cavity and inguinal canals; occasionally laparoscopy can be used to locate suspected intra-abdominal testes. The internal inguinal ring is inspected to locate the vas deferens and if it is seen to enter the canal, this indicates that the testis or atrophic remnant is within the inguinal canal.

Congenital penile abnormality such as micropenis, epispadias or exstrophy may be obvious from clinical examination. Depending on findings, appropriate investigation can include studies of androgen receptor status. However, congenital angulation of the erect penis including chordee often require examination during erection. In general if a young man says he has a bent erection this should be investigated because nearly always the problem will be confirmed.

I.3.10.4 Differential Diagnosis

When there is unilateral impalpable testis, the differential diagnosis is between testicular agenesis and intra-abdominal or impalpable inguinal testis. The finding at laparoscopy of the vas disappearing into the internal ring and the absence of the testis within the inguinal canal on MRI or ultrasound scanning is sufficient to make the diagnosis of unilateral agenesis of the testicle. If in such cases inguinal canal exploratory surgery is undertaken the vas will be found to be blind ending.

I.3.10.5 Treatment

There is at present no treatment to correct chromosomal or genetic abnormalities, although potentially this may become possible with gene transfer and germline correction (see Chap. II.4.18). However, such approaches to treatment are controversial and in some countries illegal (see p. 9). If sperm can be obtained, then IVF and where necessary ICSI techniques can be used to enable fertility. The main risk is the passage of severe, disabling or lethal chromosomal or genetic disorders to the next generation and thus any fertility treatment needs to be undertaken in the context of genetic counselling so that the couple understand the risks (if any) to the future child. Consideration also needs to be given to preimplantation diagnosis and replacement of chromosomally and genetically normal embryos. In some situations, especially when preimplantation diagnosis is impractical, unaffordable or unavailable, the best decision can be not to proceed with fertility treatments. Another possibility is amniocentesis or villous biopsy and termination of pregnancy depending on the result, but this is always a very difficult option, especially in the context of an infertile couple where the pregnancy has been hard to attain. The couple and the treating clinicians have to balance consideration of risks to the potential child with the desire of the couple to have children. The main difficulties will occur if there is a conflict of interest between the wishes of the couple and the interests of a future child. The best initial management is to give full information to the couple, who should then decide whether to proceed or not. However, where there is any increase in risk of a future child inheriting a genetic disorder before the decision is taken to proceed, it is important for the couple to appreciate fully what may be in store for their potential child and the future impact on their lives. It often helps to arrange a visit by the parents to see someone with the condition, e.g. a visit to a young adult with clinical cystic fibrosis. If the decision is taken to transfer an embryo with known chromosomal or genetic disorder the managing clinician should first seek approval from the local ethics committee.

Treatment for men with Klinefelter syndrome is directed towards recovery of sperm for fertility and consideration of androgen replacement in older age. Klinefelter syndrome is probably under-diagnosed (De Kretser, personal communication) but should be considered in all men with low sperm concentration or azoospermia who have small, firm testicles.

For men with other chromosomal disorders, apart from sperm recovery and IVF, ICSI treatment is dictated by other clinical manifestations (if any) of the disorder.

For men with Y microdeletions, the defect will be passed to sons; thus Y microdeletion analysis is desirable in men with severely damaged spermatogenesis who are seeking IVF/ICSI. Diagnostic techniques for Y microdeletions are becoming generally available but do not detect all known microdeletions. If a man is found to have microdeletions and the couple wishes to proceed with ICSI, they can be advised that microdeletions will be passed to sons but not daughters and that sons may in turn have a fertility problem but that there is no other known health consequence.

Treatment of testicular maldescent depends on the age of diagnosis, position of the testis and whether the condition is bilateral. Ideally, the condition is suspected during the examination of newborn male babies and confirmed by re-examination at 1 year of age and treated by surgical correction during the 2nd or 3rd year of life. However, this depends on adequate facilities for surgery on small children and in some situations it may be safer to defer surgery to 5–6 years of age. In general, the aim of treatment is to place the testicle within the scrotum as early as possible to give the best chance for normal development of the seminiferous tubules.

I.3.10.6 Results of Treatment

It is difficult to assess the results of fertility treatments undertaken for couples where the man has chromosomal or genetic disorders because some of these disorders are rare and facilities for preimplantation diagnosis, amniocentesis and the legality of termination vary from country to country. Also, there is a lack of information on how many couples later regret a decision to proceed with pregnancy despite a known abnormality. Ideally, clinics should collaborate with national and international data collection, including collection of information on long-term outcome and later regret. It is very difficult for clinicians to say no to requests for treatment and there is a need for evidence to underpin such decisions.

There is a lack of good information on the fertility of men who had orchiopexy in early childhood, mainly because it is very difficult to undertake long-term studies after childhood treatments. It is generally believed that orchiopexy before the age of 2 years gives the best chance of subsequent normal spermatogenesis, as this is before the onset of spermatogenesis, but there is an alternative view that damage to spermatogenesis and testicular maldescent are caused by the same factors and that orchiopexy makes little difference. A good reason for orchiopexy is to place the testicle in the scrotum so that subsequent examination is easy and any developing lumps can be detected early.

Treatment of erectile deformity is discussed in Chap. I.4 and usually the ability for penetrative intercourse can be attained, but if not fertility is possible using artificial insemination techniques.

I.3.10.7 Prevention

If early orchiopexy preserves fertility this is a good reason for treatment, but at present there is a lack of good follow-up data on babies who have had orchiopexy before the age of 2 years compared with those who have had orchiopexy at later ages.

The cause of testicular maldescent is not known but could in some cases relate to environmental pollution with endocrine disruptors and if so there may be opportunities to reduce the levels of such pollutants and preserve male fertility.

I.3.11 Acquired Testicular Damage

G. Haidl

I.3

Key Messages

- Permanent testicular damage with reduced volume or testicular atrophy is mainly caused by infectious agents.
- Although relatively rare, further events leading to testicular damage are testicular injuries and torsion.
- Early detection and treatment of causative factors may prevent or restore fertility.

I.3.11.1 Definition

Acquired testicular damage should be recorded when the abnormal spermatozoa are considered to be due to either parotitis with orchitis or orchitis with other viral or bacterial infections, or pathology possibly causing testicular damage, resulting in either a testicular volume of less than 15 ml or one of the both testes being nonpalpable. This diagnosis requires the following to be true:

- History of a pathology causing testicular damage
- At least one testis with a volume less than 15 ml or nonpalpable

I.3.11.2 Aetiology and Pathogenesis

I.3.11.2.1 Infections

Orchitis

An isolated inflammation of the testis, an orchitis, is a rare event. Most frequently it occurs in association with an epididymitis, as a so-called epididymo-orchitis. The spread of infection in orchitis is not always clear, the haematogenic and lymphogenic pathway occurs probably more frequently compared to the canalicular pathway via the epididymal duct (Weidner and Krause 1999). In contrast, epididymo-orchitis always develops by ascending infection. Orchitis can be subdivided into specific granulomatous forms in tuberculosis, syphilis, typhus or brucellosis, in viral forms such as mumps orchitis, as well as in nonspecific granulomatous orchitis of the adult, and in epididymo-orchitis caused by *Neisseria gonorrhoeae*, *Chlamydia trachomatis* or by enterobacteria. Orchitis is seen with other viral infections as well, e.g. coxsackie or herpes. In testicular tissue of infertile men, unusually high numbers of adenoassociated virus (AAV) have been observed (Schlehofer 2003). Less known are inflammatory influences on the testes by severe influenza, hepatitis or infectious mononucleosis (Rowe et al. 2000; Haidl and Weidner 2002). Autoimmune orchitis is known as an experimental model, where an orchitis is induced by active immunization with testis homogenate or bacteria (Tung and Teuscher 1995). As already pointed out, acute inflammations of the testes are normally not seen in the infertility clinic. Chronic inflammatory conditions of the testes would be expected to disrupt the normal process of spermatogenesis and cause alterations both in sperm number and quality (Purvis and Christiansen 1995). It is generally accepted that chronic infections may also be an important cause of spermatogenetic arrest (Diemer and Desjardins 1999) and testicular atrophy after mumps paramyxovirus orchitis (Weidner and Krause 1999).

I.3.11.2.2 Testicular Injury

Testicular trauma as a cause of infertility is rare. Most frequently, sporting and traffic accidents as well as accidents at work can affect the testis.

I.3.11.2.3 Testicular Torsion

Testicular torsion is a torsion of the testis and spermatic cord round the longitudinal axis due to abnormal mobility; it is a relatively infrequent cause of infertility.

I.3.11.3 Clinical and Laboratory Findings

I.3.11.3.1 Orchitis

Acute epididymitis and orchitis are painful conditions accompanied by fever and further discomforting symptoms and are usually not seen in the infertility clinic. Patients with orchitis or epididymo-orchitis in their history may show a reduced volume of the affected testis; moreover, delicate physical findings such as a slight decrease in the consistency of the testes and a thickened periorchium may be present.

Sperm parameters in the different forms of orchitis caused by virus infection or epididymo-orchitis are characterized by impairment of sperm count, motility and morphology. The occurrence of antisperm antibodies in cases of inflammatory conditions in the epididymis and testis due to disturbed blood–testis and blood–epididymis barrier is conceivable, but has – so far – not been convincingly demonstrated (Weidner et al. 1999).

Determination of virus serology in the blood may provide information about the causative virus in cases of orchitis.

I.3.11.3.2 Injury

A contused trauma can be accompanied by a haematoma and causes sharp pain as well as nausea and vomiting (see also Chap. I.7.2). In contrast, a history of minor scrotal injury is common but in most cases not relevant with regard to fertility problems. Injury should be recorded if it was accompanied by signs of tissue damage such as scrotal haematoma, haematospermia or haematuria. Subsequent testicular atrophy is a strong indication of the relevance of the traumatic incident. Severe injury, even when unilateral, may be important as it may cause disruption of the blood–testis barrier and initiate antisperm antibody production (Rowe et al. 2000).

Depending on the type and severity of the injury, highly variable semen characteristics may result.

I.3.11.3.3 Testicular Torsion

Patients with a history of testicular torsion relevant for their fertility may reveal a testicle with reduced size. Impaired semen parameters may be present as well (see also Chap. I.7.1).

I.3.11.4 Differential Diagnosis

In conditions with painful swelling of the testis, acute orchitis and epididymitis have to be considered. Testicular torsion is the most important differential diagnosis of acute epididymitis, which normally occurs only after puberty. Chronic, ongoing inflammatory processes of the testis and epididymis usually cause only minor discomfort if at all. In these cases with uncharacteristic symptoms, radiating pain from the spine or ureter, or strain in the inguinal area have to be considered. Finally, psychosomatic complaints and unspecific pain in the testis have to be differentiated from inflammatory disturbances. In patients with a history of testicular injury or torsion, further factors contributing to the abnormal semen parameters have to be excluded.

I.3.11.5 Treatment

Epididymo-orchitis

Patients with epididymo-orchitis in their history should be treated as having an idiopathic abnormality according to semen quality. The same applies to patients with a history of testicular injury or torsion. In cases of relevant amounts of antisperm antibodies, methods of assisted reproduction are recommended (Mortimer 1999).

Steroidal and nonsteroidal antiphlogistic substances have been suggested for the treatment of nonspecific chronic epididymo-orchitis (Weidner et al. 1999).

I.3.11.6 Results of Treatment

The results of idiopathic treatment will depend on the severity of the disturbance. Studies on idiopathic treatment in patients with a history of acquired damage do not exist.

The effect of antiphlogistic treatment in chronic nonspecific inflammations of the testis and epididymis with regard to fertility is not proven.

I.3.11.7 Prognosis

Following an attack of mumps orchitis, the recovery of fertility is variable; some men remain sterile and in other cases the time to recovery of sperm production may take as long as 2 years. Mumps occurring before puberty and mumps not accompanied by orchitis do not interfere with fertility (Rowe et al. 2000).

Chronic, ongoing inflammations may result in conditions known as mixed atrophy; others may even cause Sertoli-cell-only syndromes (Schuppe et al. 2001).

I.3.11.8 Prevention

Mumps orchitis can be prevented by vaccination in childhood, early diagnosis and adequate treatment of every infectious or inflammatory disease of the testis and epididymis can prevent later fertility disturbances, which is also true for early treatment of testicular torsion and severe injury.

I.3.11.9 Other

In summary, testicular injury and torsion are rare causes of male infertility. Acute inflammations and infections of the epididymis and testis, potentially leading to permanent testicular damage, can be treated effectively and thus prevent later fertility disturbances, whereas chronic silent inflammatory conditions cannot be sufficiently diagnosed by semen analysis. Generally accepted therapeutic guidelines for these disturbances are not yet available.

References

Diemer T, Desjardins C (1999) Disorders of spermatogenesis. In: Knobil E, Neill JD (eds) Encyclopedia of reproduction, vol. 4. Academic Press, San Diego, pp 546–556

Haidl G, Weidner W (2002) Epididymitis and orchitis – clinical and andrological implications. Reproduktionsmedizin 18: 61–65

Mortimer D (1999) Structured management for male factor infertility. In: Gagon C (ed) The male gamete: from basic knowledge to clinical applications. Cache River, Vienna, IL

Purvis K, Christiansen E (1995) Infection in the male reproductive tract. Impact, diagnosis and treatment in relation to male infertility. Int J Androl 16:1–13

Rowe PJ, Comhaire FH, Hargreave TB, Mahmoud AMA (2000) WHO Manual for the standardized investigation, diagnosis and management of the infertile male. Cambridge University Press, Cambridge, pp 10–11

Schlehofer JR (2003) Virus infections in disorders of the male reproductive system. Andrologia 35:157–159

Schuppe HC, Neumann NJ, Scheffzyk A, Schock-Skasa G, Hofmann N, Schill WB (2001) Inflammatory reactions in testicular biopsies of infertile men. Andrologia 33: 327–328

Tung KS, Teuscher C (1995) Mechanisms of autoimmune disease in the testis and ovary. Hum Reprod Update 1:35–50

Weidner W, Krause W (1999) Orchitis. In: Knobil E, Neill JD (eds) Encyclopedia of reproduction, vol. 3. Academic Press, San Diego, pp 92–95

Weidner W, Krause W, Ludwig M (1999) Relevance of male accessory gland infection for subsequent fertility with special focus on prostatitis. Hum Reprod Update 5:421–432

I.3.12 Cause: Varicocele

F. Comhaire, A. Mahmoud

Key Messages

- Reflux of blood in the internal spermatic vein(s) causes testicular and epididymal malfunction as a result of clinically palpable or subclinical varicocele.
- Varicocele is the most common cause of male infertility.
- The presence of varicocele must be detected in all patients with abnormal semen quality, including azoospermia.
- Palpation may fail to detect spermatic venous reflux, and contact thermography is the most accurate diagnostic technique, complemented by duplex Doppler ultrasonography.
- Interruption of reflux by retrograde transcatheter embolization or surgery must be complete, including right-sided reflux, which results in improvement of semen quality in 70% to 80% of cases.
- The natural conception rate after varicocele treatment is three- to fourfold higher than in untreated couples, and is enhanced by a holistic management of both female and male partners.

I.3.12.1 Definition

Varicocele, either palpable or subclinical, must be associated with abnormal spermatozoa in order to be accepted as a cause of infertility (Rowe et al. 2000). If a man with varicocele has normal semen analysis, the varicocele is not considered to be the cause of infertility and, obviously, treating this condition will not change his fertilizing potential. Clinical varicocele is defined as the presence of distension of the intrascrotal veins of the plexus pampiniformis, which is either a visible bulging of the scrotal skin, or easily palpable, or palpable during Valsalva manoeuvre only. Subclinical varicocele cannot be palpated, but is detected by means of technical investigations.

I.3.12.2 Aetiology and Pathogenesis

Varicocele develops as a result of impaired venous efflux from the testis (Tulloch 1952). Venous blood refluxes in the internal spermatic vein due to the absence or malfunction of valves. The refluxing blood commonly originates from the renal vein, but may derive from the peri-renal plexus through reno-spermatic bypasses. The blood contains vasoactive substances including catecholamines (Comhaire and Vermeulen 1974), causing constriction of the testicular arterioles after venoarterial counter-current exchange at the level of the pampiniform plexus. Also, accumulation of toxic substances and oxidants occurs. Inadequate function of the valves in (the lower part) of the internal spermatic vein causes increased hydrostatic pressure in the testicular venules (Shafik and Bedeir 1980), exceeding the pressure in the arterial capillaries and reducing testicular perfusion.

Varicoceles occur more commonly at the left side for anatomical reasons (Ahlberg et al. 1965), but increased hydrostatic pressure and reflux may be present on the right side as well (Comhaire et al. 1981; Gat et al. 2004).

Varicocele usually becomes evident during puberty (Steeno et al. 1976). It impairs Sertoli cell function and histology (Terquem and Dadoune 1981), with decreased support of spermatogenesis. Maturation of spermatogenic cells is impaired with decreased production of mature spermatozoa and oligozoospermia, and increased sloughing of spermatogenic cells that appear in the ejaculate as peroxidase negative round cells. Leydig cell function and histology is altered as well, with lowered testosterone production (Comhaire and Vermeulen 1975).

I.3.12.3 Clinical Findings, Technical Investigations and Laboratory Findings

In general, patients suffering from varicocele report few or no symptoms. Sometimes they may have noticed some dull feeling within the scrotum, particularly upon physical exertion. Varicocele may have been detected during school examination, but left untreated.

Physical examination should be performed in a room where the temperature is 20–22°C. The patient should stand undressed for approximately 5 min before being examined. At lower temperatures, the scrotum may retract, making palpation difficult. The patient should be standing up while the scrotum is inspected and palpated. Palpation must be performed gently in order not to provoke pain, and attention must be paid to the risk of syncope.

Varicoceles are graded into:

- Grade III: When the distended venous plexus bulges visibly through the scrotal skin and is easily palpable
- Grade II: When the intrascrotal venous distension is easily palpable but not visible

Grade III and II are usually considered as large varicoceles

- Grade I: When there is no visible or palpable distension except when the man performs the Valsalva manoeuvre
- Subclinical: Where there is no clinical varicocele but an abnormality is present upon scrotal thermography or duplex Doppler ultrasonography

Commonly, testicular volume is lower (WHO 1992) at the side of the varicocele and/or the consistency is softer. Sometimes the epididymis at the side of the varicocele is thicker and slightly more sensitive upon palpation.

Thermography of the scrotal skin can be performed by means of a tele-thermographic equipment or infrared camera (Comhaire et al. 1976). The investigation is done with the man standing up. The easiest method is through contact thermography using a specially designed flexible strip containing thermosensitive liquid crystals (WHO 1985). The crystals change colour, reflecting the temperature of the underlying skin. In normal men, the temperature of the scrotal skin does not exceed 33.5°C (Zorgniotti and Macleod 1973). Any clear asymmetrical, in case of unilateral varicocele, or symmetrical temperature increase must be recorded. In case of normal thermography, the probability of a varicocele is small.

Doppler investigations include ultrasonography or, in centres having access to the suitable apparatus, duplex Doppler. The test is performed with the man in recumbent position. The testicular artery is located in the pampiniform plexus and the patient is then requested to perform the Valsalva manoeuvre. Normally, venous efflux is increased and arterial pulsations may decrease, but no reflux of blood should occur. In case of malfunction or absence of valves on the internal spermatic vein, reflux is recorded.

Echography is not the best method to detect varicocele since distension of the veins of the pampiniform plexus may not occur in cases with grade I and subclinical varicocele, which may be overlooked by this technique.

Semen analysis reveals oligozoospermia, usually with poor sperm motility (asthenozoospermia) and a subnormal proportion of spermatozoa with normal morphology (teratozoospermia). Typically, the sperm heads tend to be elongated (tapering or leptoform heads) and the mid-piece may be broadened because of the presence of a cytoplasmic droplet. The number of round cells may be increased as a result of premature release (sloughing) of spermatogenic cells (Macleod 1965). These stain negative for peroxidase, contrary to the peroxidase-positive white blood cells. Some patients with grade I or subclinical varicoceles present a high ejaculate volume (>6 ml), which is a suggestive finding. If the ejaculate volume is below normal, this may indicate concurrent infection and deficient secretion of the accessory sex glands.

Blood analysis may reveal a relatively low testosterone concentration corresponding with impaired secretion by the cells of Leydig. An elevated serum FSH level indicates severely deficient Sertoli cell function.

I.3.12.4 Differential Diagnosis

An untrained investigator may confuse an enlarged epididymis with an expanded intrascrotal vein. Whereas the swollen epididymis will not change when the patient is recumbent, the expanded vein will collapse. With regard to the differential diagnosis, in case of increased temperature registered by thermography, inflammation of the skin or the underlying epididymis should be excluded.

I.3.12.5 Treatment

Men with varicocele but normal semen analysis should not be treated since the male factor is probably not the cause of the infertility. In fact, this has been confirmed empirically with no increase in the pregnancy rate in such couples. There is ample and reliable scientific evidence that correct treatment of men with varicocele and abnormal semen quality improves the sperm characteristics and fertilizing potential, as well as the spontaneous pregnancy rate (Dubin and Amelar 1975; Madgar et al. 1995; Hargreave and Ghosh 1998). Treatment must interrupt the reflux of blood in the internal spermatic vein and its collaterals, and should be performed bilaterally if reflux is present at both sides. Surgical treatment preferentially uses the supra-inguinal approach (Ivanissevich 1960), or can be done through laparoscopy (Kattan 2001; Sautter et al. 2002), or by means of microsurgical techniques at the neck of the scrotum (Marmar et al. 1985). Surgery must avoid damaging the testicular artery, but it may be complicated by hydrocele, requiring a second intervention.

The preferred method uses interventional radiology through the Seldinger approach. Retrograde venography from the renal veins visualizes the path of reflux and permits assessment of the internal spermatic veins of both sides. Subsequently embolization with tissue adhesive is performed through super-selective catheterization (Kunnen 1982).

Although much promoted by some authors (Tauber and Johnsen 1994; Mazzoni et al. 2002), ascending venography and venous sclerosis is not the method of first choice, because it does not follow the path of reflux, it has a relatively high complication rate (Ficarra et al. 2002) and is applied to one side only.

Concomitant pathology, such as accessory gland infection or hypoandrogenism must always be treated at the same time, and recovery of the fertilizing potential of sperm may be accelerated by the administration of a food supplement. Intrauterine insemination or, if needed, IVF/ICSI may be used if spontaneous conception fails to occur within a reasonable period of time.

I.3.12.6 Results of Treatment

In retrospective and prospective cohort studies and in treated cases of randomized trials, between 35% and 40% of couples attain spontaneous pregnancy within 12 months after treatment, and between 60% and 75% within 2 years (Madgar et al. 1995). This pregnancy rate is about three times higher than that observed in untreated controls. Meta-analysis of published randomized trials fails to reach significance in favour of treatment (Evers and Collins 2004), but the cases included are highly variable, yielding extremely variable pregnancy rates in controls. In certain studies, men with normal semen quality have been included, and the technical accuracy of surgical treatment can be questioned in some trials, with unexpectedly low pregnancy rates among treated cases (Comhaire and Mahmoud 2004).

I.3.12.7 Prognosis

Varicocele develops at pubertal age (Steeno et al. 1976). If left untreated, the degree of testicular impairment increases with the longer duration of the disease, explaining why varicocele is the most common abnormality found in couples with secondary infertility. Also, testosterone production is known to decline more rapidly in ageing men with than in those without varicocele (Comhaire and Vermeulen 1975). This may induce premature andropause and sexual dysfunction.

Several factors have been identified that determine the success rate in terms of probability of natural conception after treatment (Comhaire and Kunnen 1985). Patients with subclinical or grade I varicoceles and low total testicular volume of less than 30 ml have a relatively poor prognosis after treatment. In such patients, other factors may be involved in testicular impairment, including a genetic defect or a congenital factor. Men combining varicocele with normal total testicular volume (30 ml or more) and a serum FSH level below the median for a normal population have a high chance of full recovery of fertility and successful natural conception of up to 80% within 1 year after treatment. In cases with large varicoceles and testicular volume lower than 30 ml, and in cases with normal testicular volume and serum FSH level above median, the probability of attaining successful pregnancy is between 30% and 40%.

Concurrent pathology affecting the epididymis or an immunological factor decreases the probability of conception.

I.3.12.8 Prevention

Generally speaking, varicocele becomes manifest during puberty, and it has been suggested that treatment should be performed at that time. This would prevent the disease from causing serious and sometimes irreversible testicular damage later in life (Sayfan et al. 1997).

The decision whether or not to perform preventive treatment of varicocele in adolescents will largely depend on the risk/benefit ratio of the treatment. Clearly the benefit of any correct treatment is similar. The risk, the level of invasiveness and the cost of retrograde venography and transcatheter embolization are lower, since this treatment is performed under local anaesthesia and on an out-patient basis. Therefore, the benefit may exceed the risk, and preventive treatment seems justifiable.

I.3.12.9 Other

It must be underscored that the detection and correct treatment of varicocele is indicated in all infertile patients with abnormal semen quality. Not to do so is in conflict with the rules of good medical practice. However, it is mandatory to search and treat complementary causes of infertility, or factors exerting a negative effect, including lifestyle factors. This fits in the concept of the holistic approach of the infertile male.

References

Ahlberg NE, Bartley O, Chidekel N (1965) Retrograde contrast filling of the left gonadal vein. Acta Radiol Diagn 3:385–392

Comhaire FH, Kunnen M (1985) Factors affecting the probability of conception after treatment of subfertile men with varicocele by transcatheter embolization with Bucrylate. Fertil Steril 43:781–786

Comhaire FH, Mahmoud AM (2004) Editorial commentary. J Androl 25:771–772

Comhaire F, Vermeulen A (1974) Varicocele sterility: cortisol and catecholamines. Fertil Steril 25:88–95

Comhaire F, Vermeulen A (1975) Plasma testosterone in patients with varicocele and sexual inadequacy. J Clin Endocrinol Metab 40:824–829

Comhaire F, Monteyne R, Kunnen M (1976) The value of scrotal thermography as compared with selective retrograde venography of the internal spermatic vein for the diagnosis of "subclinical" varicocele. Fertil Steril 27:694–698

Comhaire F, Kunnen M, Nahoum C (1981) Radiological anatomy of the internal spermatic vein(s) in 200 retrograde venograms. Int J Androl 4:379–387

Dubin L, Amelar RD (1975) Varicocelectomy as therapy in male infertility: a study of 504 cases. Fertil Steril 26:217–220

Evers J, Collins J (2004) Surgery or embolisation for varicocele in subfertile men. Cochrane Database Syst Rev 3:CD000479

Ficarra V, Porcaro AB, Righetti R, Cerruto MA, Pilloni S, Cavalleri S, Malossini G, Artibani W (2002) Antegrade scrotal sclerotherapy in the treatment of varicocele: a prospective study. BJU Int 89:264–268

Gat Y, Bachar GN, Zukerman Z, Belenky A, Gornish M (2004) Varicocele: a bilateral disease. Fertil Steril 81:424–429

Hargreave T, Ghosh C (1998) Varicocele: does treatment promote male fertility? Urologe A 37:258–264

Ivanissevich O (1960) Left varicocele due to reflux; experience with 4,470 operative cases in forty-two years. J Int Coll Surg 34:742–755

Kattan S (2001) The impact of internal spermatic artery ligation during laparoscopic varicocelectomy on recurrence rate and short post operative outcome. Scand J Urol Nephrol 35:218–221

Kunnen M (1982) Nonsurgical cure of varicocele by transcatheter embolization of the internal spermatic vein with bucrylate. In: Jecht EW, Zeitler E (eds) Varicocele and male fertility. Recent advances in diagnosis and therapy. Springer, Berlin Heidelberg New York, pp 153–161

Macleod J (1965) Seminal cytology in the presence of varicocele. Fertil Steril 16:735–757

Madgar I, Weissenberg R, Lunenfeld B, Karasik A, Goldwasser B (1995) Controlled trial of high spermatic vein ligation for varicocele in infertile men. Fertil Steril 63:120–124

Marmar JL, DeBenedictis TJ, Praiss D (1985) The management of varicoceles by microdissection of the spermatic cord at the external inguinal ring. Fertil Steril 43:583–588

Mazzoni G, Minucci S, Gentile V (2002) Recurrent varicocele: role of antegrade sclerotherapy as first choice treatment. Eur Urol 41:614–618

Rowe PJ, Comhaire FH, Hargreave TB, Mahmoud AMA (2000) WHO manual for the standardized investigation, diagnosis and management of the infertile male. Cambridge University Press, Cambridge

Sautter T, Sulser T, Suter S, Gretener H, Hauri D (2002) Treatment of varicocele: a prospective randomized comparison of laparoscopy versus antegrade sclerotherapy. Eur Urol 41:398–400

Sayfan J, Siplovich L, Koltun L, Benyamin N (1997) Varicocele treatment in pubertal boys prevents testicular growth arrest. J Urol 157:1456–1457

Shafik A, Bedeir GA (1980) Venous tension patterns in cord veins. I. In normal and varicocele individuals. J Urol 123:383–385

Steeno O, Knops J, Declerck L, Adimoelja A, Van de Voorede H (1976) Prevention of fertility disorders by detection and treatment of varicocele at school and college age. Andrologia 8:47–53

Tauber R, Johnsen N (1994) Antegrade scrotal sclerotherapy for the treatment of varicocele: technique and late results. J Urol 151:386–390

Terquem A, Dadoune JP (1981) Morphological findings in varicocele: an ultrastructural study of 30 bilateral testicular biopsies. Int J Androl 4:515–531

Tulloch WS (1952) A consideration of sterility factors in the light of subsequent pregnancies: subfertility in the male. Trans Edinb Obstet Soc 52:29–34

WHO (1985) Comparison among different methods for the diagnosis of varicocele. Fertil Steril 43:575–582

WHO (1992) The influence of varicocele on parameters of fertility in a large group of men presenting to infertility clinics. Fertil Steril 57:1289–1293

Zorgniotti AW, Macleod J (1973) Studies in temperature, human semen quality, and varicocele. Fertil Steril 24:854–863

I.3.13 Infection/Inflammation of the Accessory Sex Glands

F. Comhaire, A. Mahmoud

Key Messages

- Infection of the accessory sex glands is diagnosed in a variable proportion of cases with abnormal semen quality depending on regional differences.
- The influence of infection/inflammation of the epididymis on semen quality and fertility is more important than that of infection/inflammation of the prostate or seminal vesicles.
- Whereas bacteria themselves have little influence on the fertilizing capacity of spermatozoa, changes in the function of the affected glands and reactive oxygen species generated by white blood cells damage spermatozoa.
- The diagnosis of male accessory sex gland infection is based on a combination of elements in the patient's history, clinical signs, and biological analysis of urine and semen.
- Treatment uses antibiotics and antioxidants, complemented with intrauterine insemination and/or assisted reproduction, depending on the severity and reversibility or irreversibility of damage to sperm cells.

I.3.13.1 Definition

The diagnosis of male accessory gland infection is given when semen classification is azoospermia or abnormal spermatozoa and this is considered to result from present or past infection of the accessory sex glands, or inflammatory disease of the urogenital tract (Rowe et al. 2000).

I.3.13.2 Aetiology and Physiopathology

Infection of the accessory sex glands includes epididymitis, vesiculitis and/or prostatitis, which are caused by either pathogens transmitted by sexual contact or by so-called trivial urological pathogens. Among the former, *Chlamydia trachomatis* is the most common pathogen (Keck et al. 1998), but gonococcus may also occur. The urological pathogens commonly identified are *Escherichia coli*, *Streptococcus faecalis*, *Proteus mirabilis* and pseudomonas. The role of coagulase-negative staphylococcus is uncertain, while *Staphylococcus aureus* is usually a laboratory contaminant (Rodin et al. 2003).

Infection causes inflammation characterized by the classical symptoms such as pain, swelling, and impaired function. The latter is responsible for deficient secretion of minerals, enzymes and fluids that are needed for optimal function and transport of the spermatozoa. The abnormal biochemical make-up of the seminal plasma results in decreased seminal volume, abnormal viscosity and liquefaction, abnormal pH, and impaired functional capacity of the spermatozoa. These are commonly poorly motile and may have antisperm antibodies attached of the IgG and/or IgA class, causing immunological infertility.

In addition, infection or inflammation increase the number of peroxidase-positive white blood cells (pus cells) generating reactive oxygen species that change the lipid composition of the sperm membrane, reducing its fluidity and fusogenic capacity with impaired acrosome reactivity and ability to fuse with the oolemma (Comhaire et al. 1999). Reactive oxygen species induce oxidative damage to sperm DNA, with excessive production of a.o. 8-hydroxy-2-deoxyguanosin and mutagenesis (Chen et al. 1997). Also, inflammation increases the production of a number of cytokines such as interleukin 1 (alpha and beta), interleukin 6 and 8, and tumour necrosis factor, which further impair sperm function and fertilizing capacity (Depuydt et al. 1996; Gruschwitz et al. 1996).

Chronic inflammation of the epididymis may result in (partial) obstruction of the sperm passage with oligo- or azoospermia (Dohle et al. 2003). Rupture of the blood-testis barrier from obstruction causes antisperm antibodies (Hendry 1986).

I.3.13.3 Clinical and Laboratory Findings

History taking commonly reveals one or several episodes of dysuria and/or pollakisuria, which may have disappeared spontaneously or after a short treatment with an antibiotic or urinary antiseptic. However, the patient may be unaware of any acute urinary symptoms in the past. Sometimes, the patient mentions recurrent episodes of intrascrotal pain that usually feels rather dull and is exacerbated by pressure. Ejaculatory symptoms may occur such as reduced ejaculation force or volume, painful sensation during or immediately after ejaculation, or blood staining of the ejaculate. Finally, sexual complaints may be mentioned, including decreased libido and orgasmic feeling, or even erectile dysfunction.

Clinical examination should focus on the careful palpation of the scrotal content, particularly the epididymis and vas deferens. Any swelling or nodularity should be noted, as well as pain during soft pressure. Rectal examination can be performed, but transrectal or transabdominal echography may reveal more relevant information.

General blood analysis may reveal signs of infection, such as increased number of white blood cells, increased sedimentation rate or abnormal globulin proportions upon electrophoresis. Specific tests for circulating antibodies against *Chlamydia* should be included in the routine investigation for male infertility. The laboratory may detect antisperm antibodies of the IgG class in serum.

Urine analysis may reveal bacterial infection or an increased number of white blood cells, but the analysis of urine obtained after prostate massage should be more relevant. However, the absence of urinary abnormality does not exclude male accessory gland infection, particularly epididymitis.

Semen analysis is of pivotal importance to the diagnosis. Semen must be collected as described in the section on semen analysis, in order to avoid contamination with cells and bacteria from the skin or urethra. When semen culture is performed for the counting and identification of bacteria, preparatory dilution of the sample is required, reducing the bacteriostatic capacity of seminal plasma, prostate fluid in particular. The number of round cells must be counted, and these must be differentiated into peroxidase-negative cells, mostly spermatogenetic cells, and peroxidase-positive white blood cells (WHO 1999). Also, it is mandatory to perform biochemical analysis of the seminal plasma in order to measure the markers of secretion of the sex glands, including, for example, alpha-glucosidase for the epididymides, citric acid or gamma glutamyl transferase (or calcium or zinc) for the prostate, and, possibly, fructose for the seminal vesicles.

Finally, the presence of antisperm antibodies on spermatozoa must be traced by means of, for example, the direct MAR test for both IgG and IgA (WHO 1999).

I.3.13.4 Diagnosis and Differential Diagnosis

The diagnosis is accepted in patients with abnormal semen quality – oligo- and/or asteno- and/or teratozoospermia, or azoospermia – who combine abnormalities under the following headings (Comhaire et al. 1980; Rowe et al. 2000):

A. A history of urinary infection, epididymitis, sexually transmitted disease, and/or physical signs: thickened or tender epididymis, thickened vas deferens, abnormal rectal examination
B. Abnormal urine after prostatic massage and/or detection of *Chlamydia trachomatis* in urine
C. Ejaculate abnormalities:
   - Elevated number of peroxidase-positive white blood cells
   - Culture with significant growth of pathogenic bacteria
   - Abnormal viscosity and/or abnormal biochemical composition, and/or high levels of inflammatory markers or highly elevated reactive oxygen species

The diagnosis requires either two signs from different headings, or at least two ejaculate signs in each of two subsequent semen samples. If bacteria are detected, they should be identical in urine and in semen, or in the two semen samples.

Male accessory sex gland infection may be combined with other diseases such as varicocele, in which case a lower number of white blood cells may cause complementary damage (Everaert et al. 2003), or an immunological factor, or sexual or ejaculatory dysfunction. These diseases will require adequate management and may interfere with the fertility outcome after treatment of the infection.

I.3.13.5 Treatment

The treatment of the infection should be the same as for urinary tract infections. However, abnormal secretion of the prostate results in an alkaline environment in this gland, by which antibiotics such as doxycycline are not concentrated and are therefore inefficient. The third-generation quinolones (e.g. ofloxacin and pefloxacin) are concentrated in both an alkaline and acidic milieu, and therefore do penetrate well into the diseased prostate and the seminal vesicles (Comhaire 1987). In case of streptococcus infection, the quinolones are poorly active, and treatment with amoxicillin or cephalosporins may be indicated.

Commonly, bacterial infestation is eradicated, but it may return, sometimes with a different pathogen. It may be necessary to add a second, longer-term treatment with another antibiotic.

I.3.13.6 Results of Treatment

Whereas bacteria can usually be eliminated from the genitourinary region, white blood cells may persist for several months, and functional impairment of the accessory glands is commonly irreversible. This implies that the processes impairing the fertilizing capacity of spermatozoa remain active, and that fertility is not restored. Complementary treatment with food supplements containing antioxidants may be required, and treatment similar to that of idiopathic oligozoospermia can be indicated.

In general, the success rate of antibiotic treatment of male accessory gland infection in terms of spontaneous conception is poor and not significantly better than that of placebo. Treatment aiming at the elimination of pathogens is, however, indicated for reasons of good medical practice, and in order to reduce the risk of future complications, including prostate cancer (Roberts et al. 2004).

Because oxygen damage to the sperm membrane and, most of all, DNA may persist after antibiotic treatment, intrauterine insemination and in vitro fertilization may yield poor results, and intracytoplasmic sperm injection, though generating pre-embryos, may fail in creating an ongoing pregnancy (Zorn et al. 2004). Therefore, careful complementary treatment and a holistic approach are indicated.

I.3.13.7 Prognosis

Depending on the localization of the infection or inflammation, the prognosis after treatment is variable. Whereas the effects of prostatitis and vesiculitis are less important, and the effect of treatment on fertility is rather favourable, (chronic) epididymitis usually causes substantial and irreversible damage to the quality and the fertilizing capacity of spermatozoa (Vicari 2000). Also, immunological infertility, resulting from rupture of the blood–testis barrier, is irreversible.

In view of the poor prognosis regarding the repair of fertility, prevention of infectious disease is of primordial importance.

I.3.13.8 Prevention

On the one hand, prevention of sexually transmitted disease, and its immediate treatment in positive cases, will prevent infertility in a later stage. In particular, recurrent infections with *Chlamydia* were documented to cause disastrous effects that are irreversible (Gonzales et al. 2004).

Men who smoke run a four- to fivefold higher risk of prostatitis and subsequent spread of infection to the other accessory sex glands. In addition, tobacco smoke generates surplus amounts of oxygen radicals and toxic damage to spermatozoa. Avoiding tobacco is, therefore, the most important factor in the prevention of male accessory gland infection by common urological pathogens. In addition, relatively symptom-poor episodes of urinary infection, e.g. occurring after an episode of diarrhoea, may remain untreated and ultimately develop into chronic infection/inflammation that is hard to treat, let alone cure. Therefore, any episode of urinary complaints suggestive for infection in the male must be treated adequately, in particular using quinolones, in order to avoid pathogens being harboured in the prostate gland.

References

Chen CS, Chao HT, Pan RL, Wei YH (1997) Hydroxyl radical-induced decline in motility and increase in lipid peroxidation and DNA modification in human sperm. Biochem Mol Biol Int 43:291–303

Comhaire FH (1987) Concentration of pefloxacin in split ejaculates of patients with chronic male accessory gland infection. J Urol 138:828–830

Comhaire F, Verschraegen G, Vermeulen L (1980) Diagnosis of accessory gland infection and its possible role in male infertility. Int J Androl 3:32–45

Comhaire FH, Mahmoud AM, Depuydt CE, Zalata AA, Christophe AB (1999) Mechanisms and effects of male genital tract infection on sperm quality and fertilizing potential: the andrologist's viewpoint. Hum Reprod Update 5:393–398

Depuydt CE, Bosmans E, Zalata A, Schoonjans F, Comhaire FH (1996) The relation between reactive oxygen species and cytokines in andrological patients with or without male accessory gland infection. J Androl 17:699–707

Dohle GR, van Roijen JH, Pierik FH, Vreeburg JT, Weber RF (2003) Subtotal obstruction of the male reproductive tract. Urol Res 31:22–24

Everaert K, Mahmoud A, Depuydt C, Maeyaert M, Comhaire F (2003) Chronic prostatitis and male accessory gland infection–is there an impact on male infertility (diagnosis and therapy)? Andrologia 35:325–330

Gonzales GF, Munoz G, Sanchez R, Henkel R, Gallegos-Avila G, Diaz-Gutierrez O, Vigil P, Vasquez F, Kortebani G, Mazzolli A, Bustos-Obregon E (2004) Update on the impact of Chlamydia trachomatis infection on male fertility. Andrologia 36:1–23

Gruschwitz MS, Brezinschek R, Brezinschek HP (1996) Cytokine levels in the seminal plasma of infertile males. J Androl 17:158–163

Hendry WF (1986) Clinical significance of unilateral testicular obstruction in subfertile males. Br J Urol 58:709–714

Keck C, Gerber-Schafer C, Clad A, Wilhelm C, Breckwoldt M (1998) Seminal tract infections: impact on male fertility and treatment options. Hum Reprod Update 4:891–903

Roberts RO, Bergstralh EJ, Bass SE, Lieber MM, Jacobsen SJ (2004) Prostatitis as a risk factor for prostate cancer. Epidemiology 15:93–99

Rodin DM, Larone D, Goldstein M (2003) Relationship between semen cultures, leukospermia, and semen analysis in men undergoing fertility evaluation. Fertil Steril 79 Suppl 3:1555–1558

Rowe PJ, Comhaire FH, Hargreave TB, Mahmoud AMA (2000) WHO manual for the standardized investigation, diagnosis and management of the infertile male. Cambridge University Press, Cambridge

Vicari E (2000) Effectiveness and limits of antimicrobial treatment on seminal leukocyte concentration and related reactive oxygen species production in patients with male accessory gland infection. Hum Reprod 15:2536–2544

WHO (1999) WHO laboratory manual of the examination of human semen and sperm-cervical mucus interaction. Cambridge University Press, Cambridge

Zorn B, Virant-Klun I, Vidmar G, Sesek-Briski A, Kolbezen M, Meden-Vrtovec H (2004) Seminal elastase-inhibitor complex, a marker of genital tract inflammation, and negative IVF outcome measures: role for a silent inflammation? Int J Androl 27:368–374

I.3.14 Endocrine Factors

R. Weber

Key Messages

- Male subfertility is rarely caused by endocrine diseases.
- Although hormone determination for classification of male infertility is rarely needed, follicle-stimulating hormone (FSH) and inhibin B can be considered useful markers of spermatogenesis.
- Plasma testosterone concentration needs to be measured in men with clinical signs of hypoandrogenism, but can be subnormal in men with male infertility without any clinical signs or symptoms.
- Testosterone measurement is also indicated in men combining abnormal semen quality with erectile dysfunction.
- High serum concentration of FSH (and luteinizing hormone, LH) in combination with subnormal serum testosterone concentration indicate primary (testicular) hypogonadism.
- Subnormal serum concentration of FSH, LH and testosterone is characteristic for hypogonadotrophic hypogonadism (secondary hypogonadism).
- Hypogonadotrophic hypogonadism and male subfertility is treated with gonadotrophins or pulsatile gonadotrophin-releasing hormone (GnRH, hypothalamic disorder).
- Persistent hypogonadism demands lifelong androgen substitution.
- Hyperprolactinaemia is a possible cause of hypogonadism.

I.3.14.1 Definition

The hypothalamus–pituitary–testis (HPT) axis is the most important endocrine system in the human male. High activity of the HPT axis is noticed during foetal life when the testis is developed, during the first 6 months after birth and during puberty. In adulthood, the serum gonadotrophins, testosterone and inhibin B, secreted in a pulsatile way, reflect testis function, and especially FSH and inhibin B are useful markers for spermatogenesis (Pierik 1998; 2003). Although a normal function of the HPT axis is mandatory for normal testosterone production and spermatogenesis, endocrine diseases of the axis that cause subnormal function of the testis are rare. Known endocrine causes of male subfertility comprise hypo- and hypergonadotrophic hypogonadism. The incidence rate of these endocrine problems, however, is highly dependent on the nature of specialization of the institute that a patient is attending. In a survey of 1,549 subfertile men referred to our institute, hypogonadotrophic hypogonadism (HH) was diagnosed in 3.4% of the men. Other diseases of the endocrine system such as prolactin (PRL) secreting pituitary adenomas, hyper- and hypothyroidism, hypercorticism (Cushing's disease and syndrome) may have a negative effect on the HPT axis, but infertility is seldom the presenting symptom of these diseases.

There are hardly any effects of diabetes mellitus on the HPT axis. However, the vascular and neurological complications, causing erectile and/or ejaculatory dysfunction, may contribute considerably to the reproductive capability of a diabetic man.

Medical practitioners should be aware of the (ab)use of anabolic steroids, which are used in doses 10–100 times the normal therapeutic dose to enhance performance in competitive sports (Chap. II.4.3f). The use of anabolic steroids may cause small testes, abnormal sperm parameters and infertility. In the biology of these cases, the levels of LH (and FSH) are commonly low due to suppression of the HPT. The effects of endocrine disruptors on testicular development during foetal life and eventually subnormal sperm parameters have not yet been elucidated (Weber 2002) (see Chap. II.2.3). Also, exposure to endocrine disruptors during adulthood may cause male subfertility, and evidence is increasing that endocrine disruptors may have a deleterious effect on male reproductive functions.

Recognition of HH is mandatory in infertile patients, since this diagnosis offers a rationale for treatment.

I.3.14.2 Aetiology and Pathogenesis

Kallmann syndrome (KS) is a genetic condition characterized by HH, due to disturbed hypothalamic secretion of GnRH, and anosmia (Seminara 1998; Hu 2003). Anosmia should be revealed by history taking, and confirmed (preferentially) by specific test(s). KS affects about 1 in 8,000 males. Although KS is considered as an inherited disease, familial cases of the disease are infrequent. However, the identification of the gene underlying the X-chromosome-linked form of the disease (KAL-1) has opened the way to molecular pathophysiology. During normal embryonic development, GnRH neurones migrate from the nasal olfactory epithelium to the basal hypothalamus. This migration is disturbed in embryos with X-linked KS.

HH can also be idiopathic (IHH) and is associated with impaired GnRH secretion.

Craniopharyngiomas, meningiomas and metastases of other tumours into the region of the hypothalamus can cause GnRH deficiency. Likewise, sarcoidosis, histiocytosis, tuberculosis, and haemochromatosis may cause GnRH deficiency. Finally, fractures of the base of the skull, ischaemic and haemorrhagic lesions, as well as radiotherapy can cause impairment of hypothalamic function or interrupt the hypothalamo-pituitary connection by stalk section.

HH may also be due to endocrine active and inactive adenomas of the pituitary gland; granulomatous illnesses, vascular diseases, irradiation, and trauma can have the same effect.

The principle of anabolics is based on suppression of GnRH, LH and FSH and subsequent testicular testosterone production. The circulating testosterone concentration is about 20- to 100-fold lower than the testosterone content of the seminiferous tubules. A substantial decrease of intratesticular testosterone concentration during anabolic use can impair spermatogenesis and fertility.

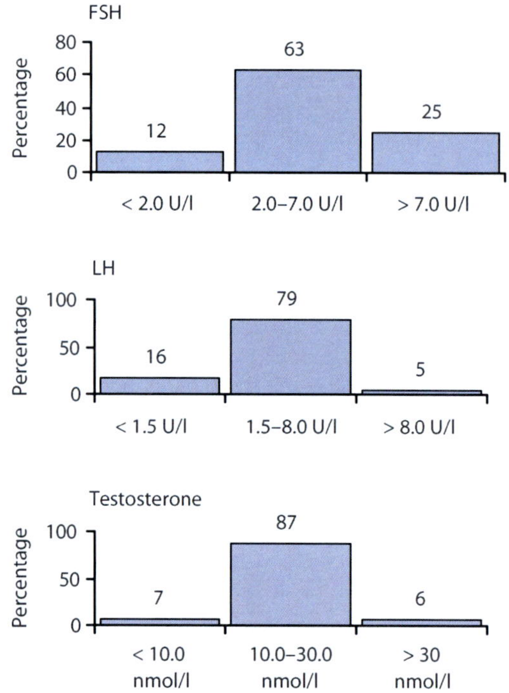

Fig. I.3.11. Percentage of 1379 subfertile men presenting with subnormal (*left bar*), normal (*middle bar*) and supranormal (*right bar*) serum concentrations of follicle-stimulating hormone (*FSH*), luteinizing hormone (*LH*) and testosterone

I.3.14.3 Clinical Findings

In order to recognize the commonly subtle symptoms of hypogonadism of infertile men, meticulous history taking plus a careful physical examination provide important clues to the origin of the problem(s). The patients may sometimes report sexual or ejaculatory dysfunction. However, when symptoms of hypogonadism are absent, additional laboratory testing is necessary. KS and IHH patients have subnormal levels of LH, FSH and testosterone. The response of LH and FSH during stimulation with GnRH can be blunted, but becomes normal after "priming" of the patient with testosterone. The response remains blunted in case of a disease of the pituitary gland (e.g. pituitary adenoma).

Most of the other diseases of the hypothalamus and/or pituitary gland, leading to HH, are not primarily diagnosed in an infertility clinic. The incidence of hyperprolactinaemia due to a micro- or macroadenoma of the pituitary gland is less than 1% of men presenting with fertility problems. Microprolactinomas and subsequently increased serum PRL concentrations are not always associated with HH. A macroprolactinoma and high concentrations of PRL not only induce HH but also impair the pituitary-thyroidal and pituitary-adrenal axes. These might not be due to the high PRL concentrations, but rather result from loss of pituitary tissue because of compression by the pituitary tumour.

Since infertility (or erectile dysfunction) is, in the majority of cases, the only reason to request medical help, it must be realized that a considerable number of these men have, besides abnormal sperm parameters, unexplained subnormal serum concentrations of LH, FSH and testosterone (Fig. I.3.11).

Supra-normal concentrations of LH and FSH (hypergonadotropism) obviously reflect a testicular disorder, but the majority of infertile men have normal serum gonadotrophins and testosterone in spite of an abnormal sperm analysis. Although the importance of hormone determinations in men with idiopathic infertility is not fully documented, it may add to a better diagnostic classification. The combination of the concentrations of inhibin B and FSH gives a reasonable insight into the level of spermatogenesis. On the other hand, testosterone and – to lesser degree – LH give a good estimate of Leydig cell function.

Routine measurement of PRL as part of the work-up of male infertility without any other symptom does not seem to be indicated. Hyperprolactinaemia can be caused by certain pituitary adenomas compressing the pituitary stalk, and this may be present in some patients with acromegaly. Further analysis of hyperprolactinaemia is always indicated, and treatment with dopamine agonists is highly efficient.

I.3.14.4 Treatment

The therapeutic approach for HH is treatment with gonadotrophins [human chorionic gonadotrophin/human menopausal gonadotrophin (hCG/hMG), FSH] or pulsatile application of GnRH. The latter uses a portable injection pump. Treatment with GnRH is useless in cases of disease of the pituitary gland.

Gonadotrophin treatment usually starts with injections of hCG, which stimulates the Leydig cell secretion of testosterone. Once the testosterone concentration in peripheral blood is normal, treatment with either pure urinary or recombinant FSH, or hMG is added to the hCG treatment. This treatment must be administered for several months and it may take up to 1 year before spermatogenesis reaches a reasonable level. In general, patients with "inborn" hypogonadotrophic hypogonadism do not attain a normal sperm concentration, but the fertilizing capacity of their semen seems to be rather good. Intrauterine insemination, or sometimes in vitro fertilization may be needed to attain pregnancy. In cases with acquired hypogonadotrophic hypogonadism, the treatment results are much better, probably because of a larger number of cells of Sertoli being present.

Once the goal of achieving fertility has been achieved, therapy has to be switched to androgen replacement. The benefit of lifelong androgen replacement therapy in case of subnormal serum testosterone concentrations in men with hypogonadotrophic hypogonadism has not yet been demonstrated, but seems to be rationalistic.

References

Hu Y, Tanriverdi F. MacColl GS, Bouloux PM (2003) Kallmann's syndrome: molecular pathogenesis. Int J Biochem Cell Biol 35:1157–1162

Pierik FH, Vreeburg JT, Stijnen T, De Jong, FH, Weber RFA (1998) Serum inhibin B as a marker of spermatogenesis. J Clin Endocrinol Metab 83:3110–3114

Pierik FH, Burdorf A, de Jong FH, Weber RFA (2003) Inhibin B: a novel markere of spermatogenesis. Ann Med 35:1–9

Seminara SB, Hayes FJ, Crowley WF Jr (1998) Gonadotropin-releasing hormone deficiency in the human (idiopathic hypogonadotropic hypogonadism and Kallmann's syndrome): pathophysiological and genetic considerations. Endocr Rev 19:521–539

Weber RFA, Pierik FH, Dohle GR, Burdorf A (2002) Environmental influences on male reproduction. BJU Int 89:143–148

I.3.15 Oligo-Astheno-Teratozoo-Spermia with No Demonstrable Cause (Idiopathic O-A-T)

F. Comhaire, A. Mahmoud

Key Messages

- In approximately one out of four cases with abnormal sperm quality and oligo- and/or astheno- and/or teratozoospermia, no causal factor can be identified.
- It is probable that a synergistic combination of internal and, mainly, external factors (lifestyle, nutrition, environment) are involved.
- In patients with idiopathic oligozoospermia and FSH that is not elevated, anti-oestrogen treatment with tamoxifen increases sperm concentration and enhances the probability of conception.
- A holistic approach of the multiple factors associated with idiopathically impaired sperm quality should be completed by nutriceutical food supplementation.
- After sperm quality has been optimized, intrauterine insemination, or – if need be – assisted reproduction, are indicated.

I.3.15.1 Definition of the Disease

The diagnosis of idiopathic oligozoospermia is given in men with normal sexual and ejaculatory function, with spermatozoa present in the ejaculate but sperm concentration lower than 20 million/ml, and in whom no other diagnosis is applicable. Idiopathic asthenozoospermia is accepted if sperm concentration is higher than 20 million/ml, but sperm motility is below the reference values, and no other diagnosis is applicable. Idiopathic teratozoospermia means that sperm concentration and motility are better than the reference values, but the proportion of spermatozoa with normal morphology is below the reference value (Rowe et al. 2000). Idiopathic cryptozoospermia is diagnosed in patients with extremely low sperm concentration, where no spermatozoa are seen in the fresh sample, but a few spermatozoa are recovered from the sediment after centrifugation, and none of the other diagnoses is applicable.

The term "idiopathic" may only be used if careful history taking, clinical examination and technical investigations have failed to detect any of the causal factors. It describes a condition diagnosed on the basis of exclusion criteria.

I.3.15.2 Aetiology and Pathogenesis

By definition, there is no known aetiological factor explaining the abnormal quality of the spermatozoa. Several hypotheses have been developed, some of which have been supported by indirect evidence. It has been postulated that some patients with idiopathic oligozoospermia may suffer from unexplained partial obstruction of sperm transport at the level of the epididymis (Jequier et al. 1983; Schoysman 1988, 1992). However, the majority of the latter patients have a history of accessory gland infection, or previous hernia repair, or cryptorchidism (Dohle et al. 2003). Also, partial obstruction has been associated with chronic sinopulmonary infections in so-called Young's syndrome (Handelsman et al. 1984). The latter has, however, no longer been reported in recent decades and seems to have disappeared spontaneously. Others have described partial obstruction in association with varicocele (Gerris et al. 1988; Belmonte and Martin 1998), but these cases must not be categorized as idiopathic. In addition, many patients with oligozoospermia related to partial obstruction present antisperm antibodies in serum, and they must be considered as suffering from immunological infertility.

In a certain number of cases, subobstruction of the epididymis has been certified by surgical exploration of the scrotal content (Gunnarsson and Olsson 1995; Hendry 1986; Schreiber et al. 1990). This type of intervention is not recommended in the work-up of cases with idiopathic oligozoospermia, because of its potential damaging effect, which may result in permanent azoospermia.

Other cases present abnormalities at the level of the rete testis that can be revealed by careful echography. Typically, the structures of the rete appear distended, possibly as a result of a defective embryonic development. In animal experiments, administering oestrogen-like substances during pregnancy can bring about this condition (Sharpe and Irvine 2004). Similarly, abnormal development of the rete and efferent ductules, causing oligo-, crypto- or azoospermia in the human male may be due to prenatal malformation resulting from the intake and accumulation of hormone disrupting substances by the mother.

Sperm production and quality are also influenced by lifestyle factors and professional as well as environmental influences, and these may even impact the fertility of the offspring (Sharpe and Franks 2002).

Nutritional factors include inappropriate calorie intake with, seldom, severe underweight (BMI <19) or, more commonly, overweight (BMI >25) or obesity (BMI >30). These conditions are associated with lower testicular volume.

Men suffering from infertility were found to consume fewer foodstuffs rich in essential fatty acids of the omega-3 group (Christophe et al. 1998), but excessive amounts of omega-6 group fatty acids. There was a direct positive correlation between the intake of 18:3-omega-3 (alpha-linolenic acid) and both sperm concentration and proportion of progressive motility. Furthermore, men with idiopathic oligozoospermia had a lower concentration of the highly poly-unsaturated fatty acids (eicosapentaenoic acid, EPA and docosahexaenoic acid, DHA) in the membrane of their spermatozoa (Zalata et al. 1998), and they showed a higher oxidative stress than normal men.

Excessive production of endogenous oestrogens by increased aromatase activity in fat tissue (Mahmoud et al. 1998), or relatively high nutritional intake of oestrogen-like hormone disrupters or heavy metals originating from the environment or the workplace, are associated with idiopathic oligozoospermia.

I.3.15.3 Clinical Findings: History, Physical Examination, Technical Investigations, Laboratory Findings

History taking usually does not reveal any relevant data. Upon physical examination, obesity may be found, and commonly testicular volume and palpation of the scrotal content are inconspicuous. Technical investigations reveal no remarkable findings. Routine blood and urine analysis do not show any abnormalities, but testosterone may be in the lower range of normal, and LH is not elevated. In spite of a low sperm concentration, serum FSH is usually not increased and serum inhibin B may be normal (Mahmoud et al. 1998).

I.3.15.4 Differential Diagnosis

It is of utmost importance to exclude all possible causal factors, since the diagnosis of idiopathic sperm deficiency is – by definition – only applicable if no other factor can be detected. Special attention must be paid to excluding small or subclinical varicoceles and subtle congenital as well as genetic factors (Chandley 1989; Chandley et al. 1989; Simpson et al. 1993).

I.3.15.5 Treatment

Surgical interventions, even those using microscopical techniques, for alleged partial obstruction of the epididymis must be considered obsolete, except if associated with the simultaneous collection of spermatozoa for ICSI (Hauser et al. 1995). Certain urologists advocate unilateral orchiectomy in case of unilateral obstruction (Hendry 1986) or nonspecific orchitis (Weidner et al. 2002). This approach does not seem acceptable in the era of assisted reproduction, particularly since the latter pathology is inaccurately defined.

Treatment should aim at correcting inappropriate nutritional habits and other factors such as smoking, taking hot baths, abusing alcohol, and a sedentary lifestyle. Counselling may be considered to relieve stress. The regular intake of a nutritional supplement containing flaxseed oil and antioxidants was demonstrated to be helpful.

If, in spite of these measures, sperm morphology remains extremely poor (less than 3%–4% spermatozoa with normal morphology), IVF using the small drop technique or complemented by ICSI is the best option to resolve the fertility problem. If, in contrast, sperm morphology is better than 4% normal forms, a treatment with the anti-oestrogen tamoxifen 20 mg/day is indicated in patients with serum levels of LH and FSH that are not elevated (Comhaire 1976). Certain authors add an androgen to the tamoxifen intake (Adamopoulos et al. 2003), but this may not be necessary in cases where the endogenous testosterone concentration significantly increases during tamoxifen intake. In general, tamoxifen treatment more than doubles sperm concentration, and improves sperm motility, but it has little effect on sperm morphology. Treatment must be given for at least 6 months in order to exert its full effect.

After a sufficient period of tamoxifen intake, when sperm characteristics have improved, intrauterine insemination may be added in order to increase the probability of conception and to shorten the time to pregnancy (Depypere et al. 1995). If this treatment fails IVF and ICSI are indicated.

I.3.15.6 Results of Treatment

Assisted reproductive technology with IVF possibly associated with ICSI results in a take-home baby rate of about 20% per attempt, and 35% after four attempts. Approximately 30%–35% of couples attain a spontaneous normal pregnancy within 6 months of treatment with tamoxifen, either or not combined with testosterone undecanoate. Three cycles of intrauterine insemination in cases with sperm characteristics exceeding the minimal requirements will produce normal pregnancies in between 40% and 50% of couples. Provided that ovarian hyperstimulation is avoided, there is no increased prevalence of multiple pregnancies (Claman et al. 2004).

I.3.15.7 Prognosis

Moderate idiopathic oligo-, astheno- or teratozoospermia may regress spontaneously when negative external causes have been eliminated. The treatment-independent pregnancy rate in such couples is better than that seen in cases with a demonstrable causal factor. The duration of infertility together with the age of the female partner (Collins and Rowe 1989) are the most important elements influencing the treatment-independent pregnancy rate and, therefore, the management of choice.

I.3.15.8 Prevention

Since idiopathic sperm deficiency seems to be related to unhealthy lifestyle and exposure to environmental influences, correcting the former and avoiding the latter may prevent the condition from occurring. Avoiding obesity, balancing the intake of essential fatty acids, refraining from tobacco smoking and recreational drugs, limiting alcohol consumption, and correcting inadequate nutritional intake of antioxidants may prevent sperm deterioration. It will take decades before environmental agents with hormone-disrupting effects will be eliminated from the environment and foodstuffs. However, the intestinal uptake of these may be reduced by probiotics providing a consortium of bacilli that absorb and metabolize several xeno-oestrogens in the gut.

I.3.15.9 Other

The approach to cases with idiopathic sperm deficiency must be tailored to each individual couple. A strategy based on the immediate implementation of assisted reproductive techniques is contrary to good medical practice. Indeed, the results of this strategy are rather poor, with ongoing pregnancy rates that are much lower than originally expected. The cost per pregnancy is extremely high, and there is increasing concern about the health of the offspring (Comhaire 2000). Except in cases with extremely poor semen quality, it is mandatory to attempt to improve the patient's natural fertility using appropriate medication and food supplementation, as well as lifestyle. The effectiveness of the latter approach has been scientifically proven beyond reasonable doubt.

References

Adamopoulos DA, Pappa A, Billa E, Nicopoulou S, Koukkou E, Michopoulos J (2003) Effectiveness of combined tamoxifen citrate and testosterone undecanoate treatment in men with idiopathic oligozoospermia. Fertil Steril 80:914–920

Belmonte IG, Martin DSM (1998) Partial obstruction of the seminal path, a frequent cause of oligozoospermia in men. Hum Reprod 13:3402–3405

Chandley AC (1989) Asymmetry in chromosome pairing: a major factor in de novo mutation and the production of genetic disease in man. J Med Genet 26:546–552

Chandley AC, Gosden JR, Hargreave TB, Spowart G, Speed RM, McBeath S (1989) Deleted Yq in the sterile son of a man with a satellited Y chromosome (Yqs). J Med Genet 26: 145–153

Christophe A, Zalata A, Mahmoud A, Comhaire F (1998) Fatty acid composition of sperm phospholipids and its nutritional implications. Middle East Fertil Soc J 3:46–53

Claman P, Wilkie V, Collins D (2004) Timing intrauterine insemination either 33 or 39 hours after administration of human chorionic gonadotropin yields the same pregnancy rates as after superovulation therapy. Fertil Steril 82:13–16

Collins JA, Rowe TC (1989) Age of the female partner is a prognostic factor in prolonged unexplained infertility: a multicenter study. Fertil Steril 52:15–20

Comhaire F (1976) Treatment of oligospermia with tamoxifen. Int J Fertil 21:232–238

Comhaire F (2000) Clinical andrology: from evidence-base to ethics. The 'E' quintet in clinical andrology. Hum Reprod 15:2067–2071

Depypere H, Milingos S, Comhaire F (1995) Intrauterine insemination in male subfertility: a comparative study of sperm preparation using a commercial Percoll kit and conventional sperm wash. Eur J Obstet Gynecol Reprod Biol 62:225–229

Dohle GR, van Roijen JH, Pierik FH, Vreeburg JT, Weber RF (2003) Subtotal obstruction of the male reproductive tract. Urol Res 31:22–24

Gerris J, Van Nueten J, Van Camp C, Gentens P, Van de Vijver I, Van Camp K (1988) Clinical aspects in the surgical treatment of varicocele in subfertile men. II. The role of the epididymal factor. Eur J Obstet Gynecol Reprod Biol 27:43–51

Gunnarsson M, Olsson AM (1995) Microsurgical correction of posttesticular obstruction. Preoperative findings and postoperative semen quality. Scand J Urol Nephrol 29:197–205

Handelsman DJ, Conway AJ, Boylan LM, Turtle JR (1984) Young's syndrome. Obstructive azoospermia and chronic sinopulmonary infections. N Engl J Med 310:3–9

Hauser R, Temple-Smith PD, Southwick GJ, McFarlane J, de Kretser DM (1995) Pregnancies after microsurgical correction of partial epididymal and vasal obstruction. Hum Reprod 10:1152–1155

Hendry WF (1986) Clinical significance of unilateral testicular obstruction in subfertile males. Br J Urol 58:709–714

Jequier AM, Crich JP, Holmes SC (1983) Incomplete obstruction of the male genital tract: a cause of oligozoospermia. Br J Urol 55:545–546

Mahmoud AM, Comhaire FH, Depuydt CE (1998) The clinical and biologic significance of serum inhibins in subfertile men. Reprod Toxicol 12:591–599

Rowe PJ, Comhaire FH, Hargreave TB, Mahmoud AMA (2000) WHO manual for the standardized investigation, diagnosis and management of the infertile male. Cambridge University Press, Cambridge

Schoysman R (1988) [Epididymal oligospermia]. Reprod Nutr Dev 28:1339–1345

Schoysman R (1992) Oligospermia associated with normal testicular function and epididymal lesions or malpositions. Acta Eur Fertil 23:117–121

Schreiber G, Zollmann C, Reiber V, Zepnick H, Lauterbach H (1990) [Severe oligozoospermia as a sequela to partial obstruction of the seminiferous tubules]. Z Urol Nephrol 83:359–365

Sharpe RM, Franks S (2002) Environment, lifestyle and infertility – an inter-generational issue. Nat Med 8 Suppl:S33-S40

Sharpe RM, Irvine DS (2004) How strong is the evidence of a link between environmental chemicals and adverse effects on human reproductive health? BMJ 328:447–451

Simpson E, Chandler P, Goulmy E, Ma K, Hargreave TB, Chandley AC (1993) Loss of the 'azoospermia factor' (AZF) on Yq in man is not associated with loss of HYA. Hum Mol Genet 2:469–471

Weidner W, Colpi GM, Hargreave TB, Papp GK, Pomerol JM, Ghosh C (2002) EAU guidelines on male infertility. Eur Urol 42:313–322

Zalata AA, Christophe AB, Depuydt CE, Schoonjans F, Comhaire FH (1998) The fatty acid composition of phospholipids of spermatozoa from infertile patients. Mol Hum Reprod 4:111–118

I.3.16 Azoospermia

G.R. Dohle

Key Messages

- Testicular dysfunction is the main cause of azoospermia.
- Testicular dysgenesis is an important cause of testicular dysfunction and can be explained by genetic and environmental factors during early foetal development.
- Obstructive azoospermia can be a treatable cause of male infertility and occurs in 15% to 20% of azoospermic men.
- Hormonal investigations, scrotal ultrasound and genetic screening are essential tools in the evaluation of the azoospermic man.

I.3.16.1 Definition

Azoospermia is the total absence of spermatozoa in the ejaculate.

Azoospermia should be distinguished from the absence of semen caused by ejaculatory disorders, such as anejaculation and retrograde ejaculation (see Chap. I.3.1). The diagnosis is made by semen analysis according to the WHO guidelines (WHO 1999); the absence of spermatozoa must be confirmed by centrifugation of the semen at 3,000 *g* for 15 min and microscopic examination of the pellet.

I.3.16.2 Introduction

Azoospermia is found in 10% of male infertility cases and is caused by a testicular insufficiency in the majority of patients. In 20%, a bilateral obstruction of the male genital tract is responsible for the azoospermia (Hendry 1994).

There has recently been renewed interest in azoospermia, mainly because of new therapeutic options for obstructive azoospermia and some cases of nonobstructive azoospermia. Through intracytoplasmic sperm injection (ICSI) (Palermo et al. 1992), combined with microsurgical epididymal sperm aspiration and testicular sperm extraction, biological parenthood can be offered to couples for whom pregnancy used to be impossible (Devroey et al. 1994). However, these techniques also raise questions about the safety of using immature spermatozoa for micromanipulation. Several congenital diseases and genetic disorders, leading to ductal obstruction or testicular failure, can be transferred to a subsequent generation through ICSI. Our knowledge of the genetics and pathophysiology of azoospermia is still limited and more research on this issue is needed. Currently the technical advances are ahead of the basic understanding of the mechanisms that lead to ductal obstruction and testicular failure.

I.3.16.2.1 Classification

A classification of azoospermia can be based on obstructive and nonobstructive forms.

Nonobstructive azoospermia can be subdivided into several aetiological categories, according to the histological pattern found on testicular biopsy. Table I.3.8 summarizes the most common causes of testicular failure.

Nonobstructive azoospermia is characterized by hypergonadotrophic hypogonadism: bilateral small testes and elevated follicle-stimulating hormone (FSH) are found. For the definitive diagnosis of testicular failure, a testicular biopsy is needed (Johnsen 1970). However, this procedure is performed only to exclude obstructive azoospermia, when physical examination and FSH are normal. Since FSH feedback is determined by the function of the Sertoli cells, maturation arrest and even some form of germinal aplasia (Sertoli-cell-only syndrome) can be present with normal FSH levels.

Obstructive azoospermia is less frequent and occurs in 15%–20% of men with azoospermia. Common causes of obstructive azoospermia are summarized in Table I.3.9.

Table I.3.8. Classification of nonobstructive azoospermia, based on the results of a testicular biopsy

1. Hypospermatogenesis
Idiopathic
Cryptorchidism
Drugs, cytotoxic therapy
Irradiation
Systemic illness
Hypogonadotrophic hypogonadism
2. Maturation arrest
Idiopathic (probably genetic of origin)
3. Germinal aplasia (Sertoli-cell-only syndrome)
Idiopathic
Cytotoxic therapy
Irradiation
Y chromosome microdeletions
Other genetic disorders
4. Seminiferous tubular sclerosis
Klinefelter's syndrome
Vascular injury/testicular torsion
Viral (mumps) orchitis

Table I.3.9. Classification of obstructive azoospermia on the basis of ductal obstruction due to congenital and acquired causes

1. Epididymal obstruction	
Congenital forms	Idiopathic epididymal obstruction
Acquired forms	Postinfective (epididymitis)
	Postsurgical (epididymal cysts)
2. Vas deferens obstruction	
Congenital forms	Congenital absence of the vas deferens
Acquired forms	Postvasectomy
	Postsurgical (hernia, scrotal surgery)
3. Ejaculatory duct obstruction	
Congenital forms	Prostatic cysts (Müllerian cysts)
Acquired forms	Postsurgical (bladder neck surgery)
	Postinfective

Men with obstructive azoospermia present with normal size testes and normal FSH. On examination, enlargement of the epididymis can be found and sometimes the vas deferens appears absent, due to congenital factors or previous inguinal or scrotal surgery. Although obstructions in primary infertile men are commonly present at the epididymal level, other sites of obstruction are the ejaculatory ducts and the vas deferens. In 25% of men with a suspected obstruction, no spermatozoa are found in the epididymis during scrotal exploration, indicating that there is an intratesticular obstruction.

I.3.16.3 Investigations

I.3.16.3.1 Semen Analysis

Additional seminal tests are alpha-glucosidase and fructose for epididymal obstruction and ejaculatory duct obstruction. Alpha-glucosidase is mainly produced by the epididymis and is significantly reduced in cases of epididymal obstruction. Fructose is produced by the seminal vesicles and is decreased in case of ejaculatory duct obstruction (EDO).

I.3.16.3.2 Hormonal Investigation

Endocrine malfunctions are more prevalent in infertile men than in the general population, but still quite uncommon. Hormonal screening can be limited to determining FSH, luteinizing hormone (LH) and testosterone levels. In men diagnosed with azoospermia or extreme oligozoospermia, it is important to distinguish between obstructive and nonobstructive causes. A criterion with reasonable predictive value for obstruction is a normal FSH with bilaterally a normal testicular volume. However, 29% of men with a normal FSH appear to have a defective spermatogenesis.

Hypergonadotrophic Hypogonadism (Elevated FSH/LH)

Hypergonadotrophic hypogonadism is a primary testicular development disorder with an elevated production of gonadotrophins. It is an isolated failure of spermatogenesis and generally not caused by a disruption of the endocrine system. The main causes are:

- Congenital: Klinefelter syndrome, anorchia, enzyme defects in the androgen synthesis, cryptorchidism
- Acquired: after orchitis, testicular torsion, castration, cytotoxic therapy

Hypogonadotrophic Hypogonadism (Deficient FSH/LH)

The main causes of low levels of gonadotrophins due to a dysfunction of the pituitary gland or hypothalamus are:

- Congenital: isolated arrest of FSH and LH secretion (Kallmann's syndrome, accompanied by anosmia), isolated arrest of LH secretion (fertile eunuch), idiopathic hypopituitarism, delayed puberty
- Acquired: generally as an expression of a more complex disorder of the pituitary gland or hypothalamus, or iatrogenic [gonadotrophin-releasing hormone (GnRH) agonists and anti-androgens]

In case hypogonadotrophic hypogonadism is suspected, the medical examination should include an MRI scan of the pituitary gland.

I.3.16.3.3 Microbiological Assessment

An indication to carry out microbiological assessment may be abnormal urine samples, urinary tract infections, male accessory gland infections (MAGIs) and sexually transmitted diseases (STDs). The clinical implication of the detection of white blood cells in a semen sample is as yet undetermined. In combination with a small ejaculate volume, this may point to a (partial) obstruction of the ejaculatory ducts caused by a (chronic) infection of the prostate or the vesicula seminalis. Genital infections may stimulate the production of spermatotoxic free oxygen radicals. Gonorrhoea and *Chlamydia trachomatis* can also cause obstruction of the tractus genitalis.

I.3.16.3.4 Genetic Evaluation

A substantial number of andrological fertility disorders, which used to be described as idiopathic male infertility, will in fact have a genetic origin. By carrying out an extensive family history and karyotype analysis, a number of these disorders can be detected. This will not only yield a diagnosis, but will also allow for appropriate genetic counselling. The latter may be very important with the advent of ICSI, since the fertility disorder and the possibly corresponding genetic defect may be transferred to the offspring.

Chromosomal abnormalities are more common in men with extreme OAT and azoospermia: the most common sex chromosome abnormality is Klinefelter syndrome (47 XXY), which affects around 10% of men diagnosed with azoospermia. Klinefelter syndrome is characterized by disproportionally long legs, gynaecomastia and hypergonadotrophic hypogonadism. Occasionally a eunuchoid phenotype is found, and at times psychological disorders. Both testicles are very small and present with tubular sclerosis. Around 60% of all patients will develop a low level of testosterone requiring androgen replacement with ageing.

In men presenting with azoospermia or extremely poor quality semen, chromosome translocations and deletions can be found which may be hereditary and may cause habitual abortion and congenital malformations in the offspring.

It is recommended that all men presenting with less than 1 million spermatozoa per millilitre, candidates for ICSI, should have at least a karyotyping performed.

Furthermore, in cases of azoospermia or severe OAT, deletions in the Y chromosome of RNS-binding proteins (DAZ, RBM and SPGY) occur and testing is advised. The prevalence of Y deletions is considerable (around 5%) in this group of patients. Identifying Y chromosome microdeletions means that the defect will be passed on to sons who will then also be infertile.

When performing ICSI with surgically retrieved sperm based on the diagnosis of a congenital bilateral absence of the vas deferens (CBAVD), both the male and the female partners should be checked for mutations in the cystic fibrosis transmembrane conductance regulator (CFTR) gene. Apart from causing cystic fibrosis, this gene is also associated with CBAVD; 85% of all males diagnosed with CBAVD also test positive for 1 or 2 CFTR gene mutations. In case the partner is a carrier of a CFTR mutation, depending on the mutation involved, there is a 25% chance of a child with CF or CBAVD. Genetic counselling is recommended in these cases.

I.3.16.3.5 Ultrasonography

When trying to locate intrascrotal defects, ultrasonography is a useful tool. In case of epididymal obstruction, dilatation and cystic lesions of the epididymis and rete testis can be found. The vas deferens can be identified easily with ultrasound.

Colour Doppler ultrasound of the scrotum can detect a varicocele in around 30% of infertile males. Testicular tumours can be found in 0.5% of infertile men and testicular microcalcifications, a potentially premalignant condition, is detected in around 5% of infertile males, especially in patients diagnosed with a history of cryptorchism (Dohle and Schröder 2000).

A transrectal ultrasonography (TRUS) is indicated in men with a low ejaculate volume (< 1.5 ml) and a history of MAGI to exclude obstruction of the ejaculatory ducts, caused by a midline prostatic cyst or a stenosis of the ejaculatory ducts which can occur after prostatitis. Ejaculatory duct obstruction is characterized by azoospermia or severe oligozoospermia with a low seminal volume and decreased levels of seminal fructose (Jarow 1996).

I.3.16.3.6 Testicular Biopsy

Indications for performing a testis biopsy are azoospermia in the presence of a normal volume of the testes and normal FSH levels. The biopsy is aimed at differentiating between testicular insufficiency and obstruction of the male genital tract. Pathological classifications are:

- The absence of tubuli seminiferi (tubular sclerosis)
- The presence of Sertoli cells only (Sertoli-cell-only syndrome)
- Maturation arrest: incomplete spermatogenesis, not beyond the spermatocyte stage
- Hypospermatogenesis: all cell types up to spermatozoa are present but there is a distinct decline in the number of reproducing spermatogonia

Carcinoma in situ of the testis can be found, especially in men with bilateral microcalcifications in the testes and in men with a history of testicular tumour.

If testicular biopsy is performed, in any case, cryopreservation of testicular tissue is highly recommended to store germ cells for later intracytoplasmic sperm injections (Fig. I.3.12).

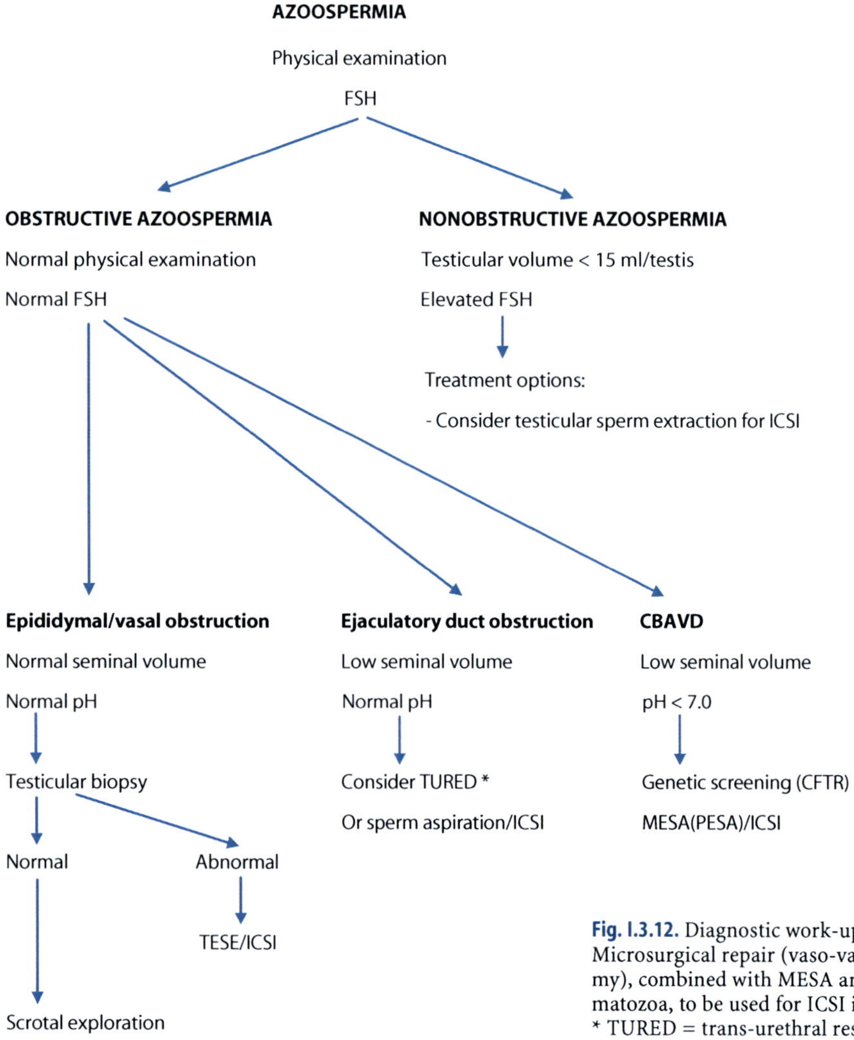

Fig. I.3.12. Diagnostic work-up of azoospermia
Microsurgical repair (vaso-vasotomy or vaso-epididymostomy), combined with MESA and cryopreservation of the spermatozoa, to be used for ICSI in case of surgical failure.
* TURED = trans-urethral resection of the ejaculatory ducts

References

Devroey P, Liu J, Nagy Z, Tournaye H, Silber SJ, Van Steirteghem AC (1994) Normal fertilization of human oocytes after testicular sperm extraction and intracytoplasmic sperm injection. Fertil Steril 62:639–641

Dohle GR, Schröder FH (2000) Ultrasonographic assessment of the scrotum. Lancet 356:1625–1626

Hendry WF (1994) Azoospermia and surgery for testicular obstruction. In: Hargreave TB (ed) Male infertility. Springer, Berlin Heidelberg New York, pp 337–363

Jarow JP (1996) Transrectal ultrasonography in the diagnosis and management of ejaculatory duct obstruction. J Androl 17:467–472

Johnsen SG (1970) Testicular biopsy score count. A method for registration of spermatogenesis in human testis: normal values and results in 335 hypogonadal males. Hormones 1:2

Palermo G, Joris H, Devroey P et al (1992) Pregnancy after intracytoplasmic injection of a single spermatozoon into an oocyte. Lancet 340:17–18

Skakkebaek NE, Rajpert-De Meyts E, Main KM (2001) Testicular dysgenesis syndrome: an increasingly common development disorder with environmental aspects. Hum Reprod 16:972–978

World Health Organization (1999) WHO laboratory manual for the examination of human semen and sperm-cervical mucus interaction, 4th edn. Cambridge University Press, Cambridge

Problem: Sexual Dysfunction I.4

I.4.1 Erectile Dysfunction

T.B. HARGREAVE

Key Messages

- Performance anxiety is a contributory cause in almost all men with erectile dysfunction (ED).
- Type 5 phosphodiesterase (PDE5) inhibitors are safe and can be used as first-line treatment for almost all men with ED.
- In older men in developed countries, vascular disease is the most common aetiological factor
- All men complaining of ED should be screened for diabetes.
- Older men attending with ED should be screened for coronary artery disease, and appropriate lifestyle modifications should be advised in addition to any other treatment.

I.4.1.1 Definition of the Disease

Erectile dysfunction (ED) is defined as failure of sufficient penile rigidity for sexual intercourse. There may be a complete lack of penile rigidity, partial rigidity or premature loss of erection. When there is premature loss of erection, the problem is categorized as ED if the loss of erection occurs before ejaculation. The severity of the problem can be scored using the International Index of Erectile Function (IIEF).

I.4.1.2 Aetiology and Pathogenesis

I.4.1.2.1 Changing Sexual Function with Age

Normal male sexual function involves penile erection, a sensation of orgasm and ejaculation of semen. The various reflexes coordinating these functions usually occur in a synchronized manner but those relating to penis erection are independent of reflexes relating to orgasm and ejaculation. Thus it is possible to have an orgasm and ejaculate without penis erection. There is a latent period following orgasm when penile stimulation is ineffective or less effective in producing repeat orgasm. There are changes in sexual function with age. In young men, erection and ejaculation can occur within 20–30 s and the latent period is short, but as men get older it takes more to stimulate erection and the later period is longer; however, sometimes older men have unrealistic expectations. The latent period varies between men, with a small proportion of men having the ability to ejaculate repeatedly with no significant latent period; this may relate to postorgasmic levels of prolactin.

I.4.1.2.2 Sexual Function and Drugs

Drugs such as alcohol, barbiturates, cocaine, heroin, methadone (Crowley and Simpson 1978) and opium can cause an initial sexual stimulation, but the chronic effect is to cause a decrease in almost all domains of sexual function, including an increase in the latent period. The adverse sexual side effects are one reason some young addicts may be persuaded to stop abuse (Palha and Esteves 2002).

I.4.1.2.3 Anatomical Problems

Anatomical problems can be congenital or acquired. It is relatively uncommon for a man with a congenital abnormality of the penis to come for medical help because of lack of penis erections; more often the problem is manifest during infancy or childhood because of an obvious visual abnormality such as hypospadias or epispadias or exstrophy. However, young men with a tight phimosis may experience pain during erection and be too embarrassed to seek medical help and may eventually present with erectile failure. Similarly, young men with an imbalance in growth between the right and left corpora cavernosa have a bent erection but again may be too embarrassed to seek help and present years later with ED. In the case of the man with erectile deformity, the situation is made worse if the first doctor does not take the problem seriously and jokes about the condition. This can happen because there is often little or nothing to find on examination of the flaccid penis and the inexperienced doctor can in these circumstances dismiss the young man's complaint as frivolous. Acquired erectile deformity associated with Peyronie's disease may be associated with ED, especially in older men, because of concomitant arterial disease. Also, men with Peyronie's may have considerable anxiety because of concern about whether the problem is a manifestation of serious disease such as cancer, and this anxiety may be sufficient to cause ED.

I.4.1.2.4 Endocrine Erectile Dysfunction

Endocrine causes include pituitary failure causing a lack of luteinizing hormone (LH) secretion. This may be a primary failure or secondary to pituitary tumour or other pituitary disease, or after head injury with severing of the pituitary stalk. ED may also occur in association with hyperprolactinaemia and a prolactinoma, or other mass lesions of the sella. Testicular failure with low testosterone output can cause ED. It is a commonly held lay opinion that lack of testosterone as men get older is the most common cause of ED and that the problem can be corrected by androgen therapy, whereas in reality ED secondary to androgen deficiency is relatively uncommon compared with vasculogenic ED. A proportion of older men are androgen-deficient, but if the onset of their androgen deficiency has been slow only a small proportion seek help with sexual function because of their lack of libido. Older men with rapid onset endocrine-mediated ED are more likely to seek help. For example, the majority of men with newly diagnosed prostate cancer who require androgen ablation therapy report loss of libido and ED (Metz et al. 1988). The response to type 5 phosphodiesterase (PDE5) inhibitor treatment is improved if partial androgen deficiency is also corrected (Aversa et al. 2003), but in men over the age of 50 before starting androgen therapy, care must be taken to exclude prostate cancer by the finding of a normal rectal examination and prostate-specific antigen (PSA) and with follow-up PSA 6 months after the start of treatment.

I.4.1.2.5 Vasculogenic Erectile Dysfunction

Vasculogenic ED is the commonest cause of erection problems in older men. The risk factors for erection problems include being overweight, high blood pressure, diabetes and smoking, and these are the same risk factors for heart attacks and strokes (Table I.4.1). In fact, the onset of ED in a man in his late forties or fifties may be an indication of circulatory impairment and good reason for the man to have his circulatory status checked, including measurement of his blood pressure, blood lipids and cholesterol. There is evidence that the onset of ED may precede a coronary thrombosis by a few years and it would seem that there is an opportunity to intervene to try to prevent coronary thrombosis.

Table I.4.1. Risk factors for coronary artery disease. The same risk factors predict erectile dysfunction (*ED*) except that ED predates coronary occlusion by approximately 5 years

Three-star risk factors
Typical anginal pain
Diabetes
Peripheral vascular disease
Two-star risk factors
Hypertension
Smoking
Total cholesterol level > 265 mg/dl (6.85 mmol/l)
High LDL (bad) cholesterol levels
One-star risk factors
Age greater than 65 years
Obesity
Sedentary lifestyle
Family history of coronary artery disease
Stress

Another vasculogenic cause of ED is venous leakage. Although the diagnosis is based on X-ray visualization of large exit veins during erection by cavernosography, the actual pathology is failure of sufficient pressure within the corporal bodies to close the venous exits through the corporal wall, often because of partial fibrosis of the corpora cavernosal muscle; thus venous leakage is a manifestation of corpora cavernosa dysfunction and not a primary venous problem.

I.4.1.2.6 Neurogenic Erectile Dysfunction

This is secondary to any condition that affects nerve pathways from the central nervous system (CNS) to the penis. These include cerebral lesions (rare), spinal cord injury including cervical spondylosis, lumbar disc and spinal dysraphism (spina bifida and associated spinal fusion disorders), injury to the pelvic plexus after pelvic trauma and after major pelvic surgery such as pelvic exenteration, injury to nerves adjacent to the prostate following radical prostatectomy and irradiation, in association with autonomic neuropathy (e.g. in diabetes), and finally in association with disease processes that affect peripheral nerves such as multiple sclerosis and diabetes.

I.4.1.2.7
Corporeal Fibrosis After Prolonged Disuse

After a long period of time without sexual or nocturnal erections, there is a replacement of corpus cavernosa muscle by scar tissue. The fibrosis is time-dependent but is one of the explanations for the aphorism "use it or lose it". Unfortunately once fibrous tissue has formed, pharmacotherapy becomes less effective and penile implant surgery may become the only alternative. It is important to avoid any significant time of failed erections and thus it often helps to prescribe PDE5 inhibitors in the postoperative period of any operation that may cause temporary impairment of erectile function, especially after radical prostatectomy but also after transurethral resection of the prostate (TURP) or other genital operations.

I.4.1.3
Clinical Findings: History, Physical Examination, Technical Investigations, Laboratory Findings

In general, younger men with ED are more likely to have psychogenic problems, whereas older men with ED are more likely to have impaired circulation. When ED is associated with endocrine or neurological conditions, the problem usually becomes evident on careful history taking. An important clue is the relatively rapid onset of ED in a younger man and in such cases care should be taken to question about possible pituitary symptoms, such as visual field disturbance, or possible neurological symptoms, such as changes in handwriting, coordination problems and other subtle symptoms. ED is more common in men with diabetes mellitus than in the general population and all men attending with ED should have routine urine testing for sugar. The initial assessment includes a general medical history, including history of all medications (whether prescribed or not) and past history. Clinical examination should include a general examination to assess endocrine state (virilization, testicular consistency, gynaecomastia) and examination of the genitalia. A history of galactorrhoea or this finding on examination is strongly indicative of a prolactinoma. There is controversy about whether rectal examination is indicated; a safe protocol is to include rectal examination on all men age 50 or over and for all men younger than 50 if there is any indication of urinary or prostatic dysfunction. A full neurological examination is indicated if there are any indicators of neurological disease but otherwise can be omitted.

In general, preservation of nocturnal and morning erections, preservation of libido and the finding of normal size and normal consistency testicles are good indicators that hormone levels are likely to be normal. In cases of suspected pituitary disease, there may be other manifestations of endocrine deficiency, visual field changes or past history of head injury. Investigations include formal assessment of visual fields, measurement of LH and follicle-stimulating hormone (FSH) and magnetic resonance imaging (MRI) scans of the pituitary fossa. Although hyperprolactinaemia is uncommon, it has been recommended that serum prolactin should be measured in all cases.

For men with suspected testicular failure, history taking is difficult because of the lack of specific symptoms; for example, complaints of general tiredness may indicate lack of androgens but can also be related to disorders as diverse as depression and cardiac insufficiency. Assessment should therefore begin with a full medical history and physical examination. Care must be taken to identify men who have been taking medication that may interfere with native androgen production. Some younger men take anabolic steroids to enhance sporting prowess and by feedback to the pituitary these may shut down the pituitary drive to the testes. If no specific disease process is identified it is helpful to ask the man to complete the Ageing Male Symptoms Score. Testosterone should be measured in a blood sample taken in the morning. If the result is low or in the lower quartile of the normal range, then the measurement should be repeated along with measurement of LH, sex hormone-binding globulin and ideally the albumin level. From these figures it is possible to calculate the free androgens; this is most easily done using the free testosterone calculator at the ISSAM website (www.issam.ch/freetesto.htm), but many laboratories will report the free androgen index. In some clinics, it is also possible to measure free testosterone but the laboratory methodology is exacting and the test is not always available or reliable. The coincidence of testosterone below the lower level of the normal range and suggestive symptoms, i.e. a high symptom score, are sufficient to warrant treatment with androgen replacement. Much more problematical is the common situation of suggestive symptoms in association with marginally low total or calculated free testosterone.

For men with suspected vasculogenic ED, chest pain or claudication should be noted and examination should include assessment of weight and blood pressure as well as assessment of lower limb nutrition and peripheral pulses. In fact, the onset of vasculogenic ED usually precedes the onset of other vascular disease by approximately 5 years and there are often no particular vascular stigmata. More often than not, men in this category are given treatment with a PDE inhibitor, and most respond well and no further investigations are undertaken. This may, however, be a lost opportunity to identify vascular disease at an earlier stage and to institute preventative therapy. There are questions about whether all men over the age of 50 with suspected vasculogenic ED should be offered an electrocardiogram (ECG) and treadmill test. More detailed investigation of the vascular component of ED can be undertaken using penile colour Doppler analysis of blood flow before and after an injection of an intracavernosal agent; however, this investigation tends to be reserved for men who fail to respond to PDE therapy.

A typical history of a man with venous leakage is premature loss of erections and often there have been several prior years of sexual inactivity. Although there is initial response to PDE5 inhibitior treatment, the premature loss of erection continues. Cavernosography and Doppler studies show adequate arterial inflow but distended penile and deep dorsal veins which continue to drain venous blood throughout the process of erection. Occasionally a single large vein can be identified. Usually cavernosography is performed with a prostaglandin injection to induce erection, but anxiety and increased sympathetic tone can give false results in terms of diagnosis of venous leakage; giving in addition to prostaglandin 2 mg of phentolamine has been reported to help distinguish true cases (Gontero et al. 2004).

Traumatic AV fistulae should be suspected in men who develop ED after pelvic injury or after urethral surgery. Diagnosis is by arteriography with selective cannulation of the internal iliac arteries.

Neurogenic ED is not usually seen in isolation from other manifestations of the neurological disorder. Thus there is almost always a history of bladder or bowel disturbance or lower limb dysfunction, etc. In general, there is no treatment to correct neurogenic ED other than time, but if the problem continues for more than 2 years after the injury there is unlikely to be any further improvement. Men with neurogenic ED may be very sensitive to pharmacological agents and injection of even small doses of papaverine can induce a priapism.

ED is more common in men with diabetes mellitus compared with the general population and is multifactorial with vascular and neurogenic components as well as impaired function of the muscle fibres in the corporal bodies. In addition to routine testing of urine for sugar, some clinics advocate fasting blood sugar measurement for all men with ED. If this policy is adopted it can conveniently be combined with morning blood sampling for testosterone and indeed lipids.

I.4.1.4 Treatment

The advent of the PDE inhibitor drugs such as sildenafil (Viagra) has revolutionized the treatment of male sexual dysfunction. These drugs, when compared with older treatments, are the first easy-to-use treatment that works well for most common ED problems. The market for these drugs is now billions of US dollars each year and this has stimulated the pharmaceutical industry to address the problem of male ED to the public by way of advertising, sexual health information, men's health publications, etc., with the result that in many countries the subject is less of a taboo compared with former times.

Whatever the cause of the ED, it is almost always associated with performance anxiety. Thus part of the stimulus towards full penis erection is the sensation of getting an erection and if there is no penile response to sexual stimulation this lack of response is worrying and this worry inhibits erections and makes the problem worse. The first-line treatment for most men with ED is a PDE inhibitor such as sildenafil (Viagra), tadalafil (Cialis) or vardenafil (Levitra) and in many cases and particularly in men over 50, a major part of the benefit of these medicines is breaking the cycle of performance anxiety by increasing penile response to sexual stimulation. Very often it is possible to reduce the dose after a few uses.

The success of PDE inhibitor therapy is such that it is being prescribed for all cases with the minimum of investigations, which is a pity because opportunities are being lost for simple health screening measures such as stick urine testing for sugar and blood pressure measurement. PDE inhibitor treatment is specific and has few side-effects (Table I.4.2). In contrast to normal prescribing practice, some andrologists recommend starting men on the maximum dose for the first few occasions of use and then, if successful, the dose can be

Table I.4.2. Some side-effects of sildenafil, tadalafil and vardenafil

Headaches (16 % of men experienced headaches which get better after an hour or two). This can occur with all three
Hot flushes may be experienced by 10 %. This can occur with all three
Dyspepsia (indigestion) 7 %. This can occur with all three
Nasal congestion 4 %. This can occur with all three
Abnormal vision 3 %. You may experience a blue tinge to objects, you may experience an increased sensation of brightness or vision may be blurred. If you experience these changes you should not drive a motor vehicle. These effects may come on within 2 h of taking sildenafil or vardenafil but are less likely with tadalafil. The altered vision may last and hour or two but not longer than 8 h (sildenafil and vardenafil)
Muscle aches and backache. More likely with tadalafil
Other side-effects include: diarrhoea 3 %, dizziness 2 %, rash 2 %
Blindness caused by anterior ischaemic optic neuropathy. It is not yet certain that this is a true side-effect but recently the USA Federal Drug Administration (FDA) has required the companies selling these medicines to include a warning in their product literature. By July 2005 the USA FDA had received reports about 43 men who have developed blindness. Of these men 38 used sildenafil, 4 used tadalafil and 1 vardenafil. This is in the context of billions of prescriptions

reduced. The rationale for this is that performance anxiety is most marked on the first few occasions but once the man sees success, there is less need for higher-dose PDE inhibitor therapy, whereas if treatment starts with the minimum dose and fails, then this reinforces performance anxiety and makes higher-dose treatment less successful. For success men need to understand what PDE inhibitor treatment does and does not do. Some men have the idea that taking the tablet will cause an erection and time must be taken to explain that the treatment only works in the context of sexual stimulation by amplifying the effect of the neural impulses from the brain. It can be described to men as similar to turning up the volume control on the radio or TV – if there is no radio or TV transmission signal then turning up the volume control is useless, and similarly if there is no sexual stimulation, taking a PDE inhibitor tablet is useless. Men also need to be made aware that the tablets do not have an immediate effect and that it takes about 1 h for absorption into the bloodstream. This absorption is delayed for up to 2 h if the tablets are taken in proximity to a large meal.

PDE inhibitors affect the neural pathway mediated by nitrous oxide as the neural transmitter. The main contraindication to PDE inhibitor treatment is concurrent use of nitrous oxide donor medicines such as sublingual glyceryl trinitrate (GTN) or nitrospray inhaler. These are prescribed to stimulate vasodilation for relief of angina and the effect of the PDE inhibitor and nitrous oxide donor medicines is cumulative and can result in a marked drop in blood pressure due to general vasodilatation. This can precipitate a coronary infarct; consequently, all prescribing literature for PDE inhibitors states that they should not be used by men who have angina and who use nitrous oxide donor medicines. There is a similar danger from the use of PDE inhibitors and the drug of abuse amyl nitrite (poppers), which is available in some nightclubs. There is also a warning about postural hypotension with the concurrent use of PDE inhibitors and alpha blockers; the latter are commonly given for relief of lower urinary tract symptoms (LUTS) in association with prostate enlargement. Older men with ED commonly have LUTS; provided care is taken, PDE inhibitors and alpha blockers can usually be taken together. Apart from these concerns, the PDE inhibitors are very safe. At the time of writing there were three of these compounds on the market with competing claims by the manufacturers. Tadalafil has been shown to have a duration of action of up to 48 h compared with roughly 12 h for the other two compounds. This suits some men particularly when there is uncertainty about the timing of any sexual activity. On the other hand and especially in the context of a long-standing relationship, the shorter but possibly stronger effect of sildenafil and vardenafil may suit other men. Both sildenafil and vardenafil have some blocking effect on PDE6, which concerns the processing of light in the retina, and can produce a temporary alteration in perception of colour vision for the duration of their action. Vardenafil is more potent than sildenafil and therefore can be taken at a lower dose. It is wise to advise men who are new to these prescriptions not to drive a car until they are sure what effect if any the treatment has on colour vision.

In the case of young men with ED and a tight phimosis, treatment is with circumcision or with PDE inhibitors. Often an explanation from the treating doctor is sufficient but follow-up is needed as formal psychosexual counselling may also be needed. Diagnosis is made by history, careful clinical examination including retracting the foreskin, and when necessary by obtaining photographs of the erect penis.

Treatment of ED in the context of diabetes is with PDE inhibitor drugs and attention to good diabetic control, usually under the care of the diabetic clinic.

Most men with partial and recent-onset ED respond to PDE inhibitor treatment. When this fails, alternative treatments include intracorporeal injections of vasoactive substances, vacuum devices and generally as a last resort surgical implantation of penile prostheses.

Until the advent of PDE inhibitors, intracorporeal injections were the most widely used treatment for ED, despite the need for men to learn to self-inject. In response to this need, nurse-led ED clinics were set up in many countries in Europe. Drugs used include papaverine, prostaglandin, phentolamine and, in France, moxysilate or combinations of these medicines. Delivery routes include intracorporeal injection and intraurethral pellet. The most universally available compound was prostaglandin because compared with papaverine there was a better safety ratio in terms of efficacy versus the risk of priapism. Particular care has to be taken when prescribing injection therapy for a man with neurogenic ED because there may be extreme sensitivity to the agent; it is therefore wise to start with a very low dose, e.g. 5 µg rather than the more usual 10 µg starting dose. The main risk of intracorporeal injections is priapism, whose treatment is described in Sect. I.7.4. Preventing priapism means ensuring that the patient understands the risk, particularly if he is self-injecting at home. If the patient plans sexual activity with a new partner in a particularly stimulating situation it is often wise for him to reduce from the dose that was found to be effective in a hospital setting. If the injection does not work it is usually because it has been injected outside or into the tunica wall rather than into the corporal muscle and the man should wait 24 h before giving himself another injection. If there is an erection that last for more than 2 h a self-help measure to reduce rigidity is to walk up and down flights of stairs because the increased blood flow into the gluteal muscles steals the blood flow from the penis; however, if the erection continues beyond 5–6 h, then the patient needs clear instructions about where to attend. This can be difficult, as priapism in this context is often in the small hours of the morning and emergency room staff may not be familiar with treatment.

Vascular surgery has been used to improve arterial inflow, to decrease venous outflow and to correct post-traumatic AV fistulae. The inferior epigastric artery has been used for revascularization, but in general the results are poor, especially in older men because of concomitant generalized vascular disease. Except in specialist centres and for selected younger men, revascularization procedures have been abandoned by most clinicians. Several years ago, the condition of venous leakage was frequently diagnosed and treated by surgery to tie the deep dorsal veins. The initial result of these operations was restoration of erection in 50% of patients, but long-term results were disappointing because the treatment was based on a misunderstanding of the underlying pathophysiology and did not correct the underlying abnormality of function of the cavernosal muscle.

Venous leakage surgery is now less commonly performed but is still sometimes used because of the 50% response rate (Katzenwadel et al. 1993), especially if cavernosography identifies a single leaking vein. Traumatic AV fistulae are rare and can be difficult to treat. Treatment options include embolization via selective catheterization via the internal iliac arteries (Fernandes Arjona et al. 2001) or surgery. Surgery involves ligation of the deep crural veins (Lue 1999), but this can be difficult and there is a risk of damage to the crural arteries.

I.4.1.4.1 Vacuum Devices

The principle is simple. The penis is placed in a cylinder which is pressed against the pubis to create an airtight seal and then this cylinder is evacuated to cause the penis to fill with blood. An elastic ring is then slipped off the cylinder onto the base of the shaft of the penis to keep the penis engorged with blood. Vacuum devices can produce sufficient rigidity for penetration but the ring has to be tight enough to prevent blood flow out of the penis and this often reduces penis sensation by nerve compression and prevents external ejaculation. These problems limit patient acceptability. Care must be taken when this device is used by men with reduced penile sensation [diabetics, paraplegics (Denil et al. 1996), etc.] because leaving the ring in position too long can cause pressure necrosis of the skin. The advantage of vacuum devices is that the patient totally controls the treatment and he does not need to involve the medical profession, as the devices are available for purchase. Most reports on efficacy predate the advent of sildenafil but even in the sildenafil era some men have been found to prefer vacuum devices (Chen et al. 2001). There is a report of combination treatment with sildenafil and vacuum therapy for men with impaired response to full-dose sildenafil and a greater proportion of men were able to achieve rigidity than with sildenafil alone (Chen et al. 2004). There is also a report of the use of a vacuum device to enhance the results after insertion of a penile prosthesis (Soderdahl et al. 1997). Vacuum devices can also been used twice daily for 15 min but without the penile constriction ring to try to improve blood flow into the penis. In some countries there are vacuum clinics but this type of use has not been validated by clinical trial.

I.4.1.4.2 Penile Prosthesis

There are two main types of penile prosthesis: inflatable and semirigid. The best result is following the use of an inflatable prosthesis because this is nearer to the natural situation with the penis semi-flaccid when the device is not inflated (Table I.4.3). The devices are implanted into the corpora cavernosa. Once this has been done, it effectively destroys the corporeal muscle. Therefore, if the device has to be removed there is no other treatment available. Consequently, these devices tend to be reserved for men who have failed with medical treatment. There are a variety of different manufacturers and prosthesis formats. The advantages and disadvantages of the inflatable versus the semirigid prosthesis are shown in Table I.4.4.

Type of prosthesis	No. of men	Follow-up (months)	Failure
Mentor Alpha 1 (Garber 1996)	150	Mean 19, range 0–65	5 (3.3%)
Ambicor (Levine et al. 2001)	131	Mean 43, range 12–73	10 (7.6%)
AMS 700cx (Carson et al. 2000)	372 (case note review)	Median 47.7, up to 134	14% at 5 years
	207 (telephone)		14%
Dura 11 malleable (Ferguson and Cespedes 2003)	94	Mean 5.7	81%

Table I.4.3. Results of penile prosthesis

Table I.4.4. Advantages and disadvantages of inflatable versus semirigid penile prostheses

	Semirigid	Inflatable
Rigidity sufficient for intercourse	Yes	There is girth as well as length expansion
Flaccidity	The prosthesis is semirigid all the time but malleable so that the penis can be folded down	Although when deflated the penis is reasonably floppy, it is not as flaccid as normal, especially when shorter prostheses are used because of a shorter penile length
Operating time	60–90 min	Depends on skill of operating team 90 min or more
Cost	Less expensive Approximately 1,000 €	More expensive Nearer 5,000 €
Mechanical failure	Older types of prosthesis used to fracture but this is now very rare	Devices can leak and there is a revision rate of approximately one in five by 10 years although with improvements in prosthesis design this problem is lessening
Noise	None	Air bubbles trapped in the cylinder can cause squeaking!
Metal parts	Many of these prostheses have a core of twisted stainless steel or silver and will set off metal detectors, e.g. airport security	In some models, the inflate/deflate pump has a metal piston but the size is not sufficient to set off metal detection equipment
Premature loss of erection	No loss of erection after ejaculation	With some types of one-part inflatable prosthesis, there can be premature loss of erection if the penis is sharply bent during intercourse
Erosion into the urethra or through the glans or skin	This is a significant risk in diabetic men with reduced sensation	The risk of erosion is much less than with rigid prostheses
Infection	The risk of perioperative infection is low because the surface of the prosthesis is smooth and operation minimal	The risk of perioperative infection is higher when multipart inflatable prostheses are used because of the more extensive incision and longer operating time
Problems if there is a subsequent need for prostate surgery	This can be a problem because the length of the prostate may prevent the use of the resectoscope other than through a perineal urethrostomy	With the device deflated transurethral resection of the prostate is usually possible
Using the device	There is nothing to learn	The patient has to learn how to use the inflate/deflate pump. For multipart inflatable devices, this is located in the scrotum; some men find the inflate/deflate process is painful

I.4.1.5 Results of Treatment

The response rates to PDE inhibitor drugs can be predicted from the pretreatment IIEF score. If the patient is having partial or unsustained erections, then the response is likely to be good, with more than 90 % of men achieving an erection sufficient for penetration and less than 2 % of men stopping treatment because of side-effects. However, if there has been a prolonged time without sexual activity and if the man has no erection, then irreversible changes such as corporal fibrosis are more likely and the results of PDE inhibitor treatment are worse. Nevertheless, because side-effects are few, it is worth trying PDE inhibitor treatment in all cases unless contraindicated by angina medication.

Most older men with ED in Europe and North America have vasculogenic ED and most respond to PDE inhibitors if they have any residual erection at all. If they do not respond, this is usually an indicator of severe circulatory impairment with or without corporeal fibrosis and although second-line treatment such as vacuum devices and injection therapy may work, there is a diminishing return in terms of response to treatment. Before the days of PDE inhibitors, the main medical treatment was injection therapy and for those men resistant to single-drug therapy, some clinicians concocted mixtures with maximal dosage of several compounds, but this type of approach resulted in reduced safety margins. The use of combinations of injections and oral agents or combinations of agents is anecdotal and in the absence of proper safety and efficacy data, this treatment remains the responsibility of the individual doctor who advocates the regimen.

Most case series results of vacuum devices predate the advent of sildenafil. Between 60 % and 80 % of men who try these devices find them helpful (Baltaci et al. 1995; Bodansky 1994). Various complications have been reported, including development of skin necrosis (Meinhardt et al. 1990), Peyronie's disease (Kim and Carson 1993), urethral bleeding, trapping of scrotal skin and cavernosal ballooning (Ganem et al. 1998).

Special care has to be taken by diabetic or paraplegic men with reduced sensation (LeRoy and Pryor 1994).

The use of implantable devices enables erections sufficient for penetration, but often men have unrealistic expectations. The best results have been reported when both partners are involved in the decision to have the implant. Of those men who do not involve their partner in their decision, approximately 25 % never use the prosthesis at all in the context of sexual intercourse.

In general it is best if men seeking ED treatment discuss their treatment plans with their partner. Difficulties arise when a man decides to seek help in the context of a long-standing partnership because restoration of sexual function is not always welcomed by their partner.

I.4.1.6 Prevention

The most common cause of ED in Western Europe and North America and as men get older is vascular disease. The same risk factors are relevant for ED as for coronary insufficiency and other vascular disease: hypertension, obesity, smoking, lack of exercise, and overeating and a high-fat diet. Men should be encouraged to adopt healthy lifestyles to minimize these risk factors. There is evidence that statins and lowering of cholesterol can prevent coronary artery disease, but it is not known whether there is also a beneficial effect on preserving erectile function.

Performance anxiety is a major factor after any surgical procedure involving the male genitalia. Postoperative problems can be prevented by giving the patient proper information about the effects of surgical procedures on sexual function and also by offering adjunctive PDE5 treatment after surgery.

References

Aversa A, Isidori AM, Spera G, Lenzi A, Fabbri A (2003) Androgens improve cavernous vasodilation and response to sildenafil in patients with erectile dysfunction. Clin Endocrinol (Oxf) 58(5)632 – 638

Baltaci S, Aydos K, Kosar A, Anafarta K (1995) Treating erectile dysfunction with a vacuum tumescence device: a retrospective analysis of acceptance and satisfaction. Br J Urol 76: 757 – 760

Bodansky HJ (1994) Treatment of male erectile dysfunction using the active vacuum assist device. Diabet Med 11:410 – 412

Braunwald E, Fauci AS, Kasper DL et al (1991) Harrison's principles of internal medicine, 15th edn. McGraw-Hill, New York, p 294

Carson CC, Mulcahy JJ, Govier FE (2000) Efficacy, safety and patient satisfaction outcomes of the AMS 700CX inflatable penile prosthesis: results of a long-term multicenter study. AMX 700CX Study Group. J Urol 164:376 – 380

Chen J, Mabjeesh NJ, Greenstein A (2001) Sildenafil versus the vacuum erection device: patient preference. J Urol 166: 1779 – 1781

Chen J, Sofer M, Kaver I, Matzkin H, Greenstein A (2004) Concomitant use of sildenafil and a vacuum entrapment device for the treatment of erectile dysfunction. J Urol 171:292 – 295

Crowley TJ, Simpson R (1978) Methadone dose and human sexual behaviour. Int J Addict 13:285 – 295

Denil J, Ohl DA, Smythe C (1996) Vacuum erection device in spinal cord injured men: patient and partner satisfaction. Arch Phys Med Rehabil 77:750 – 753

Ferguson KH, Cespedes RD (2003) Prospective long-term results and quality-of-life assessment after Dura-II penile prosthesis placement. Urology 61:437 – 441

Fernandez Arjona M, Oteros R, Zarca M, Diaz Fernandez J, Cortes I (2001) Percutaneous embolization for erectile dysfunction due to venous leakage: prognostic factors for a good therapeutic result. Eur Urol 39:15 – 19

Ganem JP, Lucey DT, Janosko EO, Carson CC (1998) Unusual complications of the vacuum erection device. Urology 51: 627 – 631

Garber BB (1996) Inflatable penile prosthesis: results of 150 cases. Br J Urol 78:933 – 935

Gontero P, Sriprasad S, Wilkins CJ, Donaldson N, Muir GH, Sidhu PS (2004) Phentolamine re-dosing during penile dynamic colour Doppler ultrasound: a practical method to abolish a false diagnosis of venous leakage in patients with erectile dysfunction. Br J Radiol 77:922 – 926

Katzenwadel A, Popken G, Wetterauer U (1993) Penile venous surgery for cavernosal venous leakage: long-term results and retrospective studies. Urol Int 50:71 – 76

Kim JH, Carson CC 3rd (1993) Development of Peyronie's disease with the use of a vacuum constriction device. J Urol 149:1314 – 1315

LeRoy SC, Pryor JL (1994) Severe penile erosion after use of a vacuum suction device for management of erectile dysfunction in a spinal cord injured patient. Case report. Paraplegia 32:120 – 123

Levine LA, Estrada CR, Morgentaler A (2001) Mechanical reliability and safety of, and patient satisfaction with the Ambicor inflatable penile prosthesis: results of a 2 center study. J Urol 166:932 – 937

Lue TF (1999) Surgery for crural venous leakage. Urology 54: 739 – 741

Meinhardt W, Kropman RF, Lycklama A, Nijeholt AA, Zwartendijk J (1990) Skin necrosis caused by use of negative pressure device for erectile impotence. J Urol 144:983

Metz R, Namer M, Adenis I et al (1988) Zoladex as primary therapy in advanced prostate cancer. A French co-operative trial. Am J Clin Oncol 11 [Suppl 20]:S112–S114

Palha AP, Esteves M (2002) A study of the sexuality of opiate addicts. J Sex Marital Ther 28:427 – 437

Soderdahl DW, Petroski RA, Mode D, Schwartz BF, Thrasher JB (1997) The use of an external vacuum device to augment a penile prosthesis. Tech Urol 3:100 – 102

I.4.2 Erectile Deformity, Including Peyronie's Disease

T.B. Hargreave

Key Messages

- Vaginal penetration is usually possible with angular deformity of less than 30°.
- In general, surgery should be reserved for men with more severe deformity.
- Men considering surgery should be warned about possible postsurgical complications, including residual deformity, bumpiness of the corporal wall, foreskin problems, loss of glans sensitivity and in older men impairment of rigidity.
- Hypospadias and downward curvature should be managed by a surgeon expert in urethral reconstructive surgery.
- Surgical correction of Peyronie's disease should be deferred until the acute painful phase has settled, usually 6 – 18 months after the onset of the condition.
- Some older men with Peyronie's disease consult because they find a lump and fear that this is cancer. In this situation, simple reassurance may be all that is needed.

I.4.2.1 Definition of the Disease

Erectile deformity is defined as an abnormal shape, direction or angulation of the rigid erect penis. The condition should be distinguished from bending or kinking because of lack of rigidity, which is one of the manifestations of erectile deficiency. The deformity may be categorized into cosmetic deformity that does not interfere with penetration (angulations less than 5° to 20°), deformity which makes penetration more difficult but not impossible (angulations between 20° and 45°) and severe deformity which makes penetration impossible (angulation of more than 45°). In general, intercourse is possible with greater degrees of upward or downward angulation than lateral angulation.

I.4.2.2 Aetiology and Pathogenesis

Deformity of erection may be congenital or acquired. Congenital downward (ventral) curvature (chordee) with or without rotational deformity occurs most commonly in association with hypospadias, more rarely without hypospadias but with congenital short urethra or very rarely with deficient ventral penile skin (webbed penis). The cause of downward bending is most often a thickened band of tissue deep to the urethra but more rarely there is no thickened band of tissue but the urethra or tunica is hypoplastic. Congenital lateral bending occurs in association with hypotrophy or very rarely aplasia of one or other corpora cavernosa.

Acquired deformity is most commonly seen in association with Peyronie's disease but also may occur after accidental and surgical trauma (e.g. gunshot wounds and botched cosmetic surgery).

I.4.2.2.1 Pathogenesis of Peyronie's Disease (Induratio Plastica, Van Buren's Disease)

There is probably more than one pathogenesis of Peyronie's disease and the word "disease" is misleading in this context. In some men, the condition is associated with Dupuytren's contracture and this may represent a disease of elastic connective tissue or unknown aetiology. However, for most men with Peyronie's disease, there is no associated Dupuytren's contracture. Sometimes there is a history of a traumatic episode, e.g. missing the vaginal orifice and pushing the erect penis against the pelvis followed by pain and sometimes bruising. In this situation the development of Peyronie's probably represents the response to a minor degree of penile fracture. In other cases, the onset is sudden and spontaneous with no obvious precipitating factors, but it may nevertheless be caused by small haemorrhages secondary to minor trauma because ageing changes have rendered the tunica albuginea more liable to trauma. There is some indication that Peyronie's may occur more frequently in older but more sexually active men, and if this is correct it supports the concept of trauma being an aetiological factor. A plaque may also develop as a complication of therapy for erectile dysfunction with intracorporeal injection of papaverine (Desai and Gingell 1988) and prostaglandin therapy (Chen et al. 1994). Whatever the initiating process, it continues with a painful inflammatory reaction and replacement of elastic tissue by hyalinized or fibrous scar tissue. As the scar tissue matures, a lump becomes apparent. Normally the scar is confined to the tunica albuginea of the corpora, but it may extend into the septum between the two corpora but it does not extend into the erectile tissue. Once a scar has formed, every time there is an erection there is excess pull at the edge of the scar and this can result in pain and further trauma to the normal cavernosal wall at the edge of the plaque and extension of the plaque. Plaques vary from a few millimetres in size to the entire dorsal shaft. Calcification may occur in the plaque as an end stage of the inflammatory process.

I.4.2.3 Clinical Findings: History, Physical Examination, Technical Investigations, Laboratory Findings

It is important to listen to the history, as there may be little to find on clinical examination of the flaccid penis, particularly in young men with a congenital abnormality. Questions should be asked about how long the man has had erectile deformity and whether there is a history of trauma. A lifelong history indicates a congenital problem. The features of Peyronie's disease include a history of painful bending of the erect penis. The pain usually resolves after 6–18 months, but pain is an indication that the inflammatory process is still active, that the process has not finished and that further bending may occur. Surgical treatment should be reserved until the active phase has resolved, otherwise further angulation can occur after the operation, which makes a second procedure necessary. Some men with Peyronie's have associated Dupuytren's contracture or a past history of surgical procedures for Dupuytren's. Often men with Peyronie's feel a lump and are concerned about the possibility of cancer. This fear rather than the degree of bending is the motivation for a percentage of men with Peyronie's disease to seek medical advice, and once reassurance is given no further treatment may be requested despite severe degrees of angulation. It is thus important when taking the patient's history to explore his motives for consultation. Other causes of angulation included failed cosmetic surgery, e.g. penis enlarging procedures such as fat injection, etc. Men who have undergone such procedures are usually embarrassed and reluctant to give details, especially if they have consulted with unqualified people, and it is important to avoid being judgemental during the consultation process.

On examination, there may be obvious problems such as hypospadias with a bifid foreskin, but the degree of downward bending caused by the associated chordee is usually much more severe than would be predicted from examination of the flaccid penis. Other more unusual findings include subcutaneous fibrosed lumps following implantation of foreign materials, inflammation surrounding liquid silicone, etc. However, more often there is no visible abnormality. In cases of Peyronie's disease, a firm to hard circumscribed plaque may be palpable, most often on the dorsal aspect of the penis, but the changes may be more subtle and it is often helpful to ask the man to demonstrate where he can feel the lump. The differential diagnosis of Peyronie's disease includes congenital curvature (no plaque palpable) and dorsal phlebitis (pain but no erectile deformity). Very rarely prostate cancer can metastasize into the corporal bodies but in this case erectile firmness is impaired, the penis remains rather turgid and there is no surface plaque to palpate but instead a general induration and the prostate feels abnormal. There is one case of penile sarcoma reported in the literature (Moore et al. 1975). Thus the man with a surface plaque in the erectile body can be confidently reassured that there is no malignancy.

If there is little to find and especially in younger men, the penis should be examined when erect. This can be done by asking the man to take photographs of his erect penis at home using a digital or Polaroid camera. Alternatively, the erect penis can be examined in the clinic after intracavernosal injection of prostaglandin or another pharmacological agent and photographs taken. Photographs should be taken from two different planes to demonstrate upwards and sideways angulation. If surgery is proposed it is important to emphasize to the patient that there is often a degree of residual bending. The degree of residual bending that may be left after surgery can be conveniently demonstrated to the patient at the same time as examination of his erect penis. The photographs may help during surgery and also provide a record of the preoperative situation in case there is any residual postoperative bending. Also, before giving prostaglandin for examination of an erect penis, it is important to obtain the patient's consent and to emphasize to him that the drug will cause an erection that may last for 1 or 2 h. He needs to attend the clinic with suitable clothing and be prepared to take time to allow the erection to subside afterwards. He needs to be warned about the small risk of priapism and given instructions that if the erection lasts for more than 1 h brisk walking up and down flights of stairs will help the erection subside.

I.4.2.3.1 Imaging

Colour Doppler and ultrasound and MRI images are helpful to confirm the diagnosis and determine the extent of Peyronie's plaques or bands of chordee tissue. MRI imaging may detect septal extension of Peyronie's plaques not seen with ultrasound (Nicolai et al. 1996) and also plaques at the base of the penis (Hauck et al. 2003). Ultrasound is better than MRI for the detection of calcification, which may be helpful in planning whether to opt for plaque incision or excision once the decision for surgery has been taken. Plaque enhancement after intravenous gadolinium-diethylenetriaminepentaacetic acid may indicate active local inflammation (Vosshenrich et al. 1995), but this has not been widely adopted to distinguish active inflammation from a mature plaque. At present this distinction is made according to whether the man is still experiencing pain or not. In general, MRI imaging does not add significantly to clinical examination supplemented with ultrasound imaging and the use of any imaging technique does not help with the decision for surgery

(Ahmed et al. 1998), which is based on the patient's wishes and disability as well as the observed deformity on examination of the erect penis. Both MRI and ultrasound imaging may help with the planning of surgery once the decision for surgery has been made, but the extra information from MRI compared with ultrasound does not at present justify the time and expense of MRI in this clinical situation.

I.4.2.4 Treatment

I.4.2.4.1 Treatment Depends on the Severity and Cause of the Problem

Medical and physical treatments have been used for Peyronie's disease particularly in the acute painful phase when surgery is not appropriate, but they have no place in the treatment of congenital deformity. Oral therapies include the anti-inflammatory agent potassium para-aminobenzoate (Potaba), colchicine, vitamin E (free oxygen radical scavenger), terfenadine (antihistamine) and tamoxifen. Local delivery by way of plaque injection has been used for verapamil (Levine et al. 2002), dexamethasone (Winter and Khanna 1975), interferon alpha 2a (Polat et al. 1997) and collagenase. Other treatments that have been advocated include irradiation (Mira et al. 1980) and lithotripsy. However, none of these nonsurgical treatments have gained wide acceptance despite positive reports from single-centre case series. There is a need for prospective randomized clinical trials to evaluate some of these treatment options, but at present it seems unlikely that any of them will truly cause an established Peyronie's scar to revert back to elastic normal tunica albuginea; therefore the main role of these treatments is likely to be early in the course of the process to arrest the process and prevent progression, which makes it extremely difficult to organize appropriate clinical trials. In general, once the painful Peyronie's process has run its 12- to 18-month course, surgery is the only option that will significantly alter angular deformity of the erect penis.

I.4.2.4.2 Minor Deformity

Minor degrees of lateral deviation (<20°) are common and usually do not interfere with penetration. They are best left alone, as the results of any corrective surgery may be no better or even worse than the original problem. Some young men with minor degrees of lateral deviation are very concerned about the problem, particularly if they have never had a sexual partner. They may be reassured by taking a thorough history and clinical examination and a clear explanation, but there may be a need for sexual counselling. In this situation, the sexual problem probably does not concern any minor lateral deviation of the erect penis but more the young man's concerns about body image and sexuality, and he may be very reluctant to accept any deformity at all. Nevertheless, a young man's desire for correction of a minor deformity has to be balanced against the risk of the operation making the deformity worse and some penile shortening.

I.4.2.4.3 More Severe Deformity Interfering with the Ability to Penetrate

If there is more severe deformity surgical treatment is the option to be considered, especially by younger men. In this situation, most men are prepared to accept a minor degree of residual deformity because it will be much better than their preoperative situation. However, not all men with penile deformity seek corrective surgical treatment. Some older men with Peyronie's disease consult because they find a lump and fear that this is cancer. In this situation, a clear explanation and reassurance may be all that is necessary.

Factors to take into consideration include the complexity and success of the surgical procedure, the rigidity of the erection and the disability caused by the deformity. In general, in younger men attempts should be made to correct all except minor degrees of erectile deformity, whereas in older men one must also take into account the quality of the rigidity. If an older man has angular deformity secondary to a Peyronie's plaque and evidence of impaired erectile rigidity there is likely to be concurrent impaired penile circulation. In general, surgery to correct angular deformity makes any erectile deficiency worse and in this situation the choice is between (1) a corrective operation and possible lack of rigidity postoperatively, despite adjuvant PDE inhibitor therapy, and if this fails the need for a second operation to insert a penile prosthesis and (2) proceeding with a penile prosthesis operation as the first surgical procedure. These choices and the risks and benefits should be discussed with the patient.

If there is downward angulation associated with hypospadias, congenital short urethra or chordee, then surgical treatment is usually undertaken in infancy to bring the urethral meatus to the end of the penis. Sometimes the correction of the chordee is inadequate and further surgery is needed, but this can be difficult because usually it is necessary to redo the urethroplasty to gain the extra urethral length and often the tissues are deficient. Such patients should be referred to a specialist centre where there is expertise in salvage urethral reconstructive surgery.

Once the decision has been taken to attempt surgical correction of angular deformity, there are two different surgical solutions: either to remove some of the wall of the corpus on the long side or to insert tissue or graft material on the short side, e.g. saphenous vein graft. In cases of Peyronie's disease, this may include plaque excision. In general, graft procedures are more complex because of uncertainty about the durability of some graft materials or the need to harvest the long saphenous vein from the upper part of the leg. If the penis is very long it is often better to shorten the long side because there are fewer complications compared with grafting procedures. Whichever method of correction is used, there is often 1 – 2 cm of shortening compared with the preoperative erect length and clear preoperative information should be given to the man about what he may expect.

Surgical access is by circumcision and degloving or by a midline ventral incision. For larger plaques, dorsal plaques and more extensive deformity, the usual surgical incision to gain access to the corpora is a circumcision and degloving of the penis and in more extensive cases buttonholing the penis through a scrotal incision. This exposure allows surgical access to the entire length of both the corpora cavernosa and the corpus spongiosum. It must be explained to the man that he will have a circular incision just under the corona and that he may have a secondary incision in the midline of the scrotum. The foreskin can be preserved or removed. If the patient chooses to retain the foreskin he needs to be aware that there is a significant chance of postoperative problems with the foreskin and there will be need for a secondary circumcision because of phimosis in a substantial proportion of cases. For ventral plaques and more minor deformity, an alternative incision is the ventral midline incision. This has the advantage that removal of the foreskin is not needed but the exposure is not as complete. Once the penis has been degloved, the degree of deformity can be reassessed with a saline-induced erection and if photographs have not already been taken it is wise to do so for comparison with post-correction photographs.

The most frequently performed surgical correction is the modified Nesbit operation for Peyronie's disease and a very similar procedure can be performed for congenital angulation due to imbalance in corporal growth. For men with Peyronie's disease, surgical correction should not be undertaken until the acute-phase painful reaction has settled; otherwise there is a risk of further progression after the operation. There are several variations in technique, including plication or double-breasting the corporeal wall with no corporeal wall excision or excising an ellipse or several ellipses of the corporeal wall. If a plication or double breasting technique is used strong nonabsorbable sutures should be used. If an ellipse or ellipses are excised either nonabsorbable or PDS sutures can be used.

It may be necessary to mobilize the neurovascular bundle. The nerves fan out towards the glans. The nearer the plaque to the glans the more lateral the mobilization has to be to avoid damage to the most lateral branches of the fanning out nerves. For ventral plaques, it may be necessary to mobilize the urethra. The plane between the urethra and the corpora is very thin and it is easy to perforate the urethral lumen, but if this is repaired at the time there is usually no consequence.

I.4.2.4.4
Nesbit Technique

Once the corpora have been exposed, the Nesbit procedure (Nesbit 1965) involves taking a wedge of tunica albuginea from the normal side. Depending on the extent of the curvature, it is often best to take several wedges. Variations in technique include making parallel incisions but not removing any tunica or simply placing nonabsorbable sutures. This latter technique sometimes produces a dramatic relapse if the sutures cut out or snap, resulting in a pinging sensation and a sudden return of the deformity; therefore, it is probably best to employ a technique that involves incising into the tunica wall. The technique I use is to take one or more wedges of tissue and use 3.0 PDS sutures to approximate the edges; this has produced consistent results (Syed 2003). A modification is thinning of the plaque with a carbide burr in association with a Nesbit procedure (Liu et al. 2003), but follow-up is needed to determine whether this produces long-term, worthwhile changes in the plaque.

I.4.2.4.5
Plaque Excision and Grafting Technique

The alternative more extensive procedure is to incise or excise the plaque and insert graft material. Possible graft materials include patches of the long saphenous vein, dermal grafts, dura, bovine pericardium or an artificial material such as Gore-Tex. As a general rule, artificial materials do not have as good elastic characteristics as vein patches and both dermal patches and dura tend to scar again over the long term. At present, the best long-term results are seen with vein patches. However, these can be tedious to harvest, as the procedure requires a separate groin incision and it may be necessary to sew several lengths of vein together to create an adequately sized patch, which lengthens the operating time. For older men with any predisposition to coronary artery disease, the use of long saphenous veins for correction of penile deformity can reduce options for coronary artery bypass surgery. Various graft techniques can be used. A long circumferential incision with forked ends can be used along with a graft of bovine pericardium (Egydio et al. 2004) or a patch created from several lengths of vein. An alternative, especially if the curvature is at several points, is to create several circumferential incisions with forked, modified H-shaped ends, and to insert several vein patches at different points. The actual best technique for a particular man depends on the hardness and extent of the plaques and the site or sites of the angulation. It can be very difficult, if not impossible, to incise and sew a vein patch into a rock-hard calcified plaque, or it may be very difficult to excise a very large plaque. The appropriate solution needs to be individually tailored for each case. There is a need for better graft materials that maintain elasticity over the long term. Tissue engineering holds promise of development of such materials (Schultheiss et al. 2004).

I.4.2.4.6 Insertion of a Penile Prosthesis

For older men with severe Peyronie's and a degree of erectile dysfunction, it can be better to insert a penile prosthesis to straighten the penis. In this situation, it still may be necessary during the surgical procedure to "fracture" the plaque after insertion of the prosthesis by inflating it and forcibly straightening the penis or to excise the plaque and insert a graft.

I.4.2.4.7 Which Technique to Use

The best technique depends on the extent and site of the plaque and whether there is any concurrent circulatory impairment and erectile deficiency. Each solution has to be tailored to the individual problem and therefore the andrologist who undertakes penile corrective surgery must be competent with a number of different operations, including Nesbit-type operations, grafting procedures and insertion of penile prostheses. Retrieval surgery after failed hypospadias repair is best dealt with by a surgeon with considerable experience and expertise in hypospadias surgery and should not be undertaken by andrologists without this expertise.

I.4.2.5 Results of Treatment

I.4.2.5.1 Nonsurgical Treatments for Peyronie's Disease

There is no evidence that nonsurgical treatments of an established Peyronie's plaque will cause regeneration of normal tunica wall elastic tissue. However, the use of the anti-inflammatory agent potassium para-aminobenzoate (Potaba) may prevent progression of the active disease (Carson 1997), but there is a lack of randomized controlled studies. It is also difficult to take because of the bulk of the dose (12 g per day) and because it can cause gastrointestinal upset. Vitamin E is also still sometimes used in the acute phase because it is an antioxidant and does no harm, but this is essentially placebo therapy. Irradiation has been abandoned. Lithotripsy gives some pain relief but after meta-analysis of the results from 17 centres, it was concluded that "pain seems to resolve faster after ESWT than during the natural history. The effect on plaque size and penile curvature is less impressive" (where ESWT is extracorporeal shock wave therapy; Hauck et al. 2004). Plaque injection with verapamil has been reported to improve pain and deformity but there is a lack of evidence from randomized controlled studies and the treatment has not been widely adopted.

I.4.2.5.2 Results of Surgery

Although standard assessment of penile curvature has been proposed (Kelami 1983), no standard assessment has been adopted and different centres have different assessment criteria. It is therefore difficult to make any comparison between results from different centres. Also, very few centres report long-term results. The literature indicates that 70–80% of men are satisfied with Nesbit-type results between 5 and 10 years postoperatively. There are fewer long-term published results after vein patch surgery, but results are similar (Table I.4.5).

Table I.4.5. Results of surgical treatments

Reference	Type of procedure	No. of men	Duration of follow-up	Result
Ralph et al. (1995)	Nesbit	359	Cases from 1977–1992	82% to 90% Satisfied
Savoca et al. (2000)	Nesbit	213	72 months, mean	88% Satisfied
Syed et al. (2003)	Nesbit	57	84 months, median	76% Satisfied
Schneider et al. (2003)	Modified Nesbit	68	25 months, mean	75% Satisfied
De Stefani et al. (2000)	Vein patch	8	Postoperative	87% Straight
Montorsi et al. (2000)	Vein patch	50	32 months, mean	80% Straight 94% Rigid
Porena et al. (2002)	Vein patch	12	1 month	83% Straight
Chang et al. (2002)	Vein patch	Review of case series	Variable	80% to 96% Straight 80% to 95% Rigid

I.4

For all surgical treatments, unwanted effects can include:

- Phimosis if the foreskin is left in situ.
- Shortening of 1–4 cm depending on the technique used. In general, grafting techniques cause less shortening. Some shortening is seen after almost all procedures. It is important to discuss shortening in the context of normal penile length because for the majority of men the simpler Nesbit-type procedure gives a good outcome, and in the context of normal penile length the amount of shortening does not interfere with partner satisfaction or the ability to penetrate.
- Residual minor angulation may occur because of fibrosis during the healing process or because of insufficient or over correction. Generally, angulation of less than 30° is compatible with vaginal penetration.
- Reduced or patchy glans sensation can occur if there is a need to mobilize the dorsal bundle as is often the case with dorsal Peyronie's plaques.
- Postoperative bumpiness, narrowing or bulging of the corporeal wall. If the preoperative deformity was very severe most men are happy to have a straight erection and will tolerate slight bumpiness of the corporeal wall, but it is wise to warn patients that there may be some residual scar tissue or that they may be able to feel the suture material.
- Postoperative deterioration in erectile rigidity. Often men with Peyronie's disease have concurrent vascular insufficiency and the trauma of operation or alteration of the intracavernosal haemodynamics (Grein and Schreiter 1996) can adversely affect this, so that although the deformity is corrected, erections are not sufficiently firm for intercourse. This outcome can be prevented by careful preoperative selection of cases and the use of a penile prosthesis instead of correctional surgery in appropriate cases.
- There is almost always considerable postoperative performance anxiety and it is good practice to make available adjuvant PDE inhibitors in the postoperative period for almost all men, irrespective of age.
- Postoperative disappointment can be reduced by good preoperative information and the avoidance of unrealistic expectations. It is not possible to attain or regain the perfect body morphology, but instead the aim of surgery is attainment or restoration of a good functional result.

I.4.2.6 Prevention

Good surgical results can be obtained by appropriate selection of treatments and by giving the patient, and if appropriate his partner, comprehensive information about what can and cannot be done as well as using adjuvant postoperative PDE inhibitor treatment.

References

Ahmed M, Chilton CP, Munson KW, Williams JH, Pallan JH, Turner G (1998) The role of colour Doppler imaging in the management of Peyronie's disease. Br J Urol 81:604–606

Carson CC (1997) Potassium para-aminobenzoate for the treatment of Peyronie's disease: is it effective? Tech Urol 3: 135–139

Chang JA, Gholami, SS Lue TF (2002) Surgical management: saphenous vein grafts. Int J Impot Res 14:375–378

Chen J, Godschalk M, Katz PG, Mulligan T (1994) Peyronie's-like plaque after penile injection of prostaglandin E1. J Urol 152:961–962

De Stefani S, Savoca G, Ciampalini S, Gattuccio I, Scieri F, Belgrano E (2000) Saphenous vein harvesting by 'stripping' technique and 'W'-shaped patch covering after plaque incision in treatment of Peyronie's disease. Int J Impot Res 12:299–230

Desai KM, Gingell JC (1988) Penile corporeal fibrosis complicating papaverine self-injection therapy for erectile impotence. Eur Urol 15:132–133

Egydio PH, Lucon AM, Arap S (2004) A single relaxing incision to correct different types of penile curvature: surgical technique based on geometrical principles. BJU Int 94:1147–1157

Grein U, Schreiter F (1996) Cavernous insufficiency after dermal graft corporoplasty; Kavernöse Insuffizienz nach Dermalgraftkorporoplastik. Urologe A 35:11–13

Hauck EW, Hackstein N, Vosshenrich R, Diemer T, Schmelz HU, Bschleipfer T, Schroeder-Printzen I, Weidner W (2003) Diagnostic value of magnetic resonance imaging in Peyronie's disease – a comparison both with palpation and ultrasound in the evaluation of plaque formation. Eur Urol 43:293–299; discussion 299–300

Hauck EW, Mueller UO, Bschleipfer T, Schmelz HU, Diemer T, Weidner W (2004) Extracorporeal shock wave therapy for Peyronie's disease: exploratory meta-analysis of clinical trials. J Urol 171:740–745

Kelami A (1983) Classification of congenital and acquired penile deviation. Urol Int 38:229–233

Levine LA, Goldman KE, Greenfield JM (2002) Experience with intraplaque injection of verapamil for Peyronie's disease. J Urol 168:621–625; discussion 625–626

Liu JH, Song XD, Wang T, Wang SG, Guo XL, Ye ZQ (2003) Experience of treating Peyronie's disease by plaque thinning with carbide burs and improved Nesbit technique. Zhonghua Nan Ke Xue 9:658–660

Mira JG, Chahbazian CM, Del Regato TA (1980) The value of radiotherapy for Peyronie's disease: presentation of 56 new case studies and review of the literature. J Radiat Oncol Biol Phys 6:161–166

Montorsi F, Salonia A, Maga T, Bua L, Guazzoni G, Barbieri L, Barbagli G, Chiesa R, Pizzini G, Rigatti P (2000) Evidence based assessment of long-term results of plaque incision and vein grafting for Peyronie's disease. J Urol 163:1704–1708

Moore SW, Wheeler JE, Hefter LG (1975) Epithelioid sarcoma masquerading as Peyronie's disease. Cancer 35:1706–1710
Nesbit RM (1965) Congenital curvature of the phallus: report of three cases with description of corrective operation J Urol 93:230–232
Nicolai M, Carriero A, De Thomasis R, Iantorno R, Longeri D, Zefferini M, Tenaglia R (1996) Dynamic magnetic resonance imaging versus dynamic echography in the staging of Peyronie's disease. Angiografia a risonanza magnetica dinamica versus ecografia dinamica nella stadiazione della malattia di La Peyronie. Arch Ital Urol Androl 68 [5 Suppl]:97–100
Polat O, Gul O, Ozbey I, Ozdikici M, Bayraktar Y (1997) Peyronie's disease: intralesional treatment with interferon alpha-2A and evaluation of the results by magnetic resonance imaging. Int Urol Nephrol 29:465–471
Porena M, Mearini L, Mearini E, Costantini E, Salomone U, Zucchi A (2002) Peyronie's disease: corporoplasty using saphenous vein patch graft. Urol Int 68:91–94
Ralph DJ, al-Akraa M, Pryor JP (1995) The Nesbit operation for Peyronie's disease: 16-year experience. J Urol 154:1362–1363
Savoca G, Trombetta C, Ciampalini S, De Stefani S, Buttazzi L, Belgrano E (2000) Long-term results with Nesbit's procedure as treatment of Peyronie's disease. Int J Impot Res 12:289–293
Schneider T, Sperling H, Schenck M, Schneider U, Rubben H (2003) Treatment of penile curvature–how to combine the advantages of simple plication and the Nesbit-procedure by superficial excision of the tunica albuginea. World J Urol 20:350–355
Schultheiss D, Lorenz RR, Meister R, Westphal M, Gabouev AI, Mertsching H, Biancosino C, Schlote N Wefer J, Winkler M, Stief CG, Jonas U (2004) Functional tissue engineering of autologous tunica albuginea: a possible graft for Peyronie's disease surgery Eur Urol 45:781–786
Syed Altaf H, Abbasi, Z, Hargeave T B (2003) Nesbit procedure for disabling Peyronies curvature: A median follow up of 84 months Urology 61:999–1003
Vosshenrich R, Schroeder-Printzen I, Weidner W, Fischer U, Funke M, Ringert RH (1995) Value of magnetic resonance imaging in patients with penile induration (Peyronie's disease). J Urol 153:1122–1125
Winter CC, Khanna R (1975) Peyronie's disease: results with dermo-jet injection of dexamethasone. J Urol 114:898–900

I.4.3 Ejaculatory Dysfunction: Premature Ejaculation, Delayed Ejaculation, Anejaculation, Low-Volume Ejaculation, Retrograde Ejaculation and Painful Ejaculation

T.B. Hargreave

Key Messages

- Premature ejaculation is the commonest cause of ejaculatory dysfunction.
- A proportion of men with premature ejaculation have lifelong oversensitivity of the ejaculatory reflex.
- If there is a lack of external ejaculation one of the first investigations is examination of the postcoital urine for spermatozoa, as this will distinguish between retrograde ejaculation and anejaculation.
- Poor urine flow and postorgasmic slow seepage of ejaculate are indicators of urethral stricture.
- Pain with ejaculation can be one of the manifestations of incomplete spinal injury.

I.4.3.1 Definition of the Disease

Ejaculatory dysfunction comprises premature ejaculation, delayed ejaculation, anejaculation, low ejaculate volume, lack of force of ejaculation, retrograde ejaculation and painful ejaculation.

I.4.3.1.1 Premature Ejaculation

Premature ejaculation is the inability to control ejaculation for a sufficient length of time during vaginal penetration. There is no definition of sufficiency and when normal human intercourse has been studied in the laboratory situation, ejaculation was found to occur in fewer than 20 coital thrusts in half of subjects (Masters and Johnson 1963).

For the purposes of scientific studies, a practical definition is an intravaginal latency time (IELT) of less than 60 s. This can be assessed with a stopwatch. There are various other assessment instruments (APA 2000; Rowland et al. 2001; Yuan et al. 2004).

I.4.3.1.2 Delayed Ejaculation

Delayed ejaculation is when excessive stimulation is required to obtain orgasm with ejaculation. This a subjective diagnosis and it is difficult to distinguish when delay becomes pathological. Overall, if the patient complains of delayed ejaculation his complaint should be taken at face value.

I.4.3.1.3
Anejaculation

Anejaculation is the complete absence of antegrade or retrograde ejaculation but with preservation of the sensation of orgasm.

I.4.3.1.4
Lack of Force of Ejaculation

This is a subjective complaint. In overt cases, there is a history of failure of any spurt of ejaculation at the time of orgasm but instead a seepage of semen for several minutes after orgasm.

I.4.3.1.5
Low Ejaculate Volume

The complaint of low ejaculate volume is self-explanatory, although most men have no idea of what normal ejaculation volume should be but nevertheless can distinguish that their ejaculate volume has diminished.

I.4.3.1.6
Retrograde Ejaculation

Retrograde ejaculation is the total or sometimes partial absence of an antegrade ejaculation and instead some or all of the semen passes back into the bladder. The semen is then subsequently voided out with the urine.

I.4.3.1.7
Painful Ejaculation

This is a painful sensation felt in the perineum, urethra or urethral meatus during and sometimes after ejaculation. It most commonly occurs with prostatitis and urethritis and often there is associated painful urination. The condition may or may not be distinguishable from orgasmic pain, which is usually neurogenic in aetiology and poorly localized.

I.4.3.2
Aetiology and Pathogenesis

I.4.3.2.1
Premature Ejaculation

Premature ejaculation may be physiological, psychological, primary lifelong or secondary to thyroid overactivity or neural or pelvic pathology.

Physiological premature ejaculation is common in the context of a young man with a new partner but usually this is self-resolving with simple reassurance. Psychological premature ejaculation can occur in association with psychosexual pathology. There is a strong correlation with anxiety (Corona et al. 2004). It was once thought that almost all premature ejaculation was psychological, but more recently the entity of primary lifelong premature ejaculation has been recognized. It is thought to be associated with diminished serotonergic neurotransmission, altered 5-HT2C or 5-HT1A receptors and higher serum leptin levels (Atmaca et al. 2002). Leptin is a hormone derived from fat cells which interacts with the serotonergic pathway in the CNS. The selective serotonin reuptake inhibitor (SSRI) antidepressant citalopram has been used to treat men with premature ejaculation and causes a decrease in CNS leptin level and conversely temporary premature ejaculation has been reported for 3–4 weeks after stopping the antidepressant citalopram (Adson and Kotlyar 2003). Further experimental studies are needed (Atmaca et al. 2003).

Secondary premature ejaculation has been reported after traumatic brain injury (Simpson et al. 2003), in association with haemodialysis (Aslan et al. 2003) and in association with prostatitis (Screponi et al. 2001).

I.4.3.2.2
Delayed Ejaculation

As men get older, there is an increasing delay in achieving ejaculation and this is a part of normal ageing. Pathological delayed ejaculation may occur as a consequence of the conditions that cause anejaculation (see the next section).

I.4.3.2.3
Anejaculation

The underlying aetiology may be psychogenic, neurogenic, drug-related or obstructive.

Neurogenic anejaculation is seen in spinal cord injury, cauda equina lesions, following retroperitoneal surgery (e.g. lymphadenectomy, aortic aneurysm, horseshoe kidney), following colorectal surgery, in association with Parkinson's disease, multiple sclerosis and diabetic autonomic neuropathy. It has been reported in a man with a prolactinoma (Rigaud et al. 1992).

Drug-related anejaculation may occur with antihypertensives, antipsychotics, antidepressants and alcohol.

Obstructive anejaculation may occur with congenital or acquired blockage of the ejaculatory ducts. There may be failure of development of the prostate or seminal vesicles or following prolonged inflammation of the prostate with fibrosis or when the prostate is replaced by tumour.

The condition may occur for social or religious reasons. Some young men learn to masturbate without ejaculation. This may be seen with orthodox Jews in order not to transgress religious laws based on the old testament story of Onan, or may be seen as a consequence of Tantric sex practices aimed at enhancing partner pleasure or for other "health" reasons. The consequence of these practices is deconditioning of the ejaculatory reflex, and ultimately this may cause anejaculation. It can also sometimes cause orgasmic pain, haematospermia and congestive prostatitis.

I.4.3.2.4 Lack of Force of Ejaculation

With ageing, there is a reduction in muscle tone of the urethral wall and one of the manifestations of this is reduced propulsion of ejaculation. It also occurs when there has been disruption of the normal urethral musculature, e.g. with urethral pathology such as stricture and diverticulum and following substitution urethroplasty.

I.4.3.2.5 Reduced Ejaculate Volume

Reduced ejaculate volume may occur because of androgen deficiency. The secretions of the prostate and seminal vesicles are androgen-dependent and ejaculate volume is a good indicator of androgen sufficiency. Also, ejaculate volume may be reduced if there is severe end-stage inflammation of the prostate and seminal vesicles.

I.4.3.2.6 Retrograde Ejaculation

Retrograde ejaculation can be caused by any condition that causes failure of bladder neck closure or an increased resistance at the apex of the prostate so that the least line of resistance to passage of semen is back into the bladder.

Neurogenic retrograde ejaculation occurs with neurological conditions that cause failure of bladder neck closure or spasticity of the pelvic floor or both. Conditions that can cause this include spinal cord injury, cauda equina lesions, spinal dysraphism, tethered spinal cord, and it can occur after anterior lumbar vertebral body fusion (particularly when a transperitoneal route is used; Sasso et al. 2003). It may follow disruption of the sympathetic chain by retroperitoneal surgery, e.g. following lymphadenectomy, sympathectomy and aortic aneurysm surgery. It may follow disruption of the pelvic plexus by pelvic surgery, including colorectal and anal surgery. It may occur with generalized neurological diseases such as multiple sclerosis and diabetic autonomic neuropathy (juvenile diabetes).

Various drugs interfere with bladder neck function. These include antihypertensives, alpha-1 adrenoreceptor antagonists, antipsychotics with an alpha-blocking effect, e.g. thioridazine and risperidone (Shiloh et al. 2001; Loh et al. 2004) and antidepressants.

Anatomical bladder neck incompetence can occur in association with congenital defects of the trigone, including hemitrigone and with ectopic ureters (Lee et al. 2000) following bladder neck surgery, bladder neck resection and prostatectomy.

Obstruction at the apex prostate can be caused by congenital abnormalities such as ectopic ureterocele, urogenital sinus remnants, membranous urethral stricture and verumontanum hyperplasia.

It has also been reported in a man with drug-resistant hypertension and a retroperitoneal phaeochromocytoma (Widjaja et al. 2000).

I.4.3.3 Clinical Findings: History, Physical Examination, Technical Investigations, Laboratory Findings

I.4.3.3.1 History

All patients should be asked about whether the problem has been lifelong or acquired. History taking should include a full history of previous illness, including psychotic or depressive illness, any injuries or operations, including neck, spinal or pelvic injuries, or operations and any urinary tract operation performed during infancy. Any urinary symptoms should be noted, including whether the urine flow is good and whether the urine stream sprays (spraying indicates disturbance of normal urethral anatomy). All prescribed medicines and any other medicines or alternative treatments should be noted. It is also important to enquire about alcohol and drugs of abuse.

In addition to the above and depending on the exact complaint, direct questions should be asked on the subjects below.

Premature Ejaculation

In acquired cases, questions should be asked about symptoms suggestive of prostatitis, including prior history of sexually transmitted infection and treatment.

Delayed Ejaculation

This is a subjective complaint. In some cases the patient may go to extreme lengths to overcome his problem, including extended use of vibrators and other mechanical stimulatory techniques. Enquiry should be made about whether the problem is getting worse, as this may indicate a progressive lesion.

Anejaculation and Retrograde Ejaculation

The history given is of a lack of external ejaculation. It should be determined whether there is a lack of orgasm, in which case the problem is one of anorgasmia, or whether orgasm is present but there is a lack of external ejaculation. The patient should be asked about nocturnal emissions. If these occur and if there is no other disease process, then the problem is more likely to be one of psychogenic anejaculation (Hovav et al. 1999). Retrograde ejaculation is the more likely diagnosis if there is a history of passage of cloudy material in the postorgasmic urine.

Lack of Force of Ejaculation

The typical history is of a lack of any spurt of ejaculation but seepage of ejaculate for several minutes after orgasm. If there is also a history of poor urine flow urethral stricture is highly likely. If there is history of perineal swelling or dampness urethral diverticulum or fistula are possibilities. There may be a past history of sexually transmitted infection or urethral instrumentation.

Reduced Ejaculate Volume

Reduced ejaculate volume may be interpreted as reduced force of ejaculation. When this is secondary to androgen insufficiency, there may be other stigmata such as reduced libido, night sweats, tiredness, etc.

Painful Ejaculation

Painful ejaculation is usually associated with urethral or prostate inflammation, whereas orgasmic pain is usually neuropathic and associated with spinal or pelvic injury. However, the conditions may be difficult to distinguish. Note should be made of any prior sexually transmitted infection and whether there is urethral pain on urination of any prostatitis-related symptoms such as suprapubic pain and frequency and urgency of urination.

I.4.3.3.2 Clinical Examination

Clinical examination should include endocrine status and examination of the genitalia. The foreskin should be retracted and the external urethral meatus inspected and note made of any inflammatory changes. Rectal examination should include an assessment of anal tone and whether there is any abnormal pain or tenderness on prostatic palpation. Neurological examination should include the testing of lower limb reflexes, plantar responses and identification of any gross sensory loss, including perianal and sacral sensation. Gentle squeezing of the testicle should produce an unpleasant sensation but if diminished this may indicate autonomic neuropathy. Assessment of anal tone is done at the same time as rectal examination. Assessment may include the cremasteric response and bulbocavernosus reflex. If any abnormality is detected referral for neurological examination is recommended.

I.4.3.3.3 Laboratory and Other Investigations

Retrograde ejaculation can be distinguished from anejaculation by the finding of sperm in the postorgasmic urine.

Sometimes it is difficult to diagnose anejaculation, particularly in men who have never masturbated. In this case, the man should be encouraged to produce a semen sample during normal intercourse but wearing a silicone condom.

Further investigations may include urethroscopy or urethrography in cases of suspected stricture. It is worth noting that urine flow rate assessment is not a reliable indicator of urethral stricture. Pelvic anatomy may be assessed by CT or MRI scan. Prostate anatomy may be assessed by transrectal ultrasound or pelvic CT or MRI. Pelvic neurophysiology can be studied using sacral evoked responses, but these neurophysiological tests are little used in clinical practice because they are not very reliable (Desai et al. 1988) and usually do not affect management.

I.4.3.4 Treatment

In all cases of ejaculatory problem, the first approach is to treat any underlying disease process, e.g. ensure good diabetic control in a man with diabetes, treat prostatitis, etc. Any medication that may be causing the problem should be stopped, if possible, or substituted. Also, treatment depends on the type of ejaculation disorder and whether the man is seeking to enable his fertility, normalize his sexual function or both. In terms of fertility, it is often appropriate at an early stage in treatment to discuss with the patient and his partner home insemination techniques and sperm retrieval techniques such as microepididymal sperm aspiration (MESA), because the treatment of the underlying ejaculatory disorder may not be successful or may take a long time. In addition, treatment depends on the nature of the ejaculatory problem.

I.4.3.4.1 Treatment of Premature Ejaculation

Treatment of premature ejaculation (PE) depends on whether it is lifelong or acquired. For acquired or recent

Table I.4.6. Treatments for nonpsychogenic premature ejaculation in order of efficacy

Simple reassurance	
Ease and squeeze technique	SSRIs are better than ease and squeeze (Abdel-Hamid et al. 2001)
Topical local anaesthetic cream or spray applied 15–20 min (but not longer) before sexual contact (Atikeler et al. 2002)	Topical anaesthetic better than placebo inert cream in double-blind trial (Busato and Galindo 2004)
On demand treatment with SSRIs Daily treatment with SSRIs or tricyclics	Meta-analysis of studies between 1973 and 2003 indicated that the overall efficacy of the SSRI paroxetine was more effective than sertraline and fluoxetine and more effective that the tricyclic clomipramine (Anafranil) (De Stefani et al. 2000)
Combination topical anaesthetic and SSRI	Combination of topical local anaesthetic and fluoxetine has been found to be more efficacious than fluoxetine alone (Atan et al. 2000)

PE, treatment can proceed in a stepwise manner (Table I.4.6), depending on the severity of the problem. For lifelong PE, the choice is between topical anaesthetic or drugs because reassurance and ease and squeeze are ineffective. At present, the main drug treatment is with selective serotonin uptake inhibitors (SSRIs) and the tricyclic clomipramine, but side-effects of drug treatment can be bothersome: sleepiness at the time of coitus with SSRIs and next day nausea with clomipramine. Drug treatment is evolving and it has been proposed that the most efficacious drug is likely to be a combination of a 5-hydroxytryptamine (5-HT)2c receptor stimulation and a 5-HT1A receptor inhibitor. Although there are no published reports in the literature, there are anecdotal reports that monoamine oxidase inhibitors are effective in some cases where SSRIs have not been effective (F. Comhaire, personal communication).

I.4.3.4.2 Treatment of Delayed Ejaculation and Anejaculation

Often it is not possible to correct any underlying abnormality, e.g. after retroperitoneal lymph node dissection, and in such cases treatment results are poor. Provided the lumbosacral segments of the spinal cord are intact, some men are helped by the use of a vibrator (Sonksen and Ohl 2002), applied at the frenulum using 100 Hz and 6,000 vibrations per minute (Everaert and Oosterlinck 1997). Electroejaculation can be used to obtain sperm and is successful in 90 % of men (Lucas et al. 1991), which has replaced the older physostigmine treatment (Blockmans and Steeno 1988). The technique of electroejaculation is described in Chap. I.3.1. Prostatic massage has been used to obtain sperm from men with psychogenic anejaculation (Hovav et al. 2000) and when possible this is logistically easier than electroejaculation, which requires general anaesthesia.

With lack of force of ejaculation, an underlying abnormality such as urethral stricture should be corrected. Older men with no underlying abnormality should be given a clear explanation about urethral laxity with ageing and the effect this has on diminished force of ejaculation and postmicturition dripping.

I.4.3.4.3 Retrograde Ejaculation

Treatments to restore antegrade ejaculation include the use of alpha receptor stimulating drugs such as ephedrine and amezinium (an antihypotensive agent) (Ichiyanagi et al. 2003) or restoration of bladder neck competence by injection of bulking agents (Nagai et al. 2004) or bladder neck surgery. However, the chance of success following the injection of bulking agents or surgical treatment has to be balanced against the risk of causing urinary tract obstruction. Treatments to enable fertility include sperm recovery from the urine, bladder washings and MESA ICSI.

I.4.3.5 Prognosis

When the ejaculatory disorder is associated with pelvic nerve injury, there may be a degree of recovery, but once 2 years has passed, little further recovery will occur. There is no recovery after spinal injury. In general, it is nearly always possible to enable fertility but restoration of normal sexual function is much less certain.

I.4.3.6 Prevention

In cases of physiological premature ejaculation in younger men, subsequent sexual dysfunction can be prevented if the problem is taken seriously and the patient is given a clear explanation of what is happening and in appropriate cases supportive therapy with topical local anaesthetic or SSRIs.

References

Abdel-Hamid IA, El Naggar EA, El Gilany AH (2001) Assessment of as needed use of pharmacotherapy and the pause-squeeze technique in premature ejaculation. Int J Impot Res 13:41–45

Adson DE, Kotlyar M (2003) Premature ejaculation associated with citalopram withdrawal. Ann Pharmacother 37:1804–1806

American Psychiatric Association (2000) American Psychiatric Association Diagnostic and statistical manual of mental disorders, 4th edn. American Psychiatric Association, Washington DC

Aslan G, Arslan D, Cavdar C, Sifil A, Esen AA, Camsari T (2003) Analysis of premature ejaculation in hemodialysis patients using the International Index of Erectile Function. Urol Int 70:59–61

Atan A, Basar MM, Aydoganli L (2000) Comparison of the efficacy of fluoxetine alone vs. fluoxetine plus local lidocaine ointment in the treatment of premature ejaculation. Arch Esp Urol 53:856–858

Atikeler MK, Gecit I, Senol FA (2002) Optimum usage of prilocaine-lidocaine cream in premature ejaculation. Andrologia 34:356–359

Atmaca M, Kuloglu M, Tezcan E, Semercioz A, Ustundag B, Ayar A (2002) Serum leptin levels in patients with premature ejaculation. Arch Androl 48:345–350

Atmaca M, Kuloglu M, Tezcan E, Ustundag B, Semercioz A (2003) Serum leptin levels in patients with premature ejaculation before and after citalopram treatment. BJU Int 91: 252–254

Blockmans D, Steeno O (1988) Physostigmine as a treatment for anejaculation with paraplegic men. Andrologia 20: 311–313

Busato W, Galindo CC (2004) Topical anaesthetic use for treating premature ejaculation: a double- blind, randomized, placebo-controlled study. BJU Int 93:1018–1021

Corona G, Petrone L, Mannucci E, Jannini EA, Mansani R, Magini A, Giommi R, Forti G, Maggi M (2004) Psycho-Biological correlates of rapid ejaculation in patients attending an andrologic unit for sexual dysfunctions. Eur Urol 46:615–622

Desai KM, Dembny K, Morgan H, Gingell JC, Prothero D (1988) neurophysiological investigation of diabetic impotence. Are sacral response studies of value? Br J Urol 61: 68–73

Everaert K, Oosterlinck W (1997) Diagnosis and treatment of psychosocial induced anejaculation or anorgasm by vibratory stimulation. Acta Urol Belg 65:59–61

Hovav Y, Dan-Goor M, Yaffe H, Almagor M (1999) Nocturnal sperm emission in men with psychogenic anejaculation. Fertil Steril 72:364–365

Hovav Y, Kafka I, Horenstein E, Yaffe H (2000) Prostatic massage as a method for obtaining spermatozoa in men with psychogenic anejaculation (letter). Fertil Steril 74:184–185

Ichiyanagi O, Sasagawa I, Suzuki Y, Matsuki S, Itoh K, Miura M, Tomita Y (2003) Successful treatment of retrograde ejaculation with amezinium. Arch Androl 49:215–217

Lee SS, Sun GH, Yu DS, Chen HI, Chang SY (2000) Giant hydronephrosis of a duplex system associated with ureteral ectopia: a cause of retrograde ejaculation. Arch Androl 45:19–23

Loh C, Leckband SG, Meyer JM, Turner E (2004) Risperidone-induced retrograde ejaculation: case report and review of the literature. Int Clin Psychopharmacol 19:111–112

Lucas MG, Hargreave TB, Edmond P, Creasey GH, McParland M, Seager SW (1991) Sperm retrieval by electro-ejaculation. Preliminary experience in patients with secondary anejaculation. Br J Urol 67:191–194

Masters WH, Johnson VE (1963) The sexual response of the human male. I. Gross anatomic considerations. Western J Surg 71:85–95

Nagai A, Nasu Y, Watanabe M, Tsugawa M, Iguchi H, Kumon H (2004) Analysis of retrograde ejaculation using color Doppler ultrasonography before and after transurethral collagen injection. Int J Impot Res 16:456–458

Rigaud P, Jacquet G, Viennet G, Bittard H (1992) A rare psychogenic anejaculation. Report of a case of prolactin adenoma (in French) Prog Urol 2:459–463

Rowland DL, Cooper SE, Schneider M (2001) Defining premature ejaculation for experimental and clinical investigations. Arch Sex Behav 30:235–253

Sasso RC, Kenneth Burkus J, LeHuec JC (2003) Retrograde ejaculation after anterior lumbar interbody fusion: transperitoneal versus retroperitoneal exposure. Spine 28:1023–1026

Screponi E, Carosa E, Di Stasi SM, Pepe M, Carruba G, Jannini EA (2001) Prevalence of chronic prostatitis in men with premature ejaculation. Urology 58:198–202

Shiloh R, Weizman A, Weizer N, Dorfman-Etrog P, Munitz H (2001) Risperidone-induced retrograde ejaculation. Am J Psychiatry 158:650

Simpson G, McCann B, Lowy M (2003) Treatment of premature ejaculation after traumatic brain injury. Brain Inj 17:723–729

Sonksen J, Ohl DA (2002) Penile vibratory stimulation and electroejaculation in the treatment of ejaculatory dysfunction. J Androl 25:324–332

Waldinger MD, Zwinderman AH, Schweitzer DH, Olivier B (2004) Relevance of methodological design for the interpretation of efficacy of drug treatment of premature ejaculation: a systematic review and meta-analysis. Int J Impot Res 16:369–381

Widjaja A, Truss MC, Rademaker J, Stief CB, von zur Muhlen A (2000) An unusual cause of retrograde ejaculation and hypertension. Scand J Urol Nephrol 34:217–218

Yuan YM, Xin ZC, Jiang H, Guo YJ, Liu WJ, Tian L, Zhu JC (2004) Sexual function of premature ejaculation patients assayed with Chinese Index of Premature Ejaculation. Asian J Androl 6:121–126

I.4.4 Orgasm Dysfunction

T.B. Hargreave

Key Messages

- Orgasm, like pain, is a sensation and is difficult to categorize objectively.
- There is an alteration in the quality of the sensation of orgasm after common surgical procedures such as transurethral resection of the prostate; men about to undergo such procedures need to be made aware of this.
- Following orgasm, there is an increase in serum prolactin and this relates to the duration of the refractory period and postorgasmic sexual behaviour.
- Postorgasmic spinal ice-pick pain following partial spinal cord transaction is difficult to treat and if present for 2 years after injury is unlikely to improve.

I.4.4.1 Definition of the Disease

Included in this category is lack of orgasm (anorgasmia), reduced or diminished orgasm, painful orgasm (odynorgasmia, dysorgasmia) and unwanted multiple orgasms.

I.4.4.1.1 Anorgasmia

Anorgasmia is the inability to reach orgasm; if the spinal cord is intact it is usually associated with anejaculation. After spinal injury and with spinal cord transaction, it may be possible to stimulate reflex ejaculation, but there is no sensation of orgasm.

I.4.4.1.2 Reduced Intensity Orgasm

Altered sensation and reduced intensity of orgasm often follows radical prostatic surgery. There are two components to this: in part the altered sensation is because of the altered anatomy and the lack of the feeling of the ejaculate passing through the prostate and urethra, but also there is reduced intensity of sensation because of damage to local neural pathways.

I.4.4.1.3 Painful Orgasm

This is defined as diffuse (not well localized) pain in the pelvic/sacral/lumbar spine area at the time and immediately following orgasm, with or without radiation or referral to the lower limbs and back. The condition may be difficult to distinguish from ejaculation-associated prostatic or urethral pain, which is better localized. A separate entity is orgasmic headaches, epileptiform aura or migraines triggered by orgasm.

I.4.4.1.4 Unwanted Multiple Orgasms

A small proportion of men experience multiple orgasms (Dunn and Trost 1989). Very occasionally, the condition is acquired secondary to prostate or seminal vesicle inflammation (van der Schoot and Ypma 2002) and sufficiently bothersome to need treatment.

I.4.4.2 Aetiology and Pathogenesis

Orgasm has been shown to induce increased prolactin levels for over 1 h in healthy males and females, and it may form a feedback regulator of dopaminergic systems and regulate the refractory period and sexual appetitive behaviour following orgasm (Kruger et al. 2003a). Furthermore, the prolactin response was found to be absent in a multiorgasmic man (Haake et al. 2002) and also short-term increases or decreases in serum prolactin have been shown to increase or decrease the refractory period, respectively (Kruger et al. 2003b). There is experimental evidence that endogenous opioids modulate the intensity of orgasm and the opiate receptor antagonist naltrexone has been shown to enhance the orgasmic response (Sathe et al. 2001), whereas heroin abuse is associated with diminished or absent orgasm. Diminished or absent orgasm has been reported following medication with SSRI antidepressants (Haberfellner and Rittmannsberger 2004) and the anticonvulsant gabapentin (Brannon and Rolland 2000) but probably occurs with many other antipsychotic drugs and is almost certainly underreported (Compton and Miller 2001). In one study, sildenafil has been shown to reduce the refractory period (Mondaini et al. 2003), but it is not known whether this is a central or peripheral action. There is a need for improved understanding of the central neuropharmacological events that regulate orgasm.

Lack of orgasm may be the result of spinal cord pathology, following fracture of the posterior pelvis with damage to the pelvis plexus, and after radical pelvic surgery, or radical prostate surgery (Table I.4.7).

Table I.4.7. Postradical prostatectomy orgasmic dysfunction

No change in orgasm	22%
Decreased orgasm	37%
Complete anorgasmia	37%
Painful orgasm (odynorgasmia, dysorgasmia)	14%

N = 239. Data from Barnas et al. (2004)

Altered sensation of orgasm may occur after pelvic fracture and as a result of pelvic and after transurethral and radical prostatic surgery (Table I.4.7) and in association with prostatic and seminal vesicle inflammatory disease. The antidepressant roboxetine has been associated with delayed orgasm and orgasmic pain (Haberfellner 2002).

Painful orgasm is reported by some men with incomplete spinal transaction, compressive spondylitic cervical myelopathy, tethered spinal cord (Jacome 1998), after pelvic fracture, after radical prostatectomy and also in association with severe prostatitis and epididymitis. There are other very rare causes; for example, this author has seen painful orgasm as the first presentation of human variant Creutzfeldt–Jakob (CJD) disease. It may also occur in men with multiple sclerosis.

I.4.4.3 Clinical Findings: History, Physical Examination, Technical Investigations, Laboratory Findings

It is difficult to obtain a good medical history about orgasm because men often lack the vocabulary to express what they feel and standardized questions and assessment instruments have not been developed. The patient should be allowed to describe his problem before he is asked additional questions.

If the problem is absent, diminished or altered orgasm, the clinical history should elicit obvious factors such as spinal cord and pelvic injury or pathology or previous pelvic or prostatic surgery. If there is radiation of the pain to the back or lower limbs, this is more suggestive of spinal cord abnormality. If there are no obvious factors, enquiry should be made about all medication and substance abuse. History of urinary frequency, lower abdominal and pelvic pain or testicular pain may indicate the diagnosis of prostatitis.

If the problem is pain it may be felt in the pelvis, lumbar spine or more rarely in other areas such as the foot or cervical spine. The pain may be very severe and has been described as ice-pick-like pain. Another type of pain that may occur is orgasm-related headache. Two varieties of headache have been described: muscle contraction headache occurring as sexual excitement increases and severe throbbing or explosive-type headache, occurring at the time of orgasm, and presumably of vascular origin, but more often than not no underlying vascular pathology can be detected.

Clinical examination should include examination of the genitalia and rectal examination with palpation of the prostate. Neurological examination should also be performed. If a neurological cause is suspected then the patient should be referred to the appropriate clinic for MRI scanning of the spine. Endocrinological assessment should include examination of the breast for galactorrhoea, basic assessment of visual fields and measurement of serum prolactin.

I.4.4.4 Treatment

I.4.4.4.1 Treatment to Improve Orgasm

If possible, the underlying cause of the problem should be treated but more often than not this is not possible. If the man is taking antidepressants these should be stopped if possible or substituted, but if this is not possible then the patient can be reassured that the orgasmic problem is likely to resolve once the antidepressant treatment is no longer needed. It is likely that medication to improve orgasm will become available as understanding of central mechanisms improves; possible options include opiate receptor antagonists.

I.4.4.4.2 Treatment for Repeated Orgasm

Repeated orgasm is a rare problem. The underlying cause of the problem should be treated, and in extreme cases this may involve surgery to remove seminal vesicles or the prostate. When no cause can be defined, it may be worth trying treatment with a drug known to diminish the orgasmic response such as a SSRI antidepressant.

I.4.4.4.3 Treatment of Orgasmic Pain

If possible the underlying cause should be treated, e.g. an operation to relieve spinal cord tethering, etc. Unfortunately, there is no satisfactory treatment for men with spinal cord or pelvic injury and those who develop postorgasmic pelvic pain, as pain-relieving medicines if given prior to sexual activity and in sufficient dose to ameliorate pain tend also to stop the desire for sexual activity, which is in any case usually inhibited by the fear of the pain. If orgasm-related pain persists for more than 2 years following spinal injury, then it is likely to be permanent.

I.4.4.4.4 Treatment of Orgasmic Headaches

Vasculogenic orgasm-associated headache has been reported to have a benign course and apart from correcting obvious factors such as hypertension, the patient can usually be reassured that there is no underlying sinister cause. Muscular spasm headaches can be helped by complimentary therapies such as massage. It is often appropriate to refer such patients to headache or migraine clinics.

References

Barnas JL, Pierpaoli S, Ladd P, Valenzuela R, Aviv N, Parker M, Waters WB, Flanigan RC, Mulhall JP (2004) The prevalence and nature of orgasmic dysfunction after radical prostatectomy. BJU Int 94:603–605

Brannon GE, Rolland PD (2000) Anorgasmia in a patient with bipolar disorder type 1 treated with gabapentin. J Clin Psychopharmacol 20:379–381

Compton MT, Miller AH (2001) Sexual side effects associated with conventional and atypical antipsychotics. Psychopharmacol Bull 35:89–108

Dunn ME, Trost JE (1989) Male multiple orgasms: a descriptive study. Arch Sex Behav 18:377–387

Haake P, Exton MS, Haverkamp J, Kramer M, Leygraf N, Hartmann U, Schedlowski M, Krueger TH (2002) Absence of orgasm-induced prolactin secretion in a healthy multi-orgasmic male subject. Int J Impot Res 14:133–135

Haberfellner EM (2002) Sexual dysfunction caused by reboxetine. Pharmacopsychiatry 35:77–78

Haberfellner EM, Rittmannsberger H (2004) Spontaneous remission of SSRI-induced orgasm delay. Pharmacopsychiatry 37:127–130

Jacome DE (1998) Masturbatory-orgasmic extracephalic pain. Headache 38:138–141

Kruger TH, Haake P, Chereath D, Knapp W, Janssen OE, Exton MS, Schedlowski M, Hartmann U (2003a) Specificity of the neuroendocrine response to orgasm during sexual arousal in men. J Endocrinol 177:57–64

Kruger TH, Haake P, Haverkamp J, Kramer M, Exton MS, Saller B, Leygraf N, Hartmann U, Schedlowski M (2003b) Effects of acute prolactin manipulation on sexual drive and function in males. J Endocrinol 179:357–365

Mondaini N, Ponchietti R, Muir GH, Montorsi F, Di Loro F, Lombardi G, Rizzo M (2003) Sildenafil does not improve sexual function in men without erectile dysfunction but does reduce the postorgasmic refractory time. Int J Impot Res 15:225–228

Sathe RS, Komisaruk BR, Ladas AK, Godbole SV (2001) Naltrexone-induced augmentation of sexual response in men. Arch Med Res 32:221–226

Van der Schoot DK, Ypma AF (2002) Seminal vesiculectomy to resolve defecation-induced orgasm. BJU Int 90:761–762

I.4.5 Abnormal Libido

B. Brosig

Key Messages

- Abnormal libido is a complex sexual dysfunction of psychosomatic aetiological origin in which somatic, psychic and cultural aspects of human sexual response interact.
- Disorders of sexual hyperarousal, often signs of paraphilias, and lack or loss of sexual arousal, a common disorder, can be distinguished.
- Clinical investigation should include, in addition to a careful evaluation of the somatic status with extensive hormonal analyses, psychodynamic interviews.
- Treatment options include drug modulation of sexual drives by hormones, individual or couple therapy or a combination of these choices.
- Patients' prognostic features are duration of symptoms, underlying individual psychopathology, resulting in psychotherapeutic restrictions and response to possible somatic treatment alternatives.

I.4.5.1 Definition

"Libido", a Latin word meaning "desire, pleasure", is used in a psychological context as a basic term for every type of psychic energy that accompanies the drives or instincts. It is mainly motivated by sexual or aggressive impulses and thus the biological bedrock of psychic functioning. In this conceptual context, "libido disorder" can be understood as a somewhat imprecise, i.e. global term, for quantitative sexual disorders that present themselves clinically either as sexual dysfunctions or absence of sexual interest or as hypersexuality. Since disorders of sexual identity or preferences in the choice of a sexual object are covered by particular chapters in this volume, the following section will focus on the areas lack or loss of sexual desire, sexual aversion, lack of sexual enjoyment and excessive sexual drive. Internationally, a set of research criteria has been implemented for the diagnosis of a libido disorder. These criteria are given in the following.

I.4.5.1.1 Diagnostic Criteria

The ICD 10 (International Classification of Diseases, Version 10, criteria of research) gives the following definitions of disorders of libido.

I.4.5.1.2 General Criteria

F52 Sexual dysfunction, not caused by organic disorder or disease
- G1. The subject is unable to participate in a sexual relationship, as he or she would wish
- G2. The dysfunction occurs frequently, but may be absent on some occasions
- G3. The dysfunction has been present for at least 6 months
- G4. The dysfunction is not entirely attributable to any of the other mental and behavioural disorders in ICD 10, physical disorders (such as endocrine disorder) or drug treatment

I.4.5.1.3 Specific Symptomatology

F52.0	Lack or loss of sexual desire
F52.1	Sexual aversion and lack of sexual enjoyment, specified as
F52.1.0	Sexual aversion or
F52.1.1	Lack of sexual enjoyment
F52.2–6	Covers different disorders of sexual function (such as failure of genital response, orgasmic dysfunction, premature ejaculation, nonorganic vaginismus, nonorganic dyspareunia), which are not part of a concept of libido disorder
F52.7	Excessive sexual drive

I.4.5.2 Epidemiology

In an overview (Spector and Carey 1990), prevalence data from 23 studies on sexual dysfunction were evaluated. It could be shown that, in clinical populations, libido disorders are commonly encountered conditions and prevalence rates are still substantial in a given general population (see Table I.4.8). Rising rates of hypoactive sexual desire disorders (HSDD), up to 50% for women and 10% for men, were reported for a Swiss clinical population (Gnirss-Bornet 2004).

In a general German population survey (Brähler et al. 2004), conducted in fall 2003, around 2.2% of all men between 14 and 54 already used sexual stimulants such as sildenafil, whereas rising percentages (up to 4.8%) for the German male population over 75 years were sexual stimulant users. Taking the limitations of this study into account, it can be deduced from these data that the prevalence rates for the loss of libido are somewhere over 2% to 5% in a general male population, depending on age, if the use of lifestyle drugs such as sildenafil is taken as operationalization.

Table I.4.8. Epidemiology of sexual dysfunctions

	Clinical Populations (%)	General Populations (%)
Female		
Anorgasmia	18–76	5–18
Low libido	51–80	11–48
Vaginismus	12–17	1– 4
Dyspareunia	3– 5	8–23
Male		
Erectile failure	36–50	3– 9
Premature ejaculation	15–46	26–36
Anorgasmia	3– 8	1–10
Low libido	16–32	NA

I.4.5.3 Aetiology and Pathogenesis

Sexual desire as a motivating force is represented in four areas of the mid-brain (hypothalamic, periaqueductal, mesocortical and thalamic representations). Lesions of the brain in these regions, thus, may be causes of altered sexual behaviour such as hypersexuality or loss of sexual motivation. There is strong evidence that there are differing gender-specific localizations for the sexual drives in male and female mammals.

Table I.4.9 summarizes the different aetiological facets of libido disorder, conceptualizing it as a complex interplay of different aetiological layers and pathogenetic pathways (Gnirss-Bornet 2004). As paramount endocrine influences on the intensity of sexual drives, androgens and prolactin were isolated as regulating factors in the short term (refractorial period; Krueger et al. 2002) as well as in the long run (Thibaut et al. 1994; Graziottin 2000; Demers 2003; Castro-Acuna et al. 2004).

Table I.4.9. Aetiological aspects of libido disorders

Biological	Psychological	Social Factors
Hormones	Stress	Gender-specific role behaviour
Age	Body image	Sexual norms
Medication	Psychic disorders and conflicts	Sexual stimuli in public
Severe somatic diseases	Deviant sexual inclinations	Emergencies

Since human sexuality is relational in its nature, social and partnership issues play, parallel to individual inhibitions or arrests in ego development, a major role in the development of a hypoactive sexual desire disorder (Apt et al. 1993; Weeks and Gambescia 2002). Normal sexual behaviour, as a consequence, depends on inner psychic developmental processes (psychic maturation) on the one hand and culture-specific pathways of socialization (sex roles, gender differences, development of sexual identity, mating behaviour) on the other (Levine 2003).

The lack of sexual desire may, in this context, be part of an individual sexual inhibition (Kernberg 1999; Gnirss-Bornet 2004) or, seen from the couple and family system, be part of a dysfunctional relationship with a partner: sexual couple collusion (Clement 1996, 2002). In long-lasting partnerships (Brosig 2002), the different aetiological causes often lead to a multifaceted clinical picture with an age-related organic decrease in sexual drive, chronic, but carefully covered and denied marital conflicts and narcissistic deficits in both partners due to midlife transition (Colarusso 1995, 1998, 1999; Euler et al. 2003).

Disorders of sexual hyperarousal or compulsive sexual behaviour (CSB) were rarely diagnosed as isolated disturbances (Meisler et al. 1998; Arbior 2004; Bancroft and Vukadinovic 2004; Schwartz 2004), in terms of sexual dysfunctions in a narrower sense (Jacobson 2003). One reason might certainly be that sexual behaviour varies substantially by individual and time. Sexual vigour is, in males, part of the male social role and labelled as a "disorder" only in cases where sexual addiction hinders or even destroys careers and humiliates personalities (the Clinton syndrome; Hirsch and Imhof 1999; Jacobson 2003; Kafka 2003; Arbior 2004; Bancroft and Vukadinovic 2004).

Compulsive sexual behaviours (Travin 1995) can be found:

1. As a symptom of obsessive-compulsive spectrum disorders
2. As a symptom of affect disorders (e.g. mania)
3. As sexual addictions
4. As sexual impulse disorders

To sum up, hypersexuality is mostly considered, if not organic in origin, a part of the personality disorders with difficulties in impulse control, such as so-called borderline states, in which sexual hyperactivity and promiscuity is a common feature (Kernberg 1997, 2001).

I.4.5.4 Clinical Findings

The diagnostic procedure should include:

- Clinical and laboratory examination including testosterone and, if applicable or necessary, expanded endocrine clarification [follicle-stimulating hormone (FSH), luteinizing hormone (LH), prolactin, oestrogens], dependent upon previous findings regarding accompanying somatic pathology (Robbins 1996).
- Careful dynamic interviews should include individual aspects of the patient concerning beliefs and attitudes in regard to sexuality (McDougall 1972), desire and moral values, quality of the current relationship and possible therapy motivation.
- As a second step towards clarification of libido disorders, a couple interview is recommended, focussing on the couple's ability or fear of intimacy, open or hidden individual or systemic conflictual themes, such as distrust, sexual or aggressive traumata, and social and financial stresses.

As previously stated, libidinal disorders rarely present themselves as isolated disturbances of only one system, nor can they be attributed to only one cause. Biological background, individual psychopathology and systemic marital dysfunction contribute with different weights to a complex clinical situation.

I.4.5.5 Therapy

Having excluded or controlled possible organic causes of the disorder, a multimodal therapeutic approach should be discussed with the patient. Treatment alternatives could, depending on the patient's motivation for treatment possibly include:

- Prescription of (lifestyle) medication such as sexual stimulants or antidepressants as a first step, often administered to enhance the patient's self-esteem and motivation (Brosig et al. 2001).
- In addition to sexual stimulants, a combination of hormonal replacement strategies (Midgley et al. 2000; Demers 2003; Castro-Acuna et al. 2004) and psychotherapeutic efforts can be suggested.
- Individual or couple counselling by an experienced therapist with a focus on either behavioural therapy of sexual dysfunction (Carey 1998) or on psychodynamic, couple-oriented therapeutic strategies (Clement 1996, 2002)
- Finally, in cases of severe individual character pathologies, psychoanalytic treatment in the form of a personal psychoanalysis (Kernberg 1976, 1977, 1989, 1991a, 1991b, 1993).

As a prominent example for behavioural strategies, structured sexual therapy (according to Masters and Johnson 1970) can be divided into six stages:

1. Touching partner without genital contact for subject's own pleasure
2. Touching partner without genital contact for both partners' pleasure
3. Touching partner with genital contact, but intercourse not permitted
4. Simultaneous touching of partner and being touched by partner with genital contact, but intercourse not permitted
5. Intercourse, but without male thrusting; initial containment brief, with lengthening periods of containment with each session
6. Vaginal containment with movement; couple practice stopping before climax.

Psychodynamic strategies, in contrast, traditionally do not focus as much as behavioural therapy on the apparent symptomatology proper. These therapeutic schools intend to clarify the motives behind sexual symptoms such as (repressed) sexual wishes for other sexual objects or other forms of sexuality. Very often, the presenting symptomatology can be seen as a defence against the impact of deeper and more complex psychic phenomena such as love and intimacy. Very often, complaints concerning the lack of sexual enjoyment are the negative of the patient's fear of real intimacy and overwhelmingly experienced sexual lust, a constellation of defences, which psychoanalysis calls perverse defence (Jacobson 2003).

A combination of psychotherapeutic efforts and drug modulation of sexual drives in paraphilias and other disorders of impulse control has been extensively reviewed and the clinical use of these cooperative strategies is successfully proven (Briken et al. 2003).

In severe cases of depression as the most important underlying factor of deficient sexual arousal, a combination of hormones and psychoactive drugs has been discussed (Sharan and Saxena 1998).

I.4.5.6 Prognosis

Positive prognostic variables include a lively sexuality of both partners before the symptomatology started, open-mindedness in sexual matters and flexible forms of personal defences in the couple. Narcissistic personal structures with schizoid character traits, long-lasting sexual abstinence and few sexual experiences during youth are negative prognostic signs for a fast relief of the symptomatology. In these latter cases, intensive psychoanalysis treatment may, in some individuals with good motivation for treatment, be the ultimate alternative for a substantial change in the above-described "undesired" sexual symptomatology.

References

Apt C, Hurlbert DF, Powell D (1993) Men with hypoactive sexual desire disorder: the role of interpersonal dependency and assertiveness. J Sex Edu Ther 19:108–116

Arbior IA (2004) Sexual addiction: concept and assessment. Sexuality Disability 22:333

Bancroft J, Vukadinovic Z (2004) Sexual addiction, sexual compulsivity, sexual impulsivity, or what? Toward a theoretical model. J Sex Res 41:225–234

Brähler E, Stirn A, Brosig B (2004) Verbreitung von Körperschmuck und Inanspruchnahme von Lifestylemedizin in Deutschland. Ergebnisse zweier Repräsentativerhebungen in Deutschland 2002 und 2003. Pressemappe

Briken P, Hill A, Berner W (2003) Pharmacotherapy of paraphilias with long-acting agonists of luteinizing hormone-releasing hormone: a systematic review. J Clin Psychiatry 64: 890–897

Brosig B (2002) Sexuality and partnership in later life. Psychotherapie Psychosomatik Medizinische Psychologie 52:367

Brosig B, Kupfer J, Niemeier V, Gieler U (2001) The "Dorian Gray Syndrome": psychodynamic need for hair growth restorers and, other "fountains of youth". Int J Clin Pharmacol Ther 39:279–283

Carey MP (1998) Cognitive-behavioral treatment of sexual dysfunctions. In: Caballo V (ed) International handbook of cognitive and behavioural treatments for psychological disorders. Pergamon/Elsevier, Oxford, pp 251–280

Castro-Acuna V, Martinez-Martinez L, Larrea F (2004) Partial androgen deficiency in the aging male. Rev Invest Clin 56: 507–512

Clement U (1996) Sexual collusion: dynamic sexually dysfunctional relationships. System Familie 9:67–73

Clement U (2002) Sex in long-term relationships: a systemic approach to sexual desire problems. Arch Sex Behav 31:241–246

Colarusso CA (1995) Traversing young adulthood – the male journey from 20 to 40. Psychoanal Inq 15:75–91

Colarusso CA (1998) A developmental line of time sense – in late adulthood and throughout the life cycle. Psychoanal Study Child 53:113–140

Colarusso CA (1999) The development of time sense in middle adulthood. Psychoanal Q 68:52–83

Demers LM (2003) Andropause: an androgen deficiency state in the ageing male. Expert Opin Pharmacother 4:183–190

Euler S, Brähler E, Brosig B (2003) Das Dorian-Gray-Syndrom als "ethnische Störung" der Spätmoderne. Psychosozial 26: 73–89

Gnirss-Bornet R (2004) Libidinal disturbances. Diagnostics and treatment. Psychotherapeutics 49:341–349

Graziottin A (2000) Libido: the biologic scenario. Maturitas 34:S9–S16

Hirsch R, Imhof J (1999) The Clinton syndrome, the President and the self-destructive nature of sexual addiction. J Subst Abuse Treat 16:353–354

Jacobson L (2003) On the use of "sexual addiction" – the case for "perversion". Contemp Psychoanal 39:107–113

Kafka MP (2003) Sex offending and sexual appetite: the clinical and theoretical relevance of hypersexual desire. Int J Offender Ther Comp Criminol 47:439–451

Kernberg OF (1976) Technical considerations in the treatment of borderline personality organization. J Am Psychoanal Assoc 24:795–829

Kernberg OF (1977) Boundaries and structure in love relations. J Am Psychoanal Assoc 25:81–114

Kernberg OF (1989) The narcissistic personality disorder and the differential diagnosis of antisocial behavior. Psychiatr Clin North Am 12:553–570

Kernberg OF (1991a) Aggression and love in the relationship of the couple. J Am Psychoanal Assoc 39:45–70
Kernberg OF (1991b) Sadomasochism, sexual excitement, and perversion. J Am Psychoanal Assoc 39:333–362
Kernberg OF (1993) The couple's constructive and destructive superego functions. J Am Psychoanal Assoc 41:653–677
Kernberg OF (1997) Sexual excitement and rage: building blocks of the drives. Forum der Psychoanalyse 13:97–118
Kernberg OF (1999) A severe sexual inhibition in the course of the psychoanalytic treatment of a patient with a narcissistic personality disorder. Int J Psychoanal 80:899–908
Kernberg OF (2001) Object relations, affects, and drives: toward a new synthesis. Psychoanal Inq 21:604–619
Krueger THC, Haake P, Exton MS, Schedlowski M, Hartmann U (2002) Prolactin secretion after orgasm: feedback mechanism for sexual drive or a reproductive reflex? Sexuologie 9:30–38
Levine SB (2003) The nature of sexual desire: a clinician's perspective. Arch Sex Behav 32:279–285
Masters WH, Johnson VE (1970) Human sexual inadequacy. Churchill, London
McDougall J (1972) Primal scene and sexual perversion. Int J Psychoanal 53:371–384
Meisler JG, Myers W, Watter D (1998) Sexual addiction: a new phenomenon? J Womens Health 7:163–165
Midgley SJ, Heather N, Best D, Henderson D, McCarthy S, Davies JB (2000) Risk behaviours for HIV and hepatitis infection among anabolic-androgenic steroid users. AIDS Care-Psychological and Socio-Medical Aspects of AIDS/HIV 12:163–170
Robbins A (1996) The effects of hormones on male sexuality: findings from clinical trials on male contraception. In: Zeidenstein S, Moore K (eds) Learning about sexuality: a practical beginning. The Population Council, International Women's Health Coalition, New York, pp 278–297
Schwartz MF (2004) Sexual addiction: an integrated approach. Arch Sex Behav 33:520
Sharan P, Saxena S (1998) Treatment-resistant depression: clinical significance, concept and management. Natl Med J India 11:69–79
Spector IP, Carey MP (1990) Incidence and prevalence of the sexual dysfunctions: a critical review of the empirical literature. Arch Sex Behav 19:389–408
Thibaut F, Cordier B, Kuhn JM (1994) Drug modulation of the libido and sexual-activity – behavior effect of GnrH analog in man. Ann Endocrinol (Paris) 55:229–233
Travin S (1995) Compulsive sexual behaviors. Psychiatric Clin North Am 18:155–169
Weeks GR, Gambescia N (2002) Hypoactive sexual desire: Integrating sex and couple therapy. Norton, New York

I.4.6 Sexual Deviation and Paraphilias

M. Beutel

Key Messages

- In order to be diagnosed as paraphilias, sexually deviant behaviours need to be persistent and cause distress or social and other impairments.
- Neuropsychiatric disorders, developmental disorders, learning history and personality dysfunction contribute to the development of sexual deviance.
- Child sexual abuse is a major health problem carrying lifelong risks for depression and post-traumatic stress disorders for the victims.
- When evaluating sexual dysfunction, it is important for the clinician to be aware of the possibility of sexual deviance and its potential transmission across generations.

I.4.6.1 Definition

Paraphilias are defined as lasting (longer than 6 months), recurrent, intense sexually arousing fantasies, sexual urges or behaviours referring to (a) non-human objects, (b) suffering or degradation of oneself or one's partner or (c) children and legal minors (American Psychiatric Association 1994). In order to justify the diagnosis of a paraphilia, this must persist for more than 6 months and cause clinically significant distress or impairment in social, vocational or other areas. Major paraphilias include:

- Exhibitionism manifests by displaying of one's own genitals towards a stranger (302.4 according to DSM-IV).
- Fetishism (302.81) requires the use of inanimate objects (e.g. female underwear or shoes) for achieving sexual arousal or satisfaction.
- Paedophilia (302.2) implies that an individual is sexually attracted to prepubescent children.
- In sexual masochism, sexual arousal is associated with real or fantasized acts of degradation, beating or enchaining or to other kinds of suffering.
- Sexual sadism (302.84) implies afflicting psychological or physical harm to the victim.
- In voyeurism (302.82), sexual arousal is associated with watching a stranger who is naked, undressing or involved in sexual activity.

I.4.6.2 Aetiology and Pathogenesis

Sexual deviance may result from neuropsychiatric dysfunction, developmental disorders, learning history and personality disorders:

- Disinhibited sexual behaviour can be a part of general behaviour disinhibition as in the case of frontal lobe lesions. Demented patients may display paraphilic behaviour (exhibitionism) and nonparaphilic hypersexuality (e.g. inappropriate sexual advances). Paraphilic behaviour also occurs secondary to a variety of neuropsychiatric disorders such as temporal lobe epilepsy, postencephalitic syndromes, etc. (Bradford et al. 2001).
- Traditional psychoanalytic theories have described perversions as a regression to an infantile drive organization when sexual impulses have not been integrated into striving for genital sexual fulfilment; other theories described perversion as an attempt at conflict resolution or narcissistic restitution by means of sexualization of other, unfulfilled needs (e.g. for closeness, self-assertion, control).
- From a behavioural point of view, sexual arousal to deviant stimuli was postulated as resulting from classical or operant conditioning linking sexual arousal to specific stimuli and conditions.
- Recent psychoanalytic theories have linked paraphilia to personality disorders. Manipulation of one's own body or sexual objects may be motivated by pent-up hatred or as a defence against longings for dependency. Sexual impulses and craving for deviant sexual activity may be split off from the usual sexual functioning which may appear normal (Cohen et al. 2002).

I.4.6.3 Paedophilia as an Example of Paraphilia

Child sexual abuse has been identified as a major public health problem with 12% of men and 17% of women reported having been sexually touched by an older person when they were children (Fagan et al. 2002). It is well documented that these experiences are frequently traumatic, carrying a high life-long risk for depression, post-traumatic stress disorders and pervasive developmental impairments (e.g. trusting relationships, body image, sexual fulfilment). It is not known, however, what proportion is due to paedophilia or other forms of sexual abuse (e.g. psychopathic deviance). Paedophilic individuals are heterogeneous regarding character, temperament and their manner of sexual expression. Paedophiles may have interacted sexually with children, may have looked at sexualized pictures of children or may have controlled their sexual urges for a considerable length of time. Sexual behaviour performed with minors may vary from fondling and genital exposure to different types of intercourse or (rarely) rape or abduction of children. There may be an attraction to males, to females or to both genders; paedophilia may or may not be limited to incest and may or may not be related exclusively to specific age groups of children.

Sexual victimization is a major risk factor for the development of sexually abusive behaviour, particularly in males (Salter et al. 2003; Wiehe 2003). For example, there is a transmission of sexually deviant behaviour across generations. Additional risk factors are affective illness, psychosocial stress (e.g. loss of relationship or status) and alcohol abuse (Fagan et al. 2002).

In a recent publication (Bosinsky 2004), a 32-year-old man had presented with erectile dysfunction after 3 years of marriage. Following treatment with a PDE-inhibitor, he was charged with sexual abuse of a boy from his neighbourhood. Only then did the medical assessment determine paedophilic masturbation fantasies since his puberty, which he had hoped to overcome by his marriage. Following restoration of his potency by medication, he had acted on his suppressed paedophilic inclination.

I.4.6.4 Diagnosis and Treatment

As in the case described in the previous section, the presence of sexual deviance may not be reported regularly by patients, as they fear that the physician will report to civil agencies. It is therefore important for the clinician to be aware of the possibility of sexual deviancy associated with complaints of sexual dysfunction.

Treatment of sexually deviant behaviour is frequently initiated following discovery and criminal charges of sexual delinquency. When psychotherapy is required by court decision, concerns are raised on behalf of the clinician (e.g. issues of treatment motivation of the offender, prognosis and responsibility). As exemplified by paedophilia, both the psychoanalytic concept of curing the paraphilia by development of insight and the behavioural conception of re-conditioning sexual orientation have been given up. Rather, paedophilia is considered as a chronic psychiatric disorder, and therapeutic efforts aim at improving self-control of harmful behaviours, at correcting cognitive and social distortion and treating social impairment. For this purpose, psychotherapy may be supplemented by medication as a sexual appetite suppressant. These include testosterone-lowering medication such as methoxyprogesterone acetate or cyproterone acetate. Overall, following psychotherapeutic treatment reduced recidivism rates (defined as re-arrest or criminal charges) were found among sexual offenders (compared to no psychotherapy; Fagan et al. 2002).

References

American Psychiatric Association (1994) Diagnostic and statistical manual of mental disorders, 4th edn. American Psychiatric Association, Washington DC
Bosinski HAG (2004) Diagnostik und Therapie sexueller Störungen. Eine interdisziplinäre Herausforderung. Urologe A 43:279–284
Bradford JMW (2001) The neurobiology, neuropharmacology, and pharmacological treatment of the paraphilias and compulsive sexual behaviour. Can J Psychiatry 46:26–34
Cohen L, Nikiforov K, Sniezyna G, Poznansky O, McGeoch P, Weaver C, King EG, Cullen K, Galynker I (2002) Heterosexual male perpetrators of childhood sexual abuse: a preliminary neuropsychiatric model. Psychiatric Quaterly 73:313–336
Fagan PJ, Wise TN, Schmidt CW, Berlin FS (2002) Pedophilia. J Am Med Assoc 288:2458–2465
Salter D, McMillan D, Richards M, Talbot T, Hodges J, Bentovim A, Hastings R, Stevenson J, Skuse D (2003) Development of sexually abusive behaviour in sexually victimised males: a longitudinal study. Lancet 361:471–476
Wiehe VR (2003) Empathy and narcissism in a sample of child abuse perpetrators and a comparison sample of foster parents. Child Abuse Neglect 27:541–555

I.5 Problem: Male Contraception

I.5.1 Controversies Regarding Postvasectomy Management

J. Shah, H. Fisch

Key Messages

- Vasectomy is among the safest, easiest, and surest methods of male sterilization, with a failure rate of only 0.05%.
- Given the finality of vasectomy, thorough preoperative counselling regarding the risks, benefits, and alternatives of the procedure is imperative.
- Every vasectomy candidate should demonstrate a clear understanding of the time delay between vasectomy and azoospermia and of the need for postoperative semen analyses to confirm azoospermia.
- A semen analysis should be obtained no sooner than 3 months after vasectomy.
- The presence of motile spermatozoa 3–6 months after vasectomy indicates vasectomy failure; an isolated finding of nonmotile spermatozoa may be normal and does not necessarily signal vasectomy failure.
- Centrifugation of azoospermic semen may detect rare nonmotile spermatozoa, but no consensus exists as to the utility of routine centrifugation.

I.5.1.1 Introduction

Despite advances in other methods of family planning over the last several decades, vasectomy has remained among the most popular forms of contraception. The safety, simplicity, and durability of the procedure make it an attractive option for patients and physicians alike. However, many controversies remain regarding the appropriate management of a patient after vasectomy. In this review, we discuss outcomes after vasectomy, focusing on timing, technical aspects, and interpretation of postvasectomy semen analysis.

I.5.1.2 Definition

Vasectomy is a form of male sterilization that involves bilateral disruption of the vas deferens to halt the transmission of spermatozoa during ejaculation. It is an outpatient procedure that can be performed in the office setting under local anaesthesia, with most patients reporting only minimal postoperative pain. Unlike many of the other methods of contraception that require continuous usage or repeat administrations, vasectomy need only be performed once for a man to be rendered durably sterile.

I.5.1.3 Prevalence

Vasectomy remains among the simplest, safest and most effective contraceptive methods available. Worldwide, it has been estimated that 5% of all couples of reproductive age (approximately 42–60 million men) depend on vasectomy as their sole contraceptive method (Liskin et al. 1992; Liu and Li 1993). This number varies widely among different countries, with the highest rate of vasectomy (23%) reported in New Zealand (Schlegel and Goldstein 1993).

In the United States, 11% of women of reproductive age rely on vasectomy for family planning (Piccinino and Mosher 1998). Those most likely to elect vasectomy as their contraceptive method of choice include women between the ages 30 and 45, married women, and those with at least a high school education (Schwingl 2000). Vasectomies are much more common in white men than in black men (14% vs 2%).

I.5.1.4
Treatment

I.5.1.4.1
Preoperative Counselling

Vasectomy can be performed under local anaesthesia with relative ease and the patient may be allowed to return to his normal level of activity within several days of the procedure. Given the finality of vasectomy, thorough preoperative counselling regarding the risks, benefits and alternatives of the procedure is imperative. In addition, patients should be given reasonable expectations regarding postoperative recovery and they should be forewarned about the need for continued postoperative management. Specifically, the patient should demonstrate a clear understanding of the time delay between vasectomy and azoospermia and of the need for postoperative semen analyses to confirm azoospermia.

In addition to understanding the need for postoperative management after vasectomy, every patient must also demonstrate a clear understanding of the potential complications that may result from the procedure. Specifically, the risk of chronic inflammation and postvasectomy pain syndrome (PVPS) should be discussed. Patients with PVPS present with intermittent or constant pain in one or both testicles after vasectomy lasting for 3 or more months. PVPS is considered relatively uncommon following vasectomy, though the incidence has been suggested to be as high as 19% in one study (Ahmed et al. 1997). The exact mechanism of PVPS remains unknown, but theories involving epididymal congestion, painful sperm granulomas, vascular stasis, and nerve impingement have been forwarded. Most patients with PVPS can be managed conservatively with reassurance, nonsteroidal anti-inflammatory drugs, scrotal support, or nerve blocks. However, patients who do not respond to these measures may need secondary surgical procedures such as vasectomy reversal (Myers et al. 1997; Nangia et al. 2000), epididymectomy (Chen and Ball 1991), or spermatic cord denervation (Ahmed et al. 1997).

For men under the age of 35 years who are desirous of a vasectomy, some urologists prefer to counsel these patients on the potential increased risk of prostate cancer later in life. Several studies published in the early 1990s reported an increased risk of prostate cancer in men having undergone vasectomy, especially in men vasectomized for 20 years or more (Mettlin et al. 1990; Rosenberg et al. 1990; Giovannucci et al. 1992). While these studies received much media attention, various large-scale studies have since shown the relationship between vasectomy and prostate cancer to be tenuous at best (Stone et al. 1994; Bernal-Delgado et al. 1998; Lesko et al. 1999). The most prudent course of action would be to make the vasectomy candidate aware of the various studies and allow him to make the final decision.

Lastly, while several realistic options for reestablishment of vasoepididymal continuity in vasectomized men do exist, vasectomy is still considered a *permanent* form of male sterilization. As such, every vasectomy candidate must consider his individual circumstances, both current and future, before arriving at the decision to proceed with vasectomy. In fact, prior to undergoing vasectomy, every patient should be made aware of the option of "fertility insurance" by means of semen cryopreservation.

The goal of preoperative counselling should not be to dissuade or scare the patient from undergoing vasectomy. It should be to provide the patient with the knowledge necessary to make a fully informed decision. If done appropriately, preoperative counselling can result in patients who are more satisfied, more compliant, and less litigious.

I.5.1.4.2
Surgical Technique

The vasectomy procedure is begun by palpation of the vas deferens through the scrotal skin. The vas is then secured with the surgeon's fingers and the scrotal skin is opened. Access to the vas deferens may be obtained using either the conventional incisional method or the no-scalpel method popularized by Li in the late 1980s (Li et al. 1991). With the conventional method, a scalpel is used to make an approximately 1-cm incision, either in the midline if a single incision is used or in each hemiscrotum if two separate incisions are used. With the no-scalpel technique, a specialized sharp forceps is used to puncture the scrotal skin.

After the vas deferens is identified, it is brought out of the scrotal incision and divided. A variable length of vas is resected and the remaining free ends are occluded using one or more methods. To accomplish vas occlusion, the cut ends may be secured with nonabsorbable suture, cautery and/or metal clips. Many urologists also interpose fascia between the cut ends to minimize the risk of vasal recanalization. The crucial step for vasectomy success is vasal occlusion; the exact method of occlusion is a matter of preference.

I.5.1.5
Results of Treatment

I.5.1.5.1
Vasectomy Success

Vasectomy is the most reliable practical method of permanent contraception. However, vasectomy failures have been reported. Most sources estimate the occurrence of undesired pregnancy following vasectomy to be approximately 1 in 2,000 cases (Smith et al. 1994; Haldar et al. 2000; Weiske 2001). This pregnancy failure rate of less than 0.1 % compares favourably to the tubal ligation failure rate of 1.85 % (Peterson et al. 1996). Vasectomy failures are divided into two categories: early and late. Early failures typically occur within the first few months following vasectomy and are attributed to unprotected intercourse prior to obtaining a negative semen analysis. A missed vas during operation can also cause early failure. Late failures may occur years to decades after vasectomy and are most often attributed to recanalization of the vas deferens. The majority of vasectomy failures are early failures in men who are ineffectively counselled regarding the delay between vasectomy and azoospermia.

I.5.1.5.2 When Should a Postvasectomy Semen Analysis Be Obtained?

Though most urologists agree on the need for a semen analysis to verify the achievement of azoospermia after vasectomy, there is no consensus on the exact timing of the postvasectomy semen analysis. Most physicians use either an arbitrarily determined time period or an arbitrary number of ejaculations before obtaining a semen analysis. In a survey of 1,800 physicians performing vasectomy in the United States in 1995, Haws et al. found that postvasectomy semen analysis was obtained at 6 weeks by 59 % of the physicians, at 7 – 9 weeks by 29 %, and after 9 weeks by 12 %.

Though most physicians obtain the postvasectomy semen analysis within 6 weeks, a review of the available literature suggests that this may be too soon. Figure I.5.1, incorporating data from 12 peer-reviewed studies, shows the rate of development of postvasectomy azoospermia plotted as a function of time. Three months after vasectomy, only 72 % of men have achieved azoospermia. Six months after vasectomy, this number improves to 85 % and by 1 year after vasectomy 99 % of men are azoospermic. This slow constant rate of development of azoospermia suggests that the number of ejaculations after vasectomy perhaps may have only a minor impact on the achievement of azoospermia.

Similarly, it has been shown that there is no association between the method of vasal occlusion or length of vas excised and azoospermia (Esho et al. 1974; Esho and Cass 1978; Haws et al. 1998; Clenney and Higgins 1999; Labrecque et al. 2003). Given the relatively slow rate of achievement of postvasectomy azoospermia, our current practice is to obtain a semen analysis no sooner than 3 months after vasectomy.

I.5.1.5.3 What Is the Significance of Spermatozoa on the Postvasectomy Semen Analysis?

Postvasectomy semen analysis may show any one of three findings: complete absence of spermatozoa (azoospermia), presence of motile spermatozoa, or presence of nonmotile spermatozoa. The presence of motile spermatozoa 3 – 6 months after vasectomy indicates vasectomy failure either due to technical error or early recanalization (Edwards 1993).

The significance of nonmotile spermatozoa on semen analysis depends on when the spermatozoa are found. In the early postvasectomy period, this finding is thought to be caused by the release of nonviable residual spermatozoa in the distal reproductive tract

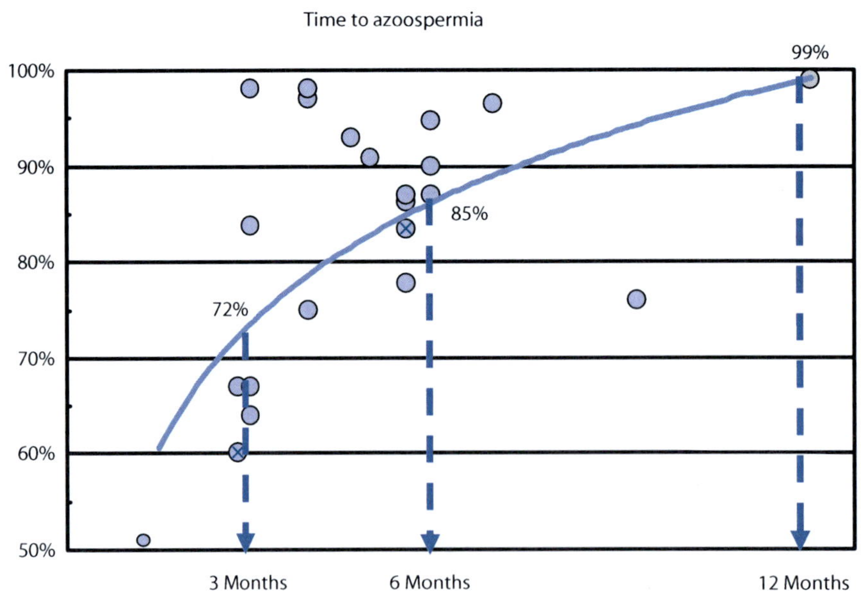

Fig. I.5.1. Rate of development of azoospermia after vasectomy. Each reference point represents data from published series on postvasectomy azoospermia at various time points. As indicated in the graph, only 72 % of men have azoospermic semen analyses 3 months after vasectomy. (Compiled from Alderman 1988; O'Brien 1995; Alcaraz 1996; Cortes 1997; DeKnijff 1997; Finger 1997; Smith 1998; Badrakumar 2000; Hancock 2002; Mason 2002; Nazerali 2002 and Barone 2003)

Table I.5.1. Rates of reappearance of rare spermatozoa in patients with previously documented azoospermia following vasectomy

	Reappearance of rare sperm	Follow-up (years)
Labrecque et al. 1998	2.2%	<1
O'Brien et al. 1995	0.6%	1
DeKnijff et al. 1997	8.0%	2
Goldstein et al. 1996	9.7%	10
Freund et al. 1989[a]	100%	2–31

[a] Freund et al. used a highly sensitive ultrafiltration and ultracentrifugation technique specifically designed to detect any trace of spermatozoa elements.

(DeKnijff et al. 1997). If found at a significant amount of time after vasectomy, nonmotile spermatozoa generally indicate recanalization of the vas deferens (Lemack and Goldstein 1996). However, it is important to understand that the isolated finding of nonmotile spermatozoa does not necessarily signal vasectomy failure. As shown in Table I.5.1, multiple investigators have reported on the reappearance of rare nonmotile spermatozoa years to decades after vasectomy in men previously documented to be azoospermic (O'Brien et al. 1995; Lemack and Goldstein 1996; DeKnijff et al. 1997). It is widely believed that the presence of a small number of nonmotile spermatozoa in vasectomized men is a normal and usual sequela of vasectomy. Additionally, it has been shown that the risk of pregnancy from nonmotile spermatozoa is only 0.05%, which is identical to the risk of pregnancy after two azoospermic semen analyses (Benger et al. 1995; Haldar et al. 2000).

The current guidelines from the British Andrology Society recommend routine centrifugation of all postvasectomy semen specimens to increase the detection of rare nonmotile spermatozoa (Hancock and McLaughlin 2002). While semen centrifugation is a useful sperm-harvesting technique for intracytoplasmic sperm injection in men with obstructive or nonobstructive azoospermia (Jaffe et al. 1998), it is not currently the clinical standard of care in the United States for postvasectomy patients. Centrifugation is a superior means to detect rare nonmotile spermatozoa, but as discussed above the presence of rare nonmotile spermatozoa after vasectomy is only of trivial significance and does not alter patient management to any degree.

I.5.1.6 Conclusion

Vasectomy remains among the safest, easiest, and surest methods of male sterilization. As such, it is one of the most popular methods of permanent contraception worldwide. However, despite the popularity of the technique itself, there has been a notable lack of consensus on the appropriate management of patients *after* vasectomy. We recommend waiting at least 3 months after vasectomy to assess azoospermia on semen analysis. A semen analysis indicating the complete absence of spermatozoa or the presence of only rare nonmotile spermatozoa is considered a marker of vasectomy success. Routine centrifugation of azoospermic semen to detect rare nonmotile spermatozoa is not currently considered the clinical standard of care in the United States.

It is clear that multiple issues must be addressed after vasectomy. In a patient's mind, the judicious handling of these issues can make the difference between a successful sterilization and an unpleasant experience. It would behove all urologists to amend our practice such that vasectomy is no longer considered a *procedure* but rather a *process*. In this context, patients may be more appropriately counselled on the facts that continued follow-up after vasectomy is essential; sterilization after vasectomy is not guaranteed; and the possibilities of spontaneous recanalization or postvasectomy pain syndrome, though small, do exist.

References

Ahmed I, Rasheed S, White C, Shaikh NA (1997) The incidence of post-vasectomy chronic testicular pain and the role of nerve stripping (denervation) of the spermatic cord in its management. Br J Urol 79:269–270

Alcaraz A, Arango O (1996) Cancer and other risks of vasectomy. Eur J Contracept Reprod Health Care 1:311–318

Alderman PM (1988) The lurking sperm. A review of failures in 8879 vasectomies performed by one physician. JAMA 259:3142–3144

Badrakumar C, Gogoi NK, Sundaram SK (2000) Semen analysis after vasectomy: when and how many? Br J Urol 86: 479–481

Barone MA, Nazerali H, Cortes M, Chen-Mok M, Pollack AE, Sokal D (2003) A prospective study of time and number of ejaculations to azoospermia after vasectomy by ligation and excision. J Urology 170:376–379

Benger JR, Swami SK, Gingell JC (1995) Persistent spermatozoa after vasectomy: a survey of British urologists. Br J Urol 76:376–379

Bernal-Delgado E, Latour-Perez J, Pradas-Arnal F, Gomez-Lopez LI (1998) The association between vasectomy and prostate cancer: a systematic review of the literature. Fertil Steril 70:191–200

Chen TF, Ball RY (1991) Epididymectomy for post-vasectomy pain: histological review. Br J Urol 68:407–413

Clenney TL, Higgins JC (1999) Vasectomy techniques. Am Fam Phys 60:137–152

Cortes M, Flick A, Barone MA, Amatya R, Pollack AE, Otero-Flores J, Juarez C, McMullen S (1997) Results of a pilot study of time to azoospermia after vasectomy in Mexico City. Contraception 56:215–222

DeKnijff DWW, Vrijhof HJEJ, Arends J, Janknegt RA (1997) Persistence or reappearance of nonmotile sperm after vasectomy: does it have clinical consequences? Fertil Steril 67:332–335

Edwards IS (1993) Earlier testing after vasectomy, based on the absence of motile sperm. Fertil Steril 59:431–436

Esho JO, Cass AS (1978) Recanalization rate following methods of vasectomy using interposition of fascial sheath of vas deferens. J Urology 120:178–179

Esho JO, Ireland GW, Cass AS (1974) Vasectomy. Comparison of ligation and Fulguration methods. Urology 3:337–338
Finger WR (1997) Time to azoospermia may be longer than often assumed. Network 18:15
Freund MJ, Weidmann JE, Goldstein M, Marmar J, Santulli R, Oliveira N (1989) Microrecanalization after vasectomy in man. J Androl 10:120–132
Giovannucci E, Tosteson TD, Speizer FE, Vessy MP, Colditz GA (1992) A long-term study of mortality in men who have undergone vasectomy. N Engl J Med 326:1392–1398
Haldar N, Cranston D, Turner E, MacKenzie I, Guillebaud J (2000) How reliable is vasectomy? Long-term follow-up of vasectomized men. Lancet 356:43–44
Hancock P, McLaughlin E for the British Andrology Society (2002) British Andrology Society guidelines for the assessment of post vasectomy semen samples (2002). J Clin Pathol 55:812–816
Haws JM, Morgan GT, Pollack AE, Koonin LM, Magnani RJ, Gargiullo PM (1998) Clinical aspects of vasectomies performed in the United States in 1995. Urology 52:685–691
Jaffe TM, Kim ED, Hoekstra TH, Lipshultz LI (1998) Sperm pellet analysis: a technique to detect the presence of sperm in men considered to have azoospermia by routine semen analysis. J Urology 159:1548–1550
Labrecque M, Hoang D, Turcot L (2003) Association between length of the vas deferens excised during vasectomy and the risk of postvasectomy recanalization. Fertil Steril 79:1003–1007
Lemack GE, Goldstein M (1996) Presence of sperm in the pre-vasectomy reversal semen analysis: incidence and implications. J Urology 155:167–169
Lesko SM, Louik C, Vezina R, Rosenberg L, Shapiro S (1999) Vasectomy and prostate cancer. J Urol 161:1848–1852
Li SQ, Goldstein M, Zhu J, Huber D (1991) The no-scalpel vasectomy. J Urology 145:341–344
Liskin I, Renoir E, Blackburn R (1992) Vasectomy – new opportunities. Population Reports [D] 5:1–23
Liu X, Li S (1993) Vasal sterilization in China. Contraception 48:255–266
Mason RG, Dodds L, Swami SK (2002) Sterile water irrigation of the distal vas deferens at vasectomy: does it accelerate clearance of sperm? A prospective randomized trial. Urology 59:424–427
Mettlin C, Natarajan M, Huben R (1990) Vasectomy and prostate cancer risk. Am J Epidemiol 132:1956–1961
Myers SA, Mershon CE, Fuchs EF (1997) Vasectomy reversal for treatment of the post-vasectomy pain syndrome. J Urol 157:518–520
Nangia AK, Mules JL, Thomas AJ (2000) Vasectomy reversal for the post-vasectomy pain syndrome: a clinical and histological evaluation. J Urol 164:1939–1342
Nazerali H, Thapa S, Hays M, Pathak LR, Pandey KR, Sokal DC (2003) Vasectomy effectiveness in Nepal: a retrospective study. Contraception 67:397–401
O'Brien TS, Cranston D, Ashwin P, Turner E, MacKenzie IZ, Gillebaud J (1995) Temporary reappearance of sperm 12 months after vasectomy. Br J Urol 76:371–372
Peterson HB, Xia Z, Hughes JM, Wilcox LS, Taylor LR, Trussel J for The US Collaborative Review of Sterilization Working Group (1996) The risk of pregnancy after tubal sterilization: findings from the US collaborative review of sterilization. Am J Obstet Gynecol 174:1161–1170
Piccinino LJ, Mosher WD (1998) Trends in contraceptive use in the United States: 1982–1995. Fam Plann Perspect 30: 4–10, 46
Rosenberg L, Palmer JR, Zauber AG, Warshauer ME, Strom BL, Harlap S, Shapiro A (1994) The relation of vasectomy to the risk of cancer. Am J Epidemiol 140:431–438
Schlegel PN, Goldstein M (1993) Vasectomy. In: Schoupe D, Haseltine FP (eds) Contraception. Springer, Berlin Heidelberg New York, pp 181–191
Schwingl PJ, Guess HA (2000) Safety and effectiveness of vasectomy. Fertil Steril 73:923–936
Smith AG, Crooks J, Singh NP, Scott R, Lloyd SN (1998) Is the timing of post-vasectomy seminal analysis important? Br J Urol 81:458–460
Smith JC, Cranston D, O'Brien T, Guillebaud J, Hindmarsh J, Turner AG (1994) Fatherhood without apparent spermatozoa after vasectomy. Lancet 344:30
Stone N, Blum DS, DeAntoni EP, Crawford ED, Schmid K, Eisenberger MA, Berger ER, Jefferson P, Staggers F, Gambert SR (1994) Prostate cancer risk factor analysis among >50,000 men in a national study of prostate-specific antigen (PSA). J Urol 151:278A
Weiske WH (2002) Vasectomy. Andrologia 33:125–134

I.5.2 Vasectomy Reversal

A. Belker

Key Messages

- The most common reason vasectomy reversal is requested is the remarriage of a divorced man.
- Either vasovasostomy or vasoepididymostomy may be required to reverse a vasectomy.
- The surgeon's choice of vasovasostomy or vasoepididymostomy depends upon many factors such as the quality of sperm in the intraoperative vas fluid, the gross appearance of the vas fluid when sperm are absent from the fluid, and the presence or absence of epididymal induration.
- Microsurgical procedures obtain results that are markedly better than the results of nonmagnified procedures.
- The success rate of vasectomy reversal decreases as the duration of the obstructive interval increases.
- The success rate of vasectomy reversal is related to the intraoperative sperm quality in the vas fluid.
- Sperm retrieval for IVF/ICSI is an alternative to vasectomy reversal that should be considered in certain situations.

I.5.2.1 Indications

The most common reason for vasectomy reversal is the desire of a man to have a child, or children, in a second or subsequent marriage. In such situations, the male partner usually has had children in a previous relationship and it is the desire of the female, who usually has not previously had children, that prompts the male to seek a vasectomy reversal. Less often, both partners have had children and simply desire to have a child in a new relationship that will be "theirs", rather than "his" or "hers" in that relationship. A relatively rare reason for vasectomy reversal is the death of a child and the desire of a couple to have another child because of that loss. Another infrequent reason for vasectomy reversal is the development of testicular or epididymal pain resulting from the vasectomy. Obstruction of the vas deferens, subsequently referred to as simply the vas, may be discovered to be the cause of azoospermia during the evaluation of a man who presents for a fertility evaluation. The obstruction of the vas in such situations almost always is the result of bilateral injury to the vas that occurred during bilateral inguinal hernia repair performed during infancy.

I.5.2.2 Contraindications

The usual contraindications to surgery, such as bleeding diatheses and general severe health problems, apply to vasectomy reversal. A reversal procedure is also contraindicated if urinary tract infection or scrotal skin infection are present. If the female partner has bilateral fallopian tube obstruction, reversal of both the fallopian tube obstruction and the vasectomy is possible. However, sperm retrieval for in vitro fertilization (IVF) with intracytoplasmic sperm injection (ICSI) (Kolettis and Thomas 1997) would be a less expensive method to achieve a pregnancy. In most centres, this alternative would be as likely, if not more likely, to produce a pregnancy than for both partners to undergo a reversal procedure.

If physical examination reveals that the patient has developed bilateral testicular atrophy, the cause of atrophy must be determined (see Chap. II.2.5). If the cause is testicular disease, correctable pituitary or hypothalamic disease, vasectomy reversal would be contraindicated.

I.5.2.3 Vasectomy Reversal Techniques

I.5.2.3.1 Vasovasostomy

Vasovasostomy is the technical name for anastomosis of the severed ends of the vas. The procedure may be performed without optical magnification (see Chap. II.4.1), but almost all authorities now agree that the results of vasovasostomy performed with the aid of microsurgery are better than the results of those procedures performed without optical magnification. A two-layer method of microsurgical vasovasostomy (see Chap. II.4.1) creates precise approximation of the mucosal edges and of the outer muscular layer edges of the vas.

I.5.2.3.2 Vasoepididymostomy

During a vasectomy reversal procedure, fluid from the testicular end of the vas is examined with a laboratory microscope. If spermatozoa are present in the fluid, vasovasostomy is performed. The absence of spermatozoa may indicate that epididymal obstruction has developed after the vasectomy (see Chap. II.4.1). In this situation, the epididymal obstruction must be bypassed by performing vasoepididymostomy, or anastomosis of the abdominal end of the vas to the epididymal tubule at a level in the epididymis above the point of obstruction. Older nonmicrosurgical methods of vasoepididymostomy relied on the creation of a fistula between openings in several loops of the epididymal tubule and the vas lumen (see Chap. II.4.1). A microsurgical method of vasoepididymostomy creates a direct connection of the edges of the epididymal tubule to the edges of the vas mucosa, with subsequent connection of the muscular layer of the vas to the edges of the epididymal tunic (see Chap. II.4.1).

As the duration of the obstructive interval, which is the elapsed time since the vasectomy, increases, an increasing percentage of men develop a back pressure-induced rupture of the epididymal tubule (Silber 1977). The subsequent leakage of spermatozoa from the epididymal tubule creates a sperm granuloma within the epididymis (Silber 1979). Because the epididymal tubule is a single, continuous tube, the obstructing sperm granuloma prevents the passage of spermatozoa beyond the point in the tubule at which the granuloma is located.

The absence of spermatozoa from the intraoperative vas fluid does not necessarily indicate that an epididymal obstruction is present. When spermatozoa are not seen in the vas fluid, the surgeon must inspect the epididymis. If a point of obstruction is clearly identified by observing dilation of the epididymal tubule above that level and collapse of the tubule below that level, then vasoepididymostomy is required. If no point of obstruction can be identified, then the surgeon may be guided by the gross appearance of the fluid that emanates from the testicular end of the vas (Belker et al. 1991) (see Chap. II.4.1).

I.5.2.4 Postoperative Care

After both vasovasostomy and vasoepididymostomy, it is recommended that a scrotal support be used and heavy physical activity be avoided for 4 weeks. Sexual intercourse should be avoided for at least 2 weeks postoperatively. Semen analyses are advised at 2- to 3-month intervals until semen parameters are stable or until a pregnancy has been achieved. The average interval until a pregnancy occurs after vasovasostomy is 1 year (Belker et al. 1991), but information about the average interval until a pregnancy occurs after vasoepididymostomy unfortunately is not available at this time.

I.5.2.5 Complications

Postoperative infection and bleeding, which may occur after any surgical procedure, fortunately are rare occurrences after vasectomy reversal. The pain that follows vasectomy reversal, whether vasovasostomy or vasoepididymostomy is required, is of brief duration and rarely requires more than oral analgesia. There has been no report of a change in sexual performance after vasectomy reversal.

I.5.2.6 Results

Numerous factors determine the success of vasectomy reversal. The most important preoperative factor that determines success is the duration of the obstructive interval (Belker et al. 1991). The rates of return of sperm to the semen and of pregnancy in the female partners, respectively, are 97% and 76% for an obstructive interval of under 3 years, 88% and 53% for 3–8 years, 79% and 44% for 9–14 years, and 71% and 30% for 15 years or longer (Belker et al. 1991). Results of the microsurgical one-layer (Schmidt 1978) and two-layer (Belker 1980) techniques are comparable (Belker et al. 1991).

An intraoperative factor that determines the success of vasovasostomy is the sperm quality in the fluid that is obtained from the testicular end of the vas. Success rates are progressively lower for vasovasostomy when the intraoperative fluid contains mainly motile sperm, mainly nonmotile sperm, mainly sperm heads (without tails), only sperm heads, or no sperm at all (Belker et al. 1991) (see Chap. II.4.1). If microsurgical vasoepididymostomy is required, the rate of return of sperm to the semen postoperatively ranges from 60% to 85% and the rate of pregnancy ranges from 20% to 44% (Matthews et al. 1995; Kim et al. 1998; Kolettis and Thomas 1997).

The success rates of both vasovasostomy and vasoepididymostomy are better when those procedures are performed microsurgically compared to the results of procedures performed without optical magnification. However, microsurgical performance of both procedures requires formal laboratory training and subsequent practice before optimal results can be expected.

I.5.2.7 Conclusions

Vasectomy reversal may require either vasovasostomy or vasoepididymostomy. The intraoperative decision regarding which procedure is required is made independently on each side. Thus, some patients may require vasovasostomy on one side and vasoepididymostomy on the other side. The results of vasectomy reversal have been improved considerably since the introduction of microsurgical methods to perform both vasovasostomy and vasoepididymostomy.

References

Belker AM (1980) Microsurgical two-layer vasovasostomy: simplified technique using hinged, folding-approximating clamp. Urology 16:376–381

Belker AM, Thomas AJ Jr, Fuchs EF, Konnak JW, Sharlip ID, Thomas AJ Jr (1991) Results of 1,469 microsurgical vasectomy reversals by the Vasovasostomy Study Group. J Urol 145: 505–511

Kim ED, Winkel E, Orejuela F, Lipshultz LI (1998) Pathological epididymal obstruction unrelated to vasectomy: results with microsurgical reconstruction. J Urol 160:2078–2080

Kolettis PN, Thomas AJ Jr (1997) Vasoepididymostomy for vasectomy reversal: a critical assessment in the era of intracytoplasmic sperm injection. J Urol 158:467–470

Matthews GJ, Schlegel PN, Goldstein M (1995) Patency following microsurgical vasoepididymostomy and vasovasostomy: temporal considerations. J Urol 154:2070–2073

Schmidt SS (1978) Vasovasostomy. Urol Clin North Am 5:585–592

Silber SJ (1977) Sperm granuloma and reversibility of vasectomy. Lancet 2:588–589

Silber SJ (1979) Epididymal extravasation following vasectomy as a cause for failure of vasectomy reversal. Fertil Steril 31:309–315

I.5.3 Male Contraception

D. Handelsman, G. Waites

I.5

Key Messages

- Men have only traditional methods (periodic abstinence, withdrawal, condoms) and vasectomy and lack reversible contraceptive methods.
- Hormonal methods based on improved progestins developed for female contraception, given orally or as implants, and combined with injectable or implantable testosterone, are closest to entering clinical practice.

I.5.3.1 Introduction

A male contraceptive aims to prevent pregnancy by reducing the number of fertile sperm in the ejaculate. At present, men have only traditional methods (periodic abstinence, withdrawal, condoms) and vasectomy but lack reliable and reversible contraceptive methods comparable to the modern female methods. Even though no new male contraceptives were introduced during the twentieth century, still one-third of all couples adopt family planning methods involving the active participation of men (United Nations 2000) and there is ample evidence from worldwide surveys that men would accept new methods (Martin et al. 2000). Hormonal methods analogous to those developed for women are those closest to entering clinical practice.

I.5.3.2 Hormonal Methods

Clinical studies employing prototype drugs have demonstrated that the hormonal approach to switching off spermatogenesis is both effective and reversible with short-term safety (Anderson and Baird 2002; Kamischke and Nieschlag 2004; Handelsman 2005). Despite available niches and popular interest, commercial development of marketable male hormonal contraceptives by the pharmaceutical industry has been slow to emerge (Handelsman 2003).

No hormonal regimen yet achieves azoospermia in all men, although testosterone administration to men in China and Indonesia gets close (WHO 1990; Gu et al. 2002). Among non-Asian men, combination regimens involving a second gonadotrophin-suppressing agent, usually a progestin, combined with testosterone achieve close to the ideal of universal suppression of spermatogenesis (Bebb et al. 1996; Handelsman et al. 1996; Meriggiola et al. 1996).

I.5.3.3 Nonhormonal Methods

Many novel nonhormonal male contraceptive approaches have been proposed. These include variations on existing physical and biochemical technologies (heat, postmeiotic and epididymal targets), and more recently the harnessing of genomic-based leads. Although the feasibility of reversibly interfering with sperm maturation in the epididymis has been established (Ford and Waites 1986; Cooper 2002), the development of a nonhormonal contraceptive drug for men remains in the preclinical stage.

I.5.3.4 Vaccines

Vaccines targeting sperm antigens involved in fertilization have long been of interest. Unlike vaccines for infection, which need not completely block the body burden of infectious agents in order for the immune system to eradicate an infection, contraceptive sperm vaccines must functionally block virtually all sperm. The lower antigenic burden achieving neutralization in women, whose oocytes are confronted by only 100–1,000 sperm once a month, suggests that a sperm vaccine is more logically targeted to women. This would also eliminate the risk of autoimmune orchitis and probably reduce the potential for immune-complex disease following immunity to normal male (but not female) antigens. Although animal models show promise, establishing the efficacy and safety of a contraceptive vaccine in humans remains a formidable challenge.

I.5.3.5 Conclusions

New male contraceptive methods would occupy niches, e.g. when delaying vasectomy, when female methods were not tolerated and during the postpartum period. Although their development has been prolonged for reasons explained elsewhere (Waites 2003), the principle of contraceptive efficacy has been established and new prototype drugs – for example, improved progestins developed for female contraception, given orally or as implants and combined with testosterone pellets, and orally active androgens, are now emerging for trial (see Chap. II.4.7).

References

Anderson RA, Baird DT (2002) Male contraception. Endocr Rev 23:735–762

Bebb RA, Anawalt BD, Christensen RB, Paulsen CA, Bremner WJ, Matsumoto AM (1996) Combined administration of levonorgestrel and testosterone induces more rapid and effective suppression of spermatogenesis than testosterone alone: a promising male contraceptive approach. J Clin Endocrinol Metab 81:757–762

Cooper TG (2002) The epididymis as a target for male contraception. In: Robaire B, Hinton BT (eds) The epididymis: from molecules to clinical practice. Kluwer Academic/Plenum, New York, pp 483–502

Ford WCL, Waites GMH (1986) Sperm maturation and the potential for contraceptive interference. In: Zatuchni GI, Goldsmith A, Spieler JM, Sciarra JJ (eds) Male contraception: advances and future prospects. Harper and Row, Philadelphia, Pa., pp 89–106

Gu YQ, Wang XH, Xu D, Peng L, Cheng LF, Huang MK, Huang ZJ, Zhang GY (2002) A multicenter contraceptive efficacy study of injectable testosterone undecanoate in healthy Chinese men. J Clin Endocrinol Metab 88:562–568

Handelsman DJ (2003) Hormonal male contraception – lessons from the East when the Western market fails. J Clin Endocrinol Metab 88:559–561

Handelsman DJ (2005) Male contraception. In: DeGroot LJ, Jameson JL (eds) Endocrinology, 5th edn. WB Saunders, Philadelphia pp 3247–3256

Handelsman DJ, Conway AJ, Howe CJ, Turner L, Mackey MA (1996) Establishing the minimum effective dose and additive effects of depot progestin in suppression of human spermatogenesis by a testosterone depot. J Clin Endocrinol Metab 81:4113–4121

Kamischke A, Nieschlag E (2004) Progress towards hormonal male contraception. Trends Pharmacol Sci 25:49–57

Martin CW, Anderson RA, Cheng L, Ho PC, van der Spuy Z, Smith KB et al (2000) Potential impact of hormonal male contraception: cross-cultural implications for development of novel preparations. Hum Reprod 15:637–645

Meriggiola MC, Bremner WJ, Paulsen CA, Valdiserri A, Incorvaia L, Motta R, Pavani A, Capelli M, Flamigni C (1996) A combined regimen of cyproterone acetate and testosterone enanthate as a potentially highly effective male contraceptive. J Clin Endocrinol Metab 81:3018–3023

United Nations (2000) Levels and trends of contraceptive use as assessed in 1998. Department of International Economic and Social Affairs, New York

Waites GMH (2003) Development of methods of male contraception: impact of the World Health Organization Task Force. Fertil Steril 80:1–15

WHO Task Force on Methods for the Regulation of Male Fertility (1990) Contraceptive efficacy of testosterone-induced azoospermia in normal men. Lancet 336: 955–959

I.5.4 Traditional Methods

D. Handelsman, G. Waites

Key Messages

- The typical 1st-year failure rates of traditional male methods (periodic abstinence, withdrawal, condoms) demonstrate that, apart from vasectomy, these methods involve high risk for contraception.
- This underlines the pressing need for men to have access to the alternative hormonal methods currently under development.

I.5.4.1 Introduction

At present, men have only traditional methods (periodic abstinence, withdrawal, condoms) and vasectomy (See Part I.5.1) and lack reliable and reversible contraceptive methods comparable to modern female methods. Nevertheless, one-third of all couples adopting family planning methods do so involving the use of these traditional methods (United Nations 2000).

I.5.4.1.1
Periodic Abstinence

Periodic abstinence for contraception is practiced by over 30 million couples worldwide (United Nations 2000). It aims to prevent pregnancy by avoiding vaginal intercourse at the expected time of ovulation, typically between days 9 and 19 of a regular menstrual cycle (WHO 1999). Periodic abstinence provides acceptable contraceptive efficacy when the timing of intercourse is strictly regulated but the failure rate rises steeply without rigid adherence to the rules. The demanding requirement, to avoid intercourse for nearly half of nonmenstrual days, is the main source of the relatively high failure rate from user error. Acceptability of this method can be enhanced with more accurate timing of the ovulatory phase than is possible by the calendar calculation (which requires a regular cycle). Evaluating indirect markers of ovulation (basal body temperature or cervical mucus changes) or more accurate but expensive urinary hormone (LH, steroids) detection methods can shorten the period of abstinence but the overall failure rates of the ovulation method (Table I.5.2) remain high (Trussell and Grummer-Strawn 1990).

I.5.4.1.2
Withdrawal

Among drug and device-free methods to prevent pregnancy, withdrawal (coitus interruptus) prior to ejaculation, is used by 40 million couples worldwide (Rogow and Horowitz 1995). Like the ovulation method, the risks of failure are primarily due to human error because of the demanding requirement of the method. As a result, the failure rates of withdrawal are relatively high and similar to those of periodic abstinence (Trussell and Kost 1987; Trussell and Grummer-Strawn 1990; Trussell and Vaughan 1999).

I.5.4.1.3
Condoms

Condoms, first described in the 16th century, are now used by over 45 million couples worldwide for pregnancy prevention (Liskin et al. 1990) and a larger number use condoms to prevent sexually transmitted diseases (STIs), including HIV. Typically, the male condom is a cylindrical sheath of latex, polyurethane or animal membranes, sometimes used in conjunction with a spermicide. Condoms are a moderately effective barrier method of contraception (Trussell et al. 1990; Trussell and Vaughan, 1999) with typical 1st year failure rates of roughly 14%, which exceed the "perfect use" failure rates of approximately 3% (Table I.5.2; Hatcher et al. 1994), a discrepancy mainly due to nonuse rather than misuse through incorrect application, damage, breakage, or slippage.

Condoms provide beneficial dual protection against pregnancy and STIs, making them ideal for unplanned sex or irregular sexual partners. By contrast, condoms are not a popular contraceptive option for couples in stable relationships because of their interference with spontaneity of lovemaking, dulling of penile sensation and cultural connotations, notably association with illicit or commercial sex. In the event of latex allergy, condoms made from polystyrene co-polymers (Rosenberg et al. 1996) are available but they have lower efficacy (Gallo et al. 2003).

Condoms provide substantial but not complete protection against STIs including HIV (Carey et al. 1999; Walsh et al. 2003; Holmes et al. 2004). Preventing STIs requires condom use on every sexual encounter, whereas reliable contraception requires only usage during mid-cycle ovulation. Consequently, condom failure rates vs STIs are always likely to exceed condom contraceptive failure rates as the major reason for failure in both settings is unreliable usage, rather than technical reasons such as breakage, slippage or porosity to infectious agents.

Table I.5.2. Typical 1st year failure rates (%), requirements and disadvantages of traditional male contraceptive options and comparison with female methods (Hatcher et al. 1994)

	Annual failure (pregnancy) rates Typical[a]	Perfect	Requirements	Disadvantages
Withdrawal	19	4	Skill and discipline	No STI protection
Abstinence with:	20	0	Regular check of fertility signs	No STI protection
Calendar method		9		
Ovulation method		3		
BBT/cervical mucus		2		
Condoms	14	3	Coitally related	Unpopular for stable couples; latex allergy
Vasectomy	0.15	0.10	Skilled practitioner	Intended irreversible
Modern reversible female methods[b]	0.1–3	0.3–1.5	Skilled practitioner	No male participation
Tubal ligation	0.4	0.4	Skilled practitioner, general anaesthetic	Intended irreversible

[a] Typical 1st year of use
[b] Includes hormonal methods and IUD

I.5.4.2 Conclusions

From the typical 1st-year failure rates of traditional male methods in Table I.5.2, it is evident that, apart from vasectomy, these methods involve high risk both when used for contraception and for protection against sexually transmitted diseases. These considerations further underline the pressing need by men to have the alternative methods currently under development (see Chap. II.4.3b).

References

Carey RF, Lytle CD, Cyr WH (1999) Implications of laboratory tests of condom integrity. Sex Transm Dis 26:216–220

Gallo MF, Grimes DA, Schulz KF (2003) Nonlatex vs. latex male condoms for contraception: a systematic review of randomized controlled trials. Contraception 68:319–326

Hatcher RA, Trussell J, Stewart F, Stewart GK, Kowal D, Guest F, Cates W Jr, Policar MS (1994) Contraceptive technology, 16th edn. Irvington, New York

Holmes KK, Levine R, Weaver M (2004) Effectiveness of condoms in preventing sexually transmitted infections. Bull World Health Organ 82:454–461

Liskin L, Wharton C, Blackburn R, Kestelman P (1990) Condoms – Now more than ever. Population Information Program, Center for Communication Programs, The Johns Hopkins University, Baltimore, Md.

Rogow D, Horowitz S (1995) Withdrawal: a review of the literature and an agenda for research. Stud Fam Plann 26:140–153

Rosenberg MJ, Waugh MS, Solomon HM, Lyszkowski AD (1996) The male polyurethane condom: a review of current knowledge. Contraception 53:141–146

Trussell J, Grummer-Strawn L (1990) Contraceptive failure of the ovulation method of periodic abstinence. Fam Plann Perspect 22:65–75

Trussell J, Kost K (1987) Contraceptive failure in the Unites States: a critical review of the literature. Stud Fam Plann 18:237–283

Trussell J, Vaughan B (1999) Contraceptive failure, method-related discontinuation and resumption of use: results from the 1995 National Survey of Family Growth. Fam Plann Perspect 31:64–72, 93

Trussell J, Hatcher RA, Cates W, Stewart FH, Kost K (1990) Contraceptive failure in the United States: an update. Stud Fam Plann 21:51–54

United Nations (2000) Levels and trends of contraceptive use as assessed in 1998. Department of International Economic and Social Affairs, New York

Walsh TL, Frezieres RG, Peacock K, Nelson AL, Clark VA, Bernstein L, Wraxall BG (2003) Use of prostate specific antigen (PSA) to measure semen exposure resulting from male condom failures: implications for contraceptive efficacy and the prevention of sexually transmitted disease. Contraception 67:139–150

WHO (1999) Annual Technical Report 1998, Special Programme of Research, Development and Research Training in Human Reproduction, Geneva, Switzerland, p 111

Problem: Reproductive Tract Infections I.6

I.6.1 Reproductive Tract Infections/ Sexually Transmitted Diseases

F.R. Ochsendorf

Key Messages

- The data on the relevance of reproductive tract infections for male infertility are conflicting.
- Depending on the local prevalence of infectious diseases and the availability of medical care, the impact is regionally different.
- Infectious agents have different modes of impairing fertility (male: organ damage, cell damage via mediators of inflammation, obstruction, binding to spermatozoa; female: pelvic inflammatory disease and tubal obstruction).
- Bacteria can often be found in semen and their mere presence appears to reflect contamination.
- The clinical relevance of the role of viruses is not known at present.
- As more past than present infections appear to be relevant for fertility, it is important to treat any infection adequately and appropriately.

I.6.1.1 Definition of the Disease

In an infection, microorganisms intrude in a macroorganism, where they attach, multiply and induce a local or systemic response. Sequelae depend on the properties of the microorganisms, the localization of this process as well as the kind and strength of the immunologic reaction.

If microorganisms are detected in the ejaculate it is difficult to decide whether these germs just colonized (attached to) the urethra or invaded the accessory glands, epididymis or testis (prostatitis is covered in Chap. I.9). Furthermore, their capacity to multiply and the extent of the body's reaction, i.e. the inflammatory response, are often impossible to assess. These factors, however, are decisive for the impairment of reproductive functions. The resulting damage of the reproductive organs persists even after spontaneous or therapeutic resolution of the infection.

Epidemiologic data link infections to male infertility. An association of age and infections as well as decreasing whole sperm counts were reported (Rolf et al. 2002). In some studies, 45 % of men attending for investigation of suspected infertility had a history of urethral discharge (Schulenburg et al. 1993; Bayasgalan et al. 2004). Others did not report relevant sexually transmitted disease (STD) histories in their patients (Oldereid et al. 1992) or could not confirm alterations of sperm characteristics after gonorrhoeic or chlamydial urethritis (Ness et al. 1997). These authors concluded their review in 1997: "Although there is tantalizing clinical and pathologic evidence for an association between STDs and infertility, . . . the current epidemiologic literature does not allow any conclusion about causality." While many reports deal with bacterial infections and STDs, information on viral infections of the reproductive tract is scarce (Dejucq and Jégou 2001). Infections and STDs have a different prevalence throughout the world. Therefore, no general comment as to the relevance of "infections" in a given population can be made.

I.6.1.2 Aetiology and Pathogenesis

Infectious agents may invade the reproductive organs via the blood, such as mumps viruses or *Mycobacterium tuberculosis* or *Mycobacterium leprae*, or by ascension via the urethra. They may impair the reproductive functions by several mechanisms (Table I.6.1).

Table I.6.2 summarizes the sexually transmitted bacterial, protozoal and fungal agents, Table I.6.3 the viruses. Depending on the site of the infection, either tissue is destroyed impairing the organ's functions, such

Table I.6.1. Possible consequences of infections of the male reproductive tract (after Dejucq and Jégou 2001)

Mechanism	Consequences
Spreading of diseases	Female disease Female infertility Infection of ova and embryo, miscarriage, embryonic and fetal abnormalities
Changes in germ cells	Male infertility/sterility
Changes in Sertoli cells	Male infertility/sterility
Changes in Leydig cells	Male infertility/sterility
Infiltration of leukocytes into the reproductive tract	T-cell-mediated response to spermatozoa and autoimmune infertility
Decrease in testosterone production	Cachexia, male infertility
Incorporation of viral genome into the germ cell genome	Risk of transmission to subsequent generations

as destruction of testicular tissue after tuberculosis or in lepromatous leprosy. Furthermore, autoimmune mechanisms could be induced (Munoz and Witkin 1995). Others, however, could not confirm a relationship between anti-sperm antibodies and the demonstration of a variety of bacteria or inflammatory signs in semen (Eggert-Kruse et al. 1998). A dysfunction of the ejaculated spermatozoa could be the result of a damage by mediators of inflammation, such as reactive oxygen species (Ochsendorf 1999). A subtotal or total obstruction of the excretory ducts could result (Dohle 2003). Some bacteria can impair motility by directly adhering to spermatozoa. This was demonstrated by very high numbers of *Escherichia coli* and ureaplasms (Bornman et al. 1992; Diemer et al. 2003; Keck et al. 1998). A significant inhibitory effect of *Candida albicans* in vitro was only detected in samples with initial germ concentrations of 2×10^7/ml (Huwe et al. 1998). A negative effect in case of mycotic vaginitis on spermatozoa motility and increased agglutination was proposed (Tuttle et al. 1977).

As bacteria can be found in high percentages of ejaculates without a detectable influence on sperm–mucus interaction, antibody formation or semen quality, seminal fluid microorganisms appear merely to be contaminants (Eggert-Kruse et al. 1992; Cottell et al. 2000).

The role of viruses is largely unknown. Viral DNA was demonstrated by nested PCR in the ejaculate of infertile men in 56% of cases [Herpes simplex virus (HSV) 49%, Epstein-Barr virus (EBV) 17%, cytomegalovirus (CMV) 7%]. Only HSV was related to low sperm count and poor motility (Kapranos et al. 2003). Others reported an incidence of 24% (El Borai et al. 1998) and 3% (Wald et al. 1999) or could not confirm the findings at all (Krause et al. 2002). Acyclovir therapy of both partners with positive HSV DNA was reported to result in pregnancies (El Borai et al. 1998; Kotronias and Kapranos 1998). A cervical herpes simplex virus infection is not a significant cause of impaired quality and penetrability of the cervical mucus (Eggert-Kruse et al. 2000).

The adeno-associated virus (AAV) was demonstrated in 38% of men with abnormal semen analyses, in 26% of testicular biopsies of infertile men and in 5% of normal semen samples. There was no difference in the incidence of human papilloma virus and CMV between the different groups (Erles et al. 2001). CMV was demonstrated in up to 5.6% of donor's semen samples cryopreserved for donor insemination (Mansat et al. 1997). CMV viral shedding did not affect semen quality (Yang et al. 1995); in other studies, the demonstration of CMV was associated with decreased concentration and motility (Torino et al. 1987). CMV was discussed as a possible causative agent of haematospermia (Komment and Poor 1983). If HPV was present in the semen the incidence of asthenozoospermia was significantly higher (Lai et al. 1997).

I.6.1.3 Clinical Findings: History, Physical Examination, Technical Investigations, Laboratory Findings

Patients may be asymptomatic or may present with clinical signs of an inflammation. The symptoms differ depending on the site of the infection: dysuria and discharge (urethritis), pain, red skin and swelling of the epididymis or testis (epididymitis, orchitis). The immunologic reaction is responsible for the strength of the clinical symptoms. Acute infections can be diagnosed by their typical clinical presentation. However, they are extremely rare in an andrological outpatient setting.

In daily practice, patients may report a prior episode of a genitourinary tract infection. If appropriate treatment was provided this infection probably was adequately treated without negative consequences. Otherwise a chronic infection may have resulted and led to tissue injury either directly or indirectly via a chronic inflammation. Sometimes a thickened epididymis could be a clinical sign of it. Some authors suggested that a chronic prostatovesiculitis could be diagnosed by transrectal ultrasound (Purvis and Christiansen 1993), whereas others showed that this method is of no use in the diagnosis of male accessory gland infection (Schipper et al. 2001). In order to prove the existence of an active infection, the responsible agent has to be found.

Chronic seminal vesiculitis can result from incomplete resolution of an acute inflammatory process. There are often no symptoms or they are the same as in chronic prostatitis, which can often be found in association (spasmodic pain during ejaculation, morning urethral discharge, haemospermia; low fructose in the ejaculate) (Farid and Hargreave 1995).

Table I.6.2. Sexually transmitted diseases: pathogenic agents, clinical findings, treatment and relevance

Disease	Pathogenic agent	Clinical findings	Physical examination	Investigation	Laboratory findings	Differential diagnosis	Treatment	Relevance for infertility
Bacteria								
Gonorrhoea	*Neisseria gonorrhoeae*	Dysuria, discharge, enlarged tender epididymis (mostly unilateral)	Urethral discharge	Urethral swab: Gram stain; culture (rapid transport, special transport medium)	Gram-negative intracellular diplococci Positive culture	Urethritis due to *Chlamydia*, *Ureaplasma* etc.	Urethritis: 1× chinolones, cephalosporins, spectinomycin, Epididymitis: longer therapy	Male + Female +
Chlamydia infection	*Chlamydia trachomatis* (D–K)	Dysuria, discharge, enlarged tender epididymis (mostly unilateral)	Urethral discharge or asymptomatic	First void urine and molecular method (PCR; LCR)	Positive DNA detection	Urethritis due to gonorrhoea	Urethritis: doxycycline 2×100 mg/day 7 days, azithromycin 1 g Epididymitis: longer	Male ? Female + Female +
Urethritis due to	*Ureaplasma urealyticum*	Dysuria, discharge	Urethral discharge or asymptomatic	Culture	High colony counts	Urethritis due to gonorrhoea or *Chlamydia*	Doxycycline 2× 100 mg/day 7 days, azithromycin 1 g	May impair motility ??
Syphilis	*Treponema pallidum*	Depending on stage: ulcer, painless lymph node enlargement, exanthema; gummatous infiltration of testicles and prostate gland	Ulcer, lymph node enlargement, skin signs, history Enlarged firm testicles or enlarged prostate	Serology (VDRL, TPHA or TPPA)	Positive culture	Depending on skin findings Testicles: tumour, benign or malignant prostate tumours	Penicillin	Co-factor for transmission of HIV Gummatous lesions: + Female +
Chancroid	*Haemophilus ducreyi*	Ulcer, lymph node painful and enlarged	Painful ulcer, painful red swollen lymph nodes	Culture, stain	Positive culture, positive stain	Syphilis	Azithromycin 1 g (and others)	–
Lymphogranuloma venereum	*Chlamydia trachomatis* (L1–L3)	Inguinal (unilateral) Lymph node enlargement, proctocolitis, fistulation	Tender lymphadenopathy	Clinical differential diagnoses, serology	Complement fixation test > 1:64	Syphilis	Doxycycline 2×100 mg 21 days	–
Granuloma inguinale	*Calymmatobacterium granulomatis*	Painless progressive ulcer	Ulceration without lymphadenopathy	Clinical differential diagnosis	Dark stained Donovan bodies in tissue crush/biopsy	Syphilis, chancroid	Doxycycline 2×100 mg > 21 days Cotrimoxazole 2×/day > 21 days	–
Protozoa								
Urethritis (prostatitis, epididymitis) due to	*Trichomonas vaginalis*	Discharge, asymptomatic or itching	Discharge	Clinical differential diagnoses	Wet mount examination of urethral discharge or urine sediment	Urethritis due to other causes	Metronidazole	? Controversial
Yeasts								
Balanitis, Urethritis due to	*Candida albicans*	Balanitis, itching	Redness, white	Clinical	Wet mount examination, culture	Contact dermatitis	Imidazole	–

I.6

Table I.6.3. Overview of the viruses found in the human genital tract/semen and abnormalities detected in the presence of virus. (*CMV* Cytomegalovirus, *EBV* Epstein–Barr virus, *HBV* hepatitis B virus, *HCV* hepatitis C virus, *HERV* human endogenous retrovirus, *HHV 8* human herpesvirus 8, *HIV* human immunodeficiency virus, *HSV* herpes simplex virus, *HTLV* human T lymphotropic virus, *LCMV* lymphocytic choriomeningitis virus)

Virus	Detected in cells	Of these organs/ secretions	Abnormalities detected in the presence of virus
HIV	Monocytes/macrophages and lymphocytes Germ cells Spermatozoa (?)	Testis Prostate Semen	Orchitis, interstitial fibrosis, lymphocyte infiltration, change in Leydig cell number, decrease in germ cell number, change in spermatogenesis; increase in testosterone at early stage of infection; decrease in AIDS Azoospermia Oligozoospermia Morphologically abnormal spermatozoa Pyospermia
CMV	Monocytes/macrophages and lymphocytes	Prostate Seminal vesicle Semen	Haematospermia Decrease in the number of CD4 cells
HBV	Monocytes/macrophages and lymphocytes Spermatozoa	Semen	
HSV 1, 2	Spermatozoa	Testis Prostate Semen	Infertility Azoospermia, oligozoospermia
Human papillomavirus	Cellular fraction (no specific cell type identified)	Prostate Semen	Asthenozoospermia Subgroup of prostate cancer (?)
Adenovirus	Cellular fraction (no specific cell type identified)	Testis Semen	Infertility Orchitis[b]
HHV 8	Mononuclear cell fraction	Prostate Semen	
Coxsackie β4 virus (?)		Epididymis	Associated with orchitis
EBV		Testis Semen ?	Orchitis[b] Testicular cancer (?)
HCV (?)	Conflicting results	Semen	
HTLV1	Contaminated lymphocytes	Semen	
Mumps	Leydig cells, germ cells (?)	Testis	Orchitis, testicular atrophy, sterility, decrease in androgen secretion, testicular cancer (?)
Parvovirus B 19		Testis	Testicular cancer (?)
Coxsackie virus A 9		Testis	Orchitis (?)

Not definitely proven to be present in testis: Bat salivary gland virus[a], Influenza virus[b], Dengue[a], LCMV[b], ECHO virus[b], Smallpox virus[b], vaccinia virus[b], rubella virus[b], chicken pox virus[b], HERV, hepatitis G.
[a] Association with significant incidence of clinical orchitis
[b] Orchitis rarely associated
Atrophy of the testis may occur after viral orchitis, but mostly unilateral, so sterility is extremely rare
For references, see Dejucq and Jégou (2001); only anomalies concerning male infertility are listed

Often the patient is asymptomatic. The ejaculates of these patients were bacterial culture-positive in between 47% (Onemu and Ibeh 2001) and 66% (Merino et al. 1995) of cases. If special conditions were used anaerobes could be detected in 99% of patients. In the latter study, however, there was no relation to impaired sperm parameters, cervical mucus penetration or later fertility (Eggert-Kruse et al. 1995). If both partners were investigated, no microorganisms were detectable in only 1%. No impairment of cervical mucus interaction was found. So the demonstration of microorganisms without symptoms of genital tract infection appears to reflect colonization and not infection (Eggert-Kruse et al. 1992). In line with this view is the observation that antibiotic treatment of asymptomatic patients with potentially pathogenic microorganisms in semen samples and/or cervical swabs did change the microbial pattern but not the ejaculate parameters (Eggert-Kruse et al. 1988).

Table I.6.2 summarizes physical/technical examinations and laboratory findings of relevant pathogenic

Table I.6.4. Synopsis of clinical presentation of patients

Microbiologic finding	History	Clinical finding	Possible interpretation	Relevance for fertility	Specific therapy
Microorganism	Remarkable	Remarkable	Infection	+	+
	Unremarkable	Remarkable	Infection	+	+
	Unremarkable	Unremarkable	Commensal	–	–
			Contamination	–	–
			Infection (?)	? +	+ If significant number of bacteria or pathogenic
No microorganism	Remarkable (for example prior discharge)	Remarkable (for example swelling/tenderness epididymis)	Chronic asymptomatic (silent) infection/inflammation	+	See MAGI
	Unremarkable	Remarkable	Chronic asymptomatic (silent) infection/inflammation??	? +	? +
	Remarkable	Unremarkable	Past infection	? +	–
			Chronic asymptomatic (silent) infection/inflammation??	? +	See MAGI

microorganisms. Table I.6.4 summarizes the clinical presentation of patients.

I.6.1.4 Differential Diagnosis

The clinical symptoms and findings do not allow a specific diagnosis. All microorganisms in Table I.6.2 can be the cause of the clinical symptoms.

The different regional prevalence of infectious diseases leads to different differential diagnosis. Indurated, enlarged, hard epididymis may be a sign of tuberculosis or bilharziasis. Enlargement of the prostate gland and clinical signs of prostatitis could be due to actinomycosis, blastomycosis, coccidioidomycosis, syphilis, or bilharziasis in some parts of the world.

I.6.1.5 Treatment

Treatment is summarized in Table I.6.2. Details can be found elsewhere (Center of Disease Control and Prevention 2002; Naber et al. 2001; Radcliffe 2001). Partner therapy is recommended.

I.6.1.6 Results of Treatment

Early treatment of an acute infection cures the disease without sequelae. The result of therapy in chronic infections depends on the damage already present at the time of treatment.

I.6.1.7 Prognosis

The prognosis is determined by the time of the first presentation of the patient, the correct diagnosis and adequate therapy. In all STDs, but especially in cases of gonorrhoea and chlamydial infections, adequate therapy of the female partner is important in order to prevent salpingitis, pelvic inflammatory disease and obstruction.

I.6.1.8 Prevention

Apparently, demonstration of microorganisms in semen samples of asymptomatic patients reflects colonization (Eggert-Kruse et al. 1992). It was concluded that more past than present infections are relevant (Gonzales et al. 2004). Therefore only adequate and early therapy of infections of the reproductive tract can prevent detrimental effects on the reproductive organs.

I.6.1.9 Other

Summarizing the available data, it appears that a large regional difference exists concerning the practical relevance of sexually transmitted infections for male infertility. In Western countries, it was concluded that, on the whole, STD infections only play a minor role with regard to male infertility (Krause and Weidner 1989) and that most of the time seminal fluid microorganisms are merely contaminants (Cottell et al. 2000). The situation in other parts of the world appears to be different. The relevance of viral infections is not completely resolved at this time.

References

Bayasgalan G, Naranbat D, Tsedmaa B, Tsogmaa B, Sukhee D, Amarjargal O, Lhagvasuren T, Radnaabazar J, Rowe PJ (2004) Clinical patterns and major causes of infertility in Mongolia. J Obstet Gynaecol Res 30:386–393

Bornman MS, Crewe-brown HH, Reif S, Mahomed MF, Broomker D, Schulenburg GW (1992) Sexually transmitted diseases (STD) in infertile males attending the andrology clinic at Ga-Rankuwa Hospital. Arch AIDS Res 6:213–220

Center of Disease Control and Prevention (2002) Sexually transmitted diseases treatment guidelines 2002. MMWR 51 (No. RR-6):1–77

Cottell E, Harrison RF, McCaffrey M, Walsh T, Mallon E, Barry-Kinsella C (2000) Are seminal fluid microorganisms of significance of merely contaminants? Fertil Steril 74:465–470

Dejucq N, Jégou B (2001) Viruses in the mammalian male genital tract and their effects on the reproductive system. Microbiol Mol Biol Rev 65:208–231

Diemer T, Huwe P, Ludwig M, Schroeder-Printzen I, Michelmann HW, Schiefer HG, Weidner W (2003) Influence of autogenous leucocytes and Escherichia coli on sperm parameters in vitro. Andrologia 35:100–105

Dohle GR (2003) Inflammatory-associated obstructions of the male genital tract. Andrologia 35:321–324

Eggert-Kruse W, Hofmann H, Gerhard I, Bilke A, Runnebaum B, Petzoldt D (1988) Effects of antimicrobial therapy on sperm-mucus interaction. Hum Reprod 3:861–869

Eggert-Kruse W, Pohl S, Naher H, Tilgen W, Runnebaum B (1992) Microbial colonization and sperm–mucus interaction: results in 1000 infertile couples. Hum Reprod 7:612–620

Eggert-Kruse W, Rohr G, Strock W, Pohl S, Schwalbach B, Runnebaum B (1995) Anaerobes in ejaculates of subfertile men. Hum Reprod Update 1:462–478

Eggert-Kruse W, Rohr G, Probst S, Rusu R, Hund M, Demirakca T, Aufenanger J, Runnebaum B, Petzoldt D (1998) Antisperm antibodies and microorganisms in genital secretions – a clinically significant relationship? Andrologia 30 [Suppl 1]: 61–71

Eggert-Kruse W, Mildenberger-Sandbrink B, Schnitzler P, Rohr G, Strowitzki T, Petzoldt D (2000) Herpes simplex virus infection of the uterine cervix–relationship with a cervical factor? Fertil Steril 73:248–257

El Borai N, LeFevre C, Inoue M, Naumova EN, Sato K, Suzuki S, Tsuji K, Yamamura M (1998) Presence of HSV-1 DNA in semen and menstrual blood. J Reprod Immunol 41:137–147

Erles K, Rohde V, Thaele M, Roth S, Edler L, Schlehofer JR (2001) DNA of adeno-associated virus (AAV) in testicular tissue and in abnormal semen samples. Hum Reprod 16:2333–2337

Farid M, Hargreave TB (1995) Infection and male infertility. In: Hargreave TB (ed) Male infertility. Springer, Berlin Heidelberg New York, pp 291–306

Gonzales GF, Munoz G, Sanchez R, Henkel R, Gallegos-Avila G, Diaz-Gutierrez O, Vigil P, Vasquez F, Kortebani G, Mazzolli A, Bustos-Obregon E (2004) Update on the impact of *Chlamydia trachomatis* infection on male fertility. Andrologia 36:1–23

Huwe P, Diemer T, Ludwig M, Liu J, Schiefer HG, Weidner W (1998) Influence of different uropathogenic microorganisms on human sperm motility parameters in an in vitro experiment. Andrologia 30 Suppl 1:55–59

Kapranos N, Petrakou E, Anastasiadou C, Kotronias D (2003) Detection of herpes simplex virus, cytomegalovirus, and Epstein-Barr virus in the semen of men attending an infertility clinic. Fertil Steril 79 [Suppl 3]:1566–1570

Keck C, Gerber-Schafer C, Clad A, Wilhelm C, Breckwoldt M (1998) Seminal tract infections: impact on male fertility and treatment options. Hum Reprod Update 4:891–903

Komment RW, Poor PM (1983) Infection by human cytomegalovirus associated with chronic hematospermia. Urology 22:617–621

Kotronias D, Kapranos N (1998) Detection of herpes simplex virus DNA in human spermatozoa by in situ hybridization technique. In Vivo 12:391–394

Krause W, Weidner W (1989) [Sexually transmitted diseases as causes of disorders of male fertility]. Z Hautkr 64:596, 599–601

Krause W, Herbstreit F, Slenzka W (2002) Are viral infections the cause of leukocytospermia? Andrologia 34:87–90

Lai YM, Yang FP, Pao CC (1997) The effect of human papillomavirus infection on sperm motility in vitro. Fertil Steril 66:1152–1155

Mansat A, Mengelle C, Chalet M, Boumzebra A, Mieusset R, Puel J, Prouhez C, Segondy M (1997) Cytomegalovirus detection in cryopreserved semen samples collected for therapeutic donor insemination. Hum Reprod 12:1663–1666

Merino G, Carranza-Lira S, Murrieta S, Rodriguez L, Cuevas E, Moran C (1995) Bacterial infection and semen characteristics in infertile men. Arch Androl 35:43–47

Munoz MG, Witkin SS (1995) Autoimmunity to spermatozoa, asymptomatic Chlamydia trachomatis genital tract infection and gamma delta T lymphocytes in seminal fluid from the male partners of couples with unexplained infertility. Hum Reprod 10:1070–1074

Naber KG, Bergman B, Bishop MC, Bjerklung-Johansen TE, Botto H, Lobel B, Cruz FJ, Selvaggy FP (2001) EAU Guidelines for the management of urinary and male genital tract infections. Eur Urol 40:576–588

Ness RB, Markovic N, Carlson CL, Coughlin MT (1997) Do men become infertile after having sexually transmitted urethritis? An epidemiologic examination. Fertil Steril 68:205–213

Ochsendorf FR (1999) Infections in the male genital tract and reactive oxygen species. Hum Reprod Update 5:399–420

Oldereid NB, Rui H, Purvis K (1992) The value of anamnestic information regarding previous genital infection in male fertility investigation. Eur J Obstet Gynecol Reprod Biol 47: 207–212

Onemu SO, Ibeh IN (2001) Studies on the significance of positive bacterial semen cultures in male fertility in Nigeria. Int J Fertil Womens Med 46:210–214

Purvis K, Christiansen E (1993) Infection in the male reproductive tract. Impact, diagnosis and treatment in relation to male infertility. Int J Androl 16:1–13

Radcliffe K (2001) European STD guidelines. Internat J STD AIDS 12 [Suppl 3]:1–102

Rolf C, Kenkel S, Nieschlag E (2002) Age-related disease pattern in infertile men: increasing incidence of infections in older patients. Andrologia 34:209–217

Schipper RA, Trum JW, Messelink EJ, van der Veen F, Kurth KH (2001) Transrectal ultrasonography in male subfertility patients: an intra- and interobserver study. Urol Res 29:57–59

Schulenburg GW, Borman MS, Reif S, Bookmer D (1993) Semen profiles in infertile African males. In: Andrology in the nineties. Int. Symposium on male infertility and assisted reproduction. Gen K, Belgium. Wyeth, The Netherlands

Torino G, Bizzarro A, Castello G, Daponte A, Fontana A, De Bellis A, Paglionico VA (1987) Cytomegalovirus and male infertility. Ann Biol Clin (Paris) 45:440–443

Tuttle JP Jr, Bannister ER, Derrick FC (1977) Interference of human spermatozoal motility and spermatozoal agglutination by Candida albicans. J Urol 118:797–799

Wald A, Matson P, Ryncarz A, Corey L (1999) Detection of herpes simplex virus DNA in semen of men with genital HSV-2 infection. Sex Transm Dis 26:1–3

Yang YS, Ho HN, Chen HF, Chen SU, Shen CY, Chang SF, Huang ES, Wu CW (1995) Cytomegalovirus infection and viral shedding in the genital tract of infertile couples. J Med Virol 45:179–182

I.6.2 HIV Infection

F.R. Ochsendorf

Key Messages

- In human semen, HIV is mainly present in leukocytes.
- HIV-infected patients often present with spermatograms within normal limits.
- With progression of the acquired immunodeficiency, testicular function is impaired, as demonstrated by pathologic semen parameters and hypogonadism.
- In serodiscordant couples, it is possible to generate HIV-free sperm samples which can be used for reproductive techniques.
- With professional handling of the infected samples, the risk for infections of the laboratory personnel is very low.

I.6.2.1 Definition of the Disease

Infection by the human immunodeficiency virus has different aspects concerning reproductive medicine: ethical issues, prevention of spread to the child, relevance for the functions of the reproductive organs and safety issues of the laboratory personnel (Ethics Committee of the American Society for Reproductive Medicine 2004).

I.6.2.2 Aetiology and Pathogenesis

In the testis of infected asymptomatic HIV-positive subjects, HIV-1 proviral DNA was detected in the nuclei of germ cells at all stages of differentiation by in situ PCR hybridization. The presence of provirus was not associated with germ cell damage, spermatogenesis was normal and a very mild local immune response was observed (Muciaccia et al. 1998). The virus was present in semen as free virus in the seminal plasma and as cell-associated virus in the leukocytes. There are conflicting data on whether the virus also infects spermatozoa (Dejucq and Jégou 2001). According to electron microscopy, HIV can attach to the surface of spermatozoa and enter these cells through the intact plasma membrane (Bagasra et al. 1994), probably by an alternative receptor (the GalAAG) (Piomboni and Baccetti 2000) or a 160-kDa sperm protein (Bandivdekar et al. 2003). Others could not confirm this (Pudney et al. 1998). Most relevant, however, are infected lymphocytes, monocytes and macrophages. (Dulioust et al. 1998), as vasectomy does not influence the amount of cell-free virus in semen (Krieger et al. 1998). Furthermore, it is possible to generate HIV-free spermatozoa fractions by washing procedures, which is an argument against infection of motile spermatozoa by this virus. In HIV patients, reduced testosterone levels were reported, which might impair testicular function (Dobs et al. 1988). Furthermore, autopsy studies reported testicular atrophy in AIDS patients (Chabon et al. 1987).

I.6.2.3 Clinical Findings: History, Physical Examination, Technical Investigations, Laboratory Findings

Many HIV-seropositive men have normal semen analyses within the WHO-defined normal range, but as the disease progresses more defects are found, particularly in strict criteria sperm morphology. Lower $CD4^+$ cell counts (<200 mm^3) were associated with significantly lower per cent motility, per cent normal sperm morphology by strict criteria, significantly more spermatids in semen, and higher percentages of teratozoospermia, oligoasthenoteratozoospermia and leukocytospermia. Healthier men, based on clinical categories, had significantly more normal-shaped spermatozoa and fewer had azoospermia, oligoasthenoteratozoospermia or leukocytospermia. In AIDS patients, grossly abnormal sperm and pyospermia was reported (Muller et al. 1998; Nicopoullos et al. 2004). Others reported reduced semen volume, reduced percentages of rapidly progressive motility, total sperm count and increased concentrations of nonspermatic cells (Dulioust et al. 2002). There were no differences in any parameter in those taking anti-retroviral medication (Nicopoullos et al. 2004).

In one sperm donor, semen could be analysed before and after HIV infection. Semen volume, sperm motility and the percentage of sperm with normal morphology were reduced after HIV positivity. A disturbed function of seminal vesicles and prostate gland could explain the decreased volume as well as the more viscous sperm found in HIV-infected subjects (Van Leeuwen et al. 2004; Dondero et al. 1996). Sperm alterations found today are attributed to effects of antiretroviral therapy (Dulioust et al. 2002; Barboza et al. 2004).

I.6.2.4 Treatment

In serodiscordant couples, assisted reproduction was successfully used. It is possible to free semen samples from HIV by certain washing procedures. Prior to use of the samples, a PCR is used to confirm that HIV is no longer present.

Antiretroviral treatment leading to low HIV-RNA serum viral load significantly improved intrauterine insemination (IUI) outcome regardless of CD4 counts, sperm parameters and stimulation regime (Nicopoullos et al. 2004).

The sperm preparation uses a gradient technique and a swim-up procedure. An aliquot of washed sperm is subsequently tested for detectable HIV RNA. In one study, about 5% of NASBA tests were positive after this procedure (Nicopoullos et al. 2004).

I.6.2.5 Results of Treatment

To date more than 300 healthy children have been born and more than 2,300 cycles of sperm washing and viral detection testing followed by IUI or in vitro fertilization/intracytoplasmic sperm injection (IVF/ICSI) worldwide have been performed, with no reported seroconversions in either partners or children (Nicopoullos et al. 2004; Semprini and Fiore 2004).

I.6.2.6 Prognosis

A viral load of less than 1,000 copies/ml and the use of antivirals were the only variables that significantly improved IUI outcome (Nicopoullos et al. 2004). Therefore, an effective antiretroviral therapy should be started prior to reproductive activities to improve the prognosis.

I.6.2.7 Prevention

It was recommended to test all gamete donors, persons who are considered at high risk for HIV infection, such as those who have a history of repeated sexually transmitted diseases, multiple sexual partners without barrier protection, bisexual behaviour or IV drug use. However, it was also recommended to encourage HIV testing for all couples who want to have children as part of responsible parenting (Ethics Committee of the American Society for Reproductive Medicine 2004).

In a serodiscordant couple, the female partner has a 0.1% to 0.2% risk of acquiring HIV per act of unprotected intercourse (Mastro et al. 1997). Attempts to conceive naturally carry a serious risk to the uninfected woman or child (Mandelbrot et al. 1997).

To date, only few occupational transmissions of HIV have been reported. In most cases, nurses and laboratory technicians accidentally inoculated themselves with a patient's blood by a needlestick or were contaminated with bloody fluid and had significant mucocutaneous exposure. If standard precautions to prevent infectious disease transmission are taken, the risk of virus transmission to lab personnel is very low.

I.6.2.8 Other

Health care providers and HIV-infected persons together share responsibility for the safety of the uninfected partner and potential offspring. They should be treated in institutions with the appropriate facilities. Alternatively, they may be advised to look to other options and consider donor sperm, adoption or not having children (Ethics Committee of the American Society for Reproductive Medicine 2004).

References

Anonymous (1983) Infertility and sexually transmitted disease: a public health challenge. Popul Rep L L114–151

Bagasra O, Farzadegan H, Seshamma T, Oakes JW, Saah A, Pomerantz RJ (1994) Detection of HIV-1 proviral DNA in sperm from HIV-1-infected men. Aids 8:1669–1674

Bandivdekar AH, Velhal SM, Raghavan VP (2003) Identification of CD4-independent HIV receptors on spermatozoa. Am J Reprod Immunol 50:322–327

Barboza JM, Medina H, Doria M, Rivero L, Hernandez L, Joshi NV (2004) Use of atomic force microscopy to reveal sperm ultrastructure in HIV patients on highly active antiretroviral therapy. Arch Androl 50:121–129

Chabon AB, Stenger AJ, Grebstaldt H (1987) Histopathology of testis in acquired immunodeficiency syndrome. Urology 29:658–663

Dejucq N, Jégou B (2001) Viruses in the mammalian male genital tract and their effects on the reproductive system. Microbiol Mol Biol Rev 65:208–231

Dobs AS, Dempsey MA, Ladenson PW, Polk PF (1988) Endocrine disorders in men infected with human immunodeficiency virus. Am J Med 84:811–816

Dondero F, Rossi T, D'Offizi G, Mazzilli F, Rosso R, Sarandrea N, Pinter E, Aiuti F (1996) Semen analysis in HIV seropositive men and in subjects at high risk for HIV infection. Hum Reprod 11:765–768

Dulioust E, Tachet A, De Almeida M, Finkielsztejn L, Rivalland S, Salmon D, Sicard D, Rouzioux C, Jouannet P (1998) Detection of HIV-1 in seminal plasma and seminal cells of HIV-1 seropositive men. J Reprod Immunol 41:27–40

Dulioust E, Du AL, Costagliola D, Guibert J, Kunstmann JM, Heard I, Juillard JC, Salmon D, Leruez-Ville M, Mandelbrot L, Rouzioux C, Sicard D, Zorn JR, Jouannet P, De Almeida M (2002) Semen alterations in HIV-1 infected men. Hum Reprod 17:2112–2118

Ethics Committee of the American Society for Reproductive Medicine (2004) Human immunodeficiency virus and infertility treatment. Fertil Steril 82 [Suppl 1]:S228–S231

Krieger JN, Nirapathpongporn A, Chaiyaporn M, Peterson G, Nikolaeva I, Akridge R, Ross SO, Coombs RW (1998) Vasectomy and human immunodeficiency virus type 1 in semen. J Urol 159:820–825; discussion 825–826

Mandelbrot L, Heard I, Henrion-Geant E, Henrion R (1997) Natural conception in HIV-negative women with HIV-infected partners. Lancet 349:850–851

Mastro TD, Kunanusont C, Dondero TJ, Wasi C (1997) Why do HIV-1 subtypes segregate among persons with different risk behaviors in South Africa and Thailand? Aids 11:113–116

Muciaccia B, Filippini A, Ziparo E, Colelli F, Baroni CD, Stefanini M (1998) Testicular germ cells of HIV-seropositive

asymptomatic men are infected by the virus. J Reprod Immunol 41:81–93
Muller CH, Coombs RW, Krieger JN (1998) Effects of clinical stage and immunological status on semen analysis results in human immunodeficiency virus type 1-seropositive men. Andrologia 30 [Suppl 1]:15–22
Nicopoullos JD, Almeida PA, Ramsay JW, Gilling-Smith C (2004) The effect of human immunodeficiency virus on sperm parameters and the outcome of intrauterine insemination following sperm washing. Hum Reprod 19:2289–2297
Piomboni P, Baccetti B (2000) Spermatozoon as a vehicle for HIV-1 and other viruses: a review. Mol Reprod Dev 56: 238–242
Pudney J, Nguyen H, Xu C, Anderson DJ (1998) Microscopic evidence against HIV-1 infection of germ cells or attachment to sperm. J Reprod Immunol 41:105–125
Semprini AE, Fiore S (2004) HIV and reproduction. Curr Opin Obstet Gynecol 16:257–262
Van Leeuwen E, Cornelissen M, De Vries JW, Lowe SH, Jurriaans S, Repping S, Van der Veen F (2004) Semen parameters of a semen donor before and after infection with human immunodeficiency virus. A case report. Hum Reprod 19:2845–2848

I.7 Problem: Emergencies in Andrology

I.7.1 Testicular Torsion

C.F. Heyns, A.J. Visser

Key Messages

- Torsion of the testis is a common emergency.
- The diagnosis is clinical and the management is emergency surgical reduction and bilateral fixation.
- A high index of suspicion is imperative in equivocal cases, and errors in management should be on the aggressive rather than the conservative side.
- Ipsilateral and contralateral orchiopexy should be performed with nonabsorbable sutures to prevent recurrent torsion.
- The testicular salvage rates correlate with the duration and the degree of torsion.
- Subfertility after torsion is well recognized but probably not of clinical importance.
- Testicular torsion remains a surgical emergency until 48 h of persistent symptoms have elapsed.
- In the presence of woody scrotal induration, testicular torsion is no longer an emergency after 24 h of persistent symptoms.
- Patients with a clinical diagnosis of intermittent or recurrent subacute torsion, and those with loss of one testis due to previous torsion, trauma or tumour, should probably undergo elective orchiopexy.
- Torsion of the testicular appendages can be managed conservatively and has no clinical importance, except that it must be distinguished from torsion of the testis.

I.7.1.1 Definition

Torsion of the testis was first described by Delasiauve in 1840 (Delasiauve 1840). The first case of torsion of a fully descended testis was reported by Langton in 1881 (Williamson 1976). In 1893, Nash first described manipulative detorsion of the testis (Nash 1893). Curling (1857) cited a case report by Rosenmerkel from Munich, who untwisted an undescended testis and fixed it in the scrotum with a stitch through the dartos tunics (Noske et al. 1998). Defontaine described the first case of operative reduction of an intrascrotal torsion in 1893 (Sparks 1971). Taylor first described extravaginal torsion in 1897 (Taylor 1897).

By 1901, Scudder was able to assemble only 32 cases from the world literature (Williamson 1976). Before 1919, only 124 cases had been reported, but between 1923 and 1930 there were 250 reported cases, probably due to wider recognition of the condition (O'Conor 1933).

We reviewed 276 articles, performed meta-analyses on the published data and reported our findings in two recent reviews, which can be consulted for the most important articles (Visser and Heyns 2003, 2004).

I.7.1.1.1 Intravaginal Torsion

Intravaginal torsion (IVT) is by far the most common type of torsion. The testis usually undergoes torsion on the last few centimetres of the spermatic cord within the tunica vaginalis. The predisposing anatomical factors are:

1. A spiral arrangement and low insertion of the fibres of the cremaster muscle.
2. A tunica vaginalis, which extends proximally around the spermatic cord – the bell-clapper deformity.
3. An abnormality of the junction of the epididymis with the testis, forming a mesorchium (Jones 1962).

Our current understanding of the mechanism and underlying anatomical abnormality can largely be credited to the work of Muschat who coined the term "bell-clapper" in 1932 when he described the findings in a case of intravaginal torsion (Muschat 1932). He postulated that during descent of the testis, the position of the scrotal organs is different in relation to the tunica vaginalis. Instead of descending posterior to the tunica vaginalis with partial covering of the descending organs, the testis and epididymis bulge into the vaginal sac and continue to descend into the sac until testis, epididymis and a portion of the spermatic cord are completely covered by the tunica vaginalis (Muschat 1932).

The term "mesorchium" has been used to describe two things:

1. The mesentery attached to the posterior aspect of the epididymis, and running vertically from the globus major to the globus minor. This arrangement is found in the normal testis, in which it acts as a stabilizing factor.
2. The thin linear attachment of the epididymis to the testis (Fig. I.7.1). This type of mesorchium may be important if the torsion occurs between the testis and the epididymis, which is a rare cause of intravaginal torsion (Jones 1962).

Intravaginal torsion is possible at three different levels:

1. The intravaginal spermatic cord may rotate and cause infarction of the testis and epididymis, which is the most common type (bell-clapper deformity).
2. The rotational plane may be through the mesorchium between the testis and epididymis, causing infarction of the testis only, while sparing the epididymis (mesorchial torsion).
3. Torsion may rarely occur through the mid epididymis, where part of the epididymis will be spared (epididymal torsion) (Parker and Robison 1971).

The bell-clapper deformity is found in 12% of autopsies, and is bilateral in 66% of these cases, suggesting that it is a common deformity in the human and more prevalent than torsion is manifest clinically (Caesar and Kaplan 1994a). In testicular torsion, the bell-clapper deformity is found in 71% to 75% of cases (Cass et al. 1980; Ransler and Allen 1982).

Mesorchial torsion is found in 9% to 25% of cases, and the abnormality is present on the contralateral side in 55% to 100% (Ransler and Allen 1982; Anderson and Williamson 1988).

Some purists prefer the term "torsion of the spermatic cord" instead of "torsion of the testis". However, from the above it is clear that torsion does not always involve the spermatic cord.

I.7.1.1.2
Extravaginal Torsion, Torsion of the Spermatic Cord, Supravaginal Torsion

Sir Astley Cooper in 1830 first noted that the entire scrotal contents of the neonate could be freely lifted out of the scrotum without tearing any tissue, and this mechanism is believed to account for the rare extravaginal torsion, which is found in neonates, where the entire testis complex twists en bloc (Williamson 1976). Jerkins et al. (1983) postulated that fixation of the testis to the scrotal wall occurs between 7 and 10 days after birth. However, fixation may take place later, since extravaginal torsion has been reported in a 5-week-old boy who was born at 36 weeks gestation (Kaufman 1984).

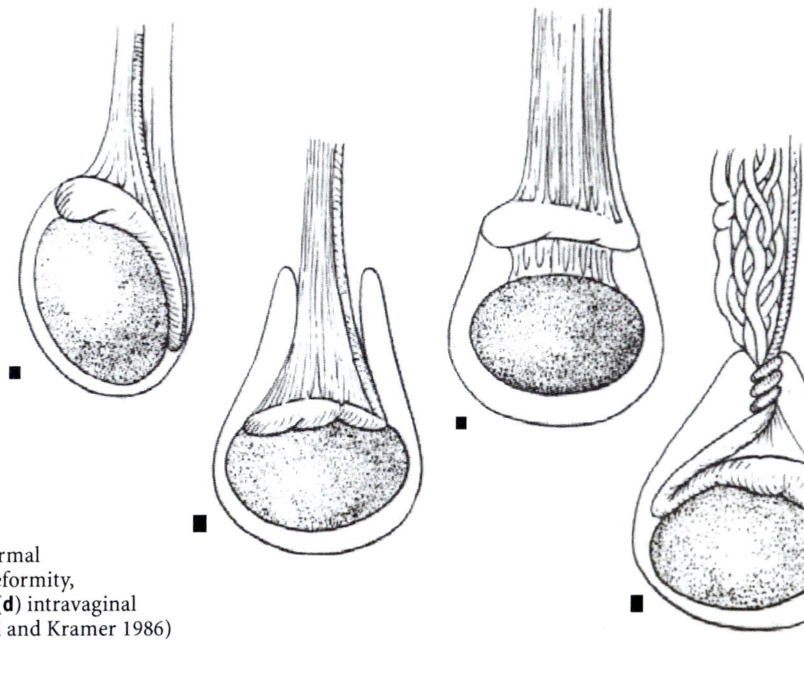

Fig. I.7.1. The anatomy of (**a**) normal attachments, (**b**) bell-clapper deformity, (**c**) abnormal mesorchium and (**d**) intravaginal torsion (Modified from Stillwell and Kramer 1986)

I.7.1.1.3 Spontaneous Detorsion

Spontaneous detorsion may occur at the time of anaesthesia or before in 10% to 25% of cases, probably due to cessation of the cremasteric spasm that maintains the torsion (Cass et al. 1980; Ransler and Allen 1982).

I.7.1.1.4 Intermittent Torsion, Subacute Torsion, Subtorsion

Van der Poel described the first case of intermittent torsion in 1895 (Schulsinger et al. 1991). Various activities are associated with intermittent torsion, including exercise, walking, sitting, standing, sleeping, coughing, leg crossing, straining at stool and coitus (Schulsinger et al. 1991).

Anderson and Williamson (1988) reported that in 76% of cases of recurrent subacute torsion, the testis had a horizontal lie on the affected side, and this anomaly was bilateral in 20%. Jones (1991) found a horizontally lying testis in 97%, and a bell-clapper deformity in 55% of patients. Cass (1982) found a bell-clapper deformity in 66% and a long mesorchium in 22% of patients with intermittent torsion.

In our meta-analysis of 521 cases of torsion of the testis from ten studies, intermittent subacute torsion accounted for 23% of all cases.

I.7.1.1.5 Torsion of Appendages

The appendix testis, a Müllerian duct remnant located at the superior pole of the testis, is the most common appendage to undergo torsion. The epididymal appendix, located on the head of the epididymis, is a Wolffian duct remnant and may also become twisted. The precise mechanism of torsion of the appendages is not clear, but it appears to be mostly restricted to the age of puberty and is usually preceded by vigorous activity or trauma. One possible mechanism is that increased oestrogen stimulation prior to the onset of puberty may cause the vestigial appendage to enlarge and strangulate (Skoglund et al. 1970b).

I.7.1.2 Aetiology and Pathogenesis

The prerequisites for intravaginal torsion include an anatomical predisposition for torsion (bell-clapper deformity or long mesorchium), an initiating force (cremasteric spasm) and a poorly understood mechanism which holds the testis in the torsed position (most probably also cremasteric spasm).

I.7.1.2.1 Intravaginal Torsion

Anatomical Predisposition

Up to 12% of the male population has an abnormal testicular attachment (bell-clapper deformity), although the occurrence of testicular torsion in the general population is much lower (Caesar and Kaplan 1994a).

Initiating Force

Cremasteric spasm associated with sleep, trauma, vigorous exercise or cold weather may be the initiating force (Williamson 1985).

Cold Weather

Several reports suggest that cold weather may predispose to torsion of the testis, probably by stimulating the cremaster fibres (Sparks 1971; Anderson and Williamson 1988; Hoshino et al. 1993). However, McCombe and Scobie (1988) found no seasonal variation in their series.

Trauma

A clear history of injury precedes torsion in 4% to 10% of cases (Anderson and Williamson 1988; Jefferson et al. 1997). Testicular trauma has been a notorious red herring in cases of missed torsion (Cos and Rabinowitz 1982). Severe blunt trauma may cause extravaginal torsion in older patients (Kursh 1981).

Exertion

Activities associated with torsion include cycling, swimming, parachuting, ice-skating, turning during sleep, sexual intercourse, football and rugby. A history of recent exercise or strenuous activity is reported in 7% to 60% of cases (Skoglund et al. 1970a; Anderson and Williamson 1988).

Sleep

Testicular torsion frequently occurs at night, often awaking the patient. It is possibly the result of a strong cremasteric reflex associated with nocturnal erections (Burgher 1998). Onset of torsion during sleep is reported in 11% to 40% of cases (Skoglund et al. 1970a; Anderson and Williamson 1988).

Puberty and Hormonal Causes

The peripubertal increase in the size of the testis relative to the spermatic cord, which imparts a greater moment to any twisting action, may contribute to torsion,

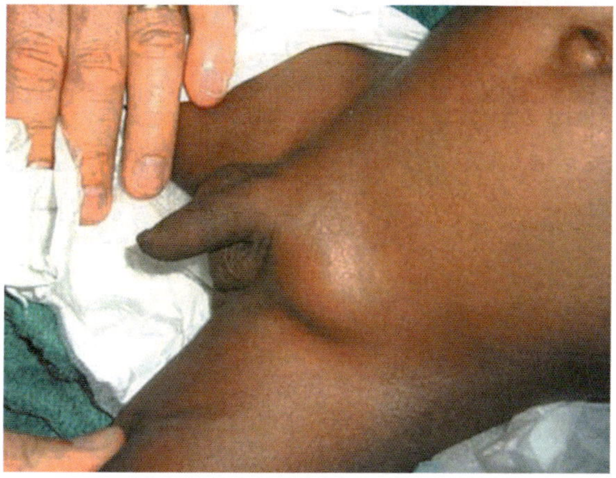

Fig. I.7.2. Torsion of an undescended testis situated in the inguinal canal, initially misdiagnosed as an incarcerated inguinal hernia

since 65% of cases affect boys between 12 and 18 years of age (Williamson 1976). Several cases have been reported of patients on human chorionic gonadotrophin (hCG) therapy undergoing torsion of the testis (Sawchuk et al. 1993; Van Glabeke et al. 1999).

Undescended Testes

Testicular torsion is ten times more likely in patients with undescended testes (Fig. I.7.2) (Williamson 1976). Before 1952, 60% of all cases of torsion of the testis were seen in undescended testes. These numbers declined with orchiopexy and currently most torsions are seen in the scrotal testis (Noske et al. 1998). Torsion in the undescended testis may be extravaginal or intravaginal (Jones 1962; Van Glabeke et al. 1999). Torsion of an intra-abdominal testis is extremely rare, with only 45 reported cases in the literature, and 65% of these patients had malignancy in the testis (Loostma and Van Der Pol 1987).

Familial

Torsion of the testis has been described in several families (Cunningham 1960; Sparks 1971; Castilla et al. 1975; Stewart and Maiti 1985; Anderson and Williamson 1988; Sinisi et al. 1993).

Polyorchidism

Witte et al. (1998) found that fewer than 100 cases of polyorchidism have been described, with their case being the ninth reported case with torsion. The left side is duplicated in 75% of cases of triorchidism (Tulchinsky and Eggli 1992). Torsion may occur in both the normal and the supernumerary testis and has been reported to be bilateral (Kajbafzadeh 1996).

I.7.1.2.2 Extravaginal/Neonatal Torsion

The most commonly accepted causes of neonatal (extravaginal) torsion are the extreme mobility of the neonatal tunica vaginalis inside the scrotum, and an active cremasteric reflex (Al-Salem 1999). Other factors are a high birth weight and trauma during difficult delivery or breech presentation. The reported mean birthweight for neonatal torsion is 3.6 kg (range, 2.9–4.2) (Guiney and McGlinchey 1981). Brandt et al. (1992) found that the birth weight was exceptionally high (3.8 kg) in their series, 60% of their cases were above the 90th percentile for birth weight, and there was also a strong correlation with multiparity. Reports of extravaginal torsion occurring in older boys have appeared, and almost half of these were associated with severe scrotal trauma (Lyon 1961; Jones 1962; Kursh 1981; Melekos et al. 1988).

I.7.1.2.3 Direction and Degree of Rotation

Torsion occurs with internal rotation (double thumbs down) in 71% to 100% of cases (Ransler and Allen 1982; Garel et al. 2000). The degree of rotation varies from 180° to 1440° (Williamson 1976). Cummings et al. found a significantly higher degree of rotation in patients 21 years or older compared to those less than 21 years of age. The mean rotation was 585° in the older group compared to 431° in the younger group (Cummings et al. 2002).

In our meta-analysis of 91 cases in the literature where the degree of torsion was specified, the median rotation was 360° and the average 480° (range 180° to 1080°) (Fig. I.7.3). The direction of rotation was seldom recorded, but in the 57 cases where it was noted, the torsion was by internal rotation in 74% and external rotation in 26%.

I.7.1.2.4 Mechanism of Infarction

When the spermatic cord is twisted, the veins in the cord are quickly obstructed due to their thin walls. Because of the tough connective tissue surrounding the spermatic cord, the swollen veins can produce sufficient pressure to shut off arterial flow, even if the twist itself has failed to occlude the artery. Initially this leads to oedema and congestion of the affected testis, which is followed by haemorrhage and infarction (Chen et al. 1983a). Arterial occlusion probably occurs with multiple twists, whereas arteriolar stasis develops secondary to venous occlusion with lesser twists (Cuckow and Frank 2000).

Experimental studies have shown that complete ces-

I.7

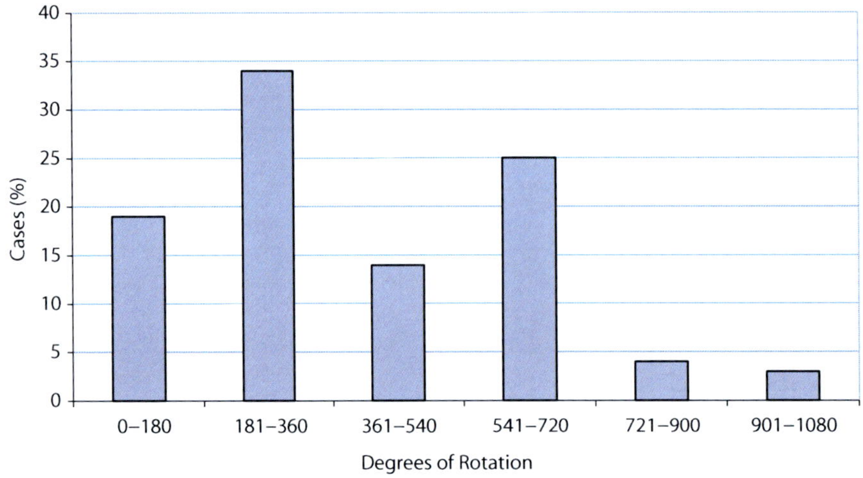

Fig. I.7.3. Degree of rotation for torsion of the testis in 91 cases from the literature

sation of arterial inflow occurs at 300° to 540° of torsion (Mevorach et al. 1991; Lee et al. 1996). Sonda and Lapides showed that three to four complete turns (1080° to 1440°) produced irreversible changes in the testis after 2 h. Torsion of 90° for periods as long as 7 days failed to cause any necrosis. Torsion of 180° demonstrated irreversible necrosis in 50 % of cases at 48 h. Torsion of 360° consistently caused necrosis within 24 h (Sonda and Lapides 1961).

Experimental studies in dogs revealed elimination of all spermatogenic and Sertoli cells by 6 h of testicular ischaemia and elimination of Leydig cells by 10 h of ischaemia (Smith 1955). In animal studies, the intratesticular pO_2 decreases within 5–7 min. If detorsion is performed within 1 h the pO_2 recovers within 15 min (Klotz et al. 1996). If the torsion is not reduced, there is usually a gradual subsidence of pain over 2–5 days, but the swelling and local tenderness persist for 10–14 days (O'Conor 1933).

The injury to the affected testis is caused by a combination of ischaemia and reperfusion. The reperfusion-induced injury only plays an important role for the first 3 h; thereafter the damage caused by ischaemia is far greater (Greenstein et al. 2001). The reperfusion injury is caused by reactive oxygen species, which arise from activation of the xanthine oxidase system in parenchymal cells, or from leukocytes that adhere to the reperfusing venule wall before undergoing diapedesis into the tissue itself (Yazawa et al. 2001).

I.7.1.3 Clinical Findings

I.7.1.3.1 Epidemiology

Torsion of the Testis

Incidence

Testicular torsion is the most common paediatric genitourinary emergency and probably the second most common surgical emergency in the adolescent age group after acute appendicitis (Rampaul and Hosking 1998). There is a ratio of approximately one testis torsion for every eight cases of acute appendicitis (Sparks 1971).

One in 158 men will have experienced torsion of the testis by the age of 25 years. The annual incidence of torsion in men below the age of 25 is 25.4/100,000. The reported incidence increased from 10.7/100,000 in 1968 to 27.0/100,000 in 1980, probably due to greater awareness (Anderson and Williamson 1988). The peak incidence occurs in the age group 15–19 years (Table I.7.1).

The relative incidence of each of the commonest causes of the acute scrotum varies from study to study. Earlier studies were based on surgical series of patients who were either hospitalized or underwent surgery, leading to a skewing of the data, with an overestimation of the incidence of testicular torsion and the belief that it was the most common cause of the acute scrotum.

Table I.7.1. Incidence of torsion per age group (Jones et al. 1986)

Age (years)	Incidence per 100,000
15–19	10.1
20–24	7.5
25–29	4.5
>30	2.0

More recent studies based on emergency department patient populations demonstrate that testicular torsion probably represents less than one-fourth of all cases presenting with acute scrotal pain (Burgher 1998). Kass et al. (1993) noted that only 29 % of cases with acute scrotum need immediate surgery. Sidler et al. (1997) performed a study of acute scrotum in boys aged less than 13 years and found testis torsion in 31 %, torsion of the testicular appendages in 31 % and epididymo-orchitis in 28 %. The acute scrotum accounted for 6 % to 10 % of the emergency abdominal surgery performed in a paediatric hospital in Paris between 1986 and 1996 (Van Glabeke et al. 1999). The incidence of testicular torsion in the presence of an acute scrotum in children ranges from 16 % to 39.5 % (Marcozzi and Suner 2001). Corbett and Simpson (2002) found that only 12 % of patients younger than 15 who presented to the emergency department with an acute scrotum had testis torsion, and of those who underwent exploration for suspected torsion, only 38 % actually had torsion of the testis.

In our meta-analysis of 5,180 patients from 50 series of acute scrotum in the paediatric and adolescent age group, epididymo-orchitis was the most common cause with a relative incidence of 30 %, followed by testicular torsion, with a relative incidence of 28 % and torsion of a testicular appendage in 23 % (Fig. I.7.3). In hospital admission series, torsion predominated with a relative incidence of 37 %, and in surgical series torsion was found in 53 % of cases. In emergency department series, torsion of the testicular appendages was the most common at 33 %, with torsion of the testis found in 22 %. In radiological series, epididymo-orchitis was the most common diagnosis (41 %) (Fig. I.7.4).

Laterality

There is a slight preponderance for the left side, with a ratio of 1.2:1, probably due to the slightly longer spermatic cord on the left (Skoglund et al. 1970a; Anderson and Williamson 1988). Up to 2 % of cases may have bilateral asynchronous torsion, although earlier studies found an incidence of 5 % to 7 %, possibly because contralateral fixation was not routinely performed (Williamson 1976). There have been several case reports of bilateral synchronous torsion (O'Conor 1933; Wasnick et al. 1981; Shefi and Haskel 1998).

In our meta-analysis of 1,971 cases of intravaginal torsion reported in the literature, 56 % were on the left and 44 % on the right (left: right ratio of 1.3:1) with 1 % being bilateral.

Age

Testicular torsion can occur at any age, but the peak incidence is at age 14, with a second smaller peak in the 1st year of life (Prater and Overdorf 1991). Intravaginal torsion has been reported in a newborn and a 77-year-old man, but 62 % of cases occur in patients between 12 and 18 years of age. Of patients with testis torsion, 89 % are below 25 years of age. Torsion is equally common in the first (14 %) and third decades (12 %) (Anderson and Williamson 1988).

In the 1st year of life, torsion of the testis is the most common cause of an acute scrotum (83 %). For 3- to 13-year-olds, the most common diagnosis is torsion of the testicular appendage. After the age of 17 years, epididymitis is the most common diagnosis (75 %) (Lewis et al. 1995).

Between 26 % and 39 % of patients with testicular torsion are older than 20 years of age and it is the second most common cause of the acute scrotum in this

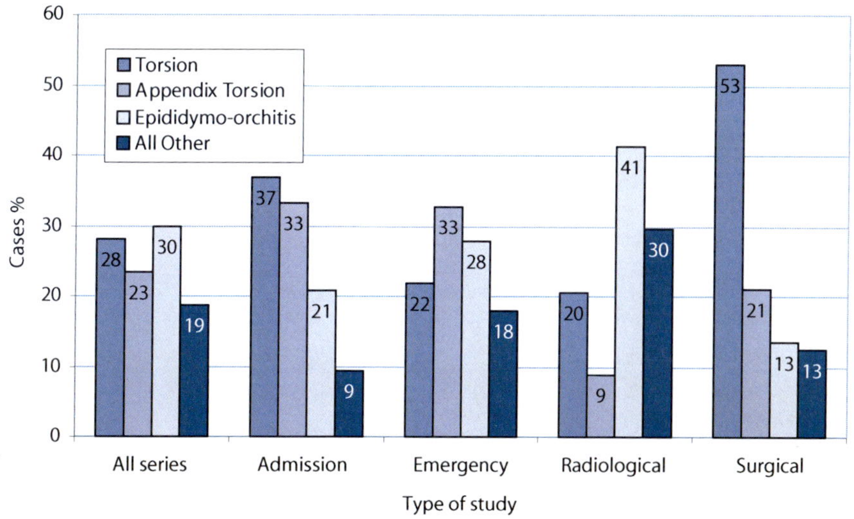

Fig. I.7.4. Relative incidence of various causes of the acute scrotum reported in 5,180 patients from 50 series in the literature

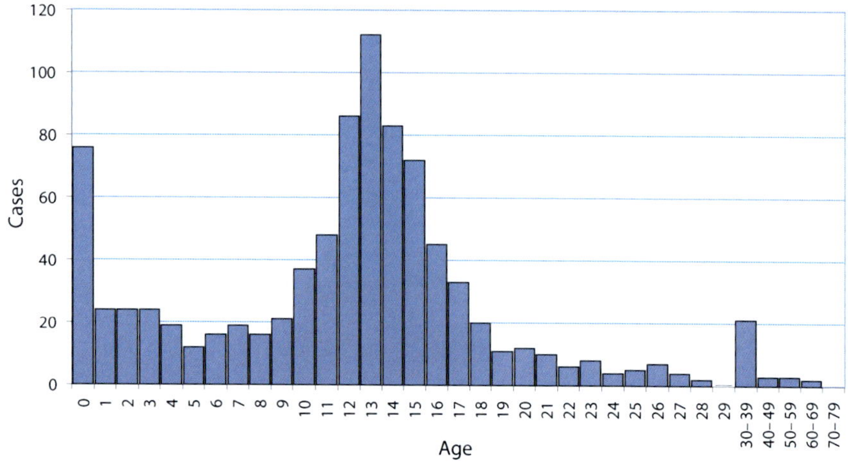

Fig. I.7.5. Age incidence for torsion of the testis in 886 cases reported in 40 series

age group after acute epididymitis (Lee et al. 1983; Witherington and Jarrell 1990). Between 5% and 9% of torsion cases are over 30 years of age (Lee et al. 1983; Watkin et al. 1996). In patients under 21 years old presenting with an acute scrotum in the emergency room, only 25% suffer from testicular torsion (Caldamone et al. 1984).

In our meta-analysis of 886 cases of testicular torsion from 40 series, the peak incidence was at 13 years, with a smaller peak in the first year (excluding the series of exclusively neonatal torsion) (Fig. I.7.5).

Torsion of the Appendages

Torsion of the testicular appendages has been reported in the first to the fifth decade, but 82% of cases occur between the ages of 7 and 14 years (Jones 1962; Williamson 1976; Holland et al. 1981). There is a peak incidence at age 11–12 years (McCombe and Scobie 1988; Hastie and Charlton 1990).

In our meta-analysis of 454 cases, the peak incidence was at age 11 years with 80% of cases being 6–13 years of age (Fig. I.7.6). In comparison, the peak incidence for testis torsion was at 13 years of age (Fig. I.7.7).

The appendix testis is involved in 92% of cases, the appendix epididymis in 7%, the vas aberrans in 0.3% and the paradidymis in 0.6% of cases (Skoglund et al. 1970b).

Both sides appear to be affected with equal frequency. Metachronous bilateral torsion of the appendages is reported in 0–11% of cases (Jones 1962; Skoglund et al. 1970b).

In our meta-analysis of 629 cases from nine studies, bilateral metachronous torsion of the appendages occurred in 2.5% of cases, and the left and right sides were affected equally.

Neonatal, Extravaginal, Supravaginal, Perinatal Torsion

Neonatal torsion is much rarer than intravaginal torsion, but over 200 cases have been reported. As many as 10% to 17% of all torsions may occur in the neonatal period (Tryfonas et al. 1994; Cuckow and Frank 2000).

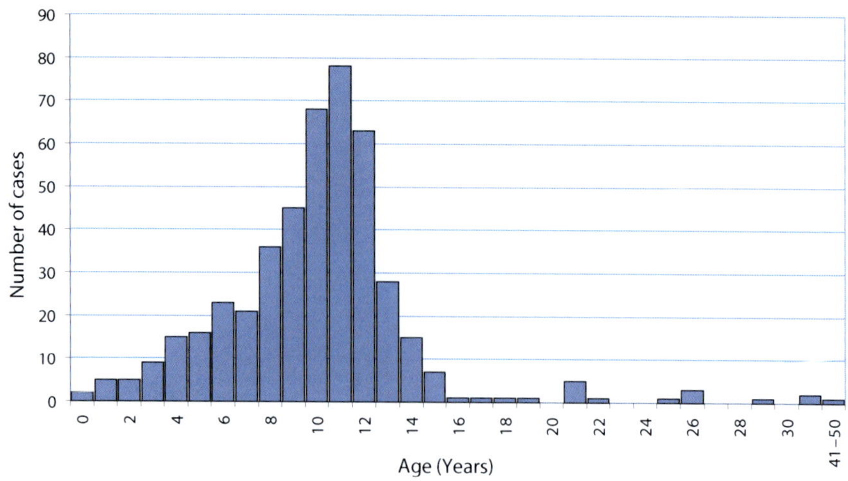

Fig. I.7.6. Age incidence for torsion of the testicular appendages in 454 cases reported in the literature

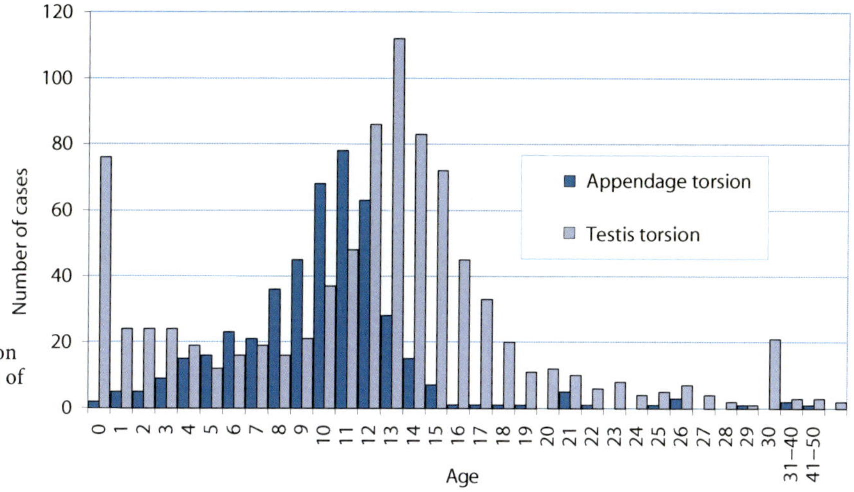

Fig. I.7.7. Age incidence for torsion of the testis compared to torsion of the appendages

Neonatal torsion can be divided into two distinct groups:

1. Prenatal (in utero torsion), which is almost exclusively extravaginal
2. Postnatal torsion, which is generally intravaginal (Das and Singer 1990; Brandt et al. 1992).

In their review of 83 cases of neonatal torsion, Das and Singer found that 72% were prenatal and 28% were postnatal. The right testis underwent torsion in 41% and the left in 38%, with 21% having bilateral torsion, while 92% had extravaginal and 8% had intravaginal torsion (Das and Singer 1990). The reported incidence of intravaginal torsion in the neonatal period ranges from 4% to 22% (Hitch et al. 1980; Das and Singer 1990; Brandt et al. 1992).

In our meta-analysis of 211 reported cases, 85% were prenatal and 15% postnatal. The right testis underwent torsion in 48% and the left in 52%, while 89% had extravaginal and 11% had intravaginal torsion. Bilateral extravaginal torsion was reported in 18%. However, this figure is probably too high, since bilateral cases may be reported more often than unilateral cases, and bilateral cases are usually operated on, whereas unilateral cases may be treated conservatively, resulting in fewer well-documented cases of unilateral torsion.

In the two largest single-institution series of postnatal torsion, there was bilateral involvement in 9% to 11% of cases (Brandt et al. 1992; Pinto et al. 1997). In our analysis of the literature, we found 37 cases of bilateral neonatal torsion, of which 19% were asynchronous.

Vanishing Testis

The term "vanishing testis" refers to testes that have become atrophic, presumably due to missed pre- or perinatal testicular torsion. It is also referred to as "testicular regression syndrome" (Belman and Rushton 2001). Turek et al. reviewed 117 cases of absent testis confirmed surgically, and found testicular remnants in the inguinal canal in 95%. The frequency of haemosiderin (30%) and calcium (35%) deposits supports the vascular accident-antenatal torsion theory, indicating that antenatal torsion must occur late in gestation, when the testis has already entered the inguinal canal (Turek et al. 1994).

In cases of acute scrotal swelling, time is of the essence. The history and physical examination should be carried out simultaneously. The most helpful aspects of the history include age, severity, duration, nausea and vomiting, previous episodes and associated activity at onset. The physical examination should be systematic, including observation followed by eliciting the cremasteric reflex on the unaffected side first, followed by the affected side. The abdomen is then examined with special attention to the inguinal canals. The scrotum is examined last, starting with the unaffected side. The scrotum is approached from inferior, examining the lower pole of the testis first and the upper pole last. The scrotum is then examined in the erect position to observe the lie of the testes. Urinalysis is performed to rule out urinary infection. At this stage the patient can be placed in one of three diagnostic categories: torsion, nontorsion or equivocal (Rabinowitz and Hulbert 1995).

I.7.1.3.2 History

Age

Testicular torsion is most common in neonates and postpubertal boys, torsion of a testicular appendage typically occurs in prepubertal boys, and epididymitis most often develops in postpubertal boys (Galejs and Kass 1999).

Onset and Severity of Pain

Pain is usually of rapid onset, with 55% to 91% of patients having acute onset pain. The sensitivity of this finding is 91%, with a specificity of 27% for torsion of the testis (Kaplan and King 1970; Van Glabeke et al. 1999). The pain is severe, and the patient appears uncomfortable. The pain may begin to diminish after 6 h (Sparks 1971). Moderate pain developing gradually over a few days is more suggestive of epididymitis or appendiceal torsion, and with either of these conditions, the patient may appear relatively comfortable except when examined (Galejs and Kass 1999).

Duration

Patients with testicular torsion tend to seek medical help earlier (median, 6 h) than with torsion of the appendix testis (median, 29–48 h) (Hastie and Charlton 1990; Watkin et al. 1996). However, up to 20% of cases with testicular torsion present after 24 h (Watkin et al. 1996).

Nonscrotal Pain

In 5–25% of patients with testicular torsion, the main or only complaint is abdominal pain (Sparks 1971; Anderson and Williamson 1988).

Nausea and Vomiting

Patients with torsion of the testis more often have nausea or vomiting at the onset of pain, while this is uncommon in torsion of the appendages (Knight and Vassy 1984). Nausea and vomiting are present in 26% to 60% of cases of torsion of the testis. Nausea has a positive predictive value of 96% and vomiting 98% for torsion, but the sensitivity is lower (nausea 69% and vomiting 60%) (Skoglund et al. 1970a; Jefferson et al. 1997).

Urinary Complaints

Urinary complaints are present in 5% to 7% of patients with testicular torsion. The symptoms are typically slight frequency and dysuria. However, urinary complaints are also found in 7% of cases with acute epididymitis (Cass et al. 1980; Anderson and Williamson 1988).

Previous Episodes (Prophetic Pain)

Between 11% and 47% of patients with torsion describe previous episodes of similar pain that lasted only a short time and resolved spontaneously, suggesting intermittent torsion with spontaneous detorsion (Skoglund et al. 1970a; Cass et al. 1980; Knight and Vassy 1984).

I.7.1.3.3 Physical Examination

Cremasteric Reflex

This is a superficial skin reflex mediated by the L1–L2 (ilioinguinal and genitofemoral) nerve roots. It is elicited by stroking the medial upper thigh, and a positive reflex results in elevation of the ipsilateral testis (Walsh et al. 1998). The reflex is normally present in 48% of newborns, 45% of boys between 1 and 30 months, and in 100% of boys between 30 months and 12 years of age (Caesar and Kaplan 1994b).

Rabinowitz reported a 100% correlation between the presence of an ipsilateral cremaster reflex and the absence of testis torsion in a series of boys with acute scrotal swelling. In those with an absent reflex, 47% had testicular torsion (Rabinowitz 1984). However, several reports have been published of confirmed torsion of the testis with a normal cremasteric reflex (Blaivas et al. 2000).

The cremasteric reflex is absent in 40% to 100% of patients with testicular torsion, but is usually present in patients with torsion of a testicular appendix. The sensitivity of an absent cremasteric reflex is 60%, with a specificity of 67% for torsion of the testis. It has a positive predictive value of 43% and a negative predictive value of 96% for torsion of the testis (Van Glabeke et al. 1999).

Drawn Up or High-Riding Testis

This sign was referred to as testis redux in older articles and may have been confused with undescended testes. A drawn up testis is present in 26% to 80% of cases of testicular torsion (Skoglund et al. 1970a; Van Glabeke et al. 1999).

Contralateral Horizontal Lie (Angell's Sign)

Between 25% and 90% of patients with torsion will have an abnormal lie of the contralateral testis, which is best seen with the patient examined in the standing position (Angell 1963; Anderson and Williamson 1988).

Ransler and Allen noted that torsion of the testis was present in 100% of patients who had both a drawn up testis and contralateral horizontal lie (Ransler and Allen 1982).

Secondary Hydrocele

This sign is found preoperatively in 52% of cases and almost always at surgery (Anderson and Williamson 1988).

Pyrexia

Pyrexia is present in 8 % to 41 % of cases with testicular torsion and is an ominous sign for testicular viability, since 50 % to 100 % of patients with testicular torsion and pyrexia will have an infarcted testis at exploration (Kaplan and King 1970; Parker and Robison 1971; Anderson and Williamson 1988; Melekos et al. 1988).

Scrotal Induration

Overlying erythema and oedema are poor prognostic signs of viability and are associated with longer duration of torsion (>12 h) (Angell 1963; Hemalatha and Rickwood 1981). This sign is present in 70 % of patients with an infarcted testis, and if it is present 78 % of testes will be infarcted (Skoglund et al. 1970a; Knight and Vassy 1984).

Prehn's Sign

When elevation of the testis relieves the pain it indicates epididymitis, and when it does not, it indicates torsion. In theory, this is analogous to elevation of a limb, where pain due to inflammation will be relieved, and pain due to ischaemia will not (Prehn 1934). However, this sign is notoriously unreliable and should not be used to make the diagnosis (Melekos et al. 1988).

Urinalysis

Urinalysis to rule out urinary tract infection is absolutely essential in cases of acute scrotum (Kass and Lundak 1997). Abnormal findings on urinalysis are present in 0 % to 10 % of cases of torsion (Skoglund et al. 1970a; Ransler and Allen 1982). Pyuria is present in approximately 50 % of patients with epididymitis, but its absence does not exclude epididymitis, nor does its presence exclude testicular torsion (Burgher 1998). However, torsion of the testis with pyuria of more than 20 leukocytes per high power field is distinctly unusual (Haynes et al. 1983).

I.7.1.3.4
Torsion of an Appendage

Tenderness limited to the upper pole suggests torsion of a testicular appendage, especially when a hard, tender nodule is palpable in this region. A small bluish discolouration may be visible through the skin in the upper pole. Dressner of Chicago coined the term “blue dot sign” in 1973 (according to Noske et al. 1998). It is virtually pathognomonic for appendiceal torsion when tenderness is also present. However, these signs are present in only 21 % of cases (McCombe and Scobie 1988). Pain is usually not severe (Jones 1962). The patients tend to present later than with torsion of the testis (Watkin et al. 1996). Meticulous transillumination may show a dark nodule at the superior pole of the testis (Skoglund et al. 1970b).

Almost all clinical aspects of testicular torsion may be present in cases of torsion of the testicular appendage, including nausea and vomiting, minor trauma, previous episodes of pain, fever, absent cremasteric reflex and abnormal urinalysis (Kaplan and King 1970). Torsion of a testicular appendage is the most commonly misdiagnosed testicular lesion, with the correct preoperative diagnosis made in only 11 % (Williamson 1976).

I.7.1.3.5
Neonatal Torsion

Prenatal Torsion

Patients present at birth with an asymptomatic scrotal swelling, which consists of a hard, swollen, nontender testis in an oedematous, dusky hemiscrotum that does not transilluminate (Das and Singer 1990). The earliest case of prenatal torsion was in a premature boy born at 32 weeks gestation with bilateral torsion, suggesting that torsion occurs around 32 weeks gestation (Ryken et al. 1990).

Postnatal Torsion

These patients present within the first 30 days of life, with symptomatic scrotal swelling and a documented normal scrotum at birth (Das and Singer 1990).

I.7.1.3.6
Clinical Diagnosis

The presence of any of the following findings strongly suggests testicular torsion.

1. An abnormal elevation of the affected testis with thickening of or a palpable twist in the spermatic cord (the high-riding testis).
2. An abnormal axis (horizontal lie) of the affected testis when the patient is examined in the standing position.
3. An abnormal position of the epididymis (anterior or lateral, instead of posterior to the testis).
4. An abnormal axis (horizontal lie) of the contralateral testis.

In approximately two-thirds of cases, the history and physical examination are sufficient to make an accurate diagnosis (Caldamone et al. 1984). The overall accuracy of the preoperative clinical diagnosis is between 60 % and 90 % (Williamson 1976; Caldamone et al. 1984). On clinical grounds, general practitioners make the correct preoperative diagnosis of torsion of the testis in 74% and specialists in 87% of cases (Watkin et al. 1996).

I.7.1.3.7 Imaging Studies

Imaging may provide useful information in cases where the diagnosis of testicular torsion is unlikely or when the duration of symptoms indicates an infarcted testis. However, the diagnosis of acute torsion should be clinical and the management urgent surgical exploration. There have been no lawsuits for negative surgical explorations, or serious morbidity after exploration of a normal testis (Cuckow and Frank 2000).

Ultrasound

Ultrasound on its own is not sufficient to evaluate the acute scrotum. Several case reports of prenatal diagnosis of neonatal torsion have appeared (Tripp and Homsy 1990; Cartwright et al. 1995). Prenatal detection is of little practical value, since the testis is already damaged and early induced labour has no role in the management.

Colour Doppler (Angiodynography)

Colour Doppler ultrasound is currently the modality of choice in equivocal cases. It is fast, cost-effective, easy to perform, widely available at all hours, and it provides anatomical information that may help distinguish other conditions that mimic testis torsion. The drawbacks are that flow is unreliably detected in small testes and at younger ages, it is operator-dependent, and the detection of flow does not rule out testis torsion (Atkinson et al. 1992; Kass et al. 1993; Steinhardt et al. 1993).

Colour Doppler ultrasound indicators of probable viability include any detectable perfusion in the affected testis and isoechogenicity without enlargement compared to the unaffected testis. Poor prognostic signs of viability include an enlarged, hypoechoic or heterogeneous testis (Burks et al. 1990; Baud et al. 1998). Baud et al. (1998) described the spiral twist sign, which is an abrupt change in spermatic cord course, size and shape below the point of torsion. Strauss et al. (1997) reported that in torsion of the testicular appendage, the swollen appendix testis lying next to the head of the epididymis produces a "Mickey Mouse" appearance on transverse view.

There have been numerous reports of false-negative cases with colour Doppler, which may be due to technical factors in the investigation, inexperience of the radiologist, difficulties in prepubertal children and the possibility that torsion may be intermittent (Allen and Elder 1995).

In our meta-analysis of 1,585 Doppler studies from 18 series, the sensitivity for torsion is 92% with a specificity of 99%. Indeterminate studies are found in 3% of cases. If the sensitivity and specificity are calculated including the indeterminate studies, the true sensitivity is 89% and the true specificity is 98%. The positive predictive value of Doppler for torsion is 96% and the negative predictive value is 98%.

Scintigraphy

Scintigraphy using technetium-99m sodium pertechnetate has been used to investigate testicular perfusion since 1973 (Nadel et al. 1973; Nakielny et al. 1984). Decreased uptake of tracer indicates ischaemia (torsion of the spermatic cord) and increased uptake may be due to epididymo-orchitis, torsion of the testicular appendages, tumour, mild trauma, or resolved torsion (Fischman et al. 1987). The halo sign is characterized by a central "cold" spot with a "hot" perimeter of markedly increased uptake of isotope and usually represents late torsion, tumour, hydrocele, abscess or haematoma (Fig. I.7.8) (Nakielny et al. 1984). The presence of the halo sign does not necessarily imply that the testis is unsalvageable (Chen et al. 1983a).

Nuclear scintigraphy is a quick and safe technique (Nakielny et al. 1984). However, its limitations include lack of availability outside usual working hours, limited

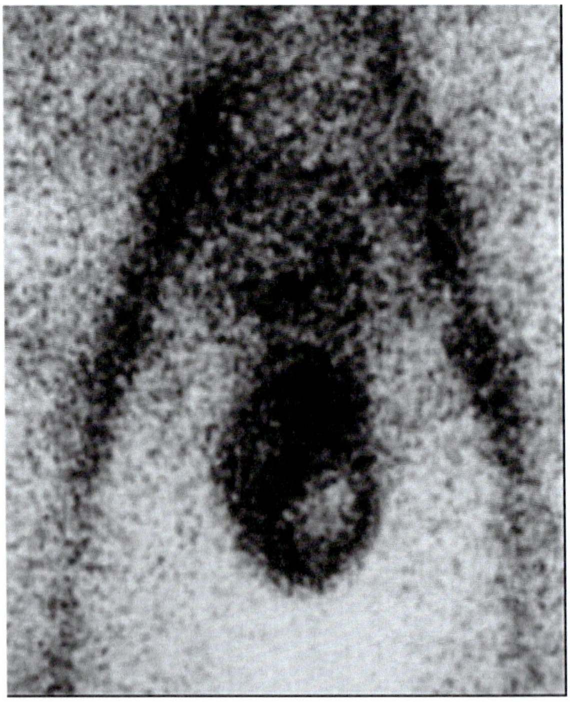

Fig. I.7.8. Nuclear scintigram showing the "halo" sign, characterized by a central "cold" spot with a "hot" perimeter of increased uptake of isotope

reliability in young children, in cases of an abnormal contralateral testis, undescended contralateral testis and in the rare cases of bilateral disease (Nakielny et al. 1984). Inability to differentiate between epididymitis and torsion of a testicular appendage and inability to detect cases in which intermittent torsion or spontaneous detorsion has occurred are further limitations (Burgher 1998).

In our meta-analysis of 527 scintigraphy studies from 12 series, the sensitivity for torsion is 97% and the specificity 99%. Indeterminate studies are found in 2% of cases. Including the indeterminate studies, the true sensitivity for torsion is 96% and the true specificity is 99%. Scintigraphy has a positive predictive value of 99% and a negative predictive value of 99% for torsion of the testis.

Magnetic Resonance Imaging

Magnetic resonance imaging (MRI) can clearly differentiate intratesticular (torsion, tumour, infarction) and extratesticular (epididymitis, appendix torsion) pathology (Fig. I.7.9) (Watanabe et al. 2000). Dynamic MRI is more expensive than colour Doppler ultrasound and less likely to have support staff during the off-hours. Its use in prepubertal male patients is limited by the need for sedation in young patients. However, more rapid and less expensive MRI techniques could change the equation in favour of MRI (Choyke 2000).

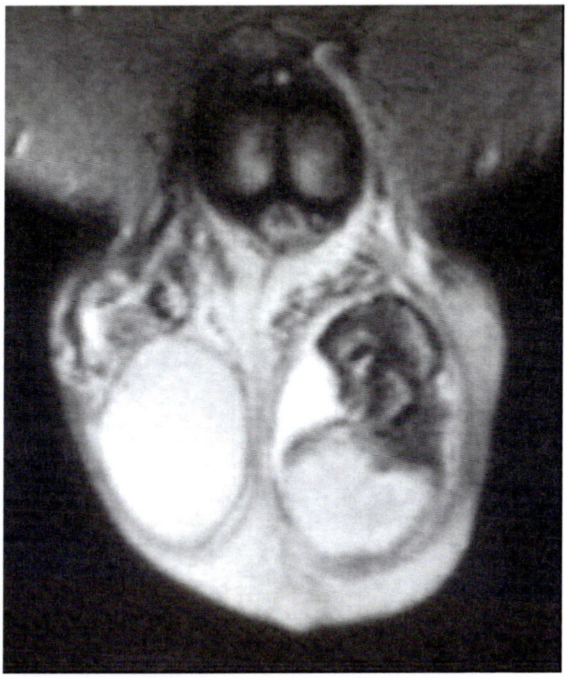

Fig. I.7.9. MRI showing torsion of the left testis

I.7.1.4 Differential Diagnosis

In 94% of cases presenting with acute scrotum, the cause would be torsion of the testis or its appendages or acute epididymitis (Knight and Vassy 1984). Although testicular torsion is the least common cause of the three, it should be the presumptive diagnosis until proven otherwise (Burgher 1998).

In the 1st year of life, torsion of the testis is the most common cause of an acute scrotum (83%). Other studies have found epididymo-orchitis in 69% and testis torsion in 31% of cases less than 1 year of age (Sidler et al. 1997). For 3- to 13-year-olds, the most common diagnosis is torsion of the testicular appendage. After the age of 17 years, epididymitis is the most common diagnosis (75%) (Lewis et al. 1995). In prepubertal boys with an acute scrotum, torsion of the testis is found in 7% to 42% of cases, with 52% to 62% of cases having a twisted appendix of the testis (Al Mufti et al. 1995; Watkin et al. 1996).

Other conditions that should be included in the differential diagnosis of the acute scrotum include orchitis, scrotal trauma, idiopathic scrotal oedema, scrotal abscess, inguinal hernia, hydrocele, Henoch Schönlein purpura, familial Mediterranean fever, testicular infarction in the absence of torsion, testis tumour and acute appendicitis (Kaplan and King 1970; Loh and Jalan 1974; Williamson 1976; Kaplan 1977; Urwin et al. 1986; Jordan 1987; Baer et al. 1989; Eshel et al. 1994; Baratelli et al. 1996; Davenport et al. 1996; Burgher 1998; Gofrit et al. 1998; Van Glabeke et al. 1999; Lee et al. 2001b).

Haemorrhage into a testicular neoplasm can present as an acute scrotum. Additionally, testicular torsion in an undescended testis may be the first manifestation of neoplastic transformation (Burgher 1998). Leukemic infiltration may also be the cause of an acute scrotum (Moharib and Krahn 1970).

Mumps orchitis usually follows the parotitis by 4–8 days. Orchitis is rarely seen in prepubertal patients, but 14% to 35% of adolescents and adults with mumps will develop orchitis. The orchitis mostly involves a single testis, but bilateral orchitis has been reported in 17% to 30% of cases. The condition usually subsides after 7–10 days. Some degree of atrophy will be present in 30% to 50% of cases. Impaired fertility has been reported in 7% to 13% of cases (Manson 1990).

Acute appendicitis may cause scrotal symptoms in the presence of a patent processus vaginalis. The same route may allow blood, pus as well as peritoneal fluid to enter the scrotal sac. This phenomenon has been reported with splenic rupture, following peritoneal dialysis and appendicitis (Mendez et al. 1998). The processus vaginalis is patent in almost all newborns, in 60%

of 1-year-olds, and possibly in up to 20% of adult males (Chen et al. 1983a).

The differential diagnosis of neonatal torsion of the testis includes hydrocele, haematocele, inguinal hernia, torsion of the appendix of the testis, epididymo-orchitis, syphilitic orchitis, idiopathic infarction of the testis, ectopic splenic or adrenal rests, meconium peritonitis with a patent processus vaginalis, tumours of the testis and birth trauma (Kaplan 2000).

I.7.1.5 Treatment

I.7.1.5.1 Intravaginal Torsion

Surgical Exploration

When the history and physical examination strongly suggest that testicular torsion is present and the duration of pain is less than 12 h, urgent surgical intervention is indicated. No imaging studies are required because they may delay treatment and thereby jeopardize testicular survival. When pain has been present for more than 12 h or the diagnosis is unclear, colour Doppler ultrasound examination can be helpful in making clinical decisions. If imaging studies are equivocal or show reduced perfusion, emergency exploration should be performed (Fig. I.7.10). It is important to remember that most patients with an acute scrotum do not have testicular torsion, only about 29% of cases with an acute scrotum require immediate surgery, and it is difficult to justify routine surgical exploration in all cases of acute scrotum (Kass et al. 1993).

Immediate surgery is indicated in all cases of acute solitary testis. All prepubertal boys with a painful, swollen scrotum should undergo immediate surgery unless Doppler examination or scintigraphy clearly demonstrates normal testicular perfusion or there is unequivocal evidence for a cause other than torsion (Haynes et al. 1983). In an editorial comment, Allen gave four sensible guidelines (Steinhardt et al. 1993):

1. Any child believed to have a reasonable likelihood of torsion should be taken to theatre immediately.
2. The diagnosis of epididymitis in early puberty should be considered highly suspect.
3. When a boy has clinical features suggesting that he does not have torsion, it would still be wise to obtain a blood flow study before rendering a final verdict.
4. No study, whether it be clinical or technological, is any better than the individual performing it.

Manual Detorsion

Despite anything that has been written to the contrary, this is a simple and very worthwhile organ-saving procedure. Because testicular torsion is usually by internal rotation, manual detorsion should first be attempted in external rotation – like opening a book. Immediate pain relief will signify proper untwisting. If manual detorsion fails in external rotation, then internal rotation should be attempted (Marcozzi and Suner 2001). The procedure can be performed without analgesia, when immediate relief of pain will indicate successful reduction. It may also be performed under sedation or with a spermatic cord block. This may be more comfortable for the patient, but successful detorsion is more difficult to judge because relief of pain cannot be used as an indicator. Even with successful detorsion, many patients will still have a partial torsion with some degree of persistent vascular impairment. Consequently, this is only a temporizing measure and should not delay the patient going to surgery for definitive repair. The procedure is reportedly successful in over 80% of attempts,

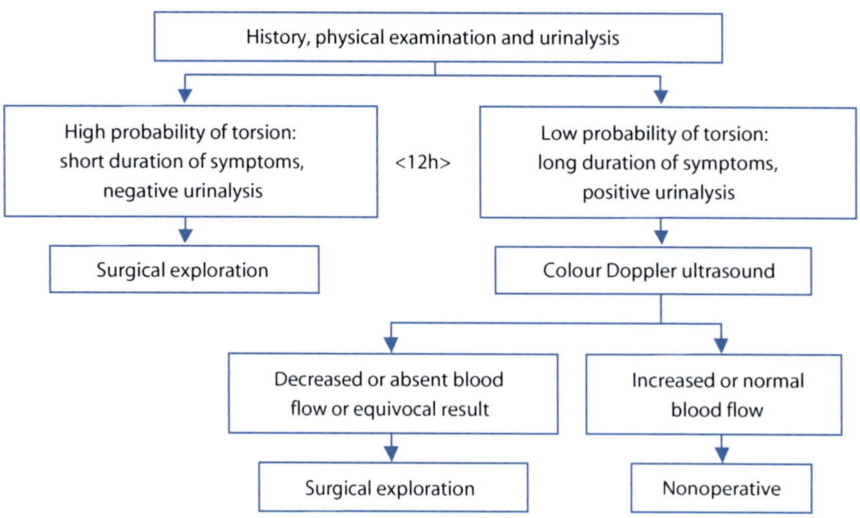

Fig. I.7.10. Management protocol for the acute scrotum (modified from Galejs and Kass 1999)

but residual twists are present in up to 28% of cases. Of the successful cases, more than 90% of testes are salvaged (Jefferson et al. 1997; Cornel and Karthaus 1999). The pitfall of partial reduction of the torsion can be avoided by monitoring the flow with Doppler ultrasound (Kiesling et al. 1984; Garel et al. 2000). Manual detorsion is probably possible in early salvageable cases only. In almost all reported successful detorsions, the duration was less than 12 h.

External Cooling

An additional measure that should be implemented as soon as testicular torsion is strongly suspected or confirmed is therapeutic cooling of the affected testicle. This is accomplished by placing an ice pack on the affected testis. A towel should be placed between the patient and the ice pack to protect the scrotum from hypothermic injury. In experimental animal studies, external cooling has been shown to preserve testicular function by 85% to 90% for up to 6 h compared to 8% to 25% in those not cooled (Miller et al. 1990). In human orchiectomy specimens, cooling the testis to 15°C extends the time before irreversible damage occurs from 2 to 6 h (Kallerhof et al. 1996). In some centres, cooling is routinely used in the emergency department prior to surgical exploration (Lewis et al. 1995).

Orchiectomy

Exploration of both scrotal compartments can usually be performed through a single small incision in the median raphe. When the torsed testis is obviously necrotic, it should be removed (Fig. I.7.11). Equivocal testes should be wrapped in a warm moist saline gauze for 5–10 min while the contralateral testis is fixed (Kass and Lundak 1997). If the testis fails to regain any pink colour after detorsion and if only black blood oozes from an incision in the tunica albuginea, and if the symptoms were present for more than 24 h, an orchiectomy is indicated. If the testis regains some mottled colour with red bleeding from an incision in the tunica albuginea and if the symptoms were present for less than 24 h, the testis should probably be preserved (Knight and Vassy 1984).

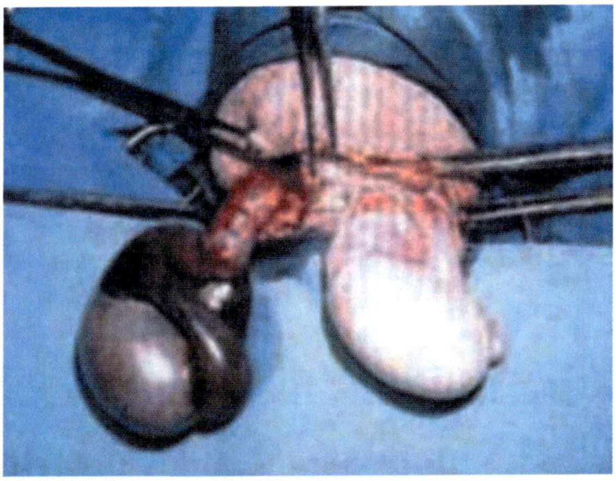

Fig. I.7.11. Torsion with gangrene of the right testis requiring orchiectomy

On the whole, conservatism is justified, because in cases of doubt the testis can be returned to the scrotum without fear of ischaemic pain or sepsis as sequelae (Jones 1962). However, it has been reported that up to 45% of obviously necrotic testes may slough and extrude through the wound or form a draining sinus when left in situ (Anderson and Williamson 1988).

Arda and Özyaylali developed a grading system for bleeding, to aid decision-making in cases of doubtful viability. After untwisting, a deep cut is made into the parenchyma and the bleeding can be graded as:

Grade 1: Sufficient bleeding
Grade 2: Insufficient bleeding but starting within 10 min
Grade 3: No bleeding within 10 min

Grades 1 and 2 testes can all be salvaged with 16% expected atrophy. Grade 3 testes will all be infarcted and should be removed (Arda and Özyaylali 2001). In spite of visual inspection and incision of the tunica albuginea for decision-making, 13% of orchiectomy specimens have histological signs of viability (Sidler et al. 1997).

Consideration should be given to simultaneous placement of a Silastic prosthesis for psychological and cosmetic reasons. It is safe to perform this at the time of exploration (Knight and Vassy 1984).

Orchiopexy

The techniques recommended for fixation of the testis include:

1. Suture fixation with three nonabsorbable sutures, preferably nylon.
2. Eversion of tunica vaginalis with dartos pouch, with or without suture fixation.
3. Window operation.

There are at least 22 reports in the English literature of recurrence after previous fixation for torsion. Absorbable sutures were used in 19 of these cases, and nonabsorbable in three (Morse and Hollabaugh 1977; May and Thomas 1980; Thurston and Whitaker 1983). Case reports have also appeared of torsion after previous orchiopexy using the dartos pouch technique (Thurston and Whitaker 1983).

The reasoning behind using absorbable sutures was that they cause a more intense inflammatory reaction with fibrosis, but they also cause a high rate of abscess formation (Morse and Hollabaugh 1977). Nonabsorbable sutures cause very little fibrosis, but their permanent nature sustains fixation. However, they may tear out of the tunics; therefore at least three sutures should be used. Silk has been shown to cause abscess formation and is more likely to extrude; therefore nylon or Prolene is the suture of choice (Thurston and Whitaker 1983).

Several studies have compared different fixation techniques in experimental animals. Morse and Hollabaugh (1977), using the window technique with silk sutures, found no case with inadequate fixation. Bellinger et al. (1989) compared fixation with absorbable or nonabsorbable sutures with dartos pouch fixation (eversion of the tunica vaginalis without any sutures) and strongly advocated the use of dartos pouch fixation with no sutures. Rodriguez and Kaplan (1988) compared suture fixation (absorbable and nonabsorbable), eversion of the tunica vaginalis (with and without a fixing suture) and chemical sclerosants (talc and tetracycline) and concluded that eversion of the tunica vaginalis was the most effective method of fixation.

Eversion of the tunica vaginalis with dartos pouch fixation produces adequate adhesion of the testis to the surrounding tissue (Rodriguez and Kaplan 1988).

The window orchiopexy is an excellent combination of suture fixation and eversion. It is fast and easy to perform and leaves a broad area of the tunica albuginea exposed for adhesion to take place with additional nonabsorbable suture fixation. An incision is made in the midline of the scrotum. The edge of the tunica vaginalis is sutured to the tunica albuginea with six interrupted 4/0 nonabsorbable sutures, creating a window of at least 1.5×2.0 cm. The other hemiscrotum is opened via the same skin incision and fixed in the same way. The incision is then closed over these two windows, leaving a broad area of the testes exposed to subcutaneous tissue (Fig. I.7.12) (Morse and Hollabaugh 1977).

Delayed Diagnosis

Urgent exploration is mandatory in all cases of testicular torsion of less than 24 h duration and in all cases where the surgeon is in doubt (Hastie and Charlton 1990). If a patient has a history of continuous pain of over 24 h duration and also has erythema and oedema of the overlying scrotal skin, the testis is usually infarcted, and the goal of exploration is to prevent subsequent contralateral torsion (Knight and Vassy 1984). Hastie and Charlton reported a strategy to reduce the number of unnecessary explorations, by observing those with a clear history of more than 24 h and a swollen erythematous scrotum. These were followed, and if they resolved over the next few days they were regarded as appendix torsion. Those that did not resolve were explored semi-electively after radiological confirmation of torsion and contralateral fixation was performed with ipsilateral orchiectomy (Hastie and Charlton 1990).

Some authors reported finding no viable testes after 48 h of symptoms (Lewis et al. 1995). Jones et al. reported an early salvage rate of 46% in patients with pain for longer than 24 h, which is much higher than reported elsewhere in the literature. Some patients with pain for longer than 24 h may be suffering from intermittent torsion of the testes and may benefit from urgent exploration despite a long acute history (Jones et al. 1986).

Several reports have appeared of testes salvaged after 3–5 days of torsion (Skoglund et al. 1970a; Chen et al. 1983b; Watkin et al. 1996). Despite these reports, it is

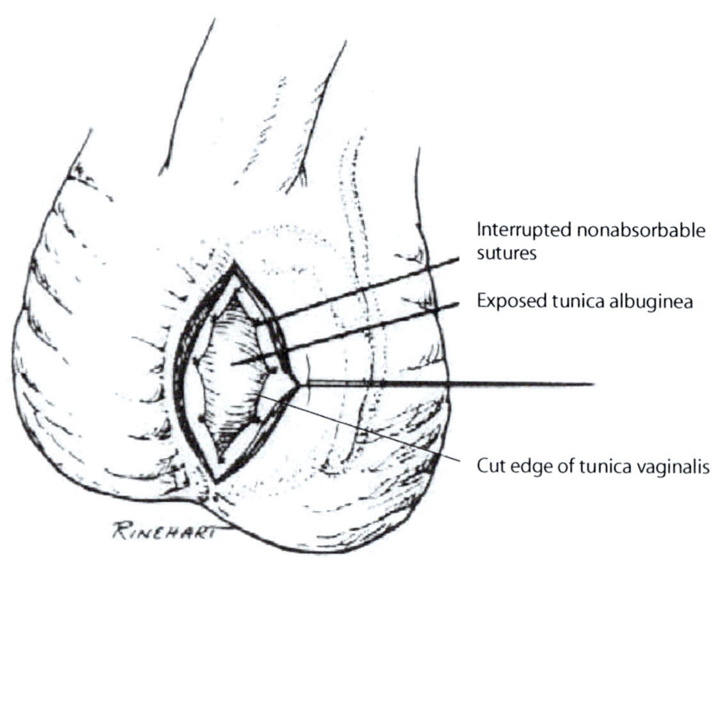

Fig. I.7.12. Surgical technique for the window orchiopexy (modified from Morse and Hollabaugh 1977)

extremely unlikely that the testis is viable if woody induration is present in cases lasting more than 24 h. Semi-elective exploration in these patients is justified. In cases with symptoms lasting up to 48 h without induration, immediate exploration is indicated. The likelihood of salvage over the long term in such cases is around 5% (Anderson and Williamson 1988).

Ipsilateral Biopsy

In a small number of cases where exploration of an acute scrotum does not yield a definite diagnosis, a testicular biopsy is indicated to rule out viral orchitis or vasculitic diseases (Knight and Vassy 1984).

I.7.1.5.2 Extravaginal Torsion

All cases of postnatal torsion should be operated on immediately. All patients with a solitary testis, and those with bilateral torsion should also be explored immediately in an all-out attempt to preserve hormonal function. Prophylactic orchiopexy should be performed in all such cases.

With regard to neonatal torsion, there is controversy about the management of unilateral cases. The arguments against operative intervention include:

1. The possibility of functional survival is remote.
2. The risk for contralateral testis torsion is very low and probably for a very short period (2–6 weeks) until the testis becomes attached to the inside of the scrotum.
3. There is an increased anaesthetic risk in newborn infants.

The arguments in favour of surgical intervention include:

1. At least 4% to 8% of neonatal torsions are intravaginal, and the only way to distinguish this is by exploration (Brandt et al. 1992). In our meta-analysis of the literature, 11% of neonatal torsions were found to be intravaginal.
2. The testis may be salvaged, although the possibility is small (Longino and Martin 1955; Guiney and McGlinchey 1981; LaQuaglia et al. 1987; Brandt et al. 1992; Pinto et al. 1997; Sidler et al. 1997; Al-Salem 1999). Our literature analysis showed that 5% of neonatal cases were salvaged at long-term follow-up.
3. Bilateral asynchronous neonatal torsion may occur, although it is rare (Kay et al. 1980; Feins 1983; LaQuaglia et al. 1987; Mishriki et al. 1992; Pinto et al. 1997; Barca et al. 1997).
4. The diagnosis is confirmed and other potential causes are excluded (e.g. tumour, hernia).
5. Even if the testis is severely damaged, some hormonal function may be preserved.
6. Leaving an infarcted testis in place may have adverse effects on the contralateral testis.

Considering these arguments, it is hard to justify conservative management if the neonate is fit for anaesthesia. The timing of surgical intervention remains in debate, but most authors recommend immediate exploration (Longino and Martin 1955; Barca et al. 1997; Pinto et al. 1997; Sidler et al. 1997; Frank and O'Brien 2002).

With regard to prenatal torsion, Brandt et al. (1992) found no viable testes and strongly believe that in utero torsion is an irreversible event best treated with early elective exploration.

Whether to use an inguinal or scrotal approach is a matter of personal preference, but the inguinal approach leaves more options open, especially in cases where the diagnosis is uncertain or where concomitant pathology is found (e.g. patent processus vaginalis). The surgical approach is also dependent on testicular position. An anterolateral or midline scrotal approach is appropriate for the twisted testis remaining within the scrotum, but where the testis has migrated into the inguinal canal, an inguinal approach with formal orchiopexy may be preferred. Transscrotal fixation of the contralateral testis should be performed. Obviously necrotic testes should be removed, but conservatism in equivocal cases is advised. Longino and Martin (1955) found no complications secondary to leaving an apparently necrotic testis in place and stated that the subsequent atrophy in such cases may be surprisingly minimal. In cases where bilateral orchiectomy was performed, hormone replacement should be initiated at the time of puberty and bilateral prosthetic testes may be implanted at school age (Barca et al. 1997).

I.7.1.5.3 Torsion of Appendages

If the diagnosis is certain, management entails several days of bed rest and scrotal elevation in an effort to minimize inflammation and oedema. Normal activity may both worsen and prolong the symptoms. Nonsteroidal anti-inflammatory drugs and analgesics are generally not helpful and thus not routinely used. The inflammation usually resolves within 2–7 days, although the testicular examination may not be completely normal for several weeks (Galejs and Kass 1999). In spite of conservative measures, 13% need surgery for persistent or recurrent pain (Holland et al. 1981). If the symptoms are still severe after 2 days, it seems reasonable to operate (Jones 1962). If a twisted appendage is found at exploration it can usually simply be excised without ligation.

Some controversy exists as to whether the contralateral side should be explored and whether all incidentally found appendages should be removed. Bilateral asynchronous torsion of the testicular appendix occurs in 1% to 4% of cases (Williamson 1976; Holland et al. 1981).

In our meta-analysis of 79 cases of torsion of the appendages which were treated conservatively, 9% failed conservative management and subsequently needed surgery. In a further analysis of 629 cases from nine studies, metachronous bilateral torsion was found in 2.5% of cases. On the whole, removing incidentally found appendages adds seconds to the operation, but exploring the contralateral side just to remove the appendages is not justified considering the insignificant risk to the contralateral side.

I.7.1.5.4 Intermittent Torsion, Subacute Torsion and Subtorsion

In a prospective study of patients with a clinical diagnosis of recurrent subacute torsion, Jones (1991) found that fixation cured 84% of their symptoms. Up to 50% of patients with acute testicular torsion have experienced previous episodes of pain, which may have been due to intermittent torsion. If elective fixation is performed on patients after resolved acute testicular pain, the overall salvage rates could improve by obviating subsequent torsion (Cass 1982). Intermittent torsion may be the cause of recurrent testicular pain, and prophylactic orchiopexy should be considered in such patients.

I.7.1.5.5 Solitary Testes

Investigation of patients with a nonpalpable testis often reveals a blind ending vas deferens leading to a nubbin of testicular remnant. These absent testes may make up 10% of patients with the initial diagnosis of cryptorchidism. The histology of these nubbins is in keeping with perinatal or silent torsion. In such cases, the contralateral testis should be fixed. Some authors even recommend fixation of all solitary testes, for instance after trauma or tumour excision, to prevent inadvertent loss of the solitary testis due to subsequent torsion (Mishriki et al. 1992; Cuckow and Frank 2000).

In patients with unilateral cryptorchidism that on exploration turns out to be monorchia, a contralateral bell-clapper deformity may be found in up to 85%; therefore fixation of the solitary testis is recommended in cases of congenital monorchia (Bellinger 1985).

I.7.1.5.6 Torsion of an Intra-abdominal Testis

Torsion of an intra-abdominal testis is extremely rare, with less than 45 reported cases. Of these patients, 65% had malignancy in the testis. The management of an acute abdominal condition in a patient with a nonpalpable testis involves immediate laparotomy to establish a diagnosis and if torsion is confirmed, untwisting of the testis and a secondary orchiopexy should be performed later to bring the testis into a scrotal position after malignancy has been excluded (Lootsma and Van der Pol 1987). Two recent case reports underline the value of laparoscopy in this setting (Lee et al. 2001; Porpiglia et al. 2001).

I.7.1.6 Results of Treatment

I.7.1.6.1 Complications of Surgery

Minor complications after scrotal exploration are reported in 2–27% of cases including postoperative fever, minor wound complications, infection, haemorrhage and haematoma (Fenner et al. 1991; Van Glabeke et al. 1999). There have been no recorded cases of mortality due to torsion of the testis or its management.

I.7.1.6.2 Recurrence after Fixation

If only ipsilateral fixation is performed and contralateral orchiopexy is omitted, 18% to 43% will experience subsequent torsion in the unfixed testis (Moharib and Krahn 1970; Skoglund et al. 1970a).

At least 22 cases of recurrent torsion after previous fixation have been reported. Absorbable sutures were used in 86% of these cases. When absorbable sutures were used, the testis was mostly mobile with no adhesions, and when adhesions were present, the testis usually twisted on the single adhesion like a pirouetting ballerina. In the three cases where nonabsorbable sutures were used (two cases silk, one case not specified), the sutures tore out completely in one case, one was intact allowing a "pirouette", and one case was fixed percutaneously and the suture was removed after 1 week (Kaplan and King 1970; Johenning 1973; Morse and Hollabaugh 1977; May and Thomas 1980; McNellis and Rabinovitch 1980; Thurston and Whitaker 1983; Knight and Vassy 1984; Kuntze et al. 1985; Steinhardt et al. 1993; Chinegwundoh 1995).

Recurrent torsion after fixation leads to necrosis or atrophy in 50% of cases (Lent and Stephani 1993).

In our meta-analysis of 22 cases of recurrent torsion,

the median time to recurrence was 21 months, and 80% occurred in the contralateral testis.

Several cases have been reported of torsion of the testis after previous surgery for undescended testis, including the dartos pouch technique. When performing orchiopexy for undescended testis, the tunica vaginalis should be everted and it is advisable to include the tunica albuginea in one of the skin sutures (Johenning 1973; Thurston and Whitaker 1983; Phipps 1987; Van Glabeke et al. 1999).

I.7.1.7 Prognosis

I.7.1.7.1 Testicular Salvage

The two most important factors determining testicular damage are the time from onset of symptoms to reduction of torsion and the degree of twisting of the cord.

Salvage Rates Relative to Era

Up to 1966, over 500 cases of torsion of the testis were reported and 90% of these cases lost the testis, 80% by immediate orchiectomy and 10% by subsequent atrophy (Sparks 1971). From 1960 to 1984, around 44% of testes were lost to torsion, 38% by orchiectomy and 6% by subsequent atrophy. In the last 5 years of this period (1980–1984), the salvage rate was 67% (Anderson and Williamson 1988).

In a 10-year study, Cass et al. found that with an aggressive surgical approach to the acute scrotum they could salvage 90% of torsion cases. However, at 6 months follow-up, only 73% of the salvaged testes were normal, while the rest had undergone atrophy (Cass et al. 1980). Tryfonas et al. surgically salvaged 72% of cases, but there was subsequent atrophy in 60% of the "salvaged" cases. True salvage was found in only 28% of cases, while the testis was totally absent in 33% of "salvaged" cases (Tryfonas et al. 1994).

The salvage rates in undescended testes undergoing torsion are poorer than in fully descended testes, with 60% to 71% requiring orchiectomy (Anderson and Williamson 1988; Nour and Mackinnon 1991).

In our meta-analysis of the literature, an increase in the overall surgical (early) salvage rates and true (long-term) salvage rates is apparent, with the early salvage rate rising from 50% in the nineteenth century to almost 80% in the late twentieth century. There is a similar rise in the true salvage rate from 0 in the nineteenth century to 65% in the 1990s (Fig. I.7.13).

Salvage Rates Relative to Duration of Torsion

The degree of subsequent atrophy is directly proportional to the duration of torsion (Krarup 1978). When the duration of torsion exceeds 4 h, some degree of testicular atrophy is almost inevitable (Thomas and Williamson 1983). Beyond 10 h of torsion, most patients had more than 50% reduction in testicular volume at follow-up (Thomas et al. 1984). Bartsch et al. (1980) found atrophy in all cases lasting longer than 8 h, ranging from 40% to 90% atrophy. Tryfonas et al. (1994) found that all cases with torsion of more than 360° and symptoms lasting more than 24 h had an absent or severely atrophic testis at follow-up.

Beyond 10 h of torsion, the chance of testicular survival is slim unless either spontaneous reduction had occurred or the degree of torsion was not more than 180°–360°. Infarction is possible as early as 4 h if the cord has twisted through several revolutions (William-

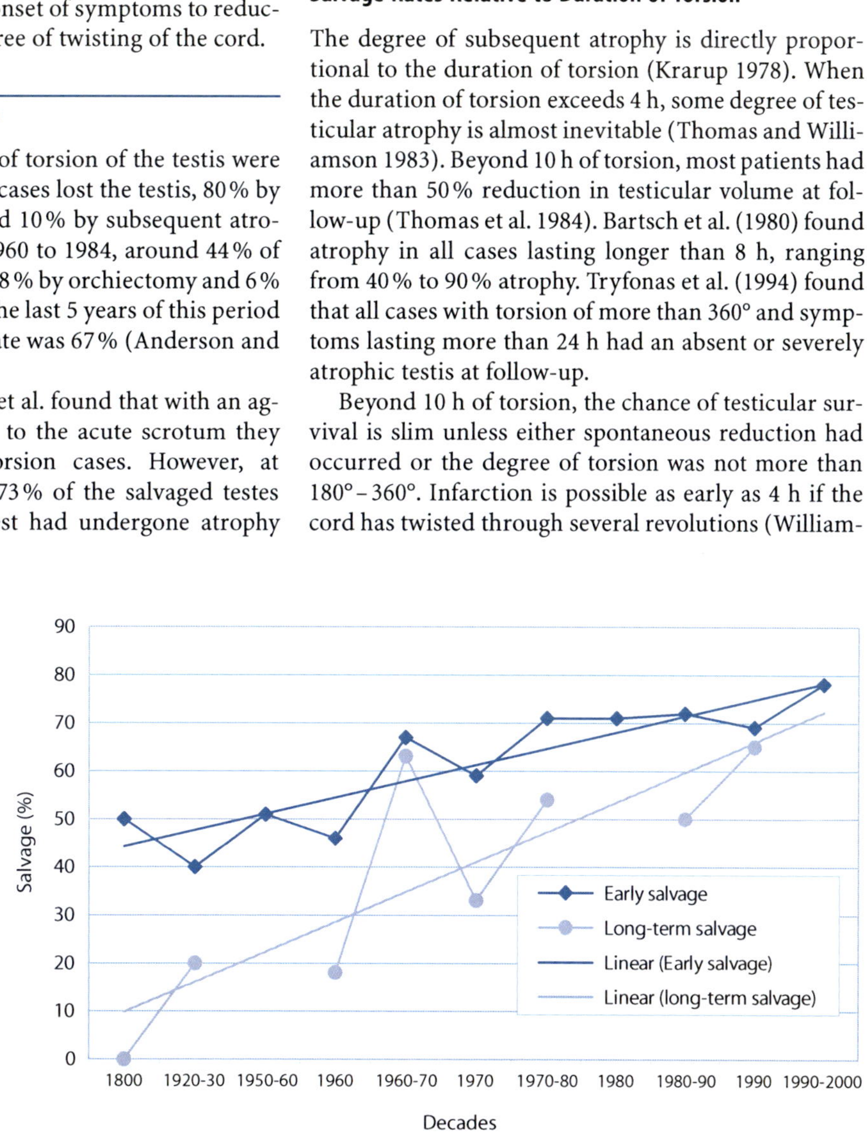

Fig. I.7.13. Early and long-term testicular salvage rates per decade from the 19th to the 21st centuries

son 1976). Whenever the testis was viable despite prolonged symptoms, the extent of the rotation did not exceed 180°, or spontaneous reduction had occurred (Anderson and Williamson 1988).

The early salvage (viable at exploration) and late salvage rates (not atrophic at follow-up) of the largest single institution series (624 cases) are shown in Table I.7.2.

In our meta-analysis of 22 series including 1,140 cases, the early testicular salvage rates relative to the duration of torsion were calculated and are shown in Table I.7.3 and Fig. I.7.14.

Table I.7.2. Testicular salvage rates in the largest published series of torsion (Anderson and Williamson 1988)

Duration of torsion (h)	Early salvage (%)	Late salvage (%)
0–6	98	98
7–12	90	89
13–18	70	59
19–24	48	31
25–48	26	5
>48	8	3

In our meta-analysis of 8 series including 535 patients, the likelihood of subsequent atrophy of a salvaged testis was calculated relative to the duration of torsion and is shown in Table I.7.4 and Fig. I.7.15.

Table I.7.3. Early testicular salvage rates relative to the duration of torsion from our meta-analysis of 1,140 cases

Duration of torsion (h)	Early salvage (%)
0–6	97
7–12	82
13–18	59
19–24	45
>24	20
>48	8

Table I.7.4. Subsequent atrophy of apparently surgically salvaged testes relative to the duration of torsion from our meta-analysis of 535 cases

Duration of torsion (h)	Likelihood of atrophy (%)
0–6	2
7–12	7
13–24	43
>24	78

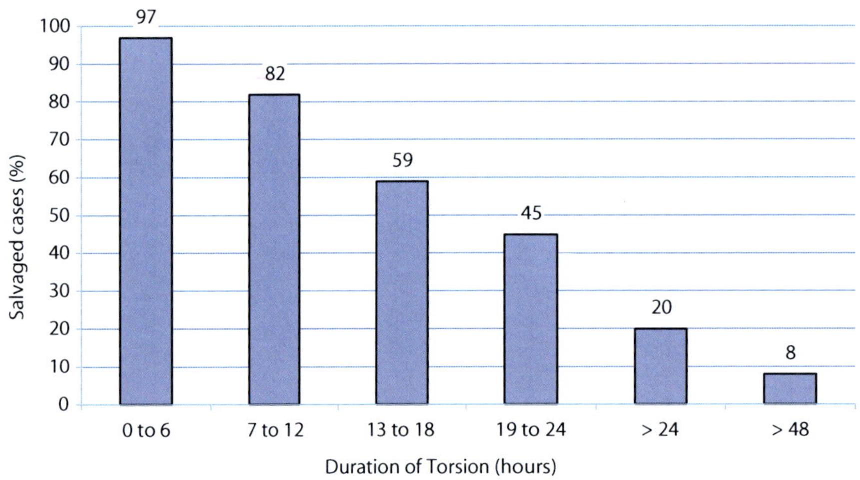

Fig. I.7.14. Early testicular salvage rates relative to the duration of torsion from our meta-analysis of 1,140 cases

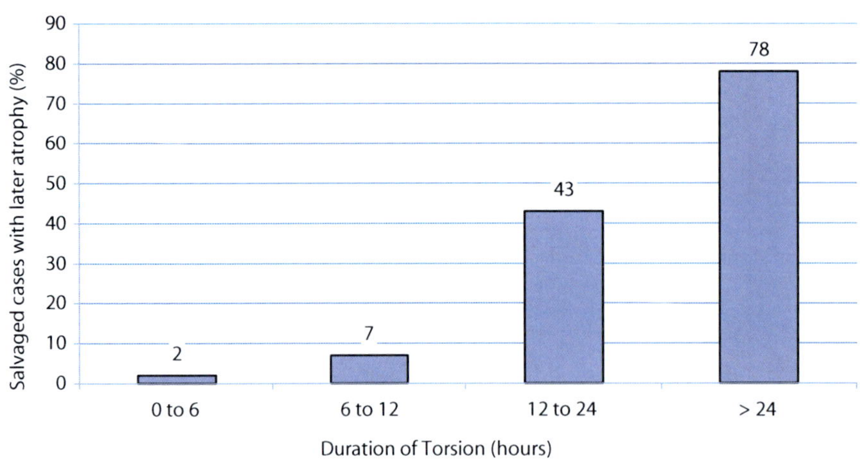

Fig. I.7.15. Subsequent atrophy of apparently surgically salvaged testes relative to the duration of torsion from our meta-analysis of 535 cases

Salvage After Neonatal Torsion

In our meta-analysis of prenatal torsion cases reported in the literature, 60% came to orchiectomy and in 34% the testis was left in place. Only 5% of all neonatal torsions were salvaged at follow-up.

I.7.1.7.2 Effect on Fertility

Many articles have been published studying the effect of torsion on fertility. The general trend is that the longer the period of untreated torsion, the worse the abnormalities in semenalysis, whether or not orchiectomy was performed. However, although testicular torsion is a common event, it is not a significant contributor to adult male infertility. It is estimated that less than 1% of males with infertility have a history of testicular torsion (Turner 1987).

Effect on Ipsilateral Testis

Findings in functional studies suggest that unilateral testicular torsion seriously interferes with subsequent spermatogenesis in about 50% of patients and produces borderline impairment in another 20%. In contrast, the exocrine function is relatively well preserved, with only a rebound rise in circulating gonadotrophins in patients with testicular atrophy (Williamson and Thomas 1984). In long-term follow-up studies, normal semenalysis is found in only 5–14% of patients after torsion of the testis (Krarup 1978; Thomas et al. 1984). Bartsch et al. found normal semen in 50% of patients studied 2.5 years after unilateral torsion and bilateral fixation. Even when detorsion and fixation was done within 4 h, the exocrine function was normal in only 50% (Bartsch et al. 1980). Subfertility, defined as sperm count of less than 20 million sperm per millilitre, is found in 36% to 39% of patients after torsion (Krarup 1978; Thomas et al. 1984).

The motile sperm count and the degree of testicular atrophy both correlate closely with the duration of torsion. Subsequent sperm counts are lower in patients with torsion of more than 8 h than those with a shorter period of torsion. Patients who have atrophy or who had undergone orchiectomy, have a significantly lower sperm count compared to those without atrophy (Krarup 1978; Thomas et al. 1984; Brasso et al. 1993).

Early detorsion and orchiopexy result in semen quality comparable to fertile controls. In patients with prolonged torsion before surgical intervention, significant deterioration in semen quality is usually found, despite removal of the torsed testis and the presence of a clinically normal contralateral testis (Andersen et al. 1992).

The majority of patients have normal luteinizing hormone (LH) and follicle-stimulating hormone (FSH), but significantly higher levels of LH and FSH are found in patients with torsion of longer than 8 h (Brasso et al. 1993). Sperm antibodies occur in 0% to 11% at the time of torsion or at later follow-up (Andersen et al. 1992; Hagen et al. 1992).

Prepubertal testes may be more resistant to the effects of torsion or have a better compensating mechanism than the older age groups. The subsequent fertility in patients after prepubertal testicular torsion where a nonviable testis was replaced in the scrotum is comparable to that of the general adult male population. After prepubertal testicular torsion, the contralateral testis undergoes normal development with normal fertility in adult life (Puri et al. 1985; Andersen et al. 1992). However, other studies found no significant differences with respect to the semen quality in patients who had torsion in the prepubertal and postpubertal period (Brasso et al. 1993).

Effect on Contralateral Testis

In older studies, it was suggested that leaving a nonviable or severely damaged testis in situ caused more damage to the contralateral testis compared to those who had an orchiectomy. In patients with symptoms lasting more than 24 h before exploration, those who underwent orchiectomy had normal semenalysis and those in whom the testis was retained had pathological semenalysis (Bartsch et al. 1980).

Contralateral testis biopsies are abnormal in 57–88% of cases after unilateral torsion. These abnormalities are apparent at the time of torsion and some pre-existing abnormalities must be present before the onset of torsion (Anderson and Williamson 1986; Hagen et al. 1991). If the contralateral biopsy is normal, semenalysis would usually also be normal. If maturation arrest is present on biopsy almost 80% will have oligozoospermia on semenalysis, and of these 40% will have raised levels of FSH (Anderson and Williamson 1986).

Hadziselimovic et al. (1998) reported that extensive apoptosis was often apparent in the germinal epithelium of the contralateral testis. They hypothesized that trauma to the blood-testis barrier initiated by torsion induces the release of apoptotic activating factors (cytokines), which cause extensive apoptosis in the contralateral germinal epithelium, leading to infertility.

The contralateral testis also deteriorates if an ipsilateral testis is damaged by various causes, including incarcerated inguinal hernia, undescended testis, varicocele, torsion, vas deferens obstruction and tumour. They all probably share a similar pathway (Andiran et al. 2000).

Several theories exist to explain bilateral exocrine failure after unilateral torsion. They include an immunologic mechanism, previous episodes of silent torsion, congenital dysplasia, release of cytokines and reflex vasoconstriction.

I.7.1.7.3
Immunologic (Sympathetic) Orchidopathy

The testis is an immunologically privileged site, and ischaemic damage may lead to breakdown of the blood–testis barrier. Antigenic material from the dying testis would be exposed to the immune system, and the resultant autoantibodies might then attack the unaffected testis. A wealth of experimental data supports this theory, but direct evidence in man is lacking (Anderson et al. 1986).

Nagler and De Vere White (1982) concluded from a study on rats that contralateral damage is mediated by immunologic events, because immunosuppression and removal of the antigenic stimulus (the necrotic testis) provided protection to the contralateral testis. Some experimental studies have supported this theory (Harrison et al. 1981; Madarikan 1987). However, other studies have indicated that autoimmune mechanisms do not play a role in contralateral testicular damage following unilateral spermatic cord torsion (Karagüzel et al. 1994a).

Mastrogiacomo found agglutinating antibodies in 20% of patients, but they were not correlated with infertility; neither were immunofluorescent antibodies. However, immobilizing antibodies were significantly correlated with infertility, especially motility changes (Mastrogiacomo et al. 1982). Zanchetta et al. (1984) found circulating antisperm autoantibodies in 13% of patients but found no correlation with exocrine or endocrine dysfunction. Fraser et al. (1985) found abnormalities of endocrine or exocrine gonadal function in 77% of patients 2–10 years after torsion, but found no evidence of testicular autoimmunization. Anderson and Williamson (1986) found minimal antisperm antibody formation and no antitestis antibodies in a prospective study of patients older than 17 years with unilateral testis torsion.

I.7.1.7.4
Preexisting Condition: Congenital Dysplasia or Intermittent Silent Torsion

Oligozoospermia after unilateral testicular torsion may be due to an underlying defect in both testes (Krarup 1978). Biopsies taken at the time of operation for suspected intermittent torsion show evidence of atrophy or peritubular fibrosis in 42% of cases (Stillwell and Kramer 1986). Biopsies of the contralateral testis, taken at the time of exploration for torsion or shortly afterwards, show evidence of pathology in 57% to 88% of cases (Anderson and Williamson 1986; Hagen et al. 1991). The histological abnormalities consist of maturation arrest, germ cell degeneration, tubular hyalinization, immature tubules and focal thickening of basement membranes. These abnormalities are present in patients with torsion of less than 24 h, indicating that they are present before the onset of torsion (Laor et al. 1990).

The anatomical abnormality predisposing the testis to torsion may be associated with a defect in spermatogenesis such as is also found in cryptorchidism. Unilateral cryptorchids are often infertile and histological abnormalities may be found in the normally descended testis. Maldescent also increases the risk of torsion tenfold (Woodhead et al. 1973). However, Thomas et al. (1984) clearly showed a correlation between the duration of torsion and total motile sperm counts, which is against the theory of preexisting testicular dysplasia as the only cause of testicular abnormalities.

I.7.1.7.5
Exploration and Contralateral Fixation

Some authors have hypothesized that exploration and fixation may cause damage to the contralateral testis (Williamson 1976). However, in experimental studies contralateral orchiopexy alone does not impair spermatogenesis (Nagler and De Vere White 1982). Pathological damage is already present at the time of exploration for torsion, and seminal abnormalities occur both in patients with and without contralateral fixation, thus making this theory unlikely (Krarup 1978).

I.7.1.7.6
Release of Cytokines

Hadziselimovic et al. (1998) hypothesized that cytokines are released from the damaged blood-testis barrier at the time of torsion or subtorsion, which induce apoptosis in the contralateral testis.

I.7.1.7.7
Reflex Vasoconstriction

The most recent theory suggests that the spermatic cord under distress induces sympathetic mediated reflex vasoconstriction of the contralateral spermatic vessels with resultant ischaemia and subsequent damage (Tanyel et al. 1989). The hypoxia resulting from the decreased blood flow has been suggested to cause contralateral testicular damage (Akgür et al. 1994; Kolettis et al. 1996; Çiftçi et al. 1997).

Nguyen et al. (1999) found a bilateral decrease in blood flow after unilateral torsion, and after detorsion there was bilateral increased blood flow. They concluded that the contralateral testicular damage was caused by the increase in perfusion after detorsion and not by the initial decrease in blood flow. Since torsion of the spermatic cord and testicular vasculature alone also causes contralateral testicular hypoxia, the testis and epididymis do not seem to be mandatory for occurrence of contralateral testicular hypoxia. The testicular artery under distress seems to be the most important structure that results in contralateral testicular hypoxia following torsion (Salman et al. 1997). Currently the most probable mechanism of contralateral injury is believed to be vasospasm through a sympathetic reflex arc, resulting in hypoxia (Altay et al. 2001).

I.7.1.8 Prevention

I.7.1.8.1 Improving Salvage Rates

To save a twisted testis, three factors are needed: prompt presentation, prompt diagnosis and referral, and immediate surgery. The last two aspects have been addressed by education of medical students and physicians, but if the patient does not present early all effort by doctors will be in vain. Our current efforts should be directed at educating the general population by whichever means possible.

Jones et al. investigated the cause of delay in presentation and operative intervention and noted a delay in seeking medical attention in 58% of cases. General practitioners made an erroneous initial diagnosis in 29% and error in management at the referral hospital was the cause in 13% (Jones et al. 1986). Any effort at the referral hospital to improve testicular salvage rates must rely on either exploration of many patients who do not have torsion or on early, accurate, noninvasive diagnosis (Haynes et al. 1983).

I.7.1.8.2 Limiting the Effects on Fertility

Several modalities have been studied in an attempt to prevent or decrease bilateral testicular damage after torsion. Many experimental treatments have been studied with varying success, but none have been implemented in clinical practice.

External cooling has been shown to delay the effect of ischaemia for a few hours (Sarica and Bakir 1999).

Treatments aimed at decreasing reperfusion injury include verapamil, surfactant, allopurinol, platelet activating factor inhibitors and hyperbaric oxygen (Akgür et al. 1994; Palmer et al. 1997; Kolski 1998; Palmer et al. 1998; Sarica et al. 1999).

Immunosuppression has been used in the form of dexamethasone, hydrocortisone, cyclosporin A and azathioprine (Madarikan 1987; Yazawa et al. 2001).

Chemical sympathectomy probably works by inhibiting the afferent impulses from the ipsilateral testis under stress and preventing contralateral hypoxia. Drugs used include capsaicin, 6-hydroxy dopamine hydrobromide, guanethidine monosulphate and nitric oxide (Karagüzel et al. 1994b; Oguzkurt et al. 1998; Dokucu et al. 2000; Sarioglu-Buke et al. 2001).

At present, the only modality used in practice, apart from surgical detorsion and fixation, is cooling of the testis on the way to the operating theatre.

I.7.1.8.3 Risk of Testicular Cancer

Chilvers et al. estimated that in men with a history of testicular torsion, there is a 3.3-fold increased risk of developing a testis tumour compared to the normal population. However, of the nine cases of testicular torsion and tumour in their series, two had simultaneous diagnosis of torsion and ipsilateral tumour and four had tumour contralateral to the torsion, indicating that torsion is unlikely to play any role in the aetiology of the tumour (Chilvers et al. 1987). Kaplan and King (1970) reported two cases of torsion of the testis where the histology showed the presence of tumour.

I.7.1.8.4 Medicolegal Litigation

As early as 1933, O'Connor reported a claim on the grounds of injury on duty resulting from testicular torsion (O'Conor 1933).

Matteson et al. reviewed medical malpractice cases resulting from torsion in New Jersey, USA, from 1979 to 1997. They found 39 cases, of which indemnity payments were made in 26, and 13 cases ended in favour of the physicians. Five cases went to trial, with only one verdict in favour of the plaintiff. The median indemnity payment was $45,000 (range $5,000–$250,000). Urologists were named most frequently, followed by emergency room physicians and general practitioners. The liabilities in paid claims included missed diagnosis, improper referral, no radiological study obtained, failure to explore, surgical error and falsified records (Matteson et al. 2001).

In a review by the Medical Protection Society of 77 claims related to torsion from 1980 to 1998, the causes for settling claims included misdiagnosis of torsion by the general practitioner based on physical examination alone, failure to arrange an urgent referral, and failure to act with the appropriate degree of urgency by the referral hospital. In cases of misdiagnosis, the physicians were misled by abdominal pain, dysuria and the age of the patient. Misdiagnosis was not considered negligent, but failure to perform further investigation was (Anthony 2002).

I.7.1.9 Conclusions

1. The acute scrotum is a common urological emergency, and testicular torsion is the third most common cause.
2. The diagnosis is clinical and the treatment is emergency exploration.
3. A high index of suspicion is imperative in equivocal cases. Doppler ultrasonography and scintigraphy may be helpful under these circumstances.
4. Errors in management should be on the aggressive rather than conservative side.
5. Ipsilateral and contralateral orchiopexy should be performed with nonabsorbable sutures to prevent recurrent torsion.
6. The two most important factors determining testicular salvage after torsion are the duration and the degree of testicular rotation.
7. Saving the ipsilateral testis requires prompt presentation by the patient, prompt diagnosis and immediate surgery.
8. Earlier diagnosis and treatment can be achieved by educating medical students and physicians, whereas improving earlier presentation requires educating the general population.
9. Contralateral testicular damage, although well documented, is perhaps not regarded seriously enough as yet.
10. Experimentally tested methods of preventing testicular damage caused by torsion still await clinical application.

References

Akgür FM, Kilinc K, Aktug T, Olguner M (1994) The effect of allopurinol pretreatment before detorting testicular torsion. J Urol 151:1715–1717

Al Mufti RA, Ogedegbe AK, Lafferty K (1995) The use of Doppler ultrasound in the clinical management of acute testicular pain. Br J Urol 76:625–627

Alfert HJ, Canning DA (1987) Testicular torsion in a 62-year-old man. J Urol 138:149–150

Allan WR, Brown RB (1966) Torsion of the testis: a review of 58 cases. BMJ 1:1396–1397

Allen TD, Elder JS (1995) Shortcomings of color Doppler sonography in the diagnosis of testicular torsion. J Urol 154:1508–1510

Al-Salem AH (1999) Intra-uterine testicular torsion: early diagnosis and treatment. BJU Int 83:1023–1025

Altaffer LF 3rd (1980) Testicular torsion in men. J Urol 123:37–38

Altay B, Hekimgil M, Kefi A, Cikili N (2001) Histopathological examination of both ipsilateral and contralateral testes with different obstructive models in prepubertal and adult rats. BJU Int 88:84–89

Anderson MJ, Dunn JK, Lipshultz LI, Coburn M (1992) Semen quality and endocrine parameters after acute testicular torsion. J Urol 147:1545–1550

Anderson JB, Williamson RC (1986) The fate of the human testes following unilateral torsion of the spermatic cord. Br J Urol 58:698–704

Anderson J, Williamson R (1988) Testicular torsion in Bristol: a 25-year review. Br J Surg 75:988–992

Anderson JB, Cooper MJ, Thomas WE, Williamson RC (1986) Impaired spermatogenesis in testes at risk of torsion. Br J Surg 73:847–849

Anderson PA, Giacomantonio JM (1985) The acutely painful scrotum in children: review of 113 consecutive cases. Can Med Assoc J 132:1153–1155

Andiran F, Okur DH, Kilinç A, Gedikoglu G, Kilinç K, Tanyel FC (2000) Do experimentally induced ipsilateral testicular torsion, vas deferens obstruction, intra-abdominal testis or venous obstruction damage the contralateral testis through a common mechanism? BJU Int 85:330–335

Angell JC (1963) Torsion of the testicle: a plea for diagnosis. Lancet 1963; 1:19–21

Anthony S (2002) Scrotal confusion: focus on diagnosis. Med Protect Soc Casebook 17:5–11

Arda IS, Özyaylali I (2001) Testicular tissue bleeding as an indicator of gonadal salvageability in testicular torsion surgery. BJU Int 87:89–92

Atallah MW, Ippolito JJ, Rubin BW (1976) Intrauterine bilateral torsion of the spermatic cord. J Urol 116:128–129

Atkinson GO Jr, Patrick LE, Ball TI Jr, Stephenson CA, Broekker BH, Woodard JR (1992) The normal and abnormal scrotum in children: evaluation with colour Doppler sonography. AJR Am J Roentgenol 158:613–617

Baer HM, Gerber WL, Kendall AR, Locke JL, Putong PB (1989) Segmental infarct of the testis due to hypersensitivity angiitis. J Urol 142:125–127

Baker L, Sigman D, Mathews R, Benson J, Docimo S (2000) An analysis of clinical outcomes using color Doppler testicular ultrasound for testicular torsion. Pediatrics 105:604–607

Baptist EC, Amin PV (1996) Perinatal testicular torsion and the hard testicle. J Perinatol 16:67–68

Barada JH, Weingarten JL, Cromie WJ (1989) Testicular salvage and age-related delay in the presentation of testicular torsion. J Urol 142:746–748

Baratelli GM, Vischi S, Mandelli PG, Gambetta GL, Visetti F, Sala EA (1996) Segmental hemorrhagic infarction of testicle. J Urol 156:1442

Barca PR, Dargallo T, Jardon JA, Estevez E, Bautista A, Varela Cives R (1997) Bilateral testicular torsion in the neonatal period. J Urol 158:1957–1959

Bartsch G, Frank S, Marberger H, Mikuz G (1980) Testicular torsion: late results with special regard to fertility and endocrine function. J Urol 124:375–378

Baud C, Veyrac C, Couture A, Ferran JL (1998) Spiral twist of the spermatic cord: a reliable sign of testicular torsion. Pediatr Radiol 28:950–954

Becker D, Burst M, Wehler M, Tauschek D, Herold C, Hahn EG (1997) Differential diagnosis of acute testicular pain using color-coded duplex ultrasonography: difference between testicular torsion and epididymitis (in German). Dtsch Med Wochenschr 122:1405–1409

Bellinger MF (1985) The blind-ending vas: the fate of the contralateral testis. J Urol 133:644–645

Bellinger MF, Abromowitz H, Brantley S, Marshall G (1989) Orchidopexy: an experimental study of the effect of surgical technique on testicular histology. J Urol 142:553–555

Belman AB, Rushton HG (2001) Is the vanished testis always a scrotal event? BJU Int 87:480–483

Bennett S, Nicholson M, Little T (1987) Torsion of the testis: why is the prognosis so poor? BMJ 294:824

Bennett S, O'Hara S, Wacksman J, Meiers H (2002) Ultrasound

findings as predictors of clinical outcomes in the acute scrotum. J Urol 167 [Suppl]:107
Bickerstaff KI, Sethia K, Murie JA (1988) Doppler ultrasonography in the diagnosis of acute scrotal pain. Br J Surg 75:238–239
Bird K, Rosenfield AT, Taylor KJ (1983) Ultrasonography in testicular torsion. Radiology 147:527–534
Blaivas M, Batts M, Lambert M (2000) Ultrasonographic diagnosis of testicular torsion by emergency physicians. Am J Emerg Med 18:198–200
Brandt MR, Sheldon CA, Wacksman J, Matthews P (1992) Prenatal testicular torsion. Principles of management. J Urol 147:670–672
Brasso K, Andersen L, Kay L, Willie-Jorgensen P, Linnet L, Egense J (1993) Testicular torsion: a follow-up study. Scand J Urol Nephrol 27:1–6
Brewer ME, Glasgow BJ (1986) Adult testicular torsion. Urology 27:356–357
Burge DM (1987) Neonatal testicular torsion and infarction: aetiology and management. BJU 59:70–73
Burgher S (1998) Acute scrotal pain. Emer Clin N Am 16: 781–809
Burks DD, Markey BJ, Burkhard TK, Balsara ZN, Haluszka MM, Canning DA (1990) Suspected testicular torsion and ischemia: evaluation with color Doppler sonography. Radiology 175:815–821
Caesar R, Kaplan G (1994a) Incidence of the bell clapper deformity in an autopsy series. Urology 44:114–116
Caesar RE, Kaplan GW (1994b) The incidence of the cremasteric reflex in normal boys. J Urol 152:779–780
Caldamone AA, Valvo JR, AltebarmakianVK, Rabinowitz R (1984) Acute scrotal swelling in children. J Pediatr Surg 19: 581–584
Calleja R, Archer TJ (1996) Bilateral testicular torsion in a neonate. BJU 78:799
Campbell MF (1948) Torsion of the spermatic cord in the newborn infant. J Ped 33:323–327
Cartwright PC, Snow BW, Reid BS, Shultz PK (1995) Color Doppler ultrasound in newborn testis torsion. Urology 45:667–670
Cass AS (1982) Elective orchiopexy for recurrent testicular torsion. J Urol 127:253–254
Cass AS, Cass BP, Veerarghavan K (1980) Immediate exploration of the unilateral acute scrotum in young male subjects. J Urol 124:829–832
Castilla EE, Sod R, Anzorena O, Texido J (1975) Neonatal testicular torsion in two brothers. J Med Genet 12:112–113
Cattolica EV (1985) Preoperative manual detorsion of the torsed spermatic cord. J Urol 133:803–805
Chen DC, Holder LE, Melloul M (1983a) Radionuclide scrotal imaging: further experience with 210 patients. Part I: Anatomy, pathophysiology, and methods. J Nucl Med 24:735–742
Chen DC, Holder LE, Melloul M (1983b) Radionuclide scrotal imaging: further experience with 210 new patients. Part II. Results and discussion. J Nucl Med 24:841–853
Chilvers CE, Pike MC, Peckham MJ (1987) Torsion of the testis: a new risk factor for testicular cancer. Br J Cancer 55:105–106
Chinegwundoh FI (1995) Acute testicular torsion following testicular fixation. BJU 76:268
Choyke PL (2000) Editorial: dynamic contrast-enhanced MR imaging of the scrotum: reality check. Radiology 217:14–15
Çiftçi AO, Müftüoglu S, Çakar N, Tanyel FC (1997) Histological evidence of decreased contralateral testicular blood flow during ipsilateral testicular torsion. BJU 80:783–786
Colt GH (1922) Torsion of the hydatid of Morgagni. Brit J Surg 9:464–465
Cooper CS, Synder OB, Hawtrey CE (1997) Bilateral neonatal testicular torsion. Clin Ped 36:653–656
Corbett H, Simpson E (2002) Management of the acute scrotum in children. Aust N Z J Surg 72:226–228
Cornel EB, Karthaus HFM (1999) Manual derotation of the twisted spermatic cord. BJU Int 83:672–674
Corriere JN (1972) Horizontal lie of the testicle: a diagnostic sign in torsion of the testis. J Urol 107:616–617
Cos LR, Rabinowitz R (1982) Trauma-induced testicular torsion in children. J Trauma 22:244–246
Cranston DW, Moisey CU (1983) The management of acute scrotum pain. Br J Surg 70:505–506
Cruickshank ME (1991) Acute scrotal pain in two brothers. BJU 68:203
Cuckow PM, Frank JD (2000) Torsion of the testis. BJU Int 86:349–353
Cummings J, Boullier J, Sekhon D, Bose B (2002) Adult testicular torsion. J Urol 167:2109–2110
Cunningham RF (1960) Familial occurrence of testicular torsion. JAMA 174:1330–1331
Das S, Singer A (1990) Controversies of perinatal torsion of the spermatic cord: a review, survey and recommendations. J Urol 143:231–233
Davenport A, Downey SE, Goel S, Maciver AG (1996) Wegener's granulomatosis involving the urogenital tract. BJU 78:354–357
Delasiauve LJF (1840) Descente tardive du testicule gauche prise pour une hernie etranglée. Rev Med Franc Étrang 1840; pp 363–375 [English abstract, Article in French]
Della Negra E, Martin M, Bernardini S, Bittard H (2000) Spermatic cord torsion in adults. Prog Urol 10:265–270 [English abstract, Article in French]
Dennis MJ, Fahim SF, Doyle PT (1987) Testicular torsion in older men. BMJ (Clin Res Ed) 294:1680
Devesa R, Munoz A, Torrents M, Comas C, Carrera JM (1998) Prenatal diagnosis of testicular torsion. Ultrasound Obstet Gynecol 11:286–288
Dewire DM, Begun FP, Lawson RK, Fitzgerald S, Foley WD (1992) Color Doppler ultrasonography in the evaluation of the acute scrotum. J Urol 147:89–91
Dokucu AI, Öztürk H, Özdemir E, Ketani A, Büyükbayram H, Yücesan S (2000) The protective effects of nitric oxide on the contralateral testis in prepubertal rats with unilateral testicular torsion. BJU Int 85:767–771
Driver CP, Losty PD (1998) Neonatal testicular torsion. BJU 82:855–858
Dunne PJ, O'Loughlin BS (2000) Testicular torsion: time is the enemy. Aust N Z J Surg 70:441–442
Eshel G, Vinograd I, Barr J, Zemmer D (1994) Acute scrotal pain complicating familial Mediterranean fever in children. Br J Surg 81:894–896
Feins NR (1983) To pex or not to pex? J Pediat Surg 18:697–698
Fenner MN, Roszhart DA, Texter JH (1991) Testicular scanning: evaluating the acute scrotum in the clinical setting. Urology 38:237–241
Festen C (1987) The acute scrotum in children (in Dutch). Ned Tijdschr Geneeskd 131:1465–1456
Fischman AJ, Palmer EL, Scott JA (1987) Radionuclide imaging of sequential torsions of the appendix testis. J Nucl Med 28:119–121
Flanigan RC, Dekernion JB, Persky L (1981) Acute scrotal pain and swelling in children. Urology 17:51–53
Foshee CH (1932) Torsion of the appendix testis. JAMA 99: 289–292
Frank J, O'Brien M (2002) Fixation of the testis. BJU Int 89: 331–333
Fraser I, Slater N, Tate C, Smart TG (1985) Testicular torsion does not cause autoimmunisation in man. Br J Surg 72:237–238
Frazier WJ, Bucy JG (1975) Manipulation of torsion of the testicle. J Urol 114:410–411

Galejs LE, Kass EJ (1999) The diagnosis and treatment of the acute scrotum. Am Fam Phys 59:817 - 824
Gandia VM, Arrizabalaga M, Leiva O, Diaz Gonzalez R (1987) Polyorchidism discovered as testicular torsion associated with an undescended atrophic contralateral testis: a surgical solution. J Urol 137:743 - 44
Garel L, Dubois J, Azzie G, Filiatrault D, Grignon A, Yazbeck S (2000) Preoperative manual detorsion of the spermatic cord with Doppler ultrasound monitoring in patients with intravaginal acute testicular torsion. Pediatr Radiol 30:41 - 44
Gofrit O, Rund D, Shapiro A, Pappo O, Landau E, Pode D (1998) Segmental testicular infarction due to sickle cell disease. J Urol 160:835 - 836
Greenstein A, Schreiber L, Matzkin H (2001) The effect of methylene blue on histological damage after spermatic cord torsion in a rat model. BJU Int 88:90 - 92
Groisman GM, Naserallah M, Bar-Maor JA (1996) Bilateral intra-uterine testicular torsion in a newborn. BJU 78:800 - 801
Guiney EJ, McGlinchey J (1981) Torsion of the testes and the spermatic cord in the newborn. Surg Gynaecol Obstet 152: 273 - 274
Hadziselimovic F, Geneto R, Emmons LR (1998) Increased apoptosis in the contralateral testes of patients with testicular torsion as a factor for infertility. J Urol 160:1158 - 1160
Hadziselimovic F, Geneto R, Emmons LR (1997) Increased apoptosis in the contralateral testis in patients with testicular torsion. Lancet 350:118
Hagen P, Buchholz M, Eigenmann J, Bandhauer K (1992) Testicular dysplasia causing disturbance of spermiogenesis in patients with unilateral torsion of the testis. Urol Int 49: 154 - 157
Hahn LC, Nadel NS, Gitter MH, Vernon A (1975) Testicular scanning: a new modality for the preoperative diagnosis of testicular torsion. J Urol 113:60 - 62
Harrison RG, Lewis-Jones DI, Moreno de Marval MJ, Connolly RC (1981) Mechanism of damage to the contralateral testis in rats with an ischaemic testis. Lancet 2:723 - 725
Hastie K, Charlton C (1990) Indications for conservative management of acute scrotal pain in children. Br J Surg 77: 309 - 311
Hawtrey CE (1998) Assessment of acute scrotal symptoms and findings. A clinician's dilemma. Urol Clin North Am 25:715 - 723
Haynes BE, Bessen HA, Haynes VE (1983) The diagnosis and management of acute scrotal conditions in boys. JAMA 249:2522 - 2527
Hemalatha V, Rickwood AM (1981) The diagnosis and management of acute scrotal conditions in boys. BJU 53:455 - 459
Hendrikx AJ, De Vries JD, Debruyne FM (1988) Differential diagnosis and therapy in acute disorders of the scrotum (in Dutch). Ned Tijdschr Geneeskd 132:1142 - 1145
Hesser U, Rosenborg M, Gierup J, Karpe B, Nystrom A, Hedenborg L (1993) Gray-scale sonography in torsion of the testicular appendages. Pediatr Radiol 23:529 - 532
Heydenrych JJ (1974) Haemoperitoneum and associated torsion of the testicle in the newborn. S Afr Med J 48:2221 - 2222
Hitch DC, Shandling B, Lilly JR (1980) Recognition of bilateral neonatal testicular torsion. Arch Dis Child 55:153 - 155
Holland JM, Graham JB, Ignatoff JM (1981) Conservative management of twisted testicular appendages. J Urol 125:213 - 214
Hollman AS, Ingram S, Carachi R, Davis C (1993) Colour Doppler imaging of the acute paediatric scrotum. Paediatr Radiol 23:83 - 87
Hoshino H, Abe T, Watanabe H, Katsuoka Y, Kawamura N (1993) Correlation between atmospheric temperature and testicular torsion. Hinyokika Kiyo 39:1031 - 1034 [English abstract, Article in Japanese]
Hubbard AE, Ayers AB, MacDonald LM, James CE (1984) In utero torsion of the testis: antenatal and postnatal ultrasonic appearances. Br J Radiol 57:644 - 646
Hughes ME, Currier SJ, Della-Giustina D (2001) Normal cremasteric reflex in a case of testicular torsion (letter). Am J Emerg Med 19:241 - 242
Ichikawa T, Kitagawa N, Shiseki Y, Sumiya H, Shimazaki J (1993) Testicular function after spermatic cord torsion. Hinyokika Kiyo 39:243 - 248 [English abstract, Article in Japanese]
Ingram S, Hollman AS, Azmy A (1993) Testicular torsion: missed diagnosis on colour Doppler sonography. Pediatr Radiol 23:483 - 484
Iuchtman M, Zoireff L, Assa J (1979) Doppler flowmeter in the differential diagnosis of the acute scrotum in children. J Urol 121:221 - 223
Jefferson RH, Perez LM, Joseph DB (1997) Critical analysis of the clinical presentation of acute scrotum: a 9-year experience at a single institution. J Urol 158:1198 - 1200
Jequier S, Patriquin H, Filiatrault D, Garel L, Grignon A, Jequier JC, Petitjeanroget T (1993) Duplex Doppler sonographic examination of the testis in prepubertal boys. J Ultrasound Med 12:317 - 322
Jerkins GR, Noe HN, Hollabaugh RS, Allen RG (1983) Spermatic cord torsion in the neonate. J Urol 129:121 - 122
Johenning PW (1973) Torsion of the previously operated testicle. J Urol 110:221 - 222
Johnson DB, Sarda R, Uehling DT (1999) Mullerian-type epithelial tumor arising within a torsed appendix testis. Urology 54:561
Jones DJ (1991) Recurrent subacute torsion: prospective study of effects on testicular morphology and function. J Urol 145:297 - 299
Jones DJ, Macreadie D, Morgans BT (1986) Testicular torsion in the armed services: twelve year review of 179 cases. Br J Surg 73:624 - 626
Jones P (1962) Torsion of the testis and its appendages during childhood. Arch Dis Child 37:214 - 226
Jordan GH (1987) Segmental hemorrhagic infarct of testicle. Urology 29:60 - 63
Kadish HA, Bolte RG (1998) A retrospective review of pediatric patients with epididymitis, testicular torsion, and torsion of testicular appendages. Pediatrics 102:73 - 76
Kajbafzadeh AM (1996) Bilateral duplication of undescended testes associated with testicular torsion. BJU 78:314 - 315
Kallerhoff M, Gross AJ, Botefur IC, Zoller G, Weidner W, Holstein AF, Ringert RH (1996) The influence of temperature on changes in pH, lactate and morphology during testicular ischaemia. BJU 78:440 - 445
Kaplan G (2000) Scrotal swelling in children. Pediatr Rev 21:311 - 314
Kaplan GW, King LR (1970) Acute scrotal swelling in children. J Urol 104:219 - 223
Kaplan GW (1977) Acute idiopathic scrotal edema. J Pediatr Surg 12:647 - 649
Karagüzel G, Gedikoglu G, Tanyel FC, Büyükpamukçu N, Hiçsönmez A (1994a) Is ipsilateral testis mandatory for contralateral testicular damage encountered following spermatic cord torsion? Urol Res 22:115 - 117
Karagüzel G, Tanyel FC, Kilinç K, Büyükpamukçu N, Hiçsönmez A (1994b) The preventive role of chemical sympathectomy on contralateral testicular hypoxic parameters encountered during unilateral testicular torsion. BJU 74:507 - 510
Kass EJ, Lundak B (1997) The acute scrotum. Pediatr Clin North Am 44:1251 - 1266
Kass EJ, Stone KT, Cacciarelli AA, Mitchell B (1993) Do all children with an acute scrotum require exploration? J Urol 150: 667 - 669

Kaufman JM (1984) Torsion of the spermatic cord in the postnatal period. J Urol 131:351–352

Kay R, Strong DW, Tank ES (1980) Bilateral spermatic cord torsion in the neonate. J Urol 123:293–294

Kiesling VJ, Schroeder DE, Pauljev P, Hull J (1984) Spermatic cord block and manual reduction: primary treatment for spermatic cord torsion. J Urol 132:921–923

Klotz T, Vorreuther R, Heidenreich A, Zumbe J, Engelmann U (1996) Testicular tissue oxygen pressure. J Urol 155:1488–1491

Knight PJ, Vassy LE (1984) The diagnosis and treatment of the acute scrotum in children and adolescents. Ann Surg 200: 664–673

Kolettis PN, Stowe NT, Inman SR, Thomas AJ (1996) Acute spermatic cord torsion alters the microcirculation of the contralateral testis. J Urol 155:350–354

Kolski JM (1998) Effect of hyperbaric oxygen therapy on testicular ischemia-reperfusion injury. J Urol 160:601–604

Krarup T (1978) The testes after torsion. Br J Urol 50:43–46

Kuntze JR, Lowe P, Ahlering TE (1985) Testicular torsion after orchidopexy. J Urol 134:1209–1210

Kursh ED (1981) Traumatic torsion of testicle. Urology 17:441–442

Laor E, Fisch H, Tennenbaum S, Sesterhenn I, Mostofi K, Reid RE (1990) Unilateral testicular torsion: abnormal histological findings in the contralateral testis – cause or effect? BJU 65:520–523

LaQuaglia M, Bauer S, Eraklis A, Feins N, Mandell J (1987) Bilateral neonatal torsion. J Urol 138:1051–1054

Lee KF, Tang YC, Leong HT (2001) Emergency laparoscopic orchidectomy for torsion of intra-abdominal testis: a case report. J R Coll Surg Edinb 46:110–112

Lee LM, Wright JE, McLoughlin MG (1983) Testicular torsion in the adult. J Urol 1983; 130:93–94

Lee FT Jr, Winter DB, Madsen FA, Zagzebski JA, Pozniak MA, Chosy SG, Scanlan KA (1996) Conventional color Doppler velocity sonography versus color Doppler energy sonography for the diagnosis of acute experimental torsion of the spermatic cord. AJR Am J Roentgenol 167:785–790

Lee Y, Huang C, Huang C (2001) Testicular infarction associated with protein S deficiency. J Urol 165:1220–1221

Lent V, Stephani A (1993) Eversion of the tunica vaginalis for prophylaxis of testicular torsion recurrences. J Urol 150: 1419–421

Lerner RM, Mevorach RA, Hulbert WC, Rabinowitz R (1990) Color Doppler US in the evaluation of acute scrotal disease. Radiology 176:355–358

Lester DB, Gummess GH (1961) Torsion of the spermatic cord in the newborn infant. J Urol 86:631–633

Levy BJ (1975) The diagnosis of torsion of the testicle using the Doppler ultrasonic stethoscope. J Urol 113:63–65

Lewis AG, Bukowski TP, Jarvis PD, Wacksman J, Sheldon CA (1995) Evaluation of acute scrotum in the emergency department. J Pediatr Surg 30:277–282

Loh HS, Jalan OM (1974) Testicular torsion in Henoch-Schönlein syndrome. BMJ 2:96–97

Londergan TA (1995) Testicular torsion in a 59-year-old man. J Urol 154:1480

Longino LA, Martin LW (1995) Torsion of the spermatic cord in the newborn infant. New Engl J Med 253:695-697

Lootsma E, Van der Pol JJ (1987) Acute abdomen caused by torsion of an undescended testis (in Dutch). Ned Tijdschr Geneeskd 131:1490–1492

Luscombe CJ, Coppinger SMV, Mountford PJ, Gadd R (1996) Diagnosing testicular torsion. BMJ 312:1358–1359

Lyon RP (1961) Torsion of the testicle in childhood: a painless emergency requiring contralateral orchiopexy. JAMA 178: 702–705

Madarikan BA (1987) Testicular salvage following spermatic cord torsion. J Pediatr Surg 22:231–234

Manson AL (1990) Mumps orchitis. Urology 36:355–358

Manson AL (1989) Traumatic testicular torsion: case report. J Trauma 29:407–408

Marcozzi D, Suner S (2001) The nontraumatic, acute scrotum. Emerg Med Clin North Am 19:547–568

Mastrogiacomo I, Zanchetta R, Graziotti P, Betterle C, Scrufari P, Lanbo A (1982) Immunological and clinical studies in patients after spermatic cord torsion. Andrologia 14:25–30

Matteson JR, Stock JA, Hanna MK, Arnold TV, Nagler HM (2001) Medicolegal aspects of testicular torsion. Urology 57:783–786; discussion 786–787

May RE, Thomas WE (1980) Recurrent torsion of the testis following previous surgical fixation. Br J Surg 67:129–130

McCombe AW, Scobie WG (1988) Torsion of scrotal contents in children. BJU 61:148–150

McNellis DR, Rabinovitch HH (1980) Repeat torsion of fixed testis. Urology 16:476–477

Melekos MD, Asbach HW, Markou SA (1988) Etiology of acute scrotum in 100 boys with regard to age distribution. J Urol 139:1023–1025

Melloul M, Paz A, Lask D, Manes A, Mukamel M (1995) The value of radionuclide scrotal imaging in the diagnosis of acute testicular torsion. BJU 76:628–631

Mendez R, Tellado M, Montero M, Rios J, Vela D, Pais E, Lafuente G, Candal J (1998) Acute scrotum: an exceptional presentation of acute nonperforated appendicitis in childhood. J Pediatr Surg 33:1435–1436

Mevorach RA, Lerner RM, Greenspan BS, Russ GA, Heckler BL, Orosz JF, Rabinowitz R (1991) Color Doppler ultrasound compared to a radionuclide scanning of spermatic cord torsion in a canine model. J Urol 145:428–433

Middleton WD, Siegel BA, Melson GL, Yates CK, Andriole GL (1990) Acute scrotal disorders: prospective comparison of color Doppler US and testicular scintigraphy. Radiology 177:177–181

Miller DC, Peron SE, Keck RW, Kropp KA (1990) Effects of hypothermia on testicular ischemia. J Urol 143:1046–1048

Milleret R (1976) Doppler ultrasound diagnosis of testicular cord torsion. J Clin Ultrasound 4:425–427

Mishriki SF, Winkle DC, Frank JD (1992) Fixation of a single testis: always, sometime or never. BJU 69:311–313

Moharib NH, Krahn HP (1970) Acute scrotum in children with emphasis on torsion of spermatic cord. J Urol 104:601–603

Morse TS, Hollabaugh RS (1977) The window orchidopexy for prevention of testicular torsion. J Pediatr Surg 12:237–240

Muschat M (1932) The pathological anatomy of testicular torsion: an explanation of its mechanism. Surg Gynecol Obstet 54:758–763

Myers NA (1961) Torsion of the spermatic cord in the neonatal period. Med J Australia 48:793–795

Nadel NS, Gitter MH, Hahn LC, Vernon AR (1973) Preoperative diagnosis of testicular torsion. Urology 1:478–479

Nagler HM, DeVere White R (1982) The effect of testicular torsion on the contralateral testis. J Urol 128:1343–1348

Naidoo VV, Boniaszczuk J, Potgieter JD, Pontin A (1994) Scrotal scintigraphy in bilateral adolescent testicular torsion. BJU 74:804–805

Nakielny RA, Thomas WE, Jackson P, Jones M, Davies ER (1984) Radionuclide evaluation of acute scrotal disease. Clin Radiol 35:125–129

Napolez A (2001) Unilateral testicular torsion in a neonate. Am J Emerg Med 19:524–525

Nash WG (1893) Acute torsion of the spermatic cord: reduction: immediate relief. BMJ 1:742–743

Nguyen L, Lievano G, Ghosh L, Radhakrishnan, Fornell L, John E (1999) Effect of unilateral testicular torsion on blood flow

and histology of contralateral testes. J Pediatr Surg 34:680–683
Nishimura K, Namba Y, Nozawa M, Sugao H, Oka T, Osafune M (1996) Clinical studies on acute scrotum-focusing on torsion of the spermatic cord. Hinyokika Kiyo 42:723–727 [English abstract, Article in Japanese]
Noske H, Kraus B, Altinkilic B, Weidner W (1998) Historical milestones regarding torsion of the scrotal organs. J Urol 159:13–16
Nour S, Mackinnon AE (1991) Acute scrotal swelling in children. J R Coll Surg Edinb 36:392–394
O'Conor VJ (1933) Torsion of the spermatic cord. Surg Gynecol Obstet 57:242–246
Oguzkurt P, Okur DH, Tanyel FC, Büyükpamukçu N, Hiçsönmez A (1998) The effects of vasodilatation and chemical sympathectomy on spermatogenesis after unilateral testicular torsion: a flow cytometric DNA analysis. BJU 82:104–108
Palmer JS, Cromie WJ, Plzak LF, Leff AR (1997) A platelet activating factor antagonist attenuates the effects of testicular ischemia. J Urol 158:1186–1190
Palmer JS, Cromie WJ, Lee RC (1998) Surfactant administration reduces testicular ischemia-reperfusion injury. J Urol 159:2136–2139
Paltiel HJ, Connolly LP, Atala A, Paltiel AD, Zurakowski D, Treves ST (1998) Acute scrotal symptoms in boys with an indeterminate clinical presentation: comparison of color Doppler sonography and scintigraphy. Radiology 207:223–231
Parker RM, Robison JR (1971) Anatomy and diagnosis of torsion of the testicle. J Urol 106:243–247
Pascoe JR, Ellenburg TV, Culbertson MR Jr, Meagher DM (1981) Torsion of the spermatic cord in a horse. J Am Vet Med Assoc 178:242–245
Patriquin HB, Yazbeck S, Trinh B, Jequier S, Burns PN, Grignon A, Filiatrault D, Garel L, Dubois J (1993) Testicular torsion in infants and children: diagnosis with Doppler sonography. Radiology 188:781–785
Perri AJ, Slachta GA, Feldman AE, Kendall AR, Karafin L (1976) The Doppler stethoscope and the diagnosis of the acute scrotum. J Urol 116:598–600
Peterson CG (1961) Testicular torsion and infarction in the newborn. J Urol 85:65–68
Phipps JH (1987) Torsion of testis following orchidopexy. BJU 59:596
Pinto KJ, Noe NH, Jerkins GR (1997) Management of neonatal testicular torsion. J Urol 158:1196–1197
Pollock WB (1981) Spermatic cord torsion in a dog. Mod Vet Pract 62:216
Porpiglia F, Destefanis P, Fiori C, Tarabuzzi R, Fontana D (2001) Laparoscopic diagnosis and management of acute intra-abdominal testicular torsion. J Urol 166:600–601
Prater JM, Overdorf BS (1991) Testicular torsion: a surgical emergency. Am Fam Physician 44:834–840
Prehn DT (1934) A new sign in the differential diagnosis between torsion of the spermatic cord and epididymitis. J Urol 32:191–200
Pryor JL, Watson LR, Day DL, Abbitt PL, Howards SS, Gonzalez R, Reinberg Y (1994) Scrotal ultrasound for evaluation of subacute testicular torsion: sonographic findings and adverse clinical implications. J Urol 151:693–697
Puri P, Barton D, O'Donnell B (1985) Prepubertal testicular torsion: subsequent fertility. J Pediatr Surg 20:598–601
Rabinowitz R, Hulbert WC Jr (1995) Acute scrotal swelling. Urol Clin North Am 22:101–105
Rabinowitz R (1984) The importance of the cremasteric reflex in acute scrotal swelling in children. J Urol 132:89–90
Rampaul MS, Hosking SW (1998) Testicular torsion: most delay occurs outside hospital. Ann R Coll Surg Engl 80:169–172
Ransler CW, Allen TD (1982) Torsion of the spermatic cord. Urol Clin North Am 9:245–250
Redman JF, Barthold SJ (1995) A technique for atraumatic scrotal pouch orchidopexy in the management of testicular torsion. J Urol 154:1511–1512
Rodriguez DD, Rodriguez WC, Rivera JJ, Rodriguez S, Otero AA (1981) Doppler ultrasound versus testicular scanning in the evaluation of the acute scrotum. J Urol 125:343–345
Rodriguez LE, Kaplan GW (1988) An experimental study of methods to produce intrascrotal testicular fixation. J Urol 139:565–567
Ryken TC, Turner JW, Haynes T (1990) Bilateral testicular torsion in a pre-term neonate. J Urol 143:102–103
Salman AB, Kilinç K, Tanyel FC (1997) Torsion of only spermatic cord in the absence of testis and/or epididymis results in contralateral testicular hypoxia. Urol Res 25:413–415
Sarica K, Bakir K (1999) Semiquantitative evaluation of testicular histology after testicular torsion: protective effect of external cooling. Urol Int 63:110–114
Sarica K, Bakir K, Yagci F, Erbagci A, Topcu O, Uysal O (1999) Unilateral testicular torsion: protective effect of verapamil on contralateral testicular histology. Urol Int 62:159–163
Sarioglu-Buke A, Erdem S, Gedikoglu G, Bingol-Kologlu M, Tanyel FC (2001) Capsaicin effectively prevents apoptosis in the contralateral testis after ipsilateral testicular torsion. BJU Int 88:787–789
Sawchuk T, Costabile RA, Howards SS, Rogers BM (1993) Spermatic cord torsion in an infant receiving human chorionic gonadotrophin. J Urol 150:1212–1213
Schneider RE, Laycob LM, Griffin WT (1973) Testicular torsion in utero. Am J Obstet Gynec 117:1126–1127
Schulsinger D, Glassberg K, Strashun A (1991) Intermittent torsion: association with horizontal lie of the testicle. J Urol 145:1053–1055
Shah SN, Miller BM, Geisler E (1992) Polyorchidism discovered as testicular torsion. Urology 39:543–544
Shefi S, Haskel Y (1998) Simultaneous bilateral testicular torsion in an adult. J Urol 159:206–207
Sheldon CA (1985) Undescended testis and testicular torsion. Surg Clin North Am 65:1303–1329
Sidler D, Brown R, Millar A, Rode H, Cywes S (1997) A 25-year review of the acute scrotum in children. S Afr Med J 87:1696–1698
Siegel M, Herman TE (1994) Special imaging casebook. Neonatal spermatic cord torsion and testicular infarction. J Perinatol 14:431–432
Sinisi AA, Di Finizio B, Lettieri F, Pasquali D, Scurini C, De Bellis A, Bellastella A (1993) Late gonadal function and autoimmunization in familial testicular torsion. Arch Androl 30:147–152
Skoglund RW, McRoberts JW, Ragde H (1970a) Torsion of testicular appendages: presentations of 43 cases and a collective review. J Urol 104:598–603
Skoglund RW, McRoberts JW, Ragde H (1970b) Torsion of the spermatic cord: a review of the literature and an analysis of 70 new cases. J Urol 104:604–607
Smith G (1955) Cellular changes from graded testicular ischemia. J Urol 73:355–362
Sonda LP, Lapides J (1961) Experimental torsion of the spermatic cord. Surg Forum 12:502–504
Sparks JP (1971) Torsion of the testis. Ann R Coll Surg Engl 49:77–91
Steinhardt G, Boyarsky S, Mackey R (1993) Testicular torsion: pitfalls of color Doppler sonography. J Urol 150:461–462
Stewart JO, Maiti AK (1985) Familial torsion of the testicle. BJU 57:190–191
Stillwell TJ, Kramer SA (1986) Intermittent testicular torsion. Pediatrics 77:908–911

Stone KT, Kass EJ, Cacciarelli AA, Gibson DP (1995) Management of suspected antenatal torsion: what is the best strategy? J Urol 153:782 – 784

Strauss S (1997) Torsion of the testicular appendages: sonographic appearance. J Ultrasound Med 16:189 – 192

Tanyel FC, Büyükpamukçu N, Hiçsönmez A (1989) Contralateral testicular blood flow during unilateral testicular torsion. BJU 63:522 – 524

Taylor MR (1897) A case of testicle strangulation at birth; castration; recovery. BMJ 1:458

Thomas WE, Williamson RC (1983) Diagnosis and outcome of testicular torsion. Br J Surg 70:213 – 216

Thomas WE, Crane GA, Cooper MJ, Lee G, Williamson RCN (1984) Testicular exocrine malfunction after torsion. Lancet 2:1357 – 360

Thompson IM, Latourette H, Chadwick S, Ross G, Lichti E (1975) Diagnosis of testicular torsion using Doppler ultrasonic flowmeter. Urology 6:706 – 707

Thurston A, Whitaker R (1983) Torsion of testis after previous testicular surgery. Br J Surg 70:217 – 230

Tripp BM, Homsy YL (1995) Prenatal diagnosis of bilateral neonatal torsion. A case report. J Urol 153:1990 – 1991

Tryfonas G, Violaki A, Tsikopoulos G, Avtzoglou P, Zioutis J, Limas C, Gregoriadis G, Badouraki M (1994) Late postoperative results in males treated for testicular torsion during childhood. J Pediatr Surg 29:553 – 556

Tulchinsky M, Eggli DF (1992) Scintigraphy of torsion in triorchidism. J Nucl Med 33:1854 – 1956

Turek PJ, Ewalt DH, Snyder HM, Snyder HM 3rd, Stampfers D, Blyth B, Huff DS, Duckett JW (1994) The absent cryptorchid testis: surgical findings and their implications for diagnosis and etiology. J Urol 151:718 – 720; discussion 720 – 721

Turner TT (1987) On unilateral testicular and epididymal torsion: no effect on the contralateral testis. J Urol 138:1285 – 1290

Urwin GH, Kehoe N, Dundas S, Fox M (1986) Testicular infarction in a patient with sickle cell trait. BJU 58:340 – 341

Van Glabeke E, Khairouni A, Larroquet M, Audry G, Gruner M (1999) Acute scrotal pain in children: results of 543 surgical explorations. Pediatr Surg Int 15:353 – 357

Visser AJ, Heyns CF (2003) Testicular function after torsion of the spermatic cord. BJU Int 92:200 – 203

Visser AJ, Heyns CF (2004) Torsion of the testis and its appendages: diagnosis and management. Afr J Urol 10:85 – 91

Vordermark JS (1984) Testicular torsion: management with ultrasonic Doppler flow detector. Urology 14:41 – 42

Walsh, PC (1998) Campbells urology, 7th edn. WB Saunders, Philadelphia, pp 2184 – 2186

Wasnick RJ, Steigman E, Macchia RJ (1981) Simultaneous bilateral torsion of the testes in a man. J Urol 125:427 – 428

Watanabe Y, Dohke M, Ohkubo K, Ishimori T, Amoh Y, Okumura A, Oda K, Hayashi T, Dodo Y, Arai Y (2000) Scrotal disorders: evaluation of testicular enhancement patterns at dynamic contrast-enhanced subtraction MR imaging. Radiology 217:219 – 227

Watkin NA, Reiger NA, Moisey CU (1996) Is the conservative management of the acute scrotum justified on clinical grounds? BJU 78:623 – 627

Weingarten JL, Garafalo FA, Cromie WJ (1990) Bilateral synchronous neonatal torsion of the spermatic cord. Urology 35:135 – 136

Whitesel JA (1971) Intrauterine and newborn torsion of spermatic cord. J Urol 106:786 – 787

Wilbert DM, Schaerfe CW, Stern WD, Strohmaier WL, Bichler KH (1993) Evaluation of the acute scrotum by color-coded Doppler ultrasonography. J Urol 149:1475 – 1477

Williamson RCN (1976) Torsion of the testis and allied conditions. Br J Surg 63:465 – 476

Williamson RCN (1985) The continuing conundrum of testicular torsion. Br J Surg 72:509 – 510

Williamson RCN, Thomas WEG (1984) Sympathetic orchiopathia. Ann R Coll Surg Engl 66:264 – 266

Witherington R, Jarrell TS (1990) Torsion of the spermatic cord in adults. J Urol 143:62 – 63

Witte M, Kim ED, Lipshultz LI (1998) Torsion in a triorchid testis. J Urol 159:1694

Woodhead DM, Pohl DR, Johnson DE (1973) Fertility of patients with solitary testes. J Urol 109:66 – 67

Yazawa H, Sasagawa I, Suzuki Y, Nakada T (2001) Glucocorticoid hormone can suppress apoptosis of rat testicular germ cells induced by testicular ischemia. Fertil Steril 75:980 – 985

Yazbeck S, Patriquin HB (1994) Accuracy of Doppler sonography in the evaluation of acute conditions of the scrotum in children. J Pediatr Surg 29:1270 – 1272

Youssef BA, Sammak BM, Al Shahed M (2000) Case report. Pre-natally diagnosed testicular torsion ultrasonographic features. Clin Radiol 55:150 – 151

Zanchetta R, Mastrogiacomo I, Graziotti P, Foresta C, Betterle C (1984) Autoantibodies against Leydig cells in patients after spermatic cord torsion. Clin Exp Immunol 55:49 – 57

Zielie PJ, Haveran LA, Fung LC (2002) Diagnosing pediatric testicular torsion with a high degree of accuracy using a clinically based protocol. J Urol 167 (Suppl) 255

Zoeller G, Ringert RH (1991) Colour-coded duplex sonography for the diagnosis of testis torsion. J Urol 146:1288 – 1290

I.7.2 Blunt Testicular Trauma

J. Vale

Key Messages

- The scrotum should be examined in all cases of major trauma to check for evidence of haematocele or the rare event of traumatic dislocation.
- Although ultrasound has become commonplace in the evaluation of the painful swollen testicle after trauma, its ability to diagnose rupture of the tunica is questionable.
- Significant scrotal swelling after trauma is a strong indication to operate regardless of ultrasound findings, as this appears to offer the greatest chance of testicular salvage.
- In the rat model, there is a significant reduction in germ cell numbers in both the traumatized and the normal contralateral testicle after significant trauma, possibly due to an immune mechanism. In this model, orchidectomy appears to be more protective of fertility than repair, but the limited human evidence to date does not support this approach.
- The current standard of care at exploration is repair of any tunical tears, with excision of any devitalized extruded testicular parenchyma.

I.7.2.1 Definition

Blunt testicular trauma is characterized by swelling, disruption or dislocation of a testicle following blunt trauma. Broadly it can be classified into:

- Contusion without significant intratesticular haematoma (minor degree of trauma).
- Significant intratesticular haematoma (moderate degree of trauma).
- Rupture of the tunica albuginea with consequent haematocele (major trauma).
- Traumatic dislocation (major, often associated with other blunt abdominal trauma).

I.7.2.2 Aetiology and Pathogenesis

Blunt testicular trauma occurs most commonly as a result of assault or sport. A significant minority (10%) occur as the result of road traffic accidents. The testicles are protected by the thighs to some extent, and their relative mobility. However, if they are trapped against the thigh or bony pelvis and severe force applied (estimated to be greater than 50 kg), rupture of the tunica albuginea may occur. This results in bleeding into the space bounded by the tunica vaginalis, and consequent haematocele. If the applied force is even greater, the tunica vaginalis may also rupture, resulting in bleeding into the groin and perineum with obvious bruising.

I.7.2.3 Diagnosis

Recognition should be straight forward from the history, and the finding of scrotal swelling with or without bruising. The exception to this is dislocation, where sometimes the testicular injury may go unnoticed in the light of other more major trauma (Ko et al. 2004). To avoid missing a dislocation, trauma specialists should have a high index of suspicion and routinely examine the scrotum in all trauma patients. The finding of an absent testicle merits cross-sectional imaging (usually a CT scan as the patient frequently has other trauma) to confirm the presence and location of the testicle. Dislocations can be manually reduced under anaesthesia in some cases, but will often require open reduction via a groin incision and fixation.

It has become commonplace to use ultrasound in the evaluation of the painful swollen testicle following trauma, often reserving exploration and repair for men with evidence of rupture of the tunica albuginea. However, how sensitive is ultrasound at making this diagnosis? Unfortunately, many of the papers advocating ultrasound cannot give us this information reliably. The researchers did not explore patients with an intact tunica on ultrasound, and thus they may have missed some cases of rupture (false negatives). Indeed, studies where exploration has proceeded regardless of the ultrasound findings suggest that ultrasound is not reliable for predicting the integrity of the tunica (Ugarte et al. 1990; Cass and Luxenberg 1991; Corrales et al. 1993; Mulhall et al. 1995). The history of ultrasound in this condition reflects the history of many emerging diagnostic tests in medicine: initial enthusiasm (1980–1990) followed by healthy realism (1995–2005). However, ultrasound using a 7.5-MHz probe is still widely used in blunt testicular trauma, and perhaps has two roles:

- To exclude or confirm any abnormality (in its broadest sense) of the testicular structure. Parenchymal heterogeneity is suggestive of intratesticular haematoma, and loss of tunical continuity is suggestive of rupture. Both of these findings indicate significant degrees of trauma and, given the unreliability of ultrasound in diagnosing rupture, should be seen as an indication for exploration if there is significant scrotal swelling.

- To exclude any co-incidental pathology such as a tumour. Obviously such a finding would have profound implications for the surgical approach.

I.7.2.4 Treatment – Conservative Versus Surgical

This is the most controversial issue in blunt testicular trauma. There are broadly two schools of thought: explore every patient with significant swelling or explore based upon sonographic evidence of rupture despite the caveats above.

To determine the best strategy, we need to define the most important end-point. This must be fertility, ideally with testicular salvage for function or, at the very least, cosmesis. Looking at fertility in the first instance, there is good evidence that unilateral trauma can have a negative impact. In the rat model, there is a significant reduction in serum inhibin B after unilateral trauma, suggesting a reduction in spermatogenesis (Ozkan et al. 2003). This is corroborated by other studies which have shown a reduction in germ cell numbers in both the traumatized and the contralateral testicle of the rat model (Srinivas et al. 2002). Some protection is achieved if the traumatized testicle is excised acutely or the rat is administered intravenous cyclosporine (Srinivas et al. 1999). The latter is consistent with an immune basis for the fertility impairment, the trauma breaking down the normal blood–testicle barrier.

If the issue is a developing immune response as a result of damage to the blood–testicle barrier, repair might not be sufficient to correct this and immediate orchiectomy might be a better option. There is conflicting evidence in this regard: in the only published human study, testicular repair and salvage does seem to protect against fertility impairment (Lin et al. 1998), but in the rat model orchiectomy appeared to be more protective (Shaul et al. 1997). Based on the current available data, repair and salvage would seem to be the treatment of choice for the ruptured testicle.

The second issue relating to immediate exploration is testicular preservation. All of the evidence suggests that the chance of testicular salvage is greater with immediate exploration, drainage of haematocele and repair of the tunica. One of the most quoted series is that of Cass and Luxenberg (1991): in 72 patients with blunt trauma, the testicular salvage rate was 94% in those explored immediately as compared to 79% in those managed conservatively in the first instance. A trend towards increased testicular salvage with early exploration was also shown by Altarac (1994), and in addition exploration reduced disability and hastened recovery.

I.7.2.4.1 Surgery for Blunt Testicular Trauma

The indication for surgery is significant scrotal swelling, regardless of any ultrasound findings. The procedure is performed through a scrotal incision, and the haematocele is drained. The testicle, epididymis and lower spermatic cord are exposed. The testicle is inspected for signs of tunical damage and any extruded testicular tissue. The latter will be devitalized and should be excised; any attempt to force such tissue back into the testicle is counterproductive as it will increase intratesticular pressure and may damage the whole testicle. The tunica is then closed using a haemostatic continuous absorbable suture such as 3/0 or 4/0 Vicryl. If the haematocele is extensive it is appropriate to leave a drain: some authors have advocated a closed drainage system such as a suction drain, others an open system such as a Penrose drain. A gauze dressing and scrotal support are applied.

I.7.2.5 Postoperative Follow-up

Trauma patients should be seen once in an out-patient setting at 4 weeks to check that everything is settling well, unless the clinical picture merits earlier review. Further follow-up and semen analysis are probably not appropriate: usually there is no preinjury semen analysis for comparison. If a patient presents subsequently with infertility he should be investigated as any other infertility case.

References

Altarac S (1994) Management of 53 cases of testicular trauma. Eur Urol 25:119–123

Cass AS, Luxenberg M (1991) Testicular injuries. Urology 37:528–530

Corrales JG, Corbel L, Cipolla B et al (1993) Accuracy of ultrasound diagnosis after blunt testicular trauma. J Urol 150: 1834–1836

Ko SF, Ng SH, Wan YL et al (2004) Testicular dislocation: an uncommon and easily overlooked complication of blunt abdominal trauma. Ann Emerg Med 43:371–375

Lin WW, Kim ED, Quesada ET et al (1998) Unilateral testicular injury from external trauma: evaluation of semen quality and endocrine parameters. J Urol 159:841–843

Mulhall JP, Gabram SG, Jacobs LM (1995) Emergency management of blunt testicular trauma. Acad Emerg Med 2: 639–643

Ozkan KU, Kucukaydin M, Muhtaroglu S et al (2003) Serum inhibin B levels reflect contralateral testicular damage following unilateral testicular trauma. Urol Int 71:73–76

Shaul DB, Xie HW, Diaz JF et al (1997) Surgical treatment of

testicular trauma: effects on fertility and testicular histology. J Paediatr Surg 32:84–87
Srinivas M, Chandrasekharam VV, Degaonkar M et al (2002) Effects of unilateral grade 1 testicular injury in the rat. Urology 60:548–551
Srinivas M, Hashim S, Mitra DK (1999) Unilateral blunt testicular trauma in pre-pubertal rats. Paediatr Surg Int 15:457–460
Ugarte R, Spaedy M, Cass AS (1990) Accuracy of ultrasound in diagnosis of rupture after blunt testicular trauma. Urology 36:253–254

I.7.3 Penile Fractures

W.D. Aiken

Key Messages

- A penile fracture is a tear in the tunica albuginea of the corpus cavernosum due to blunt trauma to the erect penis.
- Penile fractures are mostly associated with coital mishaps in which there is use of excessive coital force.
- Sudden detumescence seems to be the most useful clinical discriminator between bona fide penile fracture and rupture of penile veins, the main differential diagnosis.
- Diagnosis is usually made on clinical findings alone.
- Ultrasound and MRI may be helpful in atypical or ambiguous cases and are also useful in determining the location and extent of the tunical rupture.
- Early surgical repair results in a better functional and cosmetic outcome and a lower frequency of complications.

I.7.3.1 Definition of the Disease

A penile fracture is a catastrophic injury which occurs when there is rupture of the tunica albuginea of the corpus cavernosum following blunt trauma to the erect penis.

I.7.3.2 Aetiology and Pathogenesis

During an erection, the tunica albuginea surrounding the corpora cavernosa becomes unyielding, stretched and thinned to 0.25–0.5 mm from its 2-mm-thick measurement in the flaccid state (Bitsch et al. 1990). A penile fracture occurs when the erect penis is subjected to a sudden axial or transverse load as occurs in blunt trauma, causing a precipitous rise in intracavernosal pressure which exceeds the tensile strength of the tunica albuginea, causing it to rupture (Penson et al. 1992). In Western society, this injury most often occurs during either partner-related or autoerotic sexual activity but can also occur while rolling over in bed and in other unusual circumstances (Aiken et al. 2001; Mydlo 2001). In partner-related sexual activity, a coital mishap in which the erect penis slips out of the vagina and impinges against the perineum, adjacent proximal thigh, or pubic symphysis is the most common mechanism. Penile fracture may occur in any coital position and seems to be related to the use of excessive coital force (Eke 2002). Vigorous partner-related manual manipulation of the penis has also been reported as causing a penile fracture (Aiken et al. 2001). Attempts at achieving detumescence by forcefully manipulating the erect penis represents the most common cause of penile fracture in case series from some cultures and is thought to be due to misinformation regarding the tissues of the penis (Zargooshi 2000). In a penile fracture, the sudden rupture of the tunica albuginea causes immediate extravasation of blood from the subjacent corpus cavernosum into the surrounding tissues of the penis, resulting in interstitial haemorrhage and immediate detumescence. Buck's fascia overlying the site of tunical rupture is usually torn and the blood therefore gains access to the superficial perineal pouch and is limited by an intact Colles (dartos) fascia. In 10% to 20% of cases, there is concomitant urethral injury (Aiken et al. 2001; Mydlo 2001). Rarely, there may be complete transection of the corpus spongiosum/urethra and both corpora cavernosa, with a small bridge of tunica albuginea being preserved dorsally, deep to the penile neurovascular bundle.

I.7.3.3 Clinical Findings

I.7.3.3.1 History

Time from injury to clinical presentation is highly variable and delay is often due to embarrassment and in some instances ignorance surrounding the nature of the injury and the need for urgent medical attention. The history typically involves a clearly identifiable coital mishap or sexual misadventure with resultant blunt injury to the erect penis. At the time of injury, severe penile pain of sudden onset is experienced and a cracking or popping sound is commonly heard, which is associated with immediate detumescence along with progressive swelling, bruising and deformity of the penis. A history of urethral bleeding presenting as blood at the meatus may not always be present in cases of associated urethral laceration. Worsening penile pain and swelling on attempted voiding or an inability to void are also seen in associated urethral lacerations.

I.7.3.4 Physical Examination

The patient suspected of having a penile fracture should be examined in a professional and compassionate manner with attention given to maintaining the privacy and dignity of the patient. The external genitalia should be fully exposed and the external urethral meatus inspected for the presence of blood. In cases of marked penile swelling in which the penis is uncircumcised, some difficulty may be experienced locating the meatus to inspect it. The presence and extent of any swelling, bruising and deformity of the penis should be noted as well as any swelling and discoloration of the scrotum. The penis should be palpated in its entirety in a systematic fashion beginning distally and proceeding proximally. Diffuse swelling, ecchymosis and deformity of the penis are encountered in most instances. In cases in which Buck's fascia is fairly well preserved overlying the site of tunical rupture, a firm, smooth, tender, discrete and fixed swelling corresponding to a haematoma at the point of tunical rupture may be palpated and is referred to as the rolling sign (Naraynsingh et al. 1998). Two-thirds of tunical tears occur proximally at or close to the penoscrotal junction.

I.7.3.5 Investigations

The diagnosis of the overwhelming majority of cases of penile fracture is entirely based on clinical findings and confirmatory investigations are usually unnecessary. However, investigations may be used in an attempt to confirm an equivocal case of suspected penile fracture, to diagnose or confirm a suspected associated urethral laceration, and to demonstrate the site of tunical rupture, thereby enabling a more limited or focal surgical approach. A routine urinalysis should be done looking for the presence of red blood cells, which would suggest a possible associated urethral injury and should prompt a request for retrograde urethrography. The established investigation in the diagnosis of a penile fracture is cavernosography. This involves the injection of 50 ml of water-soluble contrast into the corpora cavernosa under X-ray control. The location of any extravasation of contrast is noted and is indicative of the site of tunical rupture. Cavernosography is limited, however, by a significant false-negative rate (Mydlo 2001) and is thought to have the potential to be damaging to erectile tissue (McAninch 2004). Ultrasonography has been reported as being helpful in localizing the site of tunical rupture (Ciciliato et al. 2002), which is advantageous when a focal approach is desired. MRI has been reported as providing precise anatomical detail in delineating the site and extent of tunical rupture, in diagnosing associated urethral injury and in distinguishing equivocal cases such as penile vein rupture from bona fide cases of tunical rupture (Uder et al. 2002). It has the advantage of being noninvasive but it is an expensive imaging modality and is not universally available.

I.7.3.6 Differential Diagnosis

The main differential diagnosis is rupture of the deep dorsal vein of the penis, which is also seen in blunt trauma to the erect penis, usually during sexual activity, presenting with immediate pain, swelling and bruising of the penis and frequently a cracking or popping sound at the time of injury (Nehru-Babu et al. 1999). Sudden detumescence is the most useful clinical discriminator for patients suspected of having a penile fracture, as immediate detumescence of the penis does not occur with dorsal vein rupture (Aiken et al. 2001). Significant swelling, bruising and deformity of the penis may be seen on examination and cavernosography, ultrasonography or MRI may be necessary to help exclude a penile fracture in these cases.

I.7.3.7 Treatment

The treatment of penile fracture has shifted from a conservative approach to one of early surgical repair of the torn tunica albuginea. This is based on many reported case series over the last two decades documenting a uniformly better outcome with surgery when compared historically with a conservative approach (Eke 2002). A subcoronal circumferential degloving incision is the one most often used and has the advantage of fully exposing the entire shaft of the penis deep to Colles' (dartos) fascia. Some surgeons advocate a limited incision, performed under local anaesthesia, directly over the site of tunical rupture (Naraynsingh et al. 1998). This requires preoperative localization of the fracture site, either through examination, which is not always reliable, or through imaging, which is unnecessary if the degloving incision is used. Tunical tears are typically oriented transversely and occur proximally close to the penoscrotal junction. Regardless of the incision used, the haematoma is evacuated, haemorrhage is controlled, and the edges of the tunical defect freshened and reapproximated with interrupted 3/0 delayed absorbable sutures, making sure the knots are inverted. In concomitant urethral injury, the urethra is primarily repaired over a 16-French silicone catheter using interrupted 4/0 absorbable sutures. Buck's fascia is closed, the degloved skin returned and a circumcision may be done at this time. Patients are discharged on the first postoperative day, sexual intercourse is prohibited for a period of 6 weeks, and patients should be reviewed at 3 months.

I.7.3.8 Results of Treatment

Potential adverse sequelae of penile fractures include erectile dysfunction, abnormal penile curvature, pain on erection and on intercourse, the presence of a penile nodule, and pulsatile diverticulum. Contemporary case series utilizing immediate surgical repair have demonstrated a uniformly better outcome with a lower reported frequency of the aforementioned adverse sequelae when compared historically to conservative treatment, suggesting that immediate surgical repair minimizes the occurrence of complications (Eke 2002).

I.7.3.9 Prognosis

The prognosis for return and maintenance of normal sexual function following penile fracture is excellent if immediate surgical repair is performed (Zargooshi 2002).

I.7.3.10 Prevention

Health education regarding the tissues of the penis is necessary in those cultures where forceful self-manipulation of the erect penis to achieve detumescence is seen, to discourage its practice (Zargooshi 2000).

References

Aiken W, Johnson L, Mayhew R, Tulloch T (2001) A ten year review of suspected penile fractures seen at two Jamaican hospitals. WIMJ 50 [Suppl 6]: 25

Bitsch M, Kromann-Andersen B, Schou J, Sjøntoft E (1990) The elasticity and the tensile strength of the tunica albuginea of the corpora cavernosa. J Urol 143:642

Ciciliato S, Bucci S, Liguori G, Marega D, Trombetta C (2002) Ultrasonographic diagnosis of penile fracture. Arch Ital Urol Androl 74:302

Eke N (2002) Fracture of the penis. Br J Surg 89:555

McAninch J (2004) Editorial comment on management of penile fracture. J Trauma 56:1140

Mydlo J (2001) Surgeon experience with penile fracture. J Urol 166:526

Naraynsingh V, Mahaaraj D, Kuruvilia T, Ramsewak R (1998) Simple repair of fractured penis. J R Coll Surg Edinb 43:97

Nehru-Babu M, Hendry D, Ai-Saffar N (1999) Rupture of the dorsal vein mimicking fracture of the penis. BJU Int 84:179

Penson D, Seftel A, Krane R, Frohrib D, Goldstein I (1992) The haemodynamic pathophysiology of impotence following blunt trauma to the erect penis. J Urol 148:1171

Uder M, Gohl D, Takahashi M, Derouet H, Defreyne L, Kramann B et al (2002) MRI of penile fracture: diagnosis and therapeutic follow-up. Eur Radiol 12:113

Zargooshi J (2000) Penile fracture in Kermanshah, Iran: report of 172 cases. J Urol 164:364

Zargooshi J (2002) Penile fracture in Kermanshah, Iran: the long term results of surgical treatment. BJU Int 89:890

I.7.4 Priapism

P. Kumar, D.J. Ralph

Key Messages

- Cavernosal blood gas analysis and colour Doppler ultrasonography aid in the diagnosis of priapism.
- Ischaemic low flow priapism is a surgical emergency, as smooth muscle necrosis and penile fibrosis are the long-term sequelae of delay in treatment.
- Aspiration of stagnant cavernosal blood and injection of sympathomimetic agents are the first stage of treatment in ischaemic priapism.
- More invasive surgical measures, including shunt formation and penile prosthesis implantation, must be considered should the first stage of treatment fail.
- Pudendal angiography and selective embolization is the treatment of choice in arterial priapism.

I.7.4.1 Definition

Priapism is defined as a pathological condition where penile erection persists beyond or is unrelated to sexual stimulation.

I.7.4.2 Aetiology and Pathogenesis

Despite advances in the knowledge of erectile pathophysiology, priapism remains a diagnostic and therapeutic enigma. Low-flow ischaemic and high-flow arterial priapism are the two main subtypes. Ischaemic priapism is most commonly idiopathic, although the condition appears to be more prevalent in certain patient groups such as patients with sickle cell disease

Table I.7.5. Causes of ischaemic priapism

Category	Subtypes
Idiopathic	
Systemic disease	Hypertension Diabetes Rheumatoid arthritis
Haematological	Sickle cell disease Thrombophilia Other haemoglobinopathies Leukaemia Myeloma
Drug therapy for erectile dysfunction	Papaverine Intracavernosal PGE1 PDE5 inhibitors Alprostadil Phentolamine
Pharmacotherapy and other drugs	Phenothiazines Selective serotonin reuptake inhibitors (SSRIs) Anticoagulants Antihypertensives Alcohol Marijuana Cocaine
Solid tumours	Bladder cancer Prostate cancer Metastatic renal cancer
Others	Total parenteral nutrition, amyloid, rabies, appendicitis

(Adeyoju 2002). Arterial priapism is due to unregulated arterial blood flow within the penis, usually secondary to a cavernosal artery laceration following penile or perineal trauma. Identification of priapism type and use of a stepwise management protocol is essential. Penile detumescence and preservation of long-term sexual function are the goals of treatment.

Although the majority of cases of ischaemic priapism are idiopathic, various systemic diseases and pharmacotherapies are associated with the condition and may give clues to the aetiology (Table I.7.5). The commonest cause of priapism is intracavernosal injection of vasoactive agents (papaverine or prostaglandin E_1).

I.7.4.3 Clinical Findings, Technical Investigations and Laboratory Findings

The duration of tumescence is indicative of the likelihood that aspiration and shunting procedures will be effective in treating ischaemic priapism. Smooth muscle damage is likely to have occurred should more than 12 h have elapsed and patients should be counselled that long-term erectile dysfunction is likely in at least 50% of patients even if initial therapy is successful (Winter 1988). Preexisting erectile dysfunction should also be elicited, as this will influence any surgical management offered.

The absence of pain would indicate that the penis is being perfused with oxygenated blood and that an arterial priapism is more likely. A history of penile or perineal trauma, most commonly during sexual activity, in the playground or on the sports field would also indicate the presence of a cavernosal or internal pudendal arterial injury causing a high-flow picture.

The spongiosum is characteristically uninvolved in priapism; hence a rigid penis with a flaccid glans is the usual finding. Penile or perineal bruising may be found in cases of prolonged priapism or where trauma is an aetiological factor. Marked tenderness of the cavernosae would indicate the priapism to be of the ischaemic type. In cases of arterial priapism, the penis may be only partially erect and firm pressure to the perineal area may effect detumescence. A full abdominal and pelvic examination including digital rectal examination should be performed, as priapism may be the result of metastatic penile deposits secondary to primary malignancy elsewhere (Schroeder-Printzen et al. 1994; Kvarstein 1996; Nezu et al. 1998).

Aspiration of blood from the cavernosae provides information that aids in the differentiation between low and high flow states (Montague et al. 2003). Analysis should include pH, pO_2, pCO_2 and blood glucose (BM) estimation. Cavernosal blood gas levels in arterial priapism are near to normal arterial saturation, whereas in ischaemic priapism hypoxia and acidosis are seen (Broderick and Harkaway 1986) (Table I.7.6).

The use of ultrasound to assess penile blood flow is safe and noninvasive. Men with arterial priapism will have high blood flow velocities within the cavernosae. Turbulent flow may be seen at the site of a traumatic cavernosal artery fistula or pseudoaneurysm. The perineum, as well as the penis itself, must be assessed, as injuries occur more commonly in the proximal portion of the penile arterial supply. Men with ischaemic priapism will have little or no blood flow within the penis.

Table I.7.6. Typical cavernosal blood gas values

	Normal flaccid penis	Ischaemic priapism	Arterial priapism
pH	7.35	<7.25	7.4
pO_2	40 mm Hg	<30 mm Hg	50–90 mm Hg
pCO_2	50 mm Hg	>60 mm Hg	40–50 mm Hg
Blood glucose (BM)	4–8	<4	6–10

I.7.4.4 Treatment

I.7.4.4.1 Management of Ischaemic Priapism

Aspiration and Injection Therapy

Two butterfly needles should be inserted into the rigid corpus and aspiration of the clotted blood attempted. This manoeuvre alone may be successful in effecting detumescence, particularly if the priapism is of very short duration. If the aspirate is heavily congealed or dry, a gentle wash out with saline should be performed. If this fails, injection of a sympathomimetic agent may aid detumescence by causing the corporeal smooth muscle to contract. The use of the α_1-agonist phenylephrine is recommended in order to minimize unwanted cardiovascular side effects (hypertension, tachycardia and arrhythmogenesis). Injections may be repeated over a 90-min period with continuous blood pressure monitoring during and for a short period after treatment. Aspiration and irrigation with sympathomimetic agents has no therapeutic role in arterial priapism.

Shunt Surgery

The aim of shunt surgery is to create an alternative venous outflow channel for blood within the corpora cavernosae, should a trial of aspiration and injection therapy be unsuccessful. Several types of shunt surgery have been described. The most common are corporoglanular shunts with the introduction of a wide-bore Tru-Cut biopsy needle or pointed scalpel via the glans penis into each cavernosum (Winter 1976; Ebbehoj 1974). The aim is to produce enough fenestrations in the intervening tunica to allow blood to leave the turgid cavernosum. The Al-Ghorab shunt is a more invasive variation where the tips of the corporeal bodies are exposed and a window made in the distal portion of each side to allow detumescence prior to glans skin closure (Wendel and Grayhack 1981). Shunt formation between the corpora cavernosae and either the proximal spongiosum or saphenous vein may be used should the distal penis be very bruised and/or oedematous. A fistula is formed between the proximal spongiosal and cavernosal bodies via a perineal incision in the cavernoso-spongiosal shunt (Quackels 1964). A cavernoso-saphenous vein shunt is the most invasive type (Grayhack et al. 1964). A length of saphenous vein is mobilized and tunnelled to the penile root where it is anastomosed to the base of the penis.

The incidence of long-term erectile dysfunction following shunt surgery is high. A recent study reported on a consecutive series of 28 patients managed with shunt surgery (Nixon et al. 2003). It was noted that up to 90% of patients described some degree of erectile dysfunction at long-term follow-up and 75% of the patients reported no spontaneous erections whatsoever.

The likelihood of sustained detumescence following shunt surgery decreases with time. The use of a cavernosal smooth muscle biopsy at the time of any surgical intervention, to determine if necrosis has already occurred, would seem a sensible option (Pryor et al. 2004). This would allow patients with prolonged ischaemic priapism who have failed to respond to medical therapies and have unviable tissue to be treated with the immediate insertion of a penile prosthesis, rather than shunt surgery, in order to minimize penile shortening and preserve sexual function.

Penile Implant Surgery

Failure to effect detumescence in ischaemic priapism using sympathomimetic agents or shunt surgery may result in cavernosal fibrosis with penile induration and shortening (Kulmala and Tamella 1995). The priapism eventually subsides with time and the resulting erectile dysfunction is likely to be severe. Placement of a penile prosthesis in the fibrotic penis can be extremely difficult and associated with higher complication rates (Douglas et al. 1990; Monga et al. 1996).

The outcome of the management of low flow priapism with the immediate insertion of a penile prosthesis has been recently reviewed (Rees et al. 2002). A series of patients with prolonged ischaemic priapism (>32 h) had failed conservative measures with aspiration and instillation of phenylephrine. Prosthesis insertion was offered to these patients as a means of relieving the painful priapism, preserving long-term sexual function and minimizing penile shortening due to fibrosis. None of the patients developed postoperative infections, the authors attributing this to the simple and rapid implant insertion. All patients were satisfied with the results of surgery, with seven out of eight patients successfully engaging in sexual intercourse at a mean follow-up of more than 1 year.

I.7.4.4.2 Management of Arterial Priapism

Visualization of the pudendal artery and its tributaries is the investigation of choice in this group of patients (Bastuba et al. 1994; Hakim et al. 1996). The exact site and nature of the vascular injury may be ascertained and targeted therapy by means of embolization carried out to effect detumescence. Long-term erectile function is preserved in these patients (Ciampalini et al. 2002). Should repeated attempts at embolization be unsuccessful or, in cases of prolonged high-flow priapism, a capsule have formed around the arteriocavernous fistula, it may be necessary to attempt open ligation of the fistula or ipsilateral feeding vessel (Riccardi et al. 1993).

In these cases, the incidence of long-term erectile dysfunction is high even with the use of intraoperative Doppler ultrasound to aid location of the fistula.

I.7.4.5 Conclusion

Urgent evaluation of the priapic patient is vital in order to identify those with ischaemic priapism. Treatment should proceed in a logical fashion with therapy aimed at the penis and any systemic disorder being carried out concurrently. Aspiration and injection therapy precedes more invasive surgical intervention. The choice of procedure depends on preexisting erectile function, duration of priapism and need for preservation of sexual function. Selective embolization for high-flow priapism is a safe, well-tolerated procedure that preserves premorbid erectile function. It is of paramount importance that patients are properly counselled as to the prognosis of priapism and the likelihood of long-term erectile dysfunction.

References

Adeyoju AB, Olujohungbe ABK, Morris J, Yardumian A, Bareford D, Akenova A, Akinyanju O, Cinkotai K, O'Reilly PH (2002) Priapism in sickle-cell disease; incidence, risk factors and complications-an international multicentre study. BJU Int 90:898–902

Bastuba MD, Saenz de Tejada I, Dinlenc CZ, Sarazen A, Krane RJ, Goldstein I (1994) Arterial priapism: diagnosis, treatment and long-term follow up. J Urol 151:1231–1237

Broderick GA, Harkaway R (1986) Pharmacological erection: time-dependent changes in the corporal environment. Int J Impot Res 6:9

Ciampalini S, Savoca G, Buttazzi L, Gattuccio I, Mucelli FP, Bertolotto M, De Stefani S, Belgrano E (2002) High-flow priapism: treatment and long-term follow-up. Urology 59:110–113

Douglas L, Fletcher H, Serjeant GR (1990) Penile prostheses in the management of impotence in sickle cell disease. Br J Urol 65:533–535

Ebbehoj J (1974) A new operation for priapism. Scand J Plast Reconstr Surg 18:241

Grayhack JT et al (1964) Venous bypass to control priapism. Invest Urol 1:509

Hakim LS, Kulaksizoglu H, Mulligan R et al (1996) Evolving concepts in the diagnosis and treatment of arterial high flow priapism. J Urol 155:541–548

Kulmala RV, Tamella TJL (1995) Effects of priapism lasting 24 h or longer caused by intracavernosal injection of vasoactive drugs. Int J Impot Res 7:131–136

Kvarstein B (1996) Bladder cancer complicated with priapism. Scan J Urol Nephrol Suppl 179:155–156

Monga M, Broderick GA, Hellstrom WJG (1996) Priapism in sickle cell disease: the case of early implantation of the penile prosthesis. Eur Urol 30:54–59

Montague DK, Jarow J et al (2003) American Urological Association guideline on the management of priapism. J Urol 170:1318–1324

Nezu FM, Dhir R, Logan TF, Lavelle J, Becich MJ (1998) Malignant priapism as the initial presentation of metastatic renal cell adenocarcinoma, with invasion of both the corpora cavernosum and spongiosum. Int J Impot Res 10:101

Nixon RG, O'Connor JL, Milam DF (2003) Efficacy of shunt surgery for refractory low flow priapism: a report on the incidence of failed detumescence and erectile dysfunction. J Urol 170:883–886

Pryor J, Akkus E, Alter G, Jordan G, Lebret T, Levine L, Mulhall J, Perovic S, Ralph DJ, Stackl W (2004) Priapism. J Sexual Med 1:116–123

Quackels R (1964) Cure of the patient suffering from priapism by cavernospongiosal anastamosis. Acta Urol Belg 32:5

Rees RW, Kalsi J, Minhas S, Peters J, Kell P, Ralph DJ (2002) The management of low-flow priapism with the immediate insertion of a penile prosthesis. Br J Urol 90:893–897

Riccardi R, Bhatt G, Cynamon J, Bakal CW, Melman A (1993) Delayed high flow priapism: pathophysiology and management. J Urol 149:119

Schroeder-Printzen I, Vosshenrich R, Weidner W, Ringert RH (1994) Malignant priapism in a patient with metastatic prostate adenocarcinoma. Urol Int 52:52–54

Wendel EF, Grayhack JT (1981) Corpora cavernosa-glans penis shunts for priapism. Surg Gynecol Obstet 153:586

Winter CC (1976) New procedure for creating fistula between glans penis and corpora cavernosa. Urology 8:389–391

Winter CC, McDowell G (1988) Experience with 105 patients with priapism: update review of all aspects. J Urol 140:980–983

I.7.5 Testicular Pain and Related Pain Syndromes

T.B. Hargreave, L. Turner-Stokes

I.7

Key Messages

- In acute pain, it is important to diagnose testicular torsion quickly, and if torsion is suspected then an exploratory operation does no significant harm, even if the diagnosis subsequently proves to be epididymo-orchitis, whereas a missed torsion results in loss of the testicle.
- It is good practice to use local anaesthetic as a supplement to general anaesthesia for all andrological surgery to ensure a pain-free postoperative recovery, as there is evidence that poor pain control may trigger chronic pain.
- The first step in the management of chronic testicular pain is to take a detailed history and complete a careful clinical examination.
- If the diagnosis is chronic testicular pain and provided ilio-inguinal pain and other pathology has been excluded, a spermatic cord denervation operation may help in up to 75 % of men, but there is a risk that further surgery can make chronic pain worse.
- Long-term management of chronic neuropathic testicular pain is best undertaken by chronic pain specialists and rehabilitation medicine experts and centres on encouraging the man to lead as normal a life as possible despite the pain.

I.7.5.1 Definition of the Disease

I.7.5.1.1 Acute Testicular Pain

Acute pain in the testicle area can occur secondary to a variety of conditions affecting the testicle and epididymis. Thus acute testicular pain is defined as the nociceptive response to local testicular or epididymal pathology.

I.7.5.1.2 Testicular Pain of Neuropathic Origin

This is defined as testicular pain caused by lesion involving the testicular nerve supply.

I.7.5.1.3 Chronic Testicular Pain and Chronic Testicular Pain Syndromes

Chronic testicular pain (orchalgia or orchiodynia) is defined as pain in the testicle and surrounding areas that has been present for more than 6 months. There is a spectrum of conditions ranging from chronic recurring epididymal pain such as may occur following vasectomy to a complete disabling chronic pain syndrome. These conditions pose a considerable management problem for both the patient and his doctor.

I.7.5.2 Aetiology and Pathogenesis

I.7.5.2.1 Acute Testicular Pain – Pathogenesis

Acute testicular pain can be caused by a variety of conditions affecting the testicle. Perhaps the commonest cause of pain is epididymo-orchitis. Other causes are torsion, bleeding into a testicular tumour or bleeding into hydroceles, epididymal cysts, and spermatoceles. Classically, testicular tumours are described as painless, but up to 40 % of patients report dull aching or heaviness.

I.7.5.2.2 Neuropathic Testicular Pain – Pathogenesis

Less commonly, testicular pain may arise from neurological injury (neuropathic pain). The nervous supply to the testicle and scrotum is complex, and in order to understand the basis for neuropathic syndromes presenting with testicular pain, it is necessary to have some understanding of the relevant neuroanatomy (Fig. I.7.16; Wesselmann et al. 1997).

- Pain sensation to the testis is supplied mainly through sympathetic fibres from T10–L1. These travel via the superior hypogastric plexus (SHP) and are then carried in the spermatic plexus along spermatic cord structures to terminate in the testis, epididymis and vas deferens.
- A second sensory supply is derived from the genito-femoral nerve (L1–L2), which takes a retroperitoneal route. The genital branch of this nerve travels down the inguinal canal to supply the cremaster, cord and tunica vaginalis.
- The posterior sacral nerves (S2–S3) provide a subsidiary supply via the sacral plexus and the

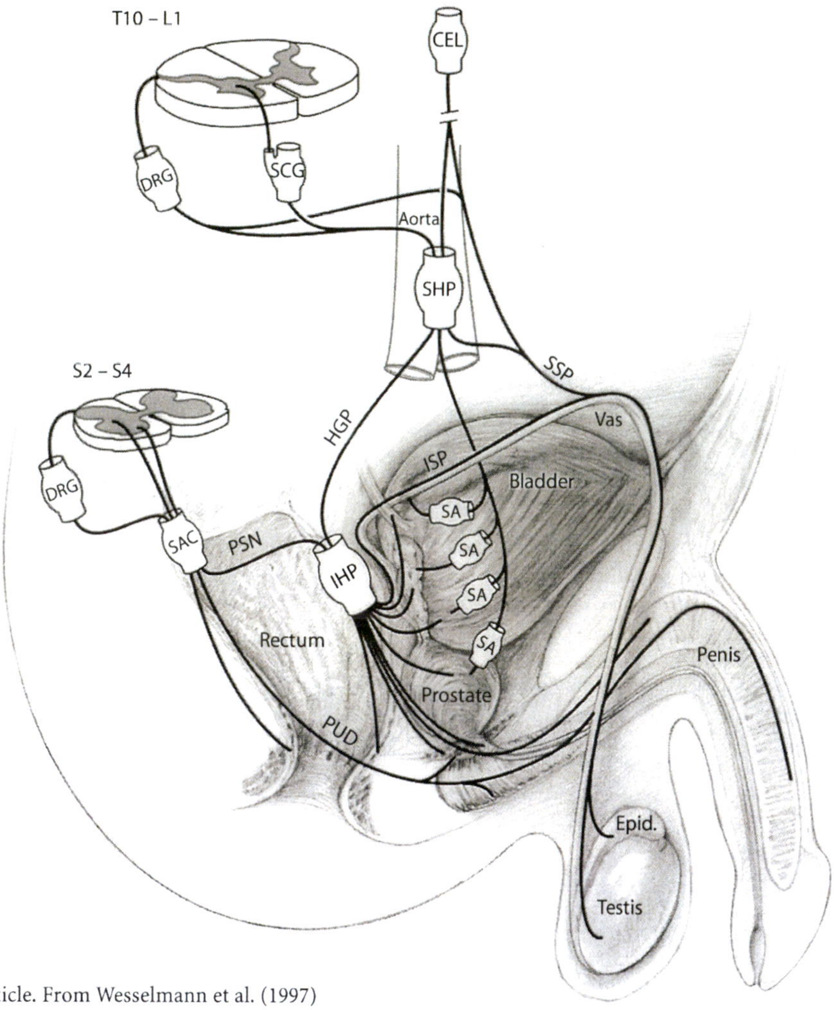

Fig. I.7.16. Innervation of the testicle. From Wesselmann et al. (1997)

pudendal nerve, to innervate a portion of the scrotum. Compression of the pudendal nerve is reported to be a cause of scrotal pain (Kim et al. 2003), which may respond on occasion to decompression.

Testicular pain of neuropathic origin may be the result of (Wesselmann et al. 1997):

- Entrapment neuropathies due to:
  - Inguinal hernias – (ilio-inguinal or genito-femoral nerve)
  - Aneurysmal dilatation of the common iliac artery (genito-femoral nerve)
  - Retroperitoneal fibrosis – testicular pain in this situation usually associated with abdominal or low back pain
  - Spinal or sacral pathology – e.g. due to a prolapsed intervertebral disc
- Local nerve damage may follow local surgical procedures, including:
  - Vasectomy
  - Hernia repair
  - Laparoscopic donor nephrectomy – Kim et al. (2003) noted ipsilateral orchalgia occurred in 14 of 145 patients (9.6 %)
- Generalized neuropathic conditions such as diabetes, alcoholic neuropathy or polyarteritis nodosa
- Referred pain – occasionally testicular pain may be referred from the hip or ureter

I.7.5.2.3 Testicular Chronic Pain Syndrome – Pathogenesis

Whilst more acute forms of pain are driven by nociceptive responses to local pathology, once pain has persisted for more than a few months, other factors come into play, such as psychological, emotional or behavioural responses, and this combination of factors may lead to a chronic pain syndrome. In this situation, the pain may no longer be relieved by simple medical or surgical interventions and a more holistic approach is required.

Chronic pain syndromes involving the limbs with somatic and autonomic nerve involvement have been recognized for many years. Alternative names to describe the various manifestations of chronic pain syndromes include causalgia, reflex sympathetic dystrophy, algodystrophy, and chronic neuropathic pain and have often been used interchangeably. The current term "complex regional pain syndrome" has been coined to emphasize the complex interaction of somatic, psychological and behavioural factors and the non-localized distribution of symptoms (Harden et al. 1999). Pain rarely follows a recognized anatomical or neuro-anatomical distribution.

In more recent years, there has been a realization that there are a number of these syndromes involving the internal organs and predominantly the autonomic nerve pathways. Examples include chronic heart pain, loin pain syndromes (Sockeel et al. 2004; Chapuis et al. 2004; Greenwell et al. 2004), chronic pelvic pain (Janicki et al. 2003), including some manifestations of chronic prostatitis. A common feature of all of these syndromes is chronic pain which is disproportionate in intensity, distribution and duration to the underlying pathology (Dunn 2000). The pain syndrome may or may not follow a triggering event such as an episode of very severe pain or an injury, which is often trivial. In addition, there may be manifestations of sympathetic overactivity, such as skin oedema, excess sweating, skin colour and temperature changes, and this has led to the term "sympathetically maintained pain", although the physiological role of the sympathetic nervous system remains unclear.

The pathology of chronic pain syndromes is not fully understood, but it is thought that there is a facilitation of pain nerve pathways at several different levels in the brain (Janig and Baron 2003), spinal cord and peripheral nerves. The process has the unfortunate result that pain signals are felt at thresholds that would not normally reach consciousness. The appreciation of pain is more extreme (hyperalgesia) and even mild stimulation is felt as pain (allodynia). In the case of chronic testicular pain, stimuli that would normally pass unnoticed such as pressure from tight underwear or sitting with legs crossed can cause noticeable discomfort or pain. Any subsequent inflammation or injury, including surgical operations, may have the effect of further facilitating pain nerve pathways and amplifying the pain. Thus any further surgery such as epididymectomy for postvasectomy epididymal pain, or even denervation operations, can make the problem very much worse.

The Relationship Between Acute and Chronic Testicular Pain

The relationship between acute and chronic testicular pain is by no means clear. In some cases, there in an identifiable triggering episode. This may be an episode of very severe pain (e.g. torsion or undertaking a vasectomy without ensuring adequate local anaesthesia) or prolonged pain, for example, from a varicocele. Alternatively there might be ischaemic damage following orchitis or orchiopexy. Not infrequently, there is an amplifying event such as a second operation, for example, epididymectomy undertaken to try to relieve minor chronic epididymal discomfort. In a typical scenario, further surgery is recommended to try to cure the source of pain and with each episode of surgery there may be a period of temporary relief but ultimately the pain recurs and is often worse. To this extent, there is always a risk that surgical procedures may amplify pain and this risk, which is unquantifiable, has to be explained to men when recommending surgical operations to try to cure testicular pain.

There is no test that defines chronic testicular pain and the assessment is based on clinical criteria. In the transition, the pain may become less well localized and there may be paraesthesia. Unlike other neuropathic pain conditions, scrotal skin oedema and skin colour changes are uncommon, probably because the innervation of the testis is entirely separate from the scrotal wall. Autonomic nerves and autonomic pain fibres travel to the testicle in close proximity to the testicular artery, vas deferens and blood vessels in the cord, whereas scrotal skin innervation is from terminal branches of the ilio-inguinal nerve. If scrotal skin oedema and colour changes are part of the clinical picture, then it is more likely that the chronic pain syndrome relates to a problem with the ilio-inguinal nerve than from a trigger in the testis.

Postvasectomy Pain

Postvasectomy pain is typically a localized tenderness or pain or extreme pain on palpation over the epididymis, and except in the most severe cases, this can often be distinguished by careful clinical examination from pain in the testicle. In approximately 25% of cases, no cause for orchalgia can be found. It has been reported to occur in up to one-third of patients, but long-lasting pain sufficient to cause the man to regret vasectomy was reported in 3 men of 172 (1.7%) who responded to the survey (McMahon et al. 1992) and in another survey in 3 out of 188 (1.6%) men who responded 10 years later [3/460 (0.7%) who were sent the questionnaire; Manikandan et al. (2004)]. These two surveys indicate that bothersome scrotal pain is more frequent than the 1 in 1,000 figure that is quoted in the literature; however, in a survey of recent prospective randomized trials of different vasectomy techniques, chronic pain was not identified as a problem (Aradhya et al. 2005), indicating that this complication may be technique-dependent. There is a need for better information about the incidence of postvasectomy bothersome chronic pain and also exploration of ways to prevent it. Some authors have suggested that pain may be prevented by leaving the testicular end of the vas unligated – the so-called open-ended vasectomy (Shapiro and Silber 1979)

I.7.5.3 Clinical Findings: History, Physical Examination, Technical Investigations, Laboratory Findings

The diagnosis of testicular pain is usually made on the basis of careful history and examination, together with basic urological investigation to reveal the causes. A practical guide to assessment is given in Box 1.

Testicular pain may be:

- Unilateral or bilateral
- Intermittent or constant
- Focal or radiating – for example to the groin, abdomen, pelvis, perineum, legs, or back

Usually there is no interference with sexual function, but pain postvasectomy is often more marked after intercourse. Testicular pain associated with infection is usually associated with urinary symptoms such as frequency or urgency or those of sexually transmitted diseases such as urethral discharge.

Assessment should routinely include a careful history, examination and urinalysis. Ultrasound of the testis is essential in acute presentations and usually worthwhile also in the chronic situation. Many men with chronic pain are worried about malignancy and a negative ultrasound scan enables the clinician to give reassurance with authority. The scan may also give diagnostic information such as the presence of a thickened epididymis with a sperm granuloma. Testicular microcalcification is a relatively frequent finding on ultrasound but although there have been some reports of an association with testicular pain (MacKinnon et al. 1990), it is a frequent finding in men who have no pain. More detailed imaging (e.g. MRI) is rarely necessary, but occasionally may serve a therapeutic purpose in providing reassurance to patient and doctor alike.

Box 1: Assessment of the patient with testicular pain – a practical guide

History:

Pain history

- Duration, character, radiation, exacerbating and relieving factors

Associated symptoms

- Lower urinary tract and bowel symptoms
- Sexual history (self assessment questionnaire can be useful and save time) (www.urologyedinburgh.co.uk/sexual_function_questionnaire.htm).

Examination

- Lying and standing examination of the testis
  1. Look for evidence of varicocele and hernia
  2. Size and tenderness of the testicles
  3. Transillumination
- Rectal examination
  1. Note pain or tenderness or any other abnormality (Chap. II.3.1)
- Peripheral nervous system – to exclude evidence of neuropathy
  1. Define any areas of hyperesthesia or any areas of sensory loss[a]
  2. evidence of motor loss or wasting
  3. examination of reflexes
- Vascular system – to exclude arteriopathy or aneurysmal dilatation
  1. Record presence of peripheral pulses and bruits
  2. Note circulatory sufficiency
  3. Bruits
- Examination of the hips, pelvis and spine
  1. Note range of movement, local tenderness in hip, pubic symphysis and sacroiliac joints
  2. Straight leg-raising

Investigations

- Routine urine analysis (sugar, blood, protein), microscopy and culture
- Ultrasound examination
  1. Testis
  2. Transrectal US
- Other procedures may include:
  1. CT or MRI scan
  2. Exclusion of inguinal hernia, injection of contrast into the peritoneal cavity and a herniogram X-ray
  3. Cord block with bupivacaine has been reported as a useful test to help select men suitable for microsurgical cord denervation

[a] Pain distribution and sensory abnormality in chronic pain syndromes typically do not follow defined nerve territories. However, assessment is complicated by the variation in the course and cutaneous innervation territories of the ilio-inguinal and genitofemoral nerves.

I.7.5.4 Differential Diagnosis

I.7.5.4.1 Differential Diagnosis of Acute Testicular Pain

The most important differential diagnosis of sudden onset acute testicular pain is between torsion (see Part I.7.1) and epididymo-orchitis. It is essential to have a high index of suspicion for torsion in the younger man who develops sudden acute testicular pain. If the differential diagnosis between torsion and epididymo-orchitis cannot be resolved with certainty by ultrasound (Dogra and Bhatt 2004), Doppler studies and clinical examination, or if there is likely to be delay in undertaking these investigations, then it is best to undertake an exploratory operation to exclude torsion. Even if an operation for suspected torsion reveals the diagnosis of epididymo-orchitis, there is unlikely to be any long-term harm, whereas failure to undertake exploratory operation and a missed diagnosis of testicular torsion results in the loss of the testicle.

I.7.5.4.2 Differential Diagnosis of Chronic Testicular Pain and Chronic Testicular Pain Syndromes

I.7

This can be very difficult and depends on the andrologist realizing all the possibilities, including causes of neuropathic pain and undertaking investigations as detailed above to exclude any treatable cause.

I.7.5.5 Treatment

I.7.5.5.1 Management of Chronic Testicular Pain (Orchalgia)

Medication for Orchalgia

In general, oral analgesia is not very helpful except in the acute postoperative period after testicular surgery. It is worth noting that there are sex differences in response to analgesics in rodents (Terner et al. 2003; Mitrovic et al. 2003) and in men (Fillingim 2002; Craft 2003), and men respond better to opioid analgesics than women; therefore household analgesics that may have been prescribed for the female partner are not necessarily the best option. For established neuropathic pain, oral medication with amitriptyline (Pilowsky and Barrow 1990; McQuay et al. 1992) and gabapentin (Gustorff et al. 2002) may help. GABA receptors are present in the testis, vas deferens (Geigerseder et al. 2003) as well as the central nervous system (Naumenko et al. 1996), and thus gabapentin may have an effect at several levels. The effect of gabapentin on fertility is not known.

Local Nerve Blockade and Ablation

Local anaesthetic blockade of sympathetic ganglia is widely used in treatment of chronic pain conditions, but generally with mixed results (Chaturvedi and Dash 2001; Hord and Oaklander 2003).

Hamza and Rowlingson (2004) reported a small series in which superior hypogastric plexus block relieved pain in 12 of 14 men with chronic testicular pain, and Yamamoto et al. (1995) reported transrectal blockade of nerves of pelvic plexus to be superior to spermatic cord nerve blockade in a further small cohort.

Pulsed radiofrequency neurotomy has been used in sacroiliac arthropathy (Ahadian 2004) and Cohen and Foster (2003) have published a case report of three men with orchalgia who were pain-free at 6 months, but none of these series provide strong evidence for effectiveness. At best, local nerve blockade may provide a temporary window of relief during which to initiate other treatments. Levine and Matkov (2001) have advocated local anaesthetic block of the spermatic cord and an initial step to identify those likely to gain from microsurgical denervation.

Intrathecal opioids and other medications have been used in other intractable chronic pain states (Kanoff 1994), as have spinal cord stimulation (Grabow et al. 2003; Kemler et al. 2004; Forouzanfar et al. 2004), acupuncture, TENS and other similar techniques. To our knowledge, there are no reported evaluations so far of the application of these techniques for chronic testicular pain.

Surgical Intervention

The place of surgical management in the context of chronic testicular pain remains a matter for debate. Surgical intervention is likely to work best for conditions where there is clear evidence of a surgically remediable cause, such as primary pathology in the testis or scrotum, or clear evidence of actual nerve entrapment, which is likely to be relieved by decompression. Treatments such as epididymectomy to remove a source of pain or denervation procedures have sometimes been advocated, but as the pain nerve pathways become more and more facilitated, ablative procedures become less and less likely to work and more and more likely to amplify the pain. Although some success has been reported following cord denervation operations, these are typically in private practice settings where there may be surgical bias towards surgical solutions. The series are generally small, and with only short-term follow-up. There are no properly controlled randomized clinical trials in the literature for any of the procedures described.

Reports of interventional procedures for testicular pain are listed in Table I.7.7.

Table I.7.7. Results of interventional procedures for chronic testicular pain

Varicocele ligation	
Ribe et al. (2002)	Improvement or resolution of pain in 22/25 men following subinguinal varicocele ligation
Yeniyol (2003)	Pain cured in 72/87
Maghraby (2002)	Pain cured in 49/58 men following laparoscopic varicocele ligation
Peterson et al. (1998)	Pain cured in 30/35 men following surgical ligation
Yaman et al. (2000)	Pain cured in 72/82 men following microsurgical subinguinal varicocele ligation
Reversal of vasectomy for post vasectomy pain	
Myers et al. (1997)	Case series ($n = 32$): reports 75% relief after first reversal procedure plus a further 10% after second procedure
Nangia et al. (2000)	Case series ($n = 13$): 69% pain-free
Microsurgical denervation of the cord	
Levine and Matkov (2001)	Complete pain relief in 25/33 testicles Selected on successful temporary spermatic cord block
Heidenreich (2001); Heidenreich et al. (2002)	Case series ($n = 35$): reports 97% success (median follow-up 31.5 months) Selected on successful temporary spermatic cord block
Devine and Schellhammer (1978)	Case report of two men
Caddedu et al. (1999)	Case series ($n = 9$). Laparoscopic denervation – pain relief in 7/9 (mean follow-up 25 months). Selected on successful temporary spermatic cord block
Choa and Swami (1992)	Case series ($n = 4$). Complete relief from pain immediately after surgery in all four cases (follow-up 2–36 months)
Nerve decompression	
Shafik (2002)	Case series ($n = 4$): Decompression of the pudendal nerve in the pudendal canal relieved pain within 1–3 weeks. Follow-up 9–14 months
Orchiectomy (orchidectomy)	
Yamamoto et al. (1995)	Three out of four men had pain relief after orchiectomy
Negri et al. (2002)	Case report of extraction and preservation of sperm in a man who had an orchiectomy. This is an option that should be considered for younger men

It must be recognized that surgery in the context of orchalgia carries a significant risk that it will make matters worse rather than better. This should be fully discussed with the patient and documented as part of the informed consent procedure. It is also important to remember that patients with chronic pain are shown to make poor decisions about risk (Apkarian et al. 2004) and this will be particularly relevant when considering the risks and benefits of further surgery.
Operations that can be considered include:

- Epididymectomy in cases of postvasectomy chronic pain, and when on clinical examination there is localized severe tenderness in the epididymis
- Varicocele ligation when there is left-sided orchalgia
- Microsurgical division of nerves in the cord to the testicle when the pain seems to be confined to the testicle

Orchiectomy is not uncommonly used when all else fails, but there are very few reported case series in the literature to define its usefulness.

Surgical denervation should probably be considered only in cases where local anaesthetic blockade of the spermatic cord has provided short-term relief (Levine and Matkov 2001). The operation of cord denervation is not standardized; some surgeons divide all structures except the testicular artery and main veins but including the vas deferens, whereas other surgeons may preserve the vas deferens and lymphatics. The procedure is best undertaken using an operating microscope, especially if lymphatics are to be preserved. It is wise to use a local anaesthetic field block with an anaesthetic such as levobupivacaine in addition to general anaesthesia, so that when the man regains consciousness immediately following his operation he feels no pain. In addition, it may be worth considering 6 weeks adjuvant postoperative gabapentin or amitriptyline; however, this is anecdotal practice and needs confirmation by clinical trial. At the 6-week postoperative review, the gabapentin can be stopped if the man has been pain-free for at least 2 weeks; otherwise it should be continued.

Interdisciplinary Pain Management for Chronic Testicular Pain Syndromes

Costabile (1991) reviewed records of 48 patients with chronic testicular pain. Between them, they had had 221 diagnostic procedures and 74 surgical procedures, in 80% of which only normal tissue was found. After 8 years, 31 were available for interview, of which 29 (93%) had pain unchanged. Schover (1990) assessed 48 men with genital pain and found that 56% met criteria for somatization, 27% met criteria for major depression, and 27% were chemically dependent. It is clear from this background that surgery is more often than not a poor treatment choice.

Once the diagnosis of a chronic testicular pain seems probable and when there is no clearly defined pathology, management changes from trying to cure the problem to helping the man come to terms with the disability and to cope with it as best he can. In the context, management is best undertaken in a multidisciplinary fashion by the urologist and the pain management team (Harden and Cole 1998). The components of an interdisciplinary approach to management are summarized in Table I.7.8.

In the presence of unremitting pain, it is common for individuals to become physically inactive. Secondary deconditioning may lead to reduced endorphin levels and heighten the experience of pain. Well-meaning family members may sometimes be oversolicitous in their care and attention, and this can result in abnormal illness behaviour, with the individual adopting an unnecessarily passive role. Sexual difficulties may place strain on partner relationships and in severe cases, excessive time off work may lead to job loss and all its accompanying disadvantages. Multiple hospital stays or surgical procedures may alert the clinician to failure of previous well-intentioned medical interventions, and any history of litigation should be noted.

Table I.7.8. Components of an interdisciplinary approach

Medical management
Reassurance that there is no life-threatening underlying cause and that increased physical activity will not be harmful
Provide continued follow-up to prevent cure seeking elsewhere and iatrogenic damage
Support any litigation/compensation claim to its resolution and conclusion
Education
Explain how emotional stress and deconditioning can increase symptom experience
Provide insight into how their own behaviours may serve to exacerbate their symptoms
Help patient to understand and accept a self-management approach
Teach relaxation techniques, breathing exercises, etc. to reverse sympathetic arousal
Psychiatry and psychology
Identify any psychological factors contributing to excessive symptoms and illness behaviours
Monitor mental state and undertake risk assessment for self-harm
Treat anxiety and depression (consider psychotropic drug management if necessary)
Teaching coping strategies, positive thought patterns to help them regain control and inhibit negative thoughts, catastrophizing, etc.
Identify and challenge secondary gain resulting in excessive illness behaviour
Identify maladaptive family behaviours and support family in encouraging individual to relinquish their sick role and do more for themselves
Physical and occupational therapy
Progressive increase in physical activity and reconditioning to build up cardiovascular fitness
Encourage recreational physical exercise and functional goals
Supported return to social, recreational and vocational activities as appropriate

Unremitting pain can be a distressing experience (Hendler 1984), which affects not only the patient (Kemler and de Vet 2000), but all others in the household (Kemler and Furnee 2002). It is important therefore to recognize and address all the emotional and psychosocial factors that contribute in each case (Stanton-Hicks 1998; Harden and Cole 1998). These may include:

- Depression, anxiety and other mood disturbance
- Anger or bitterness relating to the cause of the problem
- Fear about the underlying condition or about the future
- Sexual and relationship difficulties
- Social consequences of the problem such as inability to work and financial problems
- Litigation or other legal proceedings

The man should be encouraged to lead as normal a life as possible irrespective of his pain, and analgesics should be given in the context of encouraging the man to go out and about and work normally. The rationale is to try to distract the focus of attention from the pain.

Litigation procedures may be drawn out over a long period and may delay resolution of the pain because the man's attention is focused on the problem and its perceived cause. In some cases, it may be appropriate to work proactively with the individual and his legal advisors to bring litigation to an early conclusion and allow him to move on.

I.7.5.6 Results of Treatment

In general, if the diagnosis is chronic testicular pain, then the results of interventional treatments are reasonable, but if the diagnosis is a chronic testicular pain syndrome, then interventional treatments may make the problem worse. Unfortunately, there is no sure way other than clinical acumen to differentiate the conditions, and because of this difficulty most treatment series report failure rates of between 20% and 50% (Gray et al. 2001) (Table I.7.7). Higher success rates have been reported after microsurgical denervation procedures provided that cases are selected on the basis of a good response to a local anaesthetic nerve block.

I.7.5.7 Prognosis

I.7.5.7.1 Prevention

Prevention of Chronic Testicular Pain

Prevention of chronic pain syndromes is an important aspect of all scrotal surgery. There is some evidence that chronic pain is more likely to be triggered if there is pain in the immediate postoperative period. Therefore, it is probably good practice to use local anaesthetic field blocks in addition to general anaesthesia for all scrotal surgery. It is usually a simple extra procedure to inject 2–3 ml of 0.5% levobupivacaine into the cord at the scrotal neck during routine procedures such as hydrocele repair, epididymal cyst removal, microsurgical vasectomy reversal, etc. As is normal with administration of all local anaesthetics, care should be taken not to inject directly into a blood vessel.

I.7.5.8 Conclusion

Testicular pain shows spectrum from that caused by localized conditions that can be treated by appropriate surgery to diffuse neuropathic pain that is amplified by any surgical intervention. It is often very difficult to decide on the best management but the urologist should be aware of the possibility of making matters worse in their attempts to help men with testicular pain.

References

Ahadian FM (2004) Pulsed radiofrequency neurotomy: advances in pain medicine Curr Pain Headache Rep 8:34–40

Apkarian AV, Sosa Y, Krauss BR, Thomas PS, Fredrickson BE, Levy RE, Harden RN, Chialvo DR (2004) Chronic pain patients are impaired on an emotional decision-making task. Pain 108:129–136

Aradhya KW, Best K, Sokal DC (2005) Recent developments in vasectomy BMJ 330:296–299

Cadeddu JA, Bishoff JT, Chan DY, Moore RG, Kavoussi LR, Jarrett TW (1999) Laparoscopic testicular denervation for chronic orchalgia.[erratum appears in J Urol 1999 162:1708]. J Urol 162:733–735; discussion 735–756

Chapuis O, Sockeel P, Pallas G, Pons F, Jancovici R (2004) Thoracoscopic renal denervation for intractable autosomal dominant polycystic kidney disease-related pain. Am J Kidney Dis 43:161–163

Chaturvedi A, Dash HH (2001) Sympathetic blockade for the relief of chronic pain. J Indian Med Assoc 99:698–703

Choa RG, Swami KS (1992) Testicular denervation: a new surgical procedure for intractable testicular pain. Br J Urol 70: 417–419

Cohen SP, Foster A (2003) Pulsed radiofrequency as a treatment for groin pain and orchialgia. Urology 61:645

Costabile RA, Hahn M, McLeod DG (1991) Chronic orchialgia in the pain prone patient: the clinical perspective. J Urol 146:1571–1574

Craft RM (2003) Sex differences in drug- and non-drug-induced analgesia. Life Sci 72:2675–2688

Devine CJ, Schellhammer PF (1978) The use of microsurgical denervation of the spermatic cord for orchialgia. Trans Am Assoc Genitourin Surg 70:149–151

Dogra V, Bhatt S (2004) Acute painful scrotum. Radiol Clin North Am 42:349–363

Dunn D (2000) Chronic regional pain syndrome, type 1: Part I. AORN J 72:422–32, 435–449; quiz 452–458

Fillingim RB (2002) Sex differences in analgesic responses: evidence from experimental pain models. Eur J Anaesthesiol Suppl 26:16–24

Forouzanfar T, Kemler MA, Weber WE, Kessels AG, van Kleef M (2004) Spinal cord stimulation in complex regional pain syndrome: cervical and lumbar devices are comparably effective. Br J Anaesth 92:348–353

Geigerseder C, Doepner R, Thalhammer A, Frungieri MB, Gamel-Didelon K, Calandra RS, Kohn FM, Mayerhofer A (2003) Evidence for a GABAergic system in rodent and human testis: local GABA production and GABA receptors. Neuroendocrinology 77:314–323

Grabow TS, Tella PK, Raja SN (2003) Spinal cord stimulation for complex regional pain syndrome: an evidence-based medicine review of the literature. Clin J Pain 19:371–383

Gray CL, Powell CR Amling CL (2001) Outcomes for surgical management of orchalgia in patients with identifiable intrascrotal lesions. Eur Urol 39:455–459

Greenwell TJ, Peters JL, Neild GH, Shah PJ (2004) The outcome of renal denervation for managing loin pain haematuria syndrome. BJU Int 93:818–821

Gustorff B, Nahlik G, Spacek A, Kress HG (2002) [Gabapentin in the treatment of chronic intractable pain] Gabapentin in der Therapie chronischer therapieresistenter Schmerzen. Erste Erfahrungen bei 99 Patienten. Schmerz 16:9–14

Hamza M, Rowlingson J (2004) Management of chronic testicular pain with superior hypogastric plexus block University of Virginia, Charlottesville, VA, USA, Poster number 881, American Pain Society 2004

Harden RN, Cole PA (1998) New developments in rehabilitation of neuropathic pain syndromes. Neurol Clin 16:937–950

Heidenreich A (2001) Re: Microsurgical testicular denervation of the spermatic cord as primary surgical treatment of chronic orchialgia. J Urol 166:2322–2323

Heidenreich A, Olbert P, Engelmann UH (2002) Management of chronic testalgia by microsurgical testicular denervation. Eur Urol 41:392–397

Hendler N (1984) Depression caused by chronic pain. J Clin Psychiatry 45:30–38

Hord ED, Oaklander AL (2003) Complex regional pain syndrome: a review of evidence-supported treatment options. Curr Pain Headache Rep 7:188–196

Janicki TI (2003) Chronic pelvic pain as a form of complex regional pain syndrome. Clin Obstet Gynecol 46:797–803

Janig W Baron R (2003) Complex regional pain syndrome: mystery explained? Lancet Neurol 2:687–697

Kanoff RB (1994) Intraspinal delivery of opiates by an implantable, programmable pump in patients with chronic, intractable pain of nonmalignant origin. J Am Osteopath Assoc 94:487–493

Kemler MA, de Vet HC (2000) Health-related quality of life in chronic refractory reflex sympathetic dystrophy (complex regional pain syndrome type I). J Pain Symptom Manage 20:68–76

Kemler MA, Furnee CA (2002) The impact of chronic pain on life in the household. J Pain Symptom Manage 23:433–441

Kemler MA, De Vet HC, Barendse GA, Van Den Wildenberg FA, Van Kleef M (2004) The effect of spinal cord stimulation in patients with chronic reflex sympathetic dystrophy: two years' follow-up of the randomized controlled trial. Ann Neurol 55:13–18

Kim F, Pinto P, Su LM, Jarrett TW, Rattner LE, Montgomery R Kavoussi LR (2003) Ipsilateral orchialgia after laparoscopic donor nephrectomy. J Endourol 17:405–409

Levine LA, Matkov TG (2001) Microsurgical denervation of the spermatic cord as primary surgical treatment of chronic orchialgia. J Urol 165:1927–1929

MacKinnon J, Coz F, Diaz L (1990) [Testicular microlithiasis: echographic diagnosis of a new cause of orchialgia and infertility] Microlitiasis testicular: diagnostico ecografico de una nueva causa de orquialgia e infertilidad. Rev Chil Obstet Ginecol 55:6–9

Maghraby HA (2002) Laparoscopic varicocelectomy for painful varicoceles: merits and outcomes. J Endourol 16:107–110

Manikandan R, Srirangam SJ, Pearson E, Collins GN (2004) Early and late morbidity after vasectomy: a comparison of chronic scrotal pain at 1 and 10 years. BJU Int 93:571–574

McMahon AJ, Buckley J, Taylor A, Lloyd SN, Deane RF, Kirk D (1992) Chronic testicular pain following vasectomy. Br J Urol 70:338–339

McQuay HJ, Carroll D, Glynn CJ (1992) Low dose amitriptyline in the treatment of chronic pain. Anaesthesia 47:646–652

Mitrovic I, Margeta-Mitrovic M, Bader S Stoffel M, Jan LY, Basbaum AI (2003) Contribution of GIRK2-mediated postsynaptic signaling to opiate and alpha 2-adrenergic analgesia and analgesic sex differences. Proc Natl Acad Sci USA 100: 271–276

Myers SA, Mershon CE, Fuchs EF (1997) Vasectomy reversal for treatment of the post-vasectomy pain syndrome. J Urol 157:518–520

Nangia AK, Myles JL, Thomas AJ (2000) Vasectomy reversal for the post-vasectomy pain syndrome: a clinical and histological evaluation. J Urol 164:1939–1942

Naumenko EV, Amikishieva AV, Serova LI (1996) Role of GABAA and GABAB receptors of the brain in the negative feedback mechanism of the hypothalamohypophyseotesticular complex. Neurosci Behav Physiol 26:277–280

Negri L, Albani E, Di Rocco M, Levi-Setti PE (2002) Aspermia and chronic testicular pain after imperforate anus correction. Cryopreservation of sperm cells extracted from whole orchiectomized testis: case report. Hum Reprod 17:2935–2937

Peterson AC, Lance RS, Ruiz HE (1998) Outcomes of varicocele ligation done for pain. J Urol 159:1565–1567

Pilowsky I, Barrow CG (1990) A controlled study of psychotherapy and amitriptyline used individually and in combination in the treatment of chronic intractable, 'psychogenic' pain. Pain 40:3–19

Ribe N, Manasia P, Sarquella J, Grimaldi S, Pomerol JM (2002) Clinical follow-up after subinguinal varicocele ligation to treat pain. Arch Ital Urol Androl 74:51–53

Schover LR (1990) Psychological factores in men with genital pain. Clevel Clin J Med 57:697–670

Shafik A (2002) Re: Microsurgical denervation of the spermatic cord as primary surgical treatment of chronic orchialgia. J Urol 167:1408

Shapiro EI, Silber SJ (1979) Open-ended vasectomy, sperm granuloma, and postvasectomy orchialgia. Fertil Steril 32: 546–550

Sockeel P, Pallas P, Pons F, Jancovici R (2004) Thoracoscopic renal denervation for intractable autosomal dominant polycystic disease-related pain. Am J Kidney Dis 43:161–163

Stanton-Hicks M, Baron R, Boas R, Gordh T, Harden N, Hendler N et al (1998) Complex regional pain syndromes: guidelines for therapy. Clin J Pain 14:155–166

Terner JM, Lomas LM, Smith ES, Barrett AC, Picker MJ (2003) Pharmacogenetic analysis of sex differences in opioid antinociception in rats. Pain 106:381–391

Yamamoto M, Hibi H, Katsuno S, Miyake K (1995) Management of chronic orchialgia of unknown etiology. Int J Urol 2:47–49

Yaman O, Ozdiler E, Anafarta K, Gogus O (2000) Effect of microsurgical subinguinal varicocele ligation to treat pain. Urology 55:107–108

Yeniyol CO, Tuna A, Yener H, Zeyrek N, Tilki A (2003) High ligation to treat pain in varicocele. Int Urol Nephrol 35:65–68

Benign Lesions and Malignant Tumours of the Male Genital Tract

I.8

I.8.1 Scrotal Benign Lesions, Epididymal Cysts, Epididymal Tumours

K. Turner

Key Messages

- Most scrotal lesions can be diagnosed with a combination of clinical examination and ultrasound.
- Damage to the vas or testicular vessels is a potential hazard in all surgery on the scrotal contents. This could affect fertility and patients should be warned about it.
- Paediatric and adult hydroceles differ in aetiology.
- Excision of epididymal cysts may not resolve discomfort attributed to that cyst.

Most scrotal pathology can be diagnosed using a combination of clinical examination and ultrasound. See Fig. I.8.1.

I.8.1.1 Hydrocele

I.8.1.1.1 Definition

As the testicle descends into the scrotum during development, it takes with it a peritoneal protrusion (the processus vaginalis). The neck of the processus is usually obliterated between the deep inguinal ring and the proximal scrotum, resulting in an isolated sac of peritoneum (the tunica vaginalis) surrounding the testis. A hydrocele is an abnormal accumulation of fluid within this sac.

I.8.1.1.2 Aetiology and Pathogenesis

The causes and management of hydroceles in children differ from those in adults. Paediatric hydroceles are caused by incomplete obliteration of the processus vaginalis (see below). Adult hydroceles are generally idiopathic. However, since hydroceles can accompany testicular neoplasms, ultrasound of the scrotum should be used to confirm that the testis is normal.

I.8.1.1.3 Clinical Findings and Investigations

Adult hydroceles are fluctuant transilluminable sacs. They are confined to the scrotum and surround the testis. If the hydrocele is lax, it may be possible to palpate the testis (generally behind the hydrocele sac), but in tense hydroceles, it may not be possible to palpate the testis separately. Ultrasound is usually diagnostic.

I.8.1.1.4 Treatment

Adult hydroceles, if symptomatic, are best corrected surgically via a scrotal approach. Intrascrotal anatomy may be distorted by a hydrocele. Patients should be warned about the risk of damage to the vas or testicular vessels during hydrocele repair with consequent impairment of semen quality or fertility. There are a variety of surgical techniques, including excision of the sac, excision and reflection of the sac behind the testis and epididymis (Jaboulay's operation), and plication of the sac (Lord's procedure; Lord 1964). Whatever the technique, the patient should be warned about residual bulk on the operated side in comparison to the contralateral scrotum. There is a risk of recurrence with all approaches.

Sclerotherapy (with inflammatory agents such as phenol or tetracycline) is an alternative treatment for hydroceles (and epididymal cysts). Some surgeons have found that sclerotherapy is as efficacious as surgery, with a lower morbidity and equivalent impact on

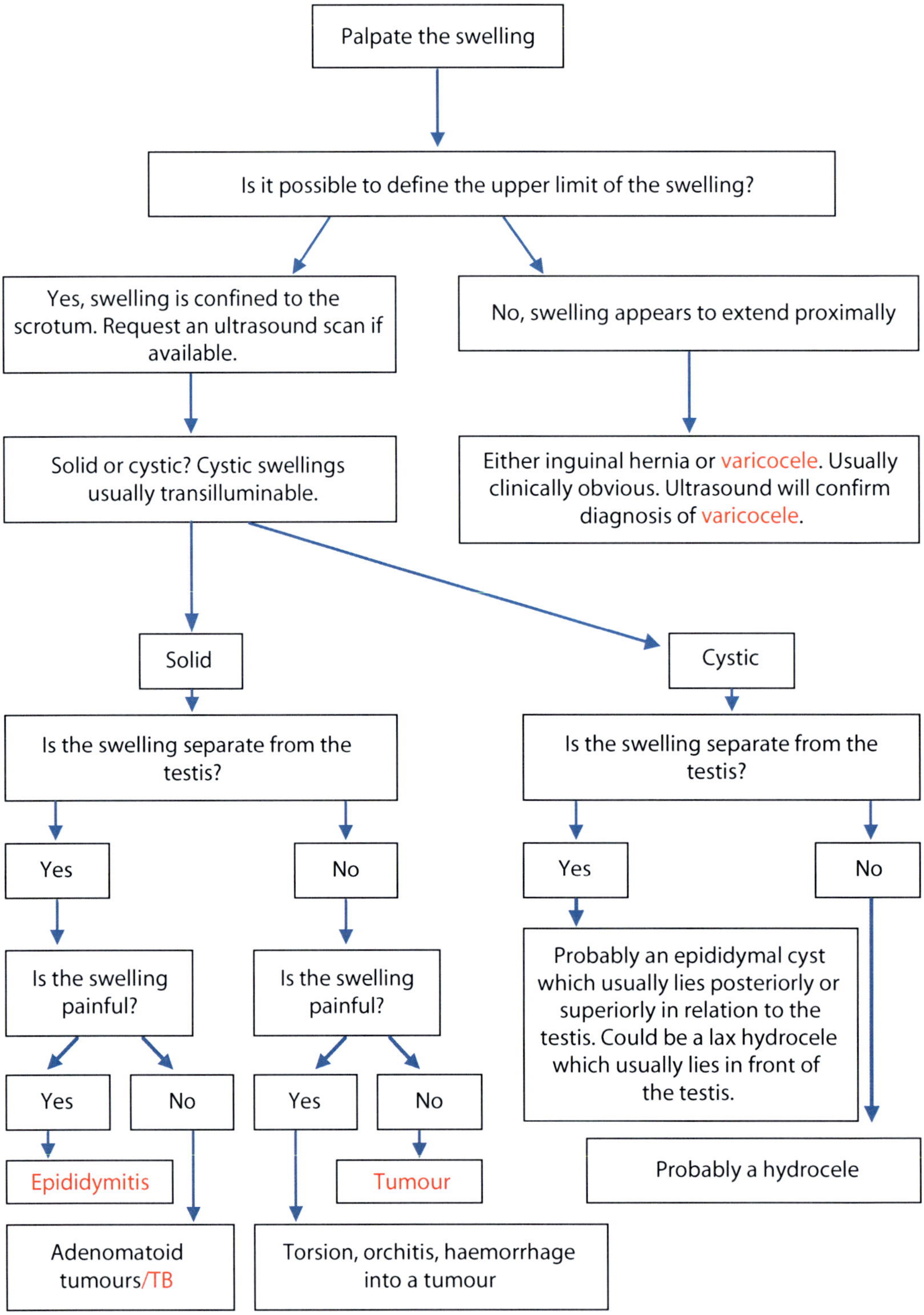

Fig. I.8.1. Flow chart for the assessment of scrotal swellings in adults. Scrotal ultrasound is almost universally available and in many centres will have been performed before the patient is assessed in secondary care. It has not replaced a careful clinical examination and the experienced clinician can often recommend management without recourse to ultrasound. Adapted with permission from Mostofi and Sesterhenn (1998)

spermatogenesis (Shan et al. 2003). Multiple injections of sclerosant may be required. Others report high recurrence rates and morbidity with sclerotherapy and advocate that it should be reserved for men where surgery carries an unacceptably high risk (Thomson and Odell 1979; Sigurdsson et al. 1994).

I.8.1.1.5 Communicating Hydrocele and Hydrocele of the Cord

Failure of the processus vaginalis to close allows intraperitoneal fluid to accumulate around the testis, resulting in a communicating hydrocele. (If the aperture of the processus is large, then an inguinal hernia may result.) Ninety per cent of communicating hydroceles resolve before a child is 1 year old and they are very rare after the age of 5 years. They usually present as painless transilluminable scrotal swellings that fluctuate in size during the day and with activity. Surgery is rarely indicated but if required then the processus is approached through a groin crease incision and is divided. The hydrocele can then be aspirated to dryness.

If a segment of the processus remains patent, then a hydrocele of the cord may result. The presenting feature is usually a mobile, painless, transilluminable mass in the line of the spermatic cord. Cord hydroceles may communicate with the peritoneal cavity (communicating hydrocele of the cord). Excision of the mass via an inguinal approach (and closure of the patent processus if the hydrocele of the cord is communicating) is usually curative.

I.8.1.2 Epididymal Cysts

I.8.1.2.1 Definition

A sperm containing cyst of the epididymis. Synonymous with spermatocele.

I.8.1.2.3 Aetiology and Pathogenesis

Epididymal cysts are very common and their incidence increases with age. In most cases, there is no obvious cause. They are more common in the progeny of women treated with diethylstilboestrol (Vohra and Morgentaler 1997). Epididymal cyst-adenomas are a feature of von Hippel-Lindau disease (Gruber et al. 1980).

I.8.1.2.4 Clinical Findings and Investigations

These cysts are usually spherical, transilluminable and distinct from the testis. They can occur anywhere in the epididymis but are most commonly located toward the head.

I.8.1.2.5 Treatment

Most are asymptomatic and once reassured most patients decline surgical intervention. Scrotal exploration and excision of the cyst may be indicated if a cyst is particularly large or if it is perceived to be the source of scrotal discomfort. Occasionally pressure on the cyst replicates a patient's pain. In all cases, patients should be warned that excision of an apparently painful cyst may not be associated with resolution of symptoms and that epididymal cysts can recur. Damage sustained by epididymal tubules during excision of an epididymal cyst may predispose to sperm granuloma formation, which itself may cause chronic discomfort. The risk of damage to the vas and testicular vessels and the possibility of consequent reduction in sperm quality and fertility should also be explained. Sclerotherapy is an alternative treatment for epididymal cysts (see above).

I.8.1.3 Epididymal Tumours

I.8.1.3.1 Clinical Features

Masses within the epididymis that do not transilluminate or are solid on ultrasound are likely to be epididymal neoplasms. They are usually painless.

I.8

I.8.1.3.2 Aetiology and Pathogenesis

Epididymal tumours are nearly always benign adenomas (adenomatoid tumours of the epididymis) (Folpe and Weiss 2000). Malignant primary epididymal neoplasms are very rare. They include leiomyosarcomas, rhabdomyosarcomas, and lymphomas (Kizer et al. 2001; Novella et al. 2001; Varzaneh et al. 2002; Maniyur et al. 2003). Metastases to the epididymis have also been described (Ozdal et al. 2002; Gaskin and Shah 2003).

I.8.1.3.3 Treatment

Surgery for solid epididymal masses should be via an inguinal approach with control of the cord before delivery of the testis. Biopsy and analysis of a frozen section may be used to differentiate benign from malignant epididymal tumours intraoperatively. The former can be excised with preservation of the testis, whilst the latter should be managed by orchiectomy (Goldstein and Waterhouse 1983).

I.8.1.4 Other Benign Epididymal Lesions: Sperm Granuloma

I.8.1.4.1 Definition

Sperm granulomas are caused by the inflammatory reaction that occurs as a consequence of sperm leakage from the urogenital tract. They consist of sperm and macrophages within epithelialized channels.

I.8.1.4.2 Aetiology and Pathogenesis

Any procedure or injury that breaches the urogenital tract and allows leakage of sperm can cause a sperm granuloma to form. The most common cause is vasectomy. The incidence after vasectomy is hard to quantify but microscopic sperm granulomas are detectable at the vasectomy site in 10 – 30 % of men who undergo vasectomy reversal.

I.8.1.4.3 Clinical Features

In most men, these granulomas are small and asymptomatic, though they can be as large as 1 – 2 cm in diameter and tender to palpation. They are probably more frequent after vasectomy performed by vasal occlusion (by suture or clip) than after vasectomy by intraluminal cautery. In men with chronic postvasectomy orchalgia, pressure on a palpable granuloma may mimic the patient's discomfort.

I.8.1.4.4 Treatment

Excision of the granuloma followed by intraluminal cautery or vasovasostomy is usually curative (Silber 1977; Schmidt 1979; Belker et al. 1992).

I.8.1.5 Other Benign Epididymal Lesions: Tuberculosis of the Epididymis

I.8.1.5.1 Aetiology and Pathogenesis

Tuberculosis of the epididymis is usually a consequence of haematogenous spread of *Mycobacterium tuberculosis*. The epididymis may be particularly vulnerable because of its rich blood supply. It may occur in association with renal TB, although frequently a renal focus can be hard to demonstrate. Involvement of the testis is rare.

I.8.1.5.2 Clinical Features

Presentation is usually with epididymal swelling (which may or may not be painful) in a man with a previous history of TB. The diagnosis is usually made by isolation of *M. tuberculosis* from the urine or semen. Where urine cultures are sterile, the bacterium may be isolated from an epididymectomy specimen from an epididymal sinus.

I.8.1.5.3 Treatment

Treatment is with antituberculous chemotherapy.

References

Belker AM, Thomas A Jr et al. (1992) Results of 1,469 microsurgical vasectomy reversals by the Vasovasostomy Study Group. J Urol Nurs 11:93 – 111

Folpe AL, Weiss SW (2000) Paratesticular soft tissue neoplasms. Semin Diagn Pathol 17:307 – 318

Gaskin DA, Shah D (2003) Bilateral epididymal metastases from primary adenocarcinoma of the prostate. West Indian Med J 52:253 – 254

Goldstein M, Waterhouse K (1983) When to use the Chevassu maneuver during exploration of intrascrotal masses. J Urol 130:1199 – 1200

Gruber MB, Healey GB et al (1980) Papillary cystadenoma of epididymis: component of von Hippel-Lindau syndrome. Urology 16:305 – 306

Kizer WS, Dykes TE et al (2001). Paratesticular spindle cell rhabdomyosarcoma in an adult. J Urol 166: 606 – 607

Lord PH (1964) A bloodless operation for the radical cure of idiopathic hydrocele. Br J Surg 51:914 – 916

Maniyur R, Anant K et al (2003). Posttransplant epididymal lymphoma: an aggressive variant. Transplantation 75:246 – 247

Novella G, Porcaro AB et al (2001) Primary lymphoma of the epididymis: case report and review of the literature. Urol Int 67:97 – 99

Ozdal OL, Yakupoglu YK et al (2002). Epididymal metastasis from gastric signet ring cell adenocarcinoma. Can J Urol 9:1498 – 1499

Schmidt SS (1979) Spermatic granuloma: an often painful lesion. Fertil Steril 31:178 – 181

Shan CJ, Lucon AM et al (2003) Comparative study of sclerotherapy with phenol and surgical treatment for hydrocele. J Urol 169:1056 – 1059

Sigurdsson T, Johansson JE et al (1994) Polidocanol sclerotherapy for hydroceles and epididymal cysts. J Urol 151:898 – 901

Silber SJ (1977) Sperm granuloma and reversibility of vasectomy. Lancet 2:588 – 589

Thomson H, Odell M (1979) Sclerosant treatment for hydroceles and epididymal cysts. BMJ 2:704 – 705

Varzaneh FE, Verghese M et al (2002) Paratesticular leiomyosarcoma in an elderly man. Urology 60:1112

Vohra S, Morgentaler A (1997) Congenital anomalies of the vas deferens, epididymis, and seminal vesicles. Urology 49: 313 – 321

I.8.2 Testicular Cancer, CIS, Microcalcifications, TNM Classification

O. Ståhl, J. Eberhard, A. Giwercman

Key Messages

- Testicular germ cell cancer (GCC) is the most common malignancy among young men. It should be suspected in each case of testicular pain and tumour.
- GCC can be prevented by screening for carcinoma-in-situ testis (CIS).
- Such screening should be considered for selected groups of patients, including those with a history of cryptorchidism, poor sperm counts or those with a unilateral GCC.
- With modern therapy, approximately 95 % of GCC patients can be cured. The question of long-term toxicity and quality of life plays, therefore, a prominent role.
- GCC per se and its treatment can have negative effects on the fertility potential of the patient. Cryopreservation of semen should be offered prior to therapy, preferably already before orchiectomy.
- GCC and its treatment may also have negative effects on Leydig cell function. GCC patients should be offered andrological counselling, both regarding their fertility and need of androgen replacement therapy.

I.8.2.1 Testicular Cancer

I.8.2.1.1 Definition of the Disease

More than 90 % of all testicular cancers in adults are of a germ cell origin – testicular germ cell cancer (TGCC) (Richie 1997). Other testicular neoplasms, such as carcinoid, lymphoma, spermatocytic seminomas, mesothelioma and Leydig- and Sertoli-cell tumours are rare and will not be discussed.

Histologically, TGCC is divided into two major subgroups, seminomas and nonseminomas, each comprising approximately 50 %. There are different classification systems: the WHO classification of germ cell tumours of the testis (Table I.8.1) (Mostofi and Sesterhenn 1998) is recommended by the European Germ Cell Cancer Consensus Group (EGCCCG) (Schmoll et al. 2004). The peak incidence of nonseminomas is in the late 20s and they are most often mixed tumours histologically. Seminomas typically present in the mid 30s. Ten per cent of GCCs are primarily located extragonadally, most commonly in the retroperitoneum or rarely primarily in the mediastinum. Cytogenetically, TGCCs are most often hyperdiploid, isochromosome 12p or other aberrations of chromosome 12 being virtually always present (Chaganti et al. 1993).

Table I.8.1. WHO classification of germ cell tumours of the testis (Mostofi and Sesterhenn 1998)

Tumours of one histological type
Seminoma
Spermatocytic seminoma
Embryonal carcinoma
Polyembryoma
Teratoma
Mature
Immature
With malignant transformation
Yolk sac tumour (endodermal sinus tumour)
Choriocarcinoma
Tumours of more than one histological type
Embryonal carcinoma with teratoma (teratocarcinoma)
Choriocarcinoma and other types
Other combinations

I.8.2.1.2 Epidemiology

TGCC is the most common malignancy among young men, but represents only 1–2 % of all malignant diseases among males. The incidence is increasing globally, with a 100 % rise every 20 years (Schmoll et al. 2004) and with a great geographical variation. The highest incidences are in Western and Northern Europe, with a peak incidence of 15/100,000 in Denmark (Richiardi et al. 2004), compared to less than 1/100,000 in African-Americans, and an even lower incidence in the Far East.

I.8.2.1.3 Aetiology and Pathogenesis

An increasing amount of evidence indicates that TGCC develops from carcinoma-in-situ (CIS) germ cells arising in early foetal life (for details see "Carcinoma-in-Situ of the Testis" below).

I.8.2.1.4 Symptoms and Clinical Findings

GCC should be suspected in men complaining of a scrotal mass or swelling, or diffuse testicular pain mimicking epididymitis or testicular torsion. Sometimes GCC is accompanied by hydrocele. Physical examination usually discloses a testicular tumour. Usually, an enlargement of testis size and tenderness is palpated; however, in some cases a small tumour can be palpated in a normal size or even atrophic gonad.

The primary site of lymph node metastases is ipsilateral retroperitoneal lymph nodes (unless the patient has undergone any surgical procedure in the inguinal region altering the lymphatic drainage of the testes). The first sign of disseminated disease is often lower back pain, caused by retroperitoneal lymph node masses. Haematological dissemination occurs primarily to the lungs, and rarely to other sites, such as liver, brain and skeleton.

I.8.2.1.5 Clinical Investigation

When a testicular tumour is suspected, an ultrasound of the testes has to be performed, separating extratesticular from intratesticular masses, of which the vast majority are malignant. If a tumour is found, a transinguinal exploration of the testis should be performed, and if a malignant tumour cannot be ruled out an orchiectomy should follow. Blood samples for measurement of serum markers, alpha fetoprotein (AFP), human chorionic gonadotrophin (βhCG) and, if available, also placenta-like alkaline phosphatase (PLAP) are obtained preoperatively. A biopsy from the contralateral testicle to exclude CIS (see "Carcinoma-in-Situ of the Testis" below) is recommended at some centres.

I.8

After the diagnosis of GCC, staging investigations, including a CT scan of the thorax, the abdomen and pelvis, follow. If the tumour markers are increased preoperatively, repetitive measurements during follow-up are used to monitor the presence of metastases. In seminomas serum levels of βhCG and PLAP are elevated in 15–20% and 50–60%, respectively. In nonseminomas βhCG and/or AFP is elevated in 60–70% of cases. Prolonged elevation of AFP and βhCG after the removal of the testicular tumour indicates disseminated disease. LDH (lactate dehydrogenase) is elevated in 70–80% in patients with disseminated GCC and might add prognostic information, especially if AFP and βhCG are normal (Table I.8.2). Due to cross-reactivity in smokers, the specificity of PLAP analysis is low, but can be used in nonsmokers with advanced seminoma.

Table I.8.2. Clinical use of tumour markers alpha-fetoprotein (*AFP*) and β human chorionic gonadotrophin (β*hCG*)

To reclassify histological seminomas to nonseminomas, AFP is elevated in nonseminomas exclusively
To detect metastasized disease
As a prognostic tool in advanced disease
To evaluate the clinical effect of therapy
For early detection of relapse
AFP can be falsely positive in case of liver disease, and rarely habitual
βhCG can be falsely positive in patients who have hypogonadism or who use marijuana

I.8.2.1.6 Staging System

There are several staging systems; the EGCCCG recommends the use of the TNM classification of the International Union Against Cancer (UICC) (2002) (Table I.8.3), with, in case of disseminated disease, a risk grouping according to the prognostic factor-based classification of the International Germ Cell Cancer Collaborative Group (IGCCG) (1997). The Royal Marsden Hospital staging system (RMH) is also widely used (Horwich 1995), and was the system most used prior to the introduction of the prognostic factor-based classification of IGCCG.

Table I.8.3. TNM classification according to UICC (Union Internationale Contre le Cancer) (2002). (*CIS* Carcinoma-in-situ)

Primary tumour (T)	
The extent of primary tumour is usually classified after radical orchiectomy, and for this reason a pathological stage is assigned	
pTX	Primary tumour cannot be assessed
pT0	No evidence of primary tumour (e.g. histologic scar in testis)
pTis	Intratubular germ cell neoplasia (CIS)
pT1	Tumour limited to the testis and epididymis without vascular/lymphatic invasion; tumour may invade into the tunica albuginea but not to the tunica vaginalis
pT2	Tumour limited to the testis and epididymis with vascular/lymphatic invasion, or tumour extending through the tunica albuginea with involvement of the tunica vaginalis
pT3	Tumour invades the spermatic cord with or without vascular/lymphatic invasion
pT4	Tumour invades the scrotum with or without vascular/lymphatic invasion
Regional lymph nodes (N)	
Clinical	
NX	Regional lymph nodes cannot be assessed
N0	No regional lymph node metastasis
N1	Metastasis with a lymph node mass 2 cm or less in greatest dimension; or multiple lymph nodes none more than 2 cm in greatest dimension
N2	Metastasis with a lymph node mass more than 2 cm but not more than 5 cm in greatest dimension; or multiple lymph nodes, any one mass greater than 2 cm but not more than 5 cm in greatest dimension
N3	Metastasis with a lymph node mass more than 5 cm in greatest dimension
Pathologic (pN)	
pNX	Regional lymph nodes cannot be assessed
pN0	No regional lymph node metastasis
pN1	Metastasis with a lymph node mass 2 cm or less in greatest dimension; and less than or equal to five nodes positive, none more than 2 cm in greatest dimension

have a negative effect on sperm number, whereas higher doses of chemotherapy or radiotherapy can induce persistent azoospermia (Petersen et al. 1994; Eberhard et al. 2004). However, for most patients receiving standard therapy the reproduction ability will return to pretreatment capacity within 2–3 years after treatment (Eberhard et al. 2004). Today we lack the means of identifying the patients who are at risk of developing permanent sterility, which is why sperm banking is recommended. Artificial reproductive techniques, such as ICSI (intracytoplasmic sperm injection) has improved chances of fatherhood for these patients.

RPLND may lead to retrograde ejaculation, even though surgical nerve sparing techniques decrease the risk.

TGCC is associated with hypogonadism, and the treatment may further decrease testosterone levels; the patients treated for TGCC should be considered as being at risk for developing androgen deficiency. Long-term side-effects also include increased risk of cardiovascular diseases and second malignancies (Huddart et al. 2003; Zagars et al. 2004).

I.8.2.1.10 Prevention

See "Carcinoma-in-Situ of the Testis" below.

I.8.2.2 Carcinoma-in-Situ of the Testis

I.8.2.2.1 Definition of the Disease

The term "carcinoma-in-situ" (CIS) of the testis refers to a characteristic histological pattern preceding all types of TGCC, except the spermatocytic seminoma. The association between CIS and subsequent development of TGCC was initially reported in 1972 by Skakkebæk (1972). In most typical cases the CIS cells are located inside the seminiferous tubules with normal-appearing Sertoli cells. In some cases, other cells of spermatogenesis, even including spermatids, can be present in tubules containing CIS. The CIS cells possess typical cellular characteristics of neoplasia with large and irregular nucleus, coarse chromatin clumps as well as often multiple nuclei (Skakkebæk 1978). The cytoplasm is abundant and glycogen-rich. Apart from the term "CIS" other designations such as "gonocytoma-in-situ", "intratubular germ cell neoplasia" and "seminoma in situ" have been applied.

I.8.2.2.2 Aetiology and Pathogenesis

The aetiology of testicular malignancy is still unknown. However, there is growing evidence indicating that CIS cells arise already during the foetal life, most likely primordial germ cells/gonocytes, at an early time point during intrauterine development (Rajpert-De Meyts et al. 1996). High risk of testicular malignancy has been found in patients with intersex conditions due to androgen insensitivity or some forms of gonadal dysgenesis. Furthermore, men with a history of cryptorchidism seem to have five to ten times increased risk of CIS and subsequently TGCC (Giwercman et al. 1993). It has been suggested that the malignant transformation from gonocytes into CIS cells is triggered by an imbalance between oestrogen and androgen effect in favour of the female sex hormones. This imbalance might be due to endogenous factors. However, it has even been hypothesized that exposure to environmental chemicals with an oestrogenic or antiandrogenic effect may increase the risk of CIS (Skakkebæk et al. 2001).

Available data indicate that having CIS implies a very high risk of subsequent development of invasive tumour. Thus, in infertile men, 70% of patients in whom CIS was diagnosed developed cancer during a 7-year follow-up. Spontaneous regression of CIS has not been reported, so it seems probable that all cases of CIS, sooner or later, progress to TGCC (Giwercman et al. 1993). The progression of CIS to invasive tumour is probably dependent on the action of sex steroids and/or gonadotrophins. CIS can progress to seminomas as well as nonseminomas.

I.8.2.2.3 Clinical Findings: History, Physical Examination, Technical Investigations, Laboratory Findings

Certain high-risk groups for development of CIS have been identified, with the numbers in parentheses indicating the percentage of individuals having CIS (Giwercman 1992):

1. Patients with unilateral TGCC (5–6% in the contralateral testis)
2. Men with a history of cryptorchidism (2–3%)
3. Infertile men with impairment of spermatogenesis (2–3% of patients with nonobstructive azoospermia)
4. Patients with extragonadal germ cell tumour (50%)
5. Intersex patients with Y chromosome (25–50%)
   The presence of CIS is usually not associated with any specific symptoms, although a few patients have registered some reduction of size and even tenderness of the testis. No tumour is palpable.

However, testicular ultrasound discloses the so-called testicular microlithiasis (TM) – multiple, uniform, nonshadowing echogenic foci in the testis (Lenz et al. 1987; von Eckardstein et al. 2001). In groups 1 and 2 above, the presence of TM was found to be associated with an approximately 20% risk of having CIS (Lenz et al. 1996; von Eckardstein et al. 2001). However, absence of TM does not exclude CIS (Lenz et al. 1996). There are no specific serum markers which can be used for diagnosing CIS.

The most reliable method for diagnosing CIS is open surgical biopsy. Since the CIS changes are in most cases spread throughout the testis, a single tissue specimen of 3 mm in diameter is very sensitive (95%) in diagnosis of CIS (Dieckmann et al. 1999). When assessed by a trained pathologist, the diagnosis can be made in standard (haematoxylin-eosin) stained specimens. However, the recognition of CIS can be facilitated by use of immunohistochemical markers such as placenta-like alkaline phosphatase or others. The sensitivity of needle biopsy or fine-needle aspiration is as yet unknown.

Screening for CIS by biopsy should be offered to the above-mentioned high-risk groups. In TGCC patients, a biopsy of the contralateral testicle may be performed, depending on local recommendations. In men with extragonadal germ cell tumour, a bilateral biopsy is recommended. As regards infertile men, with or without history of cryptorchidism, ultrasound examination can be used as prescreening and the biopsy restricted to those having TM. Intersex patients require individualized management, but the high risk of malignancy should be taken into consideration.

I.8.2.2.4
Differential Diagnosis

For a trained pathologist, the histological diagnosis of CIS does not usually imply any difficulties. Abnormal, large spermatogonia, often seen in testes of infertile men or in cryptorchid gonads, may be misinterpreted as being CIS cells. In such cases, the use of immunohistochemical markers (see above) may be helpful.

I.8.2.2.5
Treatment

The goal of the therapy of testicular CIS is prevention of TGCC and the treatment of choice depends on whether the malignancy is unilateral or bilateral.

If the malignancy is unilateral (the biopsy from the other testis should also be taken since 5–6% of cases are bilateral) – as most often seen in infertile men or in cryptorchid testes – orchiectomy is the therapy of choice. Subsequently, the usual tumour-staging procedure should be performed in order to exclude metastases, which, however, have not been reported in case of isolated testicular CIS.

In men with unilateral TGCC, harbouring CIS in the contralateral gonad, or in the rare cases of bilateral CIS, localized irradiation is recommended. Irradiation is given in fractionated doses of 2 Gy and the total dose should be between 16 and 20 Gy (Petersen et al. 2002; Schmoll et al. 2004). The advantage of using irradiation instead of orchiectomy is that the patient will keep endogenous testosterone production if the testicle is left. In more than 50% of these cases, androgen replacement will not be necessary (Petersen et al. 2002). However, radiotherapy is not recommended if the other testis is without malignancy, since the spermatogenesis becomes irreversibly destroyed by this treatment. Therefore, cryopreservation of sperm should be performed prior to irradiation for CIS.

I.8.2.2.6
Results of Treatment

In case of orchiectomy, the disease is cured and there is no risk of subsequent tumour development. Anecdotic cases of TGCC following testicular irradiation for CIS have been reported (Petersen et al. 2002). However, in such cases, the dose given was 14 Gy, and no treatment failure has been reported after 16 Gy radiation therapy.

It should be kept in mind that patients have a risk of developing Leydig cell insufficiency and consequently hypogonadism as a consequence of orchiectomy as well as testicular irradiation.

I.8.2.2.7
Prognosis

See "Results of Treatment" above.

I.8.2.2.8
Prevention

Prevention is not possible, but screening for CIS is to be considered as prevention of TGCC.

References

Beyer J, Kramar A, Mandanas R, Linkesch W, Greinix A, Droz JP, Pico JL, Diehl A, Bokemeyer C, Schmoll HJ, Nichols CR, Einhorn LH, Siegert W (1996) High-dose chemotherapy as salvage treatment in germ cell tumours: a multivariate analysis of prognostic variables. J Clin Oncol 14:2638–2645

Chaganti RS, Rodriguez E, Bosl GJ (1993) Cytogenetics of male germ-cell tumors. Urol Clin North Am 20:55–66

Classen J, Schmidberger H, Meisner C, Souchon R, Sautter-Bihl ML, Sauer R, Weinknecht S, Kohrmann KU, Bamberg M (2003) Radiotherapy for stages IIA/B testicular seminoma: final report of a prospective multicenter clinical trial. J Clin Oncol 21:1101–1106

Dieckmann KP, Souchon R, Hahn E, Loy V (1999) False-negative biopsies for testicular intraepithelial neoplasia. J Urol 162:364-368

Eberhard J, Stahl O, Giwercman Y, Cwikiel M, Cavallin-Stahl E, Lundin KB, Flodgren P, Giwercman A (2004) Impact of therapy and androgen receptor polymorphism on sperm concentration in men treated for testicular germ cell cancer: a longitudinal study. Hum Reprod 19:1418-1425

Giwercman A (1992) Carcinoma-in-situ of the testis: screening and management. Scand J Urol Nephrol 148 [Suppl]:1-47

Giwercman A, von der Maase H, Skakkebæk NE (1993) Epidemiological and clinical aspects of carcinoma in situ of the testis. Eur Urol 23:104-114

Horwich A (1995) Testicular cancer. In: Horwich A (ed) Oncology - a multidisciplinary textbook. Chapman and Hall, London pp 485-498

Huddart RA, Norman A, Shahidi M, Horwich A, Coward D, Nicholls J, Dearnaley DP (2003) Cardiovascular disease as a long-term complication of treatment for testicular cancer. J Clin Oncol 21:1513-1523

International Germ Cell Cancer Collaborative Group (1997) International Germ Cell Consensus Classification: a prognostic factor-based staging system for metastatic germ cell cancers. International Germ Cell Cancer Collaborative Group. J Clin Oncol 15:594-603

Klepp O, Dahl O, Flodgren P, Stierner U, Olsson AM, Oldbring J, Nielsson S, Daehlin L, Tornblom M, Smaland R, Starkhammar H, Abramsson L, Wist E, Raabe N, Edekling T, Cavallin-Stahl E (1997) Risk-adapted treatment of clinical stage I non-seminoma testis cancer. Eur J Cancer 7:1038-1044

Lenz S, Giwercman A, Skakkebæk NE, Bruun E, Frimodt-Møller C (1987) Ultrasound in detection of early neoplasia of the testis. Int J Androl 10:187-190

Lenz S, Skakkebæk NE, Hertel NT (1996) Abnormal ultrasonic pattern in contralateral testes in patients with unilateral testicular cancer. World J Urol 14:S55-S58

Mostofi FK, Sesterhenn IA (1998) Histological typing of testis tumours. WHO International classification of tumours. Springer, Berlin Heidelberg New York

Petersen PM, Hansen SW, Giwercman A, Rørth M, Skakkebæk NE (1994) Dose-dependent impairment of testicular function in patients treated with cisplatin-based chemotherapy for germ cell cancer. Ann Oncol 5:355-358

Petersen PM, Giwercman A, Daugaard G, Rorth M, Petersen JH, Skakkeaek NE, Hansen SW, von der Maase H (2002) Effect of graded testicular doses of radiotherapy in patients treated for carcinoma-in-situ in the testis. J Clin Oncol 20:1537-1543

Rajpert-De Meyts E, Jørgensen N, Müller J, Giwercman A, Skakkebæk NE (1996) Origin of germ cell tumours. In: Hughes IA (ed) Sex differentiation: clinical and biological aspects. Frontiers in endocrinology. Serono Symposia Publications, Rome, pp 45-54

Richiardi L, Bellocco R, Adami HO, Torrang A, Barlow L, Hakulinen T, Rahu M, Stengrevics A, Storm H, Tretli S, Kurtinaitis J, Tyczynski JE, Akre O (2004) Testicular cancer incidence in eight northern European countries: secular and recent trends. Cancer Epidemiol Biomarkers Prev 13:2157-2166

Richie JP (1997) Neoplasms of the testis. In: Walsh PC(ed) Campbell's urology. Saunders, Philadelphia, pp 2411-2452

Schmoll HJ, Souchon R, Krege S, Albers P, Beyer J, Kollmannsberger C, Fossa SD, Skakkebaek NE, de Wit R, Fizazi K, Droz JP, Pizzocaro G, Daugaard G, de Mulder PH, Horwich A, Oliver T, Huddart R, Rosti G, Paz AL, Pont O, Hartmann JT, Aass N, Algaba F, Bamberg M, Bodrogi I, Bokemeyer C, Classen J, Clemm S, Culine S, de Wit M, Derigs HG, Dieckmann KP, Flasshove M, Garcia dM, X, Gerl A, Germa-Lluch JR, Hartmann M, Heidenreich A, Hoeltl W, Joffe J, Jones W, Kaiser G, Klepp O, Kliesch S, Kisbenedek L, Koehrmann KU, Kuczyk M, Laguna MP, Leiva O, Loy V, Mason MD, Mead GM, Mueller RP, Nicolai N, Oosterhof GO, Pottek T, Rick O, Schmidberger H, Sedlmayer F, Siegert W, Studer U, Tjulandin S, von der MH, Walz P, Weinknecht S, Weissbach L, Winter E, Wittekind C (2004) European consensus on diagnosis and treatment of germ cell cancer: a report of the European Germ Cell Cancer Consensus Group (EGCCCG). Ann Oncol 15:1377-1399

Skakkebæk NE (1972) Possible carcinoma-in-situ of the testis. Lancet ii:516-517

Skakkebæk NE (1978) Carcinoma in situ of the testis: frequency and relationship to invasive germ cell tumours in infertile men. Histopathology 2:157-170

Skakkebæk NE, Rajpert-De Meyts E, Main KM (2001) Testicular dysgenesis syndrome: an increasingly common developmental disorder with environmental aspects. Hum Reprod 16:972-978

UICC (2002) UICC: TNM Classification of malignant tumours. Wiley-Liss, New York

Von Eckardstein S, Tsakmakidis G, Kamischke A, Nieschlag E (2001) Sonographic testicular microlithiasis as an indicator of premalignant conditions in normal and infertile men. J Androl 22:818-824

Warde P, Specht L, Horwich A, Oliver T, Panzarella T, Gospodarowicz M, von der Maase H (2002) Prognostic factors for relapse in stage I seminoma managed by surveillance: a pooled analysis. J Clin Oncol 20:4448-4452

Zagars GK, Ballo MT, Lee AK, Strom SS (2004) Mortality after cure of testicular seminoma. J Clin Oncol 22:640-647

I.8.3 Penile Inflammations

F.-M. Köhn

Key Messages

- Since andrologists pay special attention to the inspection and palpation of the male genital region, they should have knowledge about dermatologically relevant penile lesions.
- Inflammatory dermatoses of the penis may be symptoms of general diseases or specific alterations of the genital region.
- The differential diagnoses of penile dermatoses include infections, balanitides, neoplastic diseases, trauma, papulosquamous or systemic diseases, fixed drug reactions, allergic or irritant contact dermatitis and miscellaneous lesions.
- Some men may also be worried because they have discovered penile alterations which are physiological variations such as heterotopic sebaceous glands or pearly penile papules.

I.8.3.1 Introduction

Inflammatory dermatoses of the penis may be symptoms of general diseases or specific alterations of the genital region. The differential diagnosis includes infectious diseases or benign and malignant neoplasias. Often patients consult their physicians only if the penile disorders cause pain or affect sexual intercourse. The differential diagnoses of penile dermatoses include infections, balanitides, neoplastic diseases, trauma, papulosquamous or systemic diseases, fixed drug reactions, allergic or irritant contact dermatitis and miscellaneous lesions (English et al. 1997; Köhn et al. 1999; Buechner 2002; Bunker 2001, 2004). This section will only focus on the most important inflammatory penile diseases.

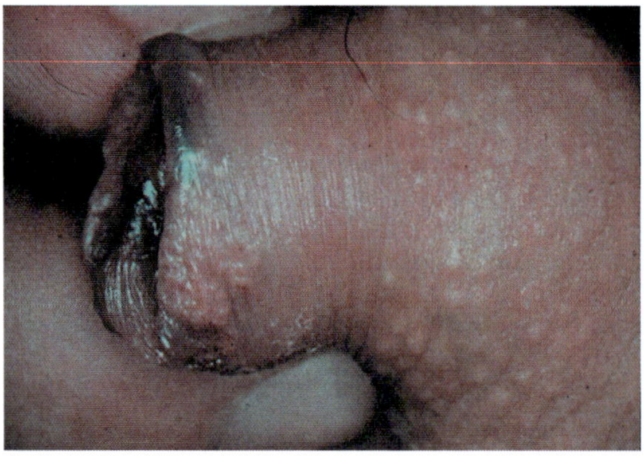

Fig. I.8.2. Heterotopic sebaceous glands

In contrast, men may also be worried because they have discovered penile alterations which are physiological variations such as heterotopic sebaceous glands (Fig. I.8.2) or pearly penile papules.

I.8.3.2 Pearly Penile Papules

I.8.3.2.1 Definition

Normal anatomic structures located at the glans penis.

I.8.3.2.2 Aetiology and Pathogenesis

Histologically, these papules are acral angiofibromas with acanthosis, dense connective tissue and a rich vascular complex (Ackerman and Kronberg 1973).

I.8.3.2.3 Clinical Findings

Pearly penile papules are skin-coloured, asymptomatic and sometimes hyperkeratotic 1- to 2-mm papules with circumferential distribution around the corona of the glans penis (Fig. I.8.3). Their incidence was found to be more than 30% (Rehbein 1977; Rufli et al. 1978).

I.8.3.2.4 Differential Diagnosis

Although pearly penile papules are typical, they are frequently misdiagnosed as condylomata or ectopic sebaceous glands.

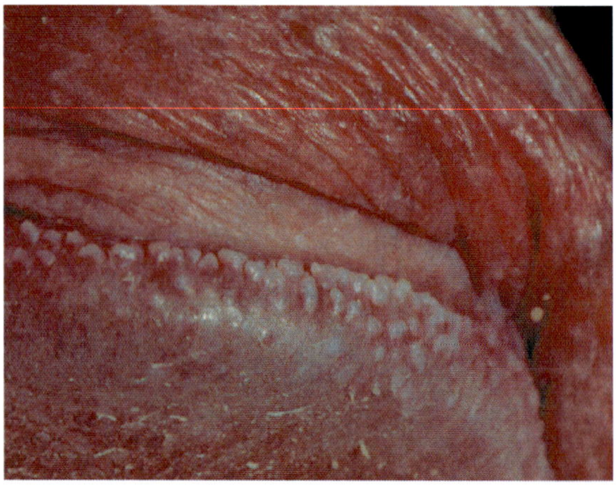

Fig. I.8.3. Pearly penile papules

I.8.3.2.5 Treatment

Treatment is not indicated and patients should be assured about the harmlessness of pearly penile papules. However, they have also been treated by carbon dioxide laser and cryosurgery (Magid and Garden 1989; Ocampo-Candiani and Cueva-Rodriguez 1996; Lane et al. 2002).

I.8.3.3 Sclerosing Lymphangitis of the Penis

I.8.3.3.1 Definition

The disease is caused by a thrombosed or sclerosed lymphatic vessel.

I.8.3.3.2 Aetiology and Pathogenesis

This disorder most often occurs after vigorous sexual activity and resolves spontaneously. However, it may also be associated with underlying sexually transmitted diseases (Rosen and Hwong 2003).

I.8.3.3.3 Clinical Findings

The typical symptom of the nonvenereal sclerosing lymphangitis is a minimally tender, indurated cord involving the coronal sulcus (Fig. I.8.4).

I.8.3.3.4 Differential Diagnosis

Sudden and almost painless cord-like induration on the penile dorsal surface is due to penile Mondor's disease which may be treated with nonsteroidal anti-inflammatory drugs (Sasso et al. 1996).

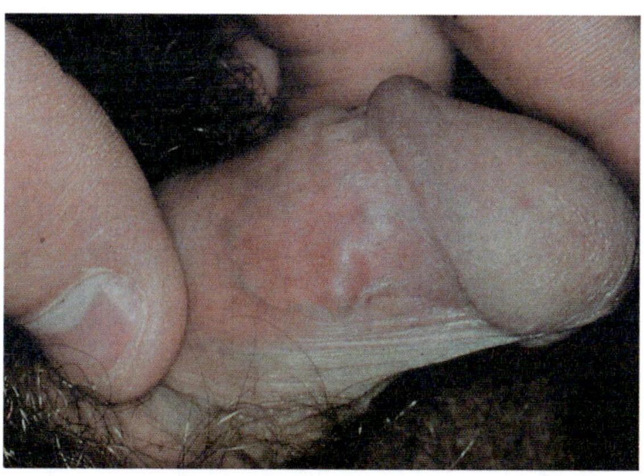

Fig. I.8.4. Sclerosing lymphangitis of the penis

I.8.3.3.5 Treatment

Treatment is usually not indicated. Topical treatment with corticosteroids is recommended in chronic cases with pain.

I.8.3.3.6 Prognosis

Self-limiting course.

I.8.3.4 Balanitis and Balanoposthitis

I.8.3.4.1 Definition

Balanoposthitis is the inflammation of the contiguous and opposing mucosa of the glans penis (balanitis) and the prepuce (posthitis, Fig. I.8.5).

I.8.3.4.2 Aetiology and Pathogenesis

The differential diagnosis of balanoposthitis includes many infectious and noninfectious diseases (Table I.8.6). Some cases of balanoposthitis cannot be classified. However, it could be demonstrated that they show common clinical and histopathological features. Balanitis was diagnosed in 11% of 2,006 patients attending a genitourinary medicine clinic (Birley et al. 1993). In the general population, the incidence of balanitis depends on whether patients are circumcised or not.

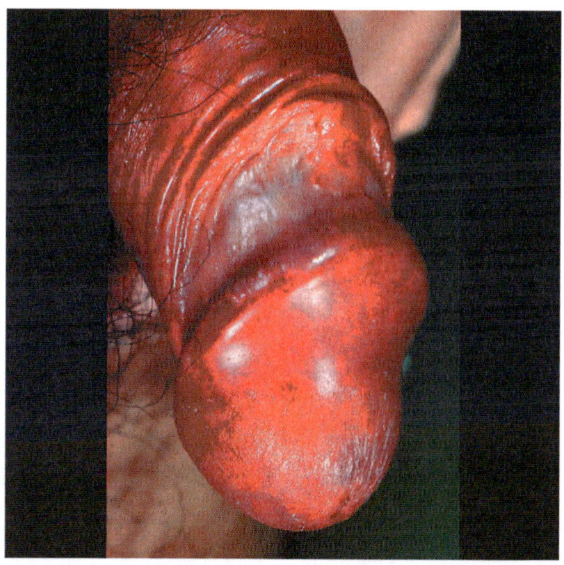

Fig. I.8.5. Acute balanoposthitis after infection with *Candida albicans* (several days after start of antimycotic treatment)

Table I.8.6. Dermatologically relevant penile infections (according to English et al. 1997; Köhn et al. 1999)

Mycotic infections	*Candida* species *Malassezia furfur* *Trichophyton rubrum* *Trichophyton mentagrophytes* *Histoplasma capsulatum* *Blastomycosis dermatitidis* *Cryptococcus neoformans* *Penicillium marneffei*
Bacterial infections	Group B β-haemolytic streptococci Group A β-haemolytic streptococci *Staphylococcus aureus* *Staphylococcus epidermidis* *Streptococcus milleri*, group HB5 *Escherichia coli* *Pseudomonas aeruginosa* *Haemophilus parainfluenza* *Klebsiella* *Enterococcus faecalis* *Proteus mirabilis* *Morganella* *Gardnerella vaginalis* *Bacteroides* species *Mycobacterium tuberculosis* *Mycobacterium celatum* *Chlamydia trachomatis* *Mycoplasma hominis* *Neisseria gonorrhoeae* *Treponema pallidum* *Haemophilus ducreyi* *Calymmatobacterium granulomatis*
Viral infections	Herpes simplex virus Human papillomavirus Varicella-zoster virus Molluscum contagiosum virus
Parasitic infections	*Entamoeba histolytica* *Trichomonas vaginalis* *Sarcoptes scabiei* *Leishmania* species

A cross-sectional study with a randomly selected group of 398 dermatology patients demonstrated that balanitis was present in 2.3% of circumcised men and in 12.5% of uncircumcised men. In patients with diabetes mellitus, balanitis occurred with a higher prevalence of 34.8% in the uncircumcised population (Fakjian et al. 1990).

The group of microorganisms causing penile lesions is heterogeneous and includes mycotic, bacterial, parasitic and viral infections (Table I.8.7). Mycotic and bacterial infections become mainly manifest as balanitis or balanoposthitis and sometimes as ulcerations or gangrene. The most frequent causes of infectious balanitis or balanoposthitis are *Candida* and *Streptococcus* species. However, anaerobes were also often found in uncircumcised men (76%) with balanoposthitis (Masfari et al. 1983). Bacteroides species were the predominant microorganisms in anaerobic balanitis (Cree et al. 1982). In tropical countries or in patients infected with human immunodeficiency virus, even rare infections of the penis have to be considered (e.g. leishmaniasis, leprosy, mycobacteriosis).

Table I.8.7. Differential diagnosis of balanitis and balanoposthitis (according to Johnson 1993, Köhn et al. 1999)

Infections
Nonspecific intertrigo
Traumatic injury
Allergic or irritant contact dermatitis
Psoriasis vulgaris
Balanitis circinata of Reiter's syndrome
Fixed drug eruption
Malignant neoplasias
Plasma cell balanitis
Lichen sclerosus et atrophicus
Pemphigus

Dermatologically relevant parasitic infections of the penis are those with *Trichomonas* and scabies. Glans penis and foreskin lesions (balanoposthitis) occurred in 34% of 46 males with trichomoniasis and were predominantly of the erosive type (Michalowski 1981).

I.8.3.4.3 Clinical Findings

Balanitis can be acute or chronic. Typical symptoms of balanitis are erythema (100%), swelling (91%), discharge (73%), dysuria (13%), bleeding (2%) and sometimes ulceration of the glans penis (1%) (Escala and Rickwood 1989). Nocturnal pruritus and erythematous, excoriated papules of the penis are typical for scabies.

I.8.3.4.4 Differential Diagnosis

The differential diagnoses are summarized in Table I.8.6.

I.8.3.4.5 Treatment

Treatment of balanoposthitis depends on aetiological agents or diseases. Therefore, antimicrobic, anti-inflammatory therapy or circumcision, especially in cases of recurrent balanoposthitis, are performed.

I.8.3.4.6 Prognosis

The prognosis depends on the aetiology of balanitis.

I.8.3.5 Lichen Sclerosus et Atrophicus

I.8.3.5.1 Definition

Lichen sclerosus et atrophicus is a chronic sclerotic process with unknown aetiology.

I.8.3.5.2 Aetiology and Pathogenesis

Traumatic factors, autoimmune disease, genetic factors and hormonal factors have been discussed.

I.8.3.5.3 Clinical Findings

The disease shows a predominant localization (83%) in the genital region and is mostly found in uncircumcised middle-aged men (Meffert et al. 1995; English et al. 1997). However, clinical examinations of 100 boys before circumcision due to phimosis demonstrated lichen sclerosus et atrophicus in 14 cases (Chalmers et al. 1984). In general, lichen sclerosus et atrophicus is found in 3.6–19% of foreskins removed for various reasons (English et al. 1997).

The disease is characterized by erythematous macules and plaques, which progress to white atrophic and sclerotic papules and plaques of the glans penis and the prepuce (Fig. I.8.6). While early lesions are asymptomatic, later patients report pruritus, burning, diminished sensation of the glans, painful erections, meatal stenosis, adhesions between prepuce and glans penis and phimosis. Haemorrhages, erosions and ulcerations may also be found in these lesions.

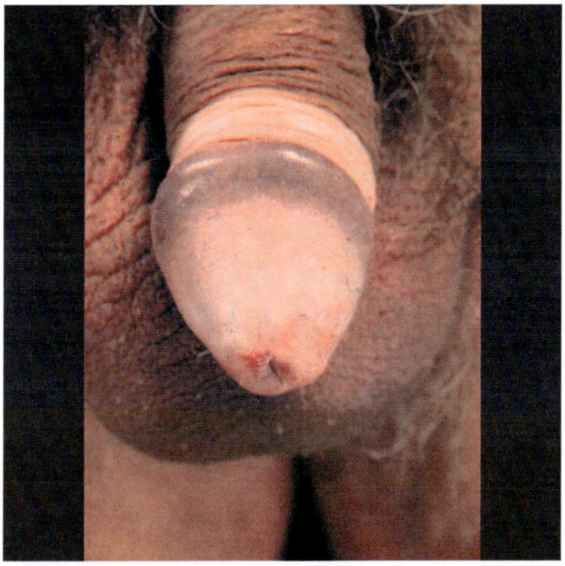

Fig. I.8.6. Lichen sclerosus et atrophicus

Lichen sclerosus was found in 68 of 207 patients with squamous cell carcinomas and giant condylomas. The preferential anatomic site of lichen sclerosus was the foreskin (Velazquez and Cubilla 2003). In contrast, 5 of 86 uncircumcised men with genital lichen sclerosus showed malignant or premalignant histopathologic features (three squamous cell carcinoma, one erythroplasia of Queyrat, one verrucous carcinoma). The average lag time from onset of lichen sclerosus was 17 years. HPV 16 infection was detected by polymerase chain reaction (PCR) in four of these patients (Nasca et al. 1999).

I.8.3.5.4 Differential Diagnosis

Vitiligo, postinflammatory hypopigmentation, posttraumatic or surgical scars, cicatrizing pemphigoid.

I.8.3.5.5 Treatment

Treatment includes circumcision, local therapy with corticosteroids (clobetasol) or immunomodulators (tacrolimus), carbon dioxide laser vaporization and topical application of antimicrobic agents in cases of superinfection (Neill and Ridley 2001). Therapy with testosterone propionate is not a generally recommended option nowadays. Patients with lichen sclerosus et atrophicus should be monitored regularly.

I.8.3.5.6 Prognosis

In rare cases, verrucous or squamous cell carcinoma can develop in lesions of lichen sclerosus et atrophicus.

I.8.3.6 Balanitis Circumscripta Plasmacellularis (Zoon's Balanitis)

I.8.3.6.1 Definition

Plasma cell balanitis is a chronic disease in uncircumcised middle-aged and older men. The prevailing histological feature is the predominance of plasma cells.

I.8.3.6.2 Aetiology and Pathogenesis

The aetiology is unknown. Poor hygiene and chronic infection with *Mycobacterium smegmatis*, physical factors such as heat, friction or trauma, unknown exogenous agents and immunological processes involving

IgE class antibodies have been postulated to play a role in the pathogenesis of Zoon's balanitis (English et al. 1997).

I.8.3.6.3
Clinical Findings

The disease appears as solitary, shiny, erythematous, smooth plaque of the glans penis and/or the prepuce (Kumar et al. 1995). Sometimes the colour is similar to that of cayenne pepper. Clinical variations with erosive and vegetative types are known (Johnson 1993). The lesion is asymptomatic with the exception of mild pruritus. The diagnosis of plasma cell balanitis has to be confirmed by biopsies and histopathological examinations. Histological findings are epidermal atrophy, loss of rete ridges, spongiosis, dense dermal infiltrate with plasma cells and scattered lymphocytes. Erythrocyte extravasation and haemosiderin deposition cannot always be found (Fig. I.8.7; Kumar et al. 1995).

I.8.3.6.4
Differential Diagnosis

The differential diagnosis of plasma cell balanitis includes erythroplasia of Queyrat, extramammary Paget's disease, fixed drug eruption, allergic contact dermatitis, psoriasis, eczema, lichen planus, lichen simplex chronicus, lichen sclerosus et atrophicus, HPV infection, Kaposi's sarcoma, secondary syphilis, *Candida* balanitis, Reiter's disease and pemphigus vulgaris.

I.8.3.6.5
Treatment

Positive effects on the disease have been reported by treatment with corticosteroids, circumcision, antimicrobic agents and carbon dioxide laser.

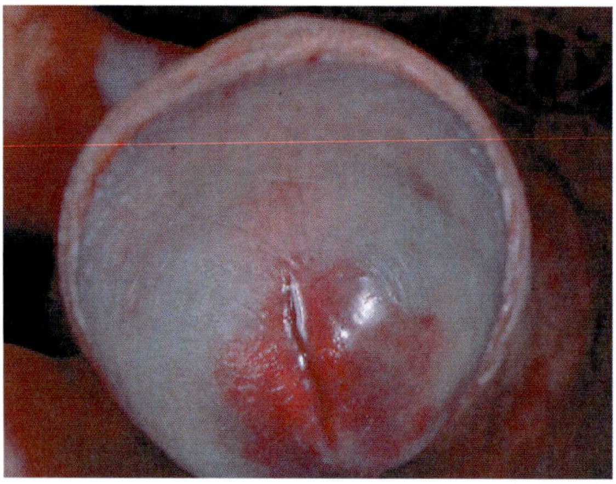

Fig. I.8.7. Balanitis circumscripta plasmacellularis (Zoon's balanitis)

I.8.3.6.6
Prognosis

Chronic disease with poor response to treatment. No association with penile cancer.

I.8.3.7
Balanitis Circinata

I.8.3.7.1
Definition

Reiter's syndrome is defined as the triad of reactive arthritis, conjunctivitis and urethritis; in addition, a variety of minor symptoms such as diarrhoea, inflammatory eye diseases and mucocutaneous lesions can be present.

I.8.3.7.2
Aetiology and Pathogenesis

The pathogenesis of this disease is not completely understood. Certain genital and gastrointestinal infections trigger the syndrome in genetically predisposed patients (HLA-B27 positivity in up to 90%). The infectious agents implicated include *Chlamydia trachomatis*, *Shigella flexneri*, *Salmonella* species, *Yersinia enterocolitica*, *Campylobacter* species, *Ureaplasma urealyticum* and *Neisseria gonorrhoeae* (Adimora et al. 1994). Genital chlamydial infections are the most frequently occurring infections associated with Reiter's syndrome (50% of male patients). The incidence and prevalence of Reiter's syndrome vary geographically. It is still speculative whether males are more commonly affected than females.

I.8.3.7.3
Clinical Findings

Most patients are between 30 and 40 years old. The incidence of Reiter's syndrome in men younger than 50 years is 3.5 per 100,000 (Michet et al. 1988). Balanitis circinata is the most common skin finding in patients with this disease; it is found in 12–70% of all patients with Reiter's syndrome (English et al. 1997). The lesions are painless and appear as serpiginous, erythematous, sometimes also erosive plaques with ragged margins (Fig. I.8.8). They are located at the glans penis in uncircumcised men. In circumcised men, the lesions are dry and scaling, resembling psoriasis (Johnson 1993). The histopathological pattern is psoriatic.

I.8.3.7.4
Differential Diagnosis

Candida balanitis.

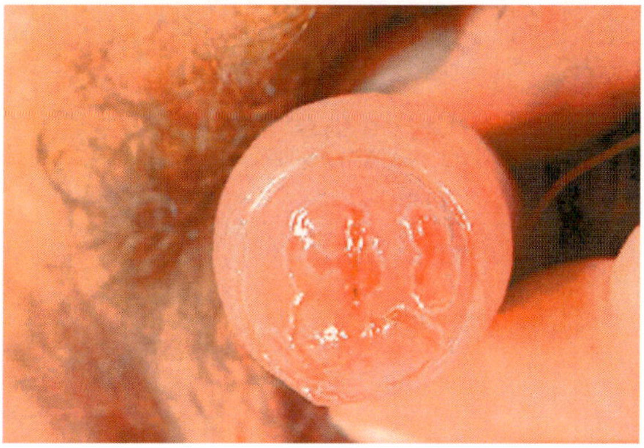

Fig. I.8.8. Balanitis circinata

I.8.3.7.5
Treatment

Treatment of first choice is local application of mild corticosteroids.

I.8.3.7.6
Prognosis

Subacute or chronic disease.

I.8.3.8
Psoriasis Vulgaris

I.8.3.8.1
Definition

Psoriasis vulgaris is a chronic relapsing skin disease with erythrosquamous lesions. In addition to lichen planus, it is the most frequently occurring systemic dermatosis with optional genital manifestation (Table I.8.8).

Table I.8.8. Papulosquamous and systemic diseases with lesions at the glans penis and prepuce (according to Johnson 1993; English et al. 1997; Köhn et al. 1999)

Psoriasis vulgaris	Dermatitis herpetiformis
Lichen planus	Henoch-Schönlein-purpura
Lichen nitidus	Wegener's granulomatosis
Seborrhoeic dermatitis	Neurofibromatosis
Atopic dermatitis	Necrobiosis lipoidica
Pityriasis rosea	Hypereosinophilic syndrome
Crohn's disease	Behçet's syndrome
Ulcerative colitis	Angiokeratoma corporis diffusum
Sarcoidosis	
Amyloidosis	Erythema multiforme
Vitiligo	Lichen sclerosus et atrophicus
Pemphigus variants	Balanitis circinata
Bullous pemphigoid	Mastocytosis

I.8.3.8.2
Aetiology and Pathogenesis

Psoriatic lesions are characterized by keratocyte proliferation (reduction of epidermal cell cycle from 311 h to 36 h) and inflammation/immune mechanisms (increased numbers of activated T cells within the altered epidermis and dermis. Early onset psoriasis is associated with class I and II HLA markers (B13, Bw57, Cw6, DR7), late onset psoriasis with A2 and B27. Trigger factors are trauma (Koebner phenomenon), (streptococcal) infections, stress and drugs (beta-adrenergic blockers). Infection with human immunodeficiency virus also seems to be a trigger for anogenital psoriasis (Weitzul and Duvic 1997).

I.8.3.8.3
Clinical Findings

The incidence of psoriasis in Western countries ranges between 1 % and 2 %. Psoriasis was diagnosed histologically in 3 % of 60 male patients attending a genitourinary medicine clinic (Hillman et al. 1992). Psoriatic lesions of the genital region occur in all age groups from infancy to the elderly. Approximately 25 – 50 % of epidemiologic studies report that genital psoriasis is present with a higher frequency in males than in females (Farber and Nall 1992). The clinical pattern of penile psoriasis varies between circumcised and uncircumcised men. While psoriatic lesions appear as well-demarcated erythematous plaques without scale in occluded skin (intact foreskin, Figs. I.8.9, I.8.10), psoriatic plaques are erythematous, with varying accumulations of scale in circumcised men (Fig. I.8.11; Johnson 1993). With the exception of optional pruritus or in-

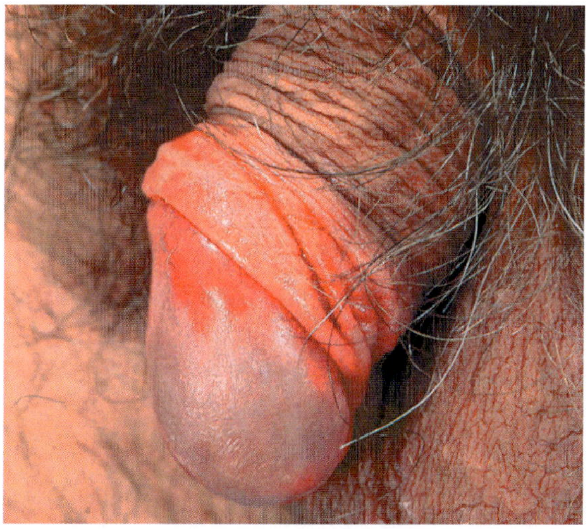

Fig. I.8.9. Psoriasis vulgaris of the penis with well-demarcated nonscaling plaques

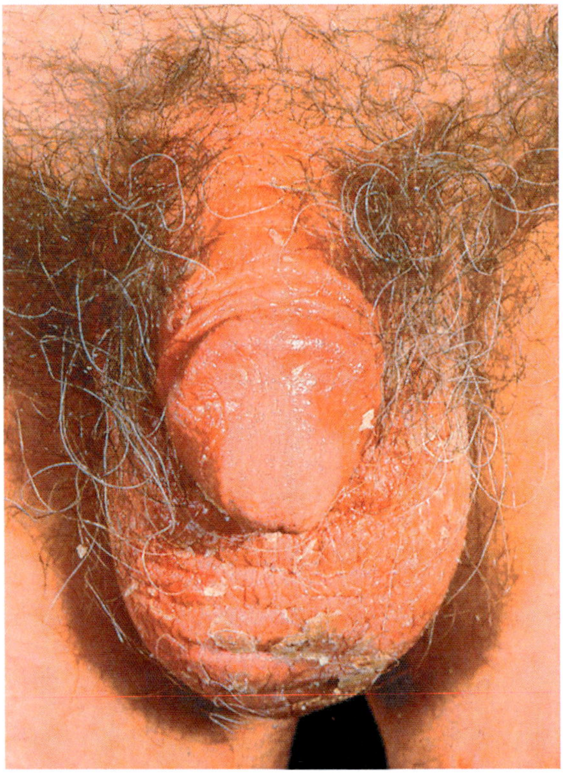

Fig. I.8.10. Psoriasis vulgaris of the penis

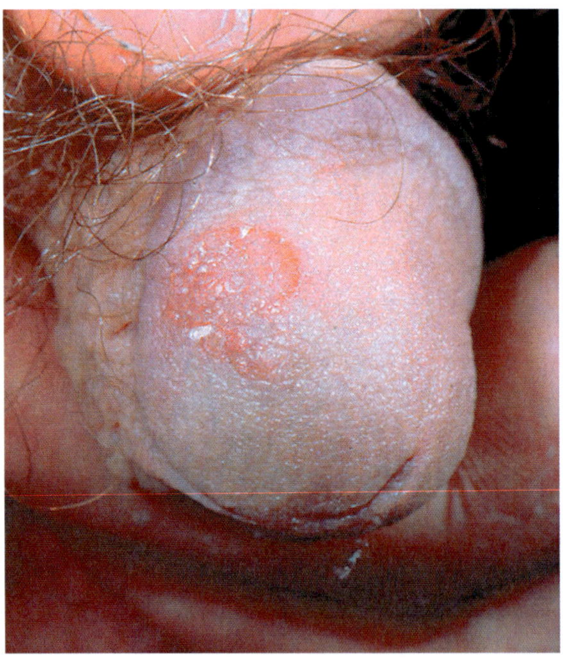

Fig. I.8.11. Psoriasis vulgaris of the penis with a scaling plaque

creased sensitivity during sexual intercourse, psoriatic lesions of the penis are asymptomatic.

I.8.3.8.4 Differential Diagnosis

Zoon' balanitis, lichen planus, erythroplasia of Queyrat and extramammary Paget's disease.

I.8.3.8.5 Treatment

Treatment includes topical application of corticosteroids, Castellani's paint or vitamin D analogues.

I.8.3.8.6 Prognosis

Chronic and relapsing disease. Genital complications associated with the therapy of psoriasis such as development of squamous cell carcinoma or genital ulcerations were demonstrated after PUVA therapy and local treatment with tazarotene, respectively (De la Brassinne and Richert 1992; Wollina 1998).

I.8.3.9 Lichen Planus

I.8.3.9.1 Definition

Lichen planus is an inflammatory dermatosis affecting both mucosal and keratinized epithelium. The male genitalia are affected in 25% of cases.

I.8.3.9.2 Aetiology and Pathogenesis

The aetiology of lichen planus is unknown. Immunologic mechanisms seem to play a major role. Association with hepatitis C has been reported (Tanei et al. 1997).

I.8.3.9.3 Clinical Findings

Penile lichen planus appears as typical polygonal, flat-topped papules with annular configuration and white striae (Figs. I.8.12, I.8.13). Erosive variants are also known. Although genital lesions are usually associated with lichen planus of other skin regions, they may develop as initial or exclusive manifestation of lichen planus. In typical cases diagnosis is made clinically; otherwise histological examinations of biopsies are necessary.

I.8

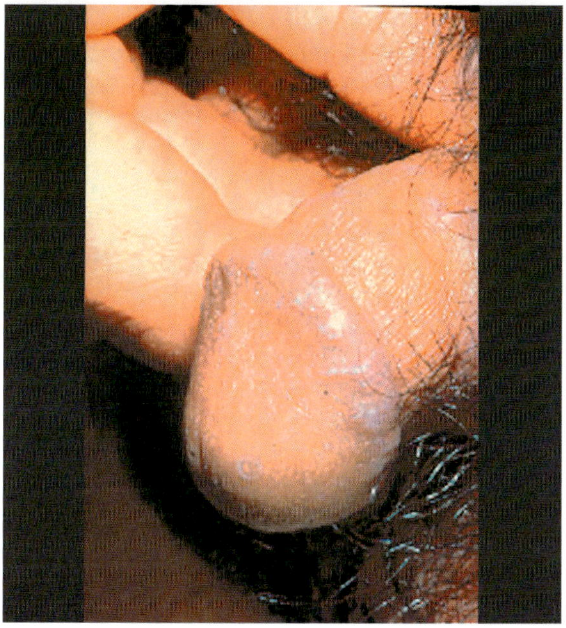

Fig. I.8.12. Penile lichen planus of the glans penis showing typical polygonal, flat-topped papules with annular configuration and white striae

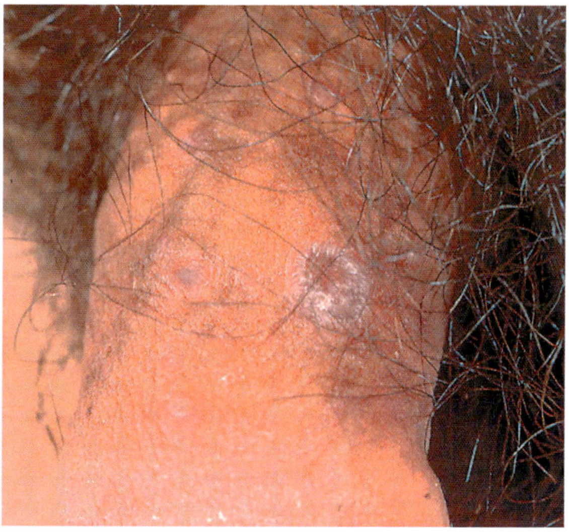

Fig. I.8.13. Penile lichen planus of the penile shaft

I.8.3.9.4 Differential Diagnosis

Psoriasis, Zoon's balanitis, lichen sclerosus, viral warts (including Bowenoid papulosis), porokeratosis.

I.8.3.9.5 Treatment

Treatment of penile lichen planus includes topical application of corticosteroids. In individual cases, erosive lesions have also been systemically treated with ciclosporin or thalidomide (Perez-Alfonzo et al. 1987; Jemec and Baadsgaard 1993).

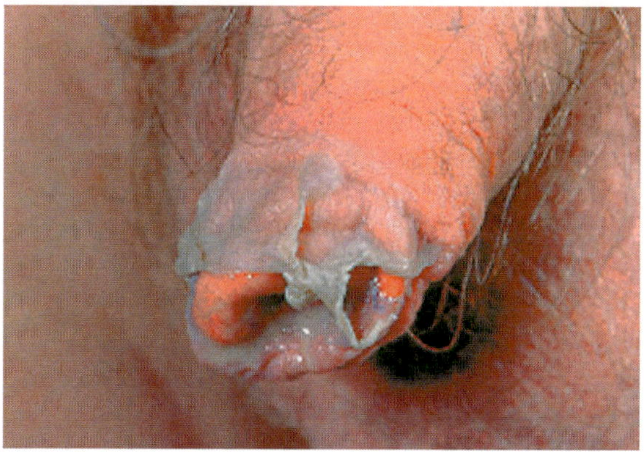

Fig. I.8.14. Fixed drug eruption with a well-demarcated erythematous macule and blistering

I.8.3.9.6 Prognosis

While spontaneous remission with postinflammatory hyperpigmentation can be expected in most cases, erosive variants of this disease may persist for decades (Johnson 1993). Squamous cell carcinoma developing in penile lichen planus is extremely rare (Leal-Khouri and Hruza 1994).

I.8.3.10 Fixed Drug Eruption

I.8.3.10.1 Definition

After sensitization to a drug, fixed drug eruptions appear as solitary or multiple well-demarcated erythematous macules or plaques, which may also develop bullae (Fig. I.8.14). The lesions typically recur at the same anatomic sites after exposure to the same drug.

I.8.3.10.2 Aetiology and Pathogenesis

Drugs causing penile fixed drug eruptions are tetracycline, doxycycline, penicillins, phenolphthalein, sulfonamides, barbiturates, salicylates, dapsone, griseofulvin, carbamazepine, dimenhydrinate, metamizole, hydroxyzine hydrochloride and colchicine. Fixed drug eruptions have also been reported after history of sexual contact with women who were found to be receiving the same medication to which their partners were hypersensitive (Zawar et al. 2004).

I.8.3.10.3 Clinical Findings

Pandhi et al. (1984) investigated fixed drug eruptions exclusively involving the genitalia of 60 male patients. The sites affected were the glans penis, coronal sulcus and preputial skin. Superficial ulceration or pigmented areas surrounded by an erythematous halo were the main clinical findings. Even ulcerations have been described.

I.8.3.10.4 Differential Diagnosis

All other differential diagnoses of acute balanitis or balanoposthitis have to be considered.

I.8.3.10.5 Treatment

Topical application of corticosteroids. Identification and withdrawal of the responsible drug.

I.8.3.10.6 Prognosis

Fixed drug eruptions heal within 2–3 weeks, leaving postinflammatory hyperpigmentation.

I.8.3.11 Other Drug-Induced Lesions of the Penis

Prolonged topical application of corticosteroids causes epithelial and dermal atrophy of the genital region (Stankler 1982). Local penile ulceration has been reported after irregular subcutaneous injection of papaverine (Borgström 1988). Penile ulcerations may also appear after use of dequalinium and in 5–28% of patients with AIDS who are treated with foscarnet, a retroviral reverse transcriptase inhibitor (Braun-Falco and Lukacs 1970; English et al. 1997). Since foscarnet is excreted unchanged in the urine, it may be responsible for an irritant contact dermatitis resulting in periurethral ulcerations. Coumarins including warfarin may induce penile necrosis (Weinberg et al. 1983). Coumarin-induced necrosis of the penis is found in patients with relative protein C deficiency and starts between the 3rd and 10th days of therapy (Barkley et al. 1989).

I.8.3.12 Allergic and Irritant Contact Dermatitis of the Penis

I.8.3.12.1 Definition

Allergic contact dermatitis is caused by a type IV, cell-mediated, delayed hypersensitivity to allergens. In contrast, irritant contact dermatitis is a nonimmunologic inflammatory reaction after exposure to a chemical or physical agent.

I.8.3.12.2 Aetiology and Pathogenesis

According to Johnson (1993), contact dermatitis of the penis may develop after hand-to-penis contact, sexual intercourse (feminine hygiene deodorant sprays and douches, lubricants containing propylene glycol) and as local manifestation of a generalized contact dermatitis. The agents causing allergic reactions depend on geographical aspects. In the United States, for example, a common cause of penile contact dermatitis are pentadecylcatechol congeners (poison ivy; Fisher 1996). Other frequently occurring allergens in condoms or rubber diaphragms are mercaptobenzothiazole, tetramethylthiuram, zinc dithiocarbamate and latex (Johnson 1993; English et al. 1997). The source of the allergen may be the condom material, the lubricant (paraben preservatives) or the spermicidal agent (Johnson 1993). Patients with spinal cord injury using rubber condom urinals have a higher chance of developing penile contact dermatitis against rubber or latex articles (Bransbury 1979). Some condoms contain local anaesthetics such as benzocaine, which is known to cause allergic contact dermatitis of the penis (Placucci et al. 1996). In contrast to allergic penile dermatitis, irritant lesions of this region occur more frequently. Irritant dermatitis was diagnosed in 72% of patients with recurrent or unresponsive balanitis (Birley et al. 1993). The most frequently occurring irritant penile dermatitis is caused by over-washing (extensive use of soaps) or over-treatment (extensive use of ointments). Diagnostic procedures include patch testing, histological and microbiological examinations.

I.8.3.12.3 Clinical Findings

Since penile vascularization is better than in most other skin regions, allergic contact dermatitis of the penis is more florid and symptomatic with erythema, oedema, microvesiculation, erosions and exudation (Fig. I.8.15). Older lesions are covered by crusts. Scratches due to intense pruritus are subject to secondary bacterial infection. Especially in cases of allergy to latex,

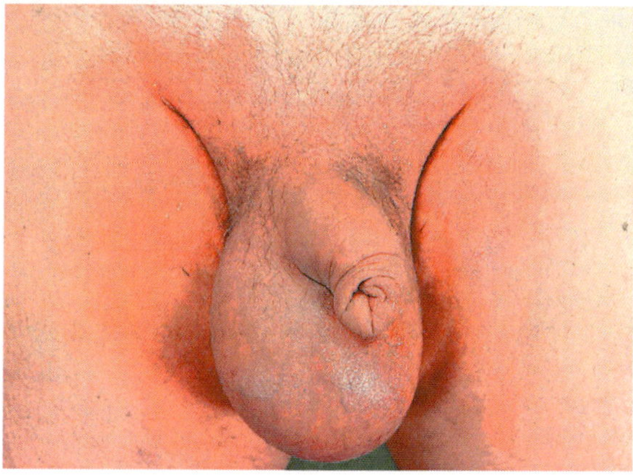

Fig. I.8.15. Acute contact dermatitis of the penis

local swelling and itching may be accompanied with systemic (urticaria) or respiratory symptoms.

I.8.3.12.4
Differential Diagnosis

All other differential diagnoses of balanitis or balanoposthitis have to be considered.

I.8.3.12.5
Treatment

Irritant or allergic penile dermatitis is treated by local application of corticosteroids or antimicrobic agents. In severe cases, corticosteroids or antihistamines are given systemically.

I.8.3.12.6
Prognosis

Men with irritant penile dermatitis had a greater lifetime incidence of atopic illness and more frequent daily genital washing with soap. For the majority (90%) of these patients, use of creams and restriction of soap washing alone reduced symptoms.

I.8.3.13
Atopic Dermatitis

I.8.3.13.1
Definition

The terms "dermatitis" and "eczema" are often used synonymously. Atopic dermatitis is one condition of atopic diathesis; other symptoms can be IgE-mediated allergies such as rhinitis, conjunctivitis or asthma, increased serum IgE-levels, dry skin (sebostasis) or familial predisposition.

I.8.3.13.2
Aetiology and Pathogenesis

Atopic dermatitis is a multifactorial disease with a genetic background, environmental and immunologic factors (IgE-mediated sensitization to a variety of allergens) and sebostasis.

I.8.3.13.3
Clinical Findings

Frequently occurring symptoms of the skin are erythema, lichenification, excoriation after scratching due to severe itching, superinfection with impetiginization. Atopic diathesis was found in more than 70% of men with irritant balanitis (Birley et al. 1993).

I.8.3.13.4
Differential Diagnosis

Seborrhoeic dermatitis, psoriasis, irritant or contact dermatitis.

I.8.3.13.5
Treatment

Atopic eczema of the penis is treated by local application of corticosteroids, immunomodulators (tacrolimus, pimecrolimus) or antimicrobic agents. In severe cases, corticosteroids, ciclosporin, antibiotics or antihistamines are given systemically.

I.8.3.13.6
Prognosis

Chronic and relapsing disease, sometimes self-limiting.

I.8.3.14
Seborrhoeic Dermatitis

I.8.3.14.1
Definition

Chronic erythrosquamous dermatosis of sebaceous follicle-rich regions of the skin (scalp, face, trunk and genital region).

I.8.3.14.2
Aetiology and Pathogenesis

Pityrosporum ovale, a commensal yeast of the epidermis and follicles, plays an important role in the pathogenesis of seborrhoeic eczema. Seborrhoeic eczema is more frequently found in men with HIV infection.

I.8.3.14.3 Clinical Findings

Typical locations of this disease are scalp, glabella, eye brows, nasolabial folds and external auditory canal, but also the genital region. Clinical symptoms are salmon-coloured erythemas with scaling.

I.8.3.14.4 Differential Diagnosis

Atopic dermatitis, psoriasis, irritant or contact dermatitis.

I.8.3.14.5 Treatment

Treatment includes local application of corticosteroids or antifungals such as imidazoles.

I.8.3.14.6 Prognosis

In most cases, mild disease; treatment is not mandatory.

References

Ackerman AB, Kronberg R (1973) Pearly penile papules. Acral angiofibromas. Arch Dermatol 108:673–675

Adimora AA, Hamilton H, Holmes KK, Sparling PF (1994) Sexually transmitted diseases. McGraw-Hill, New York

Barkley C, Badalament RA, Metz EN, Nesbitt J, Drago JR (1989) Coumarin necrosis of the penis. J Urol 141:946–948

Birley HD, Walker MM, Luzzi GA, Bell R, Taylor-Robinson D, Byrne M, Renton AM (1993) Clinical features and management of recurrent balanitis; association with atopy and genital washing. Genitourin Med 69:400–403

Borgström E (1988) Penile ulcer as complication in self-induced papaverine erections. Urology 32:416–417

Bransbury AJ (1979) Allergy to rubber condom urinals and medical adhesives in male spinal injury patients. Contact Dermatitis 5:317–323

Braun-Falco O, Lukacs I (1970) Dequalinium necrosis. Dtsch Med Wochenschr 95:1115–1117

Buechner SA (2002) Common skin disorders of the penis. BJU Int 90:498–506

Bunker CB (2001) Topics in penile dermatology. Clin Exp Dermatol 26:469–479

Bunker CB (2004) Male genital skin disease. Saunders, Edinburgh

Chalmers RJ, Burton PA, Bennett RF, Goring CC, Smith PJ (1984) Lichen sclerosus et atrophicus. A common and distinctive cause of phimosis in boys. Arch Dermatol 120: 1025–1027

Cree GE, Willis AT, Phillips KD, Brazier JS (1982) Anaerobic balanoposthitis. Br Med J Clin Res Ed 284:859–860

De la Brassinne M, Richert B (1992) Genital squamous-cell carcinoma after PUVA therapy. Dermatology 185:316–318

English JC, Laws RA, Keough GC, Wilde JL, Foley JP, Elston DM (1997) Dermatoses of the glans penis and prepuce. J Am Acad Dermatol 37:1–24

Escala JM, Rickwood AM (1989) Balanitis. Br J Urol 63:196–197

Fakjian N, Hunter S, Cole GW, Miller J (1990) An argument for circumcision. Prevention of balanitis in the adult. Arch Dermatol 126:1046–1047

Farber EM, Nall L (1992) Genital psoriasis. Cutis 50:263–266

Fisher AA (1996) Poison ivy/oak/sumac. Part II: specific features. Cutis 58:22–24

Hillman RJ, Walker MM, Harris JR, Taylor-Robinson D (1992) Penile dermatoses: a clinical and histopathological study. Genitourin Med 68:166–169

Jemec GB, Baadsgaard O (1993) Effect of cyclosporine on genital psoriasis and lichen planus. J Am Acad Dermatol 29: 1048–1049

Johnson RA (1993) Diseases and disorders of the anogenitalia of males. In: Fitzpatrick TB, Eisen AZ, Wolff K, Freedberg IM, Austen KF (eds) Dermatology in general medicine. McGraw-Hill, New York, pp 1417–1462

Köhn FM, Pflieger-Bruss S, Schill WB (1999) Penile skin diseases. Andrologia 31 [Suppl 1]:3–11

Kumar B, Sharma R, Rajagopalan M, Radotra BD (1995) Plasma cell balanitis: clinical and histopathological features-response to circumcision. Genitourin Med 71:32–34

Lane JE, Peterson CM, Ratz JL (2002) Treatment of pearly penile papules with CO2 laser. Dermatol Surg 28:617–618

Leal-Khouri S, Hruza GJ (1994) Squamous cell carcinoma developing within lichen planus of the penis. Treatment with Mohs micrographic surgery. J Dermatol Surg Oncol 20: 272–276

Magid M, Garden JM (1989) Pearly penile papules: treatment with the carbon dioxide laser. J Dermatol Surg Oncol 15:552–554

Masfari AN, Kinghorn GR, Duerden BI (1983) Anaerobes in genitourinary infections in men. Br J Vener Dis 59:255–259

Meffert JJ, Davis BM, Grimwood RE (1995) Lichen sclerosus. J Am Acad Dermatol 32:393–416

Michalowski R (1981) Trichomonal balano-posthitis. Report of 16 cases. Ann Dermatol Venereol 108:731–738

Michet CJ, Machado EB, Ballard DJ, McKenna CH (1988) Epidemiology of Reiter's syndrome in Rochester, Minnesota: 1950–1980. Arthritis Rheum 31:428–431

Nasca MR, Innocenzi D, Micali G (1999) Penile cancer among patients with genital lichen sclerosus. J Am Acad Dermatol 41:911–914

Neill SM, Ridley CM (2001) Management of anogenital lichen sclerosus. Clin Exper Dermatol 26:637–643

Ocampo-Candiani J, Cueva-Rodriguez JA (1996) Cryosurgical treatment of pearly penile papules. J Am Acad Dermatol 35:486–487

Pandhi RK, Kumar AS, Satish DA, Bhutani LK (1984) Fixed drug eruptions on male genitalia: clinical and etiologic study. Sex Transm Dis 11:164–166

Perez-Alfonzo R, Weiss E, Piquero-Martin J, Rondon-Lugo A (1987) Generalized lichen planus with erosive lesions of the penis, treated with thalidomide. Report of a case and review of the literature. Med Cutan Ibero Lat Am 15:321–326

Placucci F, Lorenzi S, La-Placa M, Vincenzi C (1996) Sensitization to benzocaine on a condom. Contact Dermatitis 34:293

Rehbein HM (1977) Pearly penile papules: incidence. Cutis 19:54–57

Rosen T, Hwong H (2003) Sclerosing lymphangitis of the penis. J Am Acad Dermatol 49:916–918

Rufli T, Eichenberger P, Heer K (1978) Papillomatosis coronae glandis. Frequency of occurrence and clinical picture. Schweiz Med Wochenschr 108:229–231

Sasso F, Gulino G, Basar M, Carbone A, Torricelli P, Alcini E (1996) Penile Mondors' disease: an underestimated pathology. Br J Urol 77:729–732

Stankler L (1982) Striae of the penis. Br J Dermatol 107:371–372
Tanei R, Ohta Y, Katsuoka K (1997) Lichen planus and Sjögren-type sicca syndrome in a patient with chronic hepatitis C. J Dermatol 24:20–27
Velazquez EF, Cubilla AL (2003) Lichen sclerosus in 68 patients with squamous cell carcinoma of the penis: frequent atypias and correlation with special carcinoma variants suggest a precancerous role. Am J Surg Pathol 27:1448–1453
Weinberg AC, Lieskovsky G, McGehee WG, Skinner DG (1983) Warfarin necrosis of the skin and subcutaneous tissue of the male external genitalia. J Urol 130:352–354
Weitzul S, Duvic M (1997) HIV-related psoriasis and Reiter's syndrome. Semin Cutan Med Surg 16:213–218
Wollina U (1998) Genital ulcers in a psoriasis patient using topical tazarotene. Br J Dermatol 138:713–714
Zawar V, Kirloskar M, Chuh A (2004) Fixed drug eruption – a sexually inducible reaction? Int J STD AIDS 15:560–563

I.8.4 Penile Cancer

I.D.C. Mitchell

Key Messages

- Rare male malignancy may have delayed presentation.
- Ninety-five per cent of malignancies are squamous cell carcinoma.
- Treatment of local disease and loco-regional nodes both need consideration in management of disease.
- Multi-modality treatment is being investigated for treatment of advanced disease.

I.8.4.1 Definition

Penile cancer is rare, with a reported incidence of around 1 per 100,000, representing 0.4–0.6% of cancers involving men in Western societies. This tumour usually affects the glans and/or prepuce of the penis. In over 90% of cases, this is a squamous cell cancer, though other tumours have been reported, for example, melanoma. It is very rare in Western countries but is more prevalent in other countries such as Brazil or India.

I.8.4.2 Aetiology and Pathogenesis

It is thought that chronic infection or inflammation gives rise to the changes that lead to malignant transformation. Associations have therefore been made with age, phimosis, viral infection, poor socioeconomic status and smoking.

It should be noted that whilst increased age is a factor, the median age of presentation is around 60 years old, and therefore this disease is not uncommon in younger men. The presence of phimosis is an extremely common finding in patients with this disease. It is felt that the conditions found under the prepuce lead to the development of the tumour. This relationship is supported when one investigates cultures that advocate early circumcision such as the Jewish faith, and here penile cancer is almost unknown. It has been noted, however, that later circumcision does not appear to offer any protection, for example as seen in the Bantu peoples of South Africa. Recent data from the SEER programme has not found any racial differences in the incidence of penile cancer between white and African-American populations. This study also did not find any differences in incidence between married men and men who have never married.

Further investigation of the pathogenesis of this tumour has found human papilloma virus (HPV) in association with this tumour. In particular, HPV types 16, 18 and 33 have been implicated.

I.8.4.3 Clinical Findings

Patients with these tumours are often described as having delayed presentation and this has been borne out by investigation. The delayed presentation may be induced by embarrassment, but also a nonretractile prepuce may hide the primary lesion. When a lesion is hidden by the prepuce, the presentation may be bleeding, foul-smelling discharge, an indurated lump arising from under the prepuce, or even by the detection of pathological inguinal nodes. The primary lesions may be ulcerative or exophytic. It is recommended that any patient who has a persistent lesion on his penis should have a biopsy taken.

In addition to the localized lesion on the penis, a significant proportion of up to 50% of patients will have palpable inguinal lymphadenopathy and accordingly the groins should be carefully examined at the time of presentation. When these nodes are histologically examined, 30–60% have been reported to be inflammatory; however, a recent study has suggested that the percentage of palpable nodes demonstrating spread is considerably higher.

There are two staging systems used to describe these tumours: Jackson (1966) and the TNM (1997), both shown in Table I.8.9.

Table I.8.9. Jackson staging and TNM classification for penile tumours

Jackson Staging – 1966	
I	Tumour confined to glans penis, or prepuce, or both
II	Tumour involves penile shaft or corpora: negative nodes
III	Tumour confined to penis, with operable inguinal lymph node metastases
IV	Tumour extends beyond penile shaft with inoperable inguinal or distant lymph nodes, or distant metastases
TNM Classification (1997)	
T – Primary tumour	
TX	Tumour cannot be assessed
T0	No evidence of primary tumour
Tis	Carcinoma in situ
Ta	Non-invasive verrucous carcinoma
T1	Tumour invades subepithelial connective tissue
T2	Tumour invades corpus spongiosum or cavernosum
T3	Tumour invades urethra or prostate
T4	Tumour invades other adjacent structures
N – regional lymph nodes	
NX	Cannot be assessed
N0	No regional lymph node metastases
N1	Tumour invades single superficial inguinal lymph node
N2	Tumour invades multiple or bilateral superficial inguinal lymph nodes
N3	Tumour invades deep inguinal or pelvic lymph nodes, unilateral or bilateral
M – distant metastases	
MX	Cannot be assessed
M0	No distant metastases
M1	Distant metastases present

I.8.4.4 Differential Diagnosis

There are a number of lesions that can mimic penile cancer and need to be excluded before making the diagnosis and carrying out definitive management. These include condylomata acuminata, Buschke-Lowenstein tumour, chancre, chancroid, lymphogranuloma venereum, granuloma inguinale and tuberculosis. These possible diagnoses reinforce the need for a pretreatment biopsy.

I.8.4.5 Treatment

When considering the management of penile cancer, it is important to consider management of the local disease and metastatic spread in conjunction, as the long-term outcome of the patient depends on each. A number of therapeutic options are available for the local management of penile cancer; the optimal treatment often will depend on a number of factors and should be tailored to each patient.

Carcinoma-in-situ has been reported to be successfully treated in a number of ways, which have included topical 5-fluorouracil, CO_2 laser, cryotherapy, Mohs' microsurgical technique (MMT) and surgical excision with skin grafting if indicated.

When one is considering the management of larger lesions, T1 and suitable T2, the concept of organ preservation has become increasingly important. This generally takes the form of conservative surgery with reconstruction or radiotherapy though MMT has its proponents. Radiotherapy has been described using three different techniques, namely mould, implant and external beam. There are significant side-effects to radiotherapy which may necessitate surgical salvage and most units currently seem to favour a surgical approach. However, when performing either a traditional partial penectomy or a reconstructive approach with split skin grafting, care must be taken to leave the patient with an adequate stump to allow proper hygiene as well as sexual function when appropriate.

Retrospective studies have shown that both these modalities can provide good local control but there are well-recognized side-effects of these treatments. It seems likely that in the future, combination approaches will be tried to reduce the morbidity of these treatments.

However, with larger tumours and T3 and T4 lesions, surgery is commonly carried out for local control, though some have advocated chemoradiotherapy as per anal cancer.

The greatest controversy and uncertainty in the management of this disease relates to the treatment of the inguinal and pelvic lymph nodes. Penile cancer is one of the few malignancies that lymphadenectomy can provide a survival benefit. This improved survival is felt to be most marked in low-volume disease (impalpable nodes); however, this procedure has significant associated morbidity and improved selection of patients for lymphadenectomy is required. There is also some doubt over the merits of carrying out pelvic lymphadenectomy in these patients, as the survival of patients with positive nodes is extremely low. Experience in the treatment of other squamous cancers such as anal or vulval cancers would suggest that multi-modality treatment would be optimal in patients with advanced disease.

Chemotherapy has only established itself in the management of penile cancer when 5-fluorouracil is used topically to treat carcinoma-in-situ; however, there is some evidence that multi-agent chemotherapy will have a role in the treatment of penile cancer. In view of the rarity of the disease, large multi-centre trials will need to be arranged to assess the validity of the use of these drugs, but the rationale seems intuitive.

I.8.4.6 Results of Treatment

It is usually possible to provide good local control for penile cancer by all approaches for early disease (Ta–T2), but for more advanced disease surgery is usually the preferred option.

The survival figures of penile cancer are summarized in Table I.8.10.

Table I.8.10. Survival figures for penile cancer. Percentages are mean 5-year survivals from various reported studies

Treatment	Survival (%) at tumour stage			
	I	II	III	IV
Surgery	65	42	27	0
Radiotherapy	68	51	21	5

Adapted from Gillenwater J, Howards S, Grayhack J, Mitchell ME (2001) Adult and Pediatric Urology, 4th edn. Lippincott, Wilkins & Williams, Philadelphia, p. 1990

I.8.4.7 Prognosis

As can be seen in the preceding section, patients with localized disease have a good prognosis; however, when there is evidence of spread (except in cases with minimal inguinal node involvement) the results of treatment are rather disappointing. Several retrospective studies have shown the presence of lymph nodal involvement has a marked impact on survival. Others have additionally demonstrated that removal of low-volume disease (prophylactic lymphadenectomy) has a survival benefit compared to the delayed treatment of clinically involved nodes. The improved survival for some patients must be balanced with considerable morbidity of lymphadenectomy. Tumour grade does have some prognostic significance. This probably reflects the propensity of poorly differentiated tumours to metastasize, but it should not be forgotten that well-differentiated tumours also metastasize.

I.8.4.8 Prevention

As has been described previously, early circumcision can prevent the development of penile cancer, but recent epidemiological studies from Scandinavia have suggested that good hygiene associated with improved socioeconomic status can lead to a decreased incidence of this disease.

I.8.4.9 Other

An increased incidence of cervical and vulval cancer has been demonstrated in partners of patients with penile cancer. This observation certainly appears to confirm that there is likely to be a common transmissible factor in the development of these diseases. Recently there has been hope expressed that vaccination against HPV will prevent cervical cancer and one would hope that a similar approach might bear fruit in preventing the development penile cancer in some patients.

I.8

I.8.5 Circumcision

C.F. Heyns, J.N. Krieger

Key Messages

- Circumcision is the most ancient surgical procedure known, and has generated more controversy than any other operation.
- Medical indications for circumcision include pathological (cicatrizing) phimosis, recurrent paraphimosis, recurrent balanitis, condylomata acuminata involving the foreskin and glans, recurrent coital injury of the prepuce, and placement of a penile prosthesis.
- Neonatal circumcision may confer a three- to sevenfold reduced risk of urinary tract infection (UTI), but the risk of UTI in an uncircumcised male infant is only about 1 %.
- The risk for acquiring sexually transmitted infections (STI), including human immunodeficiency virus (HIV), may be two to eight times higher in uncircumcised men, but there is not yet any evidence that circumcision is a cost-effective strategy to reduce the infection rate.
- Neonatal circumcision confers a threefold reduced risk of penile cancer, but almost two complications of circumcision can be expected for every case of penile cancer prevented.
- Although scientific evidence demonstrates some medical benefits of circumcision, these data are not yet sufficient to recommend routine neonatal circumcision.

I.8.5.1 Introduction

Circumcision is the oldest surgical procedure in the world, and remains one of the most controversial subjects in medicine. It has been practised for thousands of years among certain peoples on all the inhabited continents, and in Egypt the procedure can be dated back to at least 6,000 years ago (Fig. I.8.16). The Jewish practice of circumcision precedes its documentation in the Torah by over 1,000 years, and it is not a prerequisite for being Jewish. Circumcision was a common practice in pre-Islamic Arabia and is considered an external symbol of being a Muslim, but not a condition for becoming one.

The real motives for circumcision in ancient cultures are open to speculation, but theories suggest that it originated as a:

1. Rite of passage or initiation ceremony
2. Mark of defilement imposed on slaves or prisoners of war
3. Form of social control in patriarchal societies
4. Method of "pain imprinting" to enhance the child's ability for survival later in life
5. Mark of cultural identity
6. Fertility rite
7. Hygienic or preventive health intervention
8. Measure to control male sexuality
9. Rite of male bonding
   (Gairdner 1949; Kaplan 1983; Dunsmuir and Gordon 1999; Elchalal et al. 1999; Glass 1999; Goldman 1999; Goodman 1999; Hammond 1999; Rizvi et al. 1999; Lerman and Liao 2001; Alanis and Lucidi 2004).

I.8.5.2 Epidemiology of Circumcision

There are substantial differences in circumcision rates in different parts of the world, but approximately 80 % of the world's males are uncircumcised. The prevalence of neonatal circumcision is influenced by religious affiliation, country of origin, ethnicity, residential area, maternal education, socioeconomic status, type of health insurance and the attitudes of parents and physicians (Kaplan 1983; Laumann et al. 1997; Lerman and Liao 2001).

In the United States, the rate of neonatal circumcision declined from about 90 % in the 1950s to around 60–70 % in the 1980s, while recent studies have reported rates varying from 65 % to 82 %. Circumcision is very uncommon in European countries, Central and South America and Asia. In the UK, circumcision rates fell from about 30 % in 1940 to 6 % by 1975. South Korea is the only Asian country where circumcision has been widely performed since the Korean war in the 1950s, with a circumcision rate for high school boys above 90 % (Gairdner 1949; Frisch et al. 1995; Niku et al. 1995; Dunsmuir and Gordon 1999; Goldman 1999; Hammond 1999; Rickwood 1999; Quayle et al. 2003; Alanis and Lucidi 2004).

I.8.5.3 Embryology and Function of the Foreskin

Development of the prepuce begins at 8–12 weeks of intrauterine life and is usually complete by 16–20 weeks. The epithelium of the inner prepuce and glans is stratified squamous in type, with both layers

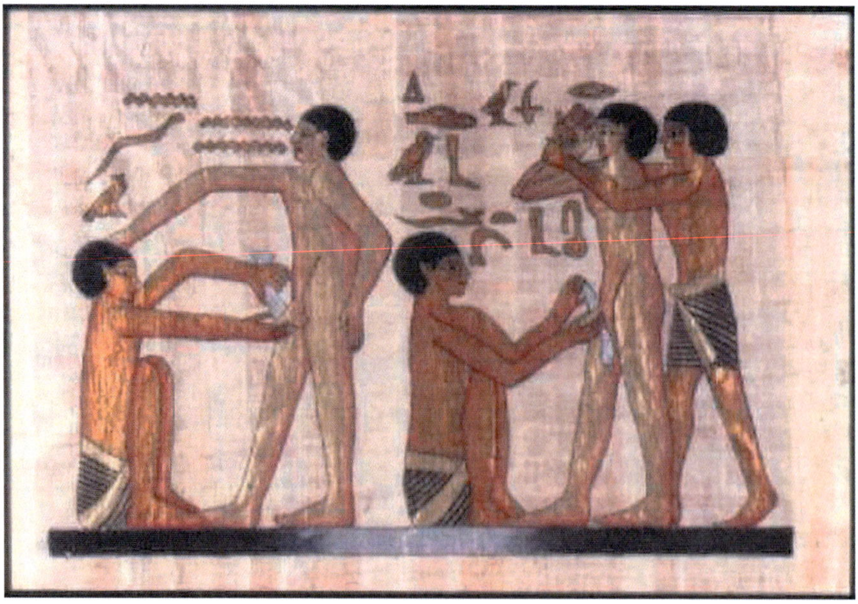

Fig. I.8.16. Modern replica on papyrus of a decoration from the tomb of Ankh-Mahor at Saqqara (2400 BCE), depicting circumcision in ancient Egypt

initially fused to each other. Separation of the prepuce from the glans begins by 24 weeks of gestation, but is usually incomplete at birth. Thus, the normal neonatal prepuce is not retractable. During the first 3–4 years of life, the prepuce and glans separate as a consequence of several processes, including growth of the penile body, accumulation of epithelial debris (smegma) and intermittent penile erections. Ventral or dorsal preputial development is usually deficient with hypospadias and epispadias, respectively (Kaplan 1983; Niku et al. 1995; Cold and Taylor 1999; Lerman and Liao 2001).

Gairdner (1949) found that the incidence of a nonretractable prepuce progressively decreased from 96% in newborns to 6% in boys aged 5–13 years. Similarly, Øster (1968) found that the foreskin was retractable in almost all boys by 17 years of age (Fig. I.8.17).

Kayaba et al. (1996) classified preputial status into five types based on retractability and found that the incidence of type V prepuce (easy exposure of the whole glans) increased from 0 in boys younger than 1 year to 63% in those 11–15 years old. A tight prepuce, defined as a stenotic ring that prevented the prepuce from being retracted, decreased from 84% at ages 0–6 months to 9% at 11–15 years.

Smegma is a white, creamy material consisting of desquamated epithelial cells which may collect under the prepuce. Male smegma contains steroids, sterols and fatty acids which may have a protective function. In boys 5–13 years old, inspissated smegma may become malodorous, which does not occur in younger boys. The production of smegma increases in quantity at the age of 12–13 years.

Uropathogenic bacteria adhere to and readily colonize the mucosal (inner) surface of the foreskin. In newborn boys, the periurethral area is colonized with aerobic bacteria, especially *Escherichia coli*, enterococci and staphylococci, but this colonization disappears during the 1st year of life. After about 5 years of age, periurethral colonization by uropathogens is found only in boys who get recurrent UTIs (Gairdner 1949; Øster 1968; American Academy of Pediatrics 1999; Cold and Taylor 1999).

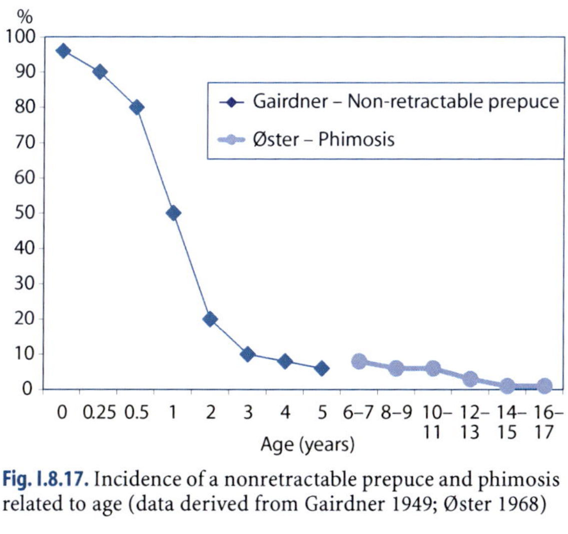

Fig. I.8.17. Incidence of a nonretractable prepuce and phimosis related to age (data derived from Gairdner 1949; Øster 1968)

The prepuce is often regarded as a redundant vestigial structure, but its functions may include:

1. Preventing meatal ulceration due to injury of the glans by contact with sodden nappies
2. Enhancing the pleasure of sexual activity by means of its sensory innervation
3. Providing lubrication for atraumatic vaginal intercourse
4. Forming part of the cutaneous mucosal immune system, because it contains Langerhans cells
5. Being a source of live human fibroblasts for cell-culture research
6. Providing tissue for genital tract reconstructive surgery
   (Gairdner 1949; Cold and Taylor 1999; Dunsmuir and Gordon 1999; Hammond 1999).

I.8.5.4 Indications for Circumcision

Indications for circumcision include:

1. Pathological phimosis
2. Recurrent paraphimosis
3. Recurrent balanitis or balanoposthitis
4. Lichen sclerosus of the penis (balanitis xerotica obliterans)
5. Condylomata acuminata (if extensive) and rare lesions such as lymphogenous cysts of the prepuce, and chronic penile lymphoedema
6. In preparation for placement of a penile prosthesis (not always necessary)
7. As part of genital reconstructive surgery for hypospadias or urethral stricture
8. Nonmedical indications: religious, cultural (parental advice), social (peer pressure), or personal (enhanced sexuality or self-image of a larger penis) (Niku et al. 1995; Cold and Taylor 1999; Kim et al. 1999; Rickwood 1999; Fink et al. 2002).

I.8.5.4.1 Pathological Phimosis

Physiological phimosis (nonretractable foreskin) seen in the infant is not an indication for circumcision. When one draws the penile shaft skin towards the base of the penis, a pinpoint opening is frequently noted, creating the impression of pathological phimosis. However, if one were to draw the prepuce distally instead, one would see that the preputial opening is quite wide and would not interfere with voiding. This is often mistakenly termed pin-hole meatus, but it is not an indication for circumcision.

True pathological phimosis is characterized by a white, scarred and/or indurated meatal orifice, with no "flowering" on attempted retraction of the foreskin. True phimosis is rare below the age of 5 years, and affects only 0.6 – 4 % of boys by the age of 17, and 0.9 % of men aged 19 – 31 years. Pathological (cicatrizing) phimosis shows histological appearances characteristic of balanitis xerotica obliterans (BXO), identical to those of vulval lichen sclerosus et atrophicus. Some authors believe that secondary phimosis may be due to attempts to retract the prepuce, causing tissue damage and scar formation, or that chronic inflammation of the foreskin may lead to scarring. True pathological phimosis that is resistant to topical corticosteroid treatment represents an absolute indication for circumcision. However, some patients may prefer to avoid steroid therapy and to proceed directly to circumcision (Gairdner 1949; Øster 1968; Kaplan 1983; Rickwood 1999; Kim et al. 1999; Larsen and Williams 1990).

I.8.5.4.2 Recurrent Paraphimosis

Paraphimosis (phimotic prepuce retracted behind the glans with swelling) is not so rare, especially on a urological service where many cases occur after procedures, but most can be managed conservatively, so that neonatal circumcision to prevent paraphimosis is not warranted. Reduction under local or general anaesthetic is almost always possible without requiring a dorsal slit. Circumcision should be considered only for the rare case experiencing recurrent episodes of paraphimosis, in patients whose paraphimosis cannot be reduced, or in uncircumcised elderly men who require intermittent or chronic bladder catheterization, and who may have a higher risk of paraphimosis (Gairdner 1949; Dunsmuir and Gordon 1999; Rickwood 1999; Lerman and Liao 2001).

I.8.5.4.3 Recurrent Balanitis/Balanoposthitis

Infection or inflammation of the glans (balanitis) and foreskin (posthitis) may occur in isolation, but simultaneous involvement of both structures (balanoposthitis) is much more common. Acute balanoposthitis is characterized by erythema and oedema of the prepuce and/or purulent discharge from the preputial orifice. Common causative organisms are *E. coli* and *Proteus vulgaris*, although in about 30 % of cases in children the preputial discharge is sterile. In adults, most cases are related to mixed infection, often including anaerobes and fungi, especially in diabetics. Posthitis may be part of an ammonia dermatitis due to urea-splitting bacteria liberating ammonia from the urea in urine. Other cases of balanoposthitis are related to contact dermatitis, fixed drug eruption, or psoriasis.

The incidence of balanoposthitis is about 3 % in uncircumcised male children, and only one-third of these experience recurrences. It occurs most often in boys between 5 and 11 years old, suggesting that it is ultimately self-limiting. In adult men, balanitis may occur five times more often in uncircumcised men, especially monilial balanitis in the setting of diabetes mellitus. However, circumcised carriers are more likely to be asymptomatic, potentially making these men a more insidious vector for the spread of yeast infections to women. Clinical experience suggests that diabetics with recurrent balanoposthitis benefit substantially from circumcision, but there are no prospective studies on the value of prophylactic circumcision in diabetic men. Zoon's balanitis may require circumcision, but topical steroid cream or carbon dioxide laser therapy are alternative treatments (Gairdner 1949; Kaplan 1983; Kayaba et al. 1996; Rickwood 1999; Van Howe 1999; Lerman and Liao 2001).

I.8.5.4.4 Penile Prosthesis

Some authors advise circumcision before placement of a semi-rigid penile prosthesis to avoid an oedematous inner-tube deformity of the subglanular skin. However, in men who prefer to remain uncircumcised, satisfactory results may be obtained after the initial preputial oedema resolves. If balanoposthitis is present, a first-stage circumcision is advised to reduce the risk of infection (Lewis and Jordan 2002).

I.8.5.5 Contraindications for Circumcision

Contraindications to performing neonatal circumcision include:

1. Prematurity, or if there is any concern about the well-being of the neonate
2. Any blood dyscrasia, haemophilia, or family history of a bleeding disorder
3. If the ventral foreskin is short or absent
4. A dorsal hood deformity
5. Hypospadias or epispadias
6. Ventral or dorsal chordee, with or without hypospadias
7. Megameatus with an intact prepuce
8. Megalourethra
9. A webbed, small or inconspicuous penis (Kaplan 1983; Niku et al. 1995; Glass 1999).

I.8.5.5.1 Redundant Prepuce

Ammonia dermatitis involving the prepuce may cause thickening of the skin, and this is often labelled a "redundant prepuce", a misnomer that may lead to unnecessary circumcision. Preputial dimensions vary little between individuals, therefore true "redundant foreskin" does not exist and the term, like "pin-hole meatus", should be discarded (Gairdner 1949; Kim et al. 1999; Rickwood 1999).

I.8.5.5.2 Ballooning of the Foreskin

A nonretractile foreskin is often associated with ballooning of the prepuce during micturition. In childhood, the condition is self-limiting, there is no evidence that it signifies urinary tract obstruction and it does not require circumcision (Gairdner 1949; Rickwood 1999; Babu et al. 2004).

I.8.5.5.3 Preputial Adhesions

Preputial adhesions are usually harmless and self-limiting and give rise to symptoms only when their breakdown results in minor episodes of inflammation. The "separation of preputial adhesions" represents unnecessary treatment (Øster J 1968; Rickwood 1999).

I.8.5.6 Complications of Circumcision

The true incidence of complications after circumcision is unknown, because the reported rates vary widely, depending on the type of study (survey vs chart review vs prospective), setting (medical facility vs community), operator (physician vs ritual circumciser), type of instrument used, definitions of specific complications, and length of follow-up. Some studies have reported a complication rate of 0.2 – 0.6% for neonatal circumcision, whereas others have mentioned figures ranging from 1.5% to 10%. The most common complications are haemorrhage, infection, meatal stenosis, frenular ulcer, buried (trapped) penis, preputial adhesions, and incomplete or inadequate circumcision (Gee and Ansell 1976; Kaplan 1983; Niku et al. 1995; Ahmed et al. 1999; Rizvi et al. 1999; Amir et al. 2000; Christakis et al. 2000; Sylla et al. 2003; Alanis and Lucidi 2004).

I.8.5.6.1 Haemorrhage

Haemorrhage is the most common complication, with a reported incidence of 0 – 35%. Most of these episodes are minor and of no clinical consequence, but fatal haemorrhage may be caused by bleeding disorders (Gairdner 1949; Kaplan 1983).

I.8.5.6.2 Infection

Wound infection is the second most common complication, with a reported incidence of 0.2 – 10%. Most of these infections are minor and of no consequence. Hesitancy and dysuria is seen in as many as 60% of older boys, and UTI may occur. Ritual circumcision in rural areas of developing countries often takes place under unsanitary conditions, which may contribute to infective complications (Kaplan 1983; Crowley and Kesner 1990; Wiswell et al. 1993; Niku et al. 1995; Senkul et al. 2004).

I.8.5.6.3 Recurrent Phimosis

When insufficient skin has been removed, the cosmetic appearance is such that the penis does not appear to have been circumcised. If there is contraction or fibrosis of the preputial ring, true recurrent phimosis can be produced, which manifests as a concealed penis (Kaplan 1983; Williams et al. 2000; Lerman and Liao 2001; Blalock et al. 2003).

I.8.5.6.4 Skin Bridge

A skin bridge between the penile shaft and the glans may tether the erect penis, with resultant pain or penile curvature. It may result from injury to the glans, or from failure to completely free the inner preputial epithelium from the glans at the time of circumcision (Kaplan 1983).

I.8.5.6.5 Meatitis/Meatal Stenosis

Meatitis and meatal ulcers probably occur because the glans is no longer protected by the prepuce from the effect of ammonia produced by bacterial action on urine, and the reported incidence is 8 – 31%. Ulcerative meatitis may lead to meatal stenosis, with a reported incidence of 5 – 10%. Meatal stenosis may also possibly result from devascularization caused by cutting of the frenular artery during circumcision (Gairdner 1949; Kaplan 1983; Niku et al. 1995; Cold and Taylor 1999; Rickwood 1999).

I.8.5.6.6
Pain

There is evidence that during and after neonatal circumcision, babies experience significant pain which can disrupt breast-feeding, mother–infant bonding and sleeping patterns (Goodman 1999; Van Howe et al. 1999; American Academy of Pediatrics 1999; Alanis and Lucidi 2004).

I.8.5.6.7
Rare Complications

Rare but serious complications may occur after circumcision, although their true incidence is unknown, because we have no denominator data. Rare but serious infective complications include septicaemia, Fournier's gangrene (necrotizing fasciitis), staphylococcal scalded skin syndrome (toxic epidermal necrolysis), meningitis, neonatal tetanus, and poststreptococcal glomerulonephritis. Tuberculosis of the penis and genital HSV-1 infection have been described after Jewish ritual circumcision in which a *mohel* (ritual circumciser) performed oral *metzitzah* (sucking on the baby's penis to stop the bleeding). Hepatitis B and C may also be transmitted during ritual circumcision.

Chordee can be produced by a dense scar on the ventrum of the penis. Both hypo- and epispadias have been produced by inadvertently splitting the glans. Epidermal inclusion cysts may be produced by the rolling-in of epidermis at the time of suturing, or by the implantation of smegma in the circumcision wound. Penile lymphoedema may occur, especially if the wound separates or becomes infected. Urinary retention may occur secondary to a tight haemostatic bandage, and may lead to urosepsis, systemic infection, renal failure or bladder rupture. Urethrocutaneous fistula may be caused by crushing the urethra with the circumcision clamp, incising it with a knife or with a suture placed for haemostasis, or by tissue damage due to electrocautery.

Amputation of the distal glans or penis with a Mogen clamp, and penile denudation or degloving injury may occur. Necrosis and slough of the glans or entire penis may result from infection, the use of solutions containing epinephrine, attempts at haemostasis with suture or cautery, prolonged use of a tourniquet or tight bandage, or using contact laser (Fig. I.8.18). Other rare complications include acute heart failure, pneumothorax, gastric rupture, pyogenic granuloma, and subglanular stricture causing a mushroom-like deformity. Death after circumcision may occur due to haemorrhage, sepsis, or anaesthesia (Gairdner 1949; King 1982; Kaplan 1983; Sotolongo et al. 1985; Crowley and Kesner 1990; Niku et al. 1995; Laumann et al. 1997; Dunsmuir and Gordon 1999; Glass 1999; Rizvi et al. 1999; Van Howe 1999; Patel et al. 2001; Ncayiyana 2003; Gesundheit et al. 2004).

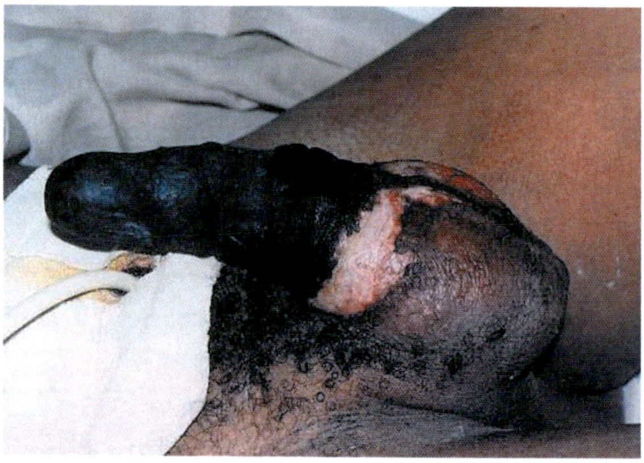

Fig. I.8.18. Gangrene of the penis probably due to use of a tourniquet after ritual circumcision in a young adult who subsequently died of systemic sepsis and multi-organ failure despite emergency penile amputation and treatment in an intensive care unit

I.8.5.7
Current Controversies About Circumcision

I.8.5.7.1
Prevention of Genital Cancer

Neonatal circumcision offers some protection against invasive penile cancer, but it has a less protective effect against carcinoma-in-situ. Circumcision after the neonatal period still carries the risk of development of penile carcinoma, while adult circumcision offers little or no protection. There appears to be at least a threefold increased risk of penile cancer in uncircumcised men, and phimosis increases this risk further. However, the estimated annual incidence of penile cancer is low, ranging from 0.1/100,000 men in Israel to 1/100,000 in the United States and 10.5/100,000 in India. Therefore, even if the risk is increased more than threefold, the likelihood of penile cancer developing in an uncircumcised man is very low. Moreover, there are alternative preventive measures, such as maintaining genital hygiene. One study estimated that circumcision decreases the number of quality-adjusted life years by a mean of 14 h, while another found a mean increase of just 10 days. It has been estimated that with neonatal circumcision almost two complications can be expected for every case of penile cancer prevented (Gairdner 1949; Kaplan 1983; Ganiats et al. 1991; Lawler et al. 1991; Frisch et al. 1995; American Academy of Pediatrics 1999; Van Howe et al. 1999; Christakis et al. 2000; Schoen et al. 2000; Lerman and Liao 2001; Alanis and Lucidi 2004).

Despite conflicting evidence, it appears that male circumcision, together with factors such as monogamy,

I.8

sexual hygiene and the use of barrier contraceptives, may reduce the incidence of cervical cancer in female partners (Niku et al. 1995; Shanta et al. 2000; Castellsague et al. 2002).

I.8.5.7.2
Prevention of Urinary Tract Infection

Bacterial adherence to the epithelial cells of the foreskin leading to periurethral colonization of the preputial sac may predispose to UTI, which may be prevented by circumcision. Recent studies, using cohort and case–control design, indicate a three- to sevenfold increased risk of UTI in uncircumcised boys, with the greatest risk in infants younger than 1 year of age. However, the absolute risk of developing a UTI in an uncircumcised male infant is low (at most about 1%). The relationship between young age at first symptomatic UTI and subsequent renal scar formation and decreased glomerular filtration is not well defined, and there is a lack of information on the sequelae of UTI in infants with a normal urogenital tract. The total cost of managing UTI in uncircumcised males may be ten times higher than for circumcised males, but there is no evidence that neonatal circumcision is a cost-effective prophylactic measure in the management of UTI in children. It has been estimated that it may take 80–100 neonatal circumcisions to prevent one UTI, while six UTIs can be prevented for every complication of circumcision endured. UTI develops more often in uncircumcised patients with vesico-ureteric reflux (VUR), because antibiotic prophylaxis is not effective in reducing bacterial colonization of the prepuce. Therefore, a persuasive case can be made for circumcision in male infants known to have major VUR or other significant structural urinary tract abnormalities. UTI may occur in up to 5% of hospitalized premature infants, suggesting that neonatal circumcision may prove beneficial in these babies, although the operative risk may be higher (Wiswell et al. 1993; American Academy of Pediatrics 1999; Rickwood 1999; Cason et al. 2000; Christakis et al. 2000; Schoen et al. 2000; Cascio et al. 2001; Alanis and Lucidi 2004; Mingin et al. 2004).

I.8.5.7.3
Prevention of Sexually Transmitted Infection

Most of the earlier studies linking uncircumcised status with STIs were not adequately adjusted for potentially confounding factors, such as race, age, socioeconomic status, level of education, number of lifetime sexual partners, frequency of sexual contacts or previous STIs, or cultural, ethnic and healthcare-seeking differences. Moreover, a substantial percentage of boys and men report their circumcision status incorrectly, and even physicians commit errors in the classification of male circumcision status, which could bias studies linking STIs to lack of circumcision. However, in recent studies there appears to be a consistent trend indicating that uncircumcised males may be two to seven times more susceptible to genital ulcer disease (GUD), i.e. herpes, syphilis and chancroid, with lymphogranuloma venereum (LGV) in some populations, while circumcised men are more prone to urethritis. The ulcerative STIs (GUD) are especially important as they are associated with breaks in the genital skin and recruitment of inflammatory cells, with a two- to fourfold increase in the rate of HIV infection and transmission. It has been proposed that, in populations in which safe sexual practices are not adhered to, routine circumcision may help to prevent STIs (Cook et al. 1994; Laumann et al. 1997; Goldman 1999; Lavreys et al. 1999; Van Howe 1999; Diseker et al. 2001; Alanis and Lucidi 2004; Reynolds et al. 2004).

I.8.5.7.4
Prevention of Human Immunodeficiency Virus Infection

Studies on the relationship between circumcision status and the risk of HIV infection have produced conflicting results, and it is possible that behavioural factors may be more important than circumcision. However, it appears likely that there is at least a two- to eightfold increased risk of HIV infection among uncircumcised men at high risk for HIV. The age at circumcision may be a critical factor, with the strongest protective effect seen in those circumcised before the age of 12, and no effect in those circumcised after the age of 20. Recommending circumcision as a public health measure for the prevention of HIV should await the results of controlled clinical trials which are at present being conducted. However, the fact that up to 30% of circumcised African men believe that circumcision protects them completely against HIV and that they could safely have sex with multiple partners, may negate any beneficial effects of removing the foreskin. Furthermore, the cost-effectiveness of circumcision as a preventive measure against HIV transmission needs to be carefully considered (Laumann et al. 1997; American Academy of Pediatrics 1999; Lavreys et al. 1999; Van Howe 1999; Quinn et al. 2000; Weiss et al. 2000; Lerman and Liao 2001; Siegfried et al. 2003; Alanis and Lucidi 2004; Reynolds et al. 2004).

I.8.5.7.5
Sexual and Psychological Consequences of Circumcision

It has been suggested that the severe pain of circumcision and the disrupted mother–infant bond may have long-lasting negative emotional consequences such as feelings of mutilation, low self-esteem, rage, resentment, depression, and a sense of violation or parental betrayal. Decreased sensitivity of the penis after adult circumcision may be perceived as favourable, giving more control over orgasm, or as an irretrievable loss. Surveys of adult men before and after circumcision found no significant difference with regard to sexual drive, erection, ejaculation or overall satisfaction, although the mean ejaculatory latency time was significantly longer (Goldman 1999; Hammond 1999; Kim et al. 1999; O'Hara and O'Hara 1999; Senkul et al. 2004).

I.8.5.7.6 Ethical and Legal Issues

Organizations for the protection of children's rights assert that neonatal circumcision is unethical, because children should not be subjected to prophylactic interventions "in their best interests" or for public health reasons when alternatives exist. It has also been suggested that offering the parents medically unnecessary surgery that will benefit the physician and hospital but not the patient is unethical. Some authors have challenged the legality of neonatal circumcision and argued that it constitutes child abuse, assault and even torture. Several countries have passed specific legislation to prohibit all forms of female genital mutilation (FGM), whereas other countries consider it illegal under existing child-abuse laws. It has been argued that courts have the duty to extend the protection against FGM to male neonatal circumcision. It has also been pointed out that proponents of the argument that FGM and male circumcision are radically different, provide no principled basis and little empirical support for treating male and female genital alteration differently (Laumann et al. 1997; Elchalal et al. 1999; Freeman 1999; Goodman 1999; Van Howe et al. 1999; Hodges et al. 2002).

I.8.5.8 Alternatives to Circumcision

I.8.5.8.1 Topical Steroids

Topical steroid treatment with betamethasone, triamcinolone, clobetasol or mometasone cream twice daily for 1 month has reported success rates of 67 – 95 % with no side-effects. Appropriate candidates are boys older than 3 years who have persistent phimosis and no evidence of infection. Topical steroids were found to be successful in 87 %, 88 % and 75 % of patients with phimosis alone, coexisting balanitis and a history of urinary tract infection, respectively. Sceptics suggest that most of these boys had physiological phimosis (unretractable foreskin), but advocates of the treatment maintain that they included only boys in whom BXO was diagnosed clinically by cicatricial phimosis (Golubovic et al. 1996; Monsour et al. 1999; Rickwood 1999; Webster and Leonard 2002; Ashfield et al. 2003).

I.8.5.8.2 Retraction of the Foreskin

Attempting to free the prepuce forcibly from the glans in small boys usually results in pain and bleeding, and runs the risk of glanular excoriation and injury, with resultant scarring and phimosis, as well as psychological trauma. Forcible retraction of the foreskin can lead to paraphimosis, and should be avoided (Gairdner 1949; Kaplan 1983; Niku et al. 1995; Cold et al. 1999; Rickwood 1999).

I.8.5.8.3 Dorsal Slit and Preputioplasty

The dorsal slit is rarely to be recommended as the cosmetic result is unsatisfactory. However, it is useful in elderly men with multiple medical problems who have severe balanoposthitis or recurrent paraphimosis. Preputioplasty may take the form either of a limited dorsal slit, with transverse suture, or longitudinal incision of the "constrictive ring" proximal to the preputial meatus, again with transverse suture. However, it has been suggested that preputioplasty is a treatment for unretractile foreskin, and not for pathological phimosis, where the operation is either ineffective from the outset, or later becomes so as the disease process restenoses the orifice (Cuckow et al. 1994; Rickwood 1999; Barber et al. 2003).

I.8.5.8.4 Uncircumcision

Surgical procedures to restore the prepuce were first described by Celsus 2,000 years ago, and several modifications have been described in the twentieth century. More recently, some members of the "genital-integrity movement" have severely criticized neonatal circumcision and have propounded the merits of uncircumcision. For the surgeon undertaking preputial restoration surgery, it is essential to carefully counsel the patient about the potential complications, cosmetic results and unusual nature of the surgery (Kaplan 1983; Brandes and McAninch 1999).

I.8.5.9 Conclusions

Male circumcision has long been used for religious and cultural reasons to provide and reinforce group identity. These differences and preferences result in wide variation in circumcision rates among different geographic areas and in various groups.

Male circumcision for specific medical indications clearly confers advantages. Well-established and generally accepted indications for male circumcision include pathological phimosis, recurrent paraphimosis, recurrent balanoposthitis, extensive condylomata acuminata, and as part of genital reconstructive surgery.

Currently, there are at least four major controversies in male circumcision:

1. The risk of genital cancer is definitely decreased by neonatal circumcision, but from the perspective of the risk-benefit ratio it is not a compelling preventive health measure.
2. The risk of UTI in boys is decreased after neonatal circumcision, and the risk-benefit ratio is better than with regard to genital cancer, but still not good enough to recommend routine neonatal circumcision.
3. The reduced risk of HIV infection is a very important question for high-risk populations and one that is under active investigation, but evidence from prospective clinical trials should be awaited before circumcision is propagated as an HIV preventive measure.
4. With regard to reduced sexual pleasure and adverse psychological effects, there is some anecdotal evidence, but this is generally not supported by well-designed prospective studies, and it remains an area of active investigation.

References

Ahmed A, Mbibi NH, Dawam D, Kalayi GD (1999) Complications of traditional male circumcision. Ann Trop Paediatr 19:113–117

Alanis MC, Lucidi RS (2004) Neonatal circumcision: a review of the world's oldest and most controversial operation. Obstet Gynecol Survey 59:379–395

American Academy of Pediatrics (1999) Task force on circumcision. Circumcision policy statement. Pediatrics 103:686–693

Amir M, Raja MH, Niaz WA (2000) Neonatal circumcision with Gomco clamp – a hospital-based retrospective study of 1000 cases. J Pak Med Assoc 50:225–227

Ashfield JE, Nickel KR, Siemens DR, MacNeily AE, Nickel JC (2003) Treatment of phimosis with topical steroids in 194 children. J Urol 169:1106–1108

Babu R, Harrison SK, Hutton KA (2004) Ballooning of the foreskin and physiological phimosis: is there any objective evidence of obstructed voiding? BJU Int 94:384–387

Barber NJ, Chappell B, Carter PG, Britton JP (2003) Is preputioplasty effective and acceptable? J R Soc Med 96:452–453

Blalock HJ, Vemulakonda V, Ritchey ML, Ribbeck M (2003) Outpatient management of phimosis following newborn circumcision. J Urol 169:2332–2324

Brandes SB, McAninch JW (1999) Surgical methods of restoring the prepuce: a critical review. BJU Int 83 [Suppl 1]: 109–113

Cascio S, Colhoun E, Puri P (2001) Bacterial colonization of the prepuce in boys with vesicoureteral reflux who receive antibiotic prophylaxis. J Pediatr 139:160–162

Cason DL, Carter BS, Bhatia J (2000) Can circumcision prevent recurrent urinary tract infections in hospitalized infants? Clin Pediatr (Phila) 39:699–703

Castellsague X, Bosch FX, Munoz N, Meijer CJ, Shah KV, de Sanjose S, Eluf-Neto J, Ngelangel CA, Chichareon S, Smith JS, Herrero R, Moreno V, Franceschi S; International Agency for Research on Cancer Multicenter Cervical Cancer Study Group (2002) Male circumcision, penile human papillomavirus infection, and cervical cancer in female partners. N Engl J Med 346:1105–1112

Cherpes TL, Meyn LA, Krohn MA, Hillier SL (2003) Risk factors for infection with herpes simplex virus type 2: role of smoking, douching, uncircumcised males, and vaginal flora. Sex Transm Dis 30:405–410

Christakis DA, Harvey E, Zerr DM, Feudtner C, Wright JA, Connell FA (2000) A trade-off analysis of routine newborn circumcision. Pediatrics 105:246–249

Cold CJ, Taylor JR (1994) The prepuce. BJU Int [Suppl 1]:34–44

Cook LS, Koutsky LA, Holmes KK (1994) Circumcision and sexually transmitted diseases. Am J Public Health 84:197–201

Crowley JP, Kesner KM (1990) Ritual circumcision (Umkwetha) among the Xhosa of the Ciskei. Br J Urol 66:318–321

Cuckow PM, Rix G, Mouriquand PD (1994) Preputial plasty: a good alternative to circumcision. J Pediatr Surg 29:561–563

Diseker RA 3rd, Lin LS, Kamb ML, Peterman TA, Kent C, Zenilman J, Lentz A, Douglas JM Jr, Rhodes F, Malotte KC, Iatesta M (2001) Fleeting foreskins: the misclassification of male circumcision status. Sex Transm Dis 28:330–335

Dunsmuir WD, Gordon EM (1999) The history of circumcision. BJU Int 83 [Suppl 1]:1–12

Elchalal U, Ben-ami B, Brzezinski A (1999) Female circumcision: the peril remains. BJU Int 83 [Suppl 1]:103–108

Fink KS, Carson CC, DeVellis RF (2002) Adult circumcision outcomes study: effect on erectile function, penile sensitivity, sexual activity and satisfaction. J Urol 167:2113–2116

Freeman MDA (1999) A child's right to circumcision. BJU Int 83 [Suppl 1]:74–78

Frisch M, Friis S, Kjaer SK, Melbye M (1995) Falling incidence of penile cancer in an uncircumcised population (Denmark 1943–90). BMJ 311:1471

Gairdner D (1949) The fate of the foreskin – a study of circumcision. BMJ 2:1433–1437

Ganiats TG, Humphrey JB, Taras HL, Kaplan RM (1991) Routine neonatal circumcision: a cost-utility analysis. Med Decis Making 11:282–293

Gee WF, Ansell JS (1976) Neonatal circumcision: a ten year overview with comparison of the Gomco clamp and the Plastibell device. Pediatrics 58:824–827

Gesundheit B, Grisaru-Soen G, Greenberg D, Levtzion-Korach O, Malkin D, Petric M, Koren G, Tendler MD, Ben-Zeev B, Vardi A, Dagan R, Engelhard D (2004) Neonatal genital herpes simplex virus type 1 infection after Jewish ritual circumcision: modern medicine and religious tradition. Pediatrics 114:259–263

Glass JM (1999) Religious circumcision: a Jewish view. BJU Int 83 [Suppl 1]:17–21

Goldman R (1999) The psychological impact of circumcision. BJU Int 83 [Suppl 1]:93–102

Golubovic Z, Milanovic D, Vukadinovic V, Rakic I, Perovic S (1996) The conservative treatment of phimosis in boys. Br J Urol 78:786–788

Goodman J (1999) Jewish circumcision: an alternative perspective. BJU Int 83 [Suppl 1]:22–27

Hammond T (1999) A preliminary poll of men circumcised in infancy and childhood. BJU Int 83 [Suppl 1]:85–92

Hodges FM, Svoboda JS, Van Howe RS (2002) Prophylactic interventions on children: balancing human rights with public health. J Med Ethics 28:10–16

Kaplan GW (1983) Complications of circumcision. Urol Clin North Am 10:543–549
Kayaba H, Tamura H, Kitajima S, Fujiwara Y, Kato T, Kato T (1996) Analysis of shape and retractability of the prepuce in 603 Japanese boys. J Urol 156:1813–1815
Kim DS, Lee JY, Pang MG (1999) Male circumcision: a South Korean perspective. BJU Int 83 [Suppl 1]:28–33
King LR (1982) Neonatal circumcision in the United States in 1982. J Urol 128:1135
Lagarde E, Dirk T, Puren A, Reathe RT, Bertran A (2003) Acceptability of male circumcision as a tool for preventing HIV infection in a highly infected community in South Africa. AIDS 17:89–95
Larsen GL, Williams SD (1990) Postneonatal circumcision: population profile. Pediatrics 85:808–812
Laumann EO, Masi CM, Zuckerman EW (1997) Circumcision in the United States: prevalence, prophylactic effects, and sexual practice. JAMA 277:1052–1057
Lavreys L, Rakwar JP, Thompson ML, Jackson DJ, Mandaliya K, Chohan BH, Bwayo JJ, Ndinya-Achola JO, Kreiss JK (1999) Effect of circumcision on incidence of human immunodeficiency virus type 1 and other sexually transmitted diseases: a prospective cohort study of trucking company employees in Kenya. J Infect Dis 180:330–336
Lawler FH, Bisoni RS, Holtgrave DR (1991) Circumcision: a decision analysis of its medical value. Fam Med 23:587–593
Lerman SE, Liao JC (2001) Neonatal circumcision. Ped Clin North Am 48:1539–1557
Mingin GC, Hinds A, Nguyen HT, Baskin LS (2004) Children with a febrile urinary tract infection and a negative radiologic workup: factors predictive of recurrence. Urology 63:562–565
Monsour MA, Rabinovitch HH, Dean GE (1999) Medical management of phimosis in children: our experience with topical steroids. J Urol 162:1162–1164
Ncayiyana DJ (2003) Astonishing indifference to deaths due to botched ritual circumcision. S Afr Med J 93:545
Niku SD, Stock JA, Kaplan GW (1995) Neonatal circumcision. Urol Clin North Am 22:57–65
O'Hara K, O'Hara J (1999) The effect of male circumcision on the sexual enjoyment of the female partner. BJU Int 83 [Suppl 1]:79–84
Øster J (1968) Further fate of the foreskin: incidence of preputial adhesions, phimosis, and smegma among Danish schoolboys. Arch Dis Childh 43:200–203
Patel HI, Moriarty KP, Brisson PA, Feins NR (2001) Genitourinary injuries in the newborn. J Pediatr Surg 36:235–239
Quayle SS, Coplen DE, Austin PF (2003) The effect of health care on circumcision rates among newborns. J Urol 170: 1533–1536
Quinn TC, Wawer MJ, Sewankambo N, Serwadda D, Li C, Wabwire-Mangen F, Meehan MO, Lutalo T, Gray RH (2000) Viral load and heterosexual transmission of human immunodeficiency virus type 1. N Engl J Med 342: 921–929
Reynolds SJ, Shepherd ME, Risbud AR, Gangakhedkar RR, Brookmeyer RS, Divekar AD, Mehendale SM, Bollinger RC (2004) Male circumcision and risk of HIV-1 and other sexually transmitted infections in India. Lancet 363:1039–1040
Rickwood AMK (1999) Medical indications for circumcision. BJU Int 83 [Suppl 1]:45–51
Rizvi SAH, Naqvi SAA, Hussain M, Hasan AS (1999) Religious circumcision: a Muslim view. BJU Int 83 [Suppl 1]:13–16
Schoen EJ, Colby CJ, Ray GT (2000) Newborn circumcision decreases incidence and costs of urinary tract infections during the first year of life. Pediatrics 105:789–793
Senkul T, IserI C, sen B, KaratemIr K, Saracoglu F, Erden D (2004) Circumcision in adults: effect on sexual function. Urology 63:155–158
Shanta V, Krishnamurthi S, Gajalakshmi CK, Swaminathan R, Ravichandran K (2000) Epidemiology of cancer of the cervix: global and national perspective. J Indian Med Assoc 98:49–52
Siegfried N, Muller M, Volmink J, Deeks J, Egger M, Low N, Weiss H, Walker S, Williamson P (2003) Male circumcision for prevention of heterosexual acquisition of HIV in men. Cochrane Database Syst Rev CD003362
Sotolongo JR jr, Hoffman S, Gribetz ME (1985) Penile denudation injuries after circumcision. J Urol 133:102–103
Sylla C, Diao B, Diallo AB, Fall PA, Sankale AA, Ba M (2003) Les complications de la circoncision. A propos de 63 cas. Prog Urol 13:266–272
Van Howe RS (1999) Does circumcision influence sexually transmitted diseases? A literature review. BJU Int 83 [Suppl 1]: 52–62
Van Howe RS, Svoboda JS, Dwyer JG, Price CP (1999) Involuntary circumcision: the legal issues. BJU Int 83 [Suppl 1]: 63–73
Webster TM, Leonard MP (2002) Topical steroid therapy for phimosis. Can J Urol 9:1492–1495
Weiss HA, Quigley MA, Hayes RJ (2000) Male circumcision and risk of HIV infection in sub-Saharan Africa: a systematic review and meta-analysis. AIDS 14:2361–2370
Williams CP, Richardson BG, Bukowski TP (2000) Importance of identifying the inconspicuous penis: prevention of circumcision complications. Urology 56:140–142
Wiswell TE, Tencer HL, Welch CA, Chamberlain JL (1993) Circumcision in children beyond the neonatal period. Pediatrics 92:791–793

Problem: Diseases of the Prostate (Infection, Benign Prostatic Hyperplasia, Cancer) I.9

I.9.1 Benign Prostatic Hyperplasia and Prostatic Cancer

S.A. McNeill, S.K.W. Leung

Key Messages

- Benign prostatic hyperplasia and prostate cancer are common conditions which increase in incidence in the ageing male.
- Both conditions may present with lower urinary tract symptoms.
- Digital rectal examination and prostate-specific antigen testing are useful methods for assessing the nature of the disease.
- Benign prostatic disease may be treated medically in many patients.
- Radical prostatectomy and radiotherapy remain the mainstay of curative treatment for organ-confined prostate cancer.

I.9.1.1 Introduction

Benign prostatic hyperplasia (BPH) and prostate cancer are two distinct diseases that commonly affect the prostate in ageing males. The prostate is a gland with accessory sexual function, located around the urethra at the base of the bladder in the male, which enlarges after puberty under the influence of testosterone. The glandular tissues of the prostate are arranged into three zones, as described in the work of McNeal (1981, 1988). The two disease processes tend to affect different areas of the gland. BPH almost exclusively affects the transition zone of the prostate, which is the region surrounding the urethra. Prostate cancer most commonly afflicts the peripheral zone of the gland, although it may also arise in the central and transition zones, which is why digital rectal examination (DRE) provides such a useful assessment of the prostate. Given the different parts of the gland preferentially affected by these diseases, it is not surprising that BPH tends to present with symptoms related to bladder outflow obstruction rather earlier than prostate cancer, whilst men with obstructive urinary symptoms caused by prostate cancer will often have advanced disease (Fig. I.9.1).

I.9.1.2 Aetiology and Pathogenesis

I.9.1.2.1 Benign Prostatic Hyperplasia

BPH is the most common benign tumour in men, which has a pathological prevalence that increases with age: 50% of men aged between 50 and 60 years are affected, and as many as 90% of men aged over 80 years (Berry et al. 1984). The aetiology of BPH is not clearly defined but is likely to involve several factors, including disordered interactions between the stroma (supporting tissues) and epithelium (glandular tissue), and their response to growth factors, androgens and oestrogens. In the absence of functioning testes, BPH does not develop. This observation led surgeons, such as Louis Mercier in 1857, to perform orchidectomy as a treatment for BPH.

The epithelial cells of the glands produce prostate-specific antigen (PSA), a kallikrein protease that is secreted into the ejaculate, where it liquefies the semen, thus promoting motility of the sperm. Consequently, the increase in epithelial tissue associated with BPH often results in a greater amount of PSA entering the serum where it can be assayed. PSA is also produced by epithelial cells which have undergone malignant change in prostate cancer, but the reader is reminded that PSA is specific to prostatic tissue and is therefore not a true marker of prostate cancer. However, the higher the PSA value, the greater the likelihood that prostatic malignancy is responsible.

The stromal tissue of the prostate consists of smooth muscle cells, fibroblasts, neuroendocrine cells, blood vessels, neural tissues and lymphatic vessels. Within the prostate and bladder neck smooth muscle, there is a rich innervation with alpha-adrenergic receptors,

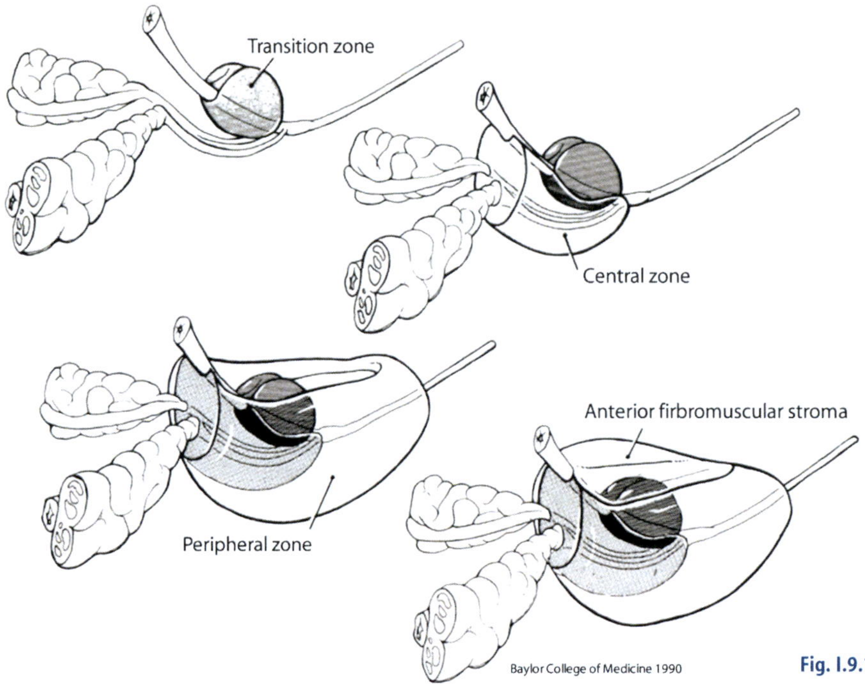

Fig. I.9.1. Zonal anatomy of the prostate

which causes closure of the bladder neck and expression of the prostatic fluid during ejaculation. Increased tone in these smooth muscles is believed to play a part in the bladder outlet obstruction associated with BPH.

I.9.1.3 Prostate Cancer

As with all cancers, the development of prostate cancer is likely to be multifactorial, and there is good evidence that genetic and dietary risk factors play a part. This is manifest by the fact that first-degree relatives of prostate cancer sufferers are themselves at three times greater risk of developing the disease, particularly if their relative develops the disease at a young age. Furthermore, prostate cancer is more common in Blacks and uncommon in Asians. There is also evidence that the Western diet, which is high in fat, increases the risk of prostate cancer (Reiter and de Kernion 2002).

The natural history of prostate cancer is often very long and thus it is possible to detect the disease when it is organ-confined and curable. Much debate centres on screening for prostate cancer using the PSA blood test, but until the results of several large, ongoing trials are available, population screening cannot be recommended.

I.9.1.4 Symptoms, Diagnosis and Treatment

The main lower urinary tract symptoms which arise as a result of bladder outlet obstruction with BPH and prostatic cancer are hesitancy (waiting for the urinary stream to commence), poor urinary flow which may be intermittent, dribbling at the end of the urinary stream (terminal dribble), urinary frequency during the day and night, and urinary urgency where the desire to pass urine is almost uncontrollable. The level of symptoms are assessed by the International Prostate Symptom Score (see Part II), whilst measurement of the urinary flow rate and postvoid residual volume measured by transabdominal ultrasound are useful for assessing the extent of bladder outlet obstruction. Benign pathology is likely if digital rectal examination of the prostate reveals a smooth gland, which is not craggy or hard, and if the serum PSA is within the normal range (see Part II). In symptomatic males, it is important to measure a serum PSA, as those with symptoms may have prostate cancer and a diagnosis of prostate cancer may alter the approach to treatment of the patient's symptoms.

If prostate cancer is suspected because of a raised PSA or an abnormal-feeling prostate on DRE, a transrectal ultrasound (TRUS) -guided biopsy, which is performed under local anaesthetic, is recommended. If a diagnosis of prostate cancer is made on TRUS-guided biopsy, then the patient may require a bone scan and MRI of the pelvis as staging investigations, prior to the optimum treatment strategy being determined for that patient at a multidisciplinary team meeting of oncologists, urological surgeons and associated clinicians and nurses. Prostate cancer is graded according to the scheme described by Gleason and Mellinger (1974), which allows it to be characterized into one of five patterns that reflect prognosis. Prostate cancer is staged according to the UICC TNM staging classification (see Part II).

I.9.1.4.1 Treatment of Benign Prostatic Hyperplasia

Medical Therapy of Benign Prostatic Hyperplasia

Whilst for many years the mainstay of therapy of BPH was the surgical removal of prostate tissue, at open operation or by transurethral resection, medical therapy has become increasingly popular over the last two decades. Alpha-adrenergic blocking agents, which specifically target the alpha-receptors in the prostate (uroselective) result in relaxation of the smooth muscle that is accompanied by an improvement in symptom scores, urinary flow and postvoid residual urine. They do not have any impact on the size of the prostate or the serum PSA.

The other class of agents commonly used are the 5-alpha-reductase inhibitors (5ARI), which inhibit the conversion of testosterone to its more active metabolite dihydrotestosterone within the prostate. This results in a reduction in the glandular volume of the prostate of 18–25% over a period of 3–6 months, which is associated with a reduction in the serum PSA of approximately 50% (McConnell et al. 1998; Roehrborn et al. 2002). Improvements in symptom scores, flow rates and a reduced incidence of acute urinary retention and surgical intervention have been observed. These effects are enhanced if an alpha-blocking agent is combined with the 5ARI (McConnell et al. 2003).

Phytotherapeutic agents are also commonly used in many European countries. Their action is thought to be mainly through 5 alpha-reductase activity.

Surgical Therapy of Benign Prostatic Hyperplasia

For patients with symptoms that are not responsive to medical therapy or who have developed complications of BPH such as refractory urinary retention, surgical removal of prostate tissue remains the treatment of choice. The various approaches to prostatectomy are outlined in Part II.

I.9.1.4.2 Treatment of Early Prostate Cancer

Early prostate cancer, where cancer is confined to the prostate and the PSA is low, can be managed with a curative intent using external beam radiotherapy, brachytherapy (implantation of radioactive pellets directly into prostate) or radical prostatectomy (surgical removal of the entire prostate and seminal vesicles). As many elderly men who are diagnosed with early prostate cancer are unlikely to die of the disease or suffer symptoms related to it, a policy of active monitoring of their prostate cancer may reasonably be adopted. Active monitoring involves regular review of the patients with PSA testing, whilst some recommend a programme of repeat prostatic biopsies.

Radiotherapy

External beam radiotherapy involves a fractionated dose of radiotherapy over a 4- to 5-week period. Using 3D conformal radiotherapy, a dose of up to 74 Gy is delivered, with reported results showing a 5-year biochemical (PSA) recurrence-free survival of up to 79% for patients with T2 disease regardless of tumour grade (Perez et al. 2002). Cystitis and proctitis, the common side effects induced by external beam radiotherapy, are less common with 3D conformal radiotherapy.

Brachytherapy involves the delivery of a dose of radiation to the prostate by the implantation of either iodine (125) or palladium (103) radioactive pellets. This has been shown to have very good biochemical progression-free survival outcomes in patients with low-risk disease [low PSA (<10)], low tumour grade (Gleason 2–6), low stage (T1–T2b) of 87% at 10 years (Grimm et al. 2001).

Radical Prostatectomy

Radical prostatectomy involves the complete surgical removal of the prostate and seminal vesicles. The reported biochemical recurrence-free survival following radical prostatectomy is related to the grade of disease reported on biopsy and the PSA at diagnosis. For those with low-grade and low-stage disease, biochemical progression-free survival rates of up to 95% have been reported at 10 years (PSA<10, Gleason 2–6, Stage T1c) (Han et al. 2001).

It will be apparent to the reader that comparing treatments for prostate cancer in terms of outcome is difficult given the impact of grade, stage and PSA on prognosis. This in turn can lead to difficulty in recommending a particular treatment to any patient. For this reason, a randomized trial of the various treatments, including active monitoring, is being undertaken in the UK (ProTecT Study) for patients with PSA detected disease (Mills et al. 2003). The outcome of this trial is eagerly awaited.

I.9.1.4.3
Treatment of Advanced Prostate Cancer

Once prostate cancer has metastasized, there is no curative therapy; however, suppression of testosterone production has been shown to cause regression of the cancer and improve survival. Whilst surgical castration was widely used in the past, chemical castration has become increasingly popular since the observations of Huggins and Hodge in 1941 of the beneficial effects of oestrogens in patients with metastatic prostate cancer. Depot injections of gonadotrophin-releasing hormone analogue have been shown to be equivalent to castration and may prolong survival for many years, depending on the grade and stage of the cancer at presentation (Albertsen et al. 1998). They act by suppressing the production of luteinizing hormone from the pituitary, which in turn causes a cessation of production of testosterone by the testes. Antiandrogens are sometimes used in combination with LHRH analogues, as they block the effect of circulating testosterone produced by the adrenal glands (maximum androgen blockade).

Chemotherapeutic strategies have had limited success in treating advanced prostate cancer thus far, but with newer agents such as Doclitaxel, improvements in outcomes are promised (Meluch et al. 2004).

References

Albertsen PC, Hanley JA, Gleason DF, Barry MJ (1998) Competing risk analysis of men aged 55 to 74 years at diagnosis managed conservatively for clinically localized prostate cancer. JAMA 280:975–980

Berry SJ, Coffey DS, Walsh PC, Ewing LL (1984) The development of human benign prostatic hyperplasia with age. J Urol 132:474–479

Gleason DF, Mellinger GT (1974) Prediction of prognosis for prostatic adenocarcinoma by combined histological grading and clinical staging. J Urol 111:58–64

Grimm PD, Blasko JD, Sylvester JE, Meier RM, Cavanagh W (2001) 10-year biochemical (prostate-specific antigen) control of prostate cancer with (125)I brachytherapy. Int J Radiat Oncol Biol Phys 51:31–40

Han M, Partin AW, Zahurak M et al (2001) Long-term biochemical disease-free and cancer-specific survival following anatomic radical retropubic prostatectomy. The 15-year Johns Hopkins experience. Urol Clin North Am 28:555-565

Huggins C, Hodges CV (1941) Studies on prostate cancer I. The effect of castration, of estrogen and of androgen injection on serum phosphatase in metastatic cancer of the prostate. Cancer Res 1:293–297

McConnell JD, Bruskewitz R et al (1998) The effect of finasteride on the risk of acute urinary retention and the need for surgical treatment among men with benign prostatic hyperplasia. Finasteride Long-Term Efficacy and Safety Study Group. N Engl J Med 338:557–563

McConnell JD, Roehrborn CG et al (2003) The long-term effect of doxazosin, finasteride, and combination therapy on the clinical progression of benign prostatic hyperplasia. N Engl J Med 349:2387–2398

McNeal JE (1981) The zonal anatomy of the prostate. Prostate 2:35–49

McNeal JE (1988) Normal histology of the prostate. Am J Surg Pathol 12:619–633

Meluch AA, Greco FA, Burris HA et al (2004) Weekly paclitaxel/estramustine phosphate plus carboplatin administered either weekly or every 4 weeks in the treatment of hormone refractory prostate cancer (HRPC): a randomised phase II trial of the Minnie Pearl Cancer Research Network. J Clin Onc 21(14S)(421s): Abstract No. 4659

Mills N, Donovan JL, Smith M et al (2003) Perceptions of equipoise are crucial to trial participation: a qualitative study of men in the ProtecT study. Control Clin Trials 24:272–282

Perez CA, Michalski JM, Mansur D, Lockett MA (2002) Three-dimensional conformal therapy versus standard radiation therapy in localized carcinoma of prostate: an update. Clin Prostate Cancer 1:97–104

Reiter RE, deKernion JB (2002) Epidemiology, etiology and prevention of prostate cancer. In: Campbell's urology, 8th edn. WB Saunders, Philadelphia

Roehrborn CG, Boyle P, Nickle JC et al (2002) Efficacy and safety of a dual inhibitor of 5-alpha-reductase types 1 and 2 (dutasteride) in men with benign prostatic hyperplasia. Urology 60:434–441

See WA, Wirth MP et al (2002) Bicalutamide as immediate therapy either alone or as adjuvant to standard care of patients with localized or locally advanced prostate cancer: first analysis of the early prostate cancer program. J Urol 168:429–435

I.9.2 Prostatitis

M.C. Bishop

Key Messages

- Acute prostatitis is a well-defined infective condition caused by standard uropathogens. Antibiotic treatment may need to be supplemented by surgery to deroof abscesses and release calculi.
- No more than 5 % of patients with chronic prostatitis have unequivocal infection in the urinary tract.
- The majority of the remainder suffer from chronic pelvic pain syndrome (CPPS; new terminology NIH Category IIIA and B).
- In a minority of CPPS cases, inflammatory cells can be identified in expressed prostatic secretion, postmassage urine, seminal fluid or in prostate biopsy samples.
- Prostatic localization tests are not recommended beyond the research clinic.
- New molecular analytical techniques are likely to clarify the link between infection, possibly by fastidious or unusual organisms, inflammation and symptoms of chronic prostatitis.
- Whatever the cause of CPPS, it is likely that treatment aimed at pain management of increasing sophistication will be required to supplement or even replace conventional treatments (antibiotics, nonsteroidal anti-inflammatory agents, alpha-blocking drugs, etc.).

I.9.2.1 Introduction

The early classification of prostatitis described four syndromes for which pelvic pain in the male was the common factor (Drach et al. 1978) (Table I.9.1). The occasional association of lower urinary tract symptoms with the common sign of prostatic tenderness was reassuring, indicating that the condition generically was due to inflammation in the prostate. Having established this commonality, it was then possible to discern that chronic prostatitis was the commonest reason for specialist urological referral in men under 50, with a prevalence in males in the same age group of approximately 10% (Schaeffer 2003). Furthermore, its devastating effect on the quality of life could be compared with unstable angina and Crohn's disease (Wenninger et al. 1996; Pewitt and Schaeffer 1997; McNaughton-Collins et al. 2000).

There was never any doubt about the diagnosis of acute bacterial prostatitis. There was a little less certainty in the criteria for chronic bacterial prostatitis as a focus for recurrent acute urinary infection (Anderson 2002). Unfortunately, the commonest categories of chronic abacterial prostatitis and prostatodynia were very loosely defined according to the presence or absence of inflammatory cells and/or bacteria in expressed prostatic secretion and/or urine passed immediately after massage or in seminal fluid. Unfortunately, the number of white blood cells and organisms diagnostic of prostatitis was never validated. Opinion was markedly divided. On the one hand, there were those who believed in the "common wisdom" dictating that a significant number of cases were caused by bacteria. However, they could not be isolated either because of inadequate bacteriological technique or as a result of the presence of fastidious organisms which eluded conventional laboratory identification. The alternative view of the sceptics was that chronic prostatitis was not a distinct entity at all (Lummus and Thompson 2001; Nickel 2000).

The later NIH classification went some way to providing a compromise and leaving the door open for further research to settle the issue. This was to use the noncom-

Table I.9.1. Classification of prostatitis. (*EPS* Expressed prostatic secretion, *PSA* prostate-specific antigen, *UTI* urinary tract infection, *WBC* white blood cell count)

Category	Name	Defining features	Old classification (Drach et al. 1978)
I	Acute bacterial prostatitis	Acute infection of prostate	Acute bacterial prostatitis
II	Chronic bacterial prostatitis (CP)	Recurrent UTI WBC and +ve culture in EPS, etc. when asymptomatic	Chronic bacterial prostatitis
IIIA	Chronic pelvic pain syndrome (CPPS) inflammatory	Symptoms of CPPS WBC in EPS/postmassage urine/ seminal fluid	Chronic nonbacterial prostatitis
IIIB	CPPS noninflammatory	Symptoms of CPPS, insignificant WBC in EPS, etc.	Prostatodynia
IV	Asymptomatic inflammatory prostatitis	No symptoms Chance finding (e.g. ↑PSA) WBC ± infection in postmassage specimens, inflammation in prostatic histology or cytology	

mittal term “chronic pelvic pain syndrome” to cover both inflammatory and noninflammatory abacterial prostatitis. An interesting new category was also defined: asymptomatic inflammatory prostatitis (Krieger et al. 1999).

It is possible that other perplexing chronic inflammatory states of the genitourinary tract having a well-defined acute phase should be considered as a continuum with prostatitis. Therefore, logically, a case could be made for considering acute and chronic cystitis, epididymo-orchitis, urethritis and prostatitis together.

I.9.2.2 Diagnosis of Prostatitis

I.9.2.2.1 Categories

Acute Prostatitis (NIH Category I)

The diagnosis of acute bacterial prostatitis is invariably straightforward. The background may be important. Patients who have undergone urethral catheterization and instrumentation or prostatic biopsy are at risk, and particularly if they are immune-compromised. They may present with pain in the lower abdomen, perineum, genitalia and lower back, a pyrexial illness and symptoms of irritative or obstructive voiding. Rectally, the prostate will be tender and even fluctuant due to abscess formation. The midstream urine specimen will show a causative organism, which with few exceptions will be a coliform with the frequency of pathogens reflecting the community from which the patient has acquired the organisms. These will invariably already populate the bowel flora. Occasionally, prostatic infection will be associated with urethritis as part of a sexually transmitted infection. The organism will then be *Gonococcus* or *Chlamydia*. Occasionally, and as in females with abacterial cystitis, several types of virus can affect the urothelium and skin simultaneously, e.g. herpes zoster. Lower urinary tract inflammation may lead to the development of systemic sepsis but rarely, generalized inflammatory symptoms may co-exist with lower urinary tract irritation as part of a named syndrome (e.g. Reiter’s, Behçet’s).

Inflammation of the prostate may cause enlargement and acute retention. Serum inflammatory markers may be grossly elevated (ESR, CRP). PSA can rise to levels of more than 100 ng/ml and it is important to understand that it may take up to 3 months after resolution of the acute prostatitis for baseline levels to be resumed (Tchetgen and Oesterling 1997).

Chronic Bacterial Prostatitis (NIH Category II)

A hallmark of a small minority of men with this condition is recurrent episodes of urinary tract infection caused by one of the standard pathogens (commonly *Escherichia coli*). There may be irritative or less often obstructive lower urinary tract symptoms and patients often complain of pain in the perineum, lower abdomen, genitalia, back and lower rectum. These men also present with exacerbations of acute urinary infection with worsening of symptoms of bladder irritation, occasionally pyrexia, abdominal and loin pain. As in acute prostatitis, standard urinary pathogens can be cultured from the midstream specimen during the episodes of UTI. Between these episodes, the prostatic origin of recurrent infection is *apparently* established by the traditional Stamey-Meares four-glass test (Meares and Stamey 1968). Here positive cultures are obtained from material which is assumed to originate in the prostate (expressed prostatic secretion, postprostatic massage urine or specimens of ejaculate). The validity of this test has always been questionable, as Koch’s postulates establishing a microbe as pathogenic are rarely fulfilled. This is discussed in more detail below.

Chronic Pelvic Pain Syndrome (NIH Category III)

The majority of patients presenting with pelvic/perineal pain do not have a history of recent urinary tract infection. There may be a wide variety of additional symptoms, much the same as are found in chronic bacterial prostatitis. In categories II–IIIB of prostatitis, the prostate is variably tender on rectal examination.

In both categories IIIA and IIIB, midstream urine specimens show normal white cell counts and insignificant bacterial colony counts on culture. The distinction between the two is based on the presence of white blood cells in expressed prostate-specific fluid and urine after prostatic massage and/or in seminal fluid. The methodology and significance of positive findings in the Stamey-Mears test and its simpler alternative is considered below.

Some enthusiastic investigators will perform transrectal ultrasound. A wide range of abnormalities may be apparent, but their validity is questionable. The significance of multifocal calcification is not settled. Occasionally prostate cancer can be diagnosed in patients presenting with pelvic pain, minimal or no elevation of the serum PSA, a tender irregular prostate and focal changes on transrectal ultrasound, which encourages the operator to perform biopsies. Investigation of lower urinary tract symptoms and haematuria will of course dictate the need for flow studies, urodynamics, cystoscopy and upper tract imaging.

Rarely prostatic pain will be referred as part of a sacral neuropathy and detailed investigation will then of course be motivated by additional clinical signs. Included in this category is the condition termed pudendal neuralgia. The mere acquisition of a diagnostic label is, for some patients, important when no proof can be advanced.

Category IV Asymptomatic Inflammatory Prostatitis

This is a relatively newly defined category in which there is evidence of inflammation, infection or both in prostate-specific specimens after massage and/or in cytological or histological investigations of prostatic biopsy specimens which have been obtained on account of elevation of the serum PSA (Potts 2000).

I.9.2.2.2 The Stamey-Meares Test

The Stamey-Meares test has been the gold standard for very many years for localizing inflammation and pathogenic organisms to the prostate. Arguably the test was first described in 1930 (Nickel 1930). The protocol is shown in Table I.9.2 and its interpretation in Table I.9.3.

Table I.9.2. Protocol for quantitative prostatic localization (Stamey-Meares). (*VB2* Premassage urine, *VB3* postmassage urine)

1. No voiding 3 h prior to test		
2. Full bladder		
3. Expose glans penis, clean with simple soap solution		
4. Void urine	First 5 – 10 ml Mid stream	VB1 VB2
5. Vigorous prostatic massage for 1 min from periphery to midline. Secretion at meatus – EPS		
6. Immediately after massage void urine	5 – 10 mol	VB3
7. VB1 – 3 and EPS immediate microscopy for WBC (N/HPF) and culture		

The test is difficult to perform. Often EPS is not obtained. False-negative findings are common. Virtually all patients labelled as chronic prostatitis will have been given antibiotics. It is quite possible that bacterial growth will be suppressed even if medication is discontinued for a month before the test is performed. Organisms other than coliforms and of doubtful significance may be cultured (e.g. Gram-positive organisms). A grave drawback is that the results may not be predictive of treatment response. Perhaps for one or more of these reasons, the test is rarely performed. A simplified "poor man's test" describing the use of pre- and postmassage urine has probably been in use unofficially as a substitute for some time (Nickel 1998) (Table I.9.2). Clearly there should be no evidence of urethritis or cystitis, which might easily co-exist with Category II prostatitis. In these circumstances, there is no alternative to treatment with an antibiotic for at least 3 days. Ideally this should not have great tissue penetration and nitrofurantoin is ideal. If chronic bacterial prostatitis is present there will still be an increase in inflammatory cells and positive bacterial culture in the postmassage urine specimen. Unfortunately, culture of the ejaculate is of uncertain significance (Weidner et al. 1991).

I.9.2.2.3 Quantitation of Symptoms

There seems little doubt that the majority of primary care physicians and possibly even urologists regard chronic prostatitis as a diagnosis made on the basis of a symptom complex and will offer standard treatment without bothering with localization studies or, if they

Table I.9.3. Interpretation of Stamey-Meares test. (*CC* Colony count, *WBC* white blood cell count)

NIH Category	TEST	VB1 Urethral urine	VB2 Bladder urine	VB3 Prostate urine	EPS Prostatic fluid	Comments
I	CC WBC	> 10^5/ml +	> 10^5/ml +	Prostatic massage contraindicated	Prostatic massage contraindicated	
II	CC WBC	Few 0	Few ±	> 10^4/ml +	> 10^4/ml +	+ recurrent UTI
IIIA	CC WBC	0 0	0 0	0 +	0 +	Occasionally bacteria cultured in VB3, EPS. No recurrent UTI
IIIB	CC WBC	0 0	0 0	0 0	0 0	
IV	CC WBC	0 0	0 0	0 +	0 +	Occasionally bacteria cultured in EPS/VB3
Cystitis (Infective)	CC WBC	> 10^5/ml	> 10^5/ml	> 10^5/ml	±> 10^5/ml	KASS count quoted but < 10^5/ml can be diagnostic VB1 → EPS can all be +ve in presence of urethritis due to contamination; therefore treat with nitrofurantoin then repeat
Urethritis	CC WBC	±> 10^5/ml +	0 +	0 +	0 0	

do perform them they are not influenced by negative results (McNaught-Collins et al. 2000). The situation is perhaps akin to the official quantitation of lower urinary tract symptoms in the IPSS score. The name implies prostatic pathology and usually BPH. However, this is by no means always the case and the score will certainly not determine a diagnosis. Nevertheless, it is immensely valuable for stratification of symptom severity and more particularly how much quality of life is affected, for epidemiology and trials of treatment. A multiplicity of questionnaires, tools, instruments and indices have been devised (Brähler et al. 1997; Nickel 1998). The common factors in all are self-assessment by the patient on the presence and degree of pain in the genitalia, perineum, rectum and abdomen. Secondly, voiding is assessed both from the point of view of obstructive and irritative symptoms. In some sexual function is assessed.

I.9.2.3 Aetiology of Chronic Prostatitis

I.9.2.3.1 An Infectious Disease?

Most prostatitis specialists feel that the majority of patients suffer from an infectious disease (Nickel 2000). Failure by a urologist to culture an organism is therefore a matter of technical inadequacy. So-called cryptic, fastidious or even nonculturable microorganisms are possible contenders (Weidner and Ludwig 2003) (Table I.9.4). One contentious issue is how long prostate-specific fluid specimens should be cultured. One group considers that EPS or semen should be cultured for 5 days rather than the conventional 2 days (Shoskes et al. 2000). In so doing, patients with white cells in EPS may in fact be shown to have organisms, too. Such patients should perhaps be classified as Category II although officially they may not have had recurrent episodes of conventional urinary tract infection.

Table I.9.4. Causes of chronic pelvic pain syndrome

Conventional uropathogens
Autoimmune reaction (? Previous bacterial infection)
Dysfunctional high pressure voiding (+ intraprostatic duct reflux)
Fastidious/nonculturable organisms/atypical bacteria
Bacterial fragments
Biofilm
Prostatic calculi
Viruses
Chemical irritation from instrumentation, catheterization, etc.
Other diagnoses
Interstitial cystitis
Carcinoma in situ of bladder
Functional somatic syndrome

There is considerable scepticism that patients without objective evidence of inflammation, i.e. Type IIIB do not have a microbial cause. The significance of inflammatory cells in EPS from patients with CPPS must be questioned when the majority of patients have no evidence of inflammation (IIIB). An important study on the histopathology in 368 biopsies from 97 patients with CPPS showed that inflammation was detectable in only 33 % of patients and this was moderate or severe in only 5 % of 97 patients who were evaluated (True et al. 1999). As asymptomatic men with positive white cells in EPS are an entity, perhaps the relationship between pain and white cells or other signs of inflammation is not causal so that the distinction between IIIA and IIIB is artificial. Even positive cultures may be questionable whilst a normal flora of the prostate is still uncertain. However, in a study of patients undergoing radical or transvesical prostatectomy, the data were more reassuring in favour of the conventional view (Hochreiter et al. 2000). Furthermore, a comprehensive analysis of specific PCR (polymerase chain reaction) for all pathogens incriminated in chronic prostatitis and of broad-spectrum PCR in prostate biopsies from men with CPPS undergoing conventional testing showed correlation of EPS white cell concentration with the presence of 16sr DNA (Krieger et al. 2003).

It is possible that the search for inflammatory cells represents a rather crude approach and a more sensitive indication of inflammation might come through the identification of cytokines and various measures of oxidative stress in EPS (Shahed and Shoskes 2000). In one such study, there was evidence of induced antioxidant enzymatic activity and of induction of the appropriate genes in symptomatic patients with positive EPS culture. However, the organisms were predominantly Gram-positive and their relevance would therefore normally be questioned. In a small number of such men, there was a detectable injury response, a favourable clinical response to antibiotics and a reduction of oxidative stress.

A variety of constituents of prostatic fluid alter their concentration rather typically in response to bacterial infection (Table I.9.5) (Weidner et al. 1997). A rise in pH can result from infection with an organism, producing urease or a fall in citric acid concentration. Theoretically this could lead to reduction in bioavailability of certain antibiotics but in practical terms this is not an issue.

Another group investigated IL1 beta and tumour necrosis factor alpha (TNFα) in prostatic secretions (Nadler et al. 2000). The levels appeared to be higher in men with Category IIIA than IIIB and in healthy controls. There was a good correlation between the presence of IL1β and TNFα but none between either and the presence of white blood cells.

It is possible that fungi might be implicated in some cases of prostatitis even if patients are not immunosup-

Table I.9.5. Changes in prostatic secretion in chronic bacterial prostatitis (NIH II)

Rise
pH, IgA, IgG, IgM
LDH5/LDH1
Fall
Specific gravity
Prostate antibacterial factor (PAF)
Cations (zinc, magnesium, calcium)
Citric acid
Enzymes (lysozyme, acid phosphatase)

From Weidner et al. (1997)

pressed (Elert et al. 2000). Specialized culture media and DNA analysis may be required to demonstrate these elusive organisms.

The small numbers of men with Category I or II prostatitis will mainly show coliform organisms of an identical type in urine and EPS. In such patients, there are a variety of potential routes of entry of bacteria into the prostate. Reflux of urine into the intraprostatic ducts is certainly feasible and has been demonstrated using appropriate imaging studies. Similarly, it is reasonable to suppose that heavy colonization of the male urethra with coliforms such as from catheterization instrumentation and anal intercourse can involve the paraurethral glands and prostate. Heterosexual transmission has also been questioned. The presence of calculi within the prostate composed of substances found in the urine but not the prostate (e.g. urate) are also indicative of reflux. Such calculi very often harbour bacteria and may be associated with biofilm, particularly if there is secondary infection from a *Proteus*. The persistence of an inflammatory process initially associated with proven bacterial infection is another fascinating conundrum and is perhaps a common factor in a family of chronic inflammatory conditions including prostatitis, epididymitis and interstitial cystitis.

I.9.2.3.2 Experimental Prostatitis

Rodent and animal models have been used to establish coliform infection of the prostate (Nickel 1997). They may provide important evidence for the origin of continuing chronic inflammation in sterile tissue from acute infective prostatitis which apparently had resolved on appropriate antibiotic treatment. Abacterial chronic prostatitis can also be induced by immunization with syngeneic prostatic tissue components. Another interesting observation in animal models is that bacterial aggregates which adhere to the ductal epithelium become covered with glycocalyx matrix, rendering them relatively resistant to host defence mechanisms and antibiotics in normal tissue concentrations.

Animal models have also allowed another principle to be established, namely that prostatic inflammation may be a consequence of dysfunctional voiding caused by obstruction combined with intraprostatic ductal reflux driving urine into the prostate gland. If the urine is infected acute bacterial prostatitis will develop, but if there has been previous infection a less severe form of chronic bacterial inflammation occurs.

Experimental prostatitis with *E. coli* is well established but there is some evidence in large animal models that *Chlamydia* can also be pathogenic. These models, and in particular the dog, have been used to demonstrate prostate secretion of various antibiotics and to study distribution and pharmacodynamics of the various agents. It was confirmed that several antibiotics, e.g. trimethoprim and quinolones, were preferentially concentrated in the duct systems. It was also shown that the intraduct compartment was likely to be very different in the inflamed gland compared with the normal uninfected gland. Infected ducts could be blocked with debris, leading to unequal distribution of antibiotics apparently present in adequate concentration in the normal gland.

There seems little doubt that animal models will offer great potential in studying the fundamental processes of bacterial invasion and adherence. It is likely that the significance of bacterial DNA fragments detectable by molecular methodology will be clarified.

I.9.2.4 Treatment

I.9.2.4.1 Conventional

Acute Prostatitis

The treatment of acute prostatitis is usually straightforward, but there is a significant risk of endotoxaemia and systemic sepsis. Initially a broad-spectrum antibiotic combination is given, if necessary intravenously, together with supportive or resuscitative measures. Blood and urine cultures should be taken and the antibiotic therapy adjusted according to the sensitivities when they become available. If the clinical response is unsatisfactory or not sustained the presence of a prostatic abscess should be considered and excluded by CT scanning. Rectal manipulations should be avoided after an initial very gentle diagnostic examination, as pressure on the inflamed gland may be extremely painful and encourage systemic spread of infection. A prostatic abscess may drain spontaneously into the urethra or rectum but is quite likely to require deroofing by transurethral resection or preferably incision with the Collins knife. Although there is little guidance from the literature, it is probably wise to continue oral antibiotic treatment for 3 weeks and to check MSU cultures monthly thereafter for 6 months. When the acute infection has settled, it is customary to investigate the urinary tract with some form of imaging. It is almost invariably normal.

Chronic Prostatitis

There is no high-quality evidence base on which to plan treatment of any category of chronic prostatitis.

Antibiotics

It is logical to give a long course of antibiotics in Category II disease, using the sensitivities from microbiological examination of the MSUs during the recurrent episodes of acute urinary infection. If these results are equivocal a clearer indication may be available from culture of EPS or postmassage urine. In the very small number of patients who hover between Category II and IIIA, i.e. those without a history of recurrent urinary infection but in whom there is clear evidence of bacterial infection in the prostate, treatment will logically be based on sensitivities.

A fluoroquinolone is recommended with a presumed Gram-negative therapeutic target (Naber et al. 2000). The new evidence from molecular bacterial analysis would suggest that tetracycline resistance is common and interestingly it is a matter of clinical experience that any initial improvement with a tetracycline-based antibiotic is not sustained (Krieger et al. 2003). Similarly, it was found that the response to antibiotic treatment in Category III patients would be predicted from the presence of bacterial genomic fragments demonstrated by 16 S recombinant real-time PCR (RTPCR) reaction (Shoskes and Shahed 2000). In other words, men with negative cultures and negative reaction could avoid prolonged courses of antibiotics and the corresponding expense and the risk of side effects. Many clinicians will, as an act of desperation, always give antibiotics in CPPS. It is possible that in the future this decision may be refined by use of these molecular techniques.

Generally speaking, there is no evidence that there is a difference in response between antibiotics with or without the addition of anti-inflammatory agents between Category IIIA and IIIB disease. The point has been well made that any benefit could be a placebo effect, particularly as it is short-lived (Weidner et al. 1999).

Prostatic Massage

Prostatic massage may be effective, particularly if undertaken under regional or general anaesthesia (Nickel et al. 1999). The logic is to open blocked ducts and disperse sequestered bacteria, allowing better antibiotic penetration. The presence of prostatic calculi may also inhibit tissue penetration and bacterial clearance, but again there is no hard evidence for this. Transurethral resection may be effective in opening up the pockets of calculi but tends to be used as a last resort, as of course the procedure has to be very radical in removing as much tissue as possible, particularly in the true glandular layer adjacent to the capsule.

Use of Alpha Blockers/Finasteride

The use of alpha-blocker agents is also controversial. Enthusiasts believe there is evidence of external urethral sphincter over-activity in patients with CP/CPPS (Barbalias 2003). However, there is no correlation between response to treatment and the presence or extent of urodynamically proven obstruction. It has even been suggested that it may be responsible for prostatic inflammation and therefore the term "painful male urethral syndrome" may be appropriate. The evidence is poor quality and therefore, as for every other agent or combination used, the trial will be empirical. The evidence for efficacy of finasteride is more convincing and perhaps underrated (Leskinen et al. 1999).

I.9.2.4.2 Alternative Treatments

The bioflavonoid quercetin was found to improve symptoms in patients with CPPS Category IIIA and B disease in a placebo-controlled trial (Shoskes et al. 1999). This naturally occurring substance has a variety of actions, including inhibition of nitric oxide, tyrosine kinase and inhibition of several inflammatory cytokines. Several studies have indicated that the levels of IL1 and TNFα in EPS and semen were higher in men with Category IIIA than IIIB disease.

Interestingly, quercetin has been shown to cause a decrease in levels of isoprostane, a marker of oxidative stress in prostatic fluid.

There are many inconsistencies in relating symptoms to the presence of white blood cells and inflammatory markers in EPS, prostatic histopathology and to the new molecular evidence for the presence of bacterial fragments. Most disturbing of all are the very considerable number of patients who can be categorized as type IV chronic prostatitis. One subgroup concerned asymptomatic patients presenting to a urology clinic for investigation of a raised PSA. Elevated white cells were found in EPS in 42% (Potts 2000). Clearly this could represent a very large number of patients in a population of middle-aged men and could be classified as a control group in the study of inflammatory markers localized to the prostate in relation to chronic pain and other symptoms which constitute the clinical diagnosis of CPPS. A recurring theme in this chapter is the lack of evidence that CPPS is a distinct entity. The point has been well made that any benefit of any of the conventional treatments could be due to placebo effect, particularly as it tends to be short-lived.

I.9.2.4.3 Psychosomatic Aspects

It is important that the clinician should not be permanently focussed upon the prostate as the source of symptoms. Almost every specialty in medicine embodies a series of painful conditions for which no cause can be found. There is undoubtedly a psychological component for any patient in whom conventional testing shows negative results and a wide range of treatments is ultimately ineffective. This is compounded by an unsympathetic, impatient approach by the clinician who may imply to the patient that his symptoms are a reflection of a weak personality or worse still malingering (Wessely et al. 1999).

In other allied specialties, gynaecology and coloproctology, very similar symptoms reflecting muscle spasm within the pelvic floor are found. It may be helpful to view all of these syndromes as one family of conditions occurring in both sexes. In principle there may be rather little difference between chronic epididymal or penile pain syndromes and vulvodynia (Fall et al. 2004). There may be more specific conditions: pudendal nerve entrapment may after all be a real condition but only if symptoms are restricted to unilateral burning sensation and lateral tenderness on rectal examination. There may be delayed pudendal nerve latency on the appropriate side and local anaesthetic may be temporarily effective. MRI scanning may demonstrate the course of pudendal and other pelvic nerves and spinal roots affected by a variety of pathological conditions. A high proportion of patients will respond, if only in the short term, to physical therapy and internal massage to effect a myofascial release of pelvic floor muscle trigger points. This physiotherapeutic technique has been shown to be effective in NIH category III patients (Potts 2003).

A whole range of allied conditions may co-exist, including irritable bowel syndrome, chronic fatigue syndrome, premenstrual pain and non-ulcer dyspepsia. Disruptions in the serotonergic pathways have been implicated. An entity termed the limbically augmented pain syndromes implies an association between treatment of refractory pain and brain functions which may be localized in the limbic system at the rostral end of the brain stem, which links the hypothalamus, pineal body, hippocampus and temporal lobe cortex. These areas control sleep and arousal, libido, aspects of memory and tolerance to stress. The corollary is that all such patients with functional somatic syndromes should be considered together.

Appropriate medication, in particular tricyclic antidepressants, stress management and biofeedback techniques, can all be effective provided they are prescribed as part of a programme planned in a specialized unit and preferably administered by a single clinician with well-developed counselling skills.

References

Anderson RU (2002) Management of chronic prostatitis – chronic pelvic pain syndrome. Urol Clin North Am 29:235–239

Barbalias GA (2003) Why alphablockers in prostatitis? Eur Urol Suppl 2:27–29

Brähler E, Wurz J, Unger U et al (1997) The Giessen Prostatitis Symptom Score. Standardisation of the questionnaire and prevalence of symptoms. J Urol 157:239

Drach GW, Fair WR, Meares EM et al (1978) Classification of benign disease as associated with prostatic pain: prostatitis or prostatodynia? J Urol 120:266–269

Elert A, Von Knobloch R, Nusser R et al (2000) Isolated candidal prostatitis. J Urol 163:244

Fall M, Baranowski AP, Fowler CJ et al (2004) EAU guidelines on chronic pelvic pain. Eur Urol 46:681–689

Hochreiter WW, Duncan JL, Schaeffer AJ (2000) Evaluation of the bacterial flora of the prostate using a 16SrRNA gene based polymerase chain reaction. J Urol 163:127–130

Krieger JN, Nyberg L, Nickel JC (1999) NIH consensus, definition and classification of prostatitis. JAMA 282:236–237

Krieger JN, Takahashi S, Riley DE (2003) Chronic prostatitis: role of uncommon organisms. Eur Urol Suppl 2:19–22

Leskinen M, Lukkarinen O, Marttila T (1999) Effects of Finasteride in patients with inflammatory chronic pelvic pain syndrome: a double blind, placebo controlled pilot study. Urology 53:502–505

Lummus WE, Thompson I (2001) Prostatitis. Emerg Med Clin North Am 19:691–707

McNaughton-Collins M, Fowler FJ, Elliott DB et al (2000a) Diagnosing and treating prostatitis: do urologists do the four glass test? Urology 55:403–407

McNaughton-Collins M, O'Leary MP, Litwin MS et al (2000b) Quality of life is impaired in men with chronic prostatitis: results from the NIH cohort study. J Urol 163 [Suppl]:23

Meares EM, Stamey TA (1968) Bacteriologic localisation patterns in bacterial prostatitis and urethritis. Invest Urol 5:492–518

Naber KG, Busch W, Focht J (2000) The German Prostatitis Study Group. Ciprofloxacin in the treatment of chronic bacterial prostatitis: prospective, non-comparative multicentre clinical trial with long term follow up. Int J Antimicrobial Agents 14:143–149

Nadler RB, Koch AE, Calhoun EA et al (2000) IL-1 beta and TNF-alpha in prostatic secretions are indicators in the evaluation of men with chronic prostatitis. J Urol 164:214–218

Nickel AC (1930) The bacteriology of chronic prostatitis and seminal vesiculitis and elective localisation of the bacteria as isolated. J Urol 24:343–346

Nickel JC (1997) The role of the animal model in the study of prostatitis. In: Bergen T (ed) Urinary tract infections. Infectiology, vol. 1. Kager, Basel, pp 89–97

Nickel JC (1998) Effective office management of chronic prostatitis. Urol Clin North Am 25:677–684

Nickel JC (2000) Chronic prostatitis: an infectious disease? Infect Urol 13:31–38

Nickel JC, Alexander R, Anderson R et al (1999) Prostatism unplugged? Prostatic massage revisited. Tech Urol 5:1–7

Pewitt EB, Schaeffer AJ (1997) Urinary tract infection in urology, including acute and chronic prostatitis. Infect Dis Clin North Am 11:623–646

Potts JM (2000) Prospective identification of national institutes of health Category IV prostatitis in men with elevated prostate specific antigen. J Urol 164:1550–1553

Potts JM (2003) Alternative approaches to the management of prostatitis: biofeedback, progressive relaxation, the concept of somatic syndromes. Eur Urol Suppl 2:34–37

Schaeffer AJ (2003) Epidemiology and demographics of prostatitis. Eur Urol Suppl 2:5–10

Shahed A, Shoskes DA (2000) Oxidative stress in prostatic fluid of men with chronic pelvic pain syndrome: correlation with bacterial growth and treatment response. J Urol 163 Suppl:24

Shoskes DA, Shahed A (2000) Presence of bacterial signal in expressed prostatic secretions predicts response to antibiotic therapy in men with chronic pelvic pain syndrome. J Urol 163 Suppl:23

Shoskes DA, Zeitlin SI, Shahed A, Rajfer J (1999) Quercetin in men with Category III chronic prostatitis: a preliminary prospective, double blind, placebo controlled trial. Urology 54:960–963

Shoskes DA, Mazurick C, Landis R et al (2000) Bacterial cultures of urine, prostatic fluid and semen of men with chronic pelvic pain syndrome: role of culture for two vs five days. J Urol 163 (Suppl):24

Tchetgen MB, Oesterling JE (1997) The effect of prostatitis, urinary retention, ejaculation and ambulation on the serum PSA. Urol Clin North Am 24:283–286

True LD, Berger RE, Rothman I et al (1999) Prostate histopathology and chronic prostatitis/chronic pelvic pain syndrome: a prospective biopsy study. J Urol 162:2014–2018

Weidner W, Ludwig M (2003) Common organisms in urogenital infections with special impact on prostatitis. Eur Urol Suppl 2:15–18

Weidner W, Jantos C, Schiefer HG et al (1991) Semen parameters in men with and without proven chronic prostatitis. Arch Androl 26:173–183

Weidner W, Ludwig M, Schiefer HG (1997) Chronic bacterial prostatitis – a clinical re-evaluation of old woes. In: Bergen T (ed) Urinary tract infections. Infectiology, vol. 1. Karger, Basel, pp 60–66

Weidner W, Ludwig M, Brähler E, Schiefer HG (1999) Outcome of antibiotic therapy with Ciprofloxacin in chronic bacterial prostatitis. Drugs 58 [Suppl 2]:103–106

Wenninger K, Heiman JR, Rothman I et al (1996) Sickness impact of chronic nonbacterial prostatitis and its correlates. J Urol 155:956–968

Wessely S, Nimnuan C, Sharpe M (1999) Functional somatic syndromes: one or many? Lancet 354:936–939

Problem: Male Breast Disorder I.10

I.10.1 Gynaecomastia and Benign Breast Hyperplasia Including Iatrogenic Causes

W. Krause

Key Messages

- Define gynaecomastia by measuring the size of the swelling.
- Look for drugs, hormones and testicular diseases.
- Consider male breast carcinoma and exclude it by mammography, in particular in men from risk families.
- Recommend surgical removal of the enlarged tissue; drug therapy is not successful.

I.10.1.1 Definition, Epidemiology

Gynaecomastia is an enlargement of the male breast. The term is derived from the Greek word "γψνε" (women) and "μαστοσ" (breast). Literally, it originally designates the female breast, and the term "andromastia" would be more correct (Leiber 1995).

There are no generally accepted clinical thresholds of gynaecomastia. It cannot be defined by means of imaging or laboratory examinations and histological signs are unknown. Niewöhner and Nuttall (1984) used a horizontal skinfold as a measure and suggested gynaecomastia, if it exceeded 2 cm (Fig. I.10.1). In our department, we followed this suggestion with two variations (Krause and Splieth 1996): if the BMI exceeded 25 kg/m^2 in the men investigated, the cut-off of the skinfold diameter was 3 cm. Irrespective of the skinfold, a gynaecomastia was assumed if the diameter of the areola mammae exceeded 3 cm.

The pathological substrate of gynaecomastia is not always an increase in glandular tissue, but an increase in fat deposits in this area also leads to an identical clinical appearance. Sometimes this is called pseudogynaecomastia or lipomastia. Although the relation of fatty and glandular tissue may be different, there is no reliable method of discrimination by clinical appearance, imaging or histological examination. (Labhardt et al. 1978). Das et al. (1995) studied 188 men with gynaecomastia by fine needle aspiration and described a pseudogynaecomastia histologically in none of them.

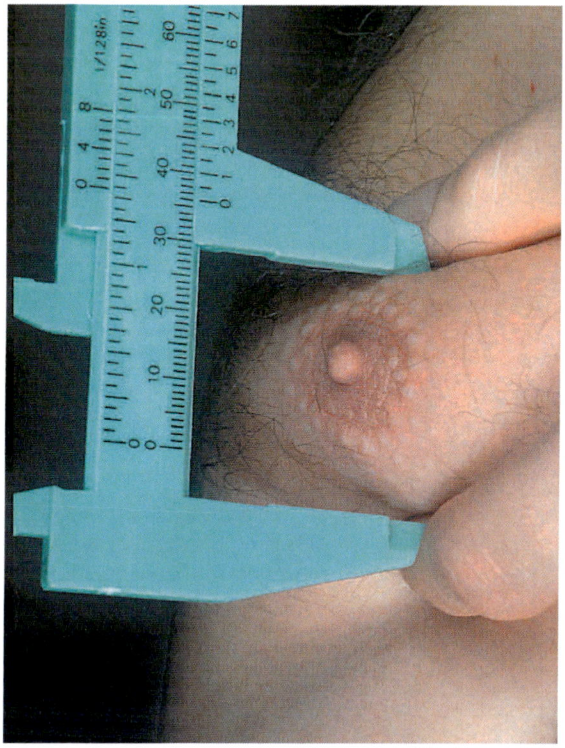

Fig. I.10.1. Measuring horizontal skinfold in gynaecomastia

A physiological gynaecomastia is found in three life periods: in the newborn, where it depends on the maternal oestrogens, in pubertal boys, where it resolves itself spontaneously, and in ageing men. The frequency in the general population is high. Niewöhner and Nuttall (1984) investigated 214 men from 27 to 92 years of age, using a horizontal skinfold as a measure. They found a gynaecomastia in 65% of these men; the percentage was higher in the men older than 50 years. They also observed a correlation with the body mass: men with a high body mass index (BMI) had a higher incidence of gynaecomastia than slender men. In a study with 115 patients in a dermatology department, gynaecomastia was observed in 32 patients (27.8%).

I.10.1.2 Aetiology and Pathogenesis

The male glandular tissue of the breast is oestrogen-susceptible. Gynaecomastia may occur with an increase of oestrogen concentrations at the cellular level because of:

- Enhanced oestrogen serum levels
- An increased on-site oestrogen metabolism or
- An increased sensitivity of the target cells

Most authors address an imbalance of androgen and oestrogen action as a pathogenic factor. Although the presence of androgen receptors in normal and pathological male breast tissue is well proven, the mechanism of an inhibiting androgen action has not been well studied up to now (Calzada et al. 2001).

Enhanced oestrogen serum levels may be the consequence of different mechanisms:

- Oestrogen-producing tumours (most frequently testicular tumours)
- Diseases with altered oestrogen metabolism (e.g. liver diseases)
- Drugs with oestrogen-like side effects (e.g. oestrogen treatment in prostatic carcinoma)
- Accidental oestrogen resorption through the skin (e.g. partner transmission of vaginal oestrogenic creams)

The increased on-site production of oestrogens by increased activity of the aromatase (conversion of androstenedione and testosterone to oestrone and oestradiol) and steroid sulphatase (conversion of oestriol sulphate to oestradiol may underlie most of the drug-induced gynaecomastias. Satoh et al. (2002) studied the effects of 29 drugs which were reported to cause gynaecomastia in vitro by incubating placental microsomes as a source of the enzymes. Table I.10.1 gives selected results of their study.

Enhanced aromatization of testosterone to oestrogens may also occur as a consequence to mutations in the aromatase gene. Isolated mutations were described by Shozu et al. (2003). An activation of the aromatase may also be the cause of gynaecomastia in diabetes mellitus (Seibel et al., 1998). A competitive inhibition of cytochrome P450 CYP3A by calcium antagonists

Table I.10.1. Drugs suspected in the literature to cause gynaecomastia (Satoh et al. 2002)

Drug	Indication	Experimental inhibition of aromatase
Allylestrenol	Nausea	
Chlormadinone acetate	Antiandrogen	12%
Cimetidine	Gastric ulcer	13%
Cyclosporin A	Immune modulator	5%
Famotidine	Gastric ulcer	
Flutamide	Antiandrogen	15%
Griseofulvin	Tinea	
Haloperidol	Schizophrenia	0
Ipriflavone	Phyto-oestrogen	
Isoniazid	Tuberculosis	
Ketoconazole	Tinea	52%
Lansoprazole	Gastric ulcer	
Manidipine	Hypertension	
Metoclopramide	Nausea	18%
Nicardipine	Hypertension	
Nifedipine	Hypertension	19%
Nisordipine	Hypertension	
Nitrendipine	Hypertension	
Omeprazole	Gastric ulcer	19%
Pilsicainide	Hypertension	
Ranitidine	Gastric ulcer	
Spironolactone	Hyperaldosteronism	23%
Sulpiride	Dopamine antagonist	
Tacrolimus	Immune modulator	0
Verapamil	Hypertension	13%

may lead to increased oestradiol levels (Ioulios et al. 2003). The mechanism leading to gynaecomastia in highly active antiretroviral therapy (HAART) for HIV infection is unclear (Jover et al. 2004).

Antiandrogens induce an imbalance of androgen and oestrogen action by blocking androgen action. The compounds are used in prostate cancer, and the incidence of gynaecomastia observed during these treatments varies between 6% and 79% (McLeod and Iversen 2000). During the treatment with bicalutamide (Casodex) in 8,113 patients, gynaecomastia occurred in 47% of cases (McLeod 2002).

Increased sensitivity to oestrogens may be the cause of unexplained gynaecomastia also in the ageing male.

Another rare cause of gynaecomastia is hyperprolactinaemia. Thresholds of prolactin levels, above which gynaecomastia occurs, are not known. The development of gynaecomastia seems to depend on individual sensitivity. It is independent of the cause of hyperprolactinaemia, which may be induced by pituitary adenoma or by drugs (Coppola and Cuomo 1998). In particular, dopamine-like drugs such as selective serotonin reuptake inhibitors are effective in this respect (Damsa et al. 2004).

I.10.1.3 Clinical Features

The term "gynaecomastia" is used in all types of increased breast volume and increased swelling of the male breast region, irrespective of the consistence and of the degree of swelling (Fig. I.10.2). Khan and Blamey (2003) discriminated two forms of gynaecomastia: a lump type and a fatty type. The former is a single firm, often retro-areolar lump, the latter is a diffuse fatty lesion in the whole breast area. The first type is more common in adolescents, the latter in elderly men. The areola may be enlarged and more heavily pigmented (Fig. I.10.3).

Neither the aetiology nor the pathological substrate can be suspected from the clinical appearance, although some authors claim to discriminate "real gynaecomastia" and "pseudogynaecomastia". An increase in glandular tissue and also an increase in fat deposits in this area lead to identical aspects. There is also no reliable histological method of discrimination. Das et al. (1995) studied 188 men with gynaecomastia by fine needle aspiration and described a pseudogynaecomastia histologically in none of them.

The gynaecomastia may be unilateral or bilateral. Bilateral breast masses indicate a low probability of cancer (Volpe et al. 1999). Pain is more common in benign gynaecomastia, but the lack of symptoms is not helpful in differential diagnosis (Giordano et al. 2002). Hyperprolactinaemia is usually associated with bilateral swelling. In most cases, the left side is more prominent.

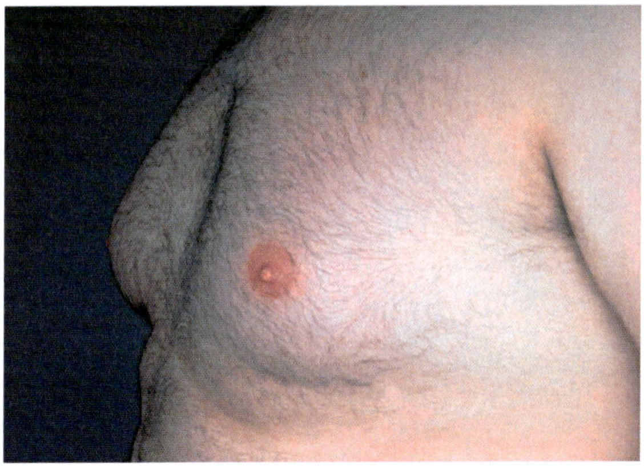

Fig. I.10.2. Gynaecomastia in the adolescent: uniform swelling of the breast surrounding and elevating the nipple

I.10.1.4 Histopathology

Correct diagnosis is impossible without histological examination of an excised tissue. The most frequent differential diagnosis was myofibroblastoma (Magro et al. 2002). Most threatening is the diagnosis of male breast cancer as a cause of breast enlargement.

Williams (1963) described two types of gynaecomastia. Type I, the florid gynaecomastia, is characterized by an increased number of ducts with irregular lumen, in some cases showing pseudolobule formation. The epithelium may have more than three layers, sometimes with small papillae. The ducts may be surrounded by cuffs of connective tissue, which is well demarcated from the normal interlobular connective tissue (Fig. I.10.4). Type II, the quiescent gynaecomastia, shows ducts with normal, unilayer epithelium, but irregular lumen and slight ectasia. No cuffs of connective tissue are seen. The stroma often shows hyalinization and no fibroblastic proliferation (Fig. I.10.5). By immunohistology, PSA immune reactivity is found in normal and hyperplastic duct epithelium in gynaecomastia, but not in male breast cancer (MBC). This may be important for differential diagnosis (Gatalica et al. 2000; Kidwai et al. 2004).

In patients with diabetes mellitus, mastopathy may be observed. There is an inflammatory reaction with

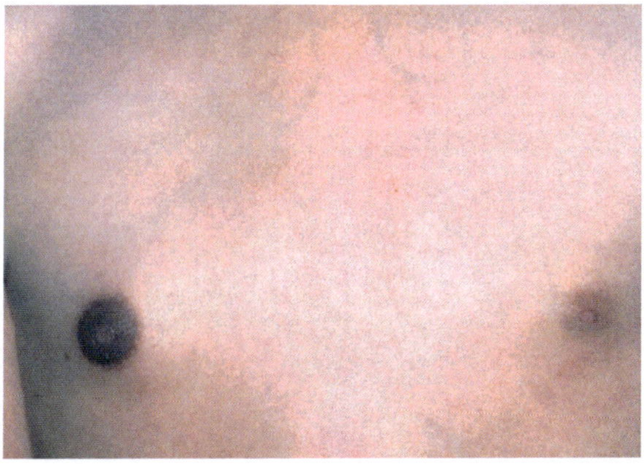

Fig. I.10.3. Enlargement and stronger pigmentation of the areola in gynaecomastia

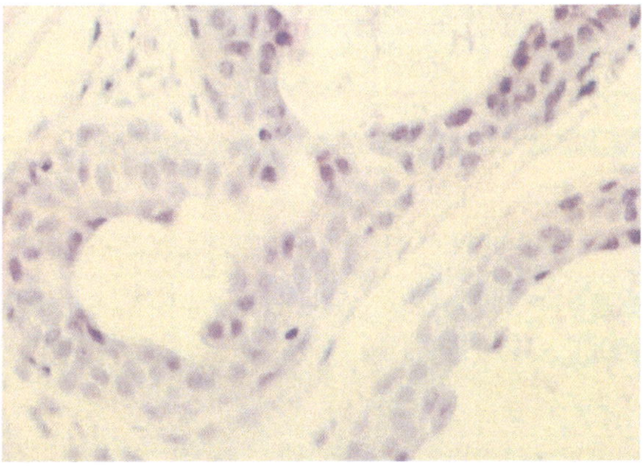

Fig. I.10.4. Histologic picture of florid gynaecomastia. The epithelium may have more than three layers, sometimes with small papillae

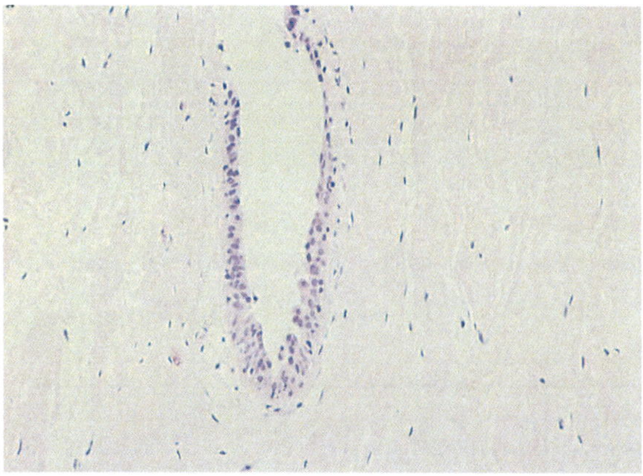

Fig. I.10.5. Histologic picture of quiescent gynaecomastia. Ducts with normal, unilayer epithelium. No cuffs of connective tissue are seen

chronic periductal and perivascular infiltrates and so-called epithelioid stromal fibroblasts within the fibrotic matrix (Hunfeld et al. 1997).

I.10.1.5 Genetic Risk Factors

Genetic causes or risk factors of gynaecomastia itself are not known. However, there is a familial occurrence. Also genetic types of hypogonadism increase the risk of gynaecomastia. In particular, genes enhancing the risk of breast cancer are important to consider in men with gynaecomastia. The most important of these genes is the *BRCA1* gene, and the combination of *BRCA1* and *BRCA2* gene mutations is responsible for approximately 80% of hereditary breast cancer risk (de Jong et al. 2002). BRCA1- and BRCA2-related proteins are produced by the normal mammary epithelium in men and women (Bernhard-Gallon et al. 2003).

I.10.1.6 Diagnostic Procedures

I.10.1.6.1 Clinical Diagnosis

In the history, drugs and diseases causing gynaecomastia have to be ruled out by standardized history taking. Oestrogens, antiandrogens and gestagens are rare, but clear causes. A number of drugs are also suspected of causing gynaecomastia (Table I.10.1). The statements are mostly based on case reports. The authors publishing this table attempted to find evidence for the efficacy of the drugs on grounds of the stimulation of the aromatase (Satoh et al. 2002).

Table I.10.2 shows the results of a small study with 115 patients suffering from gynaecomastia on the frequency of drugs. Eighteen different drugs were quoted,

Table I.10.2. Drugs indicated by the patients with (GM) and without (C) gynaecomastia (from Seibel et al. 1998)

Drug	GM	C	Odds ratio	*P*-value
Diazepam	0	2	0	1.0
Broncholytica	0	2	0	1.0
Urologica	0	2	0	1.0
Sulfonylurea	1	1	2.7	0.3
Insulin	2	0	0	0.07
Antihypertensive agents	0	3	0	0.57
Dermatica	1	2	1.30	1.0
ACE – inhibitors	2	2	2.70	0.30
Antiarrhythmic agents	0	4	0	0.55
NSAR	1	3	0.86	1.0
Allopurinol	3	2	4.19	0.13
Thyreostatica	1	4	0.63	1.0
β-blocking agents	2	3	1.77	0.61
Analgesics	2	4	1.31	0.67
Diuretics	1	5	0.50	1.0
Digitalis glycosides	1	5	0.50	1.0
Coronary dilatator	3	4	2.64	0.39
Ca-channel blocker	2	6	0.85	1.0
Cimetidine	2	2	2.70	0.30

Confidence intervals are not given, because of the low frequency of drugs indicated

but the number of patients taking the drugs was small. No patients were found taking more than two drugs (allopurinol, coronary dilators). None of the drugs was associated with a significant increase or decrease in the risk of gynaecomastia. The highest probability was found for insulin ($p = 0.07$). This may be explained by the stimulation of the aromatase in the mammary gland by insulin, thus inducing higher oestradiol levels within the tissue (Milazzo et al. 1992).

Also, a number of underlying diseases may cause the imbalance of oestrogens and androgen (Fig. I.10.6); these have to be ruled out by specific diagnostic procedures (Table I.10.3). Table I.10.4 enumerates dermatological and other diseases of the patients observed in our study. Also, none of these diseases was associated with a significant increase or decrease in the risk of

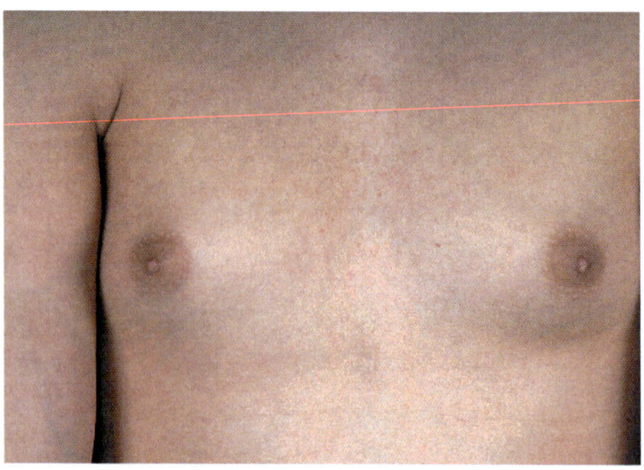

Fig. I.10.6. Gynaecomastia in a patient with Klinefelter's syndrome

Table I.10.3. Causes of gynaecomastia on the basis of oestrogen-androgen imbalance

Hypogonadism	Liver cirrhosis
Testicular tumours	HIV infection
Adrenal tumours	Malnutrition
Other tumours	Alcoholism
Renal failure	

Table I.10.4. Diseases in patients with (GM) and without (C) gynaecomastia (from Seibel et al. 1998)

Disease	GM	C	Odds ratio	Confidence interval	*P*-value
Diabetes mellitus	3	1	8.48	[0.84; 84.81]	0.065
Hyperthyreosis	1	4	0.63	[0.068; 5.92]	1.0
Liver diseases	1	6	0.35	[0.041; 2.96]	0.44
Kidney diseases	4	10	1.55	[0.42; 5.70]	0.49
Cerebral injuries	1	3	2.75	[0.52; 14.44]	0.34
Basalioma	4	18	0.48	[0.16; 1.66]	0.75
Psoriasis	5	11	1.09	[0.38; 3.81]	0.76
Allergic diseases	5	10	1.35	[0.42; 4.31]	0.75
Varicosis	2	9	0.54	[0.11; 2.68]	0.54
Dermatitis	2	7	0.72	[0.14; 3.68]	1.0
Urticaria	6	10	1.68	[0.55; 5.09]	0.26
Melanoma	1	4	0.63	[0.06; 5.92]	1.0
Erysipelas	3	1	8.48	[0.848; 84.81]	0.065
Darier's disease	1	0	0		0.278
Phimosis	2	1	2.64	[0.16; 43.60]	0.48
Psychic discomfort	1	2	1.30	[0.11; 14.92]	1.0

gynaecomastia, although a trend may be read for diabetes (OR 8.48) and erysipelas (8.48). No patients with HIV were included in our study.

I.10.1.6.2 Sonography

B-mode sonography gives unspecific results (Fig. I.10.7). The appearance of a complex cystic mass in the male breast on sonography should suggest the possibility of malignancy and therefore warrants biopsy (Yang et al. 2001).

Schinina et al. (2002) investigated patients with gynaecomastia due to HAART in HIV patients. They could not differentiate between glandular tissue and fat accumulation. They recommended magnetic resonance tomography, which successfully achieved the differentiation. However, they failed to indicate the clinical consequences of their findings.

I.10.1.6.3 Mammography

On the basis of 104 mammograms in 89 men, Merkle et al. (1996) concluded that mammography is necessary only in rare cases, when malignancy is not suspected on clinical grounds. Nevertheless, the investigation of male breast enlargement by X-rays appears to be a useful and reliable method. Appelbaum et al. (1999) described that MBC usually appeared subareolar and eccentric to the nipple. The margins of the lesions were more frequently well defined, and calcifications are less frequent and coarser than those occurring in female breast cancer (FBC). In contrast, benign gynaecomastia usually appeared as a "fan-shaped density emanating from the nipple, gradually blending into surrounding fat." However, there was substantial overlap be-

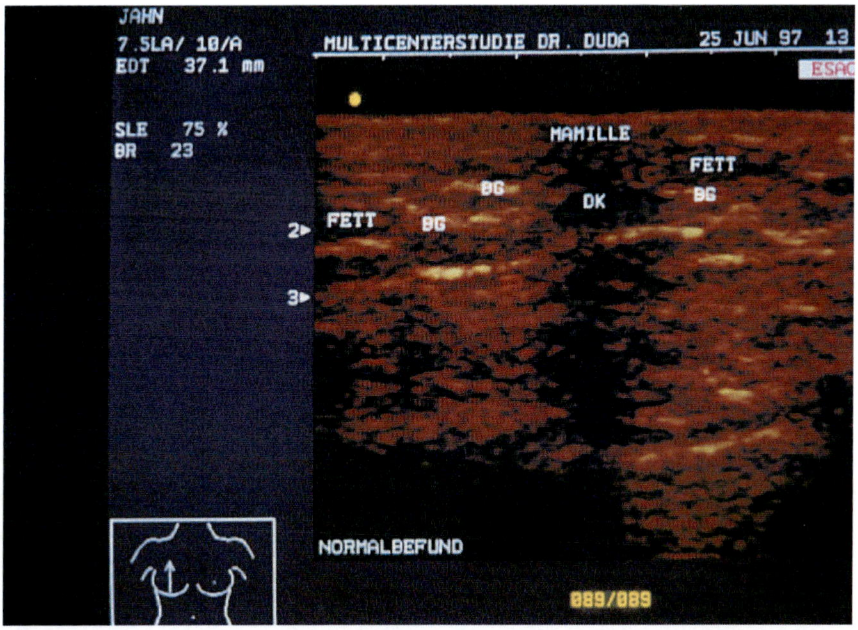

Fig. I.10.7. B-mode sonography: region of lower echogenicity with "dendritic" processus, no cysts or calcification, no distinct solid mass formation

tween these features, in particular chronic inflammation could mimic gynaecomastia.

I.10.1.6.4
Fine Needle Biopsy

Cytology of fine needle aspirates is a very reliable method for the diagnosis of breast lesions. Vetto et al. (1998) compared the results in 51 males with gynaecomastia and six cases with malignancy with histological evaluation of a biopsy. The negative predictive value and specificity for malignancy was 100 %, the positive predictive value and sensitivity was also 100 %. Mammography did not add additional diagnostic information in their series. In a case of secretory carcinoma, cytology was similar to lactational changes or a lactating adenoma (Vesoulis and Kashkari 1998).

Joshi et al. (1999) reported on fine needle aspirates from 507 men in a total group of 13,175 patients. In 393 of 507, the aspirates were satisfactory, 70 of these were positive for malignancy, 295 were negative (58 %), and 29 were inconclusive. With respect to histology as obtained after surgical intervention, FNA in this database had a sensitivity, specificity and diagnostic accuracy of 100 % for male breast lesions. Siddiqui et al. (2002), who had 614 male patients in a total of 14,026 breast fine needle aspirations, reported similar figures. The aspirates were unsatisfactory in 94 patients, 21 of which were operated on. From these 21 patients, 19 had gynaecomastia and two had cancer. They estimated 427 cases to be benign. Thirty-two were diagnosed as malignant, of these were 15 primary cancer and 17 were metastatic tumours. The overall sensitivity with respect to malignancy was 95.3 %, specificity was 100 %, and diagnostic accuracy was 98 %.

Somewhat lower numbers were reported from Westenend and Jobse (2002): the sensitivity was 100 % and the specificity 89 %. The positive predictive value of a diagnosis of malignancy, however, also was 100 %.

Pitfalls in diagnosis by fine needle aspiration cytology have to be considered, such as gynaecomastia following finasteride. There was nuclear atypia particularly and cytoplasmic vacuolization. In the subsequent excisional biopsy, no evidence of malignant change was found. With gynaecomastia in general, extreme caution should be used before rendering a cytologic diagnosis of malignancy (Zimmerman et al. 2000). When gynaecomastia occurs during systemic cytotoxic treatment, it has to be considered that histological severe cell atypia may be seen in benign tissue (Jun Yang 2002). Furthermore, histological evaluations revealed a large body of entities in gynaecomastia. Apocrine metaplasia and epithelial atypia were common findings (Amrikachi et al. 2001).

I.10

I.10.1.6.5
Discrimination Gynaecomastia – Male Breast Cancer

In general, the probability that a breast lump is a cancer is low. Gynaecomastia is not a risk factor for cancer. Olsson et al. (2002), who followed a cohort of 446 patients with gynaecomastia for 20 years and reported on the malignancies in these patients, explicitly stated that no new cases of MBC have been observed. Ambrogetti et al. (1996) reported on 748 consecutive male patients, referred for breast screening, at an average age of 50.5 years. A malignant lesion was detected in 20 patients (2.67 %). Sensitivity for nonmalignancy was 85 % for palpation, 88.8 % for mammography, 93.7 % for cytology and 100 % for ultrasound. Specificity was 95.3 %, 94 %, 95.6 % and 97.9 %, respectively. Combined palpation and mammography had 100 % sensitivity. A history of consumption of drugs known or suspected to cause gynaecomastia does not increase the probability of cancer (O'Hanlon et al. 1995). In the series of 175 men with gynaecomastia in the Daniels and Layer study (2003), at a median age of 44 years, two had testicular cancer, but no MBC was observed. As an outstandingly high percentage, Gill et al. (2000) reported on a series of 150 men, in which 58.66 % had MBC. This high percentage is due to the specific reference practice of their institution.

I.10.1.7
Prevention and Treatment

I.10.1.7.1
Pharmacological

The only drug appearing to be effective is the antioestrogenic compound tamoxifen. Mostly, it was used in adolescent gynaecomastia. Tamoxifen was effective in 83 % of patients (no controlled trial; Khan and Blamey 2003). Results of controlled trials are not available. Although side effects are rare and not severe, Doughty and Wilson (2003) emphasize that the evidence base for the treatment is small. Data are insufficient to show that tamoxifen is safe in this group of patients. Many questions remain unanswered: What effect does it have on bone growth? Does gynaecomastia come back after stopping treatment? What is the optimum duration of treatment? From the view of evidence-based medicine (EBM) the treatment cannot be recommended so far.

I.10.1.7.2
Radiotherapy

As a prevention in hormonal treatment of prostatic cancer, radiotherapy is well proven (McLeod and Iversen 2000). Tyrell et al. (2004) treated 106 men prior to the treatment with bicalutamide either by a single dose

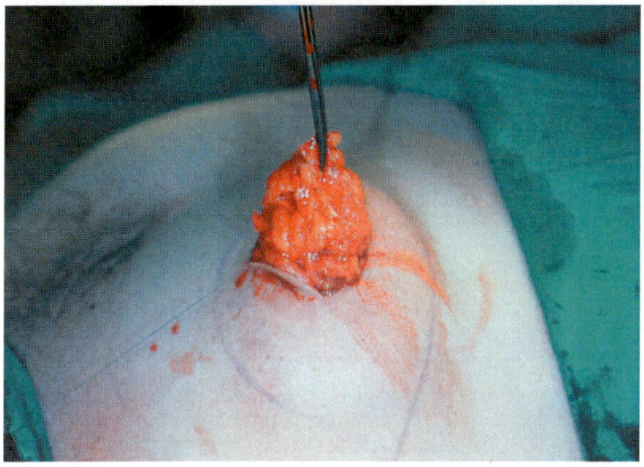

Fig. I.10.8. Surgical treatment of gynaecomastia by semicircular, intra-areolar incision and resection of tissue

of electron beam radiotherapy (10 Gy) or sham radiotherapy. The incidence of gynaecomastia was significantly lower with radiotherapy (52% vs 85%). A similar number of patients in both groups, however, experienced breast pain (83% vs 91%).

I.10.1.7.3 Surgery

The treatment of choice is surgery of the enlarged tissue. There is a great variety of procedures (Rohrich et al. 2003):

- Semicircular, intra-areolar incision and resection of tissue (Fig. I.10.8)
- Nipple transposition on a single derma flap
- Free nipple graft after excision of redundant skin and breast tissue
- Transaxillary approach
- Suction-assisted lipectomy
- Suction-assisted lipectomy, ultrasound guided

The latter is the most successful treatment from a functional and aesthetic point of view.

References

Ambrogetti D, Ciatto S, Catarzi S, Muraca MG (1996) The combined diagnosis of male breast lesions: a review of a series of 748 consecutive cases. Radiol Med (Torino) 91:356 - 359

Amrikachi M, Green LK, Rone R, Ramzy I (2001) Gynecomastia: cytologic features and diagnostic pitfalls in fine needle aspirates. Acta Cytol 45:948 - 952

Appelbaum AH, Evans GF, Levy KR, Amirkhan RH, Schumpert TD (1999) Mammographic appearances of male breast disease. Radiographics 19:559 - 568

Bernard-Gallon DJ, Dechelotte PJ, Le Corre L, Vissac-Sabatier C, Favy DA, Cravello L, De Latour MP, Bignon YJ (2003) Expression of BRCA1 and BRCA2 in male breast cancers and gynecomastias. Anticancer Res 23:661 - 667

Calzada L, Torres-Calleja J, Martinez JM, Pedron N (2001) Measurement of androgen and estrogen receptors in breast tissue from subjects with anabolic steroid-dependent gynecomastia. Life Sci 69:1465 - 1469

Coppola A, Cuomo MA (1998) Prolactinoma in the male. Physiopathological, clinical, and therapeutic features. Minerva Endocrinol 23:7 - 16

Damsa C, Bumb A, Bianchi-Demicheli F, Vidailhet P, Sterck R, Andreoli A, Beyenburg S (2004) "Dopamine-dependent" side effects of: a clinical review. J Clin Psychiatry 65:1064 - 1068

Daniels IR, Layer GT (2003) Testicular tumours presenting as gynaecomastia. Eur J Surg Oncol 29:437 - 439

Das DK, Junaid TA, Mathews SB et al (1995) Fine needle aspiration cytology diagnosis of male breast lesions. Acta Cytol 39:870 - 876

De Jong MM, Nolte IM, te Meerman GJ, van der Graaf WT, Oosterwijk JC, Kleibeuker JH, Schaapveld M, de Vries EG (2002) Genes other than BRCA1 and BRCA2 involved in breast cancer susceptibility. J Med Genet 39:225 - 242

Doughty JC, Wilson CR (2003) Tamoxifen is unproved for gynaecomastia (letter). BMJ 327:1050

Frank TS, Deffenbaugh AM, Reid JE, Hulick M, Ward BE, Lingenfelter B, Gumpper KL, Scholl T, Tavtigian SV, Pruss DR, Critchfield GC (2002) Clinical characteristics of individuals with germline mutations in BRCA1 and BRCA2: analysis of 10,000 individuals. J Clin Oncol 20:1480 - 1490

Gatalica Z, Norris BA, Kovatich AJ (2000) Immunohistochemical localization of prostate-specific antigen in ductal epithelium of male breast. Potential diagnostic pitfall in patients with gynecomastia. Appl Immunohistochem Mol Morphol 8:158 - 161

Gill MS, Kayani N, Khan MN, Hasan SH (2000) Breast diseases in males–a morphological review of 150 cases. J Pak Med Assoc 50:177 - 179

Giordano SH, Buzdar AU, Hortobagyi GN (2002) Breast cancer in men. Ann Intern Med 137:678 - 687

Hunfeld KP, Bassler R, Kronsbein H (1997) "Diabetic mastopathy" in the male breast–a special type of gynecomastia. A comparative study of lymphocytic mastitis and gynecomastia. Pathol Res Pract 193:197 - 205

Ioulios P, Charalampos M, Efrossini T (2003) The spectrum of cutaneous reactions associated with calcium antagonists: a review of the literature and the possible etiopathogenic mechanisms. Dermatol Online J 9:6

Joshi A, Kapila K, Verma K (1999) Fine needle aspiration cytology in the management of male breast masses. Nineteen years of experience. Acta Cytol 43:334 - 338

Jover F, Cuadrado JM, Roig P, Rodriguez M, Andreu L, Merino J (2004) Efavirenz-associated gynecomastia: report of five cases and review of the literature. Breast J 10:244 - 246

Jun Yang Y (2002) Gynecomastia with marked cellular atypia associated with chemotherapy. Arch Pathol Lab Med 126: 613 - 614

Khan HN, Blamey KW (2003) Endocrine treatment of physiological gynaecomastia. Tamoxifen seems to be effective. BMJ 327:301 - 302

Kidwai N, Gong Y, Sun X, Deshpande CG, Yeldandi AV, Rao MS, Badve S (2004) Expression of androgen receptor and prostate-specific antigen in male breast carcinoma. Breast Cancer Res 6:R18–R23

Krause W, Splieth B (1996) Erkrankungen der männlichen Brustdrüse. Hautarzt 47:422 - 426

Labhart A, Hedinger C, Kistler G, Müller J, et al (1978) Testis. In Labhart Klinik der inneren Sekretion, 3. Auflage, Springer, Berlin Heidelberg New York, pp 497 - 499

Leiber B (1995) Aspekte eines polyätiologischen Symptoms: Gynäkomastie. Gyne 16: 237 - 241

Llort G, Munoz CY, Tuser MP, Guillermo IB, Lluch JR, Bale AE, Franco MA (2002) Low frequency of recurrent BRCA1 and BRCA2 mutations in Spain. Hum Mutat 19:307

Magro G, Gurrera A, Scavo N, Lanzafame S, Bisceglia M (2002) Fibromatosis of the breast: a clinical, radiological and pathological study of 6 cases. Pathologica 94:238–246
Mcleod DG (2002) Emerging role of adjuvant hormonal therapy. Urology 60 [3 Suppl 1]:13–20
McLeod DG, Iversen P (2000) Gynecomastia in patients with prostate cancer: a review of treatment options. Urology 56: 713–720
Merkle E, Muller M, Vogel J, Klatt S, Gorich J, Beger HG, Brambs HJ (1996) Clinical relevance of mammography in men. Rofo Fortschr Geb Rontgenstr Neuen Bildgeb Verfahr 164:7–12
Milazzo G, Yip CC,Maddux BA, Vigneri R, Goldfine ID (1992) High-affinity insulin binding to an atypical insulin-like growth factor-I receptor in human breast cancer cells. J Clin Invest 89:899–908
Niewöhner CB, Nuttall RQ (1984) Gynecomastia in a hospitalized male population. Am J Med 77:633–638
O'Hanlon DM, Kent P, Kerin MJ, Given HF (1995) Unilateral breast masses in men over 40: a diagnostic dilemma. Am J Surg 825:170:24–26
Olsson H, Bladstrom A, Alm P (2002) Male gynecomastia and risk for malignant tumors – a cohort study. BMC Cancer 2:26
Rohrich RJ, Ha RY, Kenkel JM, Adams WP Jr (2003) Classification and management of gynecomastia: defining the role of ultrasound-assisted liposuction. Plast Reconstr Surg 111: 909–923
Satoh T, Munakata H, Fujita K, Itoh S, Itoh S, Kamataki T, Yoshizawa I (2003) Studies on the interactions between drug and estrogen. II. On the inhibitory effect of 29 drugs reported to induce gynecomastia on the oxidation of estradiol at C-2 or C-17. Biol Pharm Bull 26:695–700
Scheike O, Visfeldt J, Petersen B (1973) Male breast cancer. 4. Gynecomastia in patients with breast cancer. Arch Path Microbiol Scand A 81:359–365
Schinina V, Busi Rizzi E, Zaccarelli M, Carvelli C, Bibbolino C (2002) Gynecomastia in male HIV patients MRI and US findings. Clin Imaging 26:309–313
Seibel V, Müller HH, Krause W (1998) Die Inzidenz der Gynäkomastie bei dermatologischen Patienten. Hautarzt 49:382–387
Shozu M, Sebastia S, Takayama K, Wei-Tong Hsu, Schultz RA, Neely K, Bryant M, Bulun SE (2003) Estrogen excess associated with novel gain-of function mutation affecting the aromatase gene. New Engl J Med 348:1855–1865
Siddiqui MT, Zakowski MF, Ashfaq R, Ali SZ (2002) Breast masses in males: multi-institutional experience on fine-needle aspiration. Diagn Cytopathol 26:87–91
Tyrrell CJ, Payne H, Tammela TL, Bakke A, Lodding P, Goedhals L, Van Erps P, Boon T, Van De Beek C, Andersson SO, Morris T, Carroll K (2004) Prophylactic breast irradiation with a single dose of electron beam radiotherapy (10 Gy) significantly reduces the incidence of bicalutamide-induced gynecomastia. Int J Radiat Oncol Biol Phys 60:476–483
Vesoulis Z, Kashkari S (1998) Fine needle aspiration of secretory breast carcinoma resembling lactational changes. A case report. Acta Cytol 42:1032–1036
Vetto J, Schmidt W, Pommier R, DiTomasso J, Eppich H, Wood W, Moseson D (1998) Accurate and cost-effective evaluation of breast masses in males. Am J Surg 175:383–387
Volpe CM, Raffetto JD, Collure DW, Hoover EL, Doerr RJ (1999) Unilateral male breast masses: cancer risk and their evaluation and management. Am Surg 65:250–253
Westenend PJ, Jobse C (2002) Evaluation of fine-needle aspiration cytology of breast masses in males. Cancer 96:101–104
Williams MJ (1963) Gynecomastia. Its incidence, recognition and host characterization in 447 autopsy cases. Am J Med 34:103–112
Yang WT, Whitman GJ, Yuen EH, Tse GM, Stelling CB (2001) Sonographic features of primary breast cancer in men. AJR Am J Roentgenol 176:413–416
Zimmerman RL, Fogt F, Cronin D, Lynch R (2000) Cytologic atypia in a 53-year-old man with finasteride-induced gynecomastia. Arch Pathol Lab Med 124:625–627

I.10.2 Skin Diseases of the Male Nipple

W. Krause

Key Messages

- Skin lesions at the nipple may be part of a general skin disease.
- Tumours may be benign or malignant, in particular Paget's disease has to be considered.
- Polythelia is not associated with other general diseases.

I.10.2.1 General Skin Diseases

All the disseminated skin diseases may involve the nipple and the areola mammae. An enumeration of possibilities may be taken from any complete dermatology textbook.

I.10.2.2 Localized Inflammatory Diseases

I.10.2.2.1 Nipple Piercing

Nipple piercing may lead to mastitis. The risks in nipple piercing appear to be underestimated: they may amount to 10–20% in the months after the procedure.

I.10.2.2.2 Mammillary Eczema

Mammillary eczema, an itching and often erosive lesion, causes swelling of the nipple and areola (Fig. I.10.9). It occurs as allergic contact dermatitis after transdermal sensitization with special antigens. In this region, cosmetics, clothes and dyes, detergents, and

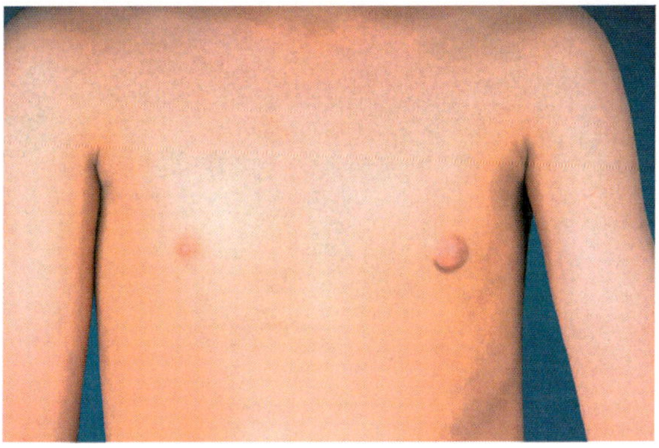

Fig. I.10.9. Mamillary eczema in a patient with atopic dermatitis

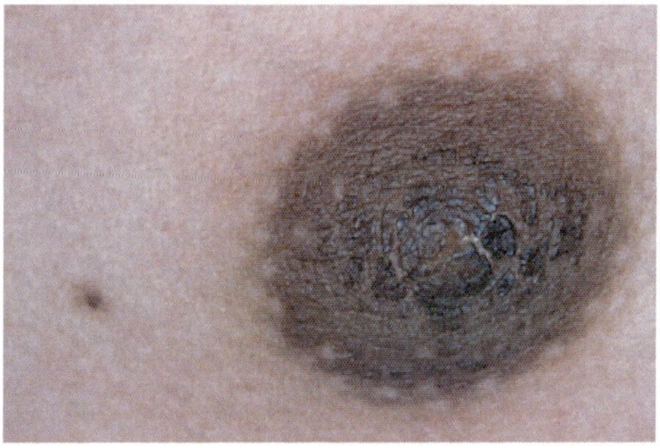

Fig. I.10.10. Nevoid hyperkeratosis: The rete ridges are markedly elongated, and the dermis in the papilla shows filiform acanthosis and hyperkeratosis with largely dilated keratin-filled spaces

scents are of relevance. Another form is part of atopic dermatitis, which is a congenital abnormal reaction of the skin to different influences.

I.10.2.2.3 Lymphadenosis Benigna Cutis

Lymphadenosis benigna cutis is a B cell lymphoma of the skin associated with *Borrelia burgdorferi* infection. Specific sites of this disease are the nipple, scrotum, and earlobe (Gissler and Heininger 2002). Usually, there are polyclonal B cells.

I.10.2.2.4 Nipple Discharge

A discharge from the nipple may indicate inflammation but also an underlying tumour. Since nipple discharge is a rare event, its diagnostic value is limited.

I.10.2.2.5 Naevoid Hyperkeratosis

Naevoid hyperkeratosis (Fig. I.10.10) was described for the first time by Tauber in 1923 (quoted from Kubota et al. 2000). Later, it was classified into three types (Kubota et al. 2000). The first type is part of epidermal naevi, the second type is associated with ichthyosis, the third is the naevoid form in young women. The rete ridges are markedly elongated, and the dermis in the papilla shows filiform acanthosis and hyperkeratosis with largely dilated keratin-filled spaces. The histological appearance resembles the "pomade crust" observed in infants resulting from intense skin care (Gartmann and Steigleder 1975).

I.10.2.3 Tumours

I.10.2.3.1 Areolar Sebaceous Hyperplasia

In the areola, areolar sebaceous hyperplasia is called Montgomery's tubercles. Although anatomically identical to sebaceous glands, these are physiologically different. Areolar sebaceous hyperplasia is different from Montgomery's hyperplasia. It occurs predominantly in women, and there are rare observations in men (Krisp and Krause 2003). It appears as whitish or yellowish plaques with a papillated surface (Fig. I.10.11). Histologically, fully differentiated sebaceous glands are observed. Treatment is not known and not necessary.

I.10.2.3.2 Benign Cutaneous Tumours

Nearly all kinds of benign cutaneous tumours have already been described at the nipple, such as melanocytic naevi (Fig. I.10.12), seborrhoeic keratosis (Fig. I.10.13), skin tags (fibroma pendulans), and venous lakes (angi-

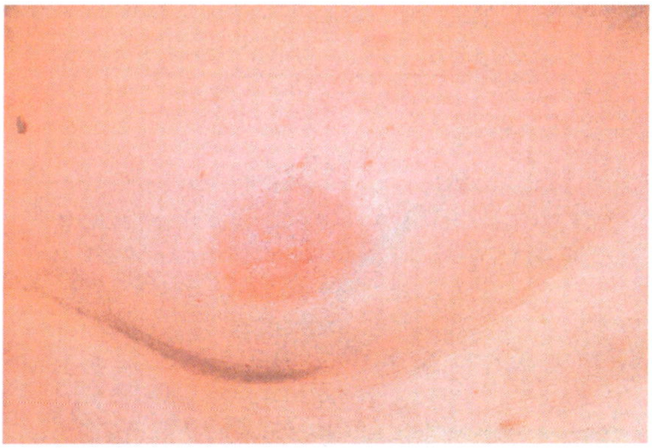

Fig. I.10.11. Areolar sebaceous hyperplasia: whitish or yellowish plaques with papillated surface

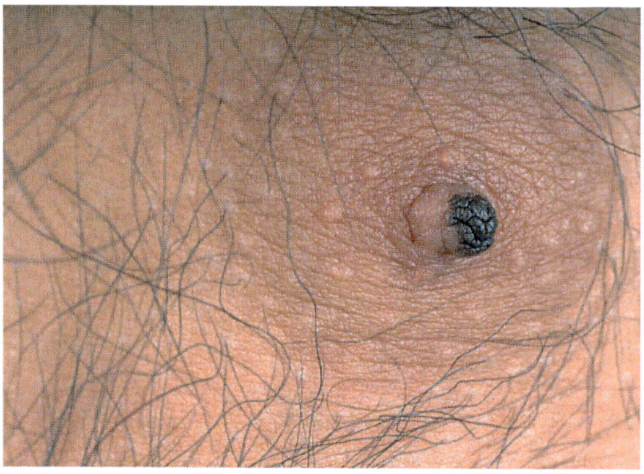

Fig. I.10.12. Melanocytic naevus (mole): brown, soft tumour, existing since childhood

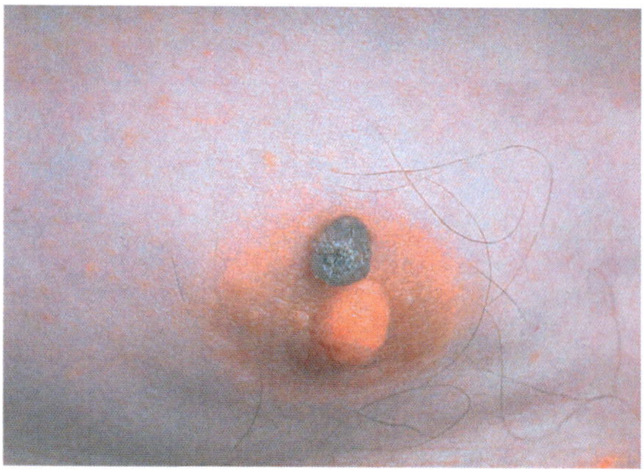

Fig. I.10.13. Seborrhoeic keratosis: flat tumour with rough, warty surface

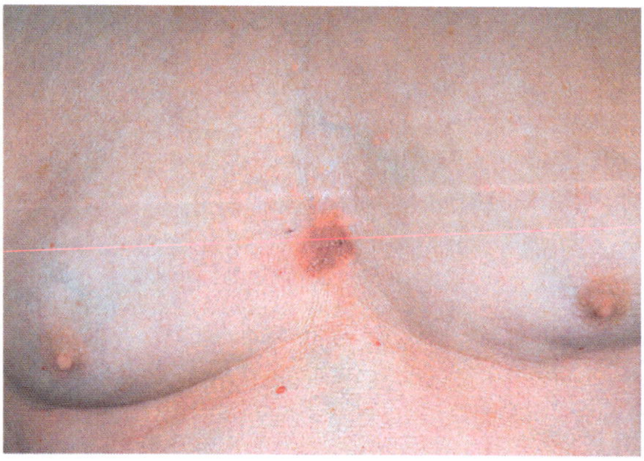

Fig. I.10.14. Basal cell carcinoma may also involve the nipple. It appears as reddish, flat tumour with minor scaling

oma senile). Clinical features and processing are identical to those in other skin areas.

Leiomyoma is a rare benign solitary skin tumour rising from smooth muscles of three types: m. arrector pili, vascular smooth muscles (angioleiomyoma) and the tunica dartos or the mamilla. Leiomyomas of the skin are usually painful, but this does not apply for those of the genital or areolar skin, although the nerve fibres are easily seen as in the other leiomyomas.

I.10.2.3.3 Basal Cell Carcinoma

Basal cell carcinoma (BCC) is the most common cancer in men (Fig. I.10.14). It usually occurs in sun-exposed skin areas, mainly in the face. The appearance on the nipple or the areola mammae is rare; Betti et al. (2003) reviewed 20 cases from the literature. The clinical appearance is similar to that of BCC of the face. An asymptomatic, flesh-colored nodule grows slowly within several months or years. Upon taking a biopsy, the typical histopathological appearance of a BCC is observed. The tumour should be surgically removed.

I.10.2.3.4 Malignant Melanoma

There is no special clinical entity of mammary malignant melanoma, but it occurs at the nipple or the mammilla by chance. The superficial spreading melanoma (SSM) may be mistaken as a benign mole for a long time. Nodular melanoma (NM) shows rapid growth in three dimensions and shows early ulceration. The diagnostic and therapeutic processing does not differ from the melanoma of other skin areas.

I.10.2.3.5 Paget's Disease

Paget's disease designates the intraepidermal spreading of cancer cells around the nipple growing out from a ductal carcinoma. The Paget cells are large, clear cells with positive immunostaining for oestrogen receptor, carcinoembryonic antigen (CEA), epithelial membrane antigen, pan-cytokeratin and human-milk fat globule protein but negative for S-100 or HMB-45 (Nakamura et al. 2001). Expression of cytokeratin-7 is characteristic for Paget cells.

Paget's disease is rarely observed in males. It has to be considered in particular in association with a breast lump. There are several reports in the literature on this disease (Desai et al. 1996; Holloway et al. 1996; Raton et al. 1998; Bodnar et al. 1999; Menet et al. 2001; Chao et al. 2003). Hayes et al. (2000) reported 43 published cases of Paget's diseases in MBC on the basis of a Medline search. In their own observation, there was the unique infiltration of skin adnexa by the malignant cells. Ottuso (2002) reported the first case of infiltrating carcinoma diagnosed on the basis of Paget's disease in the dermatological literature. As a rare variation of Paget's disease, pigmented lesions were also described. The pigmentation results from numerous melanocytes with abundant melanin in close contact with Paget's cells, possibly due to a factor similar to the proopiome-

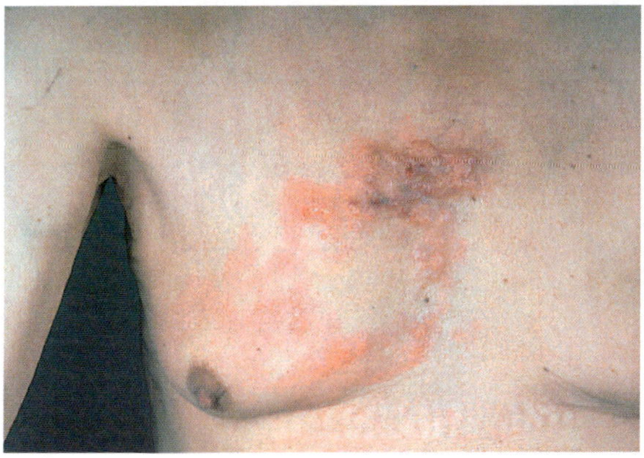

Fig. I.10.15. Carcinoma erysipelatoides: lymphatic spreading of breast carcinoma with involvement of the nipple

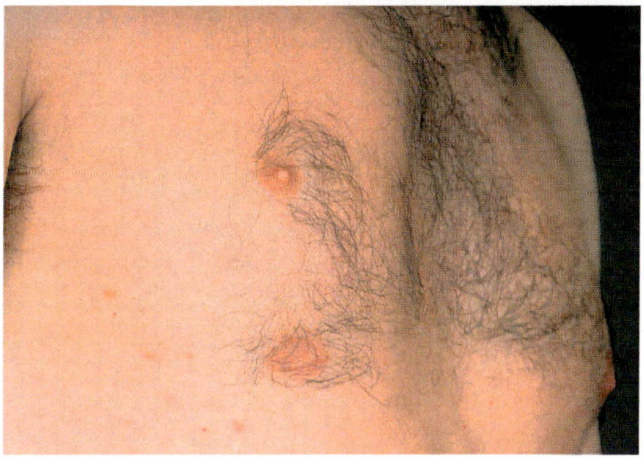

Fig. I.10.16. Polythelia: multiple areola–mamillary complexes in the adult, normal male, hirsute areola

lanocortin (POMC) peptide. These were found to be more frequent than in women (Menet et al. 2001). O'Sullivan et al. (1995) as well as Takeuchi et al. (1999) described Paget's diseases without an underlying carcinoma.

I.10.2.3.6 Breast Cancer

Inoue et al. (2003) presented a case report of a 72-year-old man with nipple enlargement accompanied by a discharge. Histopathological examination of the nipple resection revealed noninvasive intracystic papillary carcinoma of the nipple. The differential diagnosis was benign adenoma of the nipple (gynaecomastia of the nipple; Liebau et al. 1998). In our department, we observed the involvement of the nipple in carcinoma erysipelatoides (Fig. I.10.15).

As in women, male breast cancer has a genetic basis in about 10 % of cases. Mutations of the *BRCA1* and the *BRCA2* genes are responsible for the majority of genetically induced cases. Paget's disease seemed to be more frequent in *BRCA2* mutations (Neuhausen et al. 1998; Ottini et al. 2003).

I.10.2.4 Malformations

I.10.2.4.1 Aberrant Mammalian Tissue

There is a broad clinical spectrum in aberrant mammalian tissue. It occurs as (in decreasing frequency) a nipple alone (polythelia), a nipple with areola (polythelia areolaris), a nipple with adjacent glandular tissue, or a complete breast.

Polythelia is observed in up to 1 % of newborns, usually along embryonic milk lines. In most cases, this phenomenon is observed only in adulthood (Fig. I.10.16). Dermatoscopic observation (epiluminescence microscopy), which is broadly used in the diagnosis of skin diseases, in particular in pigment tumours, is also useful in an accessory nipple. Dermatoscopy reveals a central white scar-like patch with a delicate pigmented network at the periphery, which may be explained by an epidermal hyperplasia, also present in the areola mammae of the original nipple. This appearance is quite similar to that of dermatofibroma (Blum and Roehm 2003). There is also the phenomenon of intra-areolar polythelia, called paired nipples or dysplastic divided nipples (Urbani and Betti, 1996b).

Numerous publications describe the relationship between aberrant mammary tissue (AMT) and kidney–urinary tract malformations. Camacho et al. (1998) observed 72 cases in 3 years, 30 of which were men. No congenital/hereditary nephrourinary defects or sense organ disorders were found. In the literature, the association between aberrant mammary tissue and urinary tract malformations is discussed controversially. In some populations (Jewish and Hungarian), up to 40 % of children born with supernumerary nipples had malformations of the urinary tract. However, there have so far been no explanations for this association. Urbani and Betti (1996a) studied 146 patients with aberrant mammalian tissue. Kidney and urinary tract malformations were present in 11 patients with AMT (nine men, two women) and in one control. These authors are convinced that accessory mammary tissue offers an important clue for congenital and hereditary anomalies of the kidneys and urinary collecting systems.

Polythelia was also observed in Char syndrome (OMIM 169100), which consists of typical face, strabismus, and foot anomalies (Zanolli et al. 2000). There is evidence that Char syndrome is caused by missense TFAP2B (601601) defects acting in a dominant-negative manner.

I.10

I.10.2.4.2
Absence of the Nipple

Absence of the nipple occurs in Finlay-Marks syndrome (OMIM 181270), described in 1978 in a kindred with ten individuals over five generations showing an abnormality of the scalp, ears, and nipples. Although in part the scalp abnormality resembled that of aplasia cutis congenita, the syndrome appeared to be distinctive. The affected persons showed raised, firm nodules over the posterior aspect of the scalp, not covered by hair. Histologically, there was an excess of collagenous connective tissue. The nipples were rudimentary or absent. Women had virtually complete aplasia of the breasts and a small skin dimple without any pigmentation instead of the normal nipple. Dental changes included widely spaced or missing secondary teeth. The ears were cupped or folded and stood out from the head. Axillary apocrine secretion and axillary hair growth were reduced. Fingernails were brittle. Renal and urinary tract abnormalities should be regarded as part of the syndrome.

I.10.2.5
Surgical Interventions

I.10.2.5.1
Excision

The surgical excision of breast enlargement (gynaecomastia) should usually be performed through a circumareolar section with purse-string suture (see Chap. I.10.1). This creates the best aesthetic results, with few complications and little risk of relapse (Persichetti et al. 2000). An alternative surgical procedure in severe gynaecomastia is total mastectomy and free nipple grafting.

I.10.2.5.2
Reconstruction

After bilateral total loss of the nipple due to the treatment of benign and malignant tumours as well as chronic inflammations or trauma, a reconstruction for aesthetic purposes is useful. In order to calculate basic data for such a reconstruction, Beer et al. (2001) carried out a cross-sectional study on the configuration and localization of the nipple–areola complex in 100 healthy men aged 20–36 years; 91 had oval and seven had a round nipple–areola complex. Asymmetry between the right and the left side was rare. The centre of the nipple–areola complex was in the fourth intercostal space in 75% and in the fifth intercostal space in 23% of the subjects. Murphy et al. (1994) calculated the appropriate location of the new nipple from 20 healthy men as models. The average sternal notch-to-nipple measurement was determined to be 21 cm. The nipple plane was located 0.33 times the distance from the sternal notch to the pubis, and the internipple distance was 0.23 times the chest circumference. Spence (1992) reviewed technical details of reconstruction. He concluded that a satisfying reconstruction is difficult.

References

Bayramgurler D, Bilen N, Apaydin R, Ercin C (2002) Nevoid hyperkeratosis of the nipple and areola: treatment of two patients with topical calcipotriol. J Am Acad Dermatol 46: 131–133

Beer GM, Budi S, Seifert B, Morgenthaler W, Infanger M, Meyer VE (2001) Configuration and localization of the nipple-areola complex in men. Plast Reconstr Surg 108:1947–1952

Betti R, Martino P, Moneghini L, Vergani R, Tolomio E, Crosti C (2003) Basal cell carcinomas of the areola-nipple complex: case reports and review of the literature. J Dermatol 30: 822–826

Blum A, Roehm S (2003) Accessory nipple looks like dermatofibroma in dermoscopy. Arch Dermatol 139:948–949

Bodnar M, Miller OF 3rd, Tyler W (1999) Paget's disease of the male breast associated with intraductal carcinoma. J Am Acad Dermatol40:829–831

Camacho FM, Moreno-Gimenez JC, Garcia-Hernandez MJ (1998) Is aberrant mammary tissue a marker for chronic alcoholism or kidney-urinary tract malformations? Dermatology 197:132–136

Cerroni L, Hofler G, Back B, Wolf P, Maier G, Kerl H (2002) Specific cutaneous infiltrates of B-cell chronic lymphocytic leukemia (B-CLL) at sites typical for Borrelia burgdorferi infection. J Cutan Pathol 29:142–147

Chao C, Edwards MJ, Wolfson S, Sewell C, Edwards D, McMasters KM (2003) Paget's disease of the male breast: an unusual case of dermal invasion. Breast J 9:254

Desai DC, Brennan EJ Jr, Carp NZ (1996) Paget's disease of the male breast. Am Surg 62:1068–1072

Elsner E, Thewes M, Worret WI (1998) Guess What! Idiopathic hyperkeratosis and papillomatosis areolae mammae. Eur J Dermatol 8:131–132

Gartmann H, Steigleder GK (1975) Inguinale Pomaden-Kruste der Säuglinge. Z Hautkr 50:667–669

Gissler S, Heininger U (2002) Borrelia lymphocytoma ("lymphadenosis benigna cutis"). Arch Dis Child 87:12

Hayes R, Cummings B, Miller RA, Guha AK (2000) Male Paget's disease of the breast. J Cutan Med Surg 4:208–212

Holloway KB, Ramos-Caro FA, Flowers FP (1997) Paget's disease of the breast in a man with neurofibromatosis. Int J Dermatol 36:609–611

Inoue S, Kunitomo K, Okamoto H, Fujii H, Matsumoto Y (2003) A case of male noninvasive intracystic papillary carcinoma forming a tumor in the nipple duct. Breast Cancer 10:85–88

Jacobs VR, Golombeck K, Jonat W, Kiechle M (2003) Mastitis nonpuerperalis after nipple piercing: time to act. Int J Fertil Womens Med 48:226–231

Kapila K, Verma K (2003) Cytology of nipple discharge in florid gynecomastia. Acta Cytol 47:36–40

Krisp A, Krause W (2003) Areolar sebaceous hyperplasia. Acta Derm Venereol 83:61–62

Kubota Y, Koga T, Nakayama J, Kiryu H (2000) Naevoid hyperkeratosis of the nipple and areola in a man. Br J Dermatol 142:382–384

Liebau J, Machens HG, Berger A (1998) Gynecomastia of the male nipple. Ann Plast Surg 40:678–681

Lundquist K, Kohler S, Rouse RV (1999) Intraepidermal cytokeratin 7 expression is not restricted to Paget cells but is also seen in Toker cells and Merkel cells. Am J Surg Pathol 23: 212–219

Menet E, Vabres P, Brecheteau P, Bonneau-Herve F, Duport G, Levillain P, Larregue M, Babin P (2001) Pigmented Paget's disease of the male nipple. Ann Dermatol Venereol 128: 649–652

Mitxelena J, Raton JA, Bilbao I, Diaz-Perez JL (1999) Nevoid hyperkeratosis of the areola in men: response to cryotherapy. Dermatology ;199:73–74

Murphy TP, Ehrlichman RJ, Seckel BR (1994) Nipple placement in simple mastectomy with free nipple grafting for severe gynecomastia. Plast Reconstr Surg 94:818–823

Nakamura S, Ishida-Yamamoto A, Takahashi H, Hashimoto Y, Yokoo H, Iizuka H (2001) Pigmented Paget's disease of the male breast: report of a case. Dermatology 202:134–137

Neuhausen SL, Godwin AK, Gershoni-Baruch R, Schubert E, Garber J, Stoppa-Lyonnet D, Olah E, Csokay B, Serova O, Lalloo F, Osorio A, Stratton M, Offit K, Boyd J, Caligo MA, Scott RJ, Schofield A, Teugels E, Schwab M, Cannon-Albright L, Bishop T, Easton D, Benitez J, King MC, Goldgar D et al (1998) Haplotype and phenotype analysis of nine recurrent BRCA2 mutations in 111 families: results of an international study. Am J Hum Genet 62:1381–1388

O'Sullivan ST, McGreal GT, Lyons A, Burke L, Geoghegan JG, Brady MP (1994) Paget's disease of the breast in a man without underlying breast carcinoma. J Clin Pathol 47:851–852

Ottini L, Masala G, D'Amico C, Mancini B, Saieva C, Aceto G, Gestri D, Vezzosi V, Falchetti M, De Marco M, Paglierani M, Cama A, Bianchi S, Mariani-Costantini R, Palli D (2003) BRCA1 and BRCA2 mutation status and tumor characteristics in male breast cancer: a population-based study in Italy. Cancer Res 63:342–347

Ottuso P (2002) The dermatologist's role in diagnosing a rare disease – male breast cancer. Cutis 69:99–102

Persichetti P, Berloco M, Casadei RM, Marangi GF, Di Lella F, Nobili AM (2001) Gynecomastia and the complete circumareolar approach in the surgical management of skin redundancy. Plast Reconstr Surg 107:948–954

Poulain JF, Courtade S, Carmi E, Chatelain D, Denoeux JP, Lok C (2002) Genital leiomyomas of the male nipple: two cases (in French). Ann Dermatol Venereol 129 :1392–1394

Raton JA, Bilbao I, Gardeazabal J, Alvarez S, Vicente JM, Gonzalez R, Mitxelena J, Diaz-Perez JL (1998) Skin involvement in male breast carcinoma. Arch Dermatol 134:517–518

Shertz WT, Balogh K (1986) Metastasizing basal cell carcinoma of the nipple. Arch Pathol Lab Med 110:761–762

Spence RJ (1992) Bilateral reconstruction of the male nipple. Ann Plast Surg 28:288–291

Takeuchi T, Komatsuzaki M, Minesaki Y, Yokoi K, Kamide R, Niimura M, Yamada T (1999) Paget's disease arising near a male areola without an underlying carcinoma. J Dermatol 26:248–252

Tegner E, Bjornberg A (2003) Erythroderma with sparing around the nipples. Acta Derm Venereol 83:236

Urbani CE, Betti R (1996a) Accessory mammary tissue associated with congenital and hereditary nephrourinary malformations. Int J Dermatol 35:349–352

Urbani CE, Betti R (1996b) Sporadic unilateral intra-areolar polythelia. Report of an additional case and review of the literature. Acta Derm Venereol 76:156

Velasco M, Ubeda B, Autonell F, Serra C (1995) Leiomyoma of the male areola infiltrating the breast tissue. AJR Am J Roentgenol 164:511–512

Zannolli R, Mostardini R, Matera M, Pucci L, Gelb BD, Morgese G (2000) Char syndrome: an additional family with polythelia, a new finding. Am J Med Genet 95:201–203

I.10.3 Male Breast Cancer

P.S.H. Soon, J.M. Dixon

Key Messages

- Male breast cancer is rare.
- Patients most commonly present with a painless, retroareolar lump.
- Diagnosis is made by triple assessment – clinical examination, imaging and needle biopsy.
- Management is similar to that of female breast cancer

I.10.3.1 Incidence

Male breast cancer is rare, comprising less than 1 % of all breast cancers and about 1 % of all cancers in males. It also accounts for 0.1 % of all deaths from cancers in males (Memon and Donohue 1997). In the United Kingdom, less than 0.5 % of all breast cancers occur in men and breast cancer makes up 0.7 % of all male cancers (Dixon et al. 2000).

I.10.3.2 Risk Factors

Klinefelter syndrome, a congenital condition where a male inherits an extra X chromosome, resulting in the 47XXY karyotype, is the most significant risk factor for male breast cancer. Klinefelter syndrome multiplies the risk of breast cancer by 20–50 (Johnson et al. 2002).

Family history is also an important risk factor for male breast cancer. Patients with a first-degree female or male relative with breast cancer are at increased risk. SEER (surveillance, epidemiology and end results, a program run by the National Cancer Institute in the United States publishing cancer incidence and survival data from 14 population-based cancer registries and three supplemental registries covering approximately 26 % of the US population) data have shown that men with a positive family history of breast cancer have an odds ratio of 3.98 for developing breast cancer, and the risk increases with increasing numbers of first-degree

I.10

relatives, especially those with young age at diagnosis (Giordano et al. 2002).

The *BRCA2*, not the *BRCA1* gene, has been associated with male breast cancer. As in females, breast cancer in males is hormonally driven with abnormalities in oestrogen and androgen balance underpinning the risk factors. Conditions such as cirrhosis, where there is an increased serum oestrogen level due to decreased breakdown, is associated with an increased risk of male breast cancer. Obesity resulting in relative hyperoestrogenaemia, is also associated with an increased risk of male breast cancer. Gynaecomastia, which results from a relative excess of oestrogen, has been associated with male breast cancer, but any association could be due to the fact that both conditions are associated with an excess of oestrogen. Conditions causing hypoandrogenism, which include testicular trauma and infertility, are also associated with a small increased risk of breast cancer (Levi et al. 2002).

As in females, a history of chest wall irradiation also results in the risk of developing breast cancer (Memon and Donohue 1997).

Men from higher social class, single men and Jewish men are also more likely to develop breast cancer (Levi et al. 2002).

I.10.3.3 Pathology

Breast cancer in men and women differs with respect to age at diagnosis, frequency of histological types and percentage of hormone receptor expression.

Mean age of male patients with breast cancer is 60, 10 years older than for females.

Ninety per cent of male breast cancers are invasive and the remaining 10% are ductal carcinoma in situ. Most invasive breast cancers in men are ductal carcinomas; these comprise over 80% of invasive male breast cancers. It was initially thought that there were no invasive lobular carcinomas in males because of the absence of breast lobules, but a 40-year review of 229 cases of male breast cancer at the Princess Margaret hospital in Canada revealed a 2.6% incidence of invasive lobular carcinoma (Goss et al. 1999).

As in women, there is a high prevalence of hormone receptor positivity in male breast cancers; 80–90% are oestrogen-receptor positive, 70% progesterone receptor-positive and 50% androgen receptor-positive (Osborne 1998).

Prognostic factors for male breast cancer are similar to those in females. They include axillary lymph node status, tumour size, histological grade and hormone receptor status. Axillary lymph node involvement is a poor prognostic factor. A 5-year survival rate for pathological node-positive disease was 65% compared to 90% for node-negative disease in one series. The number of axillary lymph nodes involved is also an important prognostic factor, with the 10-year survival rate for patients without nodal involvement, one to three lymph nodes involved and four or more lymph nodes involved being 84%, 44% and 14%, respectively (Guinee 1993). Primary tumour size is another important prognostic factor: the 5-year survival rates are 85% for tumours under 2 cm, 63% for tumours 2–5 cm and 51% for tumours over 5 cm (Cutuli et al. 1995). Histological grade is another significant risk factor. Five-year survival rates have been reported as 76%, 66% and 43% for grades 1, 2 and 3 tumours, respectively (Ribeiro et al. 1996).

I.10.3.4 Presentation

As in women, men with breast cancer generally present with a lump (Fig. I.10.17), skin or nipple changes and blood-stained nipple discharge. Most male cancers are evident as hard, nontender lumps in the retroareolar region; the upper outer quadrant is the second most common site. In a retrospective study over 20 years from Nottingham, there were 43 male patients with breast cancer – two DCIS and 41 invasive cancers. Eighty-eight per cent (36/41) presented with a lump, three with blood-stained nipple discharge, one with pain and one with nipple deformity. Thirty-nine of the 41 had a palpable lump, with the remaining two patients having nipple discharge only (Willsher et al. 1997).

Bilateral male breast cancer is very rare. This could be due to the later onset of male breast cancer and the tendency for men to die of other causes before onset of

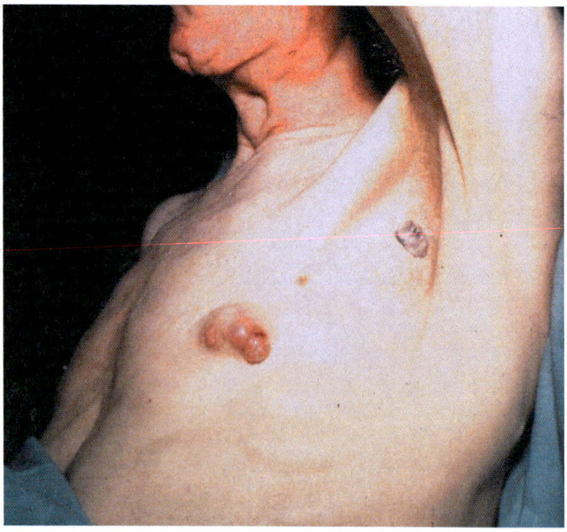

Fig. I.10.17. Picture of male patient with left breast cancer. The black mark placed in the axilla is over a palpable axillary lymph node.

I.10

contralateral breast cancer. Mammographic screening of the unaffected breast to look for contralateral cancers is not recommended in males (Goss et al. 1999).

I.10.3.5 Investigation

The main differential diagnosis of breast cancer in males is gynaecomastia; this is common in males between 5th to 8th decades. Mammography is useful in distinguishing between benign and malignant lumps (Fig. I.10.18). A carcinoma is often eccentric in the breast and has irregular, spiculated margins. Ultrasound is also valuable in helping with diagnosis and in guiding biopsy. Fine needle aspiration biopsy or core biopsy should be performed on all suspicious lumps. Core biopsy in male patients reliably diagnoses malignancy and facilitates planning of further management and avoids unnecessary operations in gynaecomastia patients (Westenend 2003). Vetto et al. (1998) looked at the cost-effectiveness of physical examination, fine needle aspiration biopsy and mammography in the assessment of breast lumps in males and concluded that mammography, in addition to physical examination and fine needle aspiration biopsy, did not add any further diagnostic information or changed management.

Once a diagnosis of breast cancer is established on biopsy, limited staging tests are usually performed. All patients should have a full blood count, liver function tests and chest X-ray. Patients with abnormal liver function tests and patients with advanced breast cancer should be considered for liver ultrasound. Bone scan should be performed in symptomatic patients or patients with advanced breast cancer.

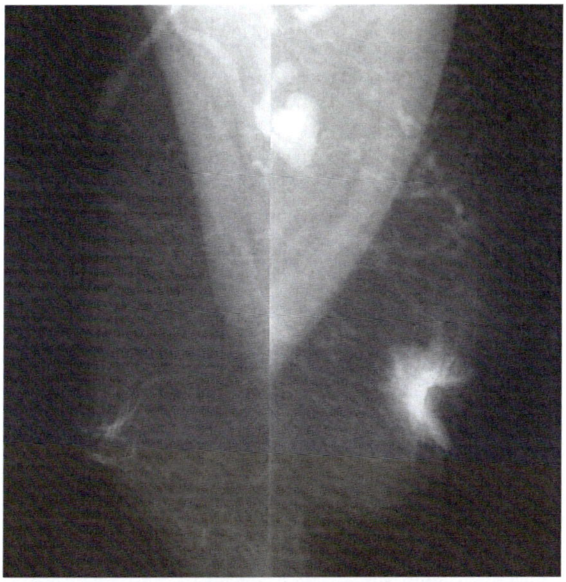

Fig. I.10.18. Bilateral mammogram of man with cancer in left breast

I.10.3.6 Management of Early Breast Cancer

Because of the rarity of male breast cancers, no randomized controlled trials have been conducted and treatment is largely based on experience with managing female breast cancers.

Surgery is the mainstay of treatment, with modified radical mastectomy (mastectomy and axillary clearance) being the most common operation. While there are no data regarding the efficacy of breast conservation surgery in males, because of the small amount of breast tissue present, lumpectomy is only an option for patients with small tumours. Though no randomized controlled study has been conducted on the use of sentinel lymph node biopsy in males with breast cancer, it is feasible to perform simple mastectomy and sentinel lymph node biopsy instead of a modified radical mastectomy. Cimmino et al. performed sentinel lymph node biopsy in six male breast cancer patients with a mean cancer size of 1.6 cm (range, 0.7–2.8 cm). A mean of 2.2 sentinel lymph nodes were identified; they used radioisotope tracer and blue dye in five patients and blue dye alone in one patient. Four of the six patients with positive sentinel lymph nodes went on to a completion axillary dissection and only one of these had further positive axillary lymph nodes. The authors concluded that sentinel lymph node biopsy can be offered as an alternative to a full axillary dissection in males with early breast cancer (Cimmino et al. 2004).

Postoperative radiotherapy is delivered to patients with locally advanced disease or tumours with presence of axillary lymph node metastases. Postoperative radiotherapy has been noted to decrease local recurrence rates but has no impact on survival (Memon and Donohue 1997). In one study of 21 patients with operable male breast cancer, it was concluded that postoperative radiotherapy is an essential part of the overall treatment strategy. Six of these 21 patients relapsed – two in the scar and four in the axilla; all the patients who relapsed had not received postoperative adjuvant radiotherapy (Schuchardt et al. 1996).

Systemic adjuvant therapy is beneficial in terms of survival for men with node-positive disease. Tamoxifen is the most frequently used systemic therapy. Ribeiro and Swindell looked at use of adjuvant tamoxifen for 1–2 years in stage 2 and operable stage 3 male breast cancer compared with historical controls. The actuarial 5-year disease-free survival of the adjuvant treated patients was 61 % compared to 44 % for historical controls, with overall survival being 56 % and 25 %, respectively (Ribeiro and Swindell 1992). Moredo Anelli et al., however, noted a 20.8 % attrition rate to adjuvant tamoxifen treatment in less than 1 year in males compared to 4% in female patients. Of 24 male patients treated with tamoxifen, 62.5% developed side effects: 29.2% experienced a decrease in libido, 25% had weight gain, 20.8% had hot flushes and mood alteration, 16.6% developed depression, 12.5% had insomnia and 4.2% had deep venous thrombosis (Moredo Anelli et al. 1994).

Chemotherapy is indicated in patients with ER-negative cancers. Treatment of node-positive male patients with surgery only yields 5-year survival rates of 16 – 57%. Patel et al. (1989) looked at adjuvant 5-fluorouracil, doxorubicin and cyclophosphamide in ten male patients with stage 2 and 3 disease and reported an estimated 5-year survival rate greater than 85%.

The MD Anderson Cancer Center recommends 5 years of tamoxifen for hormone receptor-positive tumours and offers adjuvant chemotherapy to men with node-positive disease or where the primary tumour is larger than 1 cm. Studies at the National Cancer Institute and the MD Anderson Cancer Center have shown improved outcomes with 5-year survival rates between 80% and 85% for patients with node-positive disease who have been given adjuvant chemotherapy (Giordano et al. 2002).

I.10.3.7 Management of Metastatic Breast Cancer

Systemic therapy is the mainstay of metastatic breast cancer. Orchiectomy is a highly effective form of treatment for hormone receptor-positive metastatic breast cancer. Tamoxifen, however, is the most common form of treatment as it is reversible and more acceptable to males (Giordano et al. 2002). Nevertheless, there is a high rate of treatment-limiting symptoms in these patients (Moredo Anelli et al. 1994). There have been a few reports of the use of aromatase inhibitors in patients with metastatic disease. Aromatase inhibitors appear to be less effective than tamoxifen or orchiectomy because they are only able to block about 80% of oestrogen production in males with normal testes because of the intact feedback loop (Giordano et al. 2002).

I.10.3.8 Follow-up

These patients should be followed up annually for 5 – 10 years.

I.10.3.9 Conclusion

Male breast cancer is rare. Presentation is most commonly with a painless, retroareolar lump. Diagnosis is by clinical examination, imaging and needle biopsy. Management is similar to that of female breast cancer. For early disease, surgery followed by tamoxifen with or without radiotherapy is the treatment of choice. For metastatic disease, tamoxifen or chemotherapy is indicated.

References

Cimmino VM, Degnim AC, Sabel MS, Diehl KM, Newman LA, Chang AE (2004) Efficicy of sentinel lymph node biopsy in male breast cancer. J Surg Oncol 86:74 – 77

Cutuli B, Lacroze M, Dilhuydy JM, Velten M, De Lafontan B, Marchal C, Resbeut M, Graic Y, Campana F, Moncho-Bernier V et al (1995) Male breast cancer: results of the treatments and prognostic factors in 397 cases. Eur J Cancer 31:1960 – 1964

Dixon JM, Sainsbury JRC, Rodger A (2000) Breast cancer: treatment of elderly patients and uncommon conditions. In: Dixon JM (ed) ABC of breast diseases (2nd edn.) BMJ Publishing Group, London, pp 50 – 54

Giordano SH, Buzdar AU, Hortobagyi GN (2002) Breast cancer in men. Ann Intern Med 137:678 – 687

Giordano SH, Valero V, Buzdar AU, Hortobagyi GN (2002) Efficacy of anastrozole in male breast cancer. Am J Clin Oncol 25:235 – 237

Goss PE, Reid C, Pintilie M, Lim R, Miller N (1999) Male breast carcinoma: A review of 229 patients who presented to the Princess Margaret hospital during 40 years 1955 – 1996. Cancer 85:629 – 639

Guinee VF, Olsson H, Moller T, Shallenberger RC, van den Blink JW, Peter Z, Durand M, Dische S, Cleton FJ, Zewuster R et al. (1993) The prognosis of breast cancer in males. A report of 335 cases. Cancer 71:154 – 161

Johnson KC, Pan S, Mao Y (2002) Risk factors for male breast cancer in Canada, 1994 – 1998. Eur J Cancer Prev 11:253 – 263

Levi F, Lucchini F, La Vecchia C (2002) Epidemiology of male breast cancer. Eur J Cancer Prev 11:315 – 318

Memon MA, Donohue JH (1997) Male breast cancer. Br J Surg 84:433 – 435

Moreda Anelli TF, Anelli A, Tran KN, Lebwohl DE, Borgen PI (1994) Tamoxifen administration is associated with a high rate of treatment-limiting symptoms in male breast cancer patients. Cancer 74:74 – 77

Osborne CK (1998) Tamoxifen in the treatment of breast cancer. N Engl J Med 339:1609 – 1618

Patel HZ, Buzdar AU, Hortobagyi GN (1989) Role of adjuvant chemotherapy in male breast cancer. Cancer 64:1583 – 1585

Ribeiro G, Swindell R (1992) Adjuvant tamoxifen for male breast cancer. Br J Cancer 65:252 – 254

Ribeiro G, Swindell R, Harris M, Banerjee S, Cramer A (1996) A review of the management of the male breast carcinoma based on an analysis of 420 treated cases. Breast 5:141 – 146

Schuchardt U, Seegenschmiedt MH, Kirschner MH, Renner H, Sauer R (1996) Adjuvant radiotherapy for breast carcinoma in men: A 20-year clinical experience. Am J Clin Oncol 19:330 – 336

Vetto J, Schmidt W, Pommier R, DiTomasso J, Eppich H, Wood W, Moseson D (1998) Am J Surg 175:383 – 387

Westenend PJ (2003) Core needle biopsy in male breast lesions. J Clin Pathol 56:863 – 865

Willsher PC, Leach IH, Ellis IO, Bell JA, Elston CW, Bourke JB, Blamey RW, Robertson JF (1997) Male breast cancer: pathological and immunohistochemical features. Anticancer Res 17:2335 – 2338

Problem: Male Ageing I.11

I.11.1 Neuroendocrine Regulation of Testicular Function

J.M. Kaufman

Key Messages

- Many endocrine systems change during ageing, resulting in the decreased secretion of growth hormone, dehydroepiandrosterone and testosterone.
- The circadian variability of testosterone, which is present in young men, is blunted in ageing men.
- Decreased serum concentrations of total and free testosterone result from both the decreased secretion capacity of testicular Leydig cells and the altered regulation of luteinizing hormone (LH) secretion at the hypothalamopituitary level.
- In contrast to the decreased endocrine function of the testes, Sertoli cell function and spermatogenesis are fairly well preserved in the elderly.

I.11.1.1 Definition

No physiological function remains unaffected by the ageing process, which inescapably results in diminished functional capacity and effectiveness of homeostatic regulatory mechanisms. All hormonal systems are altered to some extent by ageing, with the male gonadal axis being no exception, even though the changes are progressive and of modest amplitude compared to the rather abrupt and dramatic decrease in gonadal hormonal production that characterize climacteric transition in women.

The main hormonal changes related to androgenic action and reproductive function observed during ageing in men are summarized in Table I.11.1. These changes in healthy ageing men show considerable interindividual variation as to their pace and extent. Moreover, there is in older men a rather high prevalence of disease states and use of medication that can adversely affect sex steroid production and accentuate the age-related changes (Table I.11.2). Finally, older men can also be affected by specific diseases of the gonadal function (e.g. a prolactinoma) or still show consequences of defects of the gonadal axis that are congenital or were acquired at a younger age (e.g. Klinefelter syndrome, cryptorchidism, torsion of testis, hypogonadotrophic hypogonadism). Obviously, andrologic evaluation in an elderly man requires a thorough and broad clinical approach.

I.11.1.2 Aetiology and Pathogenesis

There is a circadian variation in serum testosterone, with amplitude of approximately 35%, the highest levels in the early morning and the lowest levels in the late afternoon (Resko and Eik-Nes 1966). This circadian rhythm is blunted in elderly men (Bremner et al. 1983; Deslypere and Vermeulen 1984; Plymate et al. 1989; Diver et al. 2003); therefore differences in serum testosterone levels between young and older men are most clearly demonstrated in studies with blood sampling performed in the morning. Such studies have shown that the mean total serum testosterone (T) level at age 65 years is about two-thirds of the mean level at age 25 (Deslypere and Vermeulen 1984; Vermeulen et al. 1996). Whereas the age-related changes in total serum T are rather subtle, they are accompanied by a progressive increase by about 1.2% per year of the serum levels of sex hormone-binding globulin (SHBG) (Vermeulen et al. 1996; Feldman et al. 2002), so that compared to the decrease of total serum T there is in fact a steeper age-related decline of the serum T fractions not bound to SHBG, i.e. the free testosterone and the so-called bio-available T (combined free T and albumin-bound T fractions) that are readily available for biological action. The population means for serum levels of free T and bio-available T are decreased by as much as 50% between age 25 and 75 years (Deslypere and Vermeulen

Table I.11.1. Ageing in men: hormonal changes related to reproduction and androgenic action; schematic representation of mean trends in healthy elderly men relative to young men

	Age-related trend	Remarks
Serum total testosterone (T)	↓	≤30% Between age 25 and 75 years; valid for (early) morning levels; in majority of subjects within range for young men; blunting of T circadian rhythm
T metabolic clearance rate (MRC)	↓	Decreased serum levels with decreased MRC indicates decreased T production
Testicular T secretion	↓	As measured in testicular vein plasma
Serum SHBG	↑↑	By about 1.2%/year
Serum FT	↓↓	Biologically active fraction; by ≥50% between age 25 and 75 years
Serum non-SHBG-bound T or bio-available T	↓↓	Biologically active fraction; by ≥50% between age 25 and 75 years
Tissue androgen concentrations	↓↓	In most tissues with some exceptions such as scrotal skin
Serum total oestradiol (E2)	→	Decreased substrate for aromatization compensated by increased aromatase activity
Serum free E2	↓	Usually ≤30% between age 25 and75 years
Serum non-SHBG-bound E2 or bio-available E2	↓	Usually ≤30% between age 25 and 75 years
Serum androstenedione	↓↓	
Serum dihydrotestosterone (DHT)	→ (↑? ↓?)	Not representative for tissue levels; unchanged according to most but not all reports
Serum DHEA (sulphate)	↓↓↓	Mainly from adrenal origin; ≥80% between age 25 and 75 years
Serum cortisol/DHEA(S) ratio	↑↑↑	Cfr. unchanged or slightly increased adrenal cortisol production
Serum luteinizing hormone (LH)	↑	In majority of subjects within range for young men
Serum follicle stimulating hormone (FSH)	↑↑	More consistent increase than for serum LH
Serum inhibin B	↓ (→)	Only modest decrease; early changes rather suggestive for testicular factors different from ageing; relatively stable in older men
Serum inhibin B/FSH	↓↓	Clear progressive decline

↑, ↑↑, ↑↑↑: limited, moderate, strong increase, respectively; ↓, ↓↓, ↓↓↓: limited, moderate, strong decrease, respectively

Table I.11.2. Some diseases and treatments that can temporarily or more permanently accentuate the age-related decline of testosterone production

Acute disease
Any acute disease state
Myocardial infarction
Acute critical illness
Chronic disease
(Morbid) obesity; insulin resistance
(Poorly controlled) diabetes mellitus
Atherosclerosis
Chronic obstructive pulmonary disease
Lung fibrosis
Asthma
Obstructive sleep apnoea
Chronic liver disease (with or without cirrhosis)
Haemochromatosis
Renal failure
Cushing syndrome
Prolactinoma
Other pituitary tumours
Habits and medication
Glucocorticoids
Neuroleptic drugs
Ketoconazole
Spironolactone
Alkylating chemotherapeutics
Opioids
Cannabinoids
Alcohol abuse

1984; Simon et al. 1992; Vermeulen et al. 1996; Ferrini and Barrett-Connor 1998). These age-related changes observed in cross-sectional studies in healthy ambulatory men have also been confirmed when assessed in a longitudinal setting (Morley et al. 1997; Zmuda et al. 1997; Harman et al. 2001; Feldman et al. 2002). Given that the metabolic clearance rate of T tends to decrease with age (Vermeulen et al. 1972), it can be assumed that the age-related decline in serum T reflects a decreased testicular T production, which has indeed been demonstrated in early studies with measurement of spermatic vein T levels (Hollander and Hollander 1958) and the T blood production rate (Kent and Acone 1966; Vermeulen et al. 1972; Giusti et al. 1975; Baker et al. 1977).

The limited information that is available on the influence of age on tissular androgen concentrations indicates that the decline in plasma T levels is paralleled by a decrease in androgen concentrations in most, albeit not in all (e.g. not in scrotal skin) tissues (Deslypere and Vermeulen 1981, 1985). Testosterone exerts direct androgenic effects through binding to the androgen receptor (AR). However, T acts as a prohormone, whereby a substantial part of the physiologic T action results from its activating metabolism in the tissues, i.e. on the one hand its 5-reduction to dihydrotestosterone (DHT), a more powerful androgen and the major androgen in the tissues from the urogenital tract, and on the other hand its aromatization to oestradiol, which exerts in men physiologically important actions through binding with the oestrogen receptor alpha and beta (ER and ER). There have been reports of unchanged (Gray et al. 1991; Vermeulen et al. 1996), decreased (Sparrow et al. 1980; Couillard et al. 2000) as well as increased (Feldman et al. 2002) DHT serum levels in ageing men. However, given that 80% of the DHT in the circulation originates from 5-reduction of testosterone in the tissues, that the 5-reductase activity is differentially regulated in different tissues (Russell and Wilson 1994) and that part of the DHT formed is metabolized locally, plasma DHT concentration should not be regarded as a reliable reflection of tissular levels.

Plasma oestradiol originates for 80% from aromatization of T and androstenedione in the tissues, i.e. in particular in (subcutaneous) fat and striated muscle, although aromatase activity is present in many tissues. Total plasma oestradiol levels in adult men do not vary substantially with age, because the age-related decline of serum concentrations of T and androstenedione, the substrate for the aromatase cytochrome P450 enzyme, is compensated by an increase in fat mass and tissue aromatase activity with age (Hemsell et al. 1974; Ferrini et al. 1998; Vermeulen et al. 2003).

The serum concentration of androstenedione shows a significant decline with age (Vermeulen 1995), the androgenic activity of androstenedione being dependent on its conversion to testosterone. Serum dehydroepiandrosterone (DHEA) and DHEA-sulphate (DHEAS) are secreted almost exclusively by the adrenals, no more than 10% of DHEA being derived from the gonads. Although the hypothesis that DHEA may have specific hormonal actions is being actively tested by several laboratories, its known hormonal actions in humans are dependent on conversion of DHEA to either T or oestrogens, and such conversion in peripheral tissues may contribute to androgenic and oestrogenic tissular activity (Labrie et al. 2003), although the contribution of DHEA(S) to the global androgenic activity in adult men is probably only marginal. The serum concentrations of both DHEA and DHEAS show a progressive and dramatic age-related decline of over 80% between age 20 and 75 years.

The end metabolites of the metabolism of endogenous androgens, i.e. androsterone, etiocholanolone and 3, 17β-diol are either glucuronidated or sulphated and excreted by the kidneys (Griffin and Wilson 1980). The serum levels and urinary excretion of androstanediol-glucuronide decrease with age, as in men the metabolite is derived for 70% from T and for 30% from DHEAS (Deslypere et al. 1982).

The age-related hormonal changes described above are mean trends for the population, but at all ages there is considerable interindividual variation, in particular for serum T levels. With ageing there is a progressive shift of the distribution of serum T towards lower values, with an increasing proportion of men presenting with serum T levels below the lower limit of the range for young men, i.e. roughly 315 ng/dl (or 11 nmol/l) for total T, approximately 6.5 ng/dl (or 0.225 nmol/l) for free T, and roughly 140 ng/dl (or 5 nmol/l) for bio-available T (Vermeulen 2001; Mahmoud et al. 2003). More than 20% of otherwise healthy men aged 65 years or older have low serum T levels compared to young men, but a majority of older men still have serum levels within the range for young men. Although the mechanisms underlying the considerable interindividual variability of serum T levels have not been fully elucidated, this variability appears to be multifactorially determined with contribution of genetic, physiological, and life-style-related factors (Kaufman and Vermeulen 1997; see Kaufman et al. 2004 for a review).

It should be emphasized that many factors intervene in the determination of T tissular action, which includes T production, T plasma protein binding and metabolic clearance rate, determinants of availability of testosterone for tissular action, the local regulation of T metabolism in the tissues, the expression of AR and/or ER, genetic variants in these receptors as well as the expression of a number of co-activators and repressors of these receptors. Many of these factors may be affected by age, and the effect of ageing may vary according to the considered tissue and physiological function. This may explain why it has not yet been clearly established whether T requirements might change with age, a clinically important issue for which the available clinical data has not yet provided a clear answer (Kaufman and Vermeulen 1997; Kaufman et al. 2004 for review).

I.11.1.2.1 Mechanisms of Decreased Serum Testosterone Levels

Some of the relevant characteristics of the gonadal axis in elderly men are summarized in Table I.11.3.

Primary testicular factors with reduced testosterone secretory capacity, altered neuroendocrine regulation of the Leydig cells and an independent increase of plasma testosterone binding capacity all contribute to the age-related changes in testosterone levels in the systemic circulation.

Primary Testicular Changes

In healthy men, ageing is accompanied by a modest decrease in testicular volume, with mean volume at age 75 years being reduced by about 30% relative to that in young men (Mahmoud et al. 2003). Studies with administration of human chorionic gonadotrophin (hCG; Longcope 1973; Rubens et al. 1974; Harman and Tsitouras 1980; Nankin et al. 1981), gonadotropin-releasing hormone (GnRH) intermittently (Mulligan et al. 1999), or biosynthetic LH following suppression of endoge-

Table I.11.3. Some reported characteristics of the gonadal axis in healthy elderly men

Testis compartment
Decreased volume (by about 30% between age 25 and 75 years)
Decreased number of Leydig cells
Decreased number of Sertoli cells
Decreased number and qualitative changes tubuli seminiferi
Decreased testosterone response to LH
Pituitary compartment
Maintained LH responsiveness to physiologic GnRH stimulation
Hypothalamic compartment
Blunted circadian rhythm of serum LH and testosterone
Decreased regularity of serum LH pulses
Unchanged or slightly increased LH pulse frequency
Decreased frequency of large amplitude LH pulses
Decreased mean LH pulse amplitude
Decreased synchrony of LH secretion with FSH and prolactin
Decreased synchrony with sleep pattern and nocturnal penile tumescence
Diminished LH response to opioid blockade (decreased opioid tone)
Increased sensitivity to sex steroid inhibitory feedback

nous LH secretion (Mulligan et al. 2001) consistently indicate that the secretory capacity of the testis for testosterone is reduced in the elderly compared to young men. This decrease in testicular secretory reserve can be attributed to a reduction in the number of Leydig cells (Harbitz 1973; Neaves et al. 1984). There is, moreover, evidence for involvement of vascular changes (Suoranta 1971) and changes in testicular steroid biosynthesis (Vermeulen and Deslypere 1986; Zirkin and Chen 2000). In accordance with the existence of primary testicular defects, mean LH levels tend to increase in ageing men (Vermeulen and Giagulli 1991; Tsitouras and Bulat 1995; Culty et al. 2002 for review).

Altered Regulation of LH Secretion

I.11

Although the combined observations of a diminished testicular reserve for testosterone secretion and of increased basal gonadotrophin levels do seem in line with the view that the age-related decline of Leydig cell function results from primary testicular dysfunction, the age-related increase in LH serum levels is of only modest amplitude and inconsistent (Morley et al. 1997), and many elderly men with serum testosterone concentrations below the range for young men do not have elevated LH levels (Vermeulen and Kaufman 2002). Moreover, the only modest increase in basal serum LH in elderly men results at least in part from a slower plasma clearance rather than from increased pituitary secretion (Kaufman et al. 1991; Bergendahl et al. 1998). In any case, in many elderly men the increase of LH is less than would be expected in the face of persistent low serum testosterone levels, which in turn indicates the existence of an altered regulation of LH secretion in these elderly men. The latter neuroendocrine changes are relevant. Indeed, whereas the experiments with direct stimulation of testicular androgen secretion revealed a diminished secretory capacity in the elderly, they also showed that elderly men usually still have a residual secretory reserve capacity that would allow many of them to substantially increase their serum testosterone levels if the pituitary LH drive is adequate.

In contrast to early reports of a delayed or diminished pituitary LH response upon stimulation with synthetic GnRH, which were based on administration of large pharmacological doses of GnRH, more recent studies assessing the pituitary LH response to in vivo administration of small, near physiological doses of synthetic GnRH have revealed a maintained (Mulligan et al. 1999) or, in line with expectations in the situation of relative hypoandrogenism, a slightly increased LH response, as measured by either immunoassay or bioassay in elderly men compared to the young (Kaufman et al. 1991). These experiments showing a preserved pituitary secretory capacity for LH thus indirectly indicate that the apparent failure of the feedback regulatory mechanisms to produce an adequate increase of serum LH in presence of persistent low testosterone levels must result from regulatory changes at the hypothalamic level.

Several changes in the neuroendocrine control of LH secretion have been documented in elderly men. First, the circadian rhythm of LH and testosterone secretion is blunted in elderly men (Bremner et al. 1983; Deslypere and Vermeulen 1984; Tenover et al. 1988; Plymate et al. 1989; Diver et al. 2003). Second, the pulsatile pattern of LH secretion is altered with increased irregularity (Pincus et al. 1997) and disruption of synchrony with the secretion of follicle-stimulating hormone (FSH) and prolactin as well as with nocturnal penile tumescence and sleep phases (Veldhuis et al. 1992, 2000; Luboshitzky et al. 2003). The LH pulse frequency remains essentially unchanged (Winters et al. 1984; Deslypere et al. 1987; Tenover et al. 1987; Urban et al. 1988) or is slightly increased (Veldhuis et al. 1992) as compared to young men, but there is a decreased frequency of large-amplitude LH pulses with a reduction of the mean LH pulse amplitude, the latter being a relevant parameter of the stimulating effect of LH pulses on Leydig cells (Deslypere et al. 1987; Veldhuis et al. 1992).

The pituitary pulsatile secretion of LH is the result of intermittent stimulation by hypothalamic GnRH, each LH pulse being the result of the release of a bolus of GnRH into the hypophyseal portal circulation. Therefore, besides the increased irregularity of LH pulses, the largely unchanged frequency of LH pulses points towards hypothalamic changes. Indeed, the frequency of the hypothalamic GnRH pulse generator is expected to increase in a state of hypoandrogenism (Plant 1986).

Given that the pituitary secretory capacity for LH is preserved in the elderly, the diminished mean LH pulse amplitude can by inference also be attributed to hypothalamic changes, with most likely a reduction in the size of the bolus of GnRH being intermittently released in the portal circulation. Although the possibility of a contribution of vascular changes in the portal circulation cannot be excluded, a reduction in the size of the intermittently released GnRH bolus can in turn be the consequence of a reduced number of GnRH neurones, a less efficient recruitment and/or synchronization of GnRH neurones, and/or a functional down-regulation of GnRH neurones by local and/or systemic factors. As to the latter, an important observation is that of a clearly increased sensitivity in elderly men to the inhibitory feedback effects of androgens (Winters et al. 1984; Deslypere et al. 1987; Mulligan et al. 1997; Winters and Atkinson 1997). This increased suppressive effect on LH secretion in the elderly has been shown for the nonaromatizable pure androgen DHT as well as for testosterone (Winters et al. 1984; Deslypere et al. 1987). It is presently not known how oestrogens are involved in the age-related alterations in the regulation of LH secretion. However, it has recently been shown that administration of an aromatase inhibitor is able to substantially raise LH and testosterone secretion in elderly men (Leder et al. 2004). The increased negative feedback effect of sex steroids in the elderly is not the consequence of an increased hypothalamic opioid tone, as the latter is rather reduced (Vermeulen et al. 1989; Mikuma et al. 1994). It has also been shown that the alterations in neuroendocrine regulation of Leydig cell function are not the consequence of abnormalities in serum leptin levels (Van den Saffele et al. 1999).

I.11.1.2.2 Increase of Plasma SHBG Binding Capacity

On the background of altered androgen secretion in the elderly as a consequence of changes at both the testicular and the hypothalamic level, the age-related increase in SHBG levels in the elderly translates into a reduction of the non-SHBG bound fraction of serum testosterone that is readily available for biological action (i.e. free T and bio-available T). This increase in SHBG occurs despite an increase in fat mass and insulin levels in the elderly, which are negative determinants of serum SHBG levels (Demoor and Goossens 1970; Haffner et al. 1993; Giagulli et al. 1994; Vermeulen et al. 1996, 2003). The mechanisms responsible for the age-associated increase in serum SHBG have yet to be unravelled. It is unlikely that the decrease in plasma T is itself responsible, since the increase in SHBG levels appears to begin at a younger age (Vermeulen et al. 1996). A possible role of the decreased activity of the somatotropic axis in the elderly is supported by indirect evidence (Erfurth et al. 1996; Pfeilschifter et al. 1996; Vermeulen et al. 1996) and needs to be further investigated.

I.11.1.2.3 Altered Spermatogenesis and Sertoli Cell Function

A decrease in mean testicular volume by about 30% in men 75 years compared to young men and a progressive increase in serum FSH (Mahmoud et al. 2003) indicate changes in spermatogenic capacity in elderly men. Nevertheless, the limited data available suggests that ageing has no major influence on sperm quality, with changes in semen parameters essentially limited to a decrease in ejaculate volume and sperm motility (Nieschlag et al. 1982; Rolf et al. 1996); the decrease of ejaculation frequency in elderly men is a confounding factor that complicates the evaluation of age-related changes.

Global testicular Sertoli cell function and spermatogenic activity, as assessed indirectly through serum inhibin B levels, appear to be well maintained in ambulatory elderly men. Indeed, it has been shown that median serum inhibin B levels show a decline at a relatively young age, with stable levels between age 35 and 79 years, and only a modest further decrease thereafter (Mahmoud et al. 2000). Nevertheless, there are age-related changes in Sertoli cell function, as the serum inhibin B levels can be maintained only at the cost of a progressive increase in the drive by pituitary FSH (Mahmoud et al. 2000). In the elderly, as in the young, serum inhibin B levels are strongly negatively associated with serum FSH, and testicular volume in older men is strongly positively associated with serum inhibin B levels and negatively with serum FSH levels. There is a sharp age-related decrease of the serum inhibin B over FSH ratio. These findings, together with the modestly reduced testicular volume, are consistent with the concept that in elderly men Sertoli cell mass is reduced (Mahmoud et al. 2003) in accordance with such a reduction described in morphologic studies (Johnson et al. 1984). Notwithstanding these testicular changes, the global Sertoli cell function is largely, albeit not fully, preserved at the cost of increased pituitary FSH stimulation. Thus, at variance with the altered neuroendocrine regulation of LH secretion, the pituitary regulation of FSH secretion appears to remain largely unchanged in the elderly.

I.11.1.2.4 Altered Adrenal Androgen Secretion

Ageing in men, as is the case in women, is accompanied by a selective and drastic decrease in plasma levels of adrenal androgens, with maintained or even increased serum cortisol levels. These changes result from a selective decrease in functional zona reticularis cells (Endoh et al. 1966). Upon stimulation with ACTH, the serum DHEA response is markedly diminished in the elderly, whereas the cortisol response is maintained compared to young men (Parker et al. 1981; Vermeulen et al. 1982). It was shown that during stimulation with ACTH, the increase in DHEAS in the elderly is proportional to the decreased basal level (Yamaji and Ibayashi 1969), which is compatible with the concept of a diminished mass of responsive cells and maintained responsiveness of the residual cells.

I.11.1.3 Clinical Findings, Technical Investigations and Laboratory Findings

History taking may reveal symptoms that are usually lumped together under the denominator of andropause or PADAM (partial androgen deficiency of the ageing male). These include psychological, physical and sexual complaints. History taking may also reveal pathology, incidents or interventions at the testicular or inguinal level having caused testicular damage or atrophy. However, symptoms similar to those described in andropause may also result from systemic diseases, and these must be excluded by general physical examination and blood tests, as well as elective imaging.

Upon physical examination, particular signs are suggestive of altered androgen secretion such as scarce pubic hair and small testicular volume. Men with varicoceles commonly present premature androgen deficiency and andropause symptoms.

The diagnosis of altered neuroendocrine functioning requires the measurement of blood hormones, including total and free testosterone, thyroid hormones and dehydroepiandrosterone sulphate.

I.11.1.4 Differential Diagnosis

The signs and symptoms of neuroendocrine alteration can be caused by systemic diseases such as obesity, diabetes, atheromatosis and cardio- as well as cerebrovascular disease, depression, and malignant tumours. Hypoandrogenism may be secondary to these and to other conditions which require preparatory treatment before any hormonal substitution is considered.

I.11.1.5 Treatment

There is an ongoing debate on the risk–benefit ratio of hormone substitution therapy in ageing men with altered neuroendocrine function. Substitution with growth hormone or dehydroepiandrosterone cannot be recommended on the basis of available scientific evidence. Tamoxifen and human chorionic gonadotrophin have been used to enhance the endogenous testosterone production, but there is insufficient evidence to sustain this treatment. The use of androgen replacement, restoring the physiological circadian variability, may be considered in particular circumstances.

I.11.1.6 Results of Treatment

Treatment aiming at the restoration of androgen concentrations observed in young men may result in amelioration of general complaints and physical condition. Fatigue, sleep disturbances, depressive mood, and impaired short-term memory have been reported to improve, and libido as well as sexual function may ameliorate. However, long-term prospective trials including a large number of cases are needed to assess the balance between some alleged beneficial effects and possible adverse effects. Hormone treatment must always be tailored to the needs of any particular patient and necessitates close follow-up.

I.11.1.7 Summary and Conclusions

Ageing in healthy men is accompanied by a progressive, individually variable decline in serum total T levels, with a sharper decline of the levels for the biologically active free T and bio-available T. These changes are underlined (1) by a diminished testicular secretory capacity resulting from a reduced mass of Leydig cells, (2) by alterations of the hypothalamic regulation of pituitary LH secretion, with increased sensitivity to sex steroid negative feedback and (3) by an independent increase in serum-binding capacity for testosterone by increased SHBG levels. As a consequence, with age there is an increasing proportion of men presenting with low serum T levels as compared to the range for young men. The prevalence of such low serum T amounts to over 20% in men 60 years and older and over 35% in men 80 years and older. Global Sertoli cell function, on the other hand, is relatively well maintained in older men, a decrease in Sertoli cell mass being compensated for by a progressive increase in FSH secretion. From the limited data available and as assessed indirectly through serum inhibin B levels, it appears that global spermatogenic activity is generally fairly well preserved in the elderly.

References

Baker HWD, Burger HG, de Kretser DM, Hudson B (1977) Endocrinology of aging: pituitary testicular axis. In: James VHT (ed) Proceedings of the Fifth International Congress of Endocrinology, pp 179–183

Bergendahl M, Aloi JA, Iranmanesh A, Mulligan TM, Veldhuis JD (1998) Fasting suppresses pulsatile luteinizing hormone

(LH) secretion and enhances orderliness of LH release in young but not older men. J Clin Endocrinol Metab 83: 1967–1975

Bremner WJ, Vitiello MV, Prinz PN (1983) Loss of circadian rhythmicity in blood testosterone levels with aging in normal men. J Clin Endocrinol Metab 56:1278–1281

Couillard C, Gagnon J, Bergeron J, Leon AS, Rao DC, Skinner JS, Wilmore JH, Despres JP, Bouchard C (2000) Contribution of body fatness and adipose tissue distribution to the age variation in plasma steroid hormone concentrations in men: The HERITAGE family study. J Clin Endocrinol Metab 85: 1026–1031

Culty M, Luo LD, Yao ZX, Chen HL, Papadopoulos V, Zirkin BR (2002) Cholesterol transport, peripheral benzodiazepine receptor, and steroidogenesis in aging Leydig cells. J Androl 23:439–447

Demoor P, Goossens JV (1970) An inverse correlation between body weight and the activity of the steroid binding globulin in human plasma. Steroidologia 1:129–136

Deslypere JP, Vermeulen A (1981) Aging and tissue androgens. J Clin Endocrinol Metab 53:430–434

Deslypere JP, Vermeulen A (1984) Leydig-cell function in normal men – effect of age, life-style, residence, diet, and activity. J Clin Endocrinol Metab 59:955–962

Deslypere JP, Vermeulen A (1985) Influence of age on steroid concentrations in skin and striated muscle in women and in cardiac muscle and lung tissue in men. J Clin Endocrinol Metab 61:648–653

Deslypere JP, Sayed A, Punjabi U, Verdonck L, Vermeulen A (1982) Plasma 5 alpha-androstane-3 alpha,17 beta-diol and urinary 5 alpha-androstane-3 alpha,17 beta-diol glucuronide, parameters of peripheral androgen action: a comparative study. J Clin Endocrinol Metab 54:386–391

Deslypere JP, Kaufman JM, Vermeulen T, Vogelaers D, Vandalem JL, Vermeulen A (1987) Influence of age on pulsatile luteinizing-hormone release and responsiveness of the gonadotrophs to sex-hormone feedback in men. J Clin Endocrinol Metab 64:68–73

Diver MJ, Imtiaz KE, Ahmad AM, Vora JP, Fraser WD (2003) Diurnal rhythms of serum total, free and bioavailable testosterone and of SHBG in middle-aged men compared with those in young men. Clin Endocrinol 58:710–717

Endoh H, Kristiansen SB, Casson PR, Buster JE, Hornsby PJ (1966) The zona reticularis is the site of biosynthesis of dehydroepiandrosterone sulphate in the adult human adrenal cortex resulting from its low expression of 3b-hydroxysteroid dehydrogenase. J Clin Endocrinol Metab 81:3558–3565

Erfurth EMT, Hagmar LE, Saaf M, Hall K (1996) Serum levels of insulin-like growth factor I and insulin-like growth factor-binding protein 1 correlate with serum free testosterone and sex hormone binding globulin levels in healthy young and middle-aged men. Clin Endocrinol 44:659–664

Feldman HA, Longcope C, Derby CA, Johannes CB, Araujo AB, Coviello AD, Bremner WJ, Mckinlay JB (2002) Age trends in the level of serum testosterone and other hormones in middle-aged men: longitudinal results from the Massachusetts Male Aging Study. J Clin Endocrinol Metab 87:589–598

Ferrini RL, Barrett-Connor E (1998) Sex hormones and age: a cross-sectional study of testosterone and estradiol and their bioavailable fractions in community-dwelling men. Am J Epidemiol 147:750–754

Giagulli VA, Kaufman JM, Vermeulen A (1994) Pathogenesis of the decreased androgen levels in obese men. J Clin Endocrinol Metab 79:997–1000

Giusti G, Gonnelli P, Borrelli D, Fiorelli G, Forti G, Pazzagli M, Serio M (1975) Age-related secretion of androstenedione, testosterone and dihydrotestosterone by human testis. Exp Geront 10:241–245

Gray A, Feldman HA, Mckinlay JB, Longcope C (1991) Age, disease, and changing sex-hormone levels in middle-aged men – results of the Massachusetts Male Aging Study. J Clin EndocrinolMetab 73:1016–1025

Griffin JE, Wilson JD (1980) The testis. In: Bondy PK, Rosenberg LE (eds) Metabolic control and disease. WB Saunders, Philadelphia, pp 1535–1538

Haffner SM, Valdez RA, Stern MP, Katz MS (1993) Obesity, body-fat distribution and sex-hormones in men. Int J Obesity 17:643–649

Harbitz TB (1973) Morphometric studies of Leydig cells in elderly men with special reference to the histology of the prostate. An analysis in an autopsy series. Acta Pathol Microbiol Scand A 81:301–314

Harman SM, Tsitouras PD (1980) Reproductive hormones in aging men. 1. Measurement of sex steroids, basal luteinizing-hormone, and Leydig-cell response to human chorionic-gonadotropin. J Clin Endocrinol Metab 51:35–40

Harman SM, Metter EJ, Tobin JD, Pearson J, Blackman MR (2001) Longitudinal effects of aging on serum total and free testosterone levels in healthy men. J Clin Endocrinol Metab 86:724–731

Hemsell DI, Grodin JM, Brenner P, Siiteri PK, McDonald PC (1974) Plasma precursors of estrogens. Correlation of the extent of conversion of plasma androstenedione to estrone with age. J Clin Endocrinol Metab 34:476–479

Hollander N, Hollander VP (1958) The microdetermination of testosterone in human spermatic vein blood. J Clin Endocrinol Metab 19:966–997

Johnson L, Zane RS, Petty CS, Neaves WB (1984) Quantification of the human Sertoli-cell population – its distribution, relation to germ-cell numbers, and age-related decline. Reprod Biol 31:785–795

Kaufman JM, Vermeulen A (1997) Declining gonadal function in elderly men. Baillieres Clin Endocrinol Metab 11:289–309

Kaufman JM, T'Sjoen G, Vermeulen A (2004) Androgens in male senescence. In: Nieschlag E, Behre HM (eds) Testosterone: action, deficiency, substitution. Cambridge University Press, Cambridge, pp 497–541

Kaufman JM, Giri M, Deslypere JM, Thomas G, Vermeulen A (1991) Influence of age on the responsiveness of the gonadotrophs to luteinizing-hormone-releasing hormone in males. J Clin Endocrinol Metab 72:1255–1260

Kent JZ, Acone AB (1966) Plasma androgens and aging. In: Vermeulen A, Exley D (eds) Androgens in normal and pathological conditions. Excerpta Medica Foundation, Amsterdam, pp 31–35

Labrie F, Belanger A, Cusan L, Candas B (2003) Physiological changes in dehydroepiandrosterone are not reflected by serum levels of active androgens and estrogens but of their metabolites: intracrinology. J Clin Endocrinol Metab 82: 2403–2409

Leder BZ, Rohrer JL, Rubin SD, Gallo J, Longcope C (2004) Effects of aromatase inhibition in elderly men with low or borderline-low serum testosterone levels. J Clin Endocrinol Metab 89:1174–1180

Longcope C (1973) Effect of human chorionic gonadotropin on plasma steroid levels in young and old men. Steroids 21: 583–590

Luboshitzky R, Shen-Orr Z, Herer P (2003) Middle-aged men secrete less testosterone at night than young healthy men. J Clin Endocrinol Metab 88:3160–3166

Mahmoud AM, Goemaere S, De Bacquer D, Comhaire FH, Kaufman JM (2000) Serum inhibin B levels in community-dwelling elderly men. Clin Endocrinol (Oxf) 53:141–147

Mahmoud AM, Goemaere S, El-Garem Y, Van Pottelbergh I, Comhaire FH, Kaufman JM (2003) Testicular volume in relation to hormonal indices of gonadal function in communi-

ty-dwelling elderly men. J Clin Endocrinol Metab 88: 179–184
Mikuma N, Kumamoto Y, Maruta H, Nitta T (1994) Role of the hypothalamic opioidergic system in the control of gonadotropin secretion in elderly men. Andrologia 26:39–45
Morley JE, Kaiser FE, Perry HM, Patrick P, Morley PMK, Stauber PM, Vellas B, Baumgartner RN, Garry PJ (1997) Longitudinal changes in testosterone, luteinizing hormone, and follicle-stimulating hormone in healthy older men. Metab Clin Exp 46:410–413
Mulligan T, Iranmanesh A, Johnson ML, Straume M, Veldhuis JD (1997) Aging alters feed-forward and feedback linkages between LH and testosterone in healthy men. Am J Physiol 42:R1407–R1413
Mulligan T, Iranmanesh A, Kerzner R, Demers LW, Veldhuis JD (1999) Two-week pulsatile gonadotropin releasing hormone infusion unmasks dual (hypothalamic and Leydig cell) defects in the healthy aging male gonadotropic axis. Eur J Endocrinol 141:257–266
Mulligan T, Iranmanesh A, Veldhuis JD (2001) Pulsatile iv infusion of recombinant human LH in leuprolide-suppressed men unmasks impoverished Leydig-cell secretory responsiveness to mid physiological LH drive in the aging male. J Clin Endocrinol Metab 86:5547–5553
Nankin HR, Lin T, Murono EP, Osterman J (1981) The aging Leydig cell. 3. Gonadotropin stimulation in men. J Androl 2:181–189
Neaves WB, Johnson L, Porter JC, Parker CR, Petty CS (1984) Leydig cell numbers, daily sperm production, and serum gonadotropin-levels in aging men. J Clin Endocrinol Metab 59:756–763
Nieschlag E, Lammers U, Freischem CW, Langer K, Wickings EJ (1982) Reproductive functions in young fathers and grandfathers. J Clin Endocrinol Metab 55:676–681
Parker L, Gral T, Perrigo V, Skowksy R (1981) Decreased adrenal androgen sensitivity to ACTH during aging. Metabolism 30:601–604
Pfeilschifter J, Scheidt-Nave C, Leidig-Bruckner G, Woitge HW, Blum WF, Wuster C, Haack D, Ziegler R (1996) Relationship between circulating insulin-like growth factor components and sex hormones in a population-based sample of 50- to 80-year-old men and women. J Clin Endocrinol Metab 81:2534–2540
Pincus SM, Veldhuis JD, Mulligan T, Iranmanesh A, Evans WS (1997) Effects of age on the irregularity of LH and FSH serum concentrations in women and men. Am J Physiol 273:E989–E995
Plant M (1986) Gonadal regulation of hypothalamic gonadotropin-releasing hormone release in primates. Endocr Rev 7:75–88
Plymate SR, Tenover JS, Bremner WJ (1989) Circadian variation in testosterone, sex hormone-binding globulin, and calculated non-sex hormone-binding globulin bound testosterone in healthy-young and elderly men. J Androl 10: 366–371
Resko JA, Eik-Nes KA (1966) Diurnal testosterone levels in peripheral plasma of human male subjects. J Clin Endocrinol Metab 26:573–576
Rolf C, Behre M, Nieschlag E (1996) Reproductive parameters of older compared to younger men of infertile couples. Int J Androl 19:135–142
Rubens R, Dhont M, Vermeulen A (1974) Further studies on Leydig cell function in old age. J Clin Endocrinol Metab 39:40–45
Russell DW, Wilson JD (1994) Steroid 5 alpha-reductase: two genes/two enzymes. Annu Rev Biochem 63:25–61
Simon D, Preziosi P, Barrettconnor E, Roger M, Saintpaul M, Nahoul K, Papoz L (1992) The influence of aging on plasma sex-hormones in men – the Telecom study. Am J Epidemiol 135:783–791
Sparrow D, Bosse R, Rowe JW (1980) The influence of age, alcohol consumption, and body build on gonadal function in men. J Clin Endocrinol Metab 51:508–512
Suoranta H (1971) Changes in the small vessels of the adult testes in relation to age and to some pathological conditions. Virchows Arch A Pathol Anat 352:765–781
Tenover JS, Matsumoto AM, Plymate SR, Bremner WJ (1987) The effects of aging in normal men on bioavailable testosterone and luteinizing hormone secretion: response to clomiphene citrate. J Clin Endocrinol Metab 65:1118–1126
Tenover JS, Matsumoto AM, Clifton DK, Bremner WJ (1988) Age related alterations in the circadian rhythms of pulsatile luteinizing hormone and testosterone secretion in healthy men. J Gerontol 43:M163–M169
Tsitouras PD, Bulat T (1995) The aging male reproductive system. Endocrinol Metab Clin North Am 24:297–315
Urban RJ, Veldhuis JD, Blizzard RM, Dufau ML (1988) Attenuated release of biologically active luteinizing hormone in healthy aging men. J Clin Invest 81:1020–1029
Van den Saffele JK, Goemaere S, De Bacquer D, Kaufman JM (1999) Serum leptin levels in healthy ageing men: are decreased serum testosterone and increased adiposity in elderly men the consequence of leptin deficiency? Clin Endocrinol 51:81–88
Veldhuis JD, Urban RJ, Lizarralde G, Johnson ML, Iranmanesh A (1992) Attenuation of luteinizing hormone secretory burst amplitude as a proximate basis for the hypoandrogenism of healthy aging in men. J Clin Endocrinol Metab 75:707–713
Veldhuis JD, Iranmanesh A, Godschalk M, Mulligan T (2000). Older men manifest multifold synchrony disruption of reproductive neurohormone outflow. J Clin Endocrinol Metab 85:1477–1486
Vermeulen A, Deslypere JP (1986) Intratesticular unconjugated steroids in elderly men. J Steroid Biochem Mol Biol 24:1079–1083
Vermeulen A, Giagulli VA (1991) Physiopathology of plasma androstanediol-glucuronide. J Steroid Biochem Mol Biol 39:829–833
Vermeulen A (2001) Androgen replacement therapy in the aging male – a critical evaluation. J Clin Endocrinol Metab 86:2380–2390
Vermeulen A (1995) Dehydroepiandrosteronesulfate and aging. Ann N Y Acad Sci 774:121–127
Vermeulen A, Verdonck L, Rubens R (1972) Testosterone secretion and metabolism in male senescence. J Clin Endocrinol Metab 34:730
Vermeulen A, Deslypere JP, Schelfhout W, Verdonck L, Rubens R (1982) Adrenocortical function in old age: response to acute adrenocorticotropin stimulation. J Clin Endocrinol Metab 54:187–191
Vermeulen A, Deslypere JP, Kaufman JM (1989) Influence of antiopioids on luteinizing hormone pulsatility in aging men. J Clin Endocrinol Metab 68:68–72
Vermeulen A, Kaufman JM, Giagulli VA (1996) Influence of some biological indexes on sex hormone-binding globulin and androgen levels in aging or obese males. J Clin Endocrinol Metab 81:1821–1826
Vermeulen A, Kaufman JM (2002) Diagnosis of hypogonadism in the aging male. Aging Male 5:170–176
Vermeulen A, Kaufman JM, Goemaere S, Van Pottelbergh I (2003) Estradiol in elderly men. Aging Male 5:98–102
Winters SJ, Atkinson L (1997) Serum LH concentrations in hypogonadal men during transdermal testosterone replacement through scrotal skin: further evidence that ageing enhances testosterone negative feedback. Clin Endocrinol 47:317–322

Winters SJ, Sherins RJ, Troen P (1984) The Gonadotropin-suppressive activity of androgen is increased in elderly men. Metab Clin Exp 33:1052–1059

Yamaji T, Ibayashi H (1969) Plasma dehydroepiandrosterone sulfate in normal and pathological conditions. J Clin Endocrinol Metab 29:273–278

Zirkin BR, Chen HL (2000) Regulation of Leydig cell steroidogenic function during aging. Biol Reprod 63:977–981

Zmuda JM, Cauley JA, Kriska A, Glynn NW, Gutai JP, Kuller LH (1997) Longitudinal relation between endogenous testosterone and cardiovascular disease risk factors in middle-aged men – A 13-year follow-up of former Multiple Risk Factor Intervention Trial participants. Am J Epidemiol 146: 609–617

I.11.2 Male Ageing: Wear and Tear

F. Comhaire, A. Mahmoud

Key Messages

- The ageing process affects the neuroendocrine and immunological systems, and free oxygen radicals cause damage to the membrane, mitochondria and DNA of body cells.
- Wear and tear damage to cells induces impaired function and increases the risk of diseases.
- The early detection and correct treatment of diseases, adaptation of nutritional habits and exercising are the cornerstones of healthy ageing.
- Cell damage can be counteracted by judicious food supplementation with particular nutraceuticals.

I.11.2.1 Definition and Pathogenesis

Although we do not get older, we live longer. This paradox summarizes the fact that the maximum life expectancy of the human species seems to be genetically limited, but that a larger proportion of the population can live up to that maximum expectancy. It seems that the number of cell divisions is limited by the loss of chromosomal material during each division, which ultimately shortens the telomeres (Morin 1997; Dhaene et al. 2000; Martens et al. 2000; Stewart et al. 2003; Baird and Kipling 2004) to such an extent that chromosomes cannot replicate and cells cannot function normally.

During the ageing process, several changes occur in the neuroendocrine system and in the immune defence mechanisms (Bruunsgaard 2002). Furthermore, organ functions decline and organ failure may occur. This, together with inherited constitution, favours the occurrence of age-related diseases.

It is not clear which factors determine the weakening cellular and organ function, but all kinds of toxins causing damage seem to be involved. These include exogenous toxins that have accumulated in the body after inhalation or from nutrition, and oxygen radicals (reactive oxygen species, ROSs) generated by endogenous metabolism. Commonly, exogenous toxins have a long half-life and they accumulate in the body, particularly in fat tissue that has a slow metabolism. Bioaccumulation and dispersion to the body from the stocks in fat tissue may hinder normal metabolism by inhibiting enzymatic processes. For instance, the apolar polychlorinated bisphenyls (PCBs) inhibit the function of the oxidoreductase Q10 which is essential for optimal energy production. Metabolism itself causes "waste" products and generates ROSs, which change the phospholipid composition of the cell membrane, decreasing the activity of membrane-bound enzymes, and which affect the three-dimensional configuration of receptors that lose some of their binding capacity. Furthermore, energy production by the lysosomes decreases, and oxidative changes of the DNA can occur, inducing mutagenesis (Knight 2000). Also, oxidative stress inducing the formation of oxidized guanosine, accelerates telomere shortening (Kawanishi and Oikawa 2004).

I.11.2.2 Clinical Findings: History, Physical Examination, Technical Investigations, Laboratory Findings

Any diseases, serious accidents or interventions leave remnants increasing the vulnerability of that particular organ or system. History taking must therefore include a full list of past as well as present medical conditions and treatments. Also, familial history is important, as this may reveal constitutional disposition for particular diseases. A systematic evaluation of the psychological status and level of activities in daily living is recommended. Careful evaluation of the physical condition must, as much as possible, assess vital systems and functions. Depending on the history and clinical findings, complementary technical investigations may be indicated, avoiding techniques with poor reliability or potential risk.

A number of blood analyses need to be performed at regular intervals in order to screen for age-related diseases, but also to evaluate the nutritional status, particularly in aged persons who depend on caretakers either in institutions or in their home.

I.11.2.3 Treatment and Prevention

Clearly, any diseases detected in ageing men need to be treated with state-of-the-art means. Thanks to the enormous improvement of techniques in anaesthesiology and surgery, interventions in the elderly carry only a slightly higher risk than in younger persons. Advanced age may, therefore, not be an excuse for not administering adequate treatment or performing surgery whenever indicated.

The early detection of age-related diseases and cancer (Mulshine 1999; Srivastava et al. 2001; Baker et al. 2004; Kelly et al. 2004; Troyer et al. 2004) should be implemented systematically, and treatment performed in as timely a fashion as possible. There is no doubt that diseases, including cancer, carry a better prognosis when detected and treated in an early stage, than if complications have occurred or curative treatment is impossible.

On the other hand, the ageing person should be encouraged to adapt his nutritional habits and reduce calorie intake (Montani et al. 2002; Patel and Finch 2002) to balance the lower level of energy expenditure. Regular physical activity adapted to the operating capacity should be stimulated (Ji 2001).

Hormone replacement therapy with testosterone should be considered in cases with hypoandrogenism, since this shifts the cytokine balance to a state of reduced inflammation and lowers total cholesterol (Malkin et al. 2004).

Finally, food supplementation using a judicious mixture of vitamins, minerals and plant extracts may reduce the burden of toxic and oxidative overload, and counteract some of their effects on DNA (Ferguson et al. 2004) and the telomeres (von Zglinicki 2000), on the cell membrane, the organs, and the vital systems (McCarty 2004).

I.11.2.4 Other

Aside from correcting endocrine deficiencies whenever present, a logical strategy to combat the consequences of ageing should pursue a holistic approach. This includes the early detection and adequate treatment of age-related diseases and cancers, the adaptation of nutrition, the encouragement of physical activities, and the judicious use of food supplements.

References

Baird DM, Kipling D (2004) The extent and significance of telomere loss with age. Ann N Y Acad Sci 1019:265 – 268

Baker SG, Kramer BS, Prorok PC (2004) Development tracks for cancer prevention markers. Dis Markers 20:97 – 102

Bruunsgaard H (2002) Effects of tumor necrosis factor-alpha and interleukin-6 in elderly populations. Eur Cytokine Netw 13:389 – 391

Dhaene K, Van Marck E, Parwaresch R (2000) Telomeres, telomerase and cancer: an up-date. Virchows Arch 437:1 – 16

Ferguson LR, Philpott M, Karunasinghe N (2004) Dietary cancer and prevention using antimutagens. Toxicology 198: 147 – 159

Ji LL (2001) Exercise at old age: does it increase or alleviate oxidative stress? Ann N Y Acad Sci 928:236 – 247

Kawanishi S, Oikawa S (2004) Mechanism of telomere shortening by oxidative stress. Ann N Y Acad Sci 1019:278 – 284

Kelly K, Alencar H, Funovics M, Mahmood U, Weissleder R (2004) Detection of invasive colon cancer using a novel, targeted, library-derived fluorescent peptide. Cancer Res 64: 6247 – 6251

Knight JA (2000) The biochemistry of aging. Adv Clin Chem 35:1 – 62

Malkin CJ, Pugh PJ, Jones RD, Kapoor D, Channer KS, Jones TH (2004) The effect of testosterone replacement on endogenous inflammatory cytokines and lipid profiles in hypogonadal men. J Clin Endocrinol Metab 89:3313 – 3318

Martens UM, Chavez EA, Poon SS, Schmoor C, Lansdorp PM (2000) Accumulation of short telomeres in human fibroblasts prior to replicative senescence. Exp Cell Res 256: 291 – 299

McCarty MF (2004) Optimizing endothelial nitric oxide activity may slow endothelial aging. Med Hypotheses 63:719 – 723

Montani JP, Antic V, Yang Z, Dulloo A (2002) Pathways from obesity to hypertension: from the perspective of a vicious triangle. Int J Obes Relat Metab Disord 26 [Suppl 2]: S28–S38

Morin GB (1997) Telomere control of replicative lifespan. Exp Gerontol 32:375 – 382

Mulshine JL (1999) Reducing lung cancer risk: early detection. Chest 116:493S-496S

Patel NV, Finch CE (2002) The glucocorticoid paradox of caloric restriction in slowing brain aging. Neurobiol Aging 23:707 – 717

Srivastava S, Verma M, Henson DE (2001) Biomarkers for early detection of colon cancer. Clin Cancer Res 7:1118 – 1126

Stewart SA, Ben Porath I, Carey VJ, O'Connor BF, Hahn WC, Weinberg RA (2003) Erosion of the telomeric single-strand overhang at replicative senescence. Nat Genet 33:492 – 496

Troyer DA, Mubiru J, Leach RJ, Naylor SL (2004) Promise and challenge: Markers of prostate cancer detection, diagnosis and prognosis. Dis Markers 20:117 – 128

Von Zglinicki T (2000) Role of oxidative stress in telomere length regulation and replicative senescence. Ann N Y Acad Sci 908:99 – 110

I.11.3 Organ Failure and Common Disease of the Ageing Male

E.J.H. Meuleman, F. Comhaire

Key Messages

- Cardiovascular disease and depression are the two major, non-cancer-related conditions that adversely affect ageing males. Both conditions are interrelated, with common urological conditions such as benign prostate hypertrophy (BPH), erectile dysfunction (ED) and late-onset hypogonadism (LOH).
- Sedentary life style, excessive food intake and lack of physical exercise are responsible for diseases such as diabetes and obesity, and the resulting metabolic syndrome and enhanced risk of all types of cancer.
- General complaints of ageing men are often considered to be part of normal ageing, whereas these complaints are in fact caused by specific and treatable as well as commonly curable diseases.
- The first goal of treatment is eliminating all causal factors detected upon extensive investigation. The second aim is symptomatic relief.

I.11.3.1 Introduction and Definition of the Disease

Men live on average 5 years less than women. This phenomenon, called gender gap, has been attributed to a difference in overall susceptibility to diseases between sexes. Also, it has been suggested that men look after themselves much less well than women do and it appears that men's coping with stressful events may be poorer because of less adaptive physiology, behaviour, and emotional tolerance (Kristenson et al. 1998; Weidner and Cain 2003).

Poor socioeconomic conditions are emerging as significant contributors to the gender gap. Men in the upper classes – those who have a good education, hold high-paying jobs, and live in comfortable neighbourhoods – live longer and healthier lives than do men in the lower classes, many of whom are members of ethnic minorities (Isaacs and Schroeder 2004). In general, education and income appear to be the most powerful predictors of mortality (Winkleby et al. 1992; Lantz et al. 1998).

In general, cardiovascular disease and depression are the two major, non-cancer-related conditions that adversely affect ageing males. Both conditions are interrelated, with common urological conditions such as benign prostate hypertrophy (BPH), erectile dysfunction (ED) and late onset hypogonadism (LOH), also known as partial androgen deficiency of the ageing male (PADAM) or andropause. On the other hand, a sedentary life style, excessive food intake and lack of physical exercise are probably responsible for diseases such as diabetes and obesity, and the resulting metabolic syndromes and enhanced risk of all types of cancer.

I.11.3.2 Aetiology and Pathogenesis

I.11.3.2.1 The Metabolic Syndrome (Syndrome X)

The metabolic syndrome was defined by Reaven (1988) and refers to a group of disorders related to the peripheral resistance to the activity of insulin. At least three of the following five risk factors should be present in order to accept the diagnosis of the metabolic syndrome (NCEP Expert Panel 2001):

1. Abdominal obesity
2. Increased fasting triglycerides
3. Low concentration of HDL cholesterol
4. Hypertension
5. Elevated fasting glycaemia

In 41 % of European men older than 55 years, the metabolic syndrome is present. The syndrome results from the interaction of genetic and lifestyle factors, particularly over-nutrition and lack of physical exercise. The X-syndrome predisposes to cardiovascular disease and type 2 diabetes mellitus (Bjorntorp 1988; Wannamethee et al. 2005).

I.11.3.2.2 Cardiovascular Disease

Until today, cardiovascular disease (CVD) has been the main cause of male death (33 %). Together with hypercholesterolaemia, hypertension and diabetes mellitus type 2, lifestyle factors and tobacco smoking in particular are the most important risk factors (NCEP Expert Panel 2001). In addition, an elevated concentration of homocysteine (Geisel et al. 2003) and an increased marker of inflammation, CRP (Ridker et al. 2001; Brandt et al. 2004), have been identified as independent risk factors. The World Health Report 2002 estimates that around 8 % of all disease burden in developed countries is caused by hypercholesterolaemia, and 11 % by elevated blood pressure. Finally, diabetes mellitus type 2, which increases the annual risk of CVD two- to fourfold (Garcia et al. 1974) occurs in 5.8% of men between 55 and 68 years of age and in 8.7% of men over 75 years (Heartstats). Diabetes not only increases the risk of CVD but also magnifies the effect of other commonly associated risk factors for CVD such as raised cholesterol levels, raised blood pressure and obesity.

I.11.3.2.3 Heart Failure

Chronic heart failure is a major disruptor of quality of life (QoL) of the ageing male with an incidence approaching 10 per 1,000 population among persons older than 65 years. Of these men, 75% have a history of hypertension, which was either undetected or has been insufficiently treated. Heart failure is a clinical syndrome arising from diverse causes. Not all patients with the condition have poorly contracting ventricular muscle, and a low ejection fraction may be due to ischaemic cardiomyopathy. Patients may suffer from uncorrected valvular disease, such as aortic stenosis or mitral regurgitation, or abnormal filling, resulting in diastolic heart failure. Many patients have at least one serious coexisting condition, in addition to advanced age (Jessup and Brozena 2003). There are reasons to believe that long-term exposure to environmental toxins may also be involved. Dioxins and (a-polar) polychlorinated polyphenyls (PCBs) present in small particles in exhaust gasses from cars (particularly those running on diesel) have been incriminated as pathogens.

I.11.3.2.4 Depression

Depression, one of the most common mental disorders, is particularly widespread among the elderly. In the USA, the prevalence of depression among community-dwelling older adults ranges from 1% to 3%, with depressive symptoms occurring in 8–16% (Blazer et al. 1987). The prevalence of depression far exceeds the frequency of Alzheimer's disease. Although depression is more common in female, unemployed, disabled persons, or persons who were never married or previously married (Alonso et al. 2004), the prevalence increases if there is chronic illness or the person is in a nursing home. It seems to be the sense of a meaningless life that is mainly responsible. According to data from clinical studies in which structured interviews were used, the reporting of somatic symptoms – somatization – by depressed patients is widespread (Simon et al. 1999). Therefore, depression frequently remains undetected (Rapp et al. 1988) and older persons in fair or poor self-reported health should especially be screened for depressive symptoms (Ried and Planas 2002).

The depression that often accompanies ischaemic heart disease, chronic lung disease, and cerebrovascular insufficiency may reflect a reduced delivery of oxygenated blood to certain regions of the brain and the regression of critical nerve cells. Moreover, current theories implicate a reduction in central nervous system serotonergic activity (Bryer et al. 1992) and the age-dependent decline of testosterone in men may be associated with symptoms of depression. It has indeed been demonstrated that hormone replacement with testosterone may produce a remarkable antidepressant effect in depressed men with low testosterone levels (Pope et al. 2003).

I.11.3.2.5 Dementia

Aside from Alzheimer's disease, senile dementia is a common pathology in elderly men. Cerebrovascular insufficiency, but also damage due to reactive oxygen species and unbalanced food intake have been identified as contributing factors. In particular, inadequate intake of polyunsaturated fatty acids of the omega 3 group has been associated with impaired memory function and progressive dementia.

I.11.3.2.6 Erectile Dysfunction

The prevalence of erectile dysfunction (ED) increases with age and has a considerable impact on QoL (Feldman et al. 1994; Fugl-Meyer et al. 1997; Stolk and Busschbach 2003). A systematic review of population-based studies shows that the prevalence of ED ranges from 2% in men younger than 40 years to 86% in men 80 years and older (Meuleman et al. 2001; Prins et al. 2002; de Boer et al. 2004). Depression, lower urinary tract symptoms (LUTS), cardiovascular disease, chronic heart failure and late-onset hypogonadism are the most common co-morbid conditions. Furthermore, ED is thought to be an early indicator of cardiovascular morbidity and mortality (Meuleman 2002; Seftel 2003).

I.11.3.2.7 Lower Urinary Tract Symptoms

Benign prostatic hyperplasia (BPH) is the main cause of lower urinary tract symptoms (LUTS) in older men. The specific biochemical event that initiates and promotes BPH has yet to be identified and characterized. Dribbling, reduced force of stream and urgency are the three most prevalent symptoms. The prevalence of LUTS increases with age: 10% of men aged 40–49 report moderate to severe symptoms compared with 44% of men over 70 (Sonke et al. 2000). Although the symptoms may adversely affect QoL and interfere with activities of daily living, only 9% of men consult a doctor because of LUTS, with a mean delay of 10 months (Stolk and Busschbach 2003). Even though the severity of LUTS is an independent risk factor for sexual dysfunction (Rosen et al. 2003), the negative impact of LUTS on QoL is not as pronounced as in ED. Nevertheless, the detection and treatment of LUTS may improve QoL (Welch et al. 2002) and may prevent acute urinary retention, surgery, incontinence, urinary tract infection, or obstructive uropathy (see Chap. II.4.3.d).

The prevalence of prostate cancer increases with age, quite remarkably at the time in life when serum testosterone in blood decreases. Prostate cancer may be detected when the patient consults because of LUTS. In an increasing proportion of cases, however, the disease is detected upon systematic screening, particularly when the prostate-specific antigen is measured in blood and/or digital rectal examination is performed (see Chap. II.3.6.). Prostate cancer is a very common finding in autopsy material of elderly men, but the disease often remains confined to the prostate. The reasons prostate cancer becomes invasive are not completely understood (see Chap. II.2.8.).

I.11.3.2.8 Late Onset Hypogonadism

With male ageing, there is a gradual decline in testosterone and an increase in sex hormone-binding globulin, resulting in a relatively greater fall in the level of free testosterone (Vermeulen et al. 1996) (partial androgen deficiency of the ageing male, or PADAM).

The clinical manifestations and the basis of the clinical part of the diagnosis of the LOH syndrome include loss of libido and erectile function; loss of lean body mass and muscle mass; reduced insulin sensitivity; decrease in bone mineral density resulting in osteoporosis; depression, irritability and diminution of mental acuity; fatigue; and vasomotor symptoms (hot flushes).

There is continuing debate about the reality of the LOH syndrome and whether the somatic and affective complaints are really related to androgen deficiency or are just physiological manifestations of ageing (Hargreave et al. 2004). Moreover, many of the symptoms that are attributed to androgen deficiency are nonspecific and may have other causes. For example, a cross-sectional study among Dutch community-dwelling older men demonstrated the adverse impact of LUTS, ED and cardiac symptoms on health status domains (Blanker et al. 2002) and community studies in Germany underline these interactions. Also, there is a relationship between failing sexual function, depression and other disease processes. Fatigue, reduced activity and increased depression scores and anxiety about sexual function are common in older men (Beute et al. 2002; Tan and Philip 1999). Based on this knowledge, it is justified to say that there is still a lack of good evidence to justify routine use of androgen replacement therapy for ageing men, although there are enormous potential benefits. First, there is a need to develop markers of the efficiency of use of testosterone as well as relying on serum testosterone levels.

I.11.3.2.9 Osteoporosis

Osteoporosis is the main cause of fractures in elderly men. Hip fractures occur at a later age in men than in women, but their prognosis is worse in men since near 50% of cases are fatal. The later occurrence of hip fractures relates to the higher peak bone mass in men than in women. Osteoporosis in men is related to the decreased testosterone production and late onset hypogonadism (Van Pottelbergh et al. 2004). In addition, the risk is significantly higher among men with elevated homocysteine concentration in blood (McLean et al. 2004; van Meurs et al. 2004), and genetic factors may be involved. The risk of fractures is particularly elevated in men treated with androgen deprivation because of prostate cancer (Shahinian et al. 2005) or patients receiving long-term corticosteroid treatment, for example, for chronic obstructive pulmonary disease (COPD) (Campbell et al. 2004).

I.11.3.3 Clinical Findings: History, Physical Examinations and Laboratory Findings

The most important message regarding organ failure and common diseases in the ageing male is that any person consulting with complaints, either in the urogenital or cardiovascular or cerebral sphere needs a thorough general investigation. History taking must include the person's previous history of diseases and treatments, present complaints and their development over time, as well as history taking related to different systems. Physical examination can only effectively be done when the man is completely undressed. The clinician must always palpate and perform careful auscultation of the entire body, assess blood circulation, measure blood pressure, perform a digital rectal examination, etc. Blood and urine analyses should be rather extensive and testing for the prostate-specific antigen (PSA), as well as a hormonal evaluation, are recommended. Imaging using radiology, echography and scanning should electively be applied depending on the findings of history taking and physical examination.

Ageing men may harbour cancer of the colon or stomach, or lung cancer, and these must be detected at an early stage to permit complete cure. Diabetes, hyperlipaemia, renal failure, anaemia, etc. need to be corrected. The cardiovascular status can be assessed by means of electrocardiography, cardioechography and cycloergometry. Bone density may need to be measured. A detailed investigation of diet and food habits may reveal unbalanced nutrition and possibly deficient intake of particular vitamins, minerals or omega-3 fatty acids.

I.11.3.4 Differential Diagnosis

Too often general complaints of ageing men are considered to be part of normal ageing, whereas these complaints are in fact caused by specific and treatable as well as commonly curable diseases. However, investigation by clinicians may be focussed on the complaints of the person, suggesting a particular organ deficiency or disease, and other diseases may be overlooked. In a series of men presenting for self-perceived andropause, over 80% showed serious pathology, whereas in no more than 20% of cases was late onset hypoandrogenism the only detectable factor (T'sjoen et al. 2003).

I.11.3.5 Treatment

Treatment must always aim at eliminating all causal factors detected upon extensive investigation. Clearly, just prescribing medication (see below) for erectile dysfunction is futile if the patient suffers from serious illness (e.g. vascular, metabolic or neurological diseases), which will remain undetected if a general evaluation is not done.

In the early 1980s, the only available treatment option for the man with ED was sex therapy, a prosthetic implant, a vacuum device or testosterone therapy, which was often inappropriate. The advent of intracavernosal injection therapy enabled stoical couples to resume sexual relationships, but many found such treatment painful and invasive (Hatzichristou et al. 2000). In 1998, the PDE5 inhibitor sildenafil was introduced as the first effective oral treatment for ED. Preferred symptomatic treatment for ED by patients consists of oral treatment (73.8%), intraurethral PGE1 (medicated urethral system for erection) (5.1%), intracavernosal injection (ICI) therapy (4.7%), vacuum erection device (5.8%) and implantation of a penile prosthesis (2.4%) (Braun et al. 2000). Based on these data, the current symptomatic ED treatment consists of a step-up program of trial and failure, ranging from noninvasive oral or mechanical treatment over intraurethral and ICI treatment to implantation of a penile prosthesis (see Chap. I.4).

The first-line treatment for men with symptomatic BPH is pharmacological, either an alpha-adrenergic-receptor antagonist (alpha-blocker), which reduces smooth-muscle tone in the prostate and bladder neck, or a 5α-reductase inhibitor, which reduces prostate volume by lowering the level of dihydrotestosterone (DHT), the primary active metabolite of testosterone in the prostate, thereby inducing epithelial atrophy (Lepor et al. 1996).

As alpha-blockers have a relatively fast onset of action in reducing symptoms (within days to weeks), they are often the first choice, particularly in men with a smaller prostate. The onset of action of 5α-reductase inhibitors which are most useful for men who have large prostates (> 40 ml) can take up to 6 months. Moreover, they reduce the long-term risk of acute urinary retention and the need for invasive therapy (McConnell et al. 1998, 2003). They also reduce the levels of PSA. Broad concern arose about the lower PSA levels as they may mask the presence of prostate cancer. However, recent evidence suggests that the ability of PSA to detect men with clinically relevant prostate cancer is not adversely affected by 5α-reductase inhibition.

The Medical Therapy of Prostatic Symptoms (MTOPS) study was conducted to determine whether combined treatment with an alpha blocker (doxasosine) and a 5α-reductase inhibitor (finasteride) would be more effective than either drug alone. The results of this study indicated that a greater delay in time to clinical progression of BPH was observed with a combination therapy than with either drug alone (risk reduction relative to placebo: doxazosin 39%, finasteride 34%, combination therapy 67%) (Tan and Philip 1999). Pharmacological treatment of LUTS due to BPH has reduced the number of surgical procedures and delayed their use. However, a quarter of men with moderate symptoms, and even more men with severe symptoms eventually need surgery. Transurethral resection of the prostate (TURP) is the standard procedure, but less invasive procedures, such as transurethral thermotherapy (TUMT) have gained prominence (de la Rosette et al. 2003).

The nonpharmaceutical approach using plant extracts should be considered as well, since its cost is lower and adverse or side effects are less common (Comhaire and Mahmoud 2004).

Osteoporosis is commonly undertreated (Meryn 2005). In fact, hormone replacement therapy with aromatizable androgens may be indicated. Supplementary nutritional calcium supply and vitamin D3, but most of all biphosphonates are the treatment of choice (Diamond 2005).

With regard to syndrome X, prevention is of pivotal importance. Treatment of affected patients commonly uses biguanides such as metformin to increase insulin sensitivity (Knowler et al. 2002).

I.11.3.6 Prevention

Whereas ageing cannot be stopped, diseases associated with it should be detected and corrected at an early stage. An unhealthy lifestyle must be corrected to promote health, by stimulating physical exercise and adaptation of nutritional habits. The regular intake of particular nutraceuticals (see Chap. II.4.15) and food supplements may decelerate cellular wear and tear and (oxidative) damage to DNA and the cell membrane. Also, nutritional supplementation with calcium and vitamin D3, as well as with vitamins B6, B9 and B12 may prevent osteoporosis, also by reducing the homocysteine level in the blood. Hormone replacement therapy may be indicated in cases of low hormone values in the blood. There is strong evidence that antioxidant supplementation with vitamin E and C, together with food supplementation with polyunsaturated fatty acids of the omega 3 group may prevent the occurrence of Alzheimer's disease (Zamaria 2004; Zandi et al. 2004).

These measures may reduce the gender gap, because there is no evident biological reason why men should not enjoy the same (healthy) life span as women.

References

Alonso J, Angermeyer MC, Bernert S, Bruffaerts R, Brugha TS, Bryson H, Girolamo G, Graaf R, Demyttenaere K, Gasquet I, Haro JM, Katz SJ, Kessler RC, Kovess V, Lepine JP, Ormel J, Polidori G, Russo LJ, Vilagut G, Almansa J, Arbabzadeh-Bouchez S, Autonell J, Bernal M, Buist-Bouwman MA, Codony M, Domingo-Salvany A, Ferrer M, Joo SS, Martinez-Alonso M, Matschinger H, Mazzi F, Morgan Z, Morosini P, Palacin C, Romera B, Taub N, Vollebergh WA (2004) Prevalence of mental disorders in Europe: results from the European Study of the Epidemiology of Mental Disorders (ESEMeD) project. Acta Psychiatr Scand Suppl 21 – 27

Beutel ME, Wiltink J, Schwarz R, Weidner W, Brähler E (2002) Complaints of the ageing male based on a representative community study. Eur Urol 41:85 – 92

Bjorntorp P (1988) Abdominal obesity and the development of noninsulin-dependent diabetes mellitus. Diabetes Metab Rev 4:615 – 622

Blanker MH, Driessen LF, Bosch JL, Bohnen AM, Thomas S, Prins A, Bernsen RM, Groeneveld FP (2002) Health status and its correlates among Dutch community-dwelling older men with and without lower urogenital tract dysfunction. Eur Urol 41:602 – 607

Blazer D, Hughes DC, George LK (1987) The epidemiology of depression in an elderly community population. Gerontologist 27:281 – 287

Brandt B, Hermann S, Straif K, Tidow N, Buerger H, Chang-Claude J (2004) Modification of breast cancer risk in young women by a polymorphic sequence in the egfr gene. Cancer Res 64:7 – 12

Braun M, Wassmer G, Klotz T, Reifenrath B, Mathers M, Engelmann U (2000) Epidemiology of erectile dysfunction: results of the 'Cologne Male Survey'. Int J Impot Res 12: 305 – 311

Bryer JB, Starkstein SE, Votypka V, Parikh RM, Price TR, Robinson RG (1992) Reduction of CSF monoamine metabolites in poststroke depression: a preliminary report. J Neuropsychiatry Clin Neurosci 4:440 – 442

Campbell IA, Douglas JG, Francis RM, Prescott RJ, Reid DM (2004) Five year study of etidronate and/or calcium as prevention and treatment for osteoporosis and fractures in patients with asthma receiving long term oral and/or inhaled glucocorticoids. Thorax 59:761 – 768

Comhaire F, Mahmoud A (2004) Preventing diseases of the prostate in the elderly using hormones and nutriceuticals. Aging Male 7:155 – 169

de Boer BJ, Bots ML, Nijeholt AA, Moors JP, Pieters HM, Verheij TJ (2004) Erectile dysfunction in primary care: prevalence and patient characteristics. The ENIGMA study. Int J Impot Res 16:358 – 364

de la Rosette JJ, Floratos DL, Severens JL, Kiemeney LA, Debruyne FM, Pilar LM (2003) Transurethral resection vs microwave thermotherapy of the prostate: a cost-consequences analysis. BJU Int 92:713 – 718

Diamond TH (2005) Pharmacotherapy of osteoporosis in men. Expert Opin Pharmacother 6:45 – 58

Feldman HA, Goldstein I, Hatzichristou DG, Krane RJ, McKinlay JB (1994) Impotence and its medical and psychosocial correlates: results of the Massachusetts Male Aging Study. J Urol 151:54 – 61

Fugl-Meyer AR, Lodnert G, Branholm IB, Fugl-Meyer KS (1997) On life satisfaction in male erectile dysfunction. Int J Impot Res 9:141 – 148

Garcia MJ, McNamara PM, Gordon T, Kannel WB (1974) Morbidity and mortality in diabetics in the Framingham population. Sixteen year follow-up study. Diabetes 23:105 – 111

Geisel J, Hennen B, Hubner U, Knapp JP, Herrmann W (2003) The impact of hyperhomocysteinemia as a cardiovascular risk factor in the prediction of coronary heart disease. Clin Chem Lab Med 41:1513 – 1517

Hargreave TB, Meuleman EJ, Weidner W (2004) Hormonal replacement therapy for aging men? The debate goes on. Eur Urol 46:155 – 161

Hatzichristou DG, Apostolidis A, Tzortzis V, Ioannides E, Yannakoyorgos K, Kalinderis A (2000) Sildenafil versus intracavernous injection therapy: efficacy and preference in patients on intracavernous injection for more than 1 year. J Urol 164:1197 – 1200

Heartstats: www.heartstats.org

Isaacs SL, Schroeder SA (2004) Class – the ignored determinant of the nation's health. N Engl J Med 351:1137 – 1142

Jessup M, Brozena S (2003) Medical progress. Heart failure. N Engl J Med 348:2007 – 2018

Knowler WC, Barrett-Connor E, Fowler SE, Hamman RF, Lachin JM, Walker EA, Nathan DM (2002) Reduction in the incidence of type 2 diabetes with lifestyle intervention or metformin. N Engl J Med 346:393 – 403

Kristenson M, Kucinskiene Z, Bergdahl B, Calkauskas H, Urmonas V, Orth-Gomer K (1998) Increased psychosocial strain in Lithuanian versus Swedish men: the LiVicordia study. Psychosom Med 60:277 – 282

Lantz PM, House JS, Lepkowski JM, Williams DR, Mero RP, Chen J (1998) Socioeconomic factors, health behaviors, and mortality: results from a nationally representative prospective study of US adults. JAMA 279:1703 – 1708

Lepor H, Williford WO, Barry MJ, Brawer MK, Dixon CM, Gormley G, Haakenson C, Machi M, Narayan P, Padley RJ (1996) The efficacy of terazosin, finasteride, or both in benign prostatic hyperplasia. Veterans Affairs Cooperative Studies Benign Prostatic Hyperplasia Study Group. N Engl J Med 335:533 – 539

McConnell JD, Bruskewitz R, Walsh P, Andriole G, Lieber M, Holtgrewe HL, Albertsen P, Roehrborn CG, Nickel JC, Wang DZ, Taylor AM, Waldstreicher J (1998) The effect of finaste-

ride on the risk of acute urinary retention and the need for surgical treatment among men with benign prostatic hyperplasia. Finasteride Long-Term Efficacy and Safety Study Group. N Engl J Med 338:557–563
McConnell JD, Roehrborn CG, Bautista OM, Andriole GL, Jr., Dixon CM, Kusek JW, Lepor H, McVary KT, Nyberg LM, Jr., Clarke HS, Crawford ED, Diokno A, Foley JP, Foster HE, Jacobs SC, Kaplan SA, Kreder KJ, Lieber MM, Lucia MS, Miller GJ, Menon M, Milam DF, Ramsdell JW, Schenkman NS, Slawin KM, Smith JA (2003) The long-term effect of doxazosin, finasteride, and combination therapy on the clinical progression of benign prostatic hyperplasia. N Engl J Med 349:2387–2398
McLean RR, Jacques PF, Selhub J, Tucker KL, Samelson EJ, Broe KE, Hannan MT, Cupples LA, Kiel DP (2004) Homocysteine as a predictive factor for hip fracture in older persons. N Engl J Med 350:2042–2049
Meryn S (2005) Undertreatment of osteoporosis in men. Arch Intern Med 165:241
Meuleman EJ (2002) Prevalence of erectile dysfunction: need for treatment? Int J Impot Res 14 (Suppl) 1:S22-S28
Meuleman EJ, Donkers LH, Robertson C, Keech M, Boyle P, Kiemeney LA (2001) [Erectile dysfunction: prevalence and effect on the quality of life; Boxmeer study]. Ned Tijdschr Geneeskd 145:576–581
NCEP Expert Panel (2001) Executive Summary of The Third Report of The National Cholesterol Education Program (NCEP) Expert Panel on Detection, Evaluation, And Treatment of High Blood Cholesterol In Adults (Adult Treatment Panel III). JAMA 285:2486–2497
Pope HG Jr, Cohane GH, Kanayama G, Siegel AJ, Hudson JI (2003) Testosterone gel supplementation for men with refractory depression: a randomized, placebo-controlled trial. Am J Psychiatry 160:105–111
Prins J, Blanker MH, Bohnen AM, Thomas S, Bosch JL (2002) Prevalence of erectile dysfunction: a systematic review of population-based studies. Int J Impot Res 14:422–432
Rapp SR, Parisi SA, Walsh DA, Wallace CE (1988) Detecting depression in elderly medical inpatients. J Consult Clin Psychol 56:509–513
Reaven GM (1988) Banting lecture 1988. Role of insulin resistance in human disease. Diabetes 37:1595–1607
Ridker PM, Stampfer MJ, Rifai N (2001) Novel risk factors for systemic atherosclerosis: a comparison of C-reactive protein, fibrinogen, homocysteine, lipoprotein(a), and standard cholesterol screening as predictors of peripheral arterial disease. JAMA 285:2481–2485
Ried LD, Planas LG (2002) Aging, health, and depressive symptoms: are women and men different? J Womens Health (Larchmt) 11:813–824
Rosen R, Altwein J, Boyle P, Kirby RS, Lukacs B, Meuleman E, O'Leary MP, Puppo P, Robertson C, Giuliano F (2003) Lower urinary tract symptoms and male sexual dysfunction: the multinational survey of the aging male (MSAM-7). Eur Urol 44:637–649
Seftel AD (2003) Erectile dysfunction in the elderly: epidemiology, etiology and approaches to treatment. J Urol 169: 1999–2007
Shahinian VB, Kuo YF, Freeman JL, Goodwin JS (2005) Risk of fracture after androgen deprivation for prostate cancer. N Engl J Med 352:154–164
Simon GE, VonKorff M, Piccinelli M, Fullerton C, Ormel J (1999) An international study of the relation between somatic symptoms and depression. N Engl J Med 341:1329–1335
Sonke GS, Kolman D, de la Rosette JJ, Donkers LH, Boyle P, Kiemeney LA (2000) [Prevalence of lower urinary tract symptoms in men and its influence on their quality of life: Boxmeer Study]. Ned Tijdschr Geneeskd 144:2558–2563
Stolk EA, Busschbach JJ (2003) Are patients and the general public like-minded about the effect of erectile dysfunction on quality of life? Urology 61:810–815
T'sjoen G, Feyen E, De Kuyper P, Comhaire F, Kaufman JM (2003) Self-referred patients in an aging male clinic: much more than androgen deficiency alone. Aging Male 6:157–165
Tan RS, Philip PS (1999) Perceptions of and risk factors for andropause. Arch Androl 43:97–103
Van Meurs JB, Dhonukshe-Rutten RA, Pluijm SM, van der KM, de Jonge R, Lindemans J, de Groot LC, Hofman A, Witteman JC, van Leeuwen JP, Breteler MM, Lips P, Pols HA, Uitterlinden AG (2004) Homocysteine levels and the risk of osteoporotic fracture. N Engl J Med 350:2033–2041
Van Pottelbergh I, Goemaere S, Zmierczak H, Kaufman JM (2004) Perturbed sex steroid status in men with idiopathic osteoporosis and their sons. J Clin Endocrinol Metab 89: 4949–4953
Vermeulen A, Kaufman JM, Giagulli VA (1996) Influence of some biological indexes on sex hormone-binding globulin and androgen levels in aging or obese males. J Clin Endocrinol Metab 81:1821–1826
Wannamethee SG, Shaper AG, Walker M (2005) Overweight and obesity and weight change in middle aged men: impact on cardiovascular disease and diabetes. J Epidemiol Community Health 59:134–139
Weidner G, Cain VS (2003) The gender gap in heart disease: lessons from Eastern Europe. Am J Public Health 93:768–770
Welch G, Weinger K, Barry MJ (2002) Quality-of-life impact of lower urinary tract symptom severity: results from the Health Professionals Follow-up Study. Urology 59:245–250
Winkleby MA, Jatulis DE, Frank E, Fortmann SP (1992) Socioeconomic status and health: how education, income, and occupation contribute to risk factors for cardiovascular disease. Am J Public Health 82:816–820
Zamaria N (2004) Alteration of polyunsaturated fatty acid status and metabolism in health and disease. Reprod Nutr Dev 44:273–282
Zandi PP, Anthony JC, Khachaturian AS, Stone SV, Gustafson D, Tschanz JT, Norton MC, Welsh-Bohmer KA, Breitner JC (2004) Reduced risk of Alzheimer disease in users of antioxidant vitamin supplements: the Cache County Study. Arch Neurol 61:82–88

Rationale

II

Understanding Normal Anatomy and Function II.1

II.1.1 Anatomy and Histology of the Male Genital Tract

A. Meinhardt

II.1.1.1 Testis and Scrotum

II.1.1.1.1 Testis

The *testis* has two major functions: the production of the male gamete, the spermatozoa, in a process called *spermatogenesis* and the synthesis and controlled release of testosterone as the main androgen, termed *steroidogenesis*. The testes are paired oval-shaped organs suspended outside the abdominal pelvic cavity resulting in a temperature 2–3 °C below the core body temperature of 37 °C. Sperm development will only progress normally at this cooler temperature. The venous plexus pampiniformis also contributes to the cooling since it is found to coil around the testicular artery to absorb heat from the arterial blood thus cooling it before it enters the gonad. Before birth the testes descend from the abdominal cavity where they develop through the inguinal canal into the scrotum. During their course they become invested by coverings derived from the serous, muscular and fibrous layers of the abdominal parietes as well as by the scrotum. Each testis is surrounded by a whitish tough fibrous capsule, the *tunica albuginea*, which contains smooth muscle cells. At the dorsal surface the tunica albuginea thickens and forms the testicular mediastinum. Here, blood and lymphatic vessels, nerves and the efferent ducts draining spermatozoa to the epididymis enter or leave the gonads. From the tunica albuginea approximately 250 fibrous trabeculae are given off centripetally subdividing the testicular parenchyma into lobules. In each lobule one to four highly convoluted *seminiferous tubules* are found, which produce sperm (Fig. II.1.1). The seminiferous tubules are continuous at both ends with other tubules, the ductuli efferentes, which transport the sperm from the testis to the ductus epididymidis.

II.1.1.1.2 Interstitial Compartment

The production of androgens and spermatozoa occurs in two discrete compartments within the testis. Spermatozoa develop within the seminiferous tubules in close association with the Sertoli cells, whereas the androgens are produced in the *Leydig cells* located in the interstitial space between the tubules (Fig. II.1.1). Besides the Leydig cells the interstitial space mainly comprises fibrocytes, blood and lymphatic vessels and a significant number of leukocytes (mainly macrophages and to a lesser extent T lymphocytes and mast cells). The Leydig cells often aggregate in small clusters around blood vessels and are rich in smooth endoplasmic reticulum, a characteristic structural feature of steroid-hormone-synthesizing cells. They have abundant pink cytoplasm with lipid, lipochrome pigment, Reinke crystalloids (hexagonal prisms by electron microscopy) as well as round nuclei with distinct nucleoli and are often associated with nerve fibres. Scattered Leydig cells are also found in the spermatic cord (funiculus spermaticus) as well as in the tunica albuginea. Leydig cells synthesize *testosterone* as the main androgen and many proteinergic factors such as growth factors, neuropeptides and cytokines. Normal Leydig cell function is dependent on luteinizing hormone (LH).

II.1.1.1.3 Scrotum

The scrotum is a cutaneous pouch that encloses the testes and the lower part of the spermatic cords. A raphe is visible on the median surface of the scrotum, which extends forward under the surface of the penis and backward as a tangible ridge along the middle line of the perineum to the anus. The external appearance of the scrotum varies under different circumstances from short and corrugated to elongated and flaccid. The scrotum consists of the following layers from outside to inside:

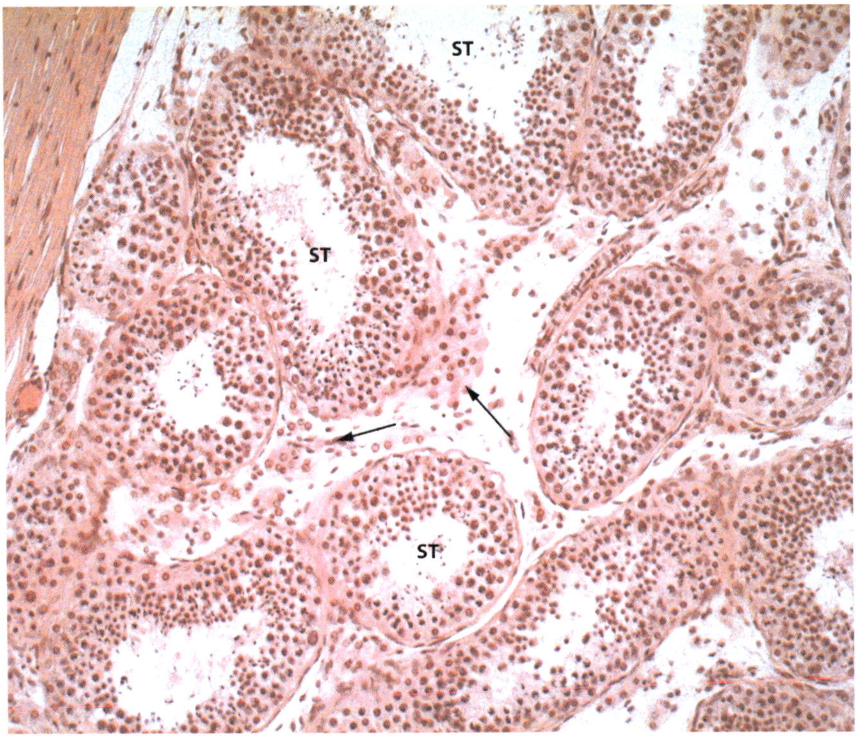

Fig. II.1.1. Histology of the human testis. The Leydig cells (*arrow*) can be seen in the interstitial space between the seminiferous tubule (*ST*). On the left the tunica albuginea is partly visible

skin (no subcutaneous fat) – tunica dartos (a thin layer of smooth muscle fibres) – the external spermatic fascia – cremaster muscle – internal spermatic fascia – tunica vaginalis [a serous membrane covering the front and sides of the testis and epididymis, composed of a visceral layer (lamina visceralis) and a parietal layer (lamina parietalis), originating from the peritoneum].

II.1.1.1.4 Vessels and Nerves

The artery supplying the testis and epididymis is the *testicular artery* which originates directly from the abdominal aorta underneath the renal artery. The testicular vein fans out to the *plexus pampiniformis* which follows the course of the testicular artery. Both vessels are found within the spermatic cord. After passage through the *inguinal canal* the veins reunite and drain on the left into the renal vein and on the right side into the inferior vena cava. The scrotum and its coverings receive their arterial blood supply via the *cremasteric artery* from the inferior epigastric and branches of the pudendal artery. The veins follow the corresponding arteries. The lymphatics of the testis end in paraaortic lymph nodes around the origin of the testicular artery (nodi lymphatici lumbales), whereas the scrotal lymphatics lead to the inguinal lymph nodes. The cremasteric muscle, the tunica dartos and the scrotal skin are innervated by the scrotal rami of the ilioinguinal nerve and by branches of the pudendal nerve.

II.1.1.2 Epididymis

The epididymis consists of a central body (corpus epididymidis), an upper enlarged extremity (caput epididymidis), and a lower pointed part, the tail (cauda epididymidis), which is continuous with the ductus deferens. The epididymis is covered by a thin fibrous tunica albuginea and is connected to the back of the testis by two small ligaments. The head of the epididymis is palpable through the skin of the scrotum and therefore accessible for clinical inspection. The rete testis at the dorsocranial part of the testis connects the seminiferous tubules with the efferent ducts in the caput of the epididymis. Approximately 6–12 *efferent ducts* converge into a single duct, the *epididymal duct*, which is highly convoluted and increases in diameter and thickness as it meanders to the ductus deferens. The convolutes are held together by fine connective tissue. The head of the epididymis contains the efferent ducts and the proximal end of the epididymal duct, whereas corpus and cauda include only the epididymal duct. Histologically the epithelium of the terminal part of the seminiferous tubules contains only Sertoli cells, and it gradually blends with the cuboidal or columnar epithelium of the *rete testis*. These epithelial cells may actually represent a continuation of the Sertoli cells that line the seminiferous tubules. The efferent ducts are characterized by a columnar epithelium of different height which gives the inner surface a wave-like appearance. The ductus epididymidis is lined with a pseudostratified stereociliated columnar epithelium which consists of ciliated tall columnar (principal) cells, narrow darker staining columnar cells, basal cells, clear cells and occasional intraepithelial lymphocytes (Fig. II.1.2). Tight junctions between neighbouring epithelial cells form a diffusion barrier. Proximally the epididymal tubules have a thin muscular coat, which becomes gradually more prominent in the corpus and particularly in the vicinity of the ductus deferens. Spermatozoa are stored within the lumen of the epididymis while they undergo a complex series of biochemical modifications to become mature sperm (Fig. II.1.2). Development and function of the epididymis depend on the luminal supply of testosterone, which is bound to a carrier protein – the androgen-binding protein (ABP), a secretory product of the Sertoli cell. The ABP–testosterone complex is transported in the ductal fluid, taken up by the epididymal epithelial cells, and metabolized to dihydrotestosterone by the activity of 5α-reductase. The epididymal epithelial cells secrete a variety of factors and enzymes that are involved in the maturation of sperm, amongst them the HE (human epididymis) proteins characteristic of the epididymis. Mature sperm are stored in the distal part of the epididymal duct until ejaculation. In times of low sexual activity excessive spermatozoa are released at a slow rate in the ductus deferens and are washed away during urination.

II.1.1.3 Spermatic Cord and Ductus Deferens

II.1.1.3.1 Spermatic Cord

The *spermatic cord (funiculus spermaticus)* extends for about 10 cm from the abdominal inguinal ring to the upper back part of the testis. The left cord is rather longer than the right, consequently the left testis hangs somewhat lower than its fellow. Embedded in fat and connective tissue, the spermatic cord contains arteries, veins, lymphatics, nerves, and the ductus deferens as the excretory duct of the epididymis. These structures are invested by the layers brought down by the testis in its descent and include from outside to inside: scrotal skin – tunica dartos – external spermatic fascia – cremaster muscle – internal spermatic fascia. The cremaster muscle serves in the regulation of testicular temperature as contraction and relaxation influence the distance between the testes and the body. The cremaster muscle is innervated by the genital branch of the genitofemoral nerve. The femoral branch in turn provides the sensory innervation of the skin of the medial surface of the thigh. Irritation of this area causes a reflective contraction of the cremaster muscle.

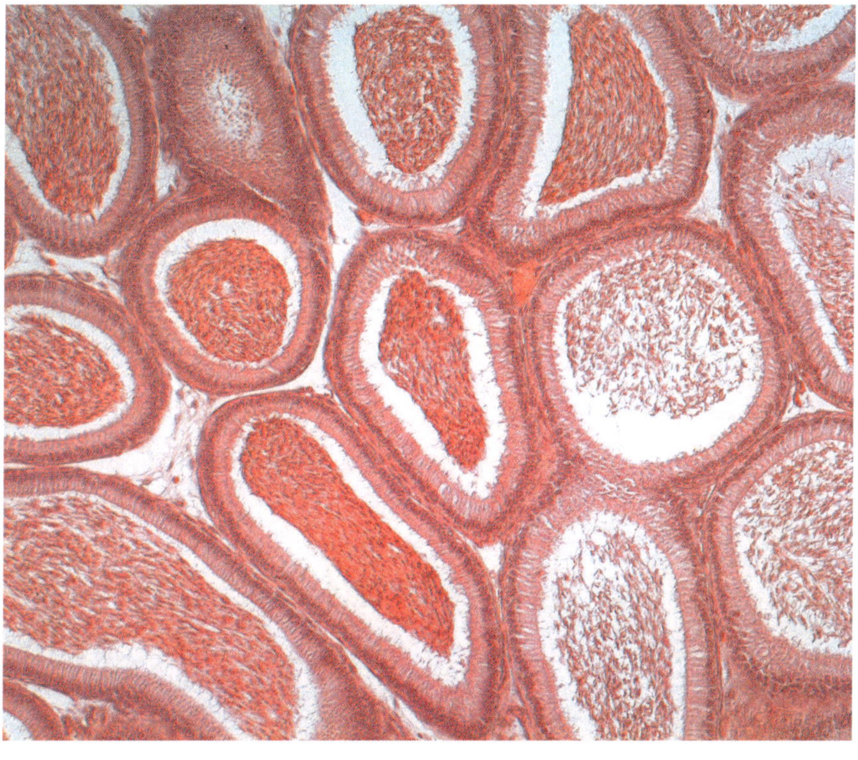

Fig. II.1.2. Cross-section showing tall columnar epithelium lining the coiled epididymal duct. The lumen is packed with spermatozoa. The tubules have a muscular coat, which plays an important role in sperm movement through the epididymis

II.1.1.3.2
Ductus Deferens

The ductus deferens is the continuation of the canal of the epididymis and is approximately 3 mm in diameter. As a constituent of the spermatic cord it traverses the inguinal canal into the pelvic cavity. Before the ductus deferens enters the prostate at its dorsal surface it enlarges to an ampulla and is subsequently joined by the duct of the seminal vesicle to form the ejaculatory duct, which passes through the prostate and opens into the prostatic portion of the urethra, close to the orifice of the prostatic utricle. The ductus deferens is palpable in the spermatic cord due to its dense wall. The adult ductus deferens is lined by pseudostratified columnar epithelium (consisting of principal cells, pencil cells, and mitochondria-enriched cells) resting on a layer of basal cells. The massive muscular coat consists of two to three massive layers of smooth muscle fibres. The external adventitia consists of connective tissue, blood vessels and nerve fibres.

II.1.1.3.3
Vessels and Nerves

The arteries of the spermatic cord comprise the testicular arteries, which divide into several branches and supply the testes and epididymis. The spermatic veins emerge from the back of the testis, and receive tributaries from the epididymis, to form a convoluted plexus, the plexus pampiniformis. Upon entering the abdomen the veins unite to form the testicular vein, which drains on the left into the left renal vein and on the right side directly into the inferior cava vein. The nerves are the genital ramus of the genitofemoral nerve, the scrotal branch of the ilioinguinal nerve, and fibres of the autonomic nervous system.

II.1.1.4
Prostate

The prostate is a firm gland about the size of a chestnut, which is placed in the pelvic cavity encircling the commencement of the urethra. Enclosed by a connective tissue capsule, it is composed of a radial array of up to 30–50 branched tubuloalveolar glands surrounded by a dense *fibromuscular stroma*. Contraction of the smooth muscle releases the contents of the prostate gland into the urethra at the time of ejaculation. The epithelium has a layer of cuboidal-to-columnar epithelium, and a second layer of basal cells (Fig. II.1.3). Most characteristic of the gland, however, is the presence of concretions which can be seen as onion-like structures in the lumen. According to embryological and histological studies, the internal structure of the human prostate is separated into four compartments: (1) the non-glandular stroma, (2) the preprostatic segment, (3) the peripheral zone and (4) the central zone. The central zone surrounds the ejaculatory ducts; it is made up of acini with a relatively simple configuration and is in-

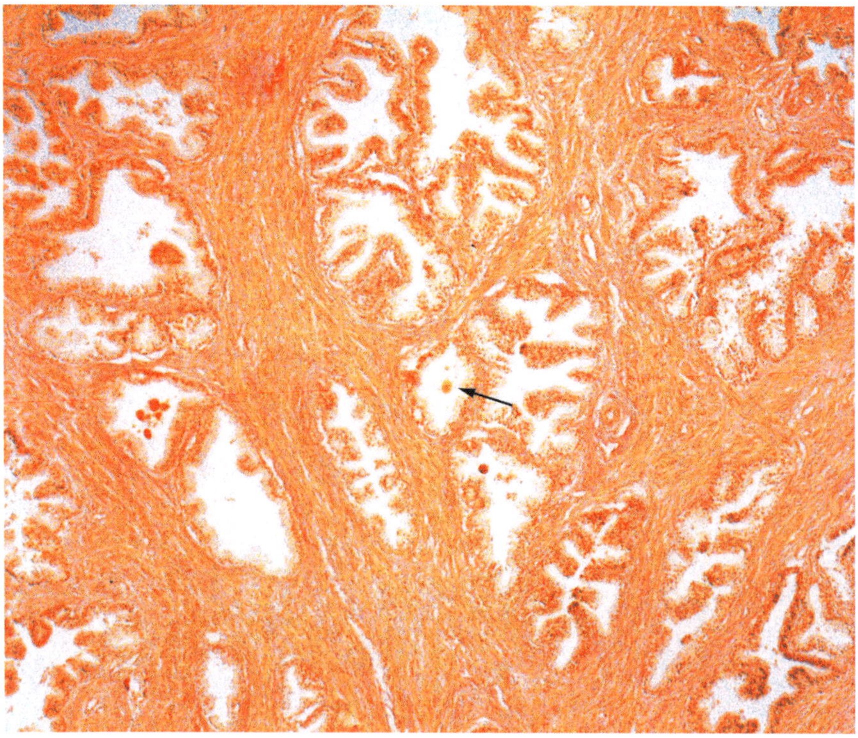

Fig. II.1.3. Cross-section through the prostate. The lumen is surrounded by a two-layered epithelium and a dense fibromuscular stroma. Occasionally concretions can be seen in the lumen (*arrow*)

II.1

serted in a wedge-like manner into the peripheral zone. The so-called preprostatic segment is the periurethral portion, which is regarded as the predilection site for the development of benign prostatic hyperplasia (BPH).

The human prostate has a dual function in that it produces a number of secretory compounds conditioning the urethral surface for sperm passage and acting on spermatozoa as well as on vesicular coagulation proteins (semen liquefaction). The secretion is lightly acid (pH 6.4) and is rich in zinc, citrate, acidic phosphatases and proteases, among which the *prostate specific antigen* is used for diagnostic purposes.

II.1.1.4.1 Vessels and Nerves

The arteries supplying the prostate are derived from the internal pudendal and inferior vesical. Its veins form the plexus vesicoprostaticus around the sides and base of the gland; they receive the dorsal vein of the penis, and end in the hypogastric veins. The prostate receives dual autonomic innervation: sympathetic from the last thoracic and lumbar roots via the hypogastric nerves, and parasympathetic via the pelvic nerves.

II.1.1.5 Seminal Vesicle, Bulbourethral Gland

II.1.1.5.1 Seminal Vesicle (Glandula Vesiculosa)

The seminal vesicles are paired, elongated, sac- or tubule-like structures surrounded by a thick coat of smooth muscle. The glands are placed between the fundus of the bladder and the rectum. The seminal vesicles have a capacity of about 3.4–4.5 ml and contribute about 60–70% of the seminal fluid. They empty separately into the posterior urethra after joining the ductus deferens. Their proximal and ampullary portions are capable of fluid reabsorption and spermatophagy (ingestion and degradation of damaged spermatozoa by epithelial cells). Each vesicle consists of a single tube, coiled upon itself and giving off several irregular diverticula, which give the gland a humpy exterior surface. The lumen is lined by one or two layers of a columnar epithelium which folds to a highly reticular pattern. The epithelium is surrounded by a muscular coat (Fig. II.1.4).

Secretory activity of the glands is a measure of testosterone supplementation to the epithelium. The secretory products of the seminal vesicles encompass

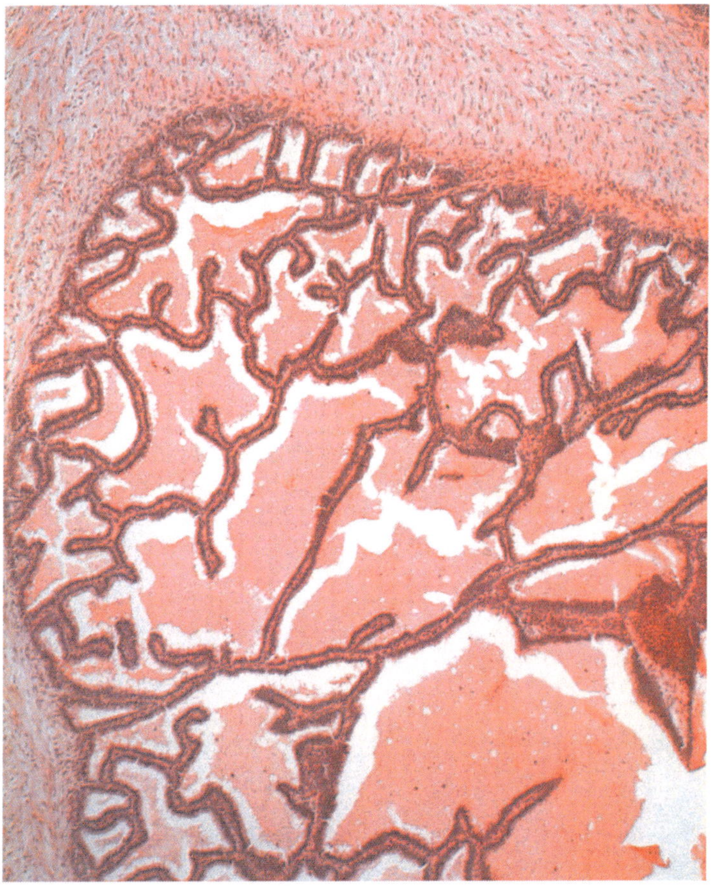

Fig. II.1.4. Histology of the seminal vesicle. The epithelium consists of one or two layers of columnar epithelial cells which fold to a characteristic highly reticular pattern. The mucosa is surrounded by a muscular coat rich in collagen and elastic fibres

ions, fructose, prostaglandins and peptides as well as proteins. In addition to plasma protein-related forms such as transferrin, lactoferrin and fibronectin, specific proteins such as *semenogelin* (52 kDa) are synthesized, the scaffold protein of semen coagulate forming the substrate of prostate specific antigen (PSA) and immunosuppressive factors. Therefore, functions of the seminal vesicles concern: (1) formation of seminal coagulum, (2) modification of sperm functions (motility, capacitation) and (3) immunosuppression.

II.1.1.5.2 Vessels and Nerves

The arteries supplying the seminal vesicle are derived from the inferior vesicle and the median rectal artery. The veins accompany the arteries and contribute to the vesicoprostatic venous plexus. The nerves are derived from the superior and inferior hypogastric plexuses. Nervous regulation of secretion is realized by cholinergic postganglionic, sympathetic (and perhaps parasympathetic) fibres, derived from the pelvic plexus. Contraction of the muscular wall occurs under the influence of excitatory adrenergic and modulatory neuropeptide Y (NPY)–encephalin–peptidergic nerve fibres.

II.1.1.5.3 Bulbourethral Gland (Cowper Gland)

The bulbourethral glands are paired, tiny, pea-sized glands situated inferiorly to the prostate. They produce a thick, clear mucus that drains into the urethra, which is released prior to ejaculation. The secretion is believed to neutralize traces of acidic urine in the urethra and to act as a lubricant.

II.1.1.6 Penis and Urethra

II.1.1.6.1 Penis

The penis and the scrotum constitute the male external genitalia. The penis consists of an attached root and a free body or shaft that ends in an enlarged sensitive tip, the glans penis, over which the skin is doubly folded to form a loosely fitted retractable case, the prepuce or foreskin. Internally, the penis comprises in essence the urethra and three spongy, erectile bodies. The two uppermost cylinders are the paired *corpora cavernosa*, the smaller lower unpaired one, which contains the urethra, is the *corpus spongiosum* (corpus cavernosum urethrae). All three masses are enclosed by a fibrous connective fascia and loose-fitting skin (Fig. II.1.5). The anterior three-quarters of the corpora cavernosa lie in close apposition, but behind this they diverge into two crura, which are firmly attached to the inferior rami of the pubic bone by two branches which are surrounded by the *ischiocavernosus muscle*. Contraction

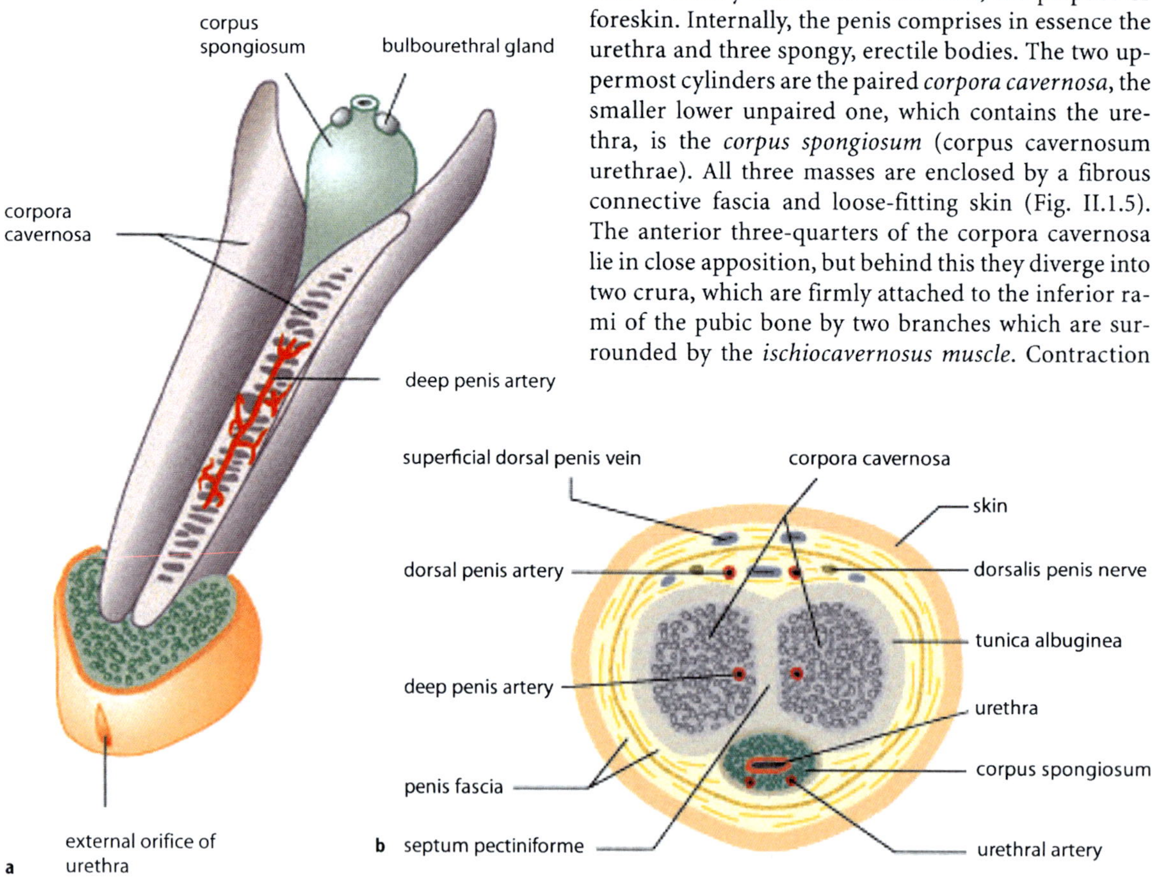

Fig. II.1.5a, b. Longitudinal and cross-sections through the penis. **a** Corpora cavernosa (*violet*) and corpus spongiosum with the glans of the penis (*green*). **b** Cross-section through the body of the penis

II.1

of this muscle results in increased tumescence of the corpora cavernosa during erection. Just before the two corpora cavernosa meet, both crura enlarge in the bulb of the corpus cavernosum penis. Each corpus cavernosum penis ends in a rounded extremity that is covered by the mushroom-shaped glans penis, which is a distal dilation of the corpus spongiosum (Fig. II.1.5). The corpora cavernosa penis are surrounded by a strong fibrous envelope, the *tunica albuginea*, forming the septum of the penis by their junction in the median plane. This is thick and complete proximally, but is imperfect distally, where it consists of a series of vertical bands arranged like the teeth of a comb; it is therefore named the *septum pectiniforme* (Fig. II.1.5). The tunica albuginea is 1 mm thick and rich in elastic fibres, which countervails a distension of the corpora cavernosa during maximal erection.

The corpus spongiosum expands at its proximal end to form the urethral bulb and is taken up in its distal course by the concave inferior side of the corpora cavernosa. The three erectile tissue cylinders are muffled by a common fascia, the fascia penis profunda. The urethra enters the bulb nearer to the upper than to the lower surface. The geminate bulbocavernosus muscle encompasses the proximal portion of the corpus spongiosum and aids in the emission of the ejaculate by compressing the urethra. The anterior end of the corpus spongiosum is dilated in the form of an obtuse cone. This expansion is termed the *glans penis* and is moulded on the anterior ends of the corpora cavernosa penis. A slit-like vertical external urethral orifice opens at the glans penis (Fig. II.1.5). The corona glandis is a flange at the base of the glans, overhanging a deep retroglandular sulcus. For descriptive purposes the penis is divided into the following regions: the root, which is connected to the periost of the pubic bone, the body and the extremity holding the glans penis.

Immediately behind the corona glandis originates the *prepuce (foreskin)* which completely covers the glans in the non-erect penis. The inner leaflet of the prepuce is covered by a stratified squamous epithelium which is slightly cornified. After birth the inner leaflet of the epidermis detaches from the prepuce and conceives flexibility, which is limited by the frenulum attached at the median inferior side of the glans.

II.1.1.6.2
Histology and Function

The *corpora cavernosa* allow the erection of the penis. They consist of a spongy tissue. The interspaces (cavernous spaces) are larger at the centre than at the periphery. They are filled with blood, and are lined by a flattened layer of cells resembling the endothelial lining of veins. The cavernous spaces are crossed by numerous fibrous trabeculae which are covered at their luminal surface by endothelial cells and contain bundles of smooth muscles and elastic fibres. They contain branches of the *Aa. helicinae* and nerves originating from the N. pudendus. The Aa. helicinae arise in numerous divisions from the A. pudenda penis, which passes through the corpus cavernosus, and branch at their distal end. Without an interposed capillary bed the Aa. helicinae open directly into the cavernous spaces. They are characterized by so-called epithelioid muscle cells located underneath the endothelium, which protrude into the lumen of the vessel.

The *corpus spongiosum* contains trabeculae that are more delicate than those in the corpora cavernosa and fewer smooth muscle cells with smaller meshes between them compared to the corpora cavernosa. Blood supply is ensured by the *A. bulbi penis*, which enters the corpus spongiosum in the bulb, and by small branches of the dorsal penis artery. Tumescence of erection is less rigid than in the corpus cavernosum to prevent obstruction of the urethra during ejaculation.

The venous blood is drained from the large central cavities in the smaller sinus at the periphery. It is collected by *venae emissariae* which pass transversally through the tunica albuginea and return the blood to the dorsal deep vein of the penis. Some veins emerge from the undersurface of the corpora cavernosa penis, receive branches from the corpus spongiosum and contribute to the deep dorsal vein after winding around the sides of the penis.

II.1.1.6.3
Vessels and Nerves

The *vena dorsalis penis profunda* is clearly visible under the skin and joins the prostatic vein plexus. The penis is traversed by numerous lymphatic vessels which are found in the skin, the glans penis and the urethra. They finally drain into the median inguinal lymph nodes. The afferent nerves are derived from the pudendal nerve via the dorsal nerve of the penis. They terminate in free endings or in specialized touch corpuscles. Parasympathetic fibres (*Nn. erigentes*) are derived from the S2–S4 segment; the sympathetic nerves originate from Th12–L2.

II.1.1.6.4
Male Urethra

The male urethra extends from the internal urethral orifice in the urinary bladder to the external urethral orifice at the end of the penis. It is approximately 20 cm in length and is divided into four portions: the *intramural, prostatic, membranous* and *cavernous portions*. The intramural portion (pars intramuralis) is 0.5–1 cm long and extends from the caudal part of the muscular wall of the bladder. It continues in the *prostatic portion* (pars prostatica), which is about 3 cm long and runs vertically through the prostate. At the posterior wall is an elevation, the colliculus seminalis, upon or within the margins of which the openings of the prostatic excretory and ejaculatory ducts are located. The *membranous portion* (pars membranacea) is 1–2 cm long and traverses the urogenital diaphragm. It is the narrowest part of the canal and is enclosed by the fibres of the sphincter urethrae muscle. The *cavernous portion* (pars cavernosa) is contained in the corpus spongiosum and represents the longest part of the urethra (15 cm). It dilates in the glans to form the fossa navicularis before it opens in the external urethral orifice. The mucosa of the male urethra shows regional differences, with the typical urothelium in the proximal portion developing a columnar pseudostratified epithelium further distally. In the fossa navicularis the columnar epithelium flattens to become cuboidal. Here, it contains glycogen, which is metabolized to lactate by the non-pathogenic lactobacilli generating an acid milieu to prevent ascending infections of the urinary tract.

Suggested Reading

Aumüller G, Seitz J (1990) Protein secretion and secretory processes in male accessory sex glands. Int Rev Cytol 121: 127–231

Benninghoff A, Drenckhahn D (2002) Anatomie. Makroskopische Anatomie, Histologie, Embryologie, Zellbiologie, Bd. 1. Urban and Fischer, Munich

II.1.2 Sexual Differentiation and Development

Y. L. Giwercman, A. Nordenskjöld

Summary

Normal sexual differentiation requires complex molecular events to take place in a precise order, and even though much knowledge has been gained in recent decades, further research is still needed to understand the pathogenesis of different disorders of sexual differentiation. For the clinician who is confronted with a child with sexual ambiguity, it is most important not to guess the sex but to initiate a proper diagnostic procedure, preferably done by a specialist team. Diagnosis generally requires a thorough clinical examination of the child and careful family history taking. The further diagnostic procedure includes cytogenetic hormonal and mutational analyses before sex assignment. Advances in molecular genetics are continuously providing tools for the detection of genetic defects and the primary diagnosis of intersex disorders. These methods may also be applied to prenatal diagnosis and carrier identification.

II.1.2.1 Introduction

Genital ambiguity is a devastating condition for parents of a newborn and an accurate diagnosis and rational sex assignment of crucial importance. Clinical diagnosis is however often difficult and knowledge of normal sexual differentiation necessary to understand these disorders. Below we describe the principles of sexual development, disorders related to different steps during sex differentiation and some helpful key points in the diagnosis of intersex disorders.

Two processes determine the phenotypic sex – sex determination as a first step followed by sex differentiation. During the first 6 weeks of normal human foetal development male and female embryos have the same phenotype although the *chromosomal sex* differs, 46, XY and 46, XX respectively. The embryo at that stage develops two bipotential gonads and two double ductal systems, the Wolffian ducts and the Müllerian ducts (Fig. II.1.6). In the sex determination step the gonad will develop to either testis or ovary according to different genetic events, thereby giving the foetus a *gonadal sex*. Classic animal studies by Alfred Jost in 1947 founded the research on mammalian sex determination (Jost 1947). Jost surgically removed the gonadal ridges, from which testes and ovaries are both derived, from developing rabbit foetuses in utero and then allowed the castrated animals to develop to term. The experiment showed that embryonic castration of male rabbits before a critical stage of development resulted in female differentiation of the internal as well as external genitalia, whereas unilateral castration resulted in female genitals unilaterally. Jost suggested that testis determining factors, i.e. locally acting hormones from the foetal testis, were essential for normal male differentiation. The testicular hormones that are essential for the male development are testosterone secreted from the testicular Leydig cells and anti-Müllerian hormone (AMH) produced by the Sertoli cells. Testosterone acts together with receptors on the Wolffian ducts thus stimulating the development of male internal genitalia, resulting in vas deferens, epididymis and the seminal vesicles. AMH acts on the cells of the Müllerian ducts, resulting in regression of these ducts and hence also preventing formation of the uterus and Fallopian tubes. In the same manner, the external genital organs in

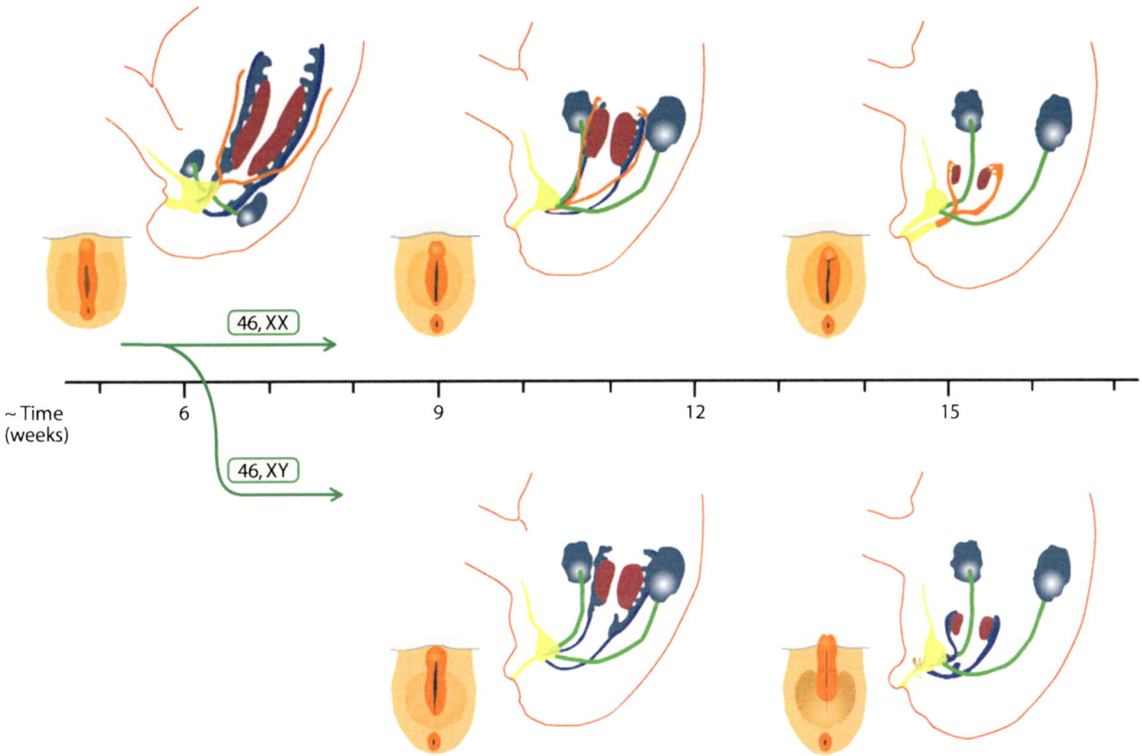

Fig. II.1.6. Development of internal genitalia. The Müllerian duct is indicated in *red* and the Wolffian in *blue*. The ureter is *green*. The urogenital sinus, the bladder, urethra and distal vagina are shown in yellow. Modified from original by Larsen, Human Embryology

males and females are identical after gestational week 6 (Fig. II.1.6). Under the androgenic influence in males the genital tubercle grows and differentiates to a penis, the urethral plate gradually closes to a urethra that opens on the tip of the glans, a scrotum is formed by fusion in the midline and the testes migrate from the initial abdominal position to the scrotum. The internal and external male genital development thereby normally constitutes the male *phenotypic sex*, together with normal puberty and fertility.

Due to this developmental cascade of events disorders of sex development in the male occur as different degrees of under-masculinization. In mild forms the boy has hypospadias with a urethral meatus located near the glans. In the most severe forms the meatus is located in the perineum. This severe form is also usually associated with a small and curved penis and often is regarded as an intersex condition. Other associated malformations are cryptorchidism and micropenis. In females, virilization causes different degrees of enlargement of the clitoris or midline closure to a urogenital sinus and scrotum. The most common cause of intersex conditions in females is congenital adrenal hyperplasia.

Based on the finding of sex chromosome abnormalities, Turner syndrome (45, XO) and Klinefelter syndrome (47, XXY) pointed to a testis-specific factor on the Y chromosome. In some male infertility patients most of the long arm of the Y chromosome was found to be lacking, whereas the short arm was duplicated (Jacobs and Ross 1966). Patients with deletion of the short arm were phenotypic females. These observations led to the conclusion that a gene or genes required for testis formation must be located on the short arm of the Y chromosome. By studying the genome of XX males with varying amounts of translocated Y chromosome material the testis-determining gene was finally cloned by Sinclair and co-workers in 1990 (Sinclair et al. 1990). The main male sex-determining factor was named SRY for the "sex-determining region of the Y chromosome", causing the indifferent gonad in males to differentiate to a testis and thereby initiating the whole cascade of events of male genital differentiation.

Besides Turner and Klinefelter syndromes, which have played crucial roles in our understanding of the importance of sex chromosomes and of testis differentiation, other disorders have also been important in defining the process of sexual differentiation thereby identifying key genes (Fig. II.1.7). Mutations in any of these genes lead to different intersex conditions with predictable phenotypes in most cases.

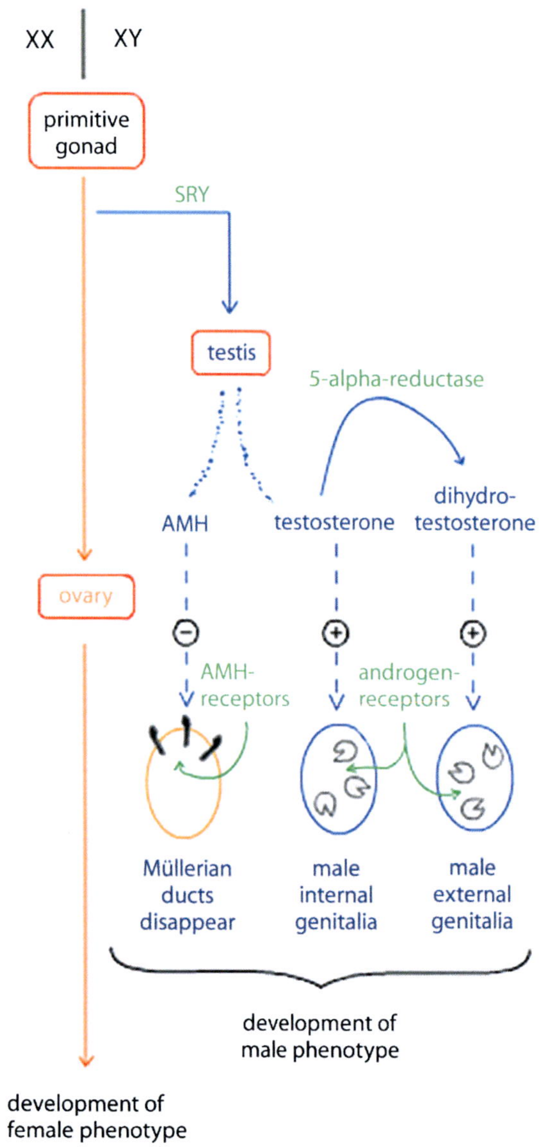

Fig. II.1.7. Schematic model of male sex differentiation

II.1.2.2 Genes Involved in Male Sex Differentiation

II.1.2.2.1 SF-1 (Steroidogenic Factor 1)

SF-1 encodes an orphan nuclear receptor protein, which is expressed in the urogenital ridge prior to differentiation of the gonad (Luo et al. 1994). SF-1 also plays a direct role in steroidogenesis by regulating the expression of steroidogenic enzymes involved in the production of testosterone. Inactivation of the mouse homologue gene results in animals lacking adrenal glands and gonads. These mice died from adrenal insufficiency shortly after birth. In 1999 the first patient with a mutation in the SF-1 gene was described (Achermann et al. 1999). This patient presented with adrenal crisis and female phenotype despite a 46, XY karyotype. As predicted from the mouse model, the phenotype was due to the absence of gonads and adrenal glands.

II.1.2.2.2 WT1 (the Wilms' Tumour 1 Gene)

WT1 was identified initially through its role as a tumour suppressor gene in Wilms' tumour or nephroblastoma, a paediatric kidney tumour (Little and Wells 1997). The normal WT1 gene product exists in different isoforms that both interact with SF-1 and promote the expression of other downstream genes, such as AMH (see below), and function by transactivation of the SRY gene (Hossain and Saunders 2001). The gene is located in the chromosomal region 11p13. Loss of this chromosomal region is seen in children with WAGR syndrome, a multigene disorder with aniridia, genital malformations, mental retardation and Wilms' tumour (Francke et al. 1979). Due to the very specific expression pattern, in both a spatially and a timely manner in the early genital ridge, gonads and kidneys, this gene was identified to cause Denys–Drash syndrome (Pelletier et al. 1991a). This unusual syndrome consists of early renal insufficiency resulting from mesangial sclerosis, gonadal dysgenesis and Wilms' tumour. In boys the syndrome is more easily recognized due to the male pseudohermaphroditism caused by the gonadal deficiency. In girls, on the other hand, only a very high grade of suspicion will reveal the diagnosis before the Wilms' tumour has already given symptoms. Therefore, this syndrome must always be suspected in small girls with renal insufficiency in order to diagnose tumours early. Mutations in this gene also seldom cause genital malformations and Wilms' tumour (Pelletier et al. 1991b).

II.1.2.2.3 SRY (Sex-Determining Region of the Y Chromosome)

SRY is the initial factor that starts the cascade of events that differentiates the bipotential gonad into a testis, leading to normal male genital differentiation. The gene is located on the short arm of the Y chromosome and consists of one exon with a central homeobox region and functions as a transcription factor (Sinclair et al. 1990). Further studies have revealed that mutations or deletions of the SRY gene cause at least 20 % of all XY females. This condition is associated with a substantial risk of gonadal tumours. A lack of normal SRY function always leads to a complete gonadal dysgenesis with streak gonads. However, all other stigmata are lacking. In addition, about 80 – 90 % of all XX males have an SRY gene translocation, usually to the X chromosome. Surprisingly, some XY female cases inherit the SRY mutation from their healthy father. The mechanism is unknown but is thought to arise through gonadal mosaicism. To add even more to the complexity of genital development, a few cases of an XX male phenotype but lacking the SRY gene have been reported, indicating that other sex reversal genes may stimulate normal male development even without SRY.

II.1.2.2.4
SOX9 (SRY-Related HMG-BOX Gene 9)

SOX9 is an autosomal gene situated on chromosome band 17q24. It is probably directly downstream of the SRY gene and is particularly important for Sertoli cell differentiation (Morais da Silva et al. 1996). It is expressed during chondrocyte differentiation and is upregulated in the male genital ridge as compared with the female. SOX9 expressed in XX gonads in a mice model gives rise to testis differentiation. Inactivating heterozygote mutations of this gene causes a syndrome called campomelic dysplasia, probably due to haploin sufficiency. This skeletal dysplasia, with characteristically bent limbs, is combined with a total gonadal dysgenesis in XY females (in 75%) or a partial dysgenesis (Foster et al. 1994).

II.1.2.2.5
DSS (Dosage-Sensitive Sex Reversal)

DSS refers to a region on the X chromosome (p21–22), which has been duplicated in some 46, XY females. This region is normally thought to be X-inactivated, since 47, XXY and 48, XXXY individuals are phenotypic males, whereas in DSS subjects, who have two active copies of the region, the function of SRY is overridden and they fail to develop testes (Bardoni et al. 1994).

II.1.2.2.6
DAX-1 (DSS-ACH Critical Region on the X Chromosome, Gene 1)

DAX-1 derives its name from its dual pathologic role in humans, i.e. DSS syndrome and adrenal hypoplasia congenital (AHC). AHC is a disease of the adrenal cortex and lethal if left untreated, due to dehydration and electrolyte imbalance because of mineralocorticoid deficit. DAX-1 is essential for the gonadal development of males but is dispensable in females. Inactivating mutations in the DAX-1 gene result in X-chromosome-linked AHC and hypogonadotrophic hypogonadism in boys (Muscatelli et al. 1994). Moreover, a testicular defect is present in AHC males, because treatment with gonadotrophins does not normalize spermatogenesis. In biopsy samples, Leydig cell hyperplasia as well as disorganization of seminiferous tubular structures is seen (Ozisik et al. 2003). However, in a female homozygous for a DAX-1 mutation, ovarian differentiation occurred (Merke et al. 1999). Over-expression of the gene, i.e. due to duplications of Xp21, causes ambiguous genitalia in 46, XY individuals, possibly by an antagonizing effect of DAX-1 on both AMH and testosterone production. The exact mechanism of DAX-1 action is not known and factors involved in DAX-1 regulation in different tissues and during development remain to be clarified.

II.1.2.2.7
MIH (Müllerian Inhibiting Hormone)

MIH, also recognized as anti-Müllerian hormone (AMH) or Müllerian inhibiting substance, is produced from the testicular Sertoli cells at 7–8 weeks of gestation, when the testis has recognizable tubules. High ipsilateral concentrations of MIH and testosterone lead to Müllerian duct regression and Wolffian duct preservation, respectively (Josso et al. 1977). Notably, there seems to be a window during development when Müllerian duct regression occurs in response to MIH between 8 and 12 weeks of gestation. Later production of MIH does not include this event. In the absence of MIH, the bilateral ducts normally develop into the internal reproductive structures of the female, and mutations in the AMH gene lead to persistent Müllerian duct syndrome in otherwise normally virilized males (Imbeaud et al. 1996). The same syndrome also occurs in about half of the total cases caused by mutations in the MIH receptor on the Müllerian ducts (Imbeaud et al. 1995).

II.1.2.2.8
17β-HSD Type 3 (17 β Hydroxysteroid Dehydrogenase)

17β-HSD type 3 is the last enzyme of the pathway of synthesis of testosterone from androstenedione in foetal testes. Deficiency of this enzyme is an autosomal recessive disorder with male pseudohermaphroditism, usually with a female phenotype but with internal male genital organs indicating a certain amount of testosterone production initially in foetal life (Geissler et al. 1994). There are three isoforms of the enzyme that probably account for the spontaneous masculinization at puberty and the initial foetal male development. The testicular form is the type 3 isoform. The syndrome can therefore be suspected in male pseudohermaphrodites with a high concentration of androstenedione exhibiting masculinization during puberty.

II.1.2.2.9
3β-HSD (3β-Hydroxysteroid Dehydrogenase)

3β-HSD isoenzymes are essential for the formation of progesterone (the precursor hormone of aldosterone) and 17-hydroxyprogesterone (17-OHP, the precursor hormone of cortisol) in the adrenal cortex. It is also essential for the formation of androstenedione, testosterone and oestrogen in the adrenal glands and gonads, thus catalysing a step in the formation of all classes of active steroid hormones. In humans, there are two 3β-HSD isoenzymes, which were chronologically designated type I and II and are encoded by the HSD3B1 and HSD3B2 genes, respectively. The HSD3B1 gene encodes the 3β-HSD isoenzyme expressed almost exclusively in the placenta and peripheral tissues, whereas the HSD3B2 gene encodes the predominant 3β-HSD isoenzyme expressed in the adrenal gland, ovary and testis. Deficiency of type II 3β-HSD is responsible for a rare form of congenital adrenal hyperplasia, causing various degrees of salt wasting in both sexes and incomplete masculinization of the external genitalia in genetic males (Simard et al. 1995). A milder, nonclassic variant of 3β-HSD deficiency has also been reported to be the cause of premature sexual hair growth in many young children and of hirsutism and menstrual disorders in a great number of adolescents and young women (Nayak et al. 1998).

II.1.2.2.10
SRD5A2 (Steroid 5α-Reductase 2)

SRD5A2 converts testosterone to the more potent dihydrotestosterone (DHT) in target organs, namely external genitalia (scrotum and penis) as well as the prostate gland. Deficiency of DHT consequently leads to insufficient development of male external organs but with normal male internal genitalia (Wilson et al. 1993). A lack of this enzyme does not have a phenotype in women. The condition is an autosomal recessively inherited form of male pseudohermaphroditism and was first described in an isolated area in the Dominican Republic (Imperato-McGinley et al. 1974). These patients will subsequently have a high testosterone/DHT ratio, accentuated after a human chorionic gonadotrophin (hCG) stimulation test that can be used for diagnostic purposes together with mutation analysis. Also in this form of male pseudohermaphroditism, there is masculinization during puberty due to an alternative isoform of the enzyme (SRD5A1). The isoenzyme is not expressed in foetal tissue and only very briefly expressed in newborn skin; however, later in life, after puberty, it is expressed in liver and skin. The remaining physical stigmata in affected individuals even after puberty include a small prostate gland, a reduced amount of body hair, lack of acne and a female temporo-frontal hairline. Due to underdevelopment of the prostate gland this disorder almost always leads to male infertility with a few exceptions (Katz et al. 1997; Nordenskjold and Ivarsson 1998). Mutational studies of affected males have shown that mutations are scattered over the five exons of the gene. Different mutations cause different degrees of impairment of the enzymatic activity due to different functional defects concerning ligand binding, co-factor binding or the half-life of the enzyme, which explains the varied severity of phenotypes of affected males (Wigley et al. 1994).

II.1.2.2.11
AR (Androgen Receptor)

The androgen insensitivity syndrome (AIS), a disorder of male sexual differentiation, is by far the most common identifiable cause of male pseudohermaphroditism (Quigley et al. 1995). AIS is an X-linked recessive disorder, thus only affecting individuals having a 46, XY karyotype. AIS is caused by an absent or dysfunctional AR and the phenotype encompasses a wide spectrum of genital ambiguities from completely female phenotype to slightly undervirilized males. Both testosterone and DHT bind to the AR and consequently any defect in the AR gene will, in the most severe cases with complete AIS (CAIS), lead to female external appearance, including female external genitalia. Generally, normal but immature testes are present and as differentiation of the embryonic Wolffian ducts occurs in response to androgens, Wolffian ducts are absent in individuals with CAIS. Müllerian ducts are usually also absent, as AMH action in the foetus is normal. Usually affected subjects lack pubic and axillary hair as well.

At puberty, the androgen resistance results in high LH levels in the circulation and subsequently an increased testosterone level. Testosterone is in turn peripherally aromatized to oestradiol, which in individuals with AIS is observed as normal breast development and feminization of the body contours. Patients with CAIS come under medical attention at various stages of life, a few being diagnosed soon after birth and some with the development of an inguinal hernia containing a testis during infancy. A portion of individuals, undiagnosed throughout childhood, present after puberty with primary amenorrhoea.

In the partial form of AIS (PAIS), the genital phenotype in affected individuals varies widely, from predominantly female appearance (cases with female external genitalia and development of pubic hair in puberty, or with slight labial fusion and/or mild clitoromegaly), to subjects with ambiguous genitalia, or cases with a predominantly male phenotype. Wolffian-duct-derived structures may be fully developed or rudimentary in PAIS, depending on residual androgen activity. Thus, the epididymes, vasa deferentia and seminal vesicles may develop to a variable extent, from rudimentary to being fully formed. At puberty, elevated LH, testosterone and oestrogen levels are observed and, as in CAIS, feminization of the breasts and body contours occurs as a result of high oestrogen levels, but in general the degree of feminization is less compared to that in individuals with CAIS.

Diagnosis of AIS requires the demonstration of a 46, XY karyotype and functional testes, which are able to synthesize and metabolize androgens normally. Once a CAIS diagnosis has been made the gonads are often removed, if possible before puberty, because of the risk of malignancy. Although some mutations were found several times in unrelated individuals, no major hotspots for mutations exist in the AR gene (AR mutation database). In situations where there is a limited family history of the disorder, precise information may be obtained only by sequencing the AR gene for the causative mutation.

II.1.2.3 Diagnosis of Sexual Ambiguity

The diagnosis of sexual ambiguity is clinically easy when the sex cannot be decided by a standard examination. It is crucial at this point not to make a guess about the sex of the child. One other immediate practical action is to take a blood sample during the first 24 h of life for testosterone investigation since that can be helpful in the final decision. The usual procedure is then to send the patient as soon as possible to a qualified team for a thorough investigation before assigning a sex to the child together with the parents. The team consists of physicians from Paediatric Endocrinology, Paediatric Surgery, Paediatric Psychiatry, Gynaecology and Clinical Genetics. The team will proceed with urgency, collecting data on heredity, making a pedigree as well as performing a thorough physical examination of the child, sometimes with ultrasound, urethrocystoscopy, laparotomy/laparoscopy and biopsy of the gonad. The single most important laboratory investigation is a karyotype and/or SRY examination. If the karyotype is 46, XX the cause is almost always congenital adrenal hyperplasia, caused by 21-hydroxylase deficiency. The further diagnostic procedure in 46, XY individuals is more complex but the above-mentioned syndromes are the most studied so far. In clinical reality, there are children with male pseudohermaphroditism (46, XY karyotype and testes with underdevelopment of the phenotypic male sex) that in the end do not have a specific molecular diagnosis before assignment to either sex. This is the ultimate future challenge for researchers in this field.

References

Achermann JC, Ito M, Hindmarsh PC, Jameson JL (1999) A mutation in the gene encoding steroidogenic factor-1 causes XY sex reversal and adrenal failure in humans. Nature Genet 22:125–126

Bardoni B, Zanaria E, Guioli G, Floridia G, Worley KC, Tononi G, Ferrante E, Chiumello G, McCabe ERB, Fraccaro M, Zuffardi O, Camerino G (1994) A dosage sensitive locus at chromosome Xp21 is involved in male to female sex reversal. Nature Genet 7:497–501

Foster JW, Dominguez-Steglich MA, Guioli S, Kwok C, Weller PA, Stevanovic M, Weissenbach J, Mansour S, Young ID, Goodfellow PN, Brook JD, Schafer AJ (1994) Campomelic dysplasia and autosomal sex reversal caused by mutations in an *SRY*-related gene. Nature 372:525–530

Francke U, Holmes LB, Atkins L, Riccardi VM (1979) Aniridia-Wilms' tumor association: evidence for specific deletion of 11p13. Cytogenet Cell Genet 24:185–192

Geissler WM, Davis DL, Wu L, Bradshaw KD, Patel S, Mendonca BB, Elliston KO, Wilson JD, Russel DW, Andersson S (1994) Male pseudohermaphroditism caused by mutations of testicular 17β-hydroxysteroid dehydrogenase 3. Nature Genet 7:34–39

Hossain A, Saunders GF (2001) The human sex-determining gene SRY is a direct target of WT1. J Biol Chem 276: 16817–16823

Imbeaud S, Faure E, Lamarre I, Mattéi M-G, di Clemente N, Tizard R, Carré-Eusèbe D, Belville C, Tragethon L, Tonkin C, Nelson J, McAuliffe M, Bidart J-M, Lababidi A, Josso N, Cate RL, Picard J-Y (1995) Insensitivity to anti-Müllerian hormone due to a mutation in the human anti-Müllerian hormone receptor. Nature Genet 11:382–388

Imbeaud S, Belville C, Messika-Zeitoun L, Rey R, di Clemente N, Josso N, Picard J-Y (1996) A 27 basepair deletion of the anti-Müllerian type II receptor gene is the most common cause of the persistent Müllerian duct syndrome. Hum Mol Genet 5:1269–1277

Imperato-McGinley J, Guerrero L, Gautier T, Peterson E (1974) Steroid 5α-reductase deficiency in man: an inherited form of male pseudohermaphroditism. Science 186:1213–1215

Jacobs PA, Ross A (1966) Structural abnormalities of the Y chromosome in man. Nature 210:352–354

Josso N, Picarf JY, Tran D (1977) The antimüllerian hormone. Rec Prog Horm Res 33:117–160

Jost A (1947) Recherches sur la differenciation sexuelle de l'embryon de lapin. Arch Anat Micr Morph Exp 36:271–315

Katz MD, Kligman I, Cai LQ, Zhu YS, Fratianni CM, Zervoudakis I, Rosenwaks Z, Imperato-McGinley J (1997) Paternity by intrauterine insemination with sperm from a man with 5-alpha-reductase-2 deficiency. N Engl J Med 336:994–997

Little M, Wells C (1997) A clinical overview of WT1 gene mutations. Human Mutat 9:209–225

Luo X, Ikeda Y, Parker KL (1994) A cell-specific nuclear receptor is essential for adrenal and gonadal development and sexual differentiation. Cell 77:481–490

Merke DP, Tajima T, Baron J, Cutler GB Jr (1999) Hypogonadotropic hypogonadism in a female caused by an X-linked recessive mutation in the DAX1 gene. N Engl J Med 340:1248–1252

Morais da Silva S, Hacker A, Harley V, Goodfellow P, Swain A, Lovell-Badge R (1996) Sox9 expression during gonadal development implies a conserved role for the gene in testis differentiation in mammals and birds. Nature Genet 14:62–68

Muscatelli F, Strom TM, Walker AP, Zanaria E, Récan D, Meindl A, Bardoni B, Guioli S, Zehetner G, Rabl W, Schwarz HP, Kaplan J-C, Camerino G, Meitinger T, Monaco AP (1994) Mutations in the *DAX-1* gene give rise to both X-linked adrenal hypoplasia congenita and hypogonadotropic hypogonadism. Nature 372:672–676

Nayak S, Lee PA, Witchel SF (1998) Variants of the type II 3beta-hydroxysteroid dehydrogenase gene in children with premature pubic hair and hyperandrogenic adolescents. Mol Genet Metab 64:184–192

Nordenskjold A, Ivarsson SA (1998) Molecular characterization of 5 alpha-reductase type 2 deficiency and fertility in a Swedish family. J Clin Endocrinol Metab 83:3236–3238

Ozisik G, Mantovani G, Achermann JC, Persani L, Spada A, Weiss J, Beck-Peccoz P, Jameson JL (2003) An alternate

translation initiation site circumvents an amino-terminal DAX1 nonsense mutation leading to a mild form of X-linked adrenal hypoplasia congenita. J Clin Endocrinol Metab 88:417–423
Pelletier J, Bruening W, Kashtan CE, Mauer SM, Manivel JC, Striegel JE, Houghton DC, Junien C, Habib R, Fouser L, Fine RN, Silverman BL, Housman D (1991a) Germline mutations in the Wilms' tumor suppressor gene disrupt urogenital development in humans. Cell 67:437–447
Pelletier J, Bruening W, Li FP, Haber DA, Glaser T, Housman DE (1991b) WT1 mutations contribute to abnormal genital system development and hereditary Wilms' tumour. Nature 353:431–434
Quigley CA, De Bellis A, Marschke KB, El-Awady MK, Wilson EM, French FS (1995) Androgen receptor defects: historical, clinical, and molecular perspectives. Endocr Rev 16:271–321
Simard J, Rheaume E, Mebarki F, Sanchez R, New MI, Morel Y, Labrie F (1995) Molecular basis of human 3 beta-hydroxysteroid dehydrogenase deficiency. J Steroid Biochem Mol Biol 53:127–138
Sinclair AH, Berta P, Palmer MS, Hawkins JR, Grittiths BL, Smith MJ, Foster JW, Frischauf A-M, Lovell-Badge R, Goodfellow PN (1990) A gene from the human sex-determining region encodes a protein with homology to a conserved DNA-binding motif. Nature 346:240–244
Wigley WC, Prihoda JS, Mowszowicz I, Mendonca BB, New MI, Wilson JD, Russel DW (1994) Natural mutagenesis study of the human steroid 5 alpha-reductase 2 isozyme. Biochemistry 33:1265–1270
Wilson JD, Griffin JE, Russell DW (1993) Steroid 5-alpha-reductase 2 deficiency. Endocr Rev 14:577–593

II.1.3 Physiology of Spermatogenesis

M. Bergmann

Summary

Spermatogenesis includes multiplication of spermatogonia, meiosis of spermatocytes and differentiation of spermatids into the male gamete, which is capable of motility and fertilizing an egg. Spermatogenesis occurs within the testicular seminiferous tubules, which consist of peritubular tissue and the seminiferous epithelium. The latter is composed of germ cells and somatic Sertoli cells. Somatic Sertoli cells divide the seminiferous epithelium into basal and adluminal compartments by inter-Sertoli cell junctional complexes protecting spermatocytes and spermatids from the immune system. They support and trigger germ cell development by mediating hormonal stimuli because they are the only cells within the epithelium possessing follicle-stimulating hormone and androgen receptors. Germ cell apoptosis is most important during pubertal establishment of the species-specific ratio of germ cells to Sertoli cells, and is increased together with spermatogenic impairment. There are six different, specific germ cell associations within the seminiferous epithelium: "stages of spermatogenesis". These stages are sequentially arranged along the length of a tubule: "wave of spermatogenesis". The duration of this wave is the "cycle of spermatogenesis". It takes 16 days; the whole process of spermatogenesis from the spermatogonium to the release of the spermatozoon takes about 70–75 days.

Spermatogenic efficiency is within the range of other primates and shows that sperm number is not limited by germ cell loss during meiosis but depends on the number of spermatogonia entering meiosis.

Spermatogenic impairment is regularly associated with Sertoli cell maturation deficiency, and incorrect DNA integrity and condensation due to failure in histone to protamine exchange may be an important factor predicting the outcome of assisted reproduction by in vitro fertilization or testicular sperm extraction/intracytoplasmic sperm injection.

II.1.3.1 Spermatogenesis

Spermatogenesis represents the entire process of germ cell development within the seminiferous epithelium of the adult testis. It can be divided into four phases and includes: (1) the proliferation and differentiation of spermatogonia, (2) meiotic divisions of spermatocytes, (3) the transformation of haploid round spermatids arising from the second meiotic division into spermatozoa (spermiogenesis), which (4) are released into the lumen of the seminiferous tubules (spermiation) (Fig. II. 1.8a, b).

II.1.3.2 Seminiferous Tubules

Seminiferous tubules have a diameter of about 180 µm and consist of peritubular tissue (lamina propria) and the seminiferous epithelium. The lamina propria (8 µm) is composed of four to five layers of contractile myofibroblasts and connective tissue. The seminiferous epithelium (80 µm) rests on a basal lamina and consists of germ cells in different developmental stages and the supporting somatic Sertoli cells, which provide an extreme cytoplasmic ramification and surround adjacent germ cells (Fig. II. 1.9a, b).

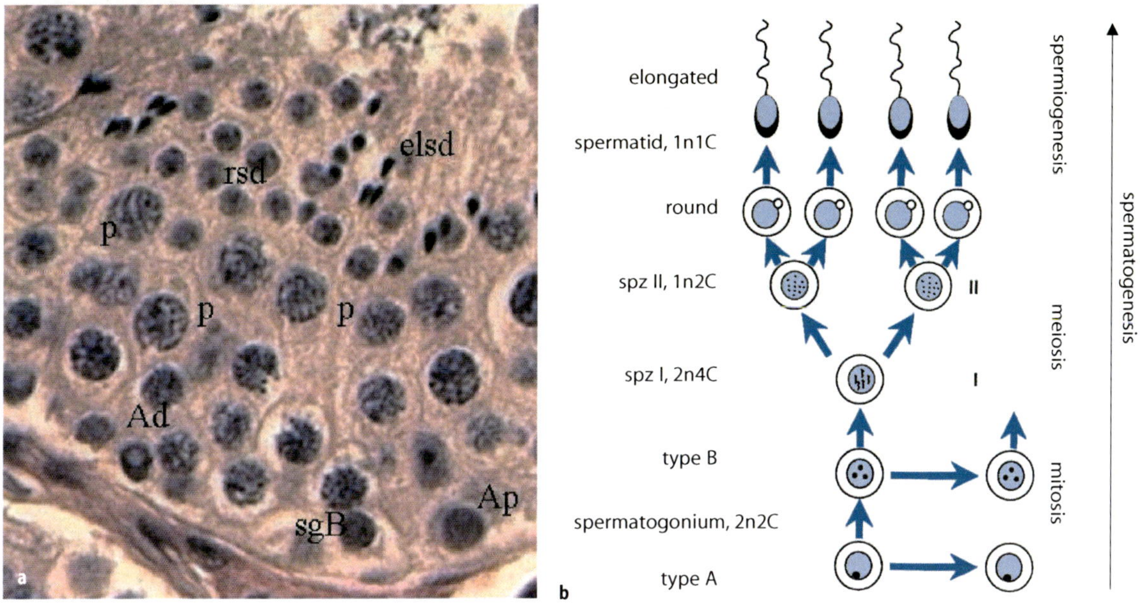

Fig. II.1.8a, b. Seminiferous epithelium and process of spermatogenesis. **a** Normal seminiferous epithelium. [*Ap* Spermatogonium type A (pale), *Ad* spermatogonium type A (dark), *sgB* spermatogonium type B, *P* primary pachytene spermatocyte, *rsd* round spermatid, *elsd* elongated spermatid.] Paraffin section, haematoxylin and eosin, primary magnification, ×40. **b** Process of spermatogenesis

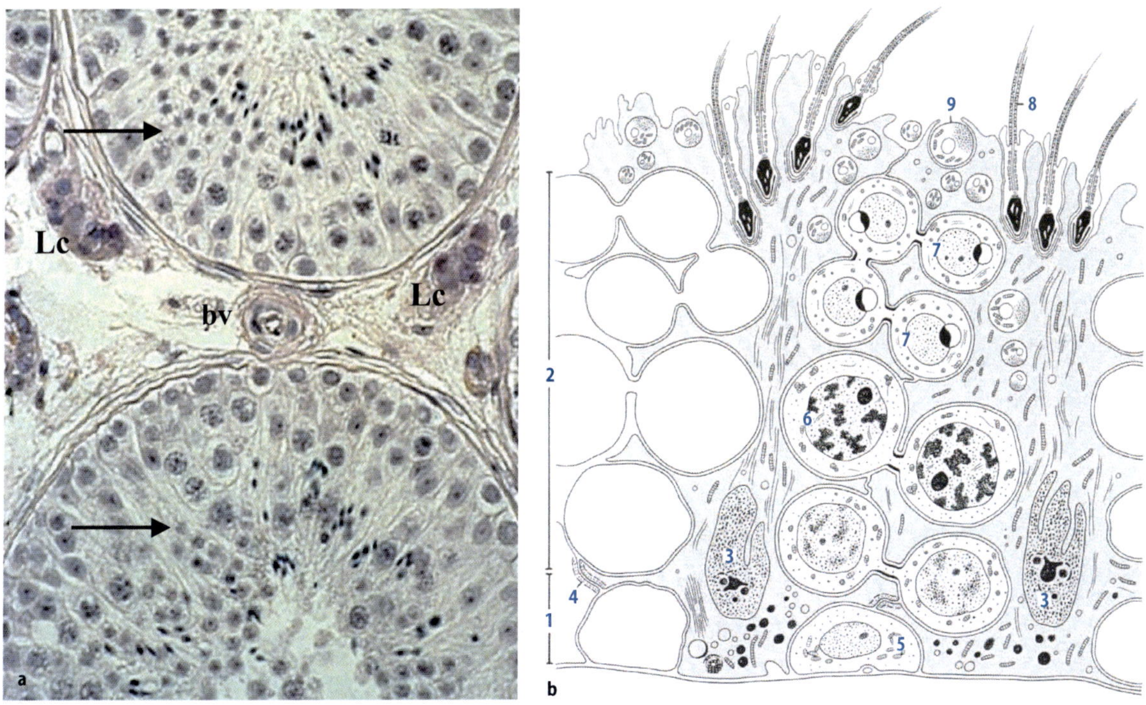

Fig. II.1.9a, b. Normal seminiferous epithelium. **a** Seminiferous tubules with intact seminiferous epithelium (*arrows*) and interstitial tissue containing blood vessels (*bv*), and Leydig cells (*Lc*); paraffin section, haematoxylin and eosin, primary magnification, ×20. **b** Schematic drawing of the seminiferous epithelium. [*1* Basal compartment, *2* adluminal compartment, *3* Sertoli cell nucleus, *4* inter-Sertoli cell junctional complex, *5* type a (pale) spermatogonium, *6* primary pachytene spermatocyte, *7* round spermatid, *8* elongated spermatid, *9* residual body.] From Holstein (1994)

II.1.3.3 Spermatogonia

Spermatogonia are the diploid (2n2 C) stem cells of spermatogenesis, and can be divided into type A and type B. They undergo mitotic divisions and thus represent the renewing stem cell population. The classification is mainly based on differences of nuclear chromatin pattern. Type A spermatogonia have an oval euchromatic nucleus in contrast to type B spermatogonia, which have a round heterochromatic nucleus. In primates including humans, type A spermatogonia are further divided into A pale (Ap) and A dark (Ad) according to their differing nuclear appearance. In contrast to Ap, Ad spermatogonia are characterized by a dark nucleus showing a light halo. A possible functional significance in respect of mitotic activity remains controversial. In non-human primates Ad spermatogonia have no or only weak proliferative activity (Schlatt and Weinbauer 1994), whereas S-phase-specific Ki-67 immunoreactivity indicating mitotic activity was found in both Ap and Ad spermatogonia by Steger et al. (1998) in the human.

It is generally agreed that type B spermatogonia are able to differentiate and enter the process of meiosis. Due to incomplete cytokinesis, type B spermatogonia remain interconnected after the last mitotic division by intercellular bridges forming cellular clones, which allow synchrony of germ cell maturation. These intercellular bridges persist until late spermiogenesis. In spermatogonia, genomic imprinting for parent-of-origin-dependent regulation of gene expression via DNA methylation takes place and is finished before the first meiotic division (Kierszenbaum 2002).

II.1.3.4 Spermatocytes/Meiosis

II.1.3.4.1 Primary Spermatocytes

II.1

Meiosis starts with DNA synthesis of type B spermatogonia which lose contact with the basal lamina (preleptotene). After completion of DNA synthesis, each chromosome consists of two chromatids (C). These cells are named primary spermatocytes, and the DNA content is tetraploid (2n4 C). Primary spermatocytes undergo the first meiotic division. The prophase of the first meiotic division takes about 1–3 weeks and is divided into several stages: the leptotene, zygotene, pachytene and diplotene stages.

The leptotene stage is characterized by DNA condensation resulting in the appearance of thin filaments within the nucleus. In the zygotene stage, condensation of chromosomes proceeds, and pairing of homologous chromosomes takes place due to the formation of the "synaptonemal complexes" which are only visible using an electron microscope. In the pachytene stage, there is an exchange of genetic material derived from maternal and paternal sources between sister chromatids of homologous chromosomes involving DNA breakage and repair in autosomes but not in the heterosomes "x" and "y". The pairing of chromosomes leads to a "crossover" of adjacent sister chromatids. When the chromosomes start to separate in the pachytene stage, these sites become visible and are termed "chiasmata". In the diplotene stage, chromosomes separate with the exception of the chiasmata sites. The end of the meiotic prophase is recognized as "diakinesis", when chromosomes shorten and the four separate chromatids become visible. Finally, the nuclear membrane disappears and chromosomes are subsequently arranged in the metaphase plate. After formation of the spindle apparatus, chromosomes move to opposite poles, but, in contrast to mitotic division, chromatids remain interconnected. Thus the number of chromosomes in resulting secondary spermatocytes is haploid, but the DNA content is still diploid (1n2 C).

II.1.3.4.2 Secondary Spermatocytes

Secondary spermatocytes undergo the second meiotic division after a short interphase of about 6 h in the human without DNA synthesis. By this division, chromatids are finally separated leading to round spermatids with a haploid number of chromosomes and DNA content (1n1 C).

II.1.3.5 Spermatids/Spermiogenesis

Early round spermatids are postmitotic cells, exhibit a nucleus with a homogenous chromatin pattern and can be identified by the perinuclear acrosome vesicle, which can easily be seen after periodic acid Schiff (PAS) reaction on formalin, or Bouin-fixed paraffin-embedded sections or at the ultrastructural level.

The transformation of conventional round cell spermatids into spermatozoa with the capacity for motility and fertilization of an egg includes a complex sequence of events: (1) formation of the acrosome, (2) condensation of the nucleus, (3) development of the sperm tail, (4) reorganization of cellular organelles such as mitochondria and centrioles and (5) reduction of the cytoplasm.

The synthesis of many acrosome-specific proteolytic enzymes starts as early as in pachytene spermatocytes. These proteins, such as proacrosin, are packed into electron-dense vesicles: proacrosomal granules (PAGs) derive from the trans-Golgi complexes. They start to fuse after completion of meiotic divisions in step1 spermatids. The growing acrosome forms a cap-like structure that covers about 30–50% of the nuclear surface (Bermudez et al. 1994).

Nuclear condensation in the human is due to replacement of about 85% of the DNA-associated lysine-rich histones by transition proteins, and finally by arginine-rich protamines. In contrast to histones, which form a loop-like association with DNA (nucleosomes), protamines are associated with the grooves of the DNA helix, leading to extreme condensation and finally to a reduction to about 10% of the original nuclear size. Transition proteins are believed to be involved in DNA repair mechanisms during histone to protamine exchange (Fig. II.1.10). Associated with the increased exchange of nuclear proteins is a decrease in and cessation of gene transcription. Thus, in spermatids gene transcription and protein translation are temporally uncoupled (for review see Steger 1999, 2001), together with the temporal storage of mRNA in spermatid-specific nucleoprotein complexes, which were described at the ultrastructural level by Holstein and Roosen-Runge (1981). The fertilization capacity of spermatozoa depends on the protamine content being adequate and the ratio of the two protamines PRM1 and PRM2 being correct (Steger et al. 2003).

The formation of the tail (flagellum) starts early in spermiogenesis. The axoneme shows the typical "9+2" structure of microtubules. This is the common pattern of eukaryotic cilia and derives from one of the pair of centrioles. These centrioles are placed in a nuclear fossa opposite the acrosome. The distal centriole gives rise to the flagellum. The other structures of the flagellum, the fibrous sheet and outer dense fibres are developed when spermiogenesis takes place.

Mitochondria from the periphery of the spermatid aggregate around the proximal part of the flagellum in a helical manner forming the latter's mid-piece. At the end, the spermatid's cytoplasm is shed by active involvement of the adjacent Sertoli cell, and this "residual body" is phagocytosed by Sertoli cells.

The events described occur either simultaneously or with a degree of overlap. For practical reasons, depending on the development and formation of the acrosome, the whole process of spermiogenesis can be divided as follows:

- Golgi phase
  Development of the acrosome vesicle
- Cap phase
  Formation of the acrosomal cap together with the start of nuclear condensation and development of the flagellum
- Acrosome phase
  Differentiation of the acrosome, and elongation of the nucleus and cell body

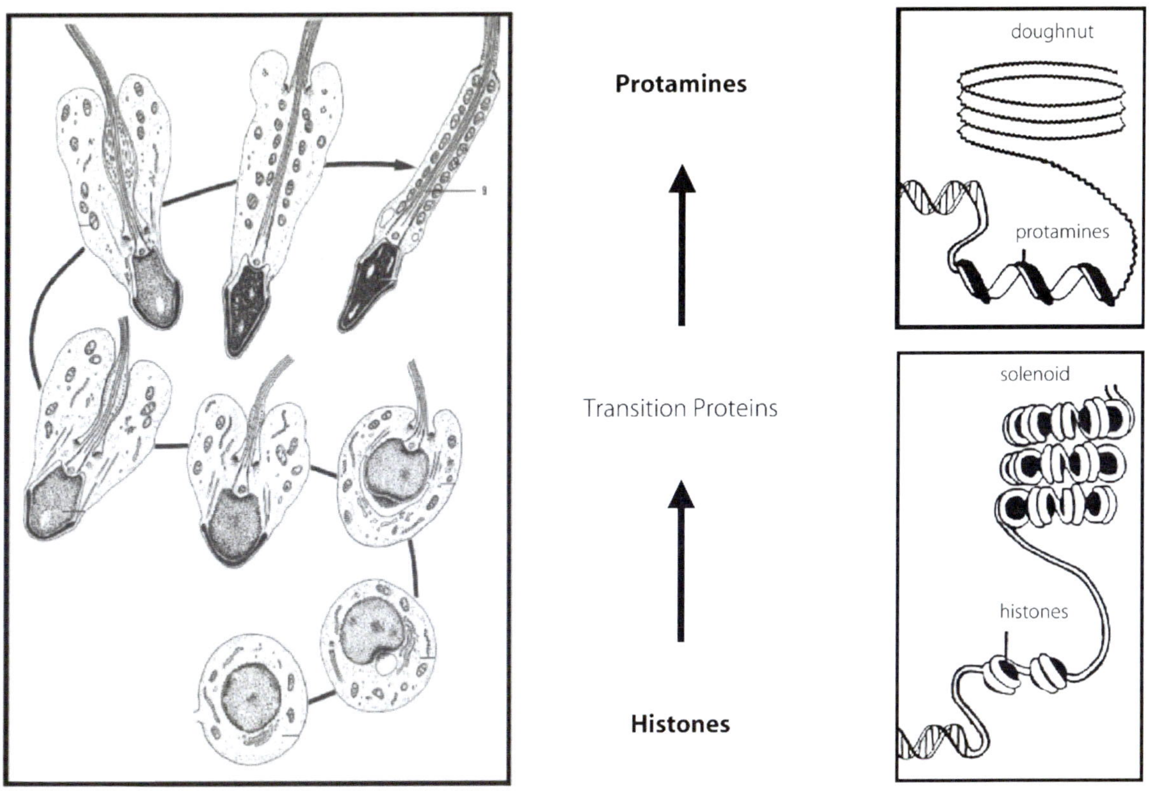

Fig. II.1.10. Schematic presentation of histone to protamine exchange

- Maturation phase
  Differentiation of the species-specific form of the acrosome and sperm head; completion of nuclear condensation, and the reduction of cytoplasm.

The release of fully differentiated spermatids into the lumen of the seminiferous tubule, which is triggered by the Sertoli cell, is termed "spermiation".

The haploid germ cell within the seminiferous epithelium is termed the "spermatid" (round, elongating, elongated). The haploid germ cell after spermiation is a "spermatozoon" (sperm).

II.1.3.6 Spermatozoon (Fig. II.1.11)

The length of the human spermatozoon measures about 60 µm. The flat and oval head (diameter: 3 µm, length: 5 µm) consists of the acrosome and the extremely condensed nucleus. The acrosome covers the head surface, and contains numerous proteolytic enzymes, i.e. hyaluronidase, collagenase, neuraminidase, phospholipase A, acrosin and others. The release of these enzymes, the so-called acrosome reaction, enables the spermatozoon to penetrate the "corona radiata" of follicle cells and the zona pellucida of the egg. Some nuclear vacuoles are common.

The flagellum measures about 55 µm in length. It possesses the central axoneme and is divided into:

- The neck/connecting piece (1 µm). It contains the basal and striated bodies and is the point of articulation between the sperm head and the flagellum.
- The mid-piece (6 µm). It contains the mitochondria and the nine doublets of microtubules, which are associated with outer dense fibres, each consisting of at least 14 polypeptides with a molecular mass ranging from 11 to 87 kDa (Henkel et al. 1994). Outer dense fibres are believed to maintain the passive elastic structure for flagellar bending and also to protect it from shearing forces during epididymal transit and ejaculation (Baltz et al. 1990). Hinsch et al. (2004) detected the voltage-dependent anion-sensitive channels VDAC2 and VDAC3 in bovine outer dense fibres, indicating their functional role in the regulation of sperm motion or sperm structural integrity.
- The principal piece (45 µm). In addition to the outer dense fibres, the flagellum contains a fibrous sheet.
- The end-piece (5 µm) only contains microtubules.

Spermatozoa acquire motility during epididymal passage and their competence for fertilization during the passage of the female genital tract (capacitation).

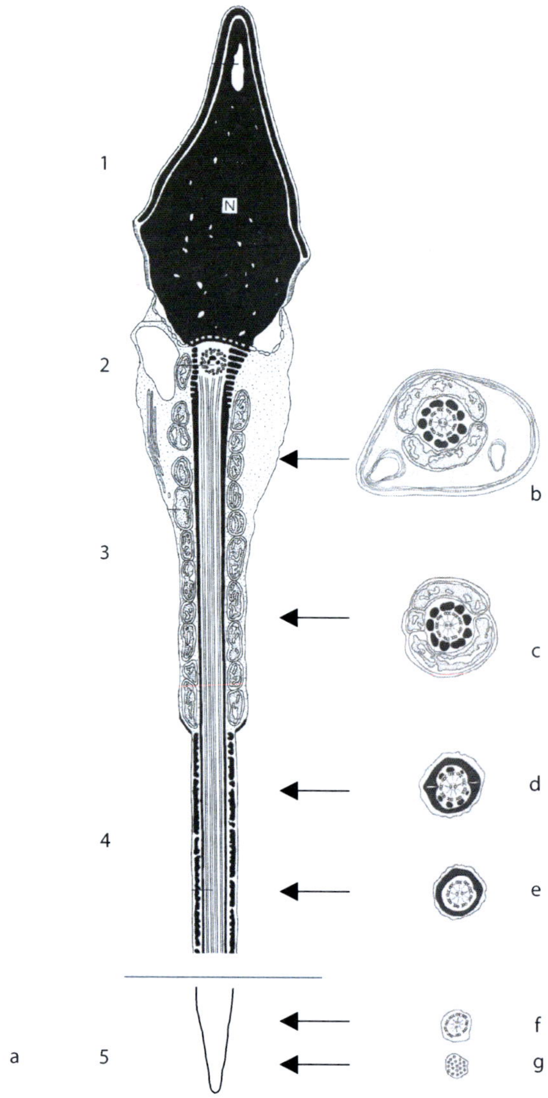

Fig. II.1.11. Schematic drawing of the human spermatozoon according to Holstein and Roosen-Runge (1981). **a** Longitudinal section showing *1* head with acrosome, *2* neck, *3* mid-piece and *4* principal piece, and *5* end-piece. **b–f** Flagellar cross sections through the **b, c** mid-piece, **d, e** principal piece, and **f** end-piece

II.1.3.7 Sertoli Cell

Sertoli cells are postmitotic somatic cells, which extend from the basement membrane of the seminiferous tubule to the lumen, providing an extreme cytoplasmic ramification, and surround adjacent germ cells (Figs. II.1.9b, II.1.12a). They are responsible for the establishment of the blood–testis barrier (BTB) within the seminiferous epithelium by inter-Sertoli cell junctional complexes. These complexes are located between the level of spermatogonia and primary spermatocytes and consist of tight junctions and gap junctions, which are associated with actin filaments and cisternae of the endoplasmic reticulum. The latter bears ribosomes on the cytoplasmic site. Tight junctions prevent diffusion through the intercellular space, which can be demonstrated by tracer application such as lanthanum or horseradish peroxidase (Bergmann et al. 1989). By this, Sertoli cells divide the seminiferous epithelium into a basal compartment (blood milieu) and an adluminal compartment (milieu of the intratubular fluid created by Sertoli cells) (Figs. II.1.9a, II.1.12b–d). The functional significance is: (1) as an immunological barrier to protect spermatocytes and spermatids from the immune system preventing autoimmune orchitis and (2) to create a specific milieu for germ cell development that differs from the normal intercellular blood-borne milieu. The BTB has to be considered as a highly dynamic structure undergoing disintegration and reconstruction during the passage of developing germ cells from the basal to the adluminal compartment.

Intercellular communication within the seminiferous epithelium occurs via inter-Sertoli cell and Sertoli-germ cell gap junctions (Fig. II.1.12d). The most important gap-junction protein is connexin 43 (Cx43) and to a lesser extent connexin 26 (Cx26), which are first expressed during puberty at the same time as the onset of spermatogenesis and the formation of the BTB (see Brehm et al. 2002).

Sertoli cells support and trigger germ cell development and differentiation by mediating the hormonal stimuli. They are known to be the only cell type within the seminiferous epithelium to express both the membrane-bound follicle-stimulating hormone (FSH) receptor (FSHR) (Böckers et al. 1994), and the nuclear androgen receptor (AR) (Van Roijen et al. 1995; Suarez-Quian et al. 1999). However, FSH and FSHR mRNA were later found in germ cells, from spermatogonia to round spermatids, by Baccetti et al. (1998). FSH expression is regulated by the steroid hormone inhibin pro-

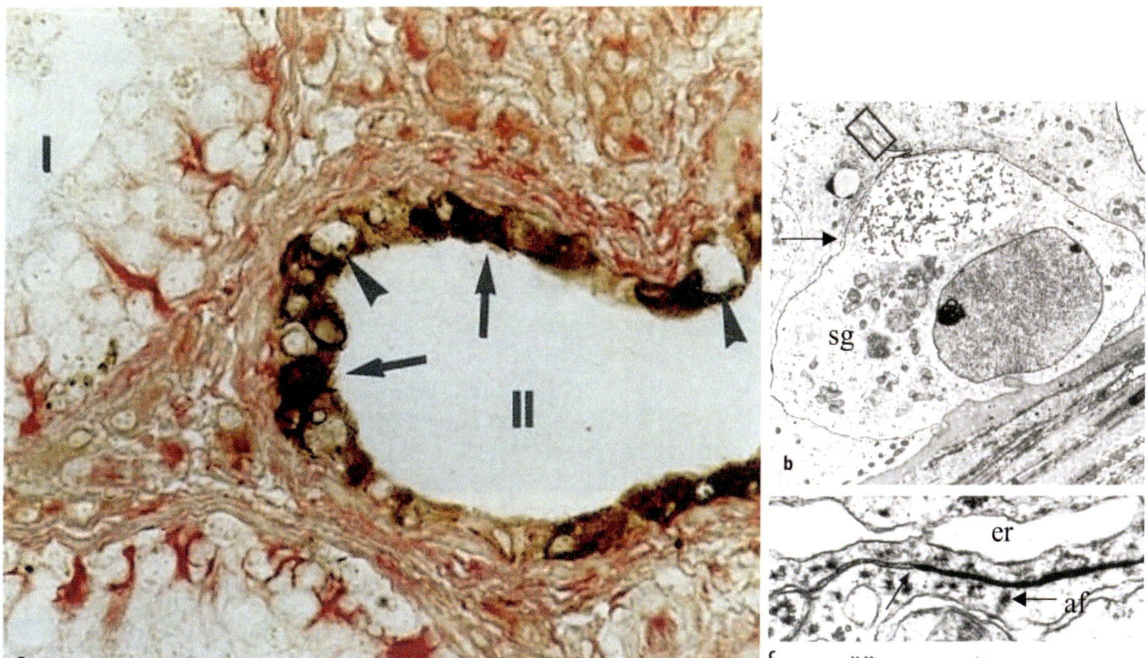

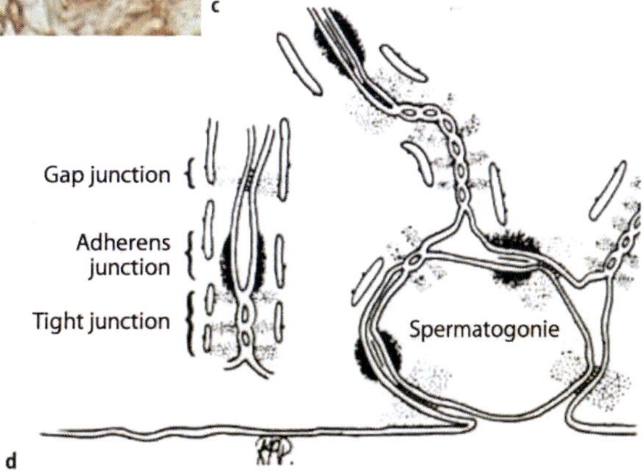

Fig. II.1.12. Sertoli cells and inter-Sertoli cell junctional complex. **a** Normal Sertoli cells within intact seminiferous epithelium showing anti-vimentin immunoreactivity (*red colour*, I) and undifferentiated Sertoli cells (*arrows*) associated with maturation arrest at the level of spermatogonia showing additional anti-cytokeratin 18 immunoreactivity (*brown colour*, II). *Arrowheads*: spermatogonia [from Bergmann and Kliesch (1994)]. **b** Electron micrograph of type A (*pale*) spermatogonium (*sg*) surrounded by electron-dense tracer lanthanum nitrate (*arrow*). **c** Magnification of rectangle in Fig. II.1.12b: showing inter-Sertoli cell junctional complexes consisting of tight junctions preventing tracer penetration (*arrow*), actin filaments (*af*) and cisternae of endoplasmic reticulum (*er*) [**b, c** from Bergmann et al. (1989)]. **d** Schematic drawing of inter-Sertoli cell junctional complex [from Pelletier and Byers (1992)]

duced by Sertoli cells. The typical cytoplasmic skeletal elements are microtubules and vimentin intermediate filaments which are responsible for Sertoli cell shape (Fig. II.1.12a) (see Bergmann and Kliesch 1994).

Sertoli cells produce numerous factors such as androgen-binding protein (ABP), which ensures high levels of testosterone in the seminal fluid within the adluminal compartment, rete testis, efferent ductules and epididymis, the iron-binding protein "transferrin" and copper-binding protein "ceruloplasmin", both necessary for germ cell differentiation (for review see De Kretser 2003). They trigger spermatogonial proliferation via the FSH-dependent stem cell factor (SCF), which binds to the tyrosine kinase receptor c-kit which is expressed by spermatogonia (Rossi et al. 2000). Their metabolism is influenced by germ cells and vice versa.

II.1.3.8 Apoptosis and Spermatogenesis

Apoptotic cell death is a prerequisite for continuous spermatogenesis, and limits the germ cell population in physiological conditions. It is most important to establish a species-specific ratio between germ cells and Sertoli cells during prespermatogenesis and especially around puberty (Heiskanen et al. 1996; Rodriguez et al. 1997). In the adult human seminiferous epithelium, apoptosis occurs at the level of spermatogonia, spermatocytes and spermatids, as a rare event (Brinkworth et al. 1997), and shows possible ethnic differences between Caucasian and Chinese men. These differences may help to explain the greater efficacy of testosterone-induced spermatogenic suppression observed in Asian compared to non-Asian men (SinhaHikim et al. 1998). However, apoptosis is increased in patients with impaired spermatogenesis (Lin et al. 1997), especially in primary spermatocytes and round spermatids associated with incomplete spermiogenic failure (Tesarik et al. 1998). Regulation of apoptosis within the seminiferous epithelium depends on the Fas/FasL system. FasL is expressed by Sertoli cells and Fas only by degenerating germ cells (Francavilla et al. 2000). The proteins of the Bcl2 family prevent apoptosis (for review see Print and Loveland 2000). It seems to be inhibited by testosterone (Singh et al. 1995) and FSH (Tesarik et al. 2000). Apoptosis of Sertoli cells under physiological conditions has not yet been reported.

II.1.3.9 Kinetics of Spermatogenesis

II.1.3.9.1 Cycle of the Seminiferous Epithelium

The seminiferous epithelium in a given cross-section shows characteristic germ cell association at different developmental stages. The type of spermatogonium is specific to the stage of meiosis and spermatid development. The series of different germ cell associations between the two appearances of the same stage was first described in the rat by LeBlond and Clermont (1952) and later by Clermont (1963) in the human as the cycle of the seminiferous epithelium. In the rat, XIV stages were defined based on 19 different steps of spermiogenesis as identified by the PAS reaction of the acrosome. The number of stages was found to differ according to the species: XII stages in the mouse or in non-human primates; VIII stages in the bull, stallion, or dog; and VI stages including eight steps of spermiogenesis in the human and great apes (Fig. II.1.13) (see Wistuba et al. 2003).

Whatever the case, stage I is defined by the occurrence of early round spermatids showing an acrosome vesicle after the second meiotic division. The last stage (VI, VIII, XII, or XIV, according to the species) is characterized by the presence of secondary spermatocytes.

In human spermatogenesis, in stage II residual bodies derived from spermatid cytoplasm are found within Sertoli cells. After stage II, spermiation takes place. Stage III is characterized by the beginning of spermatid nuclear condensation and the entry of type B spermatogonia into meiosis.

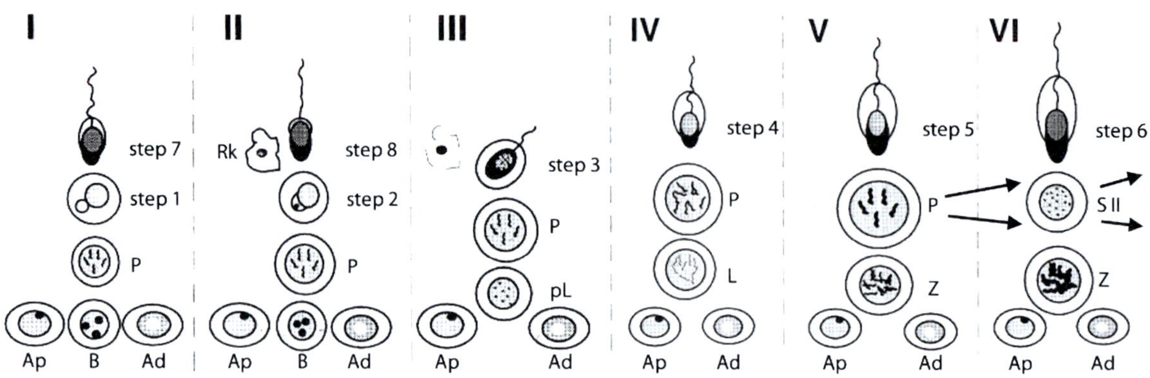

Fig. II.1.13. VI stages of spermatogenesis [from Bergmann (1998)]

Stages IV and V exhibit ongoing condensation of spermatid nuclei, and can be distinguished by the presence of leptotene primary spermatocytes in stage IV and zygotene primary spermatocytes in stage V. After stage V, pachytene primary spermatocytes undergo diakinesis and the first meiotic division takes place. The second meiotic division of secondary spermatocytes at the end of stage VI gives rise to round spermatids in stage I. In stage I, type A spermatogonia differentiate into type B spermatogonia.

These stages are arranged sequentially along the length of a tubule resulting in a "wave of spermatogenesis" in space. In contrast to most mammals investigated so far, in humans, as in the great apes, a given seminiferous tubule cross-section contains more than one stage of spermatogenesis (multi-stage arrangement vs. single-stage arrangement, i.e. in the rat) (Fig. II.1.14). This was explained by Schulze and Rheder (1984) to be the result of a helical orientation of several spirals of spermatogenic waves, but Johnson et al. (1996) demonstrated a random distribution of different stages within a given cross section. The difference between single-stage and multi-stage arrangements most likely depends on differences in the size of germ cell clones, being smaller in species with a multi-stage arrangement (for review see Luetjens et al. 2005).

The duration of this wave in time is the "cycle of spermatogenesis". In the human, this cycle takes about 16 days and the progression from spermatogonia to spermatozoa about 70–75 days, i.e. four and a half cycles (Heller and Clermont 1964).

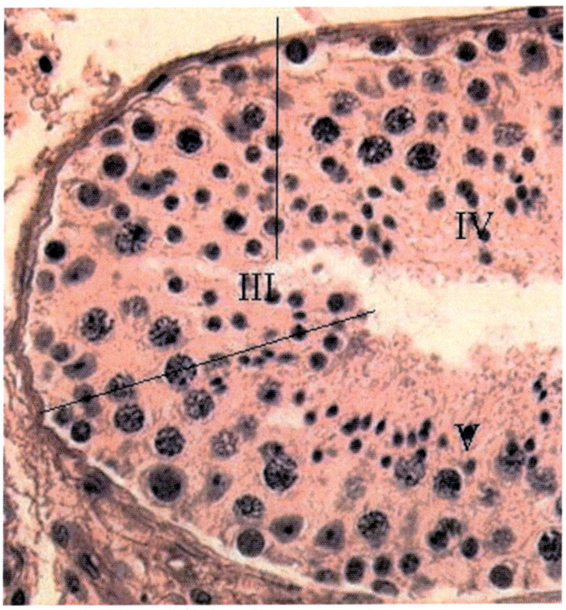

Fig. II.1.14. Multi-stage arrangement (stages II, IV, V) of normal human seminiferous epithelium, paraffin section, HE, primary magnification, ×40

II.1.3.9.2
Efficiency of Human Spermatogenesis

The efficiency of spermatogenesis depends on many factors, i.e. the absolute number of germ cells and Sertoli cells, the Sertoli cell/germ cell ratio, duration of the seminiferous cycle, germ cell loss during spermatogenesis, as well as on anatomical parameters such as the length of the seminiferous tubules or testis size resulting in different species-specific values for daily sperm production. In primates, the absolute number of germ cells is within a low range of 100–300 ml/g testis weight compared to about 530 ml/g testis weight in the rat. However, in the human, the conversion ratio from pachytene spermatocytes to round spermatids was found to be 3.5, and from round spermatids to elongated spermatids to be about 0.9 almost reaching theoretical levels of 4 and 1 respectively. These values are within the range of those for other primates as well as the rat (3.85/1.33), indicating that the efficiency of spermatogenesis in the human does not differ from that in other mammals (for review see Wistuba et al. 2003; Luetjens et al. 2005). These data also show that sperm production is not limited by germ cell loss during meiosis or spermiogenesis, but depends on the number of spermatogonia entering meiosis.

II.1.3.10
Pathophysiology of Spermatogenesis and Infertility

Impairment of spermatogenesis leading to infertility is associated with the histological appearance of hypospermatogenesis, partial or complete maturation arrest at the level of early round spermatids, primary spermatocytes or spermatogonia, to a complete loss of germ cells (Sertoli cell only syndrome = SCO) or even all cells (tubular shadows) within the seminiferous epithelium. The latter are often described as "hyalinized tubules". SCO and hyalinized tubules are often found in Klinefelter syndrome. In addition, numerous alterations of germ cell differentiation, i.e. meiotic arrest (megalospermatocytes) or impairment of spermiogenesis (multinucleated spermatids), are described (for review see Holstein et al. 1988). Interestingly, any spermatogenetic impairment is associated with a population of Sertoli cells showing signs of differentiation deficiency, including the persistence of undifferentiated nuclei, anti-Müllerian hormone secretion or the (re-)expression of foetal cytokeratin 18 intermediate filaments (Bruning et al. 1993; Bergmann and Kliesch 1994; Steger et al. 1999; Maymon et al. 2000, for review see Sharpe et al. 2003) (Fig. II.1.12a).

Impairment of spermatogenesis influences ejaculate parameters leading to a reduction of sperm density (oligo-), motility (oligo-astheno-), and an increase of abnormal morphology (oligo-astheno-teratozoospermia = OAT syndrome). There is now increasing evidence that incorrect DNA integrity and condensation due to failure during spermiogenesis (histone to protamine exchange) seems to be an important factor predicting the outcome of assisted reproduction with morphologically normal spermatozoa (Blanchard et al. 1990; Ankem et al. 2002; Steger et al. 2003) or even in globozoospermia with germ cells missing an acrosome (Vicari et al. 2002).

References

Ankem MK, Mayer E, Ward WS, Cummings KB, Barone JG (2002) Novel assay for determining DNA organization in human spermatozoa: implications for male factor infertility. Urology 59:575–578

Baccetti B, Collodel G, Constatino-Ceccarini E, Eshkol A, Gambera L, Moretti E, Strazza M, Piomboni P (1998) Localization of human follicle-stimulating hormone in the testis. FASEB J 12:1045–1054

Baltz JM, Pallini V, Burrini AG (1990) Dense fibers protect mammalian sperm against damage. Biol Reprod 43:484–491

Bergmann M (1998) Spermatogenese. In: Krause W, Weidner W (eds) Andrologie, Krankheiten der männlichen Geschlechtsorgane, Ferdinand Enke Verlag, Stuttgart, pp 9–14

Bergmann M, Kliesch S (1994) The distribution pattern of cytokeratin and vimentin immunoreactivity in testicular biopsies in infertile men. Anat Embryol 190:515–520

Bergmann M, Nashan D, Nieschlag E (1989) Pattern of compartmentation in human seminiferous tubules showing dislocation of spermatogonia. Cell Tissue Res 256:183–190

Bermudez D, Escalier D, Gallo JM, Viellefond A, Rius F, Perez-de Vargas I, Schrevel J (1994) Proacrosin as a marker of meiotic and postmeiotic germ cell differentiation: quantitative assessment of human spermatogenesis with a monoclonal antibody. J Reprod Fertil 100:567–575

Blanchard Y, Lescoat D, LeLannou D (1990) Anomalous distribution of nuclear basic proteins in round-headed human spermatozoa. Andrologia 22:549–555

Böckers T, Nieschlag E, Kreutz MR, Bergmann M (1994) Localization of follicle-stimulating hormone (FSH) immunoreactivity and hormone receptor mRNA in testicular tissue of infertile men. Cell Tissue Res 278:595–600

Brehm R, Marks A, Rey R, Kliesch S, Bergmann M, Steger K (2002) Altered expression of connexins 26 and 32 in Sertoli cells in seminiferous tubules infiltrated with carcinoma in situ. J Pathol 197:647–653

Brinkworth M, Weinbauer GF, Bergmann M, Nieschlag E (1997) Apoptosis as a mechanism of germ cell loss in elderly men. Int J Androl 20:222–228

Bruning G, Dierichs R, Stümpel C, Bergmann M (1993) Sertoli cell nuclear changes in human testicular biopsies as revealed by three dimensional reconstruction. Andrologia 25:311–316

Clermont Y (1963) The cycle of the seminiferous epithelium in man. Am J Anat 112:35–51

De Kretser DM (2003) Endocrinology of the male reproductive system. In: McLachlan R (ed) Endocrinology of male reproduction. www.endotext.com

Francavilla S, DAbrizio P, Rucci N, Silvano G, Properzi G, Straface E, Gordeschi G, Necione S, Gnessi L, Arizzi M, Ulisse S (2000) Fas and Fas ligand expression in fetal and adult human testis with normal or deranged spermatogenesis. J Clin Endocrinol Metab 85:2692–2700

Heiskanen P, Billig H, Toppari J, Kaleva M, Arsalo A, Rapola J, Dunkel L (1996) Apoptotic cell death in the normal and cryptorchid human testis: the effect of human chorionic gonadotropin on testicular germ cell survival. Pediatr Res 40: 351–356

Heller CG, Clermont Y (1964) Kinetics of the germinal epithelium in man. Rec Progr Horm Res 20:545–574

Henkel R, Stalf T, Mertens N, Miska W, Schill WB (1994) Outer dense fibers of human spermatozoa – partial characterization and possible physiological functions. Int J Androl 17:68–73

Hinsch K-B, De Pinto V, Aires VA, Schneidert X, Messina A, Hinsch E (2004) Voltage-dependent anion-selective channels VDAC2 and VDAC3 are abundant proteins in bovine outer dense fibers, a cytoskeletal component of the sperm flagellum. J Biol Chem 279:15281–15288

Holstein AF (1994) Männliche Geschlechtsorgane. In: Graumann W, Holstein AF, Sasse D, Welsch U (eds) Taschenbuch der Anatomie, vol 2. Gustav Fischer, Stuttgart

Holstein AF, Roosen-Runge EC (1981) Atlas of human spermatogenesis. Grosse, Berlin

Holstein AF, Schirren C, Roosen-Runge EC (1988) Illustrated pathology of human spermatogenesis. Grosse, Berlin

Johnson L, McKenzie KS, Snell JR (1996) Partial wave in human seminiferous tubules appears to be a random occurrence. Tissue Cell 28:127–136

Kierszenbaum AL (2002) Genomic imprinting and epigenetic reprogramming: Unearthing the garden of forking paths. Mol Reprod Dev 63:269–272

LeBlond CP, Clermont Y (1952) Definition of the stages of the cycle of the seminiferous epithelium in the rat. Ann NY Acad Sci 55:548–573

Luetjens CM, Weinbauer GF, Wistuba J (2005) Primate spermatogenesis: comparative evidence and new insights into testicular organisation, spermatogenic efficiency and endocrine control. Biol Rev Camb Philos Soc 80:475–488

Lin WW, Lamb DJ, Wheeler TM, Lippschultz L, Kim ED (1997) In situ-end-labelling of human testicular tissue demonstrates increased apoptosis in conditions of abnormal spermatogenesis. Fertil Steril 68:1065–1069

Maymon BB, Paz G, Elliott DJ, Hammel I, Kleimann SE, Yogev L, Hauser R, Botchan A, Yavetz H (2000) Maturation phenotype of Sertoli cells in testicular biopsies of azoospermic men. Hum Reprod 14:1537–1542

Pelletier RM, Byers SW (1992) The blood-testis barrier and sertoli cell junctions: structural considerations. Microsc Res Tech 20:3–33

Print C, Loveland KL (2000) Germ cell suicide: new insights into apoptosis during spermatogenesis. Bioessays 22:423–430

Rodriguez I, Ody C, Araki K, Garcia I, Vassalli P (1997) An early and massive wave of germinal cell apoptosis is required for the development of functional spermatogenesis. EMBO J 16:2262–2270

Rossi P, Sette C, Dolci S, Geremia R (2000) Role of c-kit in mammalian spermatogenesis. J Endocrinol Invest 23:609–615

Schlatt S, Weinbauer GF (1994) Immunohistochemical localization of proliferating nuclear antigen as a tool to study cell proliferation in rodent and primate testes. Int J Androl 17:214–222

Schulze W, Rheder U (1984) Organization and morphogenesis of the human seminiferous epithelium. Cell Tissue Res 237: 395–407

Sharpe RM, McKinnell C, Kivlin C, Fisher S (2003) Proliferation and functional maturation of Sertoli cells, and their relevance to disorders of testis function in adulthood. Reproduction 125:769–784

Singh J, ONeill C, Handelsman DJ (1995) Induction of spermatogenesis by androgens in gonadotropin-deficient (hpg) mice. Endocrinology 136:5311–5321

SinhaHikim AP, Wang C, Lue Y, Johnson L, Wang X-H, Swerd-

II.1

loff RS (1998) Spontaneous germ cell apoptosis in humans: evidence for ethnic differences in the susceptibility of germ cells to programmed cell death. J Clin Endocrinol Metab 83:152–156
Steger K (1999) Transcriptional and translational regulation of gene expression in haploid spermatids. Anat Embryol 199: 471–487
Steger K (2001) Haploid spermatids contain translationally repressed mRNAs. Anat Embryol 203:323–334
Steger K, Aleithe I, Behre HM, Bergmann M (1998) The proliferation of spermatogonia in normal human seminiferous epithelium: an immunohistochemical study using monoclonal antibodies against Ki-67 protein and proliferating cell nuclear antigen. Mol Hum Reprod 4:227–233
Steger K, Rey R, Louis F, Kliesch S, Behre HM, Nieschlag E, Hoepffner W, Bailey D, Marks A, Bergmann M (1999) Reversion of the differentiated phenotype and maturation block in Sertoli cells in pathological human testis. Hum Reprod 14:136–143
Steger K, Fink L, Failing K, Bohle RM, Kliesch S, Weidner W, Bergmann M (2003) Decreased protamin-1 transcript levels in testes from infertile men. Mol Hum Reprod 9:331–336
Suarez-Quian CA, Martinez-Garcia F, Nistal M, Regadera J (1999) Androgen receptor distribution in adult human testis. J Clin Endocrinol Metab 84:350–358
Tesarik J, Greco E, Cohen-Bacrie P, Mendoza C (1998) Germ cell apoptosis in men with incomplete spermiogenesis failure. Mol Hum Reprod 4:757–762
Tesarik J, Mendoza C, Greco E (2000) The effect of FSH on male germ cell survival and differentiation in vitro is mimicked by pentoxifiline but not insulin. Mol Hum Reprod 6:877–881
Van Roijen JH, Van Assen S, Van der Kwast TH, De Rooij DG, Boersma WA, Vreeburg JTM, Weber RFA (1995) Androgen receptor immunoexpression in the testes of subfertile men. J Androl 16:510–516
Vicari E, Perdichizzi A, De Palma A, Burrello N, Dàgata R, Calogero AE (2002) Globozoospermia is associated with chromatin structure abnormalities. Hum Reprod 17:2128–2133
Wistuba J, Schrod A, Greve B, Hodges JK, Aslam H, Weinbauer GF, Luetjens CM (2003) Organization of seminiferous epithelium in primates: Relationship to spermatogenic efficiency, phylogeny, and mating system. Biol Reprod 69:582–591

II.1.4 Physiology of Sexual Function

O. Baldo, I. Eardley

Summary

The parasympathetic nervous system provides the primary pro-erectile innervation of the penis. Originating from the sacral nerve roots (S2–S4) the nerves provide vasodilating innervation to the cavernosal tissue. The parasympathetic nerves release a cocktail of pro-erectile neurotransmitters, of which the most important is nitric oxide (NO), which acts on the smooth muscle cell via a second messenger system involving cyclic GMP. The sympathetic innervation mediates detumescence and originates within the thoraco-lumbar cord (T11–L2) via release of noradrenaline. Our knowledge of the pharmacology of erection has recently provided us with a number of therapeutic approaches to the treatment of erectile dysfunction. The pudendal nerve represents the somatic innervation of the penis carrying both afferent impulses from the genitalia and motor fibres to the muscles of the pelvic floor.

The erection itself is a vascular event during which the degree of erection depends upon the balance between the arterial inflow and venous outflow of the penis. Parasympathetic stimulation (with an accompanying reduction in sympathetic stimulation) results in smooth muscle relaxation in the penile arteries, relaxation of the cavernosal (trabecular) smooth muscle and closure of the venous outflow from the penis.

Ejaculation has two phases, emission and ejection, the latter usually being accompanied by orgasm. Emission involves the sequential contraction of the epididymis, vas deferens, seminal vesicles and prostate, with ejaculatory fluid being "emitted" into the posterior urethra. Ejection is accompanied by tight closure of the bladder neck, with contraction of the prostatic musculature together with a sequence of variably coordinated contractions of the bulbocavernosus, ischiocavernosus and other pelvic floor muscles. The ejaculate is propelled into the anterior urethra and beyond.

The foreskin or the prepuce is a specialized, junctional mucocutaneous tissue that marks the boundary between mucosa and skin. It may have a number of functions including one as a sensory erogenous area and there may be others, but little is actually known.

Male sexual function can be thought of as having four phases, namely desire, arousal, orgasm and resolution. This chapter will deal with the physiology of the second and third of these phases, namely arousal and orgasm. In men, the most obvious manifestation of arousal is penile erection while ejaculation usually occurs with orgasm, although they are actually separate events. This chapter will deal initially with the physiology of erection, moving on to the physiology of ejaculation and orgasm, before finishing with a brief résumé of what we know about the physiology of the foreskin.

II.1.4.1
Penile Erection

II.1.4.1.1
Neuroanatomy of Erection

The parasympathetic nervous system provides the primary pro-erectile innervation of the penis. Originating from the intermedio-lateral column of the sacral spinal cord, fibres exit via the sacral nerve roots (S2–S4) and travel in the nervi erigentes to the pelvic plexus before passing onwards in the cavernous nerves, which run alongside the prostate. These nerves provide vasodilating innervation to the cavernosal tissue. The cavernous nerve has considerable significance for surgeons, particularly in its relationship to the prostate, since it is at risk of damage during open prostatectomy. The cavernous nerve runs through the retroperitoneal space on the lateral aspect of the rectum and the bladder and then passes inferiorly and laterally towards the prostate before piercing the urogenital diaphragm just lateral to the membranous urethra (Walsh and Donker 1982). The parasympathetic nerves innervate the smooth muscle of the penile vasculature and the cavernosal sinusoids.

The sympathetic innervation mediates detumescence and originates within the thoraco-lumber cord (T11–L2). It passes via the ventral roots and the sympathetic chain to the hypogastric plexus before reaching the pelvic plexus. The postsynaptic fibres pass within cavernous nerves to the penis, where they also innervate the smooth muscle of the penile arteries and the cavernosal sinusoids.

The pudendal nerve represents the somatic innervation of the penis; it carries both afferent impulses from the genitalia via the dorsal nerve of the penis and motor fibres to the muscles of the pelvic floor including the bulbocavernosus and ischiocavernosus muscles. The cell bodies of these motor fibres lie within Onuf's nucleus, which itself is located within the sacral cord (S2–S4). The dorsal nerve of the penis is the terminal branch of the pudendal nerve and contains sensory fibres only. Lying on the dorsal aspect of the penile shaft lateral to the dorsal artery, multiple branches fan out to provide proprioceptive and sensory nerve terminals to the dorsum of the tunica albuginea and skin of the penile shaft and the glans penis.

II.1.4.1.2
Neurophysiology of Erection

There appear to be at least three ways in which an erection can be initiated. First, erections can be initiated by an erotic stimulus that may be visual, olfactory, auditory or imaginative and the stimulus is probably accompanied by cortical stimulation of the hypothalamus. These are so-called psychogenic erections. From the hypothalamus pro-erectile fibres descend in the intermediolateral column of the spinal cord to the sacral parasympathetic outflow. The second type of erection is the reflex erection that occurs in conjunction with tactile stimuli to the genitalia. Afferent impulses are carried to the spinal cord in the dorsal nerve of the penis and efferent impulses via the pelvic parasympathetic fibres. The two pathways (i.e. the central and the peripheral) can interact in order to maximize parasympathetic stimulation to the penile smooth muscle and there will also, inevitably, be simultaneous inhibition of the anti-erectile sympathetic outflow. This integration probably occurs in the spinal cord. The third mechanism of erection relates to nocturnal erections. All potent men develop several erections during the course of a night's sleep. The central neural mechanisms involved in this are not clearly understood, but must involve inhibition of the sympathetic outflow and stimulation of the parasympathetic outflow.

II.1.4.1.3
Penile Erection as a Vascular Event

An erection is a vascular event during which the degree of erection depends upon the balance between the arterial inflow and venous outflow of the penis. Parasympathetic stimulation (with an accompanying reduction in sympathetic stimulation) results in smooth muscle relaxation in the penile arteries and relaxation of the cavernosal (trabecular) smooth muscle. This causes in increased arterial inflow and accumulation of blood within the sinusoidal tissue. The resultant swelling of the cavernosal sinusoids leads to compression of the efferent sub-tunical veins against the tunica albuginea with a resultant reduction in venous outflow. This is called the veno-occlusive mechanism. The sequence of events accompanying an erection was described by (Lue et al. 1983) and is outlined in Table II.1.1.

II.1.4.1.4
Central Neuropharmacology of Erection

Our recent knowledge of the central neuropharmacology of penile erection is obtained largely from animal experiments (Giuliano and Rampin 2000). These data suggest that there are descending pro-erectile pathways that emanate from the paraventricular nucleus (PVN) and medial preoptic area (MPOA) of the hypothalamus. There are multiple cortical influences on the PVN and MPOA mediating the erotic stimuli discussed earlier. In terms of neurotransmitters, dopamine, nitric oxide (NO), alpha melanocyte-stimulating hormone (α-MSH), glutamate and adrenocorticotropic hormone (ACTH) all appear to have pro-erectile influences while gamma-aminobutyric acid (GABA) and noradrenaline (NA) appear to be inhibitory. From the hypothalamus,

Table II.1.1. Vascular physiology of erection (Lue et al. 1983)

Phase	Name	Neurophysiology	Penile vascular changes
0	Flaccid	Dominant sympathetic tone	Arterial flow is low Contracted trabecular smooth muscle Empty sinusoids Blood gases are similar to those in venous blood
1	Filling	Parasympathetic stimulation with reduced sympathetic tone	Arteriolar dilatation Massive increase in arterial flow Trabecular relaxation Sinusoidal filling without little increase in intracavernosal pressure (ICP)
2	Tumescent	Dominant parasympathetic tone	ICP rise leads to a relative fall in the arterial inflow As ICP rises above diastolic pressure, flow continues only during the systolic phase Sinusoids expand with compression of the subtunical venous plexus The penis expands to its maximal capacity
3	Full erection	Dominant parasympathetic tone	ICP equals mean systolic pressure With further blood drawn into the expanding sinusoids this causes compression of the subtunical venous plexuses leading to reduced flow into the emissary veins Blood gases equal those of the arterial blood
4	Rigid erection	Dominant parasympathetic tone with concurrent pudendal stimulation	Contraction of ischiocavernosus muscle results in a rise of ICP to greater than systolic pressure No influx of blood via the cavernous artery Veins are completely shut preventing any efflux of blood The phase continues until the muscle is fatigued and the process is reversed
5	Initial detumescence	Increased sympathetic stimulation	Smooth muscle contraction against a temporarily closed venous system Small transient rise ICP
6	Slow detumescence	Dominant sympathetic tone	Contraction of the trabecular smooth muscle Arteriolar network constricts with reduction in ICP Filling of the cavernosal venous bed
7	Fast detumescence	Dominant sympathetic tone	Rapid fall in the arterial blood flow Fall in ICP Increase in venous outflow Penile flaccidity

passing oxytocinergic pathways pass to the spinal cord from where the parasympathetic outflow originates. Dopamine may also have a pro-erectile action at this level.

There is probably a second descending pathway from the reticular formation of the medulla to the sympathetic outflow. Stimulation of this pathway will result in detumescence and current evidence suggests that the most important neurotransmitter in this system is serotonin.

There must be coordination between these two pathways, to allow reciprocal activity, but as yet the anatomical and physiological basis of the interaction is unclear.

II.1.4.1.5 Peripheral Pharmacology

The state of the smooth muscle is determined by the balance between the sympathetic (contractile) and the parasympathetic (relaxant) nervous systems, and the development of an erection requires not only an increase in the degree of parasympathetic stimulation, but also a reduction in the degree of sympathetic stimulation. Functionally, although there are minor differences, the smooth muscle of the penile arteries appears to behave similarly to the smooth muscle that lines the trabecular sinusoids. There are multiple neurotransmitters involved in the peripheral control of smooth muscle tone (Table II.1.2), but the dominant "players" are thought to be NO (smooth muscle relaxation) and NA (smooth muscle contraction) (Saenz de Tejada et al. 2004). The primary sources of the mediators are the autonomic nerves, but, as can be seen, the endothelium also plays a part, as do (to a lesser extent) circulating humoral factors.

The parasympathetic nerves that innervate the penile smooth muscle release a cocktail of pro-erectile neurotransmitters, of which the most important is NO. Synthesized by neuronal nitric oxide synthase (nNOS),

Table II.1.2. Factors influencing the state of the penile smooth muscle

Contractile factors		Relaxant factors	
Neuro-transmitter	Source	Neuro-transmitter	Source
Noradrenaline	Sympathetic nerves	Nitric oxide	Parasympathetic nerves and Endothelium
Endothelin	Endothelium	Vasoactive intestinal polypeptide	Parasympathetic nerves
Constrictor prostanoids	Endothelium	Relaxant prostanoids	Endothelium
Angiotensin II	Circulating	Acetylcholine	Parasympathetic nerves (mediated via endothelium)

and supplemented by NO from the endothelium (where it is synthesized by endothelial nitric oxide synthase or eNOS), the NO is able to enter the penile smooth muscle cell to stimulate the enzyme guanylate cyclase to produce the active second messenger, cyclic GMP (cGMP) (Fig. II.1.15). A cascade of processes ensues resulting in a fall in intracellular calcium with resultant smooth muscle relaxation (Fig. II.1.16). The action of cGMP is terminated by the enzyme phosphodiesterase type 5 (PDE5). Drugs that inhibit this enzyme, including sildenafil, tadalafil and vardenafil, will prolong the activity of cGMP and have proven to be valuable therapies in the treatment of men with erectile dysfunction.

In addition to NO, the parasympathetic nerves release vasoactive intestinal polypeptide and acetylcholine, both of which are pro-erectile. Acetylcholine appears to act (at least in part) by stimulating the eNOS within the vascular endothelium to produce NO.

The sympathetic nerves also release a cocktail of neurotransmitters including NA, while the vascular endothelium releases a number of anti-erectile substances including endothelin and various prostanoids. The action of NA upon the smooth muscle is via the alpha-1-adrenoceptor that is linked via a G protein to a membrane-bound enzyme (phospholipase C) which, in turn, initiates a series of intracellular processes, ultimately resulting in a rise of the cytoplasmic calcium and consequent smooth muscle contraction (Fig. II.1.17).

II.1.4.1.6 Pharmacological Targets for the Treatment of Erectile Dysfunction

In the past few years the use of inhibitors of phosphodiesterase type 5 (PDE5Is) has revolutionized the treatment of men with erectile dysfunction. The rationale for their use is outlined above. Although PDE5 is found in other organs (such as vascular smooth muscle, gastrointestinal smooth muscle and the nasopharyngeal mucosa), sexual stimulation results in release of NO in the penis (and not these other tissues) so there is functional selectivity for the use of these drugs to facilitate penile erection. Other approaches to the treatment of men with erectile dysfunction based upon the smooth muscle cell have included intracavernosal injections of agents that relax smooth muscle, such as prostaglandin E_1 (alprostadil) and papaverine. Alternatively, drugs that interfere with the noradrenergic smooth muscle contraction, including phentolamine (an alpha adrenoceptor blocking agent), have also been used. Modest efficacy was demonstrated with this drug both as an injectable and as an oral agent.

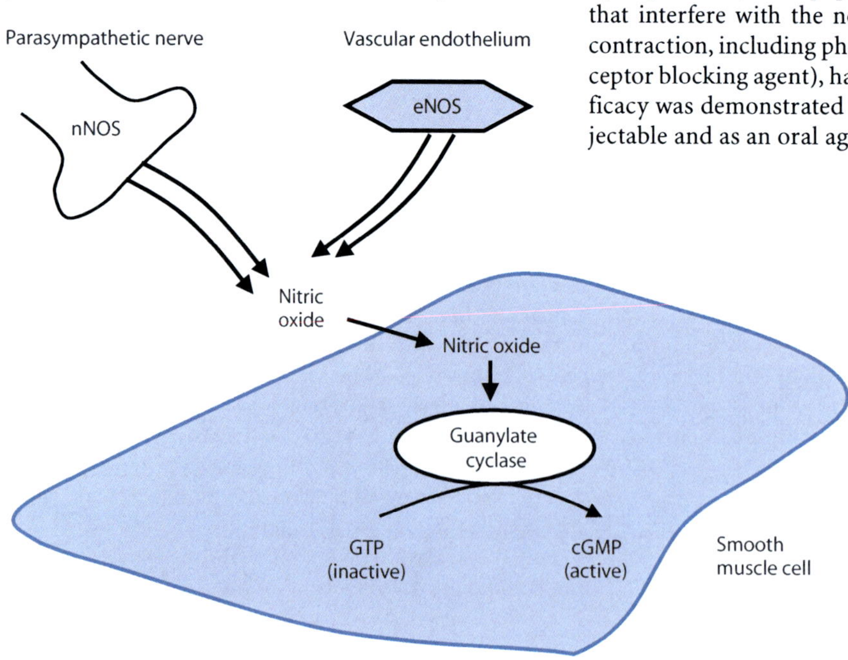

Fig. II.1.15. Diagrammatic representation of the sources of nitric oxide that lead to smooth muscle cell relaxation in the smooth muscle of the penis. Neuronal nitric oxide synthase (*nNOS*) and endothelial nitric oxide (*eNOS*) produce nitric oxide, which enters the smooth muscle cell. There it converts guanylyl triphosphate (*GTP*) to cyclic guanylyl monophosphate (*cGMP*), the active second messenger

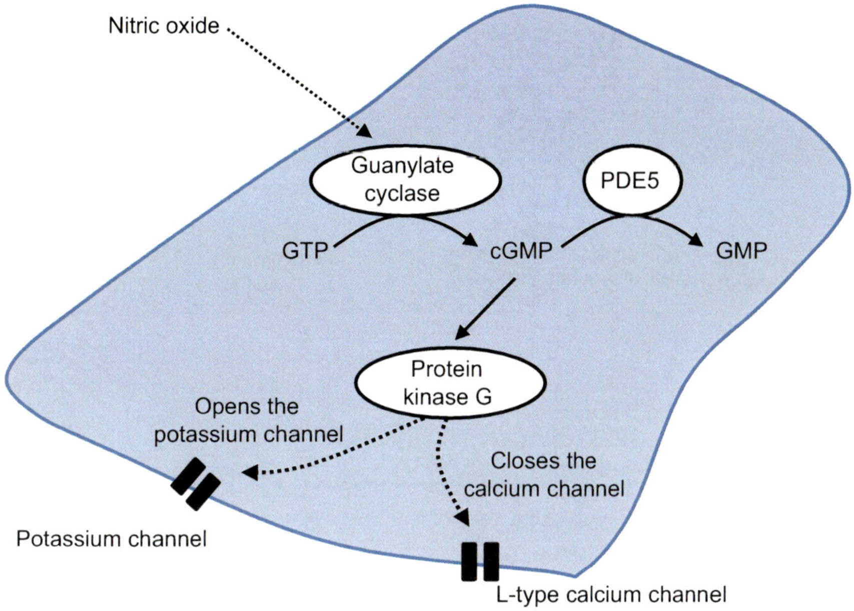

Fig. II.1.16. The intracellular actions of nitric oxide (*NO*) within the smooth muscle cell. NO stimulates guanylate cyclase to convert GTP into cGMP, the active second messenger. cGMP is broken down by phosphodiesterase type 5 (*PDE5*). cGMP stimulates protein kinase G which in turn opens the potassium channels and closes the calcium channels via a series of sequential phosphorylations. This ultimately causes a fall in the cytoplasmic calcium and smooth muscle relaxation as a consequence

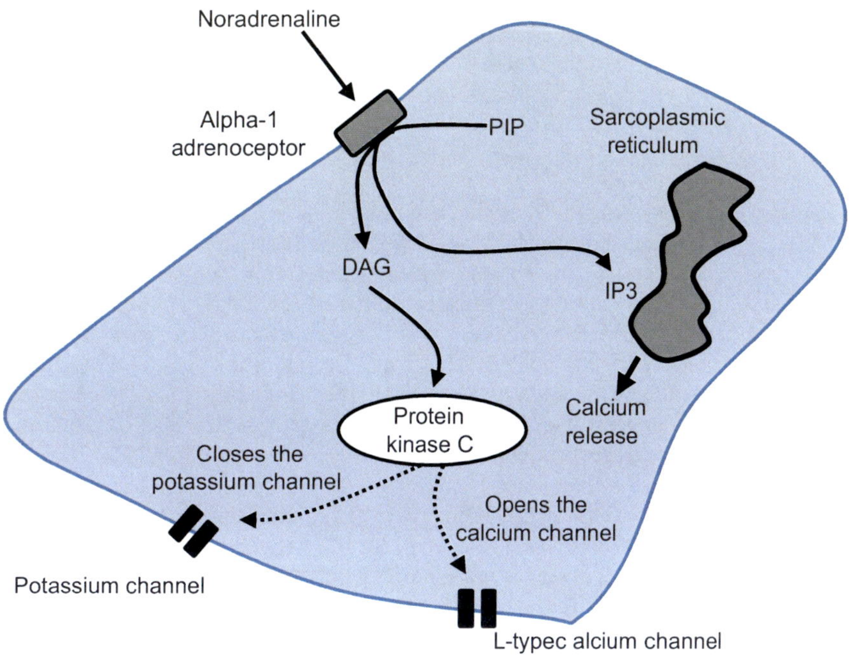

Fig. II.1.17. The actions of noradrenaline on the penile smooth muscle cell. It stimulates the cell surface alpha-1 adrenoceptor to convert phosphatidylinositol bisphosphate (*PIP*) to diacylglycerol (*DAG*) and inositol trisphosphate (*IP3*). IP3 stimulates the sarcoplasmic reticulum to release calcium into the cytoplasm and DAG stimulates protein kinase C, which in turn opens calcium channels and closes the potassium channels via a series of phosphorylations. As a result, there is a rise in the cytoplasmic calcium and smooth muscle contraction

With our increasing knowledge of the central control of penile erection, drugs that act centrally have also been tested. Apomorphine, a dopaminergic agent, has been licensed in Europe for the treatment of erectile dysfunction, although its efficacy is limited. Currently there is some interest in melanocortin analogues, which appear to stimulate erection via central pathways that may (or may not) involve the dopaminergic system.

II.1.4.2 Ejaculation and Orgasm

II.1.4.2.1 Neuroanatomy of Ejaculation

As with penile erection, our knowledge of the neuroanatomy and neurophysiology of ejaculation has largely been elucidated using animal models and our knowledge of these processes in humans is currently incomplete. We do know however that ejaculation is a reflex (Fig. II.1.18). The afferent limb begins at the sensory re-

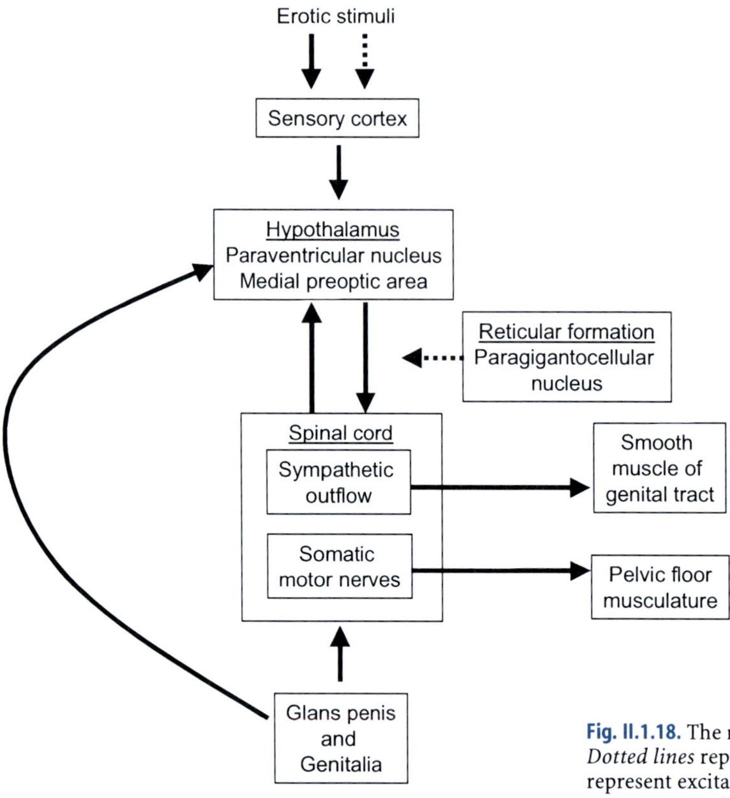

Fig. II.1.18. The neural mechanism involved in ejaculation. *Dotted lines* represent inhibitory pathways and *full lines* represent excitatory pathways

ceptors of the penis, foreskin and genitalia, and sensory fibres travel with the dorsal nerve of the penis. Somatic sensory pathways ascend in the spinal cord and are probably accompanied by sensory impulses that have travelled with the sympathetic nerves via the hypogastric plexus. The paraventricular nucleus (PVN) and the medial preoptic area (MPOA) are almost certainly the principal site in the anterior hypothalamus where the sensory inputs are integrated and where ejaculation is controlled. The PVN and MPOA receive input from the ascending sensory pathways, and also from higher centres such as the sensory cortex (McMahon et al. 2004).

From the hypothalamus, descending pathways pass to the spinal cord, and in particular to the sympathetic outflow (T12–L2). With cell bodies in the lateral columns of the grey matter, efferent fibres pass out to the sympathetic chain, which, via the hypogastric and pelvic plexus, innervate the smooth muscle of the epididymis, vas deferens, prostate, bladder neck and seminal vesicles. The paragigantocellular reticular nucleus of the medulla may have an inhibitory influence upon these descending pathways.

II.1

II.1.4.2.2 Physiology of Ejaculation

Ejaculation has two phases, emission and ejection, the latter usually being accompanied by orgasm. Emission involves the sequential contraction of the epididymis, vas deferens, seminal vesicles and prostate, with ejaculatory fluid being "emitted" into the posterior urethra. The bladder neck (or pre-prostatic sphincter) usually becomes closed at this point, thereby preventing reflux into the bladder. There is a progressive sensation of inevitability, over which there usually is some degree of voluntary control, although this is gradually lost as the degree of inevitability increases.

Ejection is accompanied by tight closure of the bladder neck, with contraction of the prostatic musculature together with a sequence of variably coordinated contractions of the bulbocavernosus, ischiocavernosus and other pelvic floor muscles. The ejaculate is propelled into the anterior urethra and beyond. Quite what happens at the striated urethral sphincter is something of a mystery; clearly it must relax for the ejaculate to pass through, but this relaxation must either be incomplete or very short lived, since men who have undergone transurethral prostatectomy (with disruption of he bladder neck) do not become incontinent at this time. There is extremely limited voluntary control of ejection.

The best explanation that we have of orgasm is that it is the sensation associated with these processes, and in particular the build up of ejaculate in the posterior urethra and the contractions of the bulbocavernosus, ischiocavernosus and the other muscles of the pelvic floor. It appears to be a spinal reflex since it can occur in those with a spinal cord injury. Clearly however, there are effects upon higher centres. For instance, there is some evidence that orgasm is accompanied by changes in cerebral blood flow, with increased perfusion in some areas (such as the right pre-frontal cortex) and decreases in others (Tiihonen et al. 1994).

II.1.4.2.3 Central Neuropharmacology of Ejaculation

Within the hypothalamus, there appears to be interplay between a number of neurotransmitters with dopamine and serotonin currently thought to be the "main players". Dopamine appears to promote ejaculation, probably via D2 receptors, while serotonin appears to be inhibitory. Which receptors are most important is unclear, but it is of clinical relevance that serotonin reuptake inhibitors (SSRIs) tend to delay ejaculation, and indeed have been used therapeutically to achieve this effect. Other neurotransmitters such as GABA, acetylcholine, noradrenaline and nitric oxide may have a role, but as with the central control of erection our knowledge is limited at this time.

II.1.4.2.4 Peripheral Pharmacology of Ejaculation

The smooth muscle of the genital tract appears to contract primarily in response to a sympathetic noradrenergic stimulus. However, other neurotransmitters are almost certainly involved, including acetylcholine, neuropeptide Y among others, and in the coming years we will learn more about the neurophysiological process involved here.

II.1.4.2.5 Pharmacological Targets for the Treatment of Premature Ejaculation

The potential use of SSRIs in the treatment of rapid ejaculation has already been alluded to. At the time of writing there are at least two SSRIs in development for the potential (on demand) treatment of premature (or rapid) ejaculation. Other approaches to this problem have included attempts to interrupt the afferent limb of the reflex arc, by the use of local anaesthetic agents applied to the glans penis. The role of PDE5Is in this condition is currently under investigation given the common coexistence of erectile dysfunction and premature ejaculation.

II.1.4.2.6 Structure and Function of the Foreskin

The foreskin or the prepuce is a specialized, junctional mucocutaneous tissue that marks the boundary between mucosa and skin (Cold and Taylor 1999). It appears at the eighth week of intrauterine life as a ring of thickened epidermis. The fused mucosa of the glans penis and the inner lining of the prepuce breaks down within the first 6 months of post-natal life and separates gradually over a period of years as a spontaneous biological process. The separation of the prepuce/glans penis mucosa is usually complete by about 17 years of age.

Structurally, the foreskin provides a transition between the epithelium of the glans penis and the normal skin of the shaft of the penis. This transition is reflected in the structural differences between the inner and the outer layers of the foreskin that have some functional significance (Table II.1.3). Between the inner and outer layers of the prepuce lies a layer of dartos muscle together with a rich vascular network.

Table II.1.3. Structural features of the prepuce

Structural feature	Inner layer of prepuce	Outer layer of prepuce
Mucosal surface	Squamous mucosal epithelium Langerhans cells are seen Melanocytes are not seen	Keratinized, stratified squamous epithelium Langerhans cells are seen Melanocytes are seen
Sensory nerve endings	Mostly free nerve endings Few encapsulated nerve endings near frenulum and coronal sulcus	Encapsulated nerve endings
Submucosal region	No hair follicles No sweat or sebaceous glands Vascular +++	Typical dermis Scattered sebaceous glands More elastic fibres than inner layer

The prepuce may have a number of functions. First it is a sensory erogenous area. However, the innervation of the glans penis provides only crude, poorly localized feelings, and indeed the only part of the body with less fine touch discrimination is the sole of the foot! However, at the junction with the outer layer of the prepuce, particularly around the frenulum, there is a change in the sensory endings (as seen on histology) and this correlates with an increased degree of discriminative sensation. Circumcision certainly seems to disturb sensation in this area.

Other possible functions include possible immunological function in the prevention of infection, via the Langerhans cells and via the presence of a wide and varied commensal community, including *Corynebacterium*, Gram-negative anaerobes, enterococci and mycobacteria. The secretions of the prostate, seminal vesicles and Littre's glands provide lubrication within the so-called preputial sac which may be of importance for lubrication during intercourse.

References

Cold CJ, Taylor JR (1999) The prepuce. BJU Int 83 [Suppl 1]: 34–44

Giuliano F, Rampin O (2000) Central control of erection and its pharmacological modification. Curr Opin Urol 10:629–633

Lue TF, Takamura T, Schmidt RA, Palubishos AJ, Tanagho EA (1983) Hemodynamics of erection in the monkey. J Urol 128:1237–1241

McMahon CG, Abdo C, Hull E, Incrocci L, Levin R, Perelman M, Rowland D, Sipski M, Stuckey B, Waldinger M, Cheng Xin Z (2004) Disorders of orgasm and ejaculation in men. In: Lue TF, Basson R, Rosen R, Giuliano F, Khoury S, Montorsi F (eds) Sexual medicine: sexual dysfunctions in men and women. Editions 21, Paris, Chap. 13

Saenz de Tejada I, Angulo J, Cellek S, Gonzalez-Cadavid NF, Heaton J, Pickard R, Simonsen U (2004) Physiology of erectile function and pathophysiology of erectile dysfunction. In: Lue TF, Basson R, Rosen R, Giuliano F, Khoury S, Montorsi F (eds) Sexual medicine: sexual dysfunctions in men and women. Editions 21, Paris, Chap. 10

Tiihonen J, Kuikka J, Kupila J, Partanen K, Vainio P et al (1994) Increase in cerebral blood flow of right prefrontal cortex in man during orgasm. Neurosci Lett 170:241–243

Walsh PC, Donker PJ (1982) Impotence following radical prostatectomy: insight into aetiology and prevention. J Urol 128:492–496

II.1.5 Endocrine Regulation

F. Comhaire, A. Mahmoud

Summary

Pulsatile secretion of luteinizing hormone releasing hormone (LHRH) by the hypothalamus stimulates the production and secretion of the gonadotrophins luteinizing hormone (LH) and follicle-stimulating hormone (FSH) by the pituitary gland. These gonadotrophins circulate in the blood to reach the testis. LH stimulates the secretion of testosterone and oestradiol by the interstitial cells of Leydig. Very high concentrations of testosterone surround the seminiferous tubules and these are required for spermatogenesis. Testosterone in blood induces puberty and virilization, and exerts feedback inhibition of LHRH and LH secretion, after aromatization and 5-alpha reduction at the hypothalamo–pituitary level. FSH binds to Sertoli cells, stimulating the production and secretion of enzymes and substances that support spermatogenesis. Depending on the intensity of spermatogenesis, the Sertoli cells secrete inhibin B into the blood, which exerts feedback inhibition of FSH secretion by the pituitary. Optimal spermatogenesis depends on adequate functioning of all aspects of the hypothalamo-pituitary-testicular axis, but can be deregulated by many internal and external factors.

II.1.5.1 Hypothalamo–Pituitary–Testicular Axis

II.1.5.1.1 Luteinizing Hormone Releasing Hormone (LHRH)

Maleness depends on the effects of androgens, mainly testosterone, which is needed for pubertal development (Hammond et al. 1979), body composition, growth, sexual function and spermatogenesis (Dufau 1988). The hypothalamic neurons produce and secrete a releasing factor called gonadotrophin releasing factor or hormone (GnRH), more commonly referred to as luteinizing hormone releasing hormone (LHRH). GnRH results in a preferred release of LH, and it seems to play a less determinant role in the secretion of follicle-stimulating hormone (FSH). However, a specific FSH-releasing hormone has not been detected (Schally et al. 1971), and the deficient secretion of GnRH results in failure to release both LH and FSH. The secretion of GnRH is not continuous, but rather pulsatile (Crowley et al. 1991). The so-called pulse generator (Kaufman et al. 1985; Knobil 1990) initiates pulsatility, which is inherent of the neuroendocrine cells of the hypothalamus (Knobil 1980; Marshall and Kelch 1986). It is under feedback control of testosterone (Matsumoto and Bremner 1984; Plant and Dubey 1984) which is converted to oestradiol by the aromatase of the hypothalamic cells. GnRH pulsatility is also influenced by neurotransmitters and endorphins (Veldhuis et al. 1984). It can be depressed in the case of extreme stress or physical exertion (MacConnie et al. 1986; Opstad 1992), serious disease conditions (Aitken et al. 1985), depression, malnutrition (Warren 1983) and abuse of "recreational drugs" (Kesner et al. 1986; Vescovi et al. 1992). The GnRH is transported through the portal veins along the pituitary stalk to the anterior lobe of the pituitary gland where it binds to the receptors on the gonadotropes. In physiological circumstances the GnRH–receptor complex is internalized and the GnRH receptor is upregulated (Clayton 1989). Continuous or high GnRH concentrations result in profound gonadotrope desensitization (Schurmeyer et al. 1984; Matsumoto et al. 1991), involving receptor downregulation (Belchetz et al. 1978; Conn and Crowley 1991). Figure II.1.19 represents a simplified summary of the hormonal regulation of testicular function and spermatogenesis.

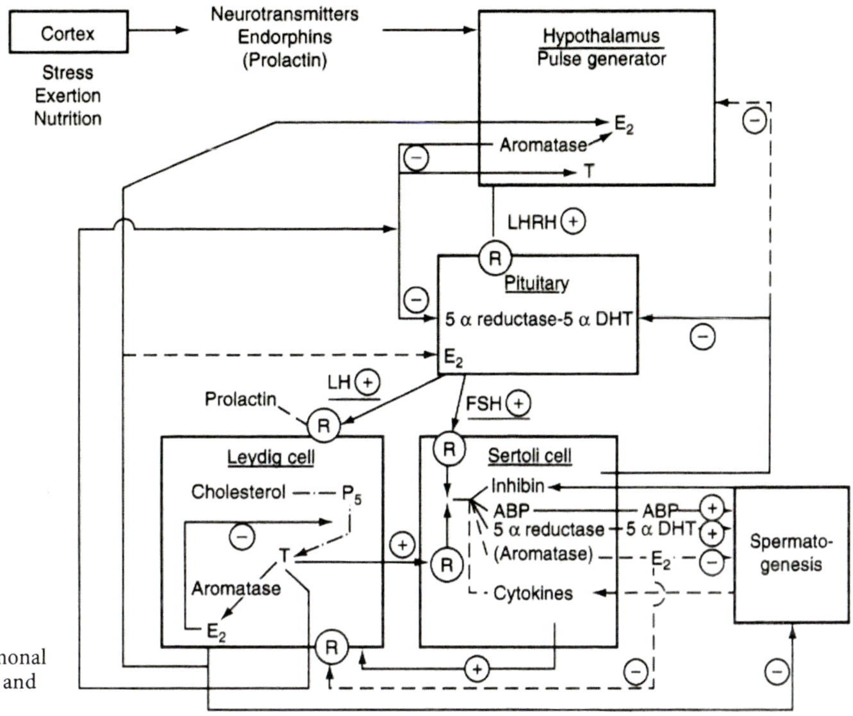

Fig. II.1.19. Summary of the hormonal regulation of testicular function and spermatogenesis

II.1.5.1.2 Luteinizing Hormone (LH)

The pituitary gonadotrophic hormones are LH and FSH, which are two structurally related glycoproteins. They are dimeric molecules composed of two dissimilar, noncovalently linked subunits: the alpha- and the beta-subunit (Nilsson et al. 1986). The alpha-subunit is common to both gonadotrophins, and shared with other hormones namely human chorionic gonadotrophin (hCG) and thyroid stimulating hormone or thyrotrophin (TSH). The specific activity of LH and FSH is determined by the beta-subunit. The secretion of LH closely follows the stimulation pattern by GnRH and is clearly pulsatile (Spratt et al. 1988), whereas this is much less clear for the secretion of FSH. The mean time interval between pulses of LH in eugonadal men is approximately 120 min. The amplitude of the LH pulses is determined by a complex interaction of several factors including the intrinsic responsiveness and the number of gonadotropes, the GnRH pulse frequency, the size of the bolus of GnRH secreted into the portal circulation along the pituitary stalk, and the time elapsed since the previous GnRH bolus. The amplitude of LH pulses in eugonadal men is highly variable within and between subjects. A remarkable diurnal variability of LH secretion is seen in pubertal boys, with strikingly higher amplitude pulses during night-time (Boyar et al. 1972). In adult men, diurnal variability is less pronounced and differs between subjects (Fehm et al. 1991).

In response to the LH stimulation, secretion of testosterone by the Leydig cells also presents a pulsatile pattern, but pulsatility is less distinct in peripheral blood (Veldhuis et al. 1987). Testosterone and oestradiol are co-secreted episodically (Winters and Troen 1986). The intra-testicular variability of the testosterone concentration is very large (Comhaire and Vermeulen 1976) and it follows the LH rhythmic secretion closely. The possible importance of the latter is unknown, but it has been speculated to serve as a kind of "pace maker" influencing the timing of the subsequent steps in spermatogenesis. A pulsatile pattern of LH secretion is not necessary for sustained testosterone secretion, since men with hypogonadotrophic hypogonadism can perfectly well be treated with injections of hCG, which cause prolonged and uninterrupted stimulation of the Leydig cells and normal male development. On the other hand, the absence of pulsatility may influence spermatogenesis, as treatment of hypogonadotrophic men with pulsatile administration of GnRH may result in better spermatogenesis than non-pulsatile treatment with gonadotrophins in some cases (Hoffman and Crowley 1982; Christiansen et al. 2002).

The secretion of LH is regulated by the feedback action of testosterone, influencing the pulse frequency of GnRH secretion (Bridges et al. 1993). Testosterone is aromatized into oestradiol by the hypothalamic neurosecretory cells, which reduces the amplitude of GnRH pulses (Santen 1975; Winters and Troen 1985). In certain models, the 5-alpha-reduced dihydrotestosterone

II.1

exerts feedback on the secretion of LH at the pituitary level, further influencing the LH secretion (Santen 1975; Canovatchel et al. 1994).

II.1.5.1.3 Follicle-Stimulating Hormone (FSH)

The pattern of secretion of FSH is less clearly pulsatile (Veldhuis et al. 1989) and FSH has a relatively long half-life. FSH binds to its receptors on the cells of Sertoli and, in synergy with testosterone, it stimulates these to produce substances that are secreted into the seminiferous tubules. These are necessary for initiating and sustaining spermatogenesis (Verhoeven 1992) (see Chap. I.3.14) in a normal qualitative and quantitative manner. Once spermatogenesis has been initiated during puberty, it can be maintained by high concentrations of testosterone alone, but sperm production will not reach a normal quantity. The Sertoli cells also secrete inhibin B (Anderson and Sharpe 2000), a glycoprotein that specifically inhibits the secretion of FSH at the pituitary level (Ying 1988; Hancock et al. 1992). Inhibin B is also implicated in the paracrine regulation of spermatogenesis and may reduce sperm production. It is debated whether FSH secretion is governed, at least in part (Hayes et al. 2001b), by feedback action of testosterone (Hayes et al. 2001a) or rather by oestradiol. The concentration of inhibin B in serum also reflects the level of spermatogenesis and its quantity. It is reduced in cases with incomplete or absent spermatogenesis (Pierik et al. 2003), and is inversely correlated with sperm concentration (Mahmoud et al. 1998).

II.1.5.1.4 Prolactin and Melatonin

The role of prolactin in endocrine regulation is complex (Bartke 1977). High concentrations of prolactin inhibit the secretion of GnRH and LH (Winters and Troen 1984) causing hypoandrogenism, whereas lower concentrations may strengthen the effect of LH on the Leydig cells through interaction with the LH receptor and androgen metabolism (Magrini et al. 1976).

Long-term melatonin administration does not alter pituitary gonadal hormone secretion in normal men. Sleep parameters are influenced by melatonin, whereas the mean nocturnal LH, FSH, testosterone and inhibin B integrated values do not change (Luboshitzky et al. 2000).

References

Aitken RJ, Sutton M, Warner P, Richardson DW (1985) Relationship between the movement characteristics of human spermatozoa and their ability to penetrate cervical mucus and zona-free hamster ooytes. J Reprod Fertil 73:441–449

Anderson RA, Sharpe RM (2000) Regulation of inhibin production in the human male and its clinical applications. Int J Androl 23:136–144

Bartke A (1977) Prolactin and the physiological regulation of the mammalian testis. In: Troen P, Nankin H (eds) The testis in normal and infertile men. Raven, New York, pp 367–378

Belchetz PE, Plant TM, Nakai Y, Keogh EJ, Knobil E (1978) Hypophysial responses to continuous and intermittent delivery of hypothalamic gonadotropin-releasing hormone. Science 202:631–633

Boyar R, Finkelstein J, Roffwarg H, Kapen S, Weitzman E, Hellman L (1972) Synchronization of augmented luteinizing hormone secretion with sleep during puberty. N Engl J Med 287:582–586

Bridges NA, Hindmarsh PC, Pringle PJ, Matthews DR, Brook CG (1993) The relationship between endogenous testosterone and gonadotrophin secretion. Clin Endocrinol (Oxf) 38:373–378

Canovatchel WJ, Volquez D, Huang S, Wood E, Lesser ML, Gautier T, Imperato-McGinley J (1994) Luteinizing hormone pulsatility in subjects with 5-alpha-reductase deficiency and decreased dihydrotestosterone production. J Clin Endocrinol Metab 78:916–921

Christiansen P, Andersson AM, Skakkebaek NE, Juul A (2002) Serum inhibin B, FSH, LH and testosterone levels before and after human chorionic gonadotropin stimulation in prepubertal boys with cryptorchidism. Eur J Endocrinol 147:95–101

Clayton RN (1989) Gonadotrophin-releasing hormone: its actions and receptors. J Endocrinol 120:11–19

Comhaire FH, Vermeulen A (1976) Testosterone concentration in the fluids of seminiferous tubules, the interstitium and the rete testis of the rat. J Endocrinol 70:229–235

Conn PM, Crowley WF Jr. (1991) Gonadotropin-releasing hormone and its analogues. N Engl J Med 324:93–103

Crowley WF Jr., Whitcomb RW, Jameson JL, Weiss J, Finkelstein JS, O'Dea LS (1991) Neuroendocrine control of human reproduction in the male. Recent Prog Horm Res 47:27–62

Dufau ML (1988) Endocrine regulation and communicating functions of the Leydig cell. Annu Rev Physiol 50:483–508

Fehm HL, Clausing J, Kern W, Pietrowsky R, Born J (1991) Sleep-associated augmentation and synchronization of luteinizing hormone pulses in adult men. Neuroendocrinology 54:192–195

Hammond GL, Koivisto M, Kouvalainen K, Vihko R (1979) Serum steroids and pituitary hormones in infants with particular reference to testicular activity. J Clin Endocrinol Metab 49:40–45

Hancock AD, Robertson DM, de Kretser DM (1992) Inhibin and inhibin alpha-chain precursors are produced by immature rat Sertoli cells in culture. Biol Reprod 46:155–161

Hayes FJ, DeCruz S, Seminara SB, Boepple PA, Crowley WFJ (2001a) Differential regulation of gonadotropin secretion by testosterone in the human male: absence of a negative feedback effect of testosterone on follicle-stimulating hormone secretion. J Clin Endocrinol Metab 86:53–58

Hayes FJ, Pitteloud N, DeCruz S, Crowley WFJ, Boepple PA (2001b) Importance of inhibin B in the regulation of FSH secretion in the human male. J Clin Endocrinol Metab 86: 5541–5546

Hoffman AR, Crowley WF Jr. (1982) Induction of puberty in men by long-term pulsatile administration of low-dose gonadotropin-releasing hormone. N Engl J Med 307:1237–1241

Kaufman JM, Kesner JS, Wilson RC, Knobil E (1985) Electrophysiological manifestation of luteinizing hormone-releasing hormone pulse generator activity in the rhesus monkey: influence of alpha-adrenergic and dopaminergic blocking agents. Endocrinology 116:1327–1333

Kesner JS, Kaufman JM, Wilson RC, Kuroda G, Knobil E (1986) The effect of morphine on the electrophysiological activity of the hypothalamic luteinizing hormone-releasing hormone pulse generator in the rhesus monkey. Neuroendocrinology 43:686–688

Knobil E (1980) The neuroendocrine control of the menstrual cycle. Recent Prog Horm Res 36:53–88

Knobil E (1990) The GnRH pulse generator. Am J Obstet Gynecol 163:1721–1727

Luboshitzky R, Levi M, Shen-Orr Z, Blumenfeld Z, Herer P, Lavie P (2000) Long-term melatonin administration does not alter pituitary-gonadal hormone secretion in normal men. Hum Reprod 15:60–65

MacConnie SE, Barkan A, Lampman RM, Schork MA, Beitins IZ (1986) Decreased hypothalamic gonadotropin-releasing hormone secretion in male marathon runners. N Engl J Med 315:411–417

Magrini B, Ebiner JR, Burckhardt P, Felber JP (1976) Study on the relationship between plasma prolactin levels and androgen metabolism in man. J Clin Endocrinol Metab 43:944–947

Mahmoud AM, Comhaire FH, Depuydt CE (1998) The clinical and biologic significance of serum inhibins in subfertile men. Reprod Toxicol 12:591–599

Marshall JC, Kelch RP (1986) Gonadotropin-releasing hormone: role of pulsatile secretion in the regulation of reproduction. N Engl J Med 315:1459–1468

Matsumoto AM, Bremner WJ (1984) Modulation of pulsatile gonadotropin secretion by testosterone in man. J Clin Endocrinol Metab 58:609–614

Matsumoto AM, Gross KM, Bremner WJ (1991) The physiological significance of pulsatile LHRH secretion in man: gonadotrophin responses to physiological doses of pulsatile versus continuous LHRH administration. Int J Androl 14:23–32

Nilsson B, Rosen SW, Weintraub BD, Zopf DA (1986) Differences in the carbohydrate moieties of the common alpha-subunits of human chorionic gonadotropin, luteinizing hormone, follicle-stimulating hormone, and thyrotropin: preliminary structural inferences from direct methylation analysis. Endocrinology 119:2737–2743

Opstad PK (1992) Androgenic hormones during prolonged physical stress, sleep, and energy deficiency. J Clin Endocrinol Metab 74:1176–1183

Pierik FH, Burdorf A, De Jong FH, Weber RF (2003) Inhibin B: a novel marker of spermatogenesis. Ann Med 35:12–20

Plant TM, Dubey AK (1984) Evidence from the rhesus monkey (*Macaca mulatta*) for the view that negative feedback control of luteinizing hormone secretion by the testis is mediated by a deceleration of hypothalamic gonadotropin-releasing hormone pulse frequency. Endocrinology 115:2145–2153

Santen RJ (1975) Is aromatization of testosterone to estradiol required for inhibition of luteinizing hormone secretion in men? J Clin Invest 56:1555–1563

Schally AV, Arimura A, Baba Y, Nair RM, Matsuo H, Redding TW, Debeljuk L (1971) Isolation and properties of the FSH and LH-releasing hormone. Biochem Biophys Res Commun 43:393–399

Schurmeyer T, Knuth UA, Freischem CW, Sandow J, Akhtar FB, Nieschlag E (1984) Suppression of pituitary and testicular function in normal men by constant gonadotropin-releasing hormone agonist infusion. J Clin Endocrinol Metab 59:19–24

Spratt DI, O'Dea LS, Schoenfeld D, Butler J, Rao PN, Crowley WF Jr. (1988) Neuroendocrine-gonadal axis in men: frequent sampling of LH, FSH, and testosterone. Am J Physiol 254:E658–E666

Veldhuis JD, Rogol AD, Samojlik E, Ertel NH (1984) Role of endogenous opiates in the expression of negative feedback actions of androgen and estrogen on pulsatile properties of luteinizing hormone secretion in man. J Clin Invest 74:47–55

Veldhuis JD, King JC, Urban RJ, Rogol AD, Evans WS, Kolp LA, Johnson ML (1987) Operating characteristics of the male hypothalamo-pituitary-gonadal axis: pulsatile release of testosterone and follicle-stimulating hormone and their temporal coupling with luteinizing hormone. J Clin Endocrinol Metab 65:929–941

Veldhuis JD, Iranmanesh A, Clarke I, Kaiser DL, Johnson ML (1989) Random and non-random coincidence between luteinizing hormone peaks and follicle-stimulating hormone, alpha subunit, prolactin, and gonadotropin-releasing hormone pulsations. J Neuroendocrinol 1:185–194

Verhoeven G (1992) Local control systems within the testis. Baillieres Clin Endocrinol Metab 6:313–333

Vescovi PP, Pedrazzoni M, Michelini M, Maninetti L, Bernardelli F, Passeri M (1992) Chronic effects of marihuana smoking on luteinizing hormone, follicle-stimulating hormone and prolactin levels in human males. Drug Alcohol Depend 30:59–63

Warren MP (1983) Effects of undernutrition on reproductive function in the human. Endocr Rev 4:363–377

Winters SJ, Troen P (1984) Altered pulsatile secretion of luteinizing hormone in hypogonadal men with hyperprolactinaemia. Clin Endocrinol (Oxf) 21:257–263

Winters SJ, Troen P (1985) Evidence for a role of endogenous estrogen in the hypothalamic control of gonadotropin secretion in men. J Clin Endocrinol Metab 61:842–845

Winters SJ, Troen P (1986) Testosterone and estradiol are co-secreted episodically by the human testis. J Clin Invest 78:870–873

Ying SY (1988) Inhibins, activins, and follistatins: gonadal proteins modulating the secretion of follicle-stimulating hormone. Endocr Rev 9:267–293

II.1.6 Immunology of the Testis and Excurrent Ducts

H.-C. Schuppe, A. Meinhardt

Summary

Immune cells are regular components of the male reproductive tract of mammals, including humans. Whereas interactions between the testis and the immune system have been a source of considerable curiosity and remained obscure for many years, there is now compelling evidence that testicular immune cells play a key role in testicular function. Located in the interstitial compartment of the normal, unaffected testis they are implicated in the mechanisms that make the testis an immunologically privileged site where germ cells are protected from autoimmune attack and foreign tissue grafts may survive for extended periods. With regard to normal development and function of the testis, both pro- and anti-inflammatory cytokines are involved in the complex interactions between testicular somatic cells and resident as well as circulating immune cells. The same cytokines experience considerable upregulation during the induction and amplification of cellular immune responses, illustrating that the testicular environment does not preclude inflammatory reactions and subsequent disturbance of spermatogenesis and steroidogenesis. Notably, active immunization with testicular tissue or adoptive transfer of specific T lymphocytes causes autoimmune orchitis in experimental animals. In men, infection and inflammation of the reproductive tract including the testes are widely accepted as important aetiological factors of infertility. Whereas symptomatic orchitis due to bacterial or viral infections is considered to be rare, a high prevalence of asymptomatic testicular inflammatory reactions is observed among infertile males.

Immune cells including macrophages, mast cells and lymphocytes are also encountered in the interstitial and peritubular tissue of the epididymis and excurrent ductal system. In contrast to the seminiferous epithelium, however, macrophages and lymphocytes are observed within the epithelium, the majority of lymphocytes being $CD8^+$ T cells. Obviously, separation of germ cell-related antigens and immune cells is not as stringent in the excurrent ducts as in the testis, but the mechanisms of local immunoregulation remain unclear. With regard to immune activation and recruitment of inflammatory cells, the epididymis appears to be more susceptible than the testis. Insults such as vasectomy are associated with a high risk of formation of antisperm antibodies.

In conclusion, immunopathological reactions in the testis and excurrent ducts should not be neglected as an underlying reason for, or co-factor of, male infertility. Further investigation of the mechanisms that regulate testicular and epididymal immune functions in health and disease may encourage the search for appropriate diagnostic and therapeutic strategies for male infertility.

II.1.6.1 Immune Privilege of the Testis

Studies in experimental animals indicate that the testis is one of very few organs of the body capable of sustaining foreign tissue grafts for extended periods of time without evidence of rejection (Head et al. 1983b; Head and Billingham 1985). Enhanced survival of allogeneic grafts was also observed after co-transplantation of testicular tissue into other sites (Bellgrau et al. 1995; Korbutt et al. 1997). This "immunological privilege" of the testis is believed to arise from the need to prevent immune responses against meiotic and haploid germ cells expressing "nonself" antigens which first appear at the time of puberty, long after the establishment of immunological self-tolerance in the perinatal period. Paradoxically, the same antigens may become targets of a vigorous autoimmune attack if activation of specific T lymphocytes is induced elsewhere in the body, e.g. after dermal injection (Tung and Teuscher 1995; Hedger 1997). Moreover, defense mechanisms including both innate and adaptive immunity are not generally impaired in the testis. This is illustrated by the obvious capacity of the testis for inflammatory responses to local and systemic infection, neoplasia as well as chemical or physical noxae (Mikuz and Damjanov 1982; Bell et al. 1987; Weidner et al. 1999; Schuppe 2002).

II.1.6.2 Immune Cells in the Testis

Immune cells are found in considerable numbers in the normal unaffected testis of mammals, including humans (El Demiry et al. 1985, 1987; Pöllänen and Niemi 1987; Hedger 1997) (Table II.1.4). Located within the interstitial compartment, they are implicated in the mechanisms that make the testis an immunologically privileged site. In addition to resident macrophages, which represent the second most abundant cell type next to Leydig cells, mast cells are regular components of interstitial and peritubular tissue (Nistal et al. 1984;

Table II.1.4. Immune cells in the normal adult human testis

Macrophages	++
Mast cells	+
Lymphocytes	(+)[a]
Natural killer (NK) cells	?
Dendritic cells	?
Granulocytes	–

Data obtained from Nistal et al. (1984), El Demiry et al. (1987), Pöllänen and Niemi (1987), Schuppe (2002)
[a] Predominantly T cells ($CD4^+$, $CD8^+$)

Gaytan et al. 1989). The number of lymphocytes in the testis is relatively small, although circulating immune cells have access to the organ, and testicular lymphatic vessels allow drainage to regional lymph nodes (Head et al. 1983a; Hedger and Meinhardt 2000). The presence of natural killer (NK) cells known to be involved in innate immune responses was reported in rodents, whereas consistent data for the human testis are not available. Moreover, dendritic cells as potential professional antigen-presenting cells and key players during induction of specific immune responses remain to be identified in the normal testis. Under physiological conditions, neither resident nor circulating immune cells are found within the seminiferous tubules and polymorphonuclear leukocytes remain completely absent.

II.1.6.2.1 Macrophages

There is substantial evidence that testicular macrophages and their functions are largely determined by the local environment (Hedger 1997, 2002). In the rat testis, two distinct subpopulations of macrophages were identified by means of the monoclonal antibodies ED1 and ED2, with 85% of the cells revealing the "resident" phenotype $ED1^-ED2^+$ (Wang et al. 1994). The number of macrophages increases during pubertal development and is partly dependent on interaction with Leydig cells (Hedger 2002). On the other hand, resident macrophages have a trophic effect on Leydig cell steroidogenesis in the adult testis (Wang et al. 1994). In mice lacking colony-stimulating factor-1, reduced numbers of testicular macrophages result in impaired spermatogenesis as a consequence of dramatically reduced testosterone levels (Cohen et al. 1999). Beyond their impact on testis-specific functions, macrophages in the testis have to be considered as potential effector cells in the first line of host defense, i.e. activating innate immune responses and thus inflammation. Notably, testicular macrophages have been shown to express major histocompatibility complex class II (MHC II) molecules essential for antigen presentation to $CD4^+$ T cells (Hedger 1997). However, the ability of freshly isolated rat testicular macrophages to release pro-inflammatory cytokines such as interleukin-1 (IL-1), IL-6 and tumour necrosis factor-α (TNF-α) is reduced in comparison with macrophages of other origin (Kern et al. 1995; Hayes et al. 1996). Available data suggest that resident macrophages in the normal adult testis mainly exert anti-inflammatory activities and participate in the regulation of steroidogenesis and spermatogenesis (Frungieri et al. 2002; Hedger 2002; Hedger and Meinhardt 2003).

II.1.6.2.2 Mast Cells

Similar to macrophages, mast cells seem to be involved in the complex local regulation of testicular function (Hedger 1997). Mast cells are known to play an important role in innate immunity as well as specific acquired immune responses and are capable of releasing a wide variety of inflammatory mediators such as tryptase and other proteases, histamine, leukotrienes, prostaglandins and cytokines (Janeway et al. 2005). In the adult human testis, mast cells can be found in the interstitium, within the lamina propria of seminiferous tubules, and in the tunica albuginea (Nistal et al. 1984; Jezek et al. 1999; Meineke et al. 2000; Schuppe 2002). Localization and different ultrastructural phenotypes of testicular mast cells suggest a functional heterogeneity.

II.1.6.2.3 Lymphocytes

Approximately 15% of the immune cells in the normal adult rat testis have been shown to be lymphocytes (Hedger 1997). Most of these lymphocytes expressed T cell markers with a predominance of $CD8^+$ T cells, whereas B cells were not detectable. Concerning the human testis, studies are scarce and only qualitative data available. Immunocytochemistry revealed few or no lymphocytes in normal peripheral testicular tissue, whereas considerable numbers of T cells were detectable within the lining epithelium ($CD8^+ > CD4^+$) and in the intertubular connective tissue ($CD4^+ > CD8^+$) of the rete testis (El-Demiry et al. 1985, 1987; Pöllänen and Niemi 1987). As in rats, B cells are largely absent. With regard to lymphocyte functions in the noninflamed testis, subpopulations of T cells and their cytokine profiles in particular remain to be characterized.

II.1.6.3 Blood–Testis Barrier

Prevention of germ cell-specific autoimmune reactions in the adult testis has long been explained solely on the basis that all germ cell-related autoantigens are segregated within the seminiferous tubules (see Table II.1.5). With the onset of meiosis during puberty, the so-called

Table II.1.5. Putative mechanisms of testicular immunoregulation

Partial segregation of germ cell-specific antigens by the blood-testis barrier
Local anergy of T lymphocytes
Apoptosis of T lymphocytes (e.g. Fas/FasL-mediated)
Suppression of T-cell-mediated immune responses by local mediators (e.g. cytokines)

Adapted from Pöllänen et al. (1997), Filippini et al. (2001)

blood-testis barrier separates the basal compartment of the seminiferous epithelium containing spermatogonia and preleptotene spermatocytes from the adluminal compartment, where meiosis and spermiogenesis occur (Lui et al. 2003; see Chaps. II.1.1, II.1.3). Morphologically, the "occluding tight junctions" between Sertoli cells render intercellular spaces impermeable to even small molecules. Thus, the microenvironment of the adluminal compartment is isolated from the vascular system and circulating immune cells. However, segregation of germ-cell-specific autoantigens by the blood-testis barrier is not complete. Autoantigenicity of the basal compartment of the seminiferous epithelium was demonstrated in rats (Yule et al. 1988; Saari et al. 1996). Moreover, barrier functions are less extensive along the rete testis and excurrent ducts (Pöllänen and Cooper 1994).

II.1.6.4 Mechanisms of Immune Tolerance in the Testis

Tissue barriers and mechanical sequestration are important but not sufficient to protect male germ cells from autoimmune attack. There is considerable evidence that multiple immunoregulatory mechanisms are involved in maintaining both tolerance towards germ cells and immune privilege within the normal adult testis (Pöllänen et al. 1997; Filippini et al. 2001) (Table II.1.5). While clonal deletion of autoreactive T lymphocytes through thymic selection during perinatal life does not control germ-cell-related autoreactivity, mechanisms of peripheral tolerance such as local anergy of T cells have been considered to play a key role (Janeway et al. 2005). Naïve T cells remain refractory to antigen-specific activation when encountering antigenic peptide:MHC complexes without antigen-independent co-stimulatory signals delivered by the same antigen-presenting cell. In line with this concept, constitutive expression of MHC molecules is found in the interstitial compartment of the testis, whereas co-stimulatory molecules such as CD80 and CD86 are absent (Tung and Teuscher 1995; Hedger 1997; Pöllänen et al. 1997). Only low constitutive expression of intercellular cell adhesion molecule-1 (ICAM-1) and vascular cell adhesion molecule-1 (VCAM-1) was reported for murine Leydig cells and Sertoli cells, whereas these adhesion molecules are restricted to the vascular endothelium in the normal human testis (Riccioli et al. 1995; Braendstrup et al. 1996; Pöllänen et al. 1997).

Avoidance of deleterious autoimmune responses can also be achieved by active suppression mediated by regulatory T (T_{reg}) cell populations (O'Garra and Vieira 2004; Janeway et al. 2005). Among $CD4^+$ effector T cells, the cytokine profile produced by T_H2 cells exerts inhibitory effects on T_H1 cells, which mediate cellular immune responses including organ-specific autoimmunity. Preliminary observations in the normal murine testis suggest functional polarization of T cells towards a T_H2 profile (Schuppe 2002). Control of inflammation in vivo has also been attributed to T_{reg} producing IL-10 or transforming growth factor-β (TGF-β) (O'Garra and Vieira 2004). Moreover, experiments with peripheral blood lymphocytes from healthy donors showed that the expansion of autoreactive T cells directed against a testis-related antigen can be suppressed by $CD4^+$ $CD25^+$ T_{reg} (Danke et al. 2004). However, the presence and possible role of $CD4^+$ $CD25^+$ T_{reg} in the testis in vivo remains to be elucidated.

A further level of protection may be afforded by activation-induced apoptosis of T lymphocytes entering the immunologically privileged testis (Table II.1.5). Recent data obtained in a mouse model indicate that memory $CD8^+$ T cells migrating into the testis are capable of mounting an immune response against foreign tissue grafts but undergo apoptosis at an increased level via upregulation of Fas (CD95) and CD30 on their surface (Dai et al. 2005). Indeed, expression of the ligand of Fas (FasL) by Sertoli cells has been implicated in maintaining testicular immune privilege as well as enhanced survival of allogeneic grafts co-transplanted with testicular tissue into other sites (Bellgrau et al. 1995; Korbutt et al. 1997). However, this hypothesis is a matter of debate and conflicting results including those from human testis studies have been reported (Francavilla et al. 2000; Kimmel et al. 2000).

Finally, immunosuppressive activity in testicular fluids has been described (Filippini et al. 2001; Hedger and Meinhardt 2003). There is evidence that locally produced mediators, i.e. cytokines, could play a key role in preventing immune activation and subsequent inflammation in the testis (Table II.1.5).

II.1.6.5 Local Factors of Testicular Immunoregulation – The Dual Role of Cytokines

Apart from overall hormonal control, precise regulation of spermatogenesis and steroidogenesis within the testis depends on numerous autocrine and paracrine mediators including growth factors and cytokines (Schlatt et al. 1997). Under physiological conditions, resident macrophages as well as nonimmune testicular

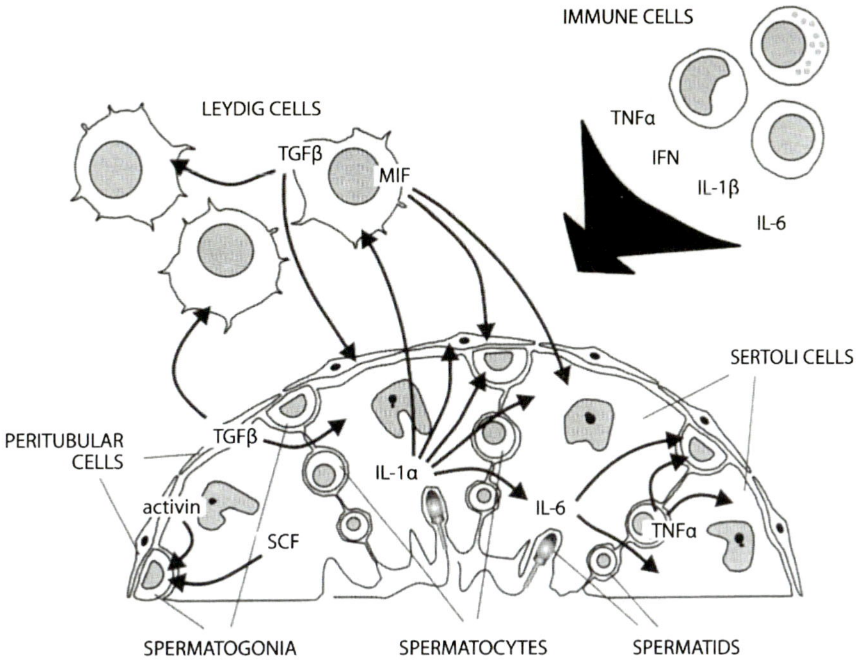

Fig. II.1.20. Synopsis of key cytokines implicated in testicular function: sites of production and potential regulatory targets. Interactions highlighted do not discriminate between sites of production under normal or inflammatory conditions. (*IL-1α* Interleukin-1α, *IL-1β* interleukin-1β, *IL-6* interleukin-6, *IFN* interferons, *MIF* macrophage migration inhibitory factor, *SCF* stem cell factor, *TGF-β* transforming growth factor-β, *TNF-α* tumour necrosis factor-α.) From Hedger and Meinhardt (2003) with permission

cells have been shown to produce both pro- and anti-inflammatory cytokines such as TNF-α, IL-1, IL-6, IL-10, interferons and members of the TGF-βfamily (Hedger and Meinhardt 2003) (Fig. II.1.20). The apparent overlap between the testicular and immune regulatory functions of these cytokines could provide the key to understanding the phenomenon of immune privilege and the processes leading to inflammation-mediated damage in the testis (see Table II.1.5).

II.1.6.5.1 Interleukin-1

The pro-inflammatory cytokine IL-1 (occurring as two isoforms: IL-1α, IL-1β) is abundantly secreted by activated macrophages, but is also inducible in other cell types (Janeway et al. 2005). In the rat testis, IL-1α is produced and secreted under physiological conditions by Sertoli cells (Syed et al. 1988; Gérard et al. 1991) (Fig. II.1.20). There is some evidence that spermatocytes and spermatids may also produce IL-1α constitutively (Haugen et al. 1994). High-affinity IL-1-binding sites and mRNA for the IL-1 signalling receptor have been found in most cells of the interstitium and seminiferous epithelium (Gomez et al. 1997). Moreover, IL-1 stimulates spermatogonial and very early (pre-leptotene) spermatocyte DNA synthesis in cultured rat seminiferous tubules (Parvinen et al. 1991). These actions indicate a role for testicular IL-1 in coordinating Sertoli and germ cell development within the seminiferous epithelium. A role in controlling steroidogenesis is indicated by the fact that IL-1 inhibits the P450 steroidogenic enzymes in adult Leydig cells in vitro (Hales et al. 1999). Recent data suggest that IL-1 generally inhibits LH-stimulated testosterone production, but can stimulate basal steroidogenesis under appropriate conditions (Svechnikov et al. 2001). In contrast to IL-1α, IL-1β does not appear to be produced in significant amounts in the normal testis (Hedger and Meinhardt 2003). However, as a third member of the family, IL-1 receptor antagonist (IL-1 RA) has been shown to be produced by mouse Sertoli cells (Zeyse et al. 2000).

II.1.6.5.2 Tumour Necrosis Factor-α

In the normal murine testis, expression of the cytotoxic immune effector molecule TNF-α has been found in pachytene spermatocytes and round spermatids (De et al. 1993) (Fig. II.1.20). Moreover, TNF-α is produced by activated testicular macrophages in vitro (Xiong and Hales 1993). Similar to IL-1, TNF-α inhibits Leydig cell steroidogenesis, and its localization to the post-meiotic germ cells also indicates possible involvement in the process of spermatogenesis (Hales et al. 1999). Observations from the human testis suggest that TNF-α might play a role in controlling the efficiency of spermatogenesis, inhibiting germ cell apoptosis by regulating the level of FasL (Pentikainen et al. 2001). With regard to testicular immunopathology, TNF-α has been implicated as a major causative agent in the development of autoimmune orchitis (Yule and Tung 1993; Suescun et al. 2003).

II.1.6.5.3
Macrophage Migration-Inhibitory Factor

The macrophage migration-inhibitory factor (MIF) is a pleiotropic protein with a wide tissue distribution participating in inflammatory responses and acting as a counter-regulator of glucocorticoid-induced immune suppression (Hedger and Meinhardt 2003). In the rat testis, MIF has been localized to the Leydig cells (Meinhardt et al. 1996) (Fig. II.1.20). Whereas testicular macrophages remain MIF negative, previously negative Sertoli cells revealed a significant compensatory MIF expression after ethane dimethane sulphonate (EDS) treatment for Leydig cell ablation (Meinhardt et al. 1999). Furthermore, MIF has been found to reduce inhibin secretion by Sertoli cells in culture and to evoke a transient increase in calcium levels in peritubular cells (Meinhardt et al. 1996; Wennemuth et al. 2000). These data support a role for MIF in the paracrine regulation of interactions between Leydig cells and the seminiferous tubule. MIF has been shown to downregulate TGF-β2 secretion in peritubular cells. Hence, upregulation of the pro-inflammatory cytokine MIF during inflammation can inhibit the immunosuppressive response of the testis (Müller et al. 2005).

II.1.6.5.4
Transforming Growth Factor-β

The TGF-β family members are dimeric cytokines with predominantly immunosuppressive and anti-inflammatory activities (Janeway et al. 2005). There are three mammalian TGF-β isoforms (1–3), which are very highly expressed by Sertoli cells, peritubular cells and Leydig cells in the foetal and immature testis, although production declines dramatically post-puberty (Mullaney and Skinner 1993) (Fig. II.1.20). The receptors for TGF-β are found in both somatic and germ cells (Caussanel et al. 1997; Goddard et al. 2000). Consequently, these cytokines have been implicated in controlling both Leydig cell and seminiferous tubule development (Hedger and Meinhardt 2003). A precise role in the adult testis has yet to be established, although TGF-β has been implicated in the immunoprotective activity of Sertoli cells and testicular immune privilege (Filippini et al. 2001). In addition to TGF-β, structurally related activins are capable of modulating pro-inflammatory cytokines such as IL-1 and IL-6 in the testis (de Kretser et al. 2001).

II.1.6.6
Inflammation of the Testis

The testicular environment does not preclude immune activation and potential damage. In fact, the recruitment of nonresident inflammatory cells into the testis indicates a profound disturbance of local immunoregulation and, thus, testicular immune privilege. Infiltrating immune cells obviously overcome the immunosuppressive influence in the testis (Hedger 1997). This is well illustrated in animal models, i.e. experimental autoimmune orchitis (EAO) (Tung and Teuscher 1995). Active immunization with homologous testis homogenates in complete Freund's adjuvant or viable syngeneic germ cells alone elicits a vigorous organ-specific immune response with characteristic deterioration of spermatogenesis ("aspermatogenesis"). The inflammatory infiltrates in EAO predominantly comprise activated T lymphocytes, accompanied by B cells and non-resident macrophages (Itoh et al. 1991; Lustig et al. 1993). Notably, TNF-α-producing $CD4^+$ Th1 cells have been implicated as key players in the development of EAO (Yule and Tung 1993; Suescun et al. 2003). In line with these results, EAO can be adoptively transferred into syngeneic recipients by $CD4^+$ T cells or testis-specific T cell lines, whereas depletion of $CD4^+$ T cells in vivo inhibits the disease (Tung and Teuscher 1995). With regard to recruitment of leukocytes, chemokines and their receptors have to be considered as crucial components (Guazzone et al. 2003).

In men, infection and inflammation of the reproductive tract including the testes are widely accepted as important aetiological factors of infertility (Rowe et al. 2000). However, acute symptomatic orchitis due to viral or bacterial infections is considered to be a rare disorder (Mikuz and Damjanov 1982; Weidner et al. 1999). On the other hand, subacute or chronic asymptomatic inflammation of the testis including noninfectious disorders may often remain obscure. Notably, testicular biopsy samples from infertile men show a high prevalence of asymptomatic inflammatory reactions with prominent peritubular infiltration of lymphocytes in a focal or multifocal pattern and characteristic signs of tubular damage in 5–15% of the cases (Suominen and Söderström 1982; Schuppe 2002). Thus, the induction of deleterious immune responses in the testis is probably not restricted to infectious agents, and a wide spectrum of aetiological factors including neoplasia, chemicals and physical trauma should be considered (Table II.1.6). Comparable to EAO in animals, severe inflammation of the human testis results in complete disruption of spermatogenesis as reflected by testicular atrophy and persistent infertility. Leydig cells in the inter-

Table II.1.6. Aetiologic factors of inflammatory reactions in the human testis

Local or systemic infection
Neoplastic disorders (seminoma, carcinoma-in-situ)
Chemical noxae
Physical factors, trauma
Other testicular disorders (e.g. congenital, early acquired)?

stitial compartment show little evidence of attrition in most patients, however bilateral orchitis may lead to failure of testicular androgen production (Mikuz and Damjanov 1982).

In line with data from animal models, a hallmark of chronic inflammatory reactions in the human testis is the infiltration of activated, inflammatory T lymphocytes ($CD4^+$, $CD8^+$), which are accompanied by increased numbers of nonresident $CD68^+$ macrophages and mast cells (El-Demiry et al. 1987; Schuppe 2002). For the latter two cell types, a shift from the interstitium to the seminiferous tubules was also reported for other testicular pathologies and has been associated with tissue remodelling and fibrosis (Meineke et al. 2000; Frungieri et al. 2002). Notably, the degree of lymphocytic infiltration correlates with characteristic signs of tubular damage including partial or complete loss of germinal epithelium, thickening of the lamina propria, and complete tubular fibrosis (Schuppe 2002).

Both predominant peritubular localization of lymphocytes and characteristic morphological changes of the seminiferous tubules resembling EAO support the concept that concomitant activation of autoreactive T cells is involved. It is unlikely, however, that deterioration of spermatogenesis results from direct T cell-mediated cytotoxicity but rather reflects the imbalance of locally produced cytokines towards a pro-inflammatory profile. Hence, impairment of Sertoli cell function and subsequent breakdown of the blood–testis barrier appear to be important features of testicular inflammatory reactions (Filippini et al. 2001).

II.1.6.7 Immunobiology and Pathology of the Excurrent Ducts

Immune cells including macrophages, mast cells and lymphocytes are not only encountered in the testis – they are also regular components of the interstitial and peritubular tissue of the epididymis and excurrent ductal system (Nistal et al. 1984; El-Demiry et al. 1985; Nashan et al. 1989; Pöllänen and Cooper 1994). In contrast to the seminiferous tubules, however, lymphocytes are also physiologically present within the epithelium of the adult rete testis, epididymis and vas deferens, most of them expressing T cell markers. In the human epididymis, lymphocytes comprise up to 12 % of the epithelial cells with increasing numbers towards the distal regions of the organ (El-Demiry et al. 1985; Yakirevich et al. 2002). The majority of the intraepithelial lymphocytes are $CD8^+$ T cells with cytotoxic properties including activated granzyme B^+ cells.

Significant differences in intraepithelial lymphocyte numbers between the normal adult epididymis and the epididymis in cryptorchidism associated with Sertoli cell only syndrome suggests that exposure of the excurrent ducts to spermatozoa or immature germ cells triggers the recruitment of T cells (Yakirevich et al. 2002). Indeed, there is considerable absorption of testicular fluid and antigenic products of sperm degradation in the excurrent ductal system. In line with this concept, macrophages containing spermatozoa or sperm fragments residing in the ductal lumen as well as cell–cell contacts between intraepithelial lymphocytes and macrophages were observed in the human epididymis (Holstein 1978; Wang and Holstein 1983). Moreover, basal cells of the epithelium have been shown to express macrophage-related antigens, and defective spermatozoa can be phagocytosed by epithelial cells (Pöllänen and Cooper 1994). On the other hand, lymphocyte-mediated cytotoxicity is unlikely to occur under physiological conditions considering that testicular germ cells as well as epididymal spermatozoa lack class I MHC molecules (Pöllänen and Cooper 1994). Thus, it has been suggested that intraepithelial $CD8^+$ T cells exert regulatory functions maintaining the immunologically privileged status of the region (Yakirevich et al. 2002).

A shorter survival time of allografts in the epididymis compared to the testis indicates, however, that the control of immune cells is less stringent in the excurrent ductal system (Kazeem 1988). With regard to barrier functions ("blood–epididymis barrier"), occlusive cell–cell junctions along the epithelium of the rete testis, epididymis and vas deferens are less extensive than those of the seminiferous epithelium (Suzuki and Nagano 1978; Pöllänen and Cooper 1994).

For the epididymis, local release of a plethora of molecules with potential immunoregulatory effects including immunoglobulins as well as components of the complement system and their inhibitors has been reported (Pöllänen and Cooper 1994). Moreover, a wide range of both pro- and anti-inflammatory cytokines was identified in human seminal plasma under physiological conditions. The cellular origin and functional significance of seminal cytokines, however, remain to be elucidated. As in the testis, cytokines could be regulators of excurrent duct functions and experience considerable upregulation during inflammation. Indeed, increased levels of pro-inflammatory cytokines such as IL-1, IL-6 or IL-8 are related to inflammatory conditions of the male genital tract (Ochsendorf 1999; see Chaps. I.3.13, II.2.4). Data from murine models suggest that high expression of IL-10 by epithelial cells is involved in local protection from autoimmune attack (Verankorva et al. 2002). Furthermore, cytokines seem to play an important role during epididymal sperm maturation. MIF is strongly expressed in the caput of the rat epididymis and has been shown to elicit the release of zinc ions from spermatozoa in vitro (Eickhoff et al. 2004). Epididymis-specific isoforms of antimicrobial defensins were shown to be involved in sperm maturation and acquisition of motility (Yenugu et al. 2004; Zhou et al. 2004).

The male excurrent ductal system appears to be more susceptible than the testis to infectious and inflammatory disorders. For example, the reported prevalence of acute infectious epididymitis exceeds by far that of symptomatic orchitis (Weidner et al. 1999; Chan and Schlegel 2002). Furthermore, the risk of immune activation and recruitment of leukocytes with subsequent autoimmunity towards spermatozoa is considered to be significantly higher in the epididymis than in the testis (Pöllänen and Cooper 1994). The formation of antisperm antibodies (ASA) is predominantly associated with insults to the genital tract such as vasectomy or other conditions of obstruction, whereas only few patients with testicular inflammatory disorders, e.g. those with a history of mumps orchitis, reveal positive antibody titres (Mazumdar and Levine 1998; Kalaydjiev et al. 2002; see Chap. I.3.4). However, the precise mechanisms underlying ASA formation in the human epididymis and the respective role of intraepithelial and interstitial lymphocytes are yet poorly defined.

References

Bell DA, Flotte TJ, Bhan AK (1987) Immunohistochemical characterization of seminoma and its inflammatory cell infiltrate. Hum Pathol 18:511–520

Bellgrau D, Gold D, Selawry H, Moore J, Franzusoff A, Duke RC (1995) A role for CD95 ligand in preventing graft rejection. Nature 377:630–632

Braendstrup O, Jensen L, Werdelin O (1996) Sertoli cells, but not tumor cells, of seminoma in situ express ICAM-1. APMIS 104:817–822

Caussanel V, Tabone E, Hendrick J-C, Dacheux F, Benahmed M (1997) Cellular distribution of transforming growth factor betas 1, 2 and 3 and their types I and II receptors during postnatal development and spermatogenesis in the boar testis. Biol Reprod 56:357–367

Chan PTK, Schlegel PN (2002) Inflammatory conditions of the male excurrent ductal system. Part I. J Androl 23:453–460

Cohen PE, Nishimura K, Zhu L, Pollard JW (1999) Macrophages: important accessory cells for reproductive function. J Leukoc Biol 66:765–72

Dai Z, Nasr IW, Reel M, Deng S, Diggs L, Larsen CP, Rothstein DM, Lakkis FG (2005) Impaired recall of CD8 memory T cells in immunologically privileged tissue. J Immunol 174:1165–1170

Danke NA, Koelle DM, Yee C, Beheray S, Kwok WW (2004) Autoreactive T cells in healthy individuals. J Immunol 172: 5967–5972

De SK, Chen HL, Pace JL, Hunt JS, Terranova PF, Enders GC (1993) Expression of tumor necrosis factor-alpha in mouse spermatogenic cells. Endocrinology 133:389–396

Eickhoff R, Baldauf C, Koyro HW, Wennemuth G, Suga Y, Seitz J, Henkel R, Meinhardt A (2004) Influence of macrophage migration inhibitory factor (MIF) on the zinc content and redox state of protein-bound sulphydryl groups in rat sperm: indications for a new role of MIF in sperm maturation. Mol Hum Reprod 10:605–611

El Demiry MI, Hargreave TB, Busuttil A, James K, Ritchie AW, Chisholm GD (1985) Lymphocyte sub-populations in the male genital tract. Br J Urol 57:769–774

El Demiry MI, Hargreave TB, Busuttil A, Elton R, James K, Chisholm GD (1987) Immunocompetent cells in human testis in health and disease. Fertil Steril 48:470–479

Filippini A, Riccioli A, Padula F, Lauretti P, D'Alessio A, De Cesaris P, Gandini L, Lenzi A, Ziparo E (2001) Control and impairment of immune privilege in the testis and in semen. Hum Reprod Update 7:444–449

Francavilla S, D'Abrizio P, Rucci N, Silvano G, Properzi G, Straface E, Cordeschi G, Necozione S, Gnessi L, Arizzi M, Ulisse S (2000) Fas and Fas ligand expression in fetal and adult human testis with normal or deranged spermatogenesis. J Clin Endocrinol Metab 85:2692–2700

Frungieri MB et al (2002) Number, distribution pattern, and identification of macrophages in the testes of infertile men. Fertil Steril 78:298–306

Gaytan F, Carrera G, Pinilla L, Aguilar R, Bellido C (1989) Mast cells in the testis, epididymis and accessory glands of the rat: effects of neonatal steroid treatment. J Androl 10:351–358

Gérard N, Syed V, Bardin W, Genetet N, Jégou B (1991) Sertoli cells are the site of interleukin-1α synthesis in rat testis. Mol Cell Endocrinol 82:R13–R16

Goddard I, Bouras M, Keramidas M, Hendrick JC, Feige JJ, Benahmed M (2000) Transforming growth factor-β receptor types I and II in cultured porcine Leydig cells: expression and hormonal regulation. Endocrinology 141:2068–2074

Gomez E, Morel G, Cavalier A, Lienard MO, Haour F, Courtens JL, Jegou B (1997) Type I and type II interleukin-1 receptor expression in rat, mouse, and human testes. Biol Reprod 56:1513–1526

Guazzone VA, Rival C, Denduchis B, Lustig L (2003) Monocyte chemoattractant protein-1 (MCP-1/CCL2) in experimental autoimmune orchitis. J Reprod Immunol 60:143–157

Hales DB, Diemer T, Hales KH (1999) Role of cytokines in testicular function. Endocrine 10:201–217

Haugen TB, Landmark BF, Josefsen GM, Hansson V, Högset A (1994) The mature form of interleukin-1α is constitutively expressed in immature male germ cells from rat. Mol Cell Endocrinol 105:R19–R23

Hayes R, Chalmers SA, Nikolic Paterson DJ, Atkins RC, Hedger MP (1996) Secretion of bioactive interleukin 1 by rat testicular macrophages in vitro. J Androl 17:41–49

Head JR, Billingham RE (1985) Immune privilege in the testis. II. Evaluation of potential local factors. Transplantation 40: 269–275

Head JR, Neaves WB, Billingham RE (1983a) Reconsideration of the lymphatic drainage of the rat testis. Transplantation 35:91–95

Head JR, Neaves WB, Billingham RE (1983b) Immune privilege in the testis. I. Basic parameters of allograft survival. Transplantation 36:423–431.

Hedger MP (1997) Testicular leukocytes: what are they doing? Rev Reprod 2:38–47

Hedger MP (2002) Macrophages and the immune responsiveness of the testis. J Reprod Immunol 57:19–34

Hedger MP, Meinhardt A (2000) Local regulation of T cell numbers and lymphocyte-inhibiting activity in interstitial tissue of the adult rat testis. J Reprod Immunol 48:69–70

Hedger MP, Meinhardt A (2003) Cytokines and the immune-testicular axis. J Reprod Immunol 58:1–26

Holstein AF (1978) Spermatophagy in the seminiferous tubules and excurrent ducts of the testis in Rhesus monkey and in man. Andrologia 10:331–352

Itoh M, Hiramine C, Tokunaga Y, Mukasa A, Hojo K (1991) A new murine model of autoimmune orchitis induced by immunization with viable syngeneic testicular germ cells alone. II. Immunohistochemical findings of fully-developed inflammatory lesion. Autoimmunity 10:89–97

Janeway CA, Travers P, Walport M, Shlomchik MJ (2005) Immunobiology: the immune system in health and disease. 6th edn. Garland, New York

Jezek D, Banek L, Hittmair A, Pezerovic-Panijan R, Goluza T, Schulze W (1999) Mast cells in testicular biopsies of infertile men with "mixed atrophy" of seminiferous tubules. Andrologia 31:203–210

Kalaydjiev S, Dimitrova D, Nenova M, Peneva S, Dikov I, Nakov L (2002) Serum sperm antibodies are not elevated after mumps orchitis. Fertil Steril 77:76–82

Kazeem AA (1988) A critical consideration of the rat epididymis as an immunologically privileged site. Scand J Immunol 27:149–156

Kern S, Robertson SA, Mau VJ, Maddocks S (1995) Cytokine secretion by macrophages in the rat testis. Biol Reprod 53:1407–1416

Kimmel SG, Ohbatake M, Kushida M, Merguerian P, Clarke ID, Kim PC (2000) Murine xenogeneic immune responses to the human testis: a presumed immune-privileged tissue. Transplantation 69:1075–1084

Korbutt GS, Elliott JF, Rajotte RV (1997) Cotransplantation of allogeneic islets with allogeneic testicular cell aggregates allows long-term graft survival without systemic immunosuppression. Diabetes 46:317–322

de Kretser DM, Loveland KL, Meehan T, O'Bryan MK, Phillips DJ, Wreford NG (2001) Inhibins, activins and follistatin: actions on the testis. Mol Cell Endocrinol 180:87–92

Lui WY, Mruk D, Lee WM, Cheng CY (2003) Sertoli cell tight junction dynamics: their regulation during spermatogenesis. Biol Reprod 68:1087–1097

Lustig L, Lourtau L, Perez R, Doncel GF (1993) Phenotypic characterization of lymphocytic cell infiltrates into the testes of rats undergoing autoimmune orchitis. Int J Androl 16:279–284

Mazumdar S, Levine AS (1998) Antisperm antibodies: etiology, pathogenesis, diagnosis, and treatment. Fertil Steril 70:799–810

Meineke V, Frungieri MB, Jessberger B, Vogt H, Mayerhofer A (2000) Human testicular mast cells contain tryptase: increased mast cell number and altered distribution in the testes of infertile men. Fertil Steril 74:239–244

Meinhardt A, Bacher M, McFarlane JR, Metz CN, Seitz J, Hedger MP, de Kretser DM, Bucala R (1996) Macrophage migration inhibitory factor production by Leydig cells: evidence for a role in the regulation of testicular function. Endocrinology 137:5090–5095

Meinhardt A, Bacher M, O'Bryan MK, McFarlane JR, Mallidis C, Lehmann C, Metz CN, de Kretser DM, Bucala R, Hedger MP (1999) A switch in the cellular localization of macrophage migration inhibitory factor in the rat testis after ethane dimethane sulfonate treatment. J Cell Sci 112:1337–1344

Mikuz G, Damjanov I (1982) Inflammation of the testis, epididymis, peritesticular membranes, and scrotum. Pathol Annu 17:101–128

Mullaney BP, Skinner MK (1993) Transforming growth factor-beta (beta 1, beta 2, and beta 3) gene expression and action during pubertal development of the seminiferous tubule: potential role at the onset of spermatogenesis. Mol Endocrinol 7:67–76

Müller R, Keng J, Rodewald M, Meinhardt A (2005) Macrophage migration inhibitory factor suppresses transforming growth factor β2 secretion in cultured rat testicular peritubular cells. Reprod Fertil Dev 17:435–438

Nashan D, Malorny U, Sorg C, Cooper T, Nieschlag E (1989) Immuno-competent cells in the murine epididymis. Int J Androl 12:85–94

Nistal M, Santamaria L, Paniagua R (1984) Mast cells in the human testis and epididymis from birth to adulthood. Acta Anat (Basel) 119:155–160

Ochsendorf FR (1999) Infections in the male genital tract and reactive oxygen species. Hum Reprod Update 5:399–420

O'Garra A, Vieira P (2004) Regulatory T cells and mechanisms of immune system control. Nature Med 10:801–805

Parvinen M, Söder O, Mali P, Froysa B, Ritzen EM (1991) In vitro stimulation of stage-specific deoxyribonucleic acid synthesis in rat seminiferous tubule segments by interleukin-1 alpha. Endocrinology 129:1614–1620

Pentikainen V, Erkkila K, Suomalainen L, Otala M, Pentikainen MO, Parvinen M, Dunkel L (2001) TNFalpha down-regulates the Fas ligand and inhibits germ cell apoptosis in the human testis. J Clin Endocrinol Metab 86:4480–4488

Pöllänen P, Cooper TG (1994) Immunology of the testicular excurrent ducts. J Reprod Immunol 26:167–216

Pöllänen P, Niemi M (1987) Immunohistochemical identification of macrophages, lymphoid cells and HLA antigens in the human testis. Int J Androl 10:37–42

Pöllänen P, Saari T, Jahnukainen K, Sainio-Pöllänen S, Verajankorva E, Martikainen M, Antola H, Hämäläinen H (1997) Mechanisms preventing an anti-germ cell immune response. In: Waites GMH, Frick J, Baker GWH (eds) Current advances in andrology. Monduzzi Editore, Bologna

Riccioli A, Filippini A, De Cesaris P, Barbacci E, Stefanini M, Starace G, Ziparo E (1995) Inflammatory mediators increase surface expression of integrin ligands, adhesion to lymphocytes, and secretion of interleukin 6 in mouse Sertoli cells. Proc Natl Acad Sci USA 92:5808–5812

Rowe PJ, Comhaire FH, Hargreave TB, Mahmoud AMA (2000) WHO manual for the standardized investigation, diagnosis and management of the infertile male. Cambridge University Press, Cambridge

Saari T, Jahnukainen K, Pöllänen P (1996) Autoantigenicity of the basal compartment of seminiferous tubules in the rat. J Reprod Immunol 31:65–79

Schlatt S, Meinhardt A, Nieschlag E (1997) Paracrine regulation of cellular interactions in the testis: factors in search of a function. Eur J Endocrinol 137:107–117

Schuppe HC (2002) Testicular inflammatory reactions in infertile men [German]. Habilitationsschrift, Fachbereich Humanmedizin, Justus-Liebig-Universität Giessen

Suescun MO, Rival C, Theas MS, Calandra RS, Lustig L (2003) Involvement of tumor necrosis factor-alpha in the pathogenesis of autoimmune orchitis in rats. Biol Reprod 68: 2114–2121

Suominen J, Söderström KO (1982) Lymphocyte infiltration in human testicular biopsies. Int J Androl 5:461–466

Suzuki F, Nagano T (1978) Regional differences of cell junctions in the excurrent duct epithelium of the rat testis as revealed by freeze fracture. Anat Rec 191:503–520

Svechnikov KV, Sultana T, Soder O (2001) Age-dependent stimulation of Leydig cell steroidogenesis by interleukin-1 isoforms. Mol Cell Endocrinol 182:193–201

Syed V, Söder O, Arver S, Lindh M, Khan S, Ritzén EM (1988) Ontogeny and cellular origin of an interleukin-1-like factor in the reproductive tract of the male rat. Int J Androl 11: 437–447

Tung KS, Teuscher C (1995) Mechanisms of autoimmune disease in the testis and ovary. Hum Reprod Update 1:35–50

Verankorva E, Pöllänen P, Hanninen A, Martikainen M, Sundström J, Antola H (2002) IL-10 is highly expressed in the cryptorchid cryptepididymal epithelium: a probable mechanism preventing immune responses against autoantigenic spermatozoa in the epididymal tubule. Int J Androl 25: 129–133

Wang J, Wreford NG, Lan HY, Atkins R, Hedger MP (1994) Leukocyte populations of the adult rat testis following removal of the Leydig cells by treatment with ethane dimethane sulfonate and subcutaneous testosterone implants. Biol Reprod 51:551–561

Wang YF, Holstein A (1983) Intraepithelial lymphocytes and macrophages in the human epididymis. Cell Tissue Res 233:517–521

Weidner W, Krause W, Ludwig M (1999) Relevance of male accessory gland infection for subsequent fertility with special focus on prostatitis. Hum Reprod Update 5:421–432

Wennemuth G, Aumüller G, Bacher M, Meinhardt A (2000) Macrophage migration inhibitory factor-induced Ca^{2+} response in rat testicular peritubular cells. Biol Reprod 62: 1632–1639

Xiong Y, Hales DB (1993) Expression, regulation, and production of tumor necrosis factor-alpha in mouse testicular interstitial macrophages in vitro. Endocrinology 133:2568–2573

Yakirevich E, Yanai O, Sova Y, Sabo E, Stein A, Hiss J, Resnick MB (2002) Cytotoxic phenotype of intra-epithelial lymphocytes in normal and cryptorchid human testicular excurrent ducts. Hum Reprod 17:275–283

Yenugu S, Hamil KG, Radhakrishnan Y, French FS, Hall SH (2004) The androgen-regulated epididymal sperm-binding protein, human beta-defensin 118 (DEFB118) (formerly ESC42), is an antimicrobial beta-defensin. Endocrinology 145:3165–3173

Yule TD, Tung KS (1993) Experimental autoimmune orchitis induced by testis and sperm antigen-specific T cell clones: an important pathogenic cytokine is tumor necrosis factor. Endocrinology 133:1098–1107

Yule TD, Montoya GD, Russell LD, Williams TM, Tung KS (1988) Autoantigenic germ cells exist outside the blood testis barrier. J Immunol 141:1161–1167

Zeyse D, Lunenfeld E, Beck M, Prinsloo I, Huleihel M (2000) Interleukin-1 receptor antagonist is produced by Sertoli cells in vitro. Endocrinology 141:1521–1527

Zhou CX, Zhang YL, Xiao L, Zheng M, Leung KM, Chan MY, Lo PS, Tsang LL, Wong HY, Ho LS, Chung YW, Chan HC (2004) An epididymis-specific beta-defensin is important for the initiation of sperm maturation. Nature Cell Biol 6:458–64

II.1.7 Male Contributions to the Biology of Conception and Fertilization

H. J. Tournaye

Summary

During the formation of spermatozoa, a process called spermatogenesis, haploid cells are formed. The development of an organism starts when this haploid cell, the spermatozoon, fertilizes an oocyte, restoring somatic diploidy. The spermatozoon does not contain just the male genome, but also a set of signals and organelles necessary for the initiation of development. Fertilization consists of four steps: gamete interaction, oocyte penetration, fusion of genetic material and activation of the oocyte's metabolism and development. However, the spermatozoon should also deliver its centrosome, which serves as a template enabling further cleavage divisions of the fertilized oocyte. Apart from the haploid genome, the spermatozoon also supplies RNA transcripts to the oocyte. However, to date their role remains speculative.

II.1.7.1 The Foreplay

II.1.7.1.1 Sperm Migration

As in most mammals, in the human too several millions of free swimming spermatozoa are left in the lower female genital tract, i.e. the upper part of the vagina, near the cervical ostium after intercourse. The cervical epithelium secretes impenetrable mucins throughout the menstrual cycle. However, in the days preceding ovulation, through the action of rising oestradiol levels from the developing follicle on the cervical epithelial cells, these mucins change their physico-chemical properties to such an extent that motile spermatozoa can eventually enter and penetrate the cervical mucus. The penetration by spermatozoa can be assessed by sperm–cervical mucus interaction tests. The cervical mucus thus acts as a primary sperm reservoir and has a filtering action. Spermatozoa with an appropriate motility pattern and adequate morphology will eventually leave the cervical mucus and continue their journey through the upper female genital tract. It has been shown that spermatozoa can be observed in the Fallopian tubes within 30 min of their deposition in the upper part of the vagina. Given a swimming speed of about 25 µm/s for a normally functional spermatozoon, it must be clear that the contractile action of the female genital tract has a beneficial effect on the migration of the spermatozoa.

II.1.7.1.2 Capacitation

Once ejaculated and in contact with the female genital tract, spermatozoa will undergo a series of physiological changes while migrating to their target, i.e. the oocyte. One of these changes is capacitation, a functional reprogramming of the spermatozoon. By interacting with the female epithelial cells and exposure to lipoproteins from the follicular fluid, the sperm surface gradually changes its functional properties mainly by lipid exchange (Therien et al. 2001). Loss of cholesterol results in an increase of plasma membrane fluidity (Go and Wolf 1985). By exposure to bicarbonate, signalling proteins become active by phosphorylation (Visconti et al. 2002) and flagellar motility becomes hyperactivated (Ho and Suarez 2001). Furthermore it has been shown in the human too that follicular fluid may exert a chemoattractive action on the free swimming spermatozoa in the female genital tract (Fabri et al. 1998; Yao et al. 2000).

II.1.7.1.3 Acrosome Reaction

Once the spermatozoon is capacitated it is able to undergo a controlled exocytosis, which in the case of the spermatozoon is called the acrosome reaction, since enzymes contained in the acrosome are released during this event. Both contact with specific receptors at the zona pellucida of the oocyte (Wassarman 1999) and progesterone secreted by the granulosa cells induce this exocytosis (Patrat et al. 2000).

II.1.7.1.4 Penetration

Only sperm that have undergone the acrosome reaction are able to penetrate the oocyte and eventually fuse with the oolemma, i.e. the egg's plasma membrane. Penetration of the zona pellucida results not only from a localized lysis by acrosomal enzymes but also from spermatozoal motility (Bedford 1998). The fusion of the oolemma with the sperm membrane is the result of binding of sperm-specific surface proteins, some belonging to the so-called ADAM family (*a* *d*isintegrin *a*nd *m*etalloprotease), with the integrin receptor on the egg's cell membrane (Bigler et al. 1997).

II.1.7.2 Paternal Contributions to Conception

II.1.7.2.1 Oocyte Activation

During fertilization, the spermatozoon provides a signal to the egg in order to resume meiosis and to start a developmental programme in the oocyte. This signalling event is called oocyte activation. Oocyte activation is an important contribution made by the spermatozoon to the initiation of embryonic development (Runft et al. 2002). For many years it was postulated that the binding of a sperm ligand to an egg receptor, possibly the above-mentioned ADAM-integrin binding, started a cascade of signals within the oocyte resulting in a release of intracellular calcium activating the fertilized egg's metabolism. This model assumes contact and fusion of the membranes of both gametes (Williams 2002). With the successful introduction of intracytoplasmic sperm injection (ICSI) (Palermo et al. 1992; Van Steirteghem et al. 1993) it became clear that alternative mechanisms may exist, since in this technique no extracellular sperm–oocyte contact is established without deficient oocyte activation. Therefore, a second model assumes the existence of intracellular, soluble sperm factors which can activate the oocyte without contact of the membranes (Swann 1993).

II.1.7.2.2 The Microtubule Organizing Centre

A centrosome is an essential requirement for a cell to divide. The centrosome acts as a template in the production of microtubules and is therefore also called the microtubule organizing centre (MTOC). After decondensation, the centrosome will bring together the pronuclei of both sperm and egg. After syngamy the centrosome will duplicate and assembly a spindle which directs the chromatids during cell cleavage (Santhanantan 1997).

In the human, centrosomal inheritance is paternal (Schatten 1994). It is the spermatozoon that supplies the centriole which will then be transformed into the centrosome after sperm-oocyte fusion (Stearns and Kirschner 1994) (Fig. II.1.21).

Once in the oocyte's cytoplasm, microtubules will elongate throughout the cytoplasm from the centrosome. This microtubular structure is called the "sperm aster" according to its morphology. It encounters the female pronucleus containing a haploid set of chromosomes after completion of meiosis. The microtubules then transport the female pronucleus towards the male pronucleus. Once pronuclear apposition is obtained, both paternal and maternal chromosomes will condense and attach aligned to the microtubules of the mitotic spindle.

Deficiencies in centriolar function are emerging as potential causes of male infertility (Asch et al. 1995; Nagy 2000; Terada et al. 2004) and fertilization failure, even after ICSI (Nijs et al. 1996; Tournaye 2000; Westlander et al. 2003). These deficiencies may also explain the high rate of chromosomal mosaicisms observed in embryos obtained after ICSI using immature spermatozoa recovered from men with deficient spermatogenesis (Silber et al. 2003; Platteau et al. 2004).

II.1.7.2.3 The Genome

A haploid set of chromosomes is the premier male contribution to fertilization and conception in mammals. Because this set includes 23 randomly derived chromosomes, a man can produce 2^{23} chromosomally different spermatozoa, i.e. 8,388,608. However, because of genetic recombination by crossing over during meiosis, there is only a infinitely small chance that two sperma-

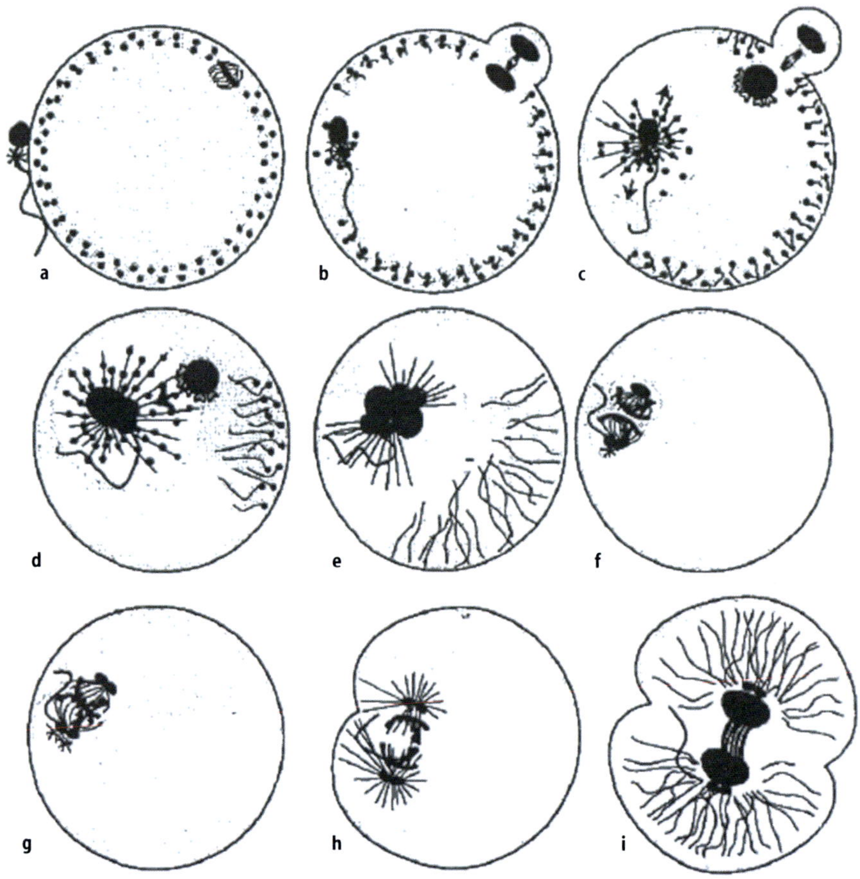

Fig. II.1.21a–i. Centrosome inheritance and microtubule organization during fertilization in humans. The mature, unfertilized oocyte has microtubules solely in the second meiotic spindle (**a**), which is arrested at metaphase, radially oriented, and, in the human, asymmetrical. The sperm introduces the centrosome (drawn as a *pinwheel* **a**). After sperm incorporation, all microtubules are radially arrayed around the sperm (**b**). Centrosome position and shape are inferred from the observed pattern of microtubules, and the size of the cell body is shown by the clearing of the cytoplasm. Microtubules are also found in the midbody of the second meiotic spindle (**b, c**). As the male and female pronuclei decondense (**c**), the sperm astral microtubules enlarge, and the male pronucleus is displaced off the cortex and into the cytoplasm. The female pronucleus moves toward the male pronucleus (**d**) as the sperm aster becomes asymmetrical. The appearance of two tufts of microtubules emanating from the region juxtapositioned between the closely apposed pronuclei (**e**) provides an indication that the centrosome splits during late interphase. The maternal and paternal chromosomes condense at prophase, during prometaphase (**f**) they move into alignment, so that by metaphase the parental genomes have united at the spindle equator (**g**). One or two small asters form at metaphase from the spindle pole associated with the sperm tail. The pronuclei remain eccentrically positioned throughout first interphase and until first mitotic anaphase (**h**). At anaphase, the mitotic asters form, enlarge and preferentially interact with the adjacent cortical region: this displaces the mitotic spindle toward the zygote centre. The cleavage furrow initially forms at this site, suggesting that sperm aster placement plays a role in the specification of the axis for first cleavage (**i**). The events after metaphase are inferred from rhesus zygotes. Defects observed in oocytes from infertile patients include failures to complete the following: (1) sperm incorporation (**a**); (2) egg activation (**a, b**); (3) sperm aster nucleation (**b**); (4) sperm aster enlargement and pronuclear decondensation (**c**); (5) migration of the female pronucleus (**d, e**); and (6) cell-cycle progression [meiosis to interphase (**a, b**) or interphase to mitosis (**e, i**)] (Reprinted from Dev Biol 165:299–335, 1994. Schatten G: The centrosome and its mode of inheritance: the reduction of the centrosome during gametogenesis and its restoration during fertilization in humans. Copyright 2006, with permission from Elsevier.)

tozoa would be genetically identical. Besides this random selection followed by recombination, a third phenomenon induces a different expression of the spermatozoal genome, i.e. genomic imprinting (Reik and Walter 2001). While random selection of chromatids and recombination are shaping the genotype, imprinting is a further modelling of the genome. The phenomenon is called imprinting because there is some imprint that is put on the oocyte's DNA or on the spermatozoal genome which marks that DNA as being maternal or paternal, and influences what the gene does in the next generation in both male and female offspring. The mark is the result of allele-specific methylation of the DNA. Paternally imprinted genes are "switched off" when passed from father to child, while maternally imprinted genes are "switched off" when passed from mother to child. Thus imprinting results in a reversible but gamete-specific marking of the genome creating a functional difference between the genetic information contributed by each parent. Usually the information from both paternal and maternal genes is actively used. However, some genes must have either a maternal or a paternal imprint in order to function. Both Prader–Willi syndrome and Angelman syndrome are examples of the imprinting concept. Both syndromes result from a deletion in the same area on chromosome 15 but if the deleted area is paternally inherited the child will develop Prader-Willi syndrome because the gene is "switched off" on the maternally inherited chromosome 15. If the deleted area is maternally inherited the child will develop Angelman syndrome because this gene is "switched off" on the paternally inherited chromosome 15.

Another example of the importance of imprinting is complete hydatidiform mole. Because of loss of the maternal genome, compensated by a duplication of the paternal genome or polyzoospermic fertilization, the embryo will only develop abnormal extraembryonic tissues. When on the other hand the genome lacks paternal input, a condition referred to as gynogenesis, the extraembryonic tissues will hardly develop, but the inner cell mass will become hypertrophic. Both conditions clearly show that although the inherited autosomes contain the same DNA sequences, they are different in terms of gene expression because of differences in allele-specific imprinting. The poor reproductive performance of cloning experiments too is yet another example of the importance of parent-specific imprinting.

Genomic imprinting changes during the life cycle of an individual. When primordial germ cells develop in the gonadal ridges during foetal life, all imprints are erased (Ueda et al. 2000). But before birth, de-novo methylation starts and imprinting is re-established (Davis et al. 2000). Although the male germ cells are imprinted even before meiosis starts, there may be concerns that imprinting is incomplete or deficient when immature gametes or gametes from men with primary testicular failure are used for assisted reproduction (Gosden et al. 2003; Lucifero et al. 2004). Although more research is urgently needed in this field, to date there is no sound evidence that assisted reproduction may increase the risk of imprinting defects.

II.1.7.3 Other Spermatozoal Attributes

II.1.7.3.1 The Sperm Mitochondria

Spermatozoa need mitochondria to generate energy for maintaining flagellar motility. Most sperm structures entering the oocyte at fertilization, i.e. fibrous sheath, microtubule doublets, outer dense fibres and the striated columns of the connecting piece, are cleared from the oocyte's cytoplasm. Mitochondria too are discarded after fertilization. After fertilization, they are submerged in the oocyte's cytoplasm diluting out the paternal mitochondrial DNA (mtDNA). The few copies of paternal mtDNA are inactivated during preimplantation embryonic development by a ubiquitin-dependent mechanism (Sutovsky et al. 1996). However, there are concerns that whenever deficient spermatozoa are used for assisted reproduction, this elimination may be incomplete and may result in mtDNA heteroplasmy (St. John et al. 2004).

II.1.7.3.2 Sperm RNA

For years it was assumed that spermatozoa did not contain mRNA as oocytes do. However, in recent years mRNAs, similar to those that are observed during spermatogenesis in the testis, have been found in mature spermatozoa (Miller et al. 2000). Mature sperm were even found to maintain a low transcriptional activity up until the acrosome reaction (Naz 1998). The role of these transcripts remains unclear, but spermatozoal mRNA has been detected in fertilized oocytes (Ostermeier et al. 2004) leading to speculation that these stored mRNA may be useful during the first steps of fertilization and maybe contribute to the paternal imprinting.

References

Asch R, Simerly C, Ord T, Ord VA, Schatten G (1995) The stages at which human fertilization arrests: microtubule and chromosome configurations in inseminated oocytes which failed to complete fertilization and development in humans. Hum Reprod 10:1897–1906

Bedford JM (1998) Mammalian fertilization misread? Sperm penetration of the eutherian zona pellucida is unlikely to be a lytic event. Biol Reprod 59:1275–1287

Bigler D, Chen M, Waters S, White JM (1997) A model for sperm-egg binding and fusion based on ADAMs and integrins. Trend Cell Biol 7:220–225

Davis TL, Yang GJ, McCarrey JR, Bartolomei MS (2000) The H19 methylation imprint is erased and re-established differentially on the parental alleles during male germ cell development. Hum Mol Genet 19:2885–2894

Fabri R, Porcu E, Lenzi A, Gandini L, Marsella T, Flamigni C (1998) Follicular fluid and human granulosa cell cultures: influence on sperm kinetic parameters, hyperactivation and acrosome reaction. Fertil Steril 69:112–117

Go KJ, Wolf DP (1985) Albumin-mediated changes in sperm sterol content during capacitation. Biol Reprod 32:145–153

Gosden R, Trasler J, Lucifero D, Faddy M (2003) Rare congenital disorders, imprinted genes, and assisted reproductive technology. Lancet 361:1975–1977

Ho HC, Suarez SS (2001) Hyperactivation of mammalian spermatozoa: function and regulation. Reproduction 122:519–526

Lucifero D, Chaillet JR, Trasler JM (2004) Potential significance of genomic imprinting defects for reproduction and assisted reproductive technology. Hum Reprod Update 10:3–18

Miller D, Briggs D, Snowden H, Hamlington J, Rollinson S, Lilford R, Krawetz SA (2000) A complex population of RNAs exists in human ejaculate spermatozoa: implications for understanding molecular aspects of spermiogenesis. Gene 237:385–392

Nagy ZP (2000) Sperm centriole dysfunction and sperm immotility. Mol Cell Endocrinol 166:59–62

Naz RK (1998) Effect of actinomycin D and cycloheximide on human sperm function. Arch Androl 41:135–142

Nijs M, Vanderzwalmen P, Vandamme B, Segal-Bertin G, Lejeune B, Segal L, van Roosendaal E, Schoysman R (1996) Fertilizing ability of immotile spermatozoa after intracytoplasmic sperm injection. Hum Reprod 11:2180–2185

Ostermeier GC, Miller D, Huntriss JD, Diamond MP, Krawetz SA (2004) Reproductive biology: delivering spermatozoon RNA to the oocyte. Nature 429:154

Palermo G, Joris H, Devroey P, Van Steirteghem AC (1992) Pregnancies after intracytoplasmic injection of single spermatozoon into an oocyte. Lancet 340(8810):17 - 18

Patrat C, Serres C, Jouannet P (2000) Induction of a sodium ion influx by progesterone in human spermatozoa. Biol Reprod 62:1380 - 1386

Platteau P, Staessen C, Michiels A, Tournaye H, Van Steirteghem A, Liebaers I, Devroey P (2004) Comparison of the aneuploidy frequency in embryos derived from testicular sperm extraction in obstructive and non-obstructive azoospermic men. Hum Reprod 19:1570 - 1574

Reik W, Walter J (2001) Genomic imprinting: parental influence on the genome. Nat Rev Genet 2:21 - 32

Runft LL, Jaffe LA, Mehlmann LM (2002) Egg activation at fertilization: where it all begins. Dev Biol 245:237 - 254

Santhanantan AH (1997) Mitosis in the human embryo: the vital role of the sperm centrosome (centriole). Histol Histopathol 12:827 - 856

Schatten G (1994) The centrosome and its mode of inheritance: the reduction of the centrosome during gametogenesis and its restoration during fertilization. Dev Biol 165:299 - 335

Silber S, Escudero T, Lenahan K, Abdelhadi I, Kilani Z, Munne S (2003) Chromosomal abnormalities in embryos derived from testicular sperm extraction. Fertil Steril 79:30 - 38

St. John JC, Lloyd R, El Shourbagy S (2004) The potential risks of abnormal transmission of mtDNA through assisted reproductive technologies. Reprod Biomed Online 8:34 - 44

Stearns T, Kirschner M (1994) In vitro reconstitution of centrosome assembly and function: the central role of gamma-tubulin. Cell 76:623 - 637

Sutovsky P, Navara CS, Schatten G (1996) Fate of the sperm mitochondria, and the incorporation, conversion, and disassembly of the sperm tail structures during bovine fertilization. Biol Reprod 55:1195 - 1205

Swann K (1993) The soluble sperm oscillogen hypothesis. Zygote 1:273 - 276

Terada Y, Nakamura S, Simerly C, Hewitson L, Murakami T, Yaegashi N, Okamura K, Schatten G (2004) Centrosomal function assessment in human sperm using heterologous ICSI with rabbit eggs: a new male factor infertility assay. Mol Reprod Dev 67:360 - 365

Therien I, Bousquet D, Manjunath P (2001) Effect of seminal phospholipid-binding proteins and follicular fluid on bovine sperm capacitation. Biol Reprod 65:41 - 51

Tournaye H (2000) Management of male infertility by assisted reproductive technologies. Baillieres Best Pract Res Clin Endocrinol Metab 14:423 - 435

Ueda T, Abe K, Miura A, Yuzuriha M, Zubair M, Noguchi M, Niwa K, Kawase Y, Kono T, Matsuda Y, Fujimoto H, Shibata H, Hayashizaki Y, Sasaki H (2000) The paternal methylation imprint of the mouse H19 locus is acquired in the gonocyte stage during foetal testis development. Genes Cells 5: 649 - 659

Van Steirteghem AC, Liu J, Joris H, Nagy Z, Janssenswillen C, Tournaye H, Derde MP, Van Assche E, Devroey P (1993) Higher success rate by intracytoplasmic sperm injection than by subzonal insemination. A report of a second series of 300 consecutive treatment cycles. Hum Reprod 8:1055 - 1060

Visconti PE, Westbrook VA, Chertihin O, Demarco I, Sleight S, Diekman AB (2002) Novel signaling pathways involved in sperm acquisition of fertilizing capacity. J Reprod Immunol 53:133 - 150

Wassarman PM (1999) Mammalian fertilization: molecular aspects of gamete adhesion, exocytosis, and fusion. Cell 96:175 - 183

Westlander G, Barry M, Petrucco O, Norman R (2003) Different fertilization rates between immotile testicular spermatozoa and immotile ejaculated spermatozoa for ICSI in men with Kartagener's syndrome: case reports. Hum Reprod 18:1286 - 1288

Williams CJ (2002) Signalling mechanisms of mammalian oocyte activation. Hum Reprod Update 8:313 - 321

Yao Y, Ho P, Yeung WS (2000) Effects of human follicular fluid on the capacitation and motility of human spermatozoa. Fertil Steril 73:680 - 686

Mechanisms of Dysfunction and Pathology II.2

II.2.1 Disorders of Prenatal Sexual Development

P. Wieacker

Summary

Male sexual differentiation and fertility are the result of a signal cascade including genetic, endocrine and cellular factors. Clinical manifestations of disorders of male sexual development are hypogonadism, intersexuality and sex reversal. They can be caused by disorders of gonadal determination and differentiation, defects of hypothalamic–pituitary–gonadal regulation and steroid hormone biosynthesis, hormone insensitivity syndromes, and anomalies of the outflow tract. After clinical examination endocrinological studies are necessary in order to delineate hypergonadotrophic hypogonadism in primary gonadal failure from hypogonadotrophic hypogonadism in hypothalamic and pituitary disorders. Genetic testing includes chromosome analysis and in an increasing number of disorders molecular genetic testing is now possible. In many instances, especially in cases of intersexuality and sex reversal, diagnostic and therapeutic management should be the result of interdisciplinary co-operation.

II.2.1.1 Introduction

Sexual development is a sequence of gonadal determination, genital differentiation and germ cell production. The principles of this developmental cascade are given in Fig. II.2.1. Chromosomal sex is established at fertilization. In the presence of a Y chromosome the bipotent gonads differentiate to testes. Genital differentiation is an endocrinological process mediated essentially by anti-Müllerian hormone (AMH) and androgens. AMH is secreted by Sertoli cells and androgens by Leydig cells and adrenal glands. AMH controls the regression of Müllerian ducts which otherwise develop to Fallopian tubes, uterus and the upper part of the vagina. Testosterone promotes the development of Wolffian ducts to vas deferens, seminal vesicles and epididymis. In the periphery, testosterone is converted to dihydrotestosterone promoting the differentiation of the prostate and external genitalia.

Disorders of sexual development can take place at the molecular, chromosomal, gonadal and somatic level leading to dissociations between these different levels.

II.2.1.2 Primary Disorders of Gonadal Development

Primary disorders of gonadal development are characterized by a hypergonadotrophic hypogonadism. They may be the result of chromosomal aberrations and gene mutations. However, in many cases the underlying defect remains unknown and cryptic rearrangements, unknown gene mutations as well as exogenous factors should be considered.

II.2.1.2.1 Klinefelter Syndrome

Klinefelter syndrome is the most frequent aberration observed in patients with azoospermia. In about 85% karyotype 47,XXY can be detected resulting from meiotic non-disjunction. The additional X chromosome is of maternal origin in slightly more than 50% (Harvey et al. 1990). In about 15% of cases mosaicism of 46,XY cells and 47,XXY cells or cells with additional X chromosomes can be observed.

Newborns with 47,XXY exhibit no significant dysmorphism. Height development is increased by the age of about 5 years. Clinical features in adults include tall stature, caused especially by the striking length of the legs, gynaecomastia in 15–30% and diminished axillary and body hair. Testes are small and show a progressive hyalinization and fibrosis of the seminiferous tubules. Leydig cells decrease in number leading to a reduced capacity for testosterone synthesis.

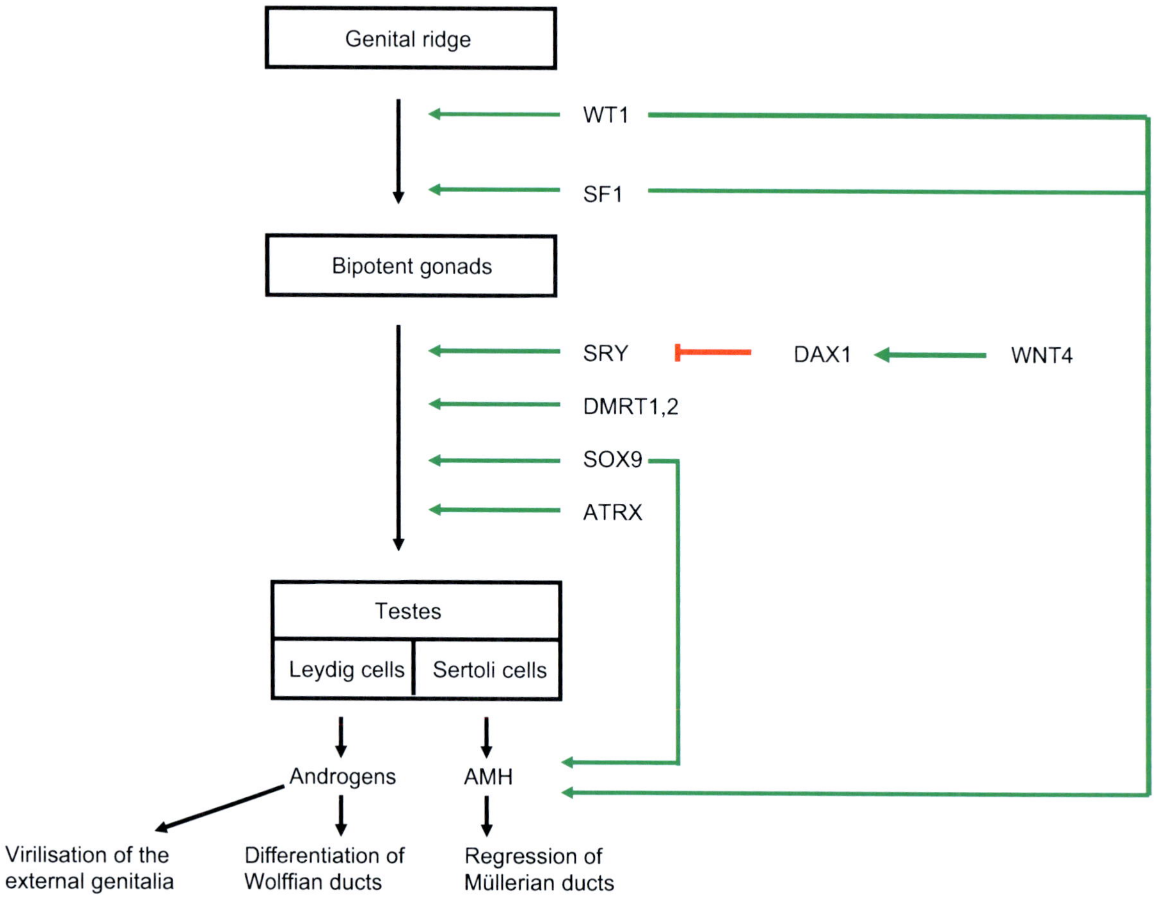

Fig. II.2.1. Cascade of male sex differentiation. *AMH* Anti-Müllerian hormone, *ATRX* alpha-thalassaemia-mental-retardation-X-linked gene, *DAX1* DSS-ACH critical region on the X chromosome, gene 1, *DMRT* doublesex- and mab-3-related transcription factor, *SF1* steroidogenic factor 1, *SOX9* SRY-related HMG-BOX gene 9, *SRY* sex-determining region of the Y chromosome, *WT1* Wilms tumour 1 gene. Stimulatory gene action (*green*) and inhibitory gene action (*red*) are shown

Without assisted reproduction, infertility is the rule. The few cases of confirmed paternity may be attributed to hidden mosaicism with 46,XY cells in the gonads. Currently, the success rate of intracytoplasmic sperm injection (ICSI) after testicular sperm extraction (TESE) in patients with Klinefelter syndrome seems to be low. Among 20 patients with 47,XXY Levron et al. (2000) could obtain testicular sperm in eight patients and pregnancy was successful in four couples. The risk of gonosomal abnormality in offspring may be about 3%. The risk of autosomal aberrations should also be considered.

II.2

II.2.1.2.2 XX Male Syndrome

XX males have a male phenotype despite a 46,XX karyotype. The incidence is about 1 in 20,000 newborn boys. Clinical features are similar to those of Klinefelter syndrome including gynaecomastia, feminine sexual hair distribution and azoospermia, but height is in the normal range. About 80% of the cases are caused by the translocation of the terminal part of Yp including SRY (sex-determining region of the Y chromosome) into the X chromosome during the paternal meiosis (Weil et al. 1994). Therefore, the gonads are testes but spermatozoa are lacking because the AZF region of Yq is absent. In about 20% of cases SRY cannot be detected. In contrast to SRY-positive XX males, SRY-negative XX males frequently exhibit genital malformations such as hypospadias or scrotum bifidum. The cause of SRY-negative XX maleness may be an inappropriate activation of the SRY-downstream cascade of testis differentiation. Jarrah et al. (2000) described an inbred kindred including SRY-negative XX maleness and XX-true hermaphroditism suggesting a monogenetic inheritance.

II.2.1.2.3 True Hermaphroditism

In true hermaphroditism the gonads comprise both testicular and ovarian structures. A few hundred cases have been reported. Separate ovaries and testes, or, more often, one or more ovotestes are present. True hermaphroditism generally presents as genital ambiguity. The gonads may be located in the abdomen, the inguinal region or the labioscrotal region. Spermatozoa are rare, but follicles are often detected. Uterus bicornis or unicornis is usually present, the latter indicating the presence of a contralateral testis or ovotestis. At puberty menstruation and breast development commonly occur. In about 60 %, the karyotype 46,XX can be detected. In about one-third of cases there is a mosaicism with a cell line containing a Y chromosome (46,XX/46,XY or 46,XX/47,XXY) or parts of it. In the minority of cases the karyotype is 46,XY (Queipo et al. 2002). The XX/XY constellation may be a chimerism resulting from the fusion of twin XX and XY embryos, whereas the XXY/XY constellation may be explained by a mosaicism after loss of an X chromosome in an XXY cell line. Most of the 46,XX cases are SRY negative and the induction of the testis development cascade downstream of SRY may be the cause. Hidden mosaicism can be the origin of XY true hermaphroditism with a cell line without a Y chromosome in parts of the gonads. In one XY case a postzygotic SRY mutation was found (Braun et al. 1993).

II.2.1.2.4 Gonadal Dysgenesis

Gonadal dysgenesis is a clinically and genetically heterogeneous disorder of gonadal differentiation. From a pathological point of view, complete and partial dysgenesis can be delineated. In complete dysgenesis gonads are degenerated to streaks consisting of connective tissue without germ cells and endocrine active cells. The phenotype is female independently from the karyotype. In contrast, partial dysgenetic gonads show residues of endocrine tissues. Therefore, in a male karyotype virilization can occur and this effect may be more pronounced at puberty. In this context gonadal dysgenesis should be delineated from testicular dysgenesis syndrome (TDS), suggested by Skakkebaek et al. (2001). TDS includes abnormal spermatogenesis, undescended testes, testicular cancer and hypospadias. Also testicular disorders such as Sertoli cell only syndrome caused by AZF deletions are not subsumed to the term gonadal dysgenesis.

From a genetic point of view gonadal dysgenesis caused by chromosomal aberrations can be delineated from XX or XY gonadal dysgenesis. Numeric aberrations are in most cases mosaics with a 45,X and a 46,XY cell line arising from postzygotic chromosome loss. The patients range in phenotype from female with classic Turner syndrome through intersex to male phenotype. In rare cases the primary cell line is 47,XXY and postzygotic loss of the Y chromosome leads to a 46,XX/47,XXY mosaicism.

Structural aberrations of the Y chromosome led to the mapping of the testis determining factor (TDF) on the short arm of the Y chromosome, because deletion of the short arm of the Y chromosome or isochromosome of the long arm of Y results in gonadal dysgenesis.

In each of XX and XY gonadal dysgenesis, syndromic or non-syndromic forms can be differentiated. In syndromic forms gonadal dysgenesis is only one feature of a complex disease, whereas in non-syndromic forms gonadal dysgenesis is the only manifestation of the disorder. In this context, it is important to remember that an extreme XY/X mosaicism may simulate XY gonadal dysgenesis if cells with gonosomal monosomy are confined to the gonads (Röpke et al. 2004).

The frequency of XY gonadal dysgenesis is about 1 in 20,000 individuals. The term Swyer syndrome should be reserved for the complete or pure form of non-syndromic XY gonadal dysgenesis. Because Leydig cells are absent, testosterone production is impaired and Wolffian ducts are absent and external genitalia are female. The absence of Sertoli cells means that AMH production is disturbed, resulting in the development of a uterus, Fallopian tubes and the upper part of the vagina. The risk of gonadal malignancy is about 30 %. In about 15 % of XY gonadal dysgenesis deletion of SRY can be detected (Cameron and Sinclair 1997). These deletions are mostly the result of a translocation of Y chromosomal material, including SRY, into the X chromosome in paternal meiosis. In a further 15 % of XY gonadal dysgenesis point mutations or insertions as well as deletions of a few nucleotides can be detected in the SRY gene. Most mutations are located in the HMG (high mobility group) domain of SRY. In this context it is noteworthy that mutations with reduced penetrance have been described. Furthermore, paternal mosaicism of SRY mutations has been demonstrated in a few cases resulting in more than one affected sibling.

The study of syndromic forms of XY gonadal dysgenesis led to the identification of further genes involved in gonadal differentiation. Genes of early gonadal development and those of testis differentiation can be delineated. Mutations of genes of early gonadal development can lead to XY or XX gonadal dysgenesis depending on the underlying karyotype.

Wilms' tumour 1 gene (WT1) in 11p13 is involved in early gonadal development and kidney differentiation. Homozygous transgenic mice for inactivating WT1 mutations are characterized by gonadal and kidney agenesis (Kreidberg et al. 1993). In humans WT1 mutations are associated with gonadal dysgenesis and glomerulopathy. Missense or stop mutations frequently cause Denys–Drash syndrome characterized by a mixed gonadal dysgenesis and ambiguous genitalia in patients with a male karyotype as well as early onset of kidney failure. In contrast, Frasier syndrome, rather caused by splice mutations in intron 9, is characterized by complete gonadal dysgenesis with female external genitalia and delayed-onset kidney failure. Furthermore, in Denys–Drash syndrome there is a high risk of Wilms' tumour and a lower risk of gonadoblastoma, whereas the opposite is true in Frasier syndrome (König et al. 1993). However, it should be considered that the two diseases show an overlap from a molecular biologic point of view. Deletions of WT1 can be part of a contiguous gene syndrome (WAGR) characterized by Wilms' tumour, aniridia, genital anomalies and mental retardation. In this syndrome, the disturbed virilization can be explained by haploinsufficiency of WT1.

A further gene involved in early gonadal development is the gene for steroidogenic factor 1 (SF-1) in 9q33, which plays an important role in adrenal development. SF-1 interacts with WT1 in order to promote AMH production and it regulates the expression of some enzymes of steroid biosynthesis. So far, only a few mutations have been reported: a heterozygous mutation in a patient affected by adrenal failure and male-to-female sex reversal, a heterozygous mutation in a female patient with adrenal failure, and a homozygous missense mutation associated with sex reversal and adrenal insufficiency (Achermann et al. 1999).

XY gonadal dysgenesis can also be caused by mutations in the SOX9 gene in 17q24.3-q25.1 (Wagner et al. 1994). Like SRY, SOX9 is a member of the HMG proteins and promotes both testis and bone development. Carriers of SOX9 mutations are afflicted by campomelic dysplasia, which is characterized by dwarfism, bowing of the limbs (especially lower limbs) and further anomalies. About two-thirds of patients with an XY karyotype are affected by male-to-female sex reversal. The gonads consist of ovarian stroma or dysgenetic testicular tissue. Mutations of SOX9 are distributed along the entire gene, but most missense mutations are localized in the HMG domain. Furthermore, a substantial number of patients have chromosome translocations with the one breakpoint in the vicinity of SOX9, suggesting a position effect. It has been assumed that SRY is a de-inhibitor of an as yet unidentified inhibitor of SOX9.

Rare cases of XY gonadal dysgenesis are inherited in an X-linked recessive trait and may be caused by duplication of the so-called dosage-sensitive sex reversal region (DSS) including the DAX1 gene in Xp21. Deletions or mutations of DAX1 cause congenital adrenal hypoplasia, hypogonadotrophic hypogonadism and azoospermia or severe oligospermia. In contrast, duplication of DAX1 is associated with male-to-female sex reversal or genital ambiguity in patients with a male karyotype (Muscatelli et al. 1994). The gonads consist of ovarian stroma with or without testicular tissue. Corresponding with gonadal histology there are variable degrees of Wolffian and Müllerian derivatives. It has been suggested that DAX1 is a dosage-dependent antagonist of SRY. However, recent analysis of Dax1 knock-out mice indicates that DAX1 per se is also important for testis determination (Meeks et al. 2003).

The study of patients with deletions of the terminal region of 9p led to the identification of DMRT1 and DMRT2 (doublesex- and mab-3-related transcription factors 1 and 2) in 9p24.3 (Raymond et al. 1998). Deletions of these genes are associated with sex reversal or genital ambiguity. Gonads turn out to be streaks or hypoplastic testes (Stumm et al. 2000). It is noteworthy that the DMRT homologue on the Z chromosome in birds is the testis-determining gene acting in a dosage-dependent mechanism. Female birds with a WZ gonosomal constellation have only one DMRT copy whereas male birds with two Z chromosomes have two DMRT copies.

A further gene involved in testis differentiation is ATRX (alpha-thalassaemia-mental-retardation-X-linked). This gene in Xq13-q21 is responsible for chromatin remodelling and has pleiotropic effects. It is involved in cognitive processes as well as sex differentiation. Recently many syndromes caused by ATRX mutations have been identified. In ATRX, Sutherland–Haan syndrome, Smith–Fineman syndrome and Juberg–Marsidi syndrome sex reversal or ambiguous genitalia can be observed. The gonads show immature testicular tissues. In an evolutionary context it is interesting that in marsupials the Y chromosome homologue ATRY is the testis-determining factor.

The "hedgehog signalling network", which plays a key role in embryonic patterning, is also involved in sexual differentiation. A mutation of Desert Hedgehog (DHH) in 12q13 has been found to be associated with partial gonadal dysgenesis and minifascicular neuropathy (Umehara et al. 2000). In testes DHH seems to control peritubular cell development, Sertoli–Leydig cell interactions and male germ line development.

Recently, mutations of the testis-specific protein-like-1 gene (TSPYL1) in 6q22-q23 have been identified as a cause of testicular dysgenesis and ambiguous genitalia in children affected by visceroautonomic dysfunction and sudden infant death (Puffenberger et al. 2004).

Autosomal aberrations have substantially contributed to the identification of genes involved in gonadal differentiation, as is the case for SRY, WT1, SOX9 and DMRT1/DMRT2. Further consistent aberrations observed in male-to-female sex reversal are the deletions 10q25-q26 (Wilkie et al. 1993) and 2q31.1-q31.3 (Slavotinek et al. 1999) or partial duplications of chromosome 1p (Wieacker et al. 1995). Some cases of 1p duplication associated with sex reversal can be explained by the duplication of WNT4 because it has been suggested that WNT4 is an agonist of DAX1 (Jordan et al. 2001).

Currently, the cause of XY gonadal dysgenesis is unknown in about 70 % of all cases including syndromic forms of gonadal dysgenesis. An important strategy in identification of the responsible genes will be the study of knock-out mice.

II.2.1.2.5
Vanishing Testes Syndrome

Vanishing testes syndrome is a heterogeneous disorder with a broad clinical spectrum reaching from agonadism to anorchia. Syndromic and non-syndromic cases can be delineated. The genital phenotype is dependent on the time of testicular regression. An early onset of testicular regression in a 46,XY embryo results in female internal and external genitalia because of the impaired production of androgens and AMH. Such cases are clinically very similar to XY gonadal dysgenesis. In the case of a later testicular regression, hypoplastic Müllerian and Wolffian structures as well as ambiguity of the external genitalia up to male external genitalia with anorchia are possible. Familial occurrence suggesting autosomal recessive inheritance has been described. It is noteworthy that affected patients of the same family can exhibit a variable phenotype including sex reversal and genital ambiguity (Wieacker et al. 2003). Furthermore, Mendonca et al. (1994) reported on agonadism in two siblings with a 46,XY and a 46,XX karyotype, respectively, suggesting also autosomal recessive inheritance of this disorder.

II.2.1.3
Disorders of Steroid Hormone Biosynthesis

Disorders of steroid hormone production are inherited in an autosomal recessive trait. Defects leading to diminished production of androgens cause male pseudohermaphroditism in the case of a male karyotype. Because gonadal differentiation is not impaired, there is normal production of AMH resulting in the absence of Müllerian structures. Defects leading to increased synthesis of androgens result in female pseudohermaphroditism in the case of a female karyotype (Fig. II.2.2).

The transport of cholesterol from the outer to the inner membrane of mitochondria is mediated by STAR (steroidogenic acute regulatory protein). Consequently, mutations of STAR are associated with a marked reduction of adrenal and gonadal steroids. Affected newborns exhibit severe adrenal failure with salt loss. Children with a male karyotype have female external genitalia or only slight features of virilization (Lin et al. 1995).

3β-Hydroxysteroid-dehydrogenase (3βHSD) is responsible for the conversion of pregnenolone to progesterone, 17-hydroxypregnenolone to 17-hydroxyprogesterone, and dehydroepiandrosterone to androstenedione. 3βHSD2 in 1p13.1 codes for the isoenzyme that is expressed in adrenal glands and gonads. Mutations of 3βHSD2 cause adrenal failure and disturbances of virilization in the case of a male karyotype. In contrast, patients with a female karyotype often show virilization of the external genitalia or hirsutism possibly caused by increased production of dehydroepiandrosterone (Pang et al. 1985).

Cytochrome P450C17 encoded by CYP17 has 17α-hydroxylase as well as 17,20-lyase activity. Mutations inactivating both domains lead to reduced levels of glucocorticoids and sex steroids, but elevated mineralocorticoids associated with hypertonia. Mutations inactivating only the 17α-hydroxylase domain result in isolated hypogonadism with female or ambiguous genitalia in the case of a male karyotype.

17β-Hydroxysteroid dehydrogenase catalyses the conversion of androstenedione to testosterone and oestrone to oestradiol. Mutations of HSD17B3 in 9q22 are associated with disturbed virilization of the external

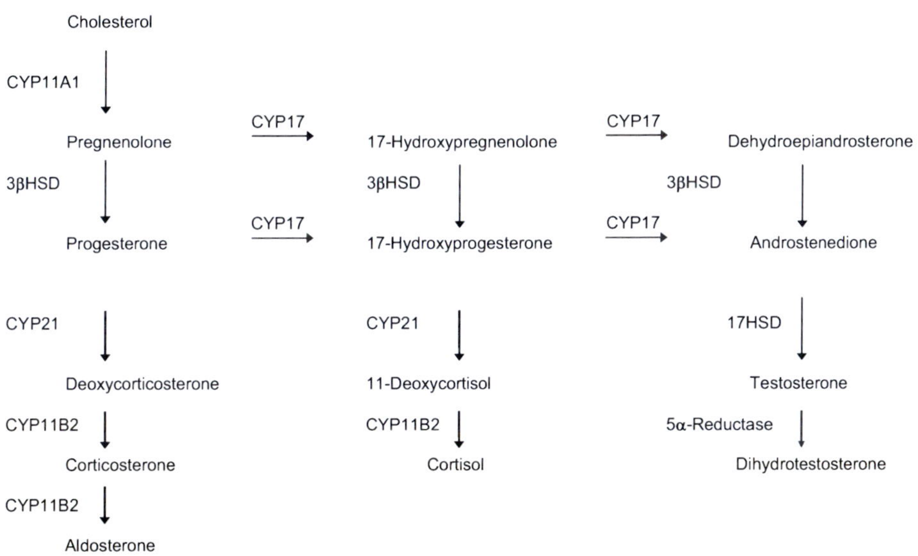

Fig. II.2.2. Important adrenal and gonadal biosynthetic pathways

genitalia, but hirsutism, clitoromegaly and voice breaking at puberty in the case of a male karyotype. After human chorionic gonadotrophin (hCG) stimulation the ratio of androstenedione to testosterone is increased (Geissler et al. 1994).

5α-Reductase is responsible for the conversion of testosterone to dihydrotestosterone. Mutations of the corresponding gene, SRD5A2 in 2p23, result in pseudovaginal perineoscrotal hypospadias (Thipgen et al. 1992). At puberty anabolic effects of testosterone are obvious and voice breaking occurs. hCG stimulation results in increased testosterone levels whereas dihydrotestosterone remains low.

Defects of 21-hydroxylase or P450C21 encoded by CYP21 in 6p21.3 are the most frequent cause of congenital adrenal hyperplasia. About 90% of CYP21 mutations are deletions or result from gene conversion. Three different clinical courses can be delineated. In congenital adrenal hyperplasia with virilization alone, the conversion of 17-hydroxyprogesterone to deoxycortisol is blocked, resulting in high levels of 17-hydroxyprogesterone and low levels of cortisol. The consequence of defective cortisol synthesis is hypersecretion of adrenocorticotropic hormone (ACTH) with resultant hyperpigmentation and overproduction of androgens leading to virilization of affected female children. In congenital adrenal hyperplasia with salt loss, the conversion of progesterone to deoxycorticosterone is also blocked. In addition to defective cortisol synthesis (with virilization in females), secretion of aldosterone is impaired and without therapy this leads to hyperkalaemia and dehydration. In late-onset adrenogenital syndrome there is a large clinical spectrum varying from ovarian dysfunction to virilization and pseudopubertas praecox. In the latter form homozygosity of mild mutations or compound heterozygosity or heterozygosity of CYP21 mutations have been detected. About 5% of cases of adrenogenital syndrome are caused by mutations of CYP11B1 encoding 11β-hydroxylase (P450C11). The impaired synthesis of cortisol results in hypersecretion of ACTH and virilization in female children. In male and female children excessive deoxycorticosterone production causes salt and water retention with hypertension.

II.2.1.4 Androgen Insensitivity

The action of androgens is mediated by binding to the androgen receptor, whose gene has been mapped to Xq12 (Wieacker et al. 1987) and was cloned in the late 1980s (Lubahn et al. 1988). Mutations of the androgen receptor gene (AR) are associated with a broad spectrum of androgen insensitivity syndromes (AIS) varying from women with female external genitalia in complete androgen insensitivity, through patients with genital ambiguity in partial androgen insensitivity, to men with male genitalia but infertility in minimal androgen insensitivity. Quigley et al. (1995) proposed a more detailed classification considering 7 grades. Grade 1 is characterized by normal male genitalia and grades 6 and 7 by a female phenotype with (grade 6) or without (grade 7) androgen-dependent effects after puberty. Grades 2–5 describe different genital manifestations of androgen insensitivity.

Complete androgen insensitivity syndrome (CAIS) with a frequency of about 1 in 20,000 is characterized by female external genitalia. The normal testis differentiation leads to undisturbed production of AMH resulting in the absence of Fallopian tubes and uterus and in a blind-ending vagina. However, in about one-third of cases rudiments of Müllerian structures are detectable. The impaired androgen action gives rise to the regression of Wolffian ducts and a maldescensus testis. The testes may be located in the abdomen, the inguinal canal, or in the labia majora. Many patients are detected in childhood because of inguinal herniae. After puberty, primary amenorrhoea, absent or sparse axillary and pubic hair, and a normal breast development are typical features of CAIS. Breast development is explained by high oestrogen levels due to peripheral aromatization of testosterone as well as the impaired androgen efficiency.

Partial AIS (PAIS) comprises a wide spectrum of clinical disorders. Incomplete testicular feminization, Lubs syndrome, Gilbert-Dreifus syndrome and Rosewater syndrome describe different manifestations of partial androgen resistance. According to the classification of Quigley et al. (1995), grade 5 is characterized by a female phenotype with mild clitoromegaly and a small degree of posterior labial fusion. In grade 4 a phallic structure in between a clitoris and a phallus, a urogenital sinus and labioscrotal folds can be observed. Grade 3 is characterized by a predominantly male phenotype including perineal hypospadias, small penis, cryptorchidism and scrotum bifidum. Individuals with grade 2 exhibit an unequivocally male phenotype with only mild effects of androgen insensitivity such as isolated hypospadias.

The risk of testicular tumours is increased in AIS patients, but it is not clear whether this risk is greater than that for patients with cryptorchidism. Dewhurst et al. (1971) have estimated the risk for malignant tumours to be in the range of 5–10%. Rutgers and Scully (1991) have found malignant tumours in 9% of cases with CAIS or PAIS.

To date more than 350 different mutations of the AR gene have been detected in patients with AIS (Gottlieb et al. 1998). Missense mutations are the most frequent and the majority of them are family-specific (Wieacker et al. 1998).

Minimal androgen insensitivity (MAIS) corresponds to grade 1 and is characterized by normal male genitalia, gynaecomastia and infertility due to azoospermia or severe oligozoospermia.

Previous androgen binding studies of genital skin fibroblasts of infertile males suggested that minimal androgen insensitivity could be a frequent cause of male infertility. However, only a few mutations have been detected in infertile men to date (Knoke et al. 1999). Yong et al. (1994) detected the missense mutation Asn727Lys in a patient with severe oligozoospermia. Interestingly, androgen therapy led to normalization of the spermiogram and restored fertility in this one patient.

II.2.1.5 Disorders of AMH Action

The AMH gene in 19p13.3 is a member of the transforming growth factor β (TGFβ) family. The regression of Müllerian ducts induced by AMH begins immediately after testicular sex is established. AMH action requires the function of AMH receptor II in 12q13. Mutations of AMH or AMHR cause persistent Müllerian duct syndrome (PMDS). Both AMH and AMHR2 mutations are inherited in an autosomal recessive fashion. Affected patients are genotypic and phenotypic males, but frequently exhibit cryptorchidism, sometimes associated with inguinal hernia. The testes are very mobile, prone to testicular torsion. The differentiation of the testes is usually normal and germ cells are present if there is no long-standing cryptorchidism. However, aplasia of the epididymis and the upper part of the vas deferens is commonly associated (Imbeaud et al. 1996).

AMH gene mutations detected in 47% of isolated PMDS are mostly family-specific and lead to very low or undetectable AMH levels. However, interpretation of AMH levels is reliable only in children because AMH production is normally repressed after puberty. In patients with AMHR2 mutations serum levels of AMH are normal. AMHR2 mutations have been detected in about 38% of isolated PMDS patients. The cause of the remaining 15% is currently unknown (Picard 2004).

II.2.1.6 Disorders of the Hypothalamic–Pituitary–Gonadal Axis

Disorders of gonadotrophin-releasing hormone (GnRH) or gonadotrophin secretion are associated with hypogonadism, but have no impact on prenatal male sexual development because foetal testosterone production is stimulated by human chorionic gonadotrophin (hCG). Therefore, among the disorders of the hypothalamic-pituitary-gonadal axis, only defects of the LH/hCG receptor will be discussed since the action of hCG is blocked by inactivating mutations of the LH receptor gene. Inactivating mutations of the LH/hCG receptor gene result in female or ambiguous external genitalia in the case of a male karyotype because of Leydig cell aplasia or hypoplasia (Kremer et al. 1995). Müllerian structures are absent because AMH production is not impaired. This is in contrast to XY-gonadal dysgenesis in which the uterus, Fallopian tubes and vagina are present. Inactivating mutations of the LH/hCG receptor gene are inherited in an autosomal recessive pattern, whereas activating mutations are dominant and cause pubertas praecox in male individuals.

II.2.1.7 Hypospadia and Undescended Testis

Hypospadia and undescended testis can be symptoms of different syndromes, but in most cases they are isolated disorders. The frequency of hypospadias is 1 in 1000 newborns. Associated malformations, especially of the urogenital tract, can be observed in about 15%. In most cases, polygenic-multifactorial inheritance is assumed, and the recurrence risk for brothers or sons is about 6–17%. However, Alléra et al. (1995) detected mutations of the androgen receptor gene in 7% of cases with severe hypospadias. In the case of a complex disorder chromosome aberrations and Mendelian disorders have to be considered.

The frequency of undescended testes is about 3–6% in newborns. Descensus testis requires androgen action, and disorders of androgen production as well as androgen insensitivity are typically associated with undescended testes. In rare instances cryptorchidism can be caused by mutations in the insulin-like-3 gene (INSL3) (Tomboc et al. 2000) or in the leucine-rich-repeat-containing G protein-coupled receptor-8 gene (L6R8) (Gorlov et al. 2002). Cryptorchidism can also be part of complex disorders. Chromosome aberrations have been detected in 2% of cryptorchidism. However, in most cases cryptorchidism seems to have a polygenic multifactorial aetiology. The recurrence risk for siblings is about 10% in the case of an isolated disorder.

References

Achermann JC, Ito M, Ito M, Hindmersch PC, Jameson JL (1999) A mutation in the gene encoding steroidogenic factor1 causes sex reversal and adrenal failure in humans. Nat Genet 22:125–126

Alléra A, Herbst MA, Griffin JE, Wilson JD, Schweikert HU, McPhaul MJ (1995) Mutations of the androgen receptor coding sequence are infrequent in patients with isolated hypospadias. J Clin Endocrinol Metab 80:2697–2699

Braun A, Kammerer S, Cleve H, Löhrs U, Schwarz HP, Kuhnle U (1993) True hermaphroditism in a 46,XY individual, caused by a postzygotic somatic point mutation in the male gonadal sex-determining locus (SRY): molecular genetics and histological findings in a sporadic case. Am J Hum Genet 52:578–585

Cameron FJ, Sinclair AH (1997) Mutations in SRY and SOX9: testis-determining genes. Hum Mut 9:388–395

Dewhurst CJ, Ferreira HP, Gillett PG (1971) Gonadal malignancy in XY females. J Obstet Gynecol Br Commonw 78:1077–1083
Geissler WMD, Davis DL, Wu L, Bradshaw KD, Patel S, Mendonca BB, Elliston KO, Wilson JD, Russel DW, Andersson S (1994) Male pseudohermaphroditism caused by mutations of testicular 17β-hydroxysteroid dehydrogenase 3. Nature Genet 7:34–39
Gorlov IPP, Kamat A, Bogatcheva, Jones E, Lamb DJ (2002) Mutations of the GREAT gene cause cryptorchidism. Hum Mol Genet 11:2309–2318
Gottlieb B, Lehvaslaiko H, Beitel LK, Lumbroso R, Pinsky L, Trifiro M (1998) The androgen receptor mutations database. Nucleic Acid Res 26:234–238
Harvey J, Jacobs PA, Hassold T, Pettay D (1990) The parental origin of 47,XXY males. Birth Defects Original Article Series 26:289–296
Imbeaud S, Belville C, Messika-Zeitoun L, Rey R, di Clemente N, Josso N, Picard JY (1996) A 27 bp-deletion of the anti-Müllerian type II receptor gene is the most frequent cause of the persistent Müllerian duct syndrome. Hum Mol Genet 5:1269–1279
Jarrah N, El-Shanti H, Khier A, Obeidat FN, Haddidi A, Ajlouni K (2000) Familial disorder of sex determination in seven individuals from three related sibships. Eur J Pediatr 159: 912–918
Jordan BK, Mohammed M, Ching ST, Delot E, Chen XN, Dewing P, Swain A, Rao PN, Elejalde BR, Vilain E (2001) Up-regulation of WNT4 signaling and dosage-sensitive sex reversal in humans. Am J Hum Genet 68:1102–1109
Knoke I, Jakubiczka S, Lehnert H, Wieacker P (1999) Mutation of the androgen receptor gene in a patient with severe oligospermia. Andrologia 31:199–201
König A, Jakubiczka S, Wieacker P, Schlösser HW, Gessler M (1993) Further evidence that imbalance of WT1 isoforms may be involved in Denys-Drash syndrome. Hum Mol Genet 2:1967–1968
Kreidberg JA, Sariola H, Lornig JM, Maeda M, Pelletier J, Housman D, Jaenisch R (1993) WT1 is required for early kidney development. Cell 74:679–691
Kremer H, Kraaj R, Toledo SPA, Post M, Fridman JB, Hayashida CY, Van Reen M, Milgrom E, Ropers HH, Marinam E, Themmen APN, Brunner HG (1995) Male pseudohermaphroditism due to a homozygous mutation in the luteinizing hormone receptor gene. Nat Genet 9:160–164
Levron J, Aviram-Goldring A, Madgar I, Raviv G, Barkai G, Dor J (2000) Sperm chromosome analysis and outcome of IVF in patients with non-mosaic Klinefelter's syndrome. Fertil Steril 74:925–929
Lin D, Sugawara T, Strauss JF, Clark BJ, Stocco DM, Saenger P, Rogol A, Miller WL (1995) Role of steroidogenic acute regulatory protein in adrenal and gonadal steroidogenesis. Science 267:1828–1831
Lubahn DB, Joseph DR, Sullivan PM, Willard HF, Wilson EM (1988) Cloning of human androgen receptor complementary DNA and localization to the X chromosome. Science 240:327–333
Meeks JJ, Weiss J, Jameson JL (2003) Dax1 is required for testis determination. Nat Genet 34:32–33
Mendonca BB, Barbosa AS, Arnhold IJ, McElreavy K, Fellous M, Moreira-Filho CA (1994) Gonadal agenesis in XX and XY sisters: evidence for the involvement of an autosomal recessive gene. Am J Med Genet 52:39–43
Muscatelli F, Strom TM, Walker AP, Zanaria E, Recan D, Meindl A, Bardoni B, Guioli S, Zehetner G, Rabl W et al (1994) Mutations in the DAX1 gene give rise to both X-linked adrenal hypoplasia congenital and hypogonadotrophic hypogonadism. Nature 372:672–676
Pang S, Lerner AJ, Stoner E, Levine LS, Oberfield SE, Engel I, New MI (1985) Late-onset adrenal steroid 3β-hydroxysteroid dehydrogenase deficiency. A cause of hirsutism in pubertal and postpubertal women. J Clin Endocrinol Metab 60:428–439
Picard JY (2004) AMH/MIS and its receptors and sexual ambiguity and persistent Müllerian derivatives. In: Epstein CJ, Erickson RP, Wynshaw-Boris A (eds) Inborn errors of development. Oxford University Press, Oxford, pp 497–501
Puffenberger EG, Hu-Lince D, Parod JM, Craig DW, Dobrin SE, Conway AR, Donarum EA, Strauss KA, Dunckley T, Cardenas JF, Melmed KR, Wright CA, Liang W, Stafford P, Flynn CR, Morton DH, Stephan DA (2004) Mapping of sudden infant death with dysgenesis of the testes syndrome (SIDDT) by a SNP genome scan and identification of TSPYL loss of function. Proc Natl Acad Sci USA 101:11689–11694
Queipo G, Zenteno JC, Pena R, Nieto K, Radillo A, Dorantes LM, Erana L, Lieberman E, Söderlund D, Jimenez AL, Ramon G, Kofman-Alfaro S (2002) Molecular analysis in true hermaphroditism: demonstration of low-level hidden mosaicism for Y-derived sequences in 46,XX cases. Hum Genet 111:278–283
Quigley CA, DeBellis A, Marschke KB, ElAwady MK, Wilson EM, French FS (1995) Androgen receptor defects: historical, clinical, and molecular perspectives. Endocr Rev 16:271–321
Raymond CS, Shamu CE, Shen MM, Seifert KJ, Hirsch B, Hodgkin J, Zarkower D (1998) Evidence for evolutionary conservation of sex-determining genes. Nature 391:691–695
Röpke A, Pelz AF, Volleth M, Schösser HW, Morlot S, Wieacker P (2004) Sex chromosomal mosaicism in the gonads of patients with gonadal dysgenesis, but normal female or male karyotypes in lymphocytes. Am J Obstet Gynecol 190:1059–1062
Rutgers JL, Scully RE (1991) The androgen insensitivity syndrome (testicular feminization): a clinicopathological study of 43 cases. Int J Gynecol Pathol 10:126–144
Skakkebaek NE, Rajpert-De Meyts E, Main KM (2001) Testicular dysgenesis syndrome: an increasingly common developmental disorder with environmental aspects. Hum Reprod 16:972–978
Slavotinek A, Schwarz C, Getty JF, Stecko O, Goodman F, Kingston H (1999) Two cases with interstitial deletions of chromosome 2 and sex reversal in one. Am J Med Genet 86: 75–81
Stumm M, Kessel-Weiner E, Pascu F, Ottolenghi C, Theile U, Wieacker P (2000) Deletion of the DM domain gene cluster in a fetus with ring chromosome 9 and sex reversal. Ped Pathol Mol Med 19:415–423
Thipgen AE, Davis DL, Milatovich A, Mendonca BB, Imperato-McGinley, Griffin JE, Francke U, Wilson JD, Russel DW (1992) Molecular genetics of 5α-reductase 2 deficiency. J Clin Invest 90:799–809
Tomboc M, Lee PE, Mitwally MF, Schneck FX, Bellinger M, Witchel SF (2000) Insulin-like 3/relaxin-like factor gene mutations are associated with cryptorchidism. J Clin Endocr Metab 85:4013–4018
Umehara F, Tate G, Itoh K, Yamaguchi N, Douchi T, Mitsuya T, Osame M (2000) A novel mutation of desert hedgehog in a patient with partial gonadal dysgenesis accompanied by minifascicular neuropathy. Am J Hum Genet 67:1302–1305
Wagner T, Wirth J, Meyer J, Zabel B, Held M, Zimmer J, Pasantes J, Bricarelli FD, Keutel J, Hustert E, Wolf U, Tommerup N, Chempp W, Scherer G (1994) Autosomal sex reversal and campomelic dysplasia are caused by mutations in and around the SRY-related gene SOX9. Cell 79:1111–1120
Weil D, Wang I, Dietrich A, Poustka A, Weissenbach J, Petit C (1994) Highly homologous loci on the X and Y chromo-

somes are hot spots for ectopic recombination leading to XX maleness. Nat Genet 7:414–419
Wieacker P, Griffin JE, Wienker T, Lopez JM, Breckwoldt M (1987) Linkage analysis with RFLPs in families with androgen resistance syndromes: evidence for close linkage between the androgen receptor locus and the DXS1 segment. Hum Genet 76:248–252
Wieacker P, Missbach D, Jakubiczka S, Albers N (1995) Sex reversal in a child with the karyotype 46,XY, dup(1) (p22.3 p32.3). Clin Genet 49:271–273
Wieacker P, Knoke I, Jakubiczka S (1998) Clinical and molecular aspects of androgen receptor defects. Exp Clin Endocrinol Diabetes 106:446–452
Wieacker P, Pfäffle R, Zabel G, Jakubiczka S (2003) Agonadismus mit phänotypischer Variabilität bei zwei Geschwistern. Reproduktionsmedizin 19:157–160
Wilkie AO, Campbell FM, Daubeney P, Grant DB, Daniels RJ, Mullarkey M, Affara NA, Fitchett M, Huson SM (1993) Complete and partial XY sex reversal associated with terminal deletion of 10q: report of 2 cases and literature review. Am J Med Genet 46:597–600
Yong EL, Ng SC, Roy AC, Yun G, Ratmann SS (1994) Pregnancy after hormonal correction of severe spermatogenic defects due to a mutation in androgen receptor gene. Lancet 344:826–827

II.2.2 Endocrine Disorders and the Role of Hormone Disrupters

A. Mahmoud, F. Comhaire

Summary

Excluding primary testicular failure and diabetes mellitus, endocrine disorders are uncommon but treatable causes of male infertility and erectile dysfunction. After treating the cause if possible, testosterone therapy induces puberty and normalizes erectile function in patients with hypogonadotrophic hypogonadism (HH). Infertility in patients with HH is treated by gonadotrophins, complemented with assisted reproductive techniques if necessary. The choice between dopamine agonists or surgery for the treatment of prolactinoma depends on tumour characteristics. The few studies available indicate that thyroid dysfunction is associated with impaired sperm quality. Recent evidence suggests that impaired spermatogenesis is associated with "subclinical" Leydig cell dysfunction. In these cases long-term follow-up of serum testosterone is recommended. The progressive increase in the incidence of male genital tract anomalies, male infertility and testicular cancer suggests a deleterious effect of environmental factors. The association of these pathologies is called "testicular dysgenesis syndrome, TDS". Many studies suggest that TDS is caused by synthetic endocrine disrupters, mostly chemicals with (anti)oestrogen-like actions (xeno-oestrogens).

II.2.2.1 Introduction

Male sexual differentiation and development (Chap. II.1.2) as well as male fertility and sexuality are under tight endocrine regulation by the hypothalamo-pituitary-testicular (HPT) axis (Chap. II.1.5). Moreover, cross talk exists between the HPT axis and other endocrine and non-endocrine organs. Any factor disturbing the HPT axis may therefore result in male gonadal dysfunction.

To complicate matters further, many exogenous substances including natural and synthetic hormonally active "endocrine or hormonal disrupters" are proven or suspected to influence male gonadal function (see below).

II.2.2.2 Endocrine Disorders

Excluding primary testicular failure (and diabetes mellitus in patients with erectile dysfunction), the incidence of endocrine abnormalities is low in patients with infertility (0.6% to 1.5%) (WHO 1987; Sigman and Jarow 1997) and erectile dysfunction (Buvat and Lemaire 1997; Earle and Stuckey 2003; Maatman and Montague 1986). Nevertheless, treatment of for example hyperprolactinaemia may result in the restoration of fertility and erectile function.

II.2.2.2.1 Hypogonadotrophic Hypogonadism (HH)

The list of causes of HH is long (Table II.2.1). A detailed description of these conditions (for example Melmed 2002) is beyond the scope of this work. Only a brief summary for the clinical andrologist and recent advances with representative references/reviews are highlighted.

Advances in molecular genetics have clarified the cause of some cases of "idiopathic" HH (Silveira et al. 2002; de Roux et al. 2003; Seminara et al. 2003).

In young patients the most common presentation of gonadotrophin deficiency is delayed puberty. Cryptorchidism, micropenis and/or hypospadias may be pre-

Table II.2.1. Causes of hypogonadotrophic hypogonadism

GnRH deficiency
Congenital and syndromic
Idiopathic
Kallmann syndrome (with anosmia/hyposmia) (Kal 1, Kal 2 gene mutations)
Prader-Willi (abnormal 15q11-q13)
Laurence-Moon
Bardet-Biedl
Septo-optic dysplasia
Adrenal hypoplasia congenita (orphan receptor DAX-1 gene mutation)
Other orphan receptor gene mutations: GPR54 (G protein-coupled receptor)
Isolated LH deficiency (fertile eunuch syndrome)
Acquired GnRH deficiency
Postpubertal idiopathic
Hypothalamic/pituitary stalk lesions:
Tumours
Craniopharyngioma
Germ cell tumours
Hamartoma
Glioma
Metastasis
Vascular, inflammatory: post infectious, irradiation, vasculitis, infarction
Head trauma and haemorrhage
Infiltrative: tuberculosis, sarcoidosis, histocytosis
Gonadotrophic deficiency
Pituitary tumour/mass: adenomas including prolactinoma, aneurysm, meningioma
Hypophysectomy
Primary empty sella
Post-infarction (pituitary apoplexy)
Pituitary infiltration/abscess: tuberculosis, haemochromatosis
Pituitary transcription factors gene mutations (HESX1, LHX3, and PROP-1)
Obesity gene mutations: leptin, leptin receptor, prohormone convertase 1 (PC1)
GnRH receptor mutations
LH, FSH β-subunit gene mutations
Immunoglobulins blocking FSH/receptor interaction? (reported in female)
Functional abnormalities
Constitutional delayed puberty
Extreme obesity, weight loss, starvation, malnutrition
Stress, extreme exercise
Medication (anabolic steroids, glucocorticoids, androgens, GnRH analogues)
Drugs, alcohol
Hyperprolactinaemia
Hypothyroidism
Systemic illnesses (e.g. renal failure, poorly controlled diabetes mellitus, severe burns)

sent from birth due to insufficient testosterone production during foetal life in congenital forms. Sexual dysfunction or infertility may be the presenting symptom of HH in adults.

The diagnosis of HH is established by finding low (or normal) gonadotrophins and low testosterone in blood of patients with infertility or erectile dysfunction. Further laboratory tests may be needed to define possible accompanying pituitary insufficiencies and appropriate imaging techniques (e.g. radiographs for bone age/quality, CT scan or better MRI for tumours and empty sella) and genetic studies will complete the diagnostic work-up. Besides treating the cause if possible, testosterone therapy is used to induce puberty and androgen replacement (see Sect. II.4.6.2, Androgens). The induction of spermatogenesis is achieved at the time when fertility is required with parenteral human menopausal gonadotrophin (hMG) with human chorionic gonadotrophin (hCG) replacing testosterone to avoid suppression of spermatogenesis (Schaison et al. 1993). Pure follicle-stimulating hormone (FSH, more expensive) may be used as an alternative to hMG but the superiority of the former remains to be demonstrated. Treatment with pulsatile gonadotrophin-releasing hormone (GnRH) in cases with GnRH deficiency is not superior to gonadotrophin treatment (Liu et al. 1988). These therapies may be combined with assisted reproductive techniques such as in vitro fertilization with intracytoplasmic sperm injection, which may allow pregnancy to occur with very low numbers of spermatozoa (AACE 2002).

Kallmann syndrome (about 1 in 10,000 live-born infants)

Kallmann syndrome is characterized by the association of hypogonadotrophic hypogonadism and anosmia/hyposmia (especially for aromatic odours). Unrelated sporadic cases occur more frequently than inherited forms (Voorhoeve and Delemarre-van de Waal 2004). Autosomal inheritance, both recessive and dominant (with incomplete penetrance), is more common than the "famous" X-linked variety (Oliveira et al. 2001). The gene underlying the X-linked form of the disease is KAL-1 (chromosome Xp22.3). It encodes a glycoprotein, anosmin-1, which is involved in the embryonic migration of GnRH-synthesizing neurons and the differentiation of the olfactory bulbs (Kottler et al. 2004). A loss-of-function mutation in the fibroblast growth factor receptor 1 gene (KAL-2, chromosome 8p11-p12) has been found to cause the autosomal dominant form (Dode et al. 2003).

Prader–Willi syndrome (1 in 10,000–16,000 live-born infants)

Prader–Willi syndrome is characterized by short stature, muscular hypotonia, excessive appetite with progressive obesity, hypogonadism, mental retardation, behavioural abnormalities, sleep disturbances and dysmorphic features (Holm et al. 1993; Burman et al. 2001).

II.2.2.2.2
Hyperprolactinaemia

Hyperprolactinaemia may be asymptomatic or present with loss of libido/erectile dysfunction accompanied by pressure symptoms if caused by a tumour, for example visual field defects. The diagnosis is based on the detection of repeatedly elevated prolactin in serum. Exclude medication, for example neuroleptics, antidepressants, antihypertensives, and systemic disease (e.g. hypothyroidism) as a cause of hyperprolactinaemia. Identification of macroprolactinaemia (large biologically inactive protein complexes) is clinically important to prevent unnecessary examinations and treatments in patients with idiopathic hyperprolactinaemia (Hattori 2003). MRI is preferred to CT due to its better definition of very small lesions in the pituitary sella and better anatomical definition prior to surgery (Di Sarno et al. 2003). The choice between treatment with dopamine agonists (e.g. bromocriptine, cabergoline) and surgery depends on the size of the tumour, its progression, its response to medical treatment, and the presence or absence of pressure on neighbouring structures (Webster 1999; Colao et al. 2004; Liu and Couldwell 2004).

II.2.2.2.3
Thyroid Disorders

Both hyper- and hypothyroidism may have an adverse effect on male gonadal function but relatively few studies are available on their effects on male reproduction (reviews: Krassas and Pontikides 2004; Meikle 2004).

In patients with hyperthyroidism, levels of total testosterone, oestradiol, sex hormone-binding globulin (SHBG), luteinizing hormone (LH) and FSH, and gonadotrophin responses to GnRH were found to be significantly greater than these levels and responses in age-matched controls, while free testosterone levels were lower (Hudson and Edwards 1992). Therefore, the free testosterone/free oestradiol ratio in hyperthyroid men is lower than normal (Hudson and Edwards 1992). Sperm parameters are frequently impaired (Hudson and Edwards 1992; Abalovich et al. 1999). These abnormalities may revert following the correction of hyperthyroidism (Hudson and Edwards 1992; Abalovich et al. 1999).

Hypothyroidism has been reported to be associated with both hypergonadotrophic (Jaya et al. 1990) and hypogonadotrophic hypogonadism (Meikle 2004). Sperm parameters, especially sperm motility, may be impaired (Corrales Hernandez et al. 1990). Thyroid hormone replacement therapy corrects the hormonal abnormalities and improves sperm parameters (Jaya et al. 1990).

Gonadal damage may follow radioactive iodine (^{131}I) treatment for thyroid cancer. Therefore, Hyer et al. (2002) advise that sperm banking should be considered in men likely to receive cumulative doses greater than 17 GBq. This assumes that patients begin with normal testicular function, therefore the threshold for sperm banking might be even lower, especially if further ^{131}I therapy is likely (Mazzaferri 2002).

II.2.2.2.4
Impaired Spermatogenesis and "Subclinical" Leydig Cell Dysfunction

A large and well-designed study by Andersson et al. (2004) indicated that spermatogenic dysfunction is often associated with impaired Leydig cell function. They showed that between 12% and 15% of men with diminished spermatogenesis had lower testosterone levels or higher LH concentrations than 97.5% of a population of fertile men. This provides substantive support for a concept developed from several smaller studies conducted over the past 30 years (Andersson et al. 2004; review: de Kretser 2004). For example, a low LH/testosterone ratio that decreased with increasing FSH levels has been reported in idiopathic infertility (Giagulli and Vermeulen 1988). These findings suggest compensated Leydig cell insufficiency in subfertile men (Giagulli and Vermeulen 1988). It is currently unknown whether disordered androgen production is a manifestation of testicular dysgenesis syndrome (see Sect. II.2.2.3) or results from disruption of local control mechanisms between the seminiferous tubules and Leydig cells (deKretser 2004). de Kretser (2004) recommends that serum testosterone levels of patients with elevated LH but with low to normal testosterone are followed up in order to commence appropriate androgen replacement if they become frankly hypogonadal.

Andersson et al. (2004) also found that serum oestradiol, and the oestradiol/testosterone ratio were elevated in infertile men compared to fertile controls. In patients with both serum inhibin B and FSH in the normal range, it was found that oligozoospermia was associated with higher serum oestradiol levels compared with normozoospermia (Mahmoud et al. 1998). An open study indicated that treatment with an aromatase inhibitor significantly improved both the hormonal imbalance in the oestradiol/testosterone ratio and the impaired sperm parameters in these patients (Raman and Schlegel 2002). These findings may also explain the improvement in sperm parameters following treatment of subfertile men with tamoxifen (see Sect. II.4.6.5.2).

II.2.2.3
The Role of Hormone Disrupters

A temporal decline of male fertility in humans and wildlife has been documented in many studies. These changes in male fertility are paralleled by an increased incidence of "endocrine-dependent" pathologies in the male including hypospadias, cryptorchidism and testicular cancer, collectively termed "testicular dysgenesis syndrome" (Skakkebaek et al. 2001, 2003). A recent study suggests that Leydig cell dysfunction may also be a component of this syndrome (Andersson et al. 2004). The incidence of other "endocrine-dependent" diseases is also on the rise, for example prostate cancer in the male and breast cancer in the female.

The "oestrogen hypothesis" has been put forward as a possible explanation for these trends. The hypothesis is that increased exposure to natural or synthetic chemicals, mainly a group of manufactured substances with oestrogen-like action (xeno-oestrogens), is responsible for the increase in these pathologies. In vitro studies suggest that some heavy metals also have an oestrogen-like action (Choe et al. 2003; Johnson et al. 2003).

Acting on the oestrogen receptor is not the only mechanism by which endocrine disrupters exert their effect. Some endocrine disrupters are (anti)androgenic such as phthalates (Fisher 2004) and/or pro-oxidants. Also, some polyaromatic hydrocarbons may inhibit their own degradation and also increase the bioavailability of intrinsic oestrogens in target tissues through the inhibition of the enzymes involved in oestrogen inactivation (Kester et al. 2002).

Inappropriate overproduction of inhibin B by Sertoli cells on exposure to environmental insults may also suppress spermatogenesis both locally (Bame et al. 1999) and via the inhibition of FSH production by the pituitary gland (Voglmayr et al. 1990; Martin et al. 1991; Lovell et al. 2000). These include oxidative stress (Comhaire and Mahmoud 2003; Richthoff et al. 2003), lead (Mahmoud et al. 2005) and some (xeno-) oestrogens (Depuydt et al. 1999; Monsees et al. 2000).

It has been shown that human spermatozoa express aryl hydrocarbon (dioxin) receptors, providing a mechanism by which environmental dioxins, polycyclic aromatic hydrocarbons and polyhalogenated biphenyls could directly influence sperm function (Khorram et al. 2004). For further details on the mechanisms of action and methods for the detection of endocrine disrupters see the review by Eertmans et al. (2003).

A large body of animal and in vitro experiments supports the endocrine disruption hypothesis. Fewer data are available from human studies. These are summarized below.

II.2

II.2.2.3.1 Cryptorchidism and Hypospadias

An increased risk of hypospadias has been reported in the sons of women exposed to diethylstilboestrol (DES) in utero [prevalence ratio 21.3 (95% confidence interval (CI) 6.5 – 70.1)] (Klip et al. 2002). A similar tendency has been reported by Roelofs et al. (2004) [odds ratio (OR) 2.6, 95% CI 0.8 – 9.1]. Both studies indicate that hypospadias is strongly associated with low birth weight, twin or triplet pregnancy, preterm delivery and use of assisted reproductive techniques.

The risk of hypospadias was found to be doubled when the mother had been exposed to chemical hazards (pesticides) during gestation (Morera et al. 2004).

A significantly increased risk of cryptorchidism but not hypospadias was found in sons of Danish women working in gardening (adjusted OR 1.67; 95% CI 1.14 – 2.47). The risks were not increased in sons of men working in farming or gardening (Weidner et al. 1998).

Paternal exposure to pesticides occupationally has also been reported to increase the risk of cryptorchidism (OR 12.79, 95% CI 2.90 – 56.43) (Wang and Wang 2002).

Significantly higher levels of heptachloroepoxide (HCE) and hexachlorobenzene (HCB) have been detected in fatty tissue of children with cryptorchidism compared to children undergoing other surgical procedures (Hosie et al. 2000).

The results of a nested case–control study on dichlorodiphenyltrichloroethane (DDT) in relation to hypospadias/cryptorchidism were inconclusive (Longnekker et al. 2002). Boys with maternal serum levels of dichlorodiphenyldichloroethylene (DDE) greater than or equal to 85.6 μg/l had adjusted OR values of 1.3 (95% CI 0.7, 2.4) for cryptorchidism, 1.2 (95% CI 0.6, 2.4) for hypospadias and 1.9 (95% CI 0.9, 4.0) for polythelia. For cryptorchidism and polythelia, the results were consistent with a modest-to-moderate association (Longnecker et al. 2002).

In a study involving 7928 boys born to mothers taking part in the Avon Longitudinal Study of Pregnancy and Childhood, mothers who were vegetarian in pregnancy had an adjusted OR of 4.99 (95% CI 2.10 – 11.88) of giving birth to a boy with hypospadias, compared with omnivores (North and Golding 2000). Since vegetarians have a greater exposure to phytoestrogens than do omnivores, these results support the possibility that phytoestrogens (possibly also xeno-oestrogens or some unrecognized nutritional deficiency) have a deleterious effect on the developing male reproductive system.

II.2.2.3.2 Puberty

In most European countries the age of onset of puberty and of menarche has been decreasing during the past few decades (Muinich Keizer and Mul 2001). This has been attributed to environmental factors, possibly xeno-oestrogens. Also, precocious puberty has been more frequently observed in immigrant or adopted foreign children living in Western Europe than in indigenous children (Parent et al. 2003). This diagnosis is still often unrecognized. It is important not to delay diagnosis and treatment so as not to compromise the final height of the patient (De Monleon 2001). Higher levels of *p,p'*-DDE have been reported in these children in Belgium (Krstevska-Konstantinova et al. 2001). It has been hypothesized that withdrawal of xeno-oestrogens, due to lower levels of exposure in Western Europe compared to land of origin, may be the cause of precocious puberty in immigrant or adopted foreign children (Krstevska-Konstantinova et al. 2001).

Although another Belgian study indicated that exposure to polychlorinated aromatic hydrocarbons (PCAH) is associated with delayed sexual maturation (Staessen et al. 2001; Den Hond et al. 2002), the methodology and conclusions of this study have been criticized (Dhooge et al. 2001; Molenberghs et al. 2003). The pubertal development of adolescents living in a suburb near two waste incinerators was compared with another control. Significantly fewer boys from the polluted area had reached the adult stages of genital development and pubic hair growth. In individual boys, a doubling of the serum concentration of certain polychlorinated biphenyl (PCB) congeners (cogners138 and 153) increased the odds of not having matured into the adult stage of genital development and male pubic hair growth by 3.5 ($p = 0.04$). Left plus right testicular volume was lower in both polluted areas than in the control area (42.4 ml vs 47.3 ml, $p = 0.005$) but was not related to the current exposure of the adolescents to PCAHs.

II.2.2.3.3 Male Infertility

There have been concerns about a low and decreasing birth rate in many industrialized countries, where up to 5–6% of children today are born after assisted reproduction (Jensen et al. 2002). Whether this decline is due to social changes or environmental factors requires further investigation, although similar trends have been observed in wildlife.

Based on a meta-analysis of publications mainly from Europe and North America, Carlsen et al. (1992) indicated that sperm concentration overall had declined by half over a 50-year period.

Carlsen's analysis has been a matter of considerable debate. In a re-analysis of this study, Swan et al. (1997) found that the decline could have been even stronger among European men. Another interpretation of Carlsen's data indicates that sperm concentration was actually increasing and started to decline only after 1980 (Becker and Berhane 1998). In accordance with the latter interpretation, necropsy data from over 20,000 Japanese men from 1948 to 1998 indicated that testicular weight showed a general increase until it started to decline in boys born after 1960. The same authors found that the age-related decline in testicular weight has greatly accelerated over that period, and that the onset of increasing testis weight of boys has occurred at a progressively younger age (Fig. II.2.3, Mori et al. 2002). This is in accordance with the observed decreased age at puberty reported in many studies.

Many studies indicate declining sperm quality in recent years in different countries in Europe and that the deterioration in sperm quality is not geographically uniform (Auger et al. 1995; Irvine et al. 1996; Paulsen et al. 1996; Van Waeleghem et al. 1996). Compared to young men from a large city in Belgium, lower sperm

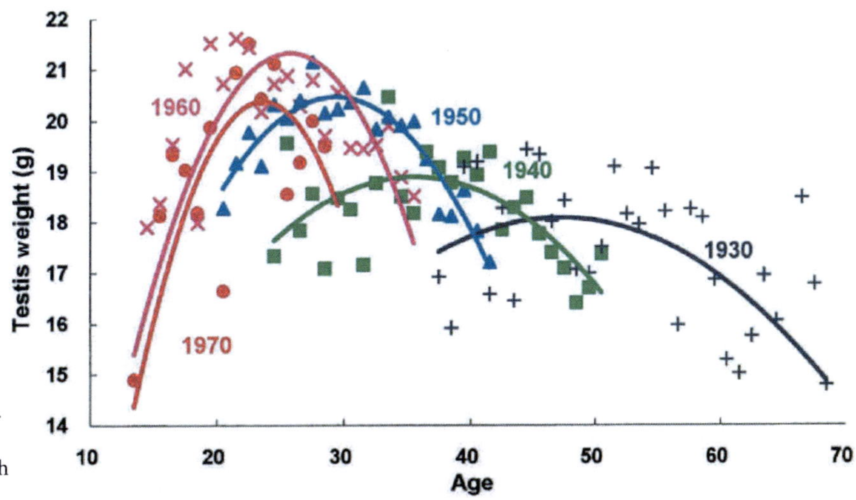

Fig. II.2.3. Evolution of testicular weight in Japanese men (reproduced from Mori et al. 2002 with permission from Blackwell)

concentration and serum testosterone levels were found in young men from an agricultural area, accompanied by higher levels of DDT in women from the same area (Dhooge et al. unpublished).

Men poisoned by PCBs and polychlorinated dibenzofurans in Taiwan (the Yucheng exposure) had increased abnormal morphology, a higher incidence of oligozoospermia, and their sperm had reduced capacity to penetrate hamster oocytes compared to controls (Hsu et al. 2003).

Data from subfertile men indicated an inverse dose–response relationship between PCB-138 and sperm concentration, motility and morphology. There was also limited evidence of an inverse relationship between both total PCBs and group 3 PCBs (cytochrome P450 enzyme inducers) and sperm motility and morphology, as well as limited evidence of an inverse association between *p,p'*-DDE and sperm motility (Hauser et al. 2003).

A population-based study from an agricultural area (Missouri, USA) identified several currently used herbicides including alachlor (30.0, 95 % CI 4.3–210), atrazine (OR 11.3, 95% CI 1.3–98.9) and the insecticide diazinon (OR 16.7, 95% CI 2.8–98.0) as associated with decreased semen quality (Swan et al. 2003).

PCBs were detected in the seminal plasma of a group of Indian infertile men but not in the controls, and the concentration of phthalate esters was significantly higher in the infertile men (Rozati et al. 2002). The same study indicated that the total motile sperm counts in infertile men were inversely proportional to their xeno-oestrogen concentrations in seminal plasma and were significantly lower than those in the respective controls (Rozati et al. 2002). Negative dose–response relations have been reported in subfertile men for monobutyl phthalate and monobenzyl phthalate in urine with one or more semen parameters (Duty et al. 2003a). Urinary monoethyl phthalate at environmental levels was found to be associated with increased DNA damage in spermatozoa (Duty et al. 2003b).

Other substances reported to be related to reduced sperm quality or fecundability include chlordecone (kepone), methamidophos, captan, 2,4-D, dibromochloropropane, ethylene dibromide, glyphosate (Cocco 2002).

Occupational exposure to ethylparathion and methamidophos seems to have a moderately adverse effect on sperm concentration and motility (Padungtod et al. 2000).

Data from the Netherlands indicate that paternal exposure to pesticides is associated with decreased fertilization and implantation rates during treatment by in vitro fertilization for infertility (Tielemans et al. 1999, 2000).

Time to pregnancy was not prolonged among couples with paternal exposure to di(2-ethylhexyl)phthalate at a mean exposure level of <0.5 mg/m^3 (Modigh et al. 2002).

II.2.2.3.4 Sex Ratio

Some data indicate a declining male proportion at birth in Europe (Martuzzi et al. 2001). Decreased male to female ratio at birth has been reported following high levels of exposure to hexachlorobenzene (Jarrell et al. 2002). Exposure of men to 2,3,7,8-tetrachlorodibenzo-para-dioxin (TCDD) in the Seveso incident in Italy (Pesatori et al. 2003) and occupational exposures (Ryan et al. 2002) was linked to a lowered male to female sex ratio in their offspring. No significant association was found between environmental pollution and the proportion of male births in Italy during the period 1989–1993 (Figa-Talamanca et al. 2003). An analysis of sex ratio over 250 years in Finland does not support the hypothesis that agricultural or industrial environmental oestrogens play any significant role in the changes in sex ratio (Vartiainen et al. 1999).

II.2.2.3.5 Prostate Cancer

Animal studies indicate that peri-natal exposure to oestrogenic compounds can result in alterations in the size of the adult prostate and increase the incidence of prostatitis (Stoker et al. 1999). Chronic inflammation of the prostate is considered a predisposing factor for prostate cancer (De Marzo et al. 2003).

A meta-analysis indicated that occupational exposure to pesticides is associated with an increased risk of prostate cancer among farmers (Keller-Byrne et al. 1997). Most of the more recent studies confirm this association.

Although the pesticide applicators from Florida were consistently and significantly healthier than the general population, prostate cancer mortality [standardized mortality ratio (SMR) 2.38, 95% CI 1.83–3.04] was significantly increased (Fleming et al. 1999).

Increased risks were found among farmers exposed to organochlorine insecticides and acaricides (OR 2.5, 95% CI 0.4–4.2), more specifically DDT (OR 2.1, 95% CI 1.2–3.8), and dicofol (OR 2.8, 95% CI 1.5–5.0), whose effects could not be well separated (Settimi et al. 2003). A pilot study indicated that oxychlordane and PCB 180 were associated with an increased risk of prostate cancer (Ritchie et al. 2003).

Prostate and testicular cancer mortality were found not to be related to estimated environmental exposure to *p,p'*-DDE in the USA (Cocco and Benichou 1998).

Moderate to high correlations were observed between pesticide sales in Brazil and prostate cancer mortality (Koifman et al. 2002).

Used amounts of atrazine and captan in central California correlated positively with the incidence of prostate cancer in black but not in white males (Mills 1998).

TCCD contamination after the Seveso accident in Italy had no effect on prostate cancer mortality (Bertazzi et al. 2001).

Hispanic farm workers with relatively high levels of exposure to organochlorine pesticides (lindane and heptachlor), organophosphate pesticides (dichlorvos), fumigants (methyl bromide), or triazine herbicides (simazine) experienced an elevated risk of prostate cancer compared to workers with lower levels of exposure (Mills and Yang 2003).

One study reported a lower than expected incidence of prostate cancer among men environmentally exposed to PCBs (Standardized Incidence Ratio=0.83; 95% CI 0.69 – 0.97) (Pavuk et al. 2004).

II.2.2.3.6 Testis Cancer

High levels of *cis*-nonachlordane have been reported in patients with testicular cancer (Hardell et al. 2003). Mothers of the same patients showed significantly increased concentrations of the sum of PCBs, hexachlorobenzene (HCB), *trans*- and *cis*-nonachlordane, and the sum of chlordanes. Among case mothers the sum of PCBs yielded an OR of 3.8 (95% CI 1.4 – 10). Odds ratios were also increased for HCB (OR 4.4, 95% CI 1.7 – 12), for *trans*-nonachlordane (OR 4.1, 95% CI 1.5 – 11) and for *cis*-nonachlordane (OR 3.1, 95% CI 1.2 – 7.8) (Hardell et al. 2003).

Moderate to high correlations were observed between pesticide sales in Brazil and infertility, as well as testis and ovarian cancer mortality (Koifman et al. 2002).

II.2.2.3.7 Serum Testosterone and Erectile Dysfunction

Exposure to environmental agents has been reported as a risk factor for erectile dysfunction in Argentine men (OR 7.1, 95% CI 1.5 – 33.0 for pesticides; OR 12.2, 95% CI 1.2 – 124.8 for solvents) (Oliva et al. 2002).

A study from Belgium indicates that andropause, otherwise termed the partial androgen deficiency of aging male (PADAM), might in part be due to excessive organochlorine pesticide accumulation (Legros et al. 2003). Males with *p,p*ĎDE >5µg/l had lower free calculated testosterone (43.3±14.1 µg/l) than males with *p,p*ĎDE <5 µg/l (59.6±23.2) (Legros et al. 2003).

References

AACE (2002) American Association of Clinical Endocrinologists Medical Guidelines for clinical practice for the evaluation and treatment of hypogonadism in adult male patients – 2002 update. Endocr Pract 8:440 – 456

Abalovich M, Levalle O, Hermes R, Scaglia H, Aranda C, Zylbersztein C, Oneto A, Aquilano D, Gutierrez S (1999) Hypothalamic-pituitary-testicular axis and seminal parameters in hyperthyroid males. Thyroid 9:857 – 863

Andersson AM, Jorgensen N, Frydelund-Larsen L, Rajpert-De Meyts E, Skakkebaek NE (2004) Impaired Leydig cell function in infertile men: a study of 357 idiopathic infertile men and 318 proven fertile controls. J Clin Endocrinol Metab 89:3161 – 3167

Auger J, Kunstmann JM, Czyglik F, Jouannet P (1995) Decline in semen quality among fertile men in Paris during the past 20 years. N Engl J Med 332:281 – 285

Bame JH, Dalton JC, Degelos SD, Good TE, Ireland JL, Jimenez-Krassel F, Sweeney T, Saacke RG, Ireland JJ (1999) Effect of long-term immunization against inhibin on sperm output in bulls. Biol Reprod 60:1360 – 1366

Becker S, Berhane K (1998) Have sperm densities declined? A reanalysis of global trend data. Environ Health Perspect 106:A420–A421

Bertazzi PA, Consonni D, Bachetti S, Rubagotti M, Baccarelli A, Zocchetti C, Pesatori AC (2001) Health effects of dioxin exposure: a 20-year mortality study. Am J Epidemiol 153: 1031 – 1044

Burman P, Ritzen EM, Lindgren AC (2001) Endocrine dysfunction in Prader-Willi syndrome: a review with special reference to GH. Endocr Rev 22:787 – 799

Buvat J, Lemaire A (1997) Endocrine screening in 1,022 men with erectile dysfunction: clinical significance and cost-effective strategy. J Urol 158:1764 – 1767

Carlsen E, Giwercman A, Keiding N, Skakkebaek NE (1992) Evidence for decreasing quality of semen during past 50 years. Br Med J 305:609 – 613

Choe SY, Kim SJ, Kim HG, Lee JH, Choi Y, Lee H, Kim Y (2003) Evaluation of estrogenicity of major heavy metals. Sci Total Environ 312:15 – 21

Cocco P (2002) On the rumors about the silent spring. Review of the scientific evidence linking occupational and environmental pesticide exposure to endocrine disruption health effects. Cad Saude Publica 18:379 – 402

Cocco P, Benichou J (1998) Mortality from cancer of the male reproductive tract and environmental exposure to the anti-androgen p,p'-dichlorodiphenyldichloroethylene in the United States. Oncology 55:334 – 339

Colao A, Vitale G, Cappabianca P, Briganti F, Ciccarelli A, De Rosa M, Zarrilli S, Lombardi G (2004) Outcome of cabergoline treatment in men with prolactinoma: effects of a 24-month treatment on prolactin levels, tumor mass, recovery of pituitary function, and semen analysis. J Clin Endocrinol Metab 89:1704 – 1711

Comhaire FH, Mahmoud A (2003) The role of food supplements in the treatment of the infertile man. Reprod Biomed Online 7:385 – 391

Corrales Hernandez JJ, Miralles Garcia JM, Garcia Diez LC (1990) Primary hypothyroidism and human spermatogenesis. Arch Androl 25:21 – 27

de Kretser DM (2004) Is spermatogenic damage associated with Leydig cell dysfunction? J Clin Endocrinol Metab 89: 3158 – 3160

De Marzo AM, Meeker AK, Zha S, Luo J, Nakayama M, Platz EA, Isaacs WB, Nelson WG (2003) Human prostate cancer precursors and pathobiology. Urology 62:55 – 62

De Monleon JV (2001) [Foreign adopted children growth follow-up]. Ann Endocrinol (Paris) 62:458 – 460

de Roux N, Genin E, Carel JC, Matsuda F, Chaussain JL, Milgrom E (2003) Hypogonadotropic hypogonadism due to loss of function of the KiSS1-derived peptide receptor GPR54. Proc Natl Acad Sci USA 100:10972 – 10976

Den Hond E, Roels HA, Hoppenbrouwers K, Nawrot T, Thijs

L, Vandermeulen C, Winneke G, Vanderschueren D, Staessen JA (2002) Sexual maturation in relation to polychlorinated aromatic hydrocarbons: Sharpe and Skakkebaek's hypothesis revisited. Environ Health Perspect 110:771–776
Depuydt CE, Mahmoud AM, Dhooge WS, Schoonjans FA, Comhaire FH (1999) Hormonal regulation of inhibin B secretion by immature rat sertoli cells in vitro: possible use as a bioassay for estrogen detection. J Androl 20:54–62
Dhooge W, Kaufman JM, Comhaire F (2001) Delayed sexual development in adolescents [letter]. Lancet 358:1816–1817
Di Sarno A, Rota F, Auriemma R, De Martino MC, Lombardi G, Colao A (2003) An evaluation of patients with hyperprolactinemia: have dynamic tests had their day? J Endocrinol Invest 26:39–47
Dode C, Levilliers J, Dupont JM, De Paepe A, Le Du N, Soussi-Yanicostas N, Coimbra RS, Delmaghani S, Compain-Nouaille S, Baverel F, Pecheux C, Le Tessier D, Cruaud C, Delpech M, Speleman F, Vermeulen S, Amalfitano A, Bachelot Y, Bouchard P, Cabrol S, Carel JC, Delemarre-van de Waal H, Goulet-Salmon B, Kottler ML, Richard O, Sanchez-Franco F, Saura R, Young J, Petit C, Hardelin JP (2003) Loss-of-function mutations in FGFR1 cause autosomal dominant Kallmann syndrome. Nat Genet 33:463–465
Duty SM, Silva MJ, Barr DB, Brock JW, Ryan L, Chen Z, Herrick RF, Christiani DC, Hauser R (2003a) Phthalate exposure and human semen parameters. Epidemiology 14:269–277
Duty SM, Singh NP, Silva MJ, Barr DB, Brock JW, Ryan L, Herrick RF, Christiani DC, Hauser R (2003b) The relationship between environmental exposures to phthalates and DNA damage in human sperm using the neutral comet assay. Environ Health Perspect 111:1164–1169
Earle CM, Stuckey BG (2003) Biochemical screening in the assessment of erectile dysfunction: what tests decide future therapy? Urology 62:727–731
Eertmans F, Dhooge W, Stuyvaert S, Comhaire F (2003) Endocrine disruptors: effects on male fertility and screening tools for their assessment. Toxicol In Vitro 17:515–524
Figa-Talamanca I, Carbone P, Lauria L, Spinelli A, Ulizzi L (2003) Environmental factors and the proportion of males at birth in Italy. Arch Environ Health 58:119–124
Fisher JS (2004) Environmental anti-androgens and male reproductive health: focus on phthalates and testicular dysgenesis syndrome. Reproduction 127:305–315
Fleming LE, Bean JA, Rudolph M, Hamilton K (1999) Mortality in a cohort of licensed pesticide applicators in Florida. Occup Environ Med 56:14–21
Giagulli VA, Vermeulen A (1988) Leydig cell function in infertile men with idiopathic oligospermic infertility. J Clin Endocrinol Metab 66:62–67
Hardell L, van Bavel B, Lindstrom G, Carlberg M, Dreifaldt AC, Wijkstrom H, Starkhammar H, Eriksson M, Hallquist A, Kolmert T (2003) Increased concentrations of polychlorinated biphenyls, hexachlorobenzene, and chlordanes in mothers of men with testicular cancer. Environ Health Perspect 111:930–934
Hattori N (2003) Macroprolactinemia: a new cause of hyperprolactinemia. J Pharmacol Sci 92:171–177
Hauser R, Chen Z, Pothier L, Ryan L, Altshul L (2003) The relationship between human semen parameters and environmental exposure to polychlorinated biphenyls and p,p'-DDE. Environ Health Perspect 111:1505–1511
Holm VA, Cassidy SB, Butler MG, Hanchett JM, Greenswag LR, Whitman BY, Greenberg F (1993) Prader-Willi syndrome: consensus diagnostic criteria. Pediatrics 91:398–402
Hosie S, Loff S, Witt K, Niessen K, Waag KL (2000) Is there a correlation between organochlorine compounds and undescended testes? Eur J Pediatr Surg 10:304–309
Hsu PC, Huang W, Yao W J Wu MH, Guo YL, Lambert GH (2003) Sperm changes in men exposed to polychlorinated biphenyls and dibenzofurans. J Am Med Assoc 289:2943–2944
Hudson RW, Edwards AL (1992) Testicular function in hyperthyroidism. J Androl 13:117–124
Hyer S, Vini L, O'Connell M, Pratt B, Harmer C (2002) Testicular dose and fertility in men following I(131) therapy for thyroid cancer. Clin Endocrinol (Oxf) 56:755–758
Irvine S, Cawood E, Richardson D, MacDonald E, Aitken J (1996) Evidence of deteriorating semen quality in the United Kingdom: birth cohort study in 577 men in Scotland over 11 years. Br Med J 312:467–471
Jarrell JF, Gocmen A, Akyol D, Brant R (2002) Hexachlorobenzene exposure and the proportion of male births in Turkey 1935–1990. Reprod Toxicol 16:65–70
Jaya KB, Khurana ML, Ammini AC, Karmarkar MG, Ahuja MM (1990) Reproductive endocrine functions in men with primary hypothyroidism: effect of thyroxine replacement. Horm Res 34:215–218
Jensen TK, Carlsen E, Jorgensen N, Berthelsen JG, Keiding N, Christensen K, Petersen JH, Knudsen LB, Skakkebaek NE (2002) Poor semen quality may contribute to recent decline in fertility rates. Hum Reprod 17:1437–1440
Johnson MD, Kenney N, Stoica A, Hilakivi-Clarke L, Singh B, Chepko G, Clarke R, Sholler PF, Lirio AA, Foss C, Reiter R, Trock B, Paik S, Martin MB (2003) Cadmium mimics the in vivo effects of estrogen in the uterus and mammary gland. Nat Med 9:1081–1084
Keller-Byrne JE, Khuder SA, Schaub EA (1997) Meta-analyses of prostate cancer and farming. Am J Ind Med 31:580–586
Kester MH, Bulduk S, van Toor H, Tibboel D, Meinl W, Glatt H, Falany CN, Coughtrie MW, Schuur AG, Brouwer A, Visser TJ (2002) Potent inhibition of estrogen sulfotransferase by hydroxylated metabolites of polyhalogenated aromatic hydrocarbons reveals alternative mechanism for estrogenic activity of endocrine disrupters. J Clin Endocrinol Metab 87: 1142–1150
Khorram O, Garthwaite M, Jones J, Golos T (2004) Expression of aryl hydrocarbon receptor (AHR) and aryl hydrocarbon receptor nuclear translocator (ARNT) mRNA expression in human spermatozoa. Med Sci Monit 10:BR135-BR138
Klip H, Verloop J, van Gool JD, Koster ME, Burger CW, van Leeuwen FE (2002) Hypospadias in sons of women exposed to diethylstilbestrol in utero: a cohort study. Lancet 359: 1102–1107
Koifman S, Koifman RJ, Meyer A (2002) Human reproductive system disturbances and pesticide exposure in Brazil. Cad Saude Publica 18:435–445
Kottler ML, Hamel A, Malville E, Richard N (2004) [GnRH deficiency: new insights from genetics]. J Soc Biol 198:80–87
Krassas GE, Pontikides N (2004) Male reproductive function in relation with thyroid alterations. Best Pract Res Clin Endocrinol Metab 18:183–195
Krstevska-Konstantinova M, Charlier C, Craen M, Du CM, Heinrichs C, de Beaufort C, Plomteux G, Bourguignon JP (2001) Sexual precocity after immigration from developing countries to Belgium: evidence of previous exposure to organochlorine pesticides. Hum Reprod 16:1020–1026
Legros JJ, Charlier C, Bouillon G, Plomteux G (2003) Partial androgen deficiency of aging male (P.A.D.A.M.) might in part be due to excessive organochlonide pesticide (OC) impregnation. Ann Endocrinol (Paris) 64:136
Liu JK, Couldwell WT (2004) Contemporary management of prolactinomas. Neurosurg Focus 16:E2
Liu L, Banks SM, Barnes KM, Sherins RJ (1988) Two-year comparison of testicular responses to pulsatile gonadotropin-releasing hormone and exogenous gonadotropins from the in-

ception of therapy in men with isolated hypogonadotropic hypogonadism. J Clin Endocrinol Metab 67:1140–1145
Longnecker MP, Klebanoff MA, Brock JW, Zhou H, Gray KA, Needham LL, Wilcox AJ (2002) Maternal serum level of 1,1-dichloro-2,2-bis(p-chlorophenyl)ethylene and risk of cryptorchidism, hypospadias, and polythelia among male offspring. Am J Epidemiol 155:313–322
Lovell TM, Knight PG, Groome NP, Gladwell RT (2000) Measurement of dimeric inhibins and effects of active immunization against inhibin alpha-subunit on plasma hormones and testis morphology in the developing cockerel. Biol Reprod 63:213–221
Maatman TJ, Montague DK (1986) Routine endocrine screening in impotence. Urology 27:499–502
Mahmoud AM, Comhaire FH, Depuydt CE (1998) The clinical and biologic significance of serum inhibins in subfertile men. Reprod Toxicol 12:591–599
Mahmoud A, Kiss P, Vanhoorne M, De Bacquer D, Comhaire F (2005) Is inhibin B involved in the toxic effect of lead on male reproduction? Int J Androl 28:150–155
Martin TL, Williams GL, Lunstra DD, Ireland JJ (1991) Immunoneutralization of inhibin modifies hormone secretion and sperm production in bulls. Biol Reprod 45:73–77
Martuzzi M, Di Tanno ND, Bertollini R (2001) Declining trends of male proportion at birth in Europe. Arch Environ Health 56:358–364
Mazzaferri EL (2002) Gonadal damage from 131I therapy for thyroid cancer. Clin Endocrinol (Oxf) 57:313–314
Meikle AW (2004) The interrelationships between thyroid dysfunction and hypogonadism in men and boys. Thyroid 14 Suppl 1:S17–S25
Melmed S (ed) (2002) The pituitary. Blackwell, Oxford
Mills PK (1998) Correlation analysis of pesticide use data and cancer incidence rates in California counties. Arch Environ Health 53:410–413
Mills PK, Yang R (2003) Prostate cancer risk in California farm workers. J Occup Environ Med 45:249–258
Modigh CM, Bodin SL, Lillienberg L, Dahlman-Hoglund A, Akesson B, Axelsson G (2002) Time to pregnancy among partners of men exposed to di(2-ethylhexyl)phthalate. Scand J Work Environ Health 28:418–428
Molenberghs G, Cuypers C, Goetghebeur EJ, Passchier WF, Pieters J (2003) Comment on sexual maturation in relation to polychlorinated aromatic hydrocarbons: Sharpe and Skakkebaek's hypothesis revisited. Environ Health Perspect 111:A202, author-3
Monsees TK, Franz M, Gebhardt S, Winterstein U, Schill WB, Hayatpour J (2000) Sertoli cells as a target for reproductive hazards. Andrologia 32:239–246
Morera AM, Asensio MJ, Chossegros L, Chauvin MA, Valmalle AF, Mouriquand P (2004) A survey of risk factors in hypospadiacs compared with controls. BJU Int 93:55–55
Mori C, Hamamatsu A, Fukata H, Koh KB, Nakamura N, Takeichi S, Kusakabe T, Saito T, Morita M, Tanihara S, Kayama F, Shiyomi M, Yoshimura J, Sagisaka K (2002) Temporal changes in testis weight during the past 50 years in Japan. Anat Sci Int 77:109–116
Muinich Keizer SM, Mul D (2001) Trends in pubertal development in Europe. Hum Reprod Update 7:287–291
North K, Golding J (2000) A maternal vegetarian diet in pregnancy is associated with hypospadias. The ALSPAC Study Team. Avon Longitudinal Study of Pregnancy and Childhood. BJU Int 85:107–113
Oliva A, Giami A, Multigner L (2002) Environmental agents and erectile dysfunction: a study in a consulting population. J Androl 23:546–550
Oliveira LM, Seminara SB, Beranova M, Hayes FJ, Valkenburgh SB, Schipani E, Costa EM, Latronico AC, Crowley WF Jr., Vallejo M (2001) The importance of autosomal genes in Kallmann syndrome: genotype-phenotype correlations and neuroendocrine characteristics. J Clin Endocrinol Metab 86:1532–1538
Padungtod C, Savitz DA, Overstreet JW, Christiani DC, Ryan LM, Xu X (2000) Occupational pesticide exposure and semen quality among Chinese workers. J Occup Environ Med 42:982–992
Parent AS, Teilmann G, Juul A, Skakkebaek NE, Toppari J, Bourguignon JP (2003) The timing of normal puberty and the age limits of sexual precocity: variations around the world, secular trends, and changes after migration. Endocr Rev 24:668–693
Paulsen CA, Berman NG, Wang C (1996) Data from men in greater Seattle area reveals no downward trend in semen quality: further evidence that deterioration of semen quality is not geographically uniform. Fertil Steril 65:1015–1020
Pavuk M, Cerhan JR, Lynch CF, Schecter A, Petrik J, Chovancova J, Kocan A (2004) Environmental exposure to PCBs and cancer incidence in eastern Slovakia. Chemosphere 54:1509–1520
Pesatori AC, Consonni D, Bachetti S, Zocchetti C, Bonzini M, Baccarelli A, Bertazzi PA (2003) Short- and long-term morbidity and mortality in the population exposed to dioxin after the Seveso accident. Ind Health 41:127–138
Raman JD, Schlegel PN (2002) Aromatase inhibitors for male infertility. J Urol 167:624–629
Richthoff J, Rylander L, Hagmar L, Giwercman A (2003) Effect of cigarette smoking on reproductive characteristics in an unselected population of young males. Reprod Biomed Online 7 [Suppl 1]: 8–9
Ritchie JM, Vial SL, Fuortes LJ, Guo H, Reedy VE, Smith EM (2003) Organochlorines and risk of prostate cancer. J Occup Environ Med 45:692–702
Roelofs L, Brouwers M, Gier RDE, Feitz W, Kiemeney B, Roeleveld N (2004) Diethylstilbestrol, risk factors and hypospadias development. BJU Int 93:55–55
Rozati R, Reddy PP, Reddanna P, Mujtaba R (2002) Role of environmental estrogens in the deterioration of male factor fertility. Fertil Steril 78:1187–1194
Ryan JJ, Amirova Z, Carrier G (2002) Sex ratios of children of Russian pesticide producers exposed to dioxin. Environ Health Perspect 110:A699–A701
Schaison G, Young J, Pholsena M, Nahoul K, Couzinet B (1993) Failure of combined follicle-stimulating hormone-testosterone administration to initiate and/or maintain spermatogenesis in men with hypogonadotropic hypogonadism. J Clin Endocrinol Metab 77:1545–1549
Seminara SB, Messager S, Chatzidaki EE, Thresher RR, Acierno JS Jr., Shagoury JK, Bo-Abbas Y, Kuohung W, Schwinof KM, Hendrick AG, Zahn D, Dixon J, Kaiser UB, Slaugenhaupt SA, Gusella JF, O'Rahilly S, Carlton MB, Crowley WF Jr., Aparicio SA, Colledge WH (2003) The GPR54 gene as a regulator of puberty. N Engl J Med 349:1614–1627
Settimi L, Masina A, Andrion A, Axelson O (2003) Prostate cancer and exposure to pesticides in agricultural settings. Int J Cancer 104:458–461
Sigman M, Jarow JP (1997) Endocrine evaluation of infertile men. Urology 50:659–664
Silveira LF, MacColl GS, Bouloux PM (2002) Hypogonadotropic hypogonadism. Semin Reprod Med 20:327–338
Skakkebaek NE, Rajpert-De Meyts E, Main KM (2001) Testicular dysgenesis syndrome: an increasingly common developmental disorder with environmental aspects. Hum Reprod 16:972–978
Skakkebaek NE, Holm M, Hoei-Hansen C, Jorgensen N, Rajpert-De Meyts E (2003) Association between testicular dysgenesis syndrome (TDS) and testicular neoplasia: evidence

from 20 adult patients with signs of maldevelopment of the testis. APMIS 111:1–9
Staessen JA, Nawrot T, Hond ED, Thijs L, Fagard R, Hoppenbrouwers K, Koppen G, Nelen V, Schoeters G, Vanderschueren D, Van Hecke E, Verschaeve L, Vlietinck R, Roels HA (2001) Renal function, cytogenetic measurements, and sexual development in adolescents in relation to environmental pollutants: a feasibility study of biomarkers. Lancet 357: 1660–1669
Stoker TE, Robinette CL, Cooper RL (1999) Perinatal exposure to estrogenic compounds and the subsequent effects on the prostate of the adult rat: evaluation of inflammation in the ventral and lateral lobes. Reprod Toxicol 13:463–472
Swan SH, Elkin EP, Fenster L (1997) Have sperm densities declined? A reanalysis of global trend data. Environ Health Perspect 105:1228–1232
Swan SH, Kruse RL, Liu F, Barr DB, Drobnis EZ, Redmon JB, Wang C, Brazil C, Overstreet JW (2003) Semen quality in relation to biomarkers of pesticide exposure. Environ Health Perspect 111:1478–1484
Tielemans E, van Kooij R, te Velde ER, Burdorf A, Heederik D (1999) Pesticide exposure and decreased fertilisation rates in vitro. Lancet 354:484–485
Tielemans E, van Kooij R, Looman C, Burdorf A, te Velde E, Heederik D (2000) Paternal occupational exposures and embryo implantation rates after IVF. Fertil Steril 74:690–695
Van Waeleghem K, De Clercq N, Vermeulen L, Schoonjans F, Comhaire F (1996) Deterioration of sperm quality in young healthy Belgian men. Hum Reprod 11:325–329
Vartiainen T, Kartovaara L, Tuomisto J (1999) Environmental chemicals and changes in sex ratio: analysis over 250 years in Finland. Environ Health Perspect 107:813–815
Voglmayr JK, Mizumachi M, Washington DW, Chen CL, Bardin CW (1990) Immunization of rams against human recombinant inhibin alpha-subunit delays, augments, and extends season-related increase in blood gonadotropin levels. Biol Reprod 42:81–86
Voorhoeve PG, Delemarre-van de Waal HA (2004) [From gene to disease; hypogonatrophic hypogonadism and anosmia: Kallmann's syndrome]. Ned Tijdschr Geneeskd 148:1142–1144
Wang J, Wang B (2002) Study on risk factors of cryptorchidism. Zhonghua Liu Xing Bing Xue Za Zhi 23:190–193
Webster J (1999) Clinical management of prolactinomas. Baillieres Best Pract Res Clin Endocrinol Metab 13:395–408
Weidner IS, Moller H, Jensen TK, Skakkebaek NE (1998) Cryptorchidism and hypospadias in sons of gardeners and farmers. Environ Health Perspect 106:793–796
WHO (1987) Towards more objectivity in diagnosis and management of male infertility. Int J Androl Suppl 7

II.2.3 Infection/Inflammation of the Male Genital Tract as Cause of Abnormal Spermatozoa

C. Depuydt, A. Mahmoud, K. Everaert

Summary

The effects of infection/inflammation of the accessory glands (MAGI) on male fertility depend on the type of pathogen, the acute versus chronic course of the disease and the organ(s) affected. The mechanisms through which MAGI impair the fertilizing capacity of spermatozoa are reasonably well understood. Damage caused by abnormal concentrations of cytokines, growth factors and reactive oxygen species alters the sperm membrane and DNA.

Antibiotic treatment commonly does not result in the restoration of accessory gland function and sperm fertilizing potential. Complementary treatment with antioxidant nutriceuticals and, sometimes, assisted reproduction may be indicated.

II.2.3.1 Introduction

Clinicians treating subfertile men are confronted with patients presenting accessory gland infection (MAGI) as a common occurrence (WHO 1987; Rowe et al. 2000). For some time MAGI has been accepted as an aetiological diagnosis if semen classification is abnormal spermatozoa, including azoospermia. According to the World Health Organization (WHO), the diagnosis of MAGI as a cause of infertility is given if a patient has abnormal spermatozoa and certain criteria are satisfied in history taking, physical examination, and in the analysis of urine and/or the ejaculate (see Chap. I.3.13). MAGI may cause couple infertility not only through its direct effects on the fertilizing capacity of the spermatozoa, but also through effects on the female partner (Eggert-Kruse et al. 1997; Rowe et al. 2000). Controversy persisting about this point of view (Tomlinson et al. 1993) may be related to problems in defining the diagnosis of MAGI, and the fact that antibiotic treatment of infertile men with MAGI commonly does not restore fertility (Comhaire et al. 1986; Branigan and Muller 1994; Yanushpolsky et al. 1995). There seems to be less disagreement about the impact of the disease in terms of the biochemistry and functional quality of the spermatozoa. Also, many of the functional abnormalities caused do not become evident upon "basic semen analysis", explaining why some authors are unable to link infection of the accessory sex glands to infertility (Comhaire et al. 1999).

Numerous different pathogens and other factors influence the degree of impairment of fertility in patients with MAGI: bacteria, viruses, white blood cells, inflammation, obstruction, site of infection and immunological factors. All of these factors are suggested to play a pathological role, but some lack proof of causality (Wolff 1998), and it has been suggested that synergistic multifactorial causality is involved (Chap. I.3.3). Finally, the term MAGI does not refer to an organ-specific disease. It does not distinguish between acute disease and chronic infection, between infection and inflammation, and between organ-specific diseases such as prostatitis and epididymitis.

II.2.3.2 Causal Factors and the Role of Cytokines

Human semen contains a repertoire of cytokines whose effects on semen quality and sperm function are still subject to investigation. It is now realized that cytokines rarely act in isolation but rather induce or inhibit other cytokines, creating a network to which the cells respond (Wilson et al. 1998). Inflammatory cytokines are produced by white blood cells (WBC), mainly macrophages, in response to foreign antigens, pathogens (infection challenge) and also in chronic inflammation (immunological activation). The initiators of infection are pathogens (Wilson et al. 1998) that may either originate from the urinary tract or be sexually transmitted (Ness et al. 1997) (see Chap. II.2.4).

II.2.3.2.1 Bacteria and Viruses

Among urinary invaders, *Escherichia coli*, *Proteus* species, *Klebsiella* and *Streptococcus* group D are common pathogens (Comhaire et al. 1980). During acute bacterial infection of the male accessory sex glands there are obvious alterations of sperm parameters, including sperm motility and morphology, fertilizing capacity, and biochemical markers of seminal plasma (Gonzales et al. 1989; Depuydt et al. 1998b; Wolff et al. 1990; Diemer et al. 2000). High counts of *E. coli* and other pathogens can cause direct damage to spermatozoa in vitro (Table II.2.2).

Other important pathogens of the urogenital tract are *Chlamydia trachomatis*, mycoplasmata, staphylococci and enterococci (Huwe et al. 1998). Evidence exists that *E. coli*, mycoplasmata and *Chlamydia trachomatis* can inhibit the acrosome reaction (Köhn et al. 1998; Jungwirth et al. 2002), however, literature fails to demonstrate a decreased fertilizing potential of spermatozoa in vivo. We have reported a decreased probability of conception following intrauterine insemination in patients with *Chlamydia trachomatis* infection (Everaert et al. 2003).

In summary, the impact of pathogens in *acute infection* is obvious, but the role of *chronic infection* remains the subject of debate (Purvis and Christiansen 1993; Huwe et al. 1998). Also, the mere presence of microorganisms in semen is an insufficient criterion for diagnosing male genital tract infection. Measurement of the concentrations of cytokines may more accurately indicate an early phase of infection/inflammation. It should also be underscored that bacterial infection is not the only factor able to induce an elevated number of white blood cells and infertility. Other factors, including the presence of a high proportion of abnormal spermatozoa, chemical and environmental toxins, as well as viral infections, can provoke a similar immunobiological reaction. The role of yeasts, other fungi and viruses has hardly been evaluated yet, because of experimental difficulties and their questionable clinical significance.

Table II.2.2. The potential impact of bacteria on fertility in patients with MAGI

	In vitro	In vivo	Comment
Gram negative	+	-	Motility and viability
Gram positive	-	-	-
Candida	±	-	Mechanical effect?
Chlamydia trachomatis	±	-	*Female factor* *More in obstructive azoospermia* *Can attach to sperm cells*
Neisseria gonorrhoeae	±	±	*Obstruction*
Ureaplasma urealyticum	±	-	*Can attach to sperm cells*

II.2.3.2.2 Inflammation

Infection, trauma, allergy, neurological damage, chemical (e.g. metabolites of tobacco smoke; Mahmoud et al. 1998b) and mechanical factors can lead to a long-lasting inflammation of the pelvic organs, which may persist after removal of the aetiological agent. This then may be related to infertility through the effects of cytokines (Pavone et al. 2000; Everaert et al. 2003).

Interleukins and growth factors are produced in response to infection and tissue damage, or by bacteria, and are proven to exert deleterious effects on the fertilizing potential of spermatozoa.

II.2.3.2.3 Cytokines

Infiltrating pathogens stimulate the production of interleukin-8 (IL-8) by macrophages (Yoshimura et al. 1987). This cytokine has been reported to exert a negative effect on the fertilizing capacity of spermatozoa (Buch et al. 1994; Rajasekaran et al. 1995). An elevated concentration in seminal plasma of IL-8 is considered a

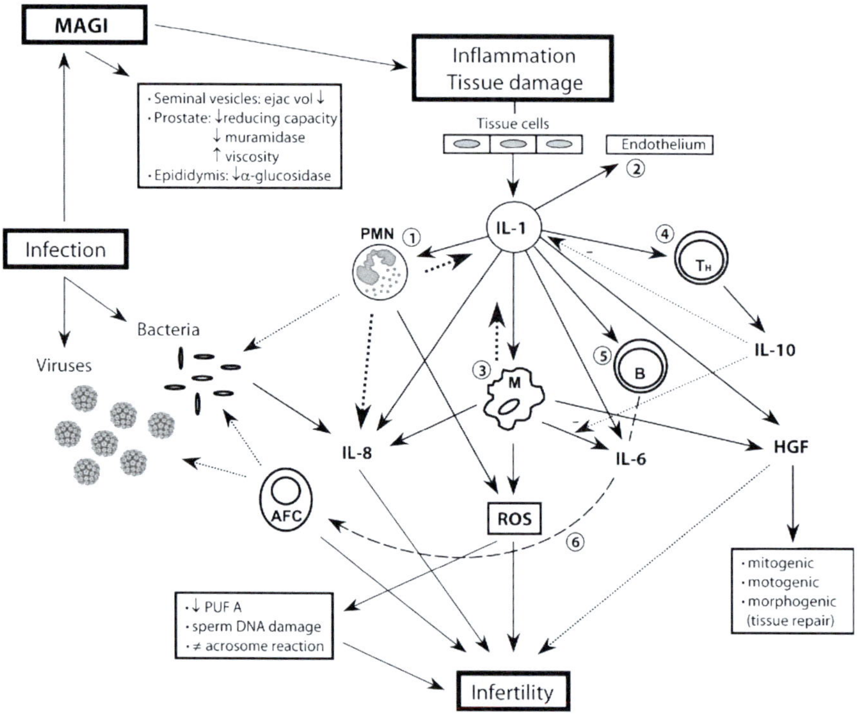

Fig. II.2.4. Composite overview of some of the effects of infection on the function of the accessory sex glands, the generation of reactive oxygen species, cytokines and hepatocyte growth factor, and the changes in sperm function (adapted from Depuydt et al. 1998b). IL-1 is produced by many cell types in response to damage, infection or antigens. It influences many cells and processes: (*1*) PMNs are metabolically activated and move towards the site of IL-1 production by chemotaxis (*dashed arrow*); (*2*) in the endothelium, adhesion molecules and procoagulants are induced, and permeability is increased. (*3*) Prostaglandin production and cytocidal activity increase in macrophages. Chemotaxis is also stimulated (*dashed arrow*). (*4*) Th cell proliferation, IL-2 receptor and cytokine production are all enhanced. (*5*) B cell proliferation and differentiation into antibody-forming cells is stimulated and regulated (*6*) by other cytokines. [*AFC* Antibody-forming cell, *B* B lymphocyte, *HGF* hepatocyte growth factor (scatter factor), *IL-1* interleukin 1, *IL-6* interleukin 6, *IL-8* interleukin 8, *IL-10* interleukin 10, *M* macrophage, *PMN* polymorphonuclear white blood cells, *PUFA* polyunsaturated fatty acids, *ROS* reactive oxygen species]

sensitive marker of silent genital infection (Eggert-Kruse et al. 2001), and for the diagnosis of MAGI (Koumantakis et al. 1998). Tissue damage caused by the infection provokes an inflammatory reaction stimulating the generation of interleukin-1 (IL-1), which induces several effects in the surrounding environment (Arend and Dayer 1995). Interleukin-1 stimulates polymorphonuclear neutrophils to secrete, amongst other substances, both IL-8 and reactive oxygen species. Interleukin-1 also stimulates macrophages, which are the major source of IL-8 and also secrete IL-6 and hepatocyte growth factor (also called scatter factor) (Depuydt et al. 1998a). Interleukin-6 interacts with B lymphocytes that become antibody-producing cells (Hirano 1998). These antibodies are directed against the invading pathogens, but they can also interfere with sperm function (Fig. II.2.4) (Depuydt et al. 1998b).

It has been documented that particular cytokines, e.g. IL-6, can cause membrane damage (Yamauchi-Takihara et al. 1995), which may decrease the functional capacity of spermatozoa. Also increased levels of IL-6 in seminal plasma were related to MAGI (Comhaire et al. 1994; Shimoya et al. 1995; Eggert-Kruse et al. 2001; Friebe et al. 2003). Over the past few years, various growth factors and cytokines have been measured in seminal plasma: hepatocyte growth factor (HGF), IL-1α, IL-1β, IL-2, IL-6, IL-8, IL-10, tumour necrosis factor-α (TNF-α), soluble TNF (sTNF) receptor types I and II, and several other soluble receptors (sR) such as sR IL-2, sR IL-6, and the IL-1 receptor antagonist (RA) (Comhaire et al. 1994; Rajasekaran et al. 1995; Depuydt et al. 1996; Gruschwitz et al. 1996; Dousset et al. 1997; Denison et al. 1999; Huleihel et al. 1999). However, studies on the effects of cytokines and growth factors on sperm function have given somewhat contradictory results (for a review see Depuydt and Comhaire 1998).

The development of appropriate cytokine networks to combat infections will depend on the nature of the infecting organism and on the genetic makeup of the individual. A number of cytokine genes have been found to present polymorphisms in noncoding regions, which can control the rate of production of the cytokine. It is assumed that these different cytokine networks may render individuals more or less resistant to particular infections (Westendorp et al. 1997). For example, men with chronic nonbacterial prostatitis/pelvic pain syndrome were more likely to express the genotype associated with low IL-10 production when compared with healthy controls (Shoskes et al. 2002).

Table II.2.3. Contact time between sperm cells and the different organs, their secretions or cellular components

Testis: 74 days
Epididymis: 7 – 14 days
Vas deferens: seconds
Seminal vesicles, prostate, urethra: seconds
Ejaculate: minutes to hours

Wolff (1995)

II.2.3.2.4
Site of Infection

The direct causality between infection and infertility strongly depends on the contact time between the inflammatory factors (e.g. white blood cells, reactive oxygen species, cytokines) and the sperm cells, which differs depending on the affected organs (Table II.2.3). In addition to differences in the contact time, there are also differences in the impairment of the secretory function. The effects of prostatitis, decreasing the secretion of muramidase, gamma glutamyl transferase, prostate specific antigen (PSA) and citric acid, and reducing liquefaction with increased viscosity, are completely different from the effects of infection of the seminal vesicles, namely decreasing the volume of the ejaculate and the fructose concentration. In epididymitis the secretion of alpha-glucosidase and carnitines is decreased, as is the production of antioxidants (Mahmoud et al. 1998a,b; Ludwig et al. 2002). So far, the mechanism by which these changes interfere with fertility has only been partially elucidated. Considering the variable effects of different locations of the infectious/inflammatory process, every effort must be made to identify the site of MAGI. For this reason, assessment of the physical and biochemical characteristics of the ejaculate is mandatory (see Chap. II.3.2).

II.2.3.3
White Blood Cells and Reactive Oxygen Species

Leukocytes in semen are identified as peroxidase-positive round cells. In addition, measuring elastase activity or reactive oxygen species (ROS) seems useful. The generation of ROS by polymorphonuclear white blood cells and/or macrophages results in altered fatty acid composition of the spermatozoon's plasma membrane (Zalata et al. 1998). Typically, the phospholipids of the spermatozoon's membrane in fertile men contain a high proportion of polyunsaturated fatty acids with a long chain, belonging to the omega-3 group, particularly docosahexaenoic acid (DHA; 22:6 ω3). In contrast, the level of DHA in the membrane of spermatozoa of men with MAGI is strongly decreased. This, together with the relatively higher proportion of saturated fatty acids in spermatozoa of MAGI patients, reduces the fluidity of the sperm membrane. As a result the (induced) acrosome reactivity and the fusogenic capacity of spermatozoa are impaired, decreasing their fertilizing potential (Zalata et al. 2004). On the other hand, high levels of ROS induce oxidative changes in the DNA of spermatozoa, e.g. by converting guanosine into 8-OH-2-deoxyguanosine, corresponding to transition mutagenesis (Loft and Poulsen 1996; Chen et al. 1997). A high concentration of oxidized DNA in spermatozoa was shown to decrease the monthly conception rate among first-pregnancy planners (Loft et al. 2003).

Although clinical MAGI commonly coincides with leukcytospermia, asymptomatic MAGI may be associated with variable concentrations of white blood cells. Also, there may be a high rate of spontaneous resolution of white blood cells from the ejaculate, and leukocytes may even exert a positive effect on fertilization (Aitken and Baker 1995; Wolff 1995; Yanushpolsky et al. 1995; Ludwig et al. 1998). These conflicting data suggest that leukocytes per se do not have a negative effect on male fertility, and that optimal levels of ROS, interleukins and growth factors produced by these leukocytes are necessary for normal sperm function (good Samaritans) (Aitken and Baker 1995). However, excessive concentrations (relative to sperm concentration) of white blood cells, possibly in synergism with other pathogenic factors, are deleterious for male fertility (see Chap. I.3.3). This provides the rationale for antioxidant treatment (Mahmoud et al. 1999; Comhaire et al. 2000).

II.2.3.4
Obstruction of Sperm Transport and Anti-Sperm Antibodies

Both acute and chronic infection and/or inflammation can cause partial or complete obstruction of sperm transport with, respectively, oligozoospermia or azoospermia. Bilateral obstruction of, especially, the epididymides is common after (recurrent) infection with *Chlamydia* or *Gonococcus* (Weidner et al. 1999). From the anatomical point of view it is easy to link complete obstruction of sperm transport with male infertility, but the impact of partial or unilateral obstruction is debatable. Complete obstruction is diagnosed in cases with azoospermia and very low alpha-glucosidase activity in seminal plasma, but the value of this marker for the diagnosis of partial obstruction remains unclear (Mahmoud et al. 1998a). Aside from the anatomical consequences of obstruction, inflammation may act as a co-factor in the aetiopathogenesis of infertility. Also, pressure-induced rupture of the epididymal duct or ductuli efferentes will disrupt the blood–testis barrier (Witkin 1988), activating an immunological defence reaction and inducing the production of anti-sperm antibodies (Munoz and Witkin 1995; Witkin et al. 1995) (see Chap. I.3.7).

References

Aitken RJ, Baker HWC (1995) Seminal leucocytes: passengers, terrorists or good Samaritans? Hum Reprod 10:1736–1739

Arend WP, Dayer JM (1995) Inhibition of the production and effects of interleukin-1 and tumor necrosis factor alpha in rheumatoid arthritis. Arthritis Rheum 38:151–160

Branigan EF, Muller CH (1994) Efficacy of treatment and recurrence rate of leukocytospermia in infertile men with prostatitis. Fertil Steril 62:580–584

Buch JP, Kolon TF, Maulik N, Kreutzer DL, Das DK (1994) Cytokines stimulate membrane lipid peroxidation of human sperm. Fertil Steril 62:186–188

Chen CS, Chao HT, Pan RL, Wei YH (1997) Hydroxyl radical-induced decline in motility and increase in lipid peroxidation and DNA modification in human sperm. Biochem Mol Biol Int 43:291–303

Comhaire F, Verschraegen G, Vermeulen L (1980) Diagnosis of accessory gland infection and its possible role in male infertility. Int J Androl 3:32–45

Comhaire FH, Rowe PJ, Farley TM (1986) The effect of doxycycline in infertile couples with male accessory gland infection: a double blind prospective study. Int J Androl 9:91–98

Comhaire F, Bosmans E, Ombelet W, Punjabi U, Schoonjans F (1994) Cytokines in semen of normal men and of patients with andrological diseases. Am J Reprod Immunol 31:99–103

Comhaire FH, Mahmoud AMA, Depuydt CE, Zalata AA, Christophe AB (1999) Mechanisms and effects of male genital tract infection on sperm quality and fertilizing potential: the andrologist's viewpoint. Hum Reprod Update 5:393–398

Comhaire FH, Christophe AB, Zalata AA, Dhooge WS, Mahmoud AM, Depuydt CE (2000) The effects of combined conventional treatment, oral antoxidants and essential fatty acids on sperm biology in subfertile men. Prostaglandins Leukot Essent Fatty Acids 63:159–165

Denison FC, Grant VE, Calder AA, Kelly RW (1999) Seminal plasma components stimulate interleukin-8 and interleukin-10 release. Mol Hum Reprod 5:220–226

Depuydt CE, Comhaire FH (1998) Role of cytokines and other growth factors in sperm function. Modern ART in the 2000s: andrology in the nineties: the proceedings of an International Symposium on Male Infertility and Assisted Reproduction (Studies in profertility series; v. 8), p 165–175

Depuydt CE, Bosmans E, Zalata A, Schoonjans F, Comhaire FH (1996) The relation between reactive oxygen species and cytokines in andrological patients with or without male accessory gland infection. J Androl 17:699–707

Depuydt CE, De Potter CR, Zalata A, Baekelandt E, Bosmans E, Comhaire FH (1998a) Levels of hepatocyte growth factor/scatter factor (HGF/SF) in seminal plasma of patients with andrological diseases. J Androl 19:175–182

Depuydt C, Zalata A, Christophe A, Mahmoud A, Comhaire F (1998b) Mechanisms of sperm deficiency in male accessory gland infection. Andrologia 30:29–33

Diemer T, Ludwig M, Huwe P, Hales DB, Weidner W (2000) Influence of urogenital infection on sperm function. Curr Opin Urol 10:39–44

Dousset B, Hussenet F, Daudin M, Bujan L, Foliguet B, Nabet P (1997) Seminal cytokine concentrations (IL-1beta, IL-2, IL-6, sR IL-2, sR IL-6), semen parameters and blood hormonal status in male infertility. Hum Reprod 12:1476–1479

Eggert-Kruse W, Rohr G, Demirakca T, Rusu R, Naher H, Petzoldt D, Runnebaum B (1997) Chlamydial serology in 1303 asymptomatic subfertile couples. Hum Reprod 12:1464–1475

Eggert-Kruse W, Boit R, Rohr G, Aufenanger J, Hund M, Strowitzki T (2001) Relationship of seminal plasma interleukin (IL)-8 and IL-6 with semen quality. Hum Reprod 16:517–528

Everaert K, Mahmoud A, Depuydt C, Maeyaert M, Comhaire F (2003) Chronic prostatitis and male accessory gland infection – is there an impact on male infertility (diagnosis and therapy)? Andrologia 35:325–330

Friebe K, Bohring C, Skrzypek J, Krause W (2003) Levels of interleukin-6 and interleukin-8 in seminal fluid of men attending an andrological clinic. Andrologia 35:126–129

Gonzales GF, Garcia-Hjarles MA, Gutierrez R, Guerra-Garcia R (1989) The secretory activity of the seminal vesicles and its relationship to sperm motility: effects of infection in the male reproductive tract. Int J Androl 12:286–294

Gruschwitz MS, Brezinschek R, Brezinschek HP (1996) Cytokine levels in the seminal plasma of infertile males. J Androl 17:158–163

Hirano T (1998) Interleukin 6 and its receptor: ten years later. Int Rev Immunol 16:249–284

Huleihel M, Lunenfeld E, Horowitz S, Levy A, Potashnik G, Mazor M, Glezerman M (1999) Expression of IL-12, IL-10, PGE2, sIL-2R and sIL-6R in seminal plasma of fertile and infertile men. Andrologia 31:283–288

Huwe P, Diemer T, Ludwig M, Liu J, Schiefer HG, Weidner W (1998) Influence of different uropathogenic microorganisms on human sperm motility parameters in an in vitro experiment. Andrologia 30:55–59

Jungwirth A, Straberger A, Esterbauer B, Fink K, Schmeller N (2003) Acrosome reaction in chlamydia positive and negative patients. Andrologia 35:314–316

Köhn FM, Erdman I, Oeda T, El Mulla KF, Schiefer HG, Schill WB (1998) Influence of urogenital infections on sperm function. Andrologia 30:73–80

Koumantakis E, Matalliotakis I, Kyriakou D, Fragouli Y, Relakis K (1998) Increased levels of interleukin-8 in human seminal plasma. Andrologia 30:339–343

Loft S, Poulsen HE (1996) Cancer risk and oxidative DNA damage in man. J Mol Med 74:297–312

Loft S, Kold-Jensen T, Hjollund NH, Giwercman A, Gyllemborg J, Ernst E, Olsen J, Scheike T, Poulsen HE, Bonde JP (2003) Oxidative DNA damage in human sperm influences time to pregnancy. Hum Reprod 18:1265–1272

Ludwig M, Kümmel C, Schroeder-Printzen I, Ringert RH, Weidner W (1998) Evaluation of seminal plasma parameters in patients with chronic prostatitis or leucocytospermia. Andrologia 30:41–47

Ludwig M, Vidal A, Diemer T, Pabst W, Failing K, Weidner W (2002) Seminal secretory capacity of the male accessory glands in chronic pelvic pain syndrome (CPPS)/chronic prostatitis with special focus on the new prostatitis classification. Eur Urol 42:24–28

Mahmoud AM, Geslevich J, Kint J, Depuydt C, Huysse L, Zalata A, Comhaire FH (1998a) Seminal plasma alpha-glucosidase activity and male infertility. Hum Reprod 13:591–595

Mahmoud AM, Schoonjans F, Zalata AA, Comhaire FH (1998b) The effect of male smoking on semen quality, reducing capacity, reactive oxygen species, and spontaneous and assisted conception rates. Andrology in the Nineties, Gent, Belgium, April 22–25, 13

Mahmoud AM, Comhaire FH, Christophe AB (1999) Oral antioxidants and male infertility. Hum Reprod 14:1028–1033

Munoz MG, Witkin SS (1995) Autoimmunity to spermatozoa, asymptomatic *Chlamydia trachomatis* genital tract infection and gamma delta T lymphocytes in seminal fluid from the male partners of couples with unexplained infertility. Hum Reprod 10:1070–1074

Ness RB, Markovic N, Carlson CL, Coughlin MT (1997) Do men become infertile after having sexually transmitted urethritis? An epidemiologic examination. Fertil Steril 68:205–213

Pavone C, Caldarera E, Liberti P, Miceli V, Di Trapani D, Serretta V, Porcu M, Pavone-Macaluso M (2000) Correlation between chronic prostatitis syndrome and pelvic venous disease: a survey of 2,554 urological outpatients. Eur Urol 37:400–403

Purvis K, Christiansen E (1993) Infection in the male reproductive tract. Impact, diagnosis and treatment in relation to male infertility. Int J Androl 16:1–13

Rajasekaran M, Hellstrom WJ, Naz RK, Sikka SC (1995) Oxidative stress and interleukins in seminal plasma during leukocytospermia. Fertil Steril 64:166–171

Rowe PJ, Comhaire FH, Hargreave TB, Mahmoud AM (2000) World Health Organization manual for the standardized investigation, diagnosis and management of the infertile male, 1st edn. Cambridge University Press, Cambridge

Shimoya K, Matsuzaki N, Ida N, Okada T, Taniguchi T, Sawai K, Itoh S, Ohashi K, Saji F, Tanizawa O (1995) Detection of monocyte chemotactic and activating factor (MCAF) and interleukin (IL)-6 in human seminal plasma and effect of leukospermia on these cytokine levels. Am J Reprod Immunol 34:311–316

Shoskes DA, Albakri Q, Thomas K, Cook D (2002) Cytokine polymorphisms in men with chronic prostatitis/chronic pelvic pain syndrome: association with diagnosis and treatment response. J Urol 168:331–335

Tomlinson MJ, Barratt CLR, Cooke ID (1993) Prospective study of leukocytes and leukocyte subpopulations in semen suggests they are not a cause of male infertility. Fertil Steril 60:1069–1075

Weidner W, Krause W, Ludwig M (1999) Relevance of male accessory gland infection for subsequent fertility with special focus on prostatitis. Hum Reprod 5:421–432

Westendorp RG, Langermans JA, Huizinga TW, Verweij CL, Sturk A (1997) Genetic influence on cytokine production in meningococcal disease. Lancet 28; 349(9069):1912–1913

WHO (1987) Towards more objectivity in diagnosis and management of male infertility. Int J Androl [Suppl 7] 19–33

Wilson M, Seymour R, Henderson B (1998) Bacterial perturbation of cytokine networks. Infect Immun 66:2401–2409

Witkin SS (1988) Mechanisms of active suppression of the immune response to spermatozoa. Am J Reprod Immunol Microbiol 17:61–64

Witkin SS, Kligman I, Bongiovanni AM (1995) Relationship between asymptomatic male genital tract exposure to *Chlamydia trachomatis* and an autoimmune response to spermatozoa. Hum Reprod 10:2952–2955

Wolff H (1995) The biological significance of white blood cells in semen. Fertil Steril 63:1143–1157

Wolff H (1998) Methods for the determination of male genital tract inflammation. Andrologia 30:35–39

Wolff H, Politch JA, Martinez A, Haimovici F, Hill JA, Anderson DJ (1990) Leucocytospermia is associated with poor semen quality. Fertil Steril 53:528–536

Yamauchi-Takihara K, Ihara Y, Ogata A, Yoshizaki K, Azuma J, Kishimoto T (1995) Hypoxic stress induces cardiac myocyte-derived interleukin-6. Circulation 91:1520–1524

Yanushpolsky EH, Politch JA, Hill JA, Anderson DJ (1995) Antibiotic therapy and leucocytospermia: a prospective, randomised, controlled study. Fertil Steril 63:142–147

Yoshimura T, Matsushima K, Oppenheim JJ, Leonard JJ (1987) Neutrophil chemotactic factor produced by lipopolysaccharide (LPS)- stimulated human blood mononuclear leukocytes: partial characterization and separation from interleukin 1 (IL 1). J Immunol 139:788–793

Zalata AA, Christophe A, Depuydt CE, Schoonjans F, Comhaire FH (1998) White blood cells cause oxidative damage to the fatty acid composition of phospholipids of human spermatozoa. Int J Androl 21:154–162

Zalata AA, Ahmed AH, Allamaneni SS, Comhaire FH, Agarwal A (2004) Relationship between acrosin activity of human spermatozoa and oxidative stress. Asian J Androl 6:313–318

II.2.4 Urethritis, Sexually Transmitted Diseases (STD), Acquired Immunodeficiency Syndrome (AIDS)

F. R. Ochsendorf

Summary

According to the present data, urethritis poses no problem for male fertility. In chronic infections, for example gonorrhoea, urethral strictures and epididymo-orchitis are possible. *Chlamydia trachomatis* and *Neisseria gonorrhoeae* can lead to pelvic inflammatory disease of the female partner and tubal obstruction. Depending on the local prevalence some sexually transmitted disease (STD) agents can impair male fertility if not adequately treated. Any STD increases the chance of transmission of human immunodeficiency virus (HIV). HIV infection is associated with infectious semen and the risk of transmission of the virus. Men who are seropositive only and do not have full-blown AIDS often present with normal semen parameters. Their endocrine and exocrine testicular functions are, however, impaired with progression of the acquired immunodeficiency. Reproduction in HIV-serodiscordant couples is possible by special sperm washing procedures and testing of the samples prior to assisted reproductive techniques.

II.2.4.1 Introduction

A common feature shared by STD is that the causative microorganisms are labile in inanimate environments. Therefore, they are only transmitted via intimate contact. They are summarized in Table II.2.4 and Chap. I.6.1. Due to their shared mode of transmission, several of these agents may be transferred together, so the diagnosis of one STD prompts the search for others.

II.2

Table II.2.4. The most common microorganisms causing urethritis, their diagnoses and treatment. The percentages are taken from the literature; in case of strong variance, the maximal and minimal numbers are given in parentheses (from Gall et al. 1999; Elsner et al. 1987; Heise 2001; Kohl 2001)

Microorganism and incubation time	Frequency (%)	Detection method	Therapy
Neisseria gonorrhoea 1–6 (–14) days	[0] 0.4 – 9– [18]	Culture (Thayer-Martin selective medium; fast transport!); DNA hybridization (first-void urine)	Once: spectinomycin 2 g or ceftriaxone 0.25 g i.m. alternatively (p.o.): cefixim 400 mg or ciprofloxacin 500 mg or ofloxacin 400 mg or azithromycin 1 g
C. trachomatis 7–21 days	[6] 15–26	Ag-detection (direct immunofluorescence, EIA), DNA amplification (PCR; LCR)	Once: azithromycin 1 × 1000 mg or 7 days: doxycycline 2 × 100 mg; alternative: (7 days p.o.): tetracyclines 4 × 500 mg or erythromycin 4 × 500 mg or ofloxacin 2 × 300 mg
Mycoplasma	10–21	Culture (special medium)	As *Chlamydia*
Ureaplasma urealyticum	15–17		
Mycoplasma hominis	4–6		
Mycoplasma genitalium (Deguchi and Maeda 2002)	18–45	Special culture (no routine method available)	7 days doxycycline 2 × 100 mg/day; alternative: macrolides, new chinolone
Pathogenic bacteria (*Enterococcus*, beta-haemolysing streptococci, *E. coli*, *Staphylococcus aureus*)	[4] – 20–31	Culture	According to antibiogram
Trichomonas vaginalis 4 days to 3 weeks	0.4–1	Urine sediment of first-void urine	Once metronidazole 2 g p.o. or tinidazole 2 g p.o.
Herpes simplex	Single cases	Only if no therapeutic effect: culture, antigen detection or PCR	Aciclovir 5 × 200 mg p.o. 5–7 days
Candida	Single cases 3	Only if no therapeutic effect: culture	Topical imidazole derivative; alternative: p.o.: fluconazole 1 × 150 mg p.o. or ketoconazole 2 × 200 mg 5 days
No agent demonstrable	-26		
Possible causes:			
False-negative test		Repetition of microbiologic tests, history	
Functional irritation			
Traumatic urethritis			
Tumours of the urethra		Urologic diagnostics (urethroscopy)	
HPV infection			
General disease		History	

STDs can lead to pelvic inflammatory disease (Ankum et al. 1996), ectopic pregnancy, infertility, chronic pelvic pain, genital lesions, genital neoplasms, adverse pregnancy outcomes, immune system dysfunction, liver disease, gonococcal sepsis and even death; so, they have a considerable impact on the health of men and women. Even if the disease does not cause definite impairment of sperm parameters, for example *Chlamydia trachomatis* infections in men, it may be transferred to the female partner and so has considerable impact in women, such as pelvic inflammatory disease resulting in tubal occlusion (Sulak 2003).

II.2

There are studies reporting a positive history concerning STDs in 45% of infertile patients (Schulenburg et al. 1993), while others did not find associations between prior urethral discharge or dysuria and subsequent semen quality (Oldereid et al. 1992). A higher percentage of STD agents was reported in infertile men and women than in controls (Rodriguez et al. 2001). It is likely that the prevalence of STDs, the availability of health services, and the time and mode of STD treatment in a given population are all factors influencing the role of these infections in male infertility (Cates et al. 1985; De Schryver and Meheus 1990; Bambra 1999; Jansen et al. 2003; Orroth et al. 2003; Bayasgalan et al. 2004). There are several reviews addressing these questions in more detail (Keck et al. 1998; Comhaire et al. 1999; Paavonen and Eggert-Kruse 1999; Sulak 2003).

II.2.4.2 Urethritis

II.2.4.2.1 Pathogens

Urethritis can be caused by several pathogens (Table II.2.4; Elsner et al. 1987; Gall et al. 1999; Heise 2001; Kohl 2001; Deguchi and Maeda 2002). The most relevant are gonorrhoea, *Chlamydia trachomatis*, *Ureaplasma urealyticum*, *Mycoplasma genitalium*, *Trichomonas vaginalis* (Table II.2.4). Urethritis caused by mechanical trauma is unrelated to infertility. Ascension of gonococci is estimated to occur in about 1% of infected patients.

II.2.4.2.2 Clinical Presentation

The symptoms are variable. In acute urethritis, the patient notices a urethral discharge and dysuria. Others have no symptoms or are symptom-free throughout the day and only notice a drop of pus in the morning prior to the first voiding of urine. Sometimes the glans or meatus urethrae may present with some redness as a sign of inflammation.

II.2.4.2.3 Diagnosis

The demonstration of >15 granulocytes in the sediment of the first 3 ml of urine (400× magnification) is regarded as pathognomonic for an acute inflammation of the urethra (Schiefer 1998). The definite diagnosis is made by demonstration of the pathogenic agent [culture, direct immunofluorescence, enzyme immunoassay (EIA) and nowadays molecular methods such as polymerase chain reaction (PCR) or ligase chain reaction (LCR); see Table II.2.4]. These tests have different sensitivities and specificities (Watson et al. 2002).

II.2.4.2.4 Relevance

The question of whether urethritis leads to male infertility is discussed controversially. It is biologically plausible that gonorrhoea and/or *Chlamydia* could cause male infertility. There is clinical and pathologic evidence linking these pathogens to urethritis, linking urethritis to epididymo-orchitis, and linking epididymo-orchitis to infertility. A retrospective analyses of the literature, however, could not substantiate whether these pathogens alter sperm characteristics. Methodological problems were thought to be responsible (Ness et al. 1997). As yet there are no prospective controlled studies definitely proving this association. Urethral stricture is another possible complication of urethritis, mainly due to gonococci (Bewes 1973).

Gonorrhoea

The seroprevalence of *N. gonorrhoeae* ranged from 3% to 31% in different risk groups (study in Mexico; Cravioto Mdel et al. 2003). These rates are different in other countries (Dougan et al. 2004).

Especially in Africa infertility due to tubal obstruction appears to be a relevant issue (Meheus et al. 1986). In men urethral strictures may occur (Osoba 1981; Fievet et al. 1987). Most strictures are seen in the posterior urethra, where fibrosis and narrowing may extend from a short length of under 5 mm to well over 10 cm. A wide variety of initial complaints and complications occurs. When the patient presents in acute retention or with a history of difficult micturition, the diagnosis is easy. However, when stricture is the underlying cause of perianal abscess, gangrene of the scrotum caused by extravasation, uraemia or hypertension, hernia or rectal prolapse, urinary infection, or elephantiasis of scrotum with multiple fistulae, diagnosis may be difficult. A careful history is helpful, particularly if previous gonorrhoea is involved. The definite diagnosis is made be urethrography and urethroscopy (Bewes 1973). In Western countries such as Scotland, however, gonorrhoea is not a relevant cause of urethral strictures (McMillan et al. 1994). It was proposed that a decline in subfertility in Sweden could be attributed to the eradication of gonorrhoea (Akre et al. 1999), a view not shared by others (Jensen et al. 2000).

In men with asymptomatic gonorrhoea no differences in spermatogram parameters were found before and after treatment in comparison to a control group, with the exception of lowered citrate concentrations (Perez-Plaza et al. 1982). However, a follow-up investigation of men with proven fertility after having had gonorrhoeal urethritis and unilateral epididymo-orchitis showed that 2 years later only 21% produced semen considered adequate for conception. Although the lesions were clinically confined to one testis, testicular biopsy samples showed damage in both testes. So gonorrhoea can lead to oligo- and azoospermia (Osegbe 1991). Others reported an increased incidence of antisperm antibodies after gonococcal urethritis (Shahmanesh et al. 1986). Gonococci survive cryopreservation in liquid nitrogen, which has to be taken into account for the screening of sperm donors (Sherman and Rosenfeld 1975; Glander et al. 1986).

During routine semen analyses of asymptomatic males no screening for gonococci routinely takes place in a low prevalence setting. It was reported that dilution of semen (1:2 with saline) enhances the detection rates of *N. gonorrhoeae* (undiluted: 0 positive; diluted: 9/68 positive; Vicari et al. 1986). The same authors reported positive gonorrhoea cultures in 111/785 (14%) men in an andrologic outpatient clinic (Vicari et al. 1991). So the screening apparently has to be adjusted to local prevalence of the disease.

The relevance of *N. gonorrhoeae* lies in its capacity to lead to urethral strictures and testicular damage as a consequence of epididymo-orchitis in the male as well as ductal inflammation and obstruction in the female.

Chlamydia trachomatis

The role of *Chlamydia trachomatis* as a cause of male infertility is discussed controversially (Krause and Bohring 2003; Gonzales et al. 2004). There is no doubt that *Chlamydia trachomatis* is a frequent pathogen in male genital inflammation and that this organism is rarely present in healthy men. *Chlamydia trachomatis* causes inflammation of the male urethra and the epididymis. However, it remains unresolved and unclear whether it causes prostatitis and infections of the seminal vesicles (Weidner et al. 1999, 2002).

Chlamydia trachomatis antigen or DNA is easily demonstrable in urethral swabs and the urine. The sensitivities of DNA amplification techniques (LCR, PCR, gene probe) in first-void urine were higher (85–96%) than in cervical swabs (84–88%; the same will hold true for urethral swabs) and yielded better results than an EIA (urine 38%, swab 65%). Especially in low prevalence populations the molecular methods are more effective at detecting asymptomatic chlamydial infections than conventional tests (Watson et al. 2002). *Chlamydia trachomatis*, however, cannot be reproducibly demonstrated in secretions of the male accessory glands, including semen.

Serologic studies can be useful in epidemiologic investigations. In these studies an association was found between the detection of immunotype-specific *C. trachomatis* antibodies and subfertility both in men and women. So a previous *C. trachomatis* infection appears to be associated with subfertility in male or female partners of a given couple (Karinen et al. 2004).

The role of *Chlamydia* serology as a marker of recent infection is a matter of debate. Former investigations used tests that could not discriminate between *C. trachomatis* and *C. pneumoniae*. Different test systems yielded conflicting results. Thus determination of chlamydial antibodies in serum or semen does not conclusively indicate a current infection with *C. trachomatis*. The profile of these antibodies after treatment is unknown. Some authors found higher antibody prevalences of *Chlamydia trachomatis* antibodies in infertile men and associations with heat-shock proteins (Schuppe et al. 2003), others with inflammatory markers (Wolff et al. 1991; Ochsendorf et al. 1999).

II.2

Observations are available indicating that *Chlamydia* can enter human spermatozoa (Erbengi 1993), that they may induce antibody production (Shahmanesh et al. 1986; Soffer et al. 1990; Witkin et al. 1995a, b) and may be associated with oxidative stress (Segnini et al. 2003) and inflammation (Hosseinzadeh et al. 2004). However, there are no conclusive studies showing that men infected with *C. trachomatis* are less fertile than uninfected men (literature in Krause and Bohring 2003). Furthermore, sperm functions are not impaired (Vigil et al. 2002). So sperm apparently act as vehicles to transport the pathogen to the female.

There is no question that male genital chlamydial infections are a threat to female genital organs, because *C. trachomatis* infection of the female genital organs may be deleterious to female fertility mainly due to tubal occlusion. This has been repeatedly demonstrated (Eggert-Kruse et al. 1990, 1996; Paavonen and Eggert-Kruse 1999; Krause and Bohring 2003; Mardh 2004). So *C. trachomatis* primarily has to be regarded as a threat to female infertility.

Mycoplasmas

Mycoplasmas include *Mycoplasma hominis*, *Ureaplasma urealyticum* and *Mycoplasma genitalium*. While the first two germs can colonize the urethra without causing symptoms, the latter was suspected to be a major cause of urethritis and possibly cervicitis (Uuskula and Kohl 2002). It was suggested that female partners should be screened for these microorganisms in order to detect them in the male genital tract (Trum et al. 2000). The incidence of *U. urealyticum* in the semen of fertile and infertile men was reported to range between 7 and 42% (Reichart et al. 2000). A higher incidence was reported in the semen of infertile men (38% to 9% in controls) (dXu et al. 1997). *U. urealyticum* was suspected to cause chronic prostatitis (Badalyan et al. 2003). *U. urealyticum* and *M. genitalium* can attach to spermatozoa, be transported in the female genital tract and can cause female genital disease (Taylor-Robinson 2002; Svenstrup et al. 2003).

In in vitro fertilization (IVF) programmes *M. hominis* was found in 2–12% and *U. urealyticum* in 17–29% in semen (Hill 1990; Witkin et al. 1995b). The demonstration of a mycoplasma infection was not related to a change in sperm parameters (Soffer et al. 1990) or poorer IVF outcome if prior treatment with tetracyclines had been performed (Witkin et al. 1995a, b). It was suggested, however, that this infection can cause embryo loss without necessarily affecting semen quality. One possible mechanism is unstable chromatin. In vitro incubation resulted in time- and dose-dependent chromatin decondensation and DNA damage of sperm cells. In vivo these effects could be reduced by doxycycline therapy (Reichart et al. 2000).

Thus *U. urealyticum* may cause infertility via deleterious effects on sperm chromatin and DNA, leading to impairment of embryo development. The exact role of these microorganisms, however, has still to be elucidated.

Trichomonas vaginalis

Protozoan infections of the male genital tract are rare and only a few species of parasites are involved (Martinez-Garcia et al. 1996). *T. vaginalis* is the most common agent (~120 million new cases worldwide; Crosignani et al. 1992). Recently it was shown that the incidence in men may be underestimated if only one specimen was used to screen for this agent. Compared to first-void urine and urethral swabs, semen proved to be the most sensitive single specimen (in 25% only semen positive) for the detection of *T. vaginalis* (Kaydos-Daniels et al. 2004). In areas with a high prevalence of trichomoniasis, the addition of metronidazole to the syndromic management of male urethritis is recommended (Price et al. 2003). In women no differences in the detection rates of *T. vaginalis* between fertile and infertile women were reported (Okonofua et al. 1995). However, it was stressed that trichomoniasis may play a role in the development of cervical neoplasia, postoperative infections and adverse pregnancy outcomes, and as a factor in atypical pelvic inflammatory disease and infertility (Soper 2004).

A higher seminal contamination with *Trichomonas* was found in infertile men compared to fertile men (47% to 30%) as well as a higher viscosity and sperm agglutination. A significant improvement in semen characteristics was found in 50% of patients 1 month after treatment with metronidazole (Bornman et al. 1992b). Others could not confirm detrimental effects of *T. vaginalis* on sperm motility (Daly et al. 1989). No detrimental effects on sperm–mucus interaction were found (Eggert-Kruse et al. 1987). *T. vaginalis* does not survive cryopreservation of spermatozoa (Glander et al. 1986).

Trichomoniasis might cause reversible infertility in men, although the actual role of *T. vaginalis* infection in infertility has not yet been clearly defined (Martinez-Garcia et al. 1996; Soper 2004).

II.2.4.3 STD

Agents that are sexually transmitted are summarized in Chap. I.6.1, Table II.2.4. Some agents are not listed there as they are not associated with male infertility such as scabies or human papilloma virus infections. STDs are reviewed in several publications (Moskowitz and Mellinger 1992; Radcliffe 2001; Center of Disease Control and Prevention 2002; Sulak 2003). It was concluded that STDs are less important for men than for women with regard to fertility (Westrom 1994). Studies on large cohorts of men showed that there is no increased rate of antisperm antibody production in men attending STD clinics (Hargreave et al. 1984). So this mechanism appears not to be relevant.

The prevalence of STDs differs worldwide with higher incidences in developing countries (De Schryver and Meheus 1990). Furthermore the pattern changes from year to year, with a decrease in the 1990s during the HIV epidemic and a current rise in incidence (Dougan et al. 2004).

About two-thirds of STDs affect individuals younger than 25 (Braverman 2000). This sexually active population may have long-term negative sequelae, such as infertility, chronic pelvic pain and cancer; so, educational strategies are needed for their prevention (Wilken and Rosler 1985; Stone 1990; Workowski et al. 2002). This is sometimes hampered by fragmented responsibilities for STD and infertility services (Hardon 2003).

Human papilloma virus was demonstrated on the skin of about 13% of men attending an infertility clinic as well as in the semen of men with and without genital warts (Green et al. 1991; Pakendorf et al. 1998). Transmission from the woman to the man appears to be rather inefficient. HPV type 16 DNA and RNA (25% and 8% of randomly selected patients) as well as type 18 DNA and RNA (46% and 21%) were detected in sperm cells (literature in Dejucq and Jégou 2001). The incidence of asthenozoospermia was reported to be significantly higher in patients with HPV in their semen (Lai et al. 1997).

Syphilis incidence in an andrological outpatient department was reported to be 3–8% in South Africa (Bornman et al. 1992a). This is important from an epidemiological point of view: even if *Treponema pallidum* does not directly impair male infertility it demonstrates that patients are at risk for other STDs, especially HIV infection.

Today one main impact of STDs is their potential to increase the rate of HIV transmission. This has been clearly proven and reviewed. Therefore, the treatment of STDs is not only relevant to the prevention of long-term negative consequences for fertility but also to the prevention of HIV spread (Passey 1996; Ping et al. 2000; Aral 2001; Pilcher et al. 2004).

Finally, STD agents have to be taken into account during assisted reproductive techniques (Diani 1999) and in sperm donor programmes. Again the regional variation of STDs explains the large variations in reported incidences (Craig et al. 1997; Olatunbosun et al. 1998; Wortley et al. 1998).

II.2.4.4 HIV

The first reports about unusual deaths in homosexual men were published in 1981. Within months an acquired immunodeficiency was identified. In 1983 a virus as the probable cause of this acquired immunodeficiency syndrome (AIDS) was isolated and in the following years the causal link was proven (literature in: Hoffmann and Kamps 2004 or www.HIV.net, www.hivmedicine.com). One main goal is the prevention of further spread of the disease. At present, intravaginal topical formulations of anti-HIV agents or microbicides to prevent the mucosal and perinatal HIV transmission are being developed. These agents should be capable of attacking HIV from different routes: directly inactivating HIV, preventing HIV from attaching to, entering or replicating in susceptible target cells as well as prevention of dissemination from target cells present in semen or the host cells that line the vaginal wall (D'Cruz and Uckun 2004).

In the first years of the HIV epidemic problems other than reproduction had to be addressed. The wish for an own child was opposed by concerns about possible infections of the partner as well as the prognosis of the disease. Today, HIV infection is a chronic disease, so couples will be seen in greater numbers for preconception counselling. This involves a multidisciplinary approach to ensure that a couple is fully informed. The criteria to offer treatment or not should be based on the same criteria that are applied to couples who are affected by other chronic diseases. Medical treatment is dependent on the unique circumstances of each couple (Williams et al. 2003).

It is possible to help couples by using different methods of assisted reproduction. Until the middle of 2003 more than 1800 couples were treated in about 4500 cycles and about 500 children were born in Europe (Sonnenberg-Schwan 2004).

Infection with HIV has different influences on reproductive medicine: the function of the reproductive organs, ethical issues, prevention of spread to the child and safety issues for the laboratory personnel (Ethics Committee of the American Society for Reproductive Medicine 2004).

II.2.4.4.1 Effects of HIV on the Function of Male Reproductive Organs

Testis

The most relevant sources of HIV in the male reproductive tract are infected leukocytes (lymphocytes, monocytes, macrophages) (Dulioust et al. 1998). Vasectomy does not influence the amount of free virus in seminal plasma (Krieger et al. 1998). Controversy surrounds whether the virus also infects spermatozoa (Dejucq and Jégou 2001).

II.2

It was shown that testicular macrophages express CD4, CCR5 and CXCR4 thus allowing entry of HIV into these cells and providing a reservoir (Habasque et al. 2002).

Proviral DNA was detected in the nuclei of germ cells at all stages of differentiation in the testes of HIV-positive men by in situ PCR hybridization. The presence of provirus was not associated with germ cell damage, spermatogenesis was normal and a very mild local immune response was observed (Muciaccia et al. 1998b). According to electron microscopy, HIV can attach to the surface of spermatozoa and enter these cells through the intact plasma membrane (Bagasra et al. 1994) probably by an alternative receptor (the GalAAG) (Piomboni and Baccetti 2000) or a 160-kDa sperm protein (Bandivdekar et al. 2003). Others could not confirm this (Pudney et al. 1998). It is possible to generate HIV-free spermatozoa fractions by washing procedures, which is an argument against infection of motile spermatozoa by this virus (Semprini and Fiore 2004). In prostate and testis tissues T lymphocytes were the predominant cells infected with HIV-1. So it was concluded that HIV-1 in seminal plasma is derived from the prostate, while HIV-1-infected cells in semen originate mostly from the rete testis and epididymis (Paranjpe et al. 2002).

Several endocrine and testicular dysfunctions have been reported in men infected with HIV, depending, in part, on the stage of the disease. Hypogonadism was shown to be common in HIV disease. It was suggested that the weight loss observed in full-blown AIDS may be a result of lowered testosterone levels (Dobs et al. 1988; Villette et al. 1990; Schurmeyer et al. 1997). A significant association was observed between testicular atrophy and body mass index (BMI) ($P = 0.0496$). Thus, underweight patients with HIV infection were 3.52 times more likely to have testicular atrophy than those with acceptable body weight (Mhawech et al. 2001).

Studies showing that testosterone replacement in HIV-infected patients with weight loss and low testosterone levels can improve muscle mass, effort-dependent strength, lean body mass and other symptoms of hypogonadism are in favour of this argument (Bhasin et al. 1998; Bhasin and Javanbakht 1999). If reproduction is planned, however, it has to be taken into account that reversible azoospermia may result from testosterone therapy (Pena et al. 2003). Furthermore it was shown that about one-third of HIV-infected men attending gyms used anabolic steroids (Bolding et al. 2002).

In AIDS patients orchitis, hypogonadism, oligozoospermia or azoospermia have been reported (Dobs et al. 1988; Pudney and Anderson 1991; Poretsky et al. 1995). Furthermore in some cases testicular germ cell tumours or lymphoma were found. The incidence of testis tumours was 57 times higher than the average US incidence (0.2% in 3015 HIV-positive men to 0.0035% in the normal population; Tessler and Catanese 1987).

Discussed mechanisms for the mode of action of HIV on the testis include unspecific accompanying deterioration of functions due to the chronic debilitating illness and cachexia of the patients or synergistic effects of opportunistic infections such as cytomegalovirus (CMV), *Mycobacterium avium-intracellulare* or *Toxoplasma gondii* in the testis. As only every third patient had such infections but demonstrable testis changes, these infections were probably not the main cause (De Paepe et al. 1990). A change in the hypothalamic-pituitary axis, initially discussed (Dobs et al. 1988), could not be confirmed in later studies (Schlienger and Lang 1989; Poretsky et al. 1995). Elevated luteinizing hormone (LH) and follicle-stimulating hormone (FSH) levels, found in some patients, suggest a primary testicular failure (Croxson et al. 1989).

Autopsy studies reported testicular atrophy in AIDS patients (Chabon et al. 1987). The hypogonadism probably results from a decrease in Leydig cell number and a lymphocyte infiltration and fibrosis of the interstitial testicular tissue (Dalton and Harcourt-Webster 1991; Pudney and Anderson 1991). In the testis several changes were described and a classification system for them was proposed (De Paepe and Waxman 1989; Yoshikawa et al. 1989). The authors found Sertoli cell only syndrome (42%), germ cell generation (27%), peritubular fibrosis associated with tubular hyalinization (15%), maturation arrest (12 5) and normal appearance (3%). In addition, spermatogenic arrest at various points, degenerating germ cells and block in the epididymis were described by others (Shevchuk et al. 1998). Prolonging the survival by antiretroviral drug therapy was associated with a shift in the histologic findings toward more pronounced loss of germ cells (Shevchuk et al. 1999).

Thus it appears that direct local action may be responsible for this observed damage within the gonads. There are several lines of evidence for this statement: Da Silva et al. 1990 detected the HIV p17 protein in the testis by immunohistochemistry. Later, HIV-infected cells of the lymphocytic/monocytic type were found in the seminiferous tubules and interstitium of the testis as well as semen (Pudney and Anderson 1991). With PCR HIV-1 DNA was found within testicular germ cells in spermatogonia, spermatocytes and some spermatids (Nuovo et al. 1994). Others demonstrated the presence of HIV DNA in the nuclei of spermatogonia and germ cells at all stages of differentiation (Muciaccia et al. 1998a,b). The mere presence of the provirus was not associated with impaired spermatogenesis in asymptomatic HIV-positive men. In AIDS patients, however, spermatogenesis was arrested and only few infected spermatogonia and spermatocytes were found (Muciaccia et al. 1998a). In about 25–33% of the residual germ cells in the testes of AIDS patients, HIV DNA could be found but not in the testes of adolescent boys who had acquired HIV in utero (Shevchuk et al. 1998).

So the HIV infection impairs exocrine and endocrine testicular functions with progression of the disease.

Ejaculate

In symptomless HIV-positive men semen parameters within the normal range are found. With progress of the disease more defects are found, particularly in strict criteria of sperm morphology. Lower CD4+ cell counts (<200 mm^3) were associated with significantly lower motility, lower than normal sperm morphology by strict criteria, more spermatids in semen, and higher percentages of teratozoospermia, oligoasthenoteratozoospermia and leukocytospermia. Healthier men, based on clinical categories, had significantly more normal-shaped spermatozoa and fewer had azoospermia, oligoasthenoteratozoospermia or leukocytospermia. In AIDS patients, grossly abnormal sperm and pyospermia was reported (Muller et al. 1998; Nicopoullos et al. 2004). There were no differences in any parameters in those taking antiretroviral medication (Nicopoullos et al. 2004).

Others reported reduced semen volume, lower percentages of rapidly progressive motility, total sperm count and increased concentrations of non-spermatic cells (Dulioust et al. 2002).

In one sperm donor semen was analysed before and after HIV infection. Semen volume, sperm motility and the percentage of sperm with normal morphology were reduced after HIV positivity. A disturbed function of seminal vesicles and prostate gland could explain the decreased volume as well as the more viscous semen found in HIV-infected subjects (Dondero et al. 1996; Van Leeuwen et al. 2004). Sperm alterations found today are attributed to effects of antiretroviral therapy (Dulioust et al. 2002; Barboza et al. 2004).

II.2.4.4.2 Ethical Issues

A recent update on the ethical issues associated with reproduction in HIV-positive patients concluded that HIV infection is not yet curable, but treatable. It has to be classified as a chronic disease due to the significant advances in HIV treatment, which delay the onset of AIDS in many, but not all, infected persons. The potential for HIV-positive persons to have uninfected children and not transmit the virus to their partners has been substantially enhanced. So both HIV-infected persons and health-care providers share responsibility for the safety of the uninfected partner and the potential offspring. It was recommended that couples requesting assistance should have their own genetically related child seek care at institutions with the facilities that can provide the most effective evaluation, treatment and follow-up. As an alternative, donor semen, adoption or not having children have to be considered (Ethics Committee of the American Society for Reproductive Medicine 2004).

II.2.4.4.3 Reproduction in Discordant Couples

In a serodiscordant couple the female partner has a 0.1–0.2% risk of acquiring HIV per act of unprotected intercourse (Mastro et al. 1997). This is dependent on the viral load in semen: it was calculated that the probability of HIV-1 transmission is 1/100 when semen contains 100,000 copies of HIV RNA and 3/10,000 with 1000 copies of HIV RNA in semen (Chakraborty et al. 2001). So attempts to conceive naturally carry a serious risk for the uninfected woman or child (Mandelbrot et al. 1997). The problems and unresolved questions of assisted reproduction in this situation are reviewed elsewhere (Englert et al. 2004).

During the initial consultation both partners should be counselled. This should include: information concerning diagnostics, therapy options, information on the psychosocial and economic situation and future perspectives of the couple, the family, and support through families and friends. It has to be stressed that the chances of HIV transmission are extremely improbable, but not impossible, and that a successful result of therapy, i.e. birth of a healthy child, cannot be guaranteed. Also the alternatives, i.e. the decisions of not having children, adoption or donor semen, have to be discussed.

If the couple opts for reproductive measures, an interdisciplinary approach is recommended (general medical diagnostics including infectiology, gynaecologic and andrologic workup). Contact with an experienced centre with facilities for sperm preparation and HIV testing has to be established. The costs and insurance coverage of the planned procedures, which are different everywhere, have to be considered.

Psychosocial counselling is very important. Up to one-third then decide against children. If not discussed properly frustrations could lead to unprotected intercourse. In addition, comorbidities, such as drug abuse, can be detected (Sonnenberg-Schwan 2004).

HIV Infection of the Man

Depending on the semen quality spermatozoa can be used for intrauterine insemination, IVF or intracytoplasmic sperm injection (ICSI). The semen has to be washed free of HIV and the success of this procedure has to be controlled prior to use (Hanabusa et al. 2000; Dunne et al. 2003; Weigel 2003; Bujan et al. 2004; Garrido et al. 2004; Nicopoullos et al. 2004). Potent antiretroviral therapy decreases the HIV load in semen and thus can be additionally used (Vernazza et al. 2000; Williams et al. 2003).

II.2

The spermatozoa are prepared using a gradient technique such as Puresperm (Nicadon, Sweden), which is diluted to 45% and 90% using a semen buffer medium. The ejaculate is layered over the prepared density gradients and centrifuged at 200 g at room temperature for 20 min. The supernatant is then aspirated, the sperm pellet removed, resuspended in fresh media and centrifuged again for 10 min. The washing procedure is repeated twice more. Then a swim-up procedure is done. An aliquot of washed spermatozoa is subsequently tested for detectable HIV RNA [for example, a nucleic acid-based sequence amplification (NASBA) assay such as Biomérieux]. In one study about 5% of NASBA tests were positive after this procedure (Nicopoullos et al. 2004).

HIV Infection of the Woman

Here a self-insemination could be tried at the optimum time point of the cycle. An inverted spermicide-free condom, a cervical cap, a vaginal applicator or a syringe may be used.

If assisted reproduction is necessary the experience to date points to a limited success rate (Ohl et al. 2003).

II.2.4.4.4 Safety Issues of the Laboratory Personnel

Only a few occupational transmissions of HIV have been reported. If standard precautions to prevent infectious disease transmission are taken, the risk of virus transmission to lab personnel is very small. In most cases nurses and laboratory technicians accidentally inoculated themselves with a patient's blood by a needlestick or were contaminated with bloody fluid and had significant mucocutaneous exposure (http://www.cdc.gov/niosh/topics/bbp/emergnedl.html, http://www.cdc.gov/ncidod/hip/Needle/needle.htm).

References

Akre O, Cnattingius S, Bergstrom R, Kvist U, Trichopoulos D, Ekbom A (1999) Human fertility does not decline: evidence from Sweden. Fertil Steril 71:1066–1069

Ankum WM, Mol BW, Van der Veen F, Bossuyt PM (1996) Risk factors for ectopic pregnancy: a meta-analysis. Fertil Steril 65:1093–1099

Aral SO (2001) Sexually transmitted diseases: magnitude, determinants and consequences. Int J STD AIDS 12:211–215

Badalyan RR, Fanarjyan SV, Aghajanyan IG (2003) Chlamydial and ureaplasmal infections in patients with nonbacterial chronic prostatitis. Andrologia 35:263–265

Bagasra O, Farzadegan H, Seshamma T, Oakes JW, Saah A, Pomerantz RJ (1994) Detection of HIV-1 proviral DNA in sperm from HIV-1-infected men. Aids 8:1669–1674

Bambra CS (1999) Current status of reproductive behaviour in Africa. Hum Reprod Update 5:1–20

Bandivdekar AH, Velhal SM, Raghavan VP (2003) Identification of CD4-independent HIV receptors on spermatozoa. Am J Reprod Immunol 50:322–327

Barboza JM, Medina H, Doria M, Rivero L, Hernandez L, Joshi NV (2004) Use of atomic force microscopy to reveal sperm ultrastructure in HIV-patients on highly active antiretroviral therapy. Arch Androl 50:121–129

Bayasgalan G, Naranbat D, Tsedmaa B, Tsogmaa B, Sukhee D, Amarjargal O, Lhagvasuren T, Radnaabazar J, Rowe PJ (2004) Clinical patterns and major causes of infertility in Mongolia. J Obstet Gynaecol Res 30:386–393

Bewes PC (1973) Urethral stricture. Trop Doct 3:77–81

Bhasin S, Javanbakht M (1999) Can androgen therapy replete lean body mass and improve muscle function in wasting associated with human immunodeficiency virus infection? J Parent Enteral Nutr Suppl 23:195–201

Bhasin S, Storer TW, Asbel-Sethi N, Kilbourne A, Hay R, Sinha-Hiski I, Shen R, Arver S, Beall G (1998) Effects of testosterone replacement with a nongenital, transdermal system, Androderm, in human immunodeficiency virus infected men with low testosterone levels. J Clin Endocrinol Metab 83:3155–3162

Bolding G, Sherr L, Elford J (2002) Use of anabolic steroids and associated health risks among gay men attending London gyms. Addiction 97:195–203

Bornman MS, Mokonoto JR, Mohamed MF, Boomker D, Reif S, Crewe-Brown HH (1992a) Syphilis serology in men at an andrology clinic in South Africa. Arch AIDS Res 6:71–72

Bornman MS, Grobler L, Boomker D, Mahomed MF, Schulenburg GW, Reif S, Crewe-Brown HH (1992b) Is *Trichomonas vaginalis* a cause of male infertility? Prog Reprod Biol Med 15:94

Braverman PK (2000) Sexually transmitted diseases in adolescents. Med Clin North Am 84:869–889, vi-vii

Bujan L, Daudin M, Matsuda T, Righi L, Thauvin L, Berges L, Izopet J, Berrebi A, Massip P, Pasquier C (2004) Factors of intermittent HIV-1 excretion in semen and efficiency of sperm processing in obtaining spermatozoa without HIV-1 genomes. Aids 18:757–766

Cates W, Farley TM, Rowe PJ (1985) Worldwide patterns of infertility: is Africa different? Lancet 2:596–598

Center of Disease Control and Prevention (2002) Sexually transmitted diseases treatment guidelines 2002. MMWR Morb Mortal Wkly Rep 51 (No. RR-6):1–77

Chabon AB, Stenger AJ, Grebstaldt H (1987) Histopathology of testis in acquired immunodeficiency syndrome. Urology 29:658–663

Chakraborty H, Sen PK, Helms RW, Vernazza PL, Fiscus SA, Eron JJ, Patterson BK, Coombs RW, Krieger JN, Cohen MS (2001) Viral burden in genital secretions determines male-to-female sexual transmission of HIV-1: a probabilistic empiric model. Aids 15:621–627

Comhaire FH, Mahmoud AM, Depuydt CE, Zalata AA, Christophe AB (1999) Mechanisms and effects of male genital tract infection on sperm quality and fertilizing potential: the andrologist's viewpoint. Hum Reprod Update 5:393–398

Craig JM, Barratt CL, Kinghorn GR (1997) Semen donors and STD screening. Genitourin Med 73:280–283

Cravioto Mdel C, Matamoros O, Villalobos-Zapata Y, Pena O, Garcia-Lara E, Martinez M, Castelo J, Sifuentes-Osornio J (2003) [Prevalence of anti-Chlamydia trachomatis and anti-Neisseria gonorrhoeae antibodies in Mexican populations]. Salud Publica Mex 45 (Suppl 5):S681–S689

Crosignani PG, Diczfalusy E, Newton J, Rubin B (1992) Sexually transmitted diseases. Hum. Reprod. 7: 1330

Croxson TS, Chapman WE, Miller LK, Levitt CD, Senie R, Zumoff B (1989) Changes in the hypothalamic-hypopituitary-gonadal axis in human immunodeficiency-virus infected homosexual men. J Clin Endocrinol Metabol 68:317–321

D'Cruz OJ, Uckun FM (2004) Clinical development of microbicides for the prevention of HIV infection. Curr Pharm Des 10:315–336

da Silva M, Shevchuk MM, Cronin WJ, Armenakas NA, Tannenbaum M, Fracchia JA, Ioachim HL (1990) Detection of HIV-related protein in testes and prostates of patients with AIDS. Am J Clin Pathol 93:196–201

Dalton AD, Harcourt-Webster JN (1991) The histopathology of testis and epididymis in AIDS – a post-mortem study. J Pathol 163:47–52

Daly JJ, Sherman JK, Green L, Hostetler TL (1989) Survival of *Trichomonas vaginalis* in human semen. Genitourin Med 65:106

De Paepe ME, Waxman M (1989) Testicular atrophy in AIDS: a study on 57 autopsy cases. Hum Pathol 20:210–214

De Paepe ME, Guerri C, Waxman M (1990) Opportunistic infections of the testis in acquired immunodeficiency syndrome. Mt Sinai J Med 57:25–29

De Schryver A, Meheus A (1990) Epidemiology of sexually transmitted diseases: the global picture. Bull World Health Organ 68:639–654

Deguchi T, Maeda S (2002) *Mycoplasma genitalium*: another important pathogen of nongonococcal urethritis. J Urol 167:1210–1217

Dejucq N, Jégou B (2001) Viruses in the mammalian male genital tract and their effects on the reproductive system. Microbiol Mol Biol Rev 65:208–231

Diani F (1999) Sexually-transmitted diseases and assisted reproduction techniques. Clin Exp Obstet Gynecol 26:131–132

Dobs AS, Dempsey MA, Ladenson PW, Polk PF (1988) Endocrine disorders in men infected with human immunodeficiency virus. Am J Med 84:811–816

Dondero F, Rossi T, D'Offizi G, Mazzilli F, Rosso R, Sarandrea N, Pinter E, Aiuti F (1996) Semen analysis in HIV seropositive men and in subjects at high risk for HIV infection. Hum Reprod 11:765–768

Dougan S, Brown AE, Logan LE, Patel B, Munro HL, Evans BG, Gill ON (2004) Epidemiology of HIV in young people in England, Wales and Northern Ireland. Commun Dis Public Health 7:15–23

Dulioust E, Tachet A, De Almeida M, Finkielsztejn L, Rivalland S, Salmon D, Sicard D, Rouzioux C, Jouannet P (1998) Detection of HIV-1 in seminal plasma and seminal cells of HIV-1 seropositive men. J Reprod Immunol 41:27–40

Dulioust E, Du AL, Costagliola D, Guibert J, Kunstmann JM, Heard I, Juillard JC, Salmon D, Leruez-Ville M, Mandelbrot L, Rouzioux C, Sicard D, Zorn JR, Jouannet P, De Almeida M (2002) Semen alterations in HIV-1 infected men. Hum Reprod 17:2112–2118

Dunne AL, Mitchell F, Allen KM, Baker HW, Garland S, Clarke GN, Mijch A, Crowe SM (2003) Analysis of HIV-1 viral load in seminal plasma samples. J Clin Virol 26:239–245

dXu C, Sun GF, Zhu YF, Wang YF (1997) The correlation of *Ureaplasma urealyticum* infection with infertility. Andrologia 29:219–226

Eggert-Kruse W, Gerhard I, Hofmann H, Runnebaum B, Petzoldt D (1987) Influence of microbial colonization on sperm-mucus interaction in vivo and in vitro. Hum Reprod 2:301–308

Eggert-Kruse W, Gerhard I, Naher H, Tilgen W, Runnebaum B (1990) Chlamydial infection – a female and/or male infertility factor? Fertil Steril 53:1037–1043

Eggert-Kruse W, Buhlinger-Gopfarth N, Rohr G, Probst S, Aufenanger J, Naher H, Runnebaum B (1996) Antibodies to *Chlamydia trachomatis* in semen and relationship with parameters of male fertility. Hum Reprod 11:1408–1417

Elsner P, Hartmann AA, Wecker I (1987) [Condylomata acuminata-associated STD infections of the urethra of the male. A comparative epidemiologic study]. Hautarzt 38:26–30

Englert Y, Lesage B, Van Vooren JP, Liesnard C, Place I, Vannin AS, Emiliani S, Delbaere A (2004) Medically assisted reproduction in the presence of chronic viral diseases. Hum Reprod Update 10:149–162

Erbengi T (1993) Ultrastructural observations on the entry of *Chlamydia trachomatis* into human spermatozoa. Hum Reprod 8:416–421

Ethics Committee of the American Society for Reproductive Medicine (2004) Human immunodeficiency virus and infertility treatment. Fertil Steril 82 (Suppl 1):S228–231

Fievet JP, Courbon X, Cazenave JC, Barnaud P (1987) [Urethral stricture in Africa. Urologic complication of sexually transmitted diseases in the male in Africa]. Med Trop (Mars) 47:265–272
Gall H, Beckert H, Meier-Ewert H, Tummers U, Pust RA, Peter RU (1999) [Pathogen spectrum of urethritis in the man]. Hautarzt 50:186–193
Garrido N, Meseguer M, Bellver J, Remohi J, Simon C, Pellicer A (2004) Report of the results of a 2 year programme of sperm wash and ICSI treatment for human immunodeficiency virus and hepatitis C virus serodiscordant couples. Hum Reprod 19:2581–2586
Glander HJ, Rytter M, Baumann L, Schonborn C (1986) Risk of transmission of sexually transmitted diseases by cryopreserved semen. Andrologia 18:323–325
Gonzales GF, Munoz G, Sanchez R, Henkel R, Gallegos-Avila G, Diaz-Gutierrez O, Vigil P, Vasquez F, Kortebani G, Mazzolli A, Bustos-Obregon E (2004) Update on the impact of *Chlamydia trachomatis* infection on male fertility. Andrologia 36:1–23
Green J, Monteiro E, Bolton VN, Sanders P, Gibson PE (1991) Detection of human papillomavirus DNA by PCR in semen from patients with and without penile warts. Genitourin Med 67:207–210
Habasque C, Aubry F, Jegou B, Samson M (2002) Study of the HIV-1 receptors CD4, CXCR4, CCR5 and CCR3 in the human and rat testis. Mol Hum Reprod 8:419–425
Hanabusa H, Kuji N, Kato S, Tagami H, Kaneko S, Tanaka H, Yoshimura Y (2000) An evaluation of semen processing methods for eliminating HIV-1. Aids 14:1611–1616
Hardon A (2003) Reproductive health care in The Netherlands: would integration improve it? Reprod Health Matters 11: 59–73
Hargreave TB, Harvey J, Elton RA, McMillan A (1984) Serum agglutinating and immobilising sperm antibodies in men attending a sexually transmitted diseases clinic. Andrologia 16:111–115
Heise H (2001) Gonorrhö. In: Petzoldt D, Gross G (eds) Diagnostik und Therapie sexuell übertragbarer Krankheiten. Springer, Berlin Heidelberg New York, pp 31–38
Hill AC (1990) Mycoplasmas, a review of surveys examining human genital infections and experimental infection in mice with special reference to in vitro fertilization. Lijec Vjesn 112:358–360
Hoffmann C, Kamps BS (2004) HIV.NET 2004. Steinhäuser
Hosseinzadeh S, Eley A, Pacey AA (2004) Semen quality of men with asymptomatic chlamydial infection. J Androl 25:104–109
Jansen HA, Morison L, Mosha F, Changalucha J, Todd J, Obasi A, Rusizoka M, Mayaud P, Munguti K, Mabey D, Grosskurth H, Hayes R (2003) Geographical variations in the prevalence of HIV and other sexually transmitted infections in rural Tanzania. Int J STD AIDS 14:274–280
Jensen TK, Keiding N, Scheike T, Slama R, Spira A (2000) Declining human fertility? Fertil Steril 73:421–423
Karinen L, Pouta A, Hartikainen AL, Bloigu A, Paldanius M, Leinonen M, Saikku P, Jarvelin MR (2004) Association between *Chlamydia trachomatis* antibodies and subfertility in the Northern Finland Birth Cohort 1966 (NFBC 1966), at the age of 31 years. Epidemiol Infect 132:977–984
Kaydos-Daniels SC, Miller WC, Hoffman I, Price MA, Martinson F, Chilongozi D, Namakwha D, Gama S, Phakati S, Cohen MS, Hobbs MM (2004) The use of specimens from various genitourinary sites in men, to detect *Trichomonas vaginalis* infection. J Infect Dis 189:1926–1931
Keck C, Gerber-Schafer C, Clad A, Wilhelm C, Breckwoldt M (1998) Seminal tract infections: impact on male fertility and treatment options. Hum Reprod Update 4:891–903
Kohl PK (2001) Urethritis des Mannes. In: Petzoldt D, Gross G (eds) Diagnostik und Therapie sexuell übertragbarer Krankheiten. Springer, Berlin Heidelberg New York, pp 119–125
Krause W, Bohring C (2003) Male infertility and genital chlamydial infection: victim or perpetrator? Andrologia 35:209–216
Krieger JN, Nirapathpongporn A, Chaiyaporn M, Peterson G, Nikolaeva I, Akridge R, Ross SO, Coombs RW (1998) Vasectomy and human immunodeficiency virus type 1 in semen. J Urol 159:820–825; discussion 825–826
Lai YM, Yang FP, Pao CC (1997) The effect of human papillomavirus infection on sperm motility in vitro. Fertil Steril 66:1152–1155
Mandelbrot L, Heard I, Henrion-Geant E, Henrion R (1997) Natural conception in HIV-negative women with HIV-infected partners. Lancet 349:850–851
Mardh PA (2004) Tubal factor infertility, with special regard to chlamydial salpingitis. Curr Opin Infect Dis 17:49–52
Martinez-Garcia F, Regadera J, Mayer R, Sanchez S, Nistal M (1996) Protozoan infections in the male genital tract. J Urol 156:340–349
Mastro TD, Kunanusont C, Dondero TJ, Wasi C (1997) Why do HIV-1 subtypes segregate among persons with different risk behaviors in South Africa and Thailand? Aids 11:113–116
McMillan A, Pakianathan M, Mao JH, Macintyre CC (1994) Urethral stricture and urethritis in men in Scotland. Genitourin Med 70:403–405
Meheus A, Reniers J, Colletet M (1986) Determinants of infertility in Africa. Afr J Sex Transmiss Dis 2:31–35
Mhawech P, Onorato M, Uchida T, Borucki MJ (2001) Testicular atrophy in 80 HIV-positive patients: a multivariate statistical analysis. Int J STD AIDS 12:221–224
Moskowitz MO, Mellinger BC (1992) Sexually transmitted diseases and their relation to male infertility. Urol Clin North Am 19:35–45
Muciaccia B, Filippini A, Ziparo E, Colelli F, Baroni CD, Stefanini M (1998a) Testicular germ cells of HIV-seropositive asymptomatic men are infected by the virus. J Reprod Immunol 41:81–93
Muciaccia B, Uccini S, Filippini A, Ziparo E, Paraire F, Baroni CD, Stefanini M (1998b) Presence and cellular distribution of HIV in the testes of seropositive subjects: an evaluation by in situ PCR hybridization. FASEB J 12:151–163
Muller CH, Coombs RW, Krieger JN (1998) Effects of clinical stage and immunological status on semen analysis results in human immunodeficiency virus type 1-seropositive men. Andrologia 30 (Suppl. 1):15–22
Ness RB, Markovic N, Carlson CL, Coughlin MT (1997) Do men become infertile after having sexually transmitted urethritis? An epidemiologic examination. Fertil Steril 68:205–213
Nicopoullos JD, Almeida PA, Ramsay JW, Gilling-Smith C (2004) The effect of human immunodeficiency virus on sperm parameters and the outcome of intrauterine insemination following sperm washing. Hum Reprod 19:2289–2297
Nuovo GJ, Becker J, Simsir A, Margiotta M, Khalife G, Shevchuk M (1994) HIV-1 nucleic acids localize to the spermatogonia and their progeny. A study by polymerase chain reaction in situ hybridization. Am J Pathol 144:1142–1148
Ochsendorf FR, Ozdemir K, Rabenau H, Fenner T, Oremek R, Milbradt R, Doerr HW (1999) Chlamydia trachomatis and male infertility: chlamydia-IgA antibodies in seminal plasma are *C. trachomatis* specific and associated with an inflammatory response. J Eur Acad Dermatol Venereol 12: 143–152

Ohl J, Partisani M, Wittemer C, Schmitt MP, Cranz C, Stoll-Keller F, Rongieres C, Bettahar-Lebugle K, Lang JM, Nisand I (2003) Assisted reproduction techniques for HIV serodiscordant couples: 18 months of experience. Hum Reprod 18:1244–1249

Okonofua FE, Ako-Nai KA, Dighitoghi MD (1995) Lower genital tract infections in infertile Nigerian women compared with controls. Genitourin Med 71:163–168

Olatunbosun OA, Chizen DR, Pierson RA (1998) Screening of potential semen donors for sexual transmitted diseases. West Afr J Med 17:19–24

Oldereid NB, Rui H, Purvis K (1992) The value of anamnestic information regarding previous genital infection in male fertility investigation. Eur J Obstet Gynecol Reprod Biol 47:207–212

Orroth KK, Korenromp EL, White RG, Changalucha J, de Vlas SJ, Gray RH, Hughes P, Kamali A, Ojwiya A, Serwadda D, Wawer MJ, Hayes RJ, Grosskurth H (2003) Comparison of STD prevalences in the Mwanza, Rakai, and Masaka trial populations: the role of selection bias and diagnostic errors. Sex Transm Infect 79:98–105

Osegbe DN (1991) Testicular function after unilateral bacterial epididymo-orchitis. Eur Urol 19:204–208

Osoba AO (1981) Sexually transmitted diseases in tropical Africa. A review of the present situation. Br J Vener Dis 57: 89–94

Paavonen J, Eggert-Kruse W (1999) *Chlamydia trachomatis*: impact on human reproduction. Hum Reprod Update 5: 433–447

Pakendorf UW, Bornman MS, Du Plessis DJ (1998) Prevalence of human papilloma virus in men attending the infertility clinic. Andrologia 30:11–14

Paranjpe S, Craigo J, Patterson B, Ding M, Barroso P, Harrison L, Montelaro R, Gupta P (2002) Subcompartmentalization of HIV-1 quasispecies between seminal cells and seminal plasma indicates their origin in distinct genital tissues. AIDS Res Hum Retroviruses 18:1271–1280

Passey M (1996) Issues in the management of sexually transmitted diseases in Papua New Guinea. P N G Med J 39: 252–260

Pena JE, Thornton MH Jr., Sauer MV (2003) Reversible azoospermia: anabolic steroids may profoundly affect human immunodeficiency virus-seropositive men undergoing assisted reproduction. Obstet Gynecol 101:1073–1075

Perez-Plaza M, Padron RS, Mas J, Peralta H (1982) Semen analyses in men with asymptomatic genital gonorrhoea. Int J Androl 5:6–10

Pilcher CD, Tien HC, Eron JJ, Jr., Vernazza PL, Leu SY, Stewart PW, Goh LE, Cohen MS (2004) Brief but efficient: acute HIV infection and the sexual transmission of HIV. J Infect Dis 189:1785–1792

Ping LH, Cohen MS, Hoffman I, Vernazza P, Seillier-Moiseiwitsch F, Chakraborty H, Kazembe P, Zimba D, Maida M, Fiscus SA, Eron JJ, Swanstrom R, Nelson JA (2000) Effects of genital tract inflammation on human immunodeficiency virus type 1 V3 populations in blood and semen. J Virol 74:8946–8952

Piomboni P, Baccetti B (2000) Spermatozoon as a vehicle for HIV-1 and other viruses: a review. Mol Reprod Dev 56: 238–242

Poretsky L, Can S, Zumoff B (1995) Testicular dysfunction in human immunodeficiency virus-infected men. Metabolism 44:946–953

Price MA, Zimba D, Hoffman IF, Kaydos-Daniels SC, Miller WC, Martinson F, Chilongozi D, Kip E, Msowoya E, Hobbs MM, Kazembe PN, Cohen MS (2003) Addition of treatment for trichomoniasis to syndromic management of urethritis in Malawi: a randomized clinical trial. Sex Transm Dis 30:516–522

Pudney J, Anderson D (1991) Orchitis and human immunodeficiency virus type 1 infected cells in reproductive tissues from men with the acquired immune deficiency syndrome. Am J Pathol 139:149–160

Pudney J, Nguyen H, Xu C, Anderson DJ (1998) Microscopic evidence against HIV-1 infection of germ cells or attachment to sperm. J Reprod Immunol 41:105–125

Radcliffe K (2001) European STD Guidelines. Internat J STD AIDS 12 (Suppl. 3):1–102

Reichart M, Kahane I, Bartoov B (2000) In vivo and in vitro impairment of human and ram sperm nuclear chromatin integrity by sexually transmitted *Ureaplasma urealyticum* infection. Biol Reprod 63:1041–1048

Rodriguez R, Hernandez R, Fuster F, Torres A, Prieto P, Alberto J (2001) [Genital infection and infertility]. Enferm Infecc Microbiol Clin 19:261–266

Schiefer HG (1998) Microbiology of male urethroadnexitis: diagnostic procedures and criteria for aetiologic classification. Andrologia 30 (Suppl. 1):7–13

Schlienger JL, Lang JM (1989) [Endocrine consequences of infection by human immunodeficiency virus (HIV)]. Pathol Biol (Paris) 37:921–926

Schulenburg GW, Bornman MS, Reif S, Bookmer D (1993) Semen profiles in infertile African males. In: Andrology in the nineties. International symposium on male infertility and assisted reproduction. Genk, Belgium. Wyeth, The Netherlands

Schuppe HC, Pichlmeier U, Schenk BI, Bottcher M (2003) Antibodies to Chlamydia trachomatis heat shock protein (cHSP60) and major outer membrane protein (MOMP) in men with impaired fertility. Clin Lab 49:273–275

Schurmeyer TH, Mueller V, von zur Muhlen V, Schmidt RE (1997) Endocrine testicular function in HIV-infected outpatients. Eur J Med Res 2:275–281

Segnini A, Camejo MI, Proverbio F (2003) *Chlamydia trachomatis* and sperm lipid peroxidation in infertile men. Asian J Androl 5:47–49

Semprini AE, Fiore S (2004) HIV and reproduction. Curr Opin Obstet Gynecol 16:257–262

Shahmanesh M, Stedronska J, Hendry WF (1986) Antispermatozoal antibodies in men with urethritis. Fertil Steril 46:308–311

Sherman JK, Rosenfeld J (1975) Importance of frozen-stored human semen in the spread of gonorrhea. Fertil Steril 26:1043–1047

Shevchuk MM, Nuovo GJ, Khalife G (1998) HIV in testis: quantitative histology and HIV localization in germ cells. J Reprod Immunol 41:69–79

Shevchuk MM, Pigato JB, Khalife G, Armenakas NA, Fracchia JA (1999) Changing testicular histology in AIDS: its implication for sexual transmission of HIV. Urology 53:203–208

Soffer Y, Ron-El R, Golan A, Herman A, Caspi E, Samra Z (1990) Male genital mycoplasmas and *Chlamydia trachomatis* culture: its relationship with accessory gland function, sperm quality, and autoimmunity. Fertil Steril 53:331–336

Sonnenberg-Schwan U (2004) HIV and wish for a child. In: Hoffman C, Kamps BS (eds) HIV.NET 2004. Steinhäuser, pp 589–594

Soper D (2004) Trichomoniasis: under control or undercontrolled? Am J Obstet Gynecol 190:281–290

Stone KM (1990) Avoiding sexually transmitted diseases. Obstet Gynecol Clin North Am 17:789–799

Sulak PJ (2003) Sexually transmitted diseases. Semin Reprod Med 21:399–413

Svenstrup HF, Fedder J, Abraham-Peskir J, Birkelund S, Christiansen G (2003) *Mycoplasma genitalium* attaches to human spermatozoa. Hum Reprod 18:2103–2109

Taylor-Robinson D (2002) *Mycoplasma genitalium* – an update. Int J STD AIDS 13:145–151

Tessler AN, Catanese A (1987) AIDS and germ cell tumors of testis. Urology 30:203–204
Trum JW, Pannekoek Y, Spanjaard L, Bleker OP, Van Der Veen F (2000) Accurate detection of male subclinical genital tract infection via cervical culture and DNA hybridization assay of the female partner. Int J Androl 23:43–45
Uuskula A, Kohl PK (2002) Genital mycoplasmas, including *Mycoplasma genitalium*, as sexually transmitted agents. Int J STD AIDS 13:79–85
Van Leeuwen E, Cornelissen M, De Vries JW, Lowe SH, Jurriaans S, Repping S, Van der Veen F (2004) Semen parameters of a semen donor before and after infection with human immunodeficiency virus. A case report. Hum Reprod 19:2845–2848
Vernazza PL, Troiani L, Flepp MJ, Cone RW, Schock J, Roth F, Boggian K, Cohen MS, Fiscus SA, Eron JJ (2000) Potent antiretroviral treatment of HIV-infection results in suppression of the seminal shedding of HIV. The Swiss HIV Cohort Study. Aids 14:117–121
Vicari E, Mongioi A, Speciale A, Caccamo F, Calogero A, Gulizia S, Pellegrino MB, Macchi M, D'Agata R (1986) Enhancing detection of gonococcus in ejaculates of adult males using sperm dilution. Arch Androl 16:19–23
Vicari E, Di Mauro C, Caruso V, Mongioi A (1991) [Antibiotic therapy in infertile subjects with chronic gonococcal infections: measurement of sperm output]. Arch Ital Urol Nefrol Androl 63:315–321
Vigil P, Morales P, Tapia A, Riquelme R, Salgado AM (2002) *Chlamydia trachomatis* infection in male partners of infertile couples: incidence and sperm function. Andrologia 34:155–161
Villette JM, Bourin P, Doimel C, Mansour I, Fiet J, Boudou P, Dreux C, Roue R, Debord M, Levi F (1990) Circadian variations in plasma levels of hypophyseal, adrenocortical and testicular hormones in men infected with human immunodeficiency virus. J Clin Endocrinol Metab 70:572–577
Watson EJ, Templeton A, Russell I, Paavonen J, Mardh PA, Stary A, Pederson BS (2002) The accuracy and efficacy of screening tests for *Chlamydia trachomatis*: a systematic review. J Med Microbiol 51:1021–1031
Weidner W, Krause W, Ludwig M (1999) Relevance of male accessory gland infection for subsequent fertility with special focus on prostatitis. Hum Reprod Update 5:431–432
Weidner W, Diemer T, Huwe P, Rainer H, Ludwig M (2002) The role of *Chlamydia trachomatis* in prostatitis. Int J Antimicrob Agents 19:466–470
Weigel M (2003) [German-Austrian guidelines for diagnosis and treatment of HIV-discordant couples who wish to have children]. Dtsch Med Wochenschr 128 (Suppl 1):S32–S35
Westrom LV (1994) Sexually transmitted diseases and infertility. Sex Transm Dis 21:S32–S37
Wilken H, Rosler EM (1985) [Prevention of sterility]. Zentralbl Gynakol 107:593–604
Williams CD, Finnerty JJ, Newberry YG, West RW, Thomas TS, Pinkerton JV (2003) Reproduction in couples who are affected by human immunodeficiency virus: medical, ethical, and legal considerations. Am J Obstet Gynecol 189:333–341
Witkin SS, Kligman I, Bongiovanni AM (1995a) Relationship between an asymptomatic male genital tract exposure to *Chlamydia trachomatis* and an autoimmune response to spermatozoa. Hum Reprod 10:2952–2955
Witkin SS, Kligman I, Grifo JA, Rosenwaks Z (1995b) *Ureaplasma urealyticum* and *Mycoplasma hominis* detected by the polymerase chain reaction in the cervices of women undergoing in vitro fertilization: prevalence and consequences. J Assist Reprod Genet 12:610–614
Wolff H, Neubert U, Zebhauser M, Bezold G, Korting HC, Meurer M (1991) *Chlamydia trachomatis* induces an inflammatory response in the male genital tract and is associated with altered semen quality. Fertil Steril 55:1017–1019
Workowski KA, Levine WC, Wasserheit JN (2002) U.S. Centers for Disease Control and Prevention guidelines for the treatment of sexually transmitted diseases: an opportunity to unify clinical and public health practice. Ann Intern Med 137:255–262
Wortley PM, Hammett TA, Fleming PL (1998) Donor insemination and human immunodeficiency virus transmission. Obstet Gynecol 91:515–518
Yoshikawa Y, Truong LW, Fraire AE, Kim HS (1989) The spectrum of histopathology in the testis in acquired immunodeficiency syndrome. Mod Pathol 2:233–238

II.2.5 Disorders of Blood Flow: Arterial and Venous/ Sexual Dysfunction and Varicocele

G. M. Colpi, M. Mancini, G. Piediferro, F. I. Scroppo

Summary

- Endothelial damage is the key disorder in vasculogenic organic erectile dysfunction (ED).
- Middle-aged men with ED should be screened for vasculogenic risk factors.
- Our improved understanding of endothelial damage will facilitate the development of a marker of endothelial damage, which, if developed, could have a significant impact on the diagnosis of men's vascular disorders.
- Varicocele alters the dynamics of testicular circulation and this, in turn, damages spermatogenesis and endocrine function of the testis.
- In cases of testicular torsion there is reduced blood flow in the contralateral side due to a sympathetic reflex arising from the testicular artery under distress.
- Anomalies of testicular circulation are six times more frequent in men who have had orchiopexy for testicular maldescent compared with normal men. Although some of this may be intrinsic some of this vascular damage is iatrogenic.

II.2.5.1 Erectile Dysfunction and Vascular Disease

II.2.5.1.1 Summary

Vascular penile dysfunction has been attributed to reduced arterial inflow and excessive venous leakage but the role of venous leakage in the aetiology is now doubted. Reduced arterial inflow may be both the cause and consequence of endothelial damage. Endothelial function impairment is one of the initiating events in atherosclerosis. So far, no reliable marker of early endothelial damage has been validated in erectile dysfunction (ED). At present, risk factors are the most important elements for identifying men with early atherosclerosis.

II.2.5.1.2 Pathogenesis of Penile Vascular Damage

A multifactorial origin is now generally accepted for ED. In many ED patients, the main cause is vascular disease. Vascular involvement is ultimately due to mechanical and biochemical factors.

Arterial flow in cavernosal arteries is crucial in order to obtain a good erection. To support this mechanism, luminal, endothelial and muscular integrity are essential. Thereafter, trabecular tissue relaxation is regulated by paracrine contracting and relaxing factors. Finally, penile pressure should be counterbalanced by the albuginea wall, leading to venous compression. Arterial flow loss results in venous leakage.

Although smooth muscle loss was found in men classified as having venous leakage (Nehra et al. 1996) it is now thought that venous leakage is a consequence of vasculogenic ED rather than a causative factor.

Conversely, atherosclerotic damage of penile large vessels resulting in blood flow loss and pressure decline in corpora cavernosa has been shown as a pathogenetic mechanism. Trabecular fibrosis with reduced numbers of elastic fibres and increased collagen compounds hinder rigid erection (Persson et al. 1989; Jevtich et al. 1990; Wespes et al. 1991). The ultrastructural changes occurring within the corpora cavernosa are similar to what is observed in the wall of the thinnest penile arteries (Ferrini et al. 2004). Ischaemic processes increase reactive oxygen species (ROS), stimulating transforming growth factor-β_1 (TGF-β_1) accumulation and fibroblastic proliferation.

The main factor counterbalancing this phenomenon is production of inducible nitric oxide synthase (iNOS) by smooth muscle cells (SMCs). Nitric oxide (NO) scavenges ROS, thus inhibiting collagen deposition. The damage caused by atherosclerosis results in this protective role being lost.

Therefore, arterial flow decline initiates histological and functional damage, and is the key disorder to be searched for in organic ED. Vascular damage may involve both large and small vessels.

II.2.5.1.3 Large and Small Vessel Damage

Involvement of large vessels in atherosclerosis is part of the extensive structural damage caused to the penile shaft.

In the past, slowly progressive ED was considered to be typical of vascular disease.

As early as 1988, Little and coworkers had shown that obstructive damage of small lower limb arteries correlated with increased risk of myocardial infarction.

Cavernosal arteries, the most important functional vessels in the penis, have a smaller diameter than coronary arteries (1–2 mm and 3–4 mm, respectively). In the presence of systemic atherosclerosis, a critical obstruction (>50%) of cavernosal arteries can become symptomatic as ED, at first without any thoracic discomfort. Therefore, ED could be the first marker of atherosclerosis, preceding cardiac or limb symptoms. Sixty-seven per cent of patients with coronary artery disease experienced some ED more than 3 years before their heart disease (Montorsi et al. 2003). Moreover, even only partially impaired penile arterial circulation is thought to be bound to evolve into severe permanent ED. Pritzker (1999) presented penile circulation as a window to the hearts of men.

The wide variability of peak systolic velocities in the different segments of the penile arterial tree means that the latter must be studied by careful echo Doppler ultrasound investigation, which can also identify any damage in small vessels. Observation of the latter and their variations over time is crucial in order to understand the state of health of the penile circulation. Measurement of cavernosal peak systolic velocity in a flaccid state can still be predictive of vascular damage, to be confirmed by dynamic echo Doppler (Mancini et al. 2000a, b). Reduced penile arterial ramification and increased vascular communications between dorsal and cavernosal arteries are reported to be markers of initial damage (Mancini et al. 1996; Sarteschi et al. 1998).

Ischaemia and reperfusion phenomena may modify the circulation, especially in a dynamic structure such as the penis. This was also confirmed following chronic treatments with vasodilators, which may promote circulation remodelling (Mancini et al. 2004).

Vascular damage is a dynamic process, and for diagnosing early changes markers of endothelial function are needed, as these early changes cannot be detected with echo Doppler ultrasound. Damage to the endothelium is caused by inflammatory processes and these result in plaque formation. Thus plaque evolution is the result of the interaction of various inflammatory mediators. The vascular endothelium has a fast metabolism, with high oxygen consumption (Intaglietta et al. 1996; Tsai et al. 1998). Recently, uric acid was considered important in reducing endothelial remodelling and nitric oxide production (Kanellis and Kang 2005).

II.2.5.1.4 Endothelial Damage

For artery dilatability, a cornerstone role is played by normal endothelial function. Endothelial cell activation is one of the initiating events in atherosclerosis. Some systemic diseases are classically linked to ED. Hypertension, hyperlipidaemia and hypogonadism are strong predictors of ED (Barrett-Connor 2004; Corona et al. 2004; Fung et al. 2004). They all target and damage the vascular tree, and act through endothelial damage.

The main actors are endothelin and nitric oxide. Endothelin-1 was found to be increased in ED, and in the presence of cardiovascular risk factors compared to control men (Bocchio et al. 2004).

NOS is essential for vascular activation. An improved erection was obtained by elevating intracavernosal NOS by L-arginine administration (Gonzales-Cadavid and Rajfer 2000).

In hypercholesterolaemic men, lower cholesterol levels improved erectile function (Saltzman et al. 2004). NO production seems to be the main factor responsible for this effect. NO-dependent vasodilatation was obtained in hypercholesterolaemic patients with critical limb ischaemia after L-arginine administration (Bode-Boger et al. 1996).

Experimental internal iliac arterial ligation in rats decreased the number of nerve fibres containing neuronal NOS (Li et al. 2004).

In hypertensive rats, neurogenic vascular relaxation following electrical stimulation was also reduced. Impaired neurogenic NO release was hypothesized (Ushiyama et al. 2004).

The involvement of K(ATP) channels in penile artery relaxation also suggests a possible role – in hypertensive or diabetic patients – for the drugs that are used in these diseases (i.e. glibenclamide or some diuretics), which can modify blood potassium (Ruiz Rubio 2004).

In vascular physiology, a new role seems to be played by testosterone. The ability of cavernosal arteries to dilate was reduced in neurogenic or vasculogenic impotent men, and this appears to be linked to bio-available testosterone (Virag et al. 2004). Circulating testosterone modulates central and peripheral triggers, promoting erection. In hypogonadic men, testosterone supplementation improves arterial blood flow in cavernosal arteries as recorded by echo Doppler ultrasound (Cavallini et al. 2004; Foresta 2004).

To obtain this result, functional integrity of the vascular endothelium is essential. The importance of endocrine factors in the penis was confirmed by Vignozzi et al. (2005), who described reduced immunolocalization of phosphodiesterase type 5 (PDE5) in the human penis in hypogonadotrophic hypogonadism.

In conclusion, cavernosal insufficiency and metabolic disorders lead to a common pathogenetic factor, i.e. endothelial disruption. More than 92.1% of patients with ED present at least one risk factor for atherosclerosis (El Sakka et al. 2004). Early diagnosis of metabolic disease causing ED could be a very cost-effective method of identifying men at risk for coronary artery occlusion. At present there is no validated marker for endothelial damage and the best that can be done is to screen men according to risk factors. However, if a validated endothelial marker could be developed then this could provide longer lead times for the instigation of effective treatment to modify risk and improve both penile and cardiac circulation. Our improved understanding of the mechanisms of vasculogenic ED holds the promise that such markers will be identified.

II.2.5.2 Varicocele

II.2.5.2.1 Summary

There is general agreement concerning varicocele-induced spermatogenetic damage and consequently impaired semen quality. The main pathophysiological theories currently relate to alterations in temperature, haemodynamics, and reactive oxidative species and antioxidant concentrations. The key connections between vascular abnormalities and their gonadal effects seem to be endocrine and genetic.

II.2.5.2.2 Pathogenesis of Varicocele

Varicocele usually occurs on the left because of the anatomical predisposition of the internal spermatic vein, which, on this side, drains into the renal vein at right angle, thus being exposed to an increase in venous pressure. Varicocele occurs in 15% (8–23%) of the general population (Chan and Goldstein 2002). It has been suggested that varicocele should be considered as a bilateral disease because of its high bilateral prevalence (80.7%) (Gat et al. 2004). Pathogenetic factors are still under debate (Hargreave 1993) and the following possibilities must be mentioned:

A. Theory by Coolsaet (1980)

This theory is based on the association between the lack of competent valves and the "nutcracker phenomenon" (which is created when a vein passes at the level of the origin of an artery) proximally (type I, effect of the origin of the superior mesenteric artery on the left renal vein), distally (type II, effect of the left common iliac artery on the left common iliac vein), or in a mixed site (type III, combination of the two previous ones). Flow reduction in the proximal segment of the left renal vein correlates with the reduction of the aortomesenteric angle, thus confirming the proximal nutcracker phenomenon theory: flow reversal during the Valsalva manoeuvre occurs in veins of diameter >3 mm, which are statistically associated with a reduction in the superior aortomesenteric angle (Graif et al. 2000). Pallwein et al. (2001) underlined the high frequency of the proximal nutcracker phenomenon, as detected by echo Doppler ultrasound of the renal vein and pampiniform plexus in recurrent varicoceles.

B. Theory by Sigmund et al. (1987)

By examining patients with varicocele using bidirectional echo Doppler ultrasound, clinical examination and retrograde venography, Sigmund distinguished two haemodynamic types of reflux: "stop-type" (where reflux is blocked by competent valves above communicating veins in the plexus) and "shunt-type" (where reflux falls below communicating veins because of valvular incompetence, and therefore blood flows into the cremasteric and deferential veins).

C. Theory by Shafik (1991)

Whatever the primary cause, it is venous hypertension that originates the changes found in spermatic veins. Three stages are identified:

1. "Compensated stage", where veins react to a hypertensive state by thickening their walls without dilating, and there is no venous stasis because of the good propulsion mechanism created by muscular hypertrophy of the tunica media.
2. "Concealed stage", where the muscular wall of the tunica media collapses, although no varicosity is developed.
3. "Manifest varicocele", where venous hypertension will cause hyalinization of the venous wall, with development of varicosity.

D. Puberty-Induced Arteriovenous Discrepancy

Puberty-induced arteriovenous discrepancy in the testicular region.

E. Presence of Anastomoses

Presence of anastomoses between the internal spermatic artery and the vena cava, and/or the common iliac vein, and/or the capsular veins of the kidney, and/or the renal vein, while the hypothesized arteriovenous anastomoses between the testicular artery and pampiniform plexus are interpreted as vasa vasorum upon electron microscopy.

F. Venous Drainage Obstruction

Venous drainage obstruction from a retroperitoneal mass.

II.2.5.2.3 Vessel-Induced Spermatogenetic Damage

The pathophysiological theory of the damage to spermatogenesis induced by varicocele currently relates to hyperthermia of the scrotum (Zorgniotti 1980), resulting from a slow down in testicular and peritesticular blood flow. A high intratesticular temperature causes partial or complete spermatogenetic arrest and may lead to increased production of morphologically abnormal sperm with impaired motility (Dada et al. 2003).

The degree of scrotal hyperthermia is not related to the calibre of the varicocele, but to its intrascrotal passage: a varicocele confined to the spermatic cord will lead to scarcely detrimental circumscribed hyperthermia, while a peritesticular varicocele will lead to generalized hyperthermia of the scrotum (Hamm et al. 1986). These observations were confirmed by studies conducted during varicocele microsurgery by means of microcirculation flowmetry and testicular temperature measurements by microsensors (Tritto et al. 2001).

From a clinical point of view, measuring the reflux to the testes that increases with intra-abdominal pressure – classified as type III reflux – is a diagnostic criterion in order to prevent misdiagnosis of a varicocele and unnecessary surgery (Tashi et al. 2001), as suggested by the evidence that normal-sized testicular veins in healthy subjects show a remarkably high incidence of reflux induced by the Valsalva manoeuvre (Kocakoc et al. 2001). Stagnation of blood in microcirculation vessels may cause local hypoxia and ischaemia, which lead to spermatogenic disorders (Chakraborty et al. 1985) and may also induce increased testicular vascular permeability, as shown by the volume density percentages of polymorphonuclear leukocytes per testicular blood vessel (Salama et al. 2003). These data suggest the importance of hydrostatic pressure in the pathogenesis of varicocele-induced testicular damage.

In addition, Tarhan et al. (2003) showed significantly decreased testicular arterial blood flow in men with varicocele, as well as significant positive correlations between left testicular artery blood flow, sperm concentration and left testicular volume. Following decreased testicular arterial blood flow, impaired spermatogenesis may result from defective metabolism in the microcirculatory bed. In grade 3 varicoceles, significantly increased vasoconstrictive reactivity and decreased endothelial function were shown as compared to grade 1 varicoceles, indicating that endothelial dysfunction develops at high grades of varicocele (Yildiz et al. 2003). In surgically induced varicocele, microvascular testicular blood flow dropped, and its vasomotion was inhibited once the left renal vein was partially ligated, as studied by laser Doppler flowmetry (Salama et al. 2001).

II.2.5.2.4 Vessel-Induced Endocrine and Genetic Damage

Higher scrotal temperature was shown to be accompanied by reduced Leydig cell density and Sertoli cell hypofunction (Rodriguez-Rigau et al. 1978), and these negative effects increased depending on varicocele duration and severity.

Testosterone synthesis, whose role in spermatogenesis is well known, is blocked in some particular enzymatic steps, as shown by an increased 17-hydroxyprogesterone:testosterone ratio (Hampl et al. 1992). Decreased synthesis is accompanied by an even weaker local action of testosterone, due to decreased production of androgen binding protein in hyperthermic conditions (Hagenas et al. 1978). This reduced synthesis and local binding of testosterone is thought to be further fostered by a reduction in luteinizing hormone (LH) receptors on Leydig cells, which is induced by varicoceles as a function of time (Kazama 1995).

Furthermore, studies on the DNA of varicocele patients showed higher meiotic non-disjunction rates in both seminal fluid and testicular biopsy samples. DNA damage appears to be related to high levels of seminal ROS and lower total antioxidant capacity (Saleh et al. 2003) due to biological and clinical changes such as impaired microcirculation, venous stasis, hypoxia, leukocyte activation, and cellular necrosis (Mazzilli et al. 1994).

The hypothesis that renal and adrenal metabolites enhance varicocele-induced testicular damage has also been taken into account: the flow of retrograde adrenal metabolites itself is responsible for increased follicle-stimulating hormone (FSH) levels, decreased testosterone levels and structural abnormalities upon testicular histology (Camoglio et al. 2004).

II.2

II.2.5.3 Testicular Torsion

II.2.5.3.1 Summary

Testicular torsion is a urologic emergency caused by twisting of the spermatic cord which, if not treated promptly, results in ischaemic necrosis of the testis that may even require orchiectomy. It is also responsible for parenchymal changes in the contralateral testis. In response to ischaemia, acute biochemical changes appear in both gonads within the first hour. Consequently, semen anomalies occur in nearly 25% of affected patients. Prompt diagnosis and emergency exploration of the scrotum within 6 h increase the chances of saving the twisted testis.

II.2.5.3.2 Oxidative Stress

Spermatic cord torsion is also responsible for reduced blood supply and lower relative oxygen content in the contralateral testis, albeit to a lesser extent (Salman et al. 1998); this is due to a sympathetic reflex arising from the testicular artery under distress (Karaguzel et al. 1994; Salman et al. 1997). The extent of the ischaemic damage depends on the degree of artery compression, and the lapse of time between the event and surgical correction. Several authors have tried to determine a minimum time of damage, often using animal models. During a 720-degree spermatic cord torsion in adult male rats, ipsilateral arterial flow was reduced by 94%, and 1 h of ischaemia alone is sufficient to cause a marked reduction in spermatogenesis in the twisted testis (Turner and Brown 1993). A flow reduction also occurs in the contralateral internal spermatic artery, and can be quantified at around 40% 2 h after torsion. In an attempt to reduce hydraulic resistance, vasomotion of the microcirculation of the contralateral testis is increased (Kolettis et al. 1996). In response to ischaemia, acute biochemical changes that are the expression of oxidative stress, such as increased lactic acid, hypoxanthine and lipid peroxidation product levels, appear in both gonads as early as in the first hour (Akgur et al. 1993, 1994), while the activities of the free radical scavenger enzymes superoxide dismutase (SOD) and catalase start to decrease. A significant increase in glutathione-s-transferase and hydrogen peroxide levels in rat testes occurs after 6 h of ischaemia in the twisted testis, and after 24 h in the contralateral (untwisted) testis; histology shows changes such as a high proportion of collapsed arterioles, thickening of the basement membrane, tubular fibrosis, reduced Johnsen score and ultrastructural changes in Leydig cells (Ciftci et al. 1997; Savas et al. 2002). Cell apoptosis increases from 1 h to 24 h of ischaemia, and this phenomenon is clearly connected with oxidative stress. In the first 6 h of ischaemia, all types of germ cells, without distinction, are subjected to it. As ischaemia continues, it affects predominantly spermatids and spermatocytes, and damage progresses centrifugally, starting from the seminiferous tubules located centrally within the gonad (Chaki et al. 2003).

II.2.5.3.3 Ischaemia-Reperfusion Injury

Following detorsion, blood flow to both testes is significantly increased, which gives rise to what is referred to as "ischaemia–reperfusion injury" (Nguyen et al. 1999; Filho et al. 2004). Different mechanisms are involved, but an essential role is played by lipid peroxidation of plasma membranes; this is caused by overproduction of ROS, which are generated in particular during reperfusion. Following unilateral testicular torsion, the extent of the contralateral reperfusion injury, as measured in terms of SOD and catalase activities, is also dependent on the time elapsed from twisting, and, in adult male Wistar rats, it takes on significant values after 6 h. The stages of the spermatogenetic cycle that are most sensitive to the effects of testicular torsion on the contralateral testis are stages IV–XI, i.e. those associated with low antioxidant capabilities (Vigueras et al. 2004). The role of orchiectomy would be to provide protection from contralateral histological changes due to reperfusion, and some authors stress the importance of removing a damaged testis in order to minimize any repercussions on fertility (Sarica et al. 1997). In order to minimize membrane peroxidation due to reperfusion, vitamin E-like oxidants – to be given in the acute phase – are also being studied (Romeo et al. 2004).

II.2.5.3.4 Clinical Evidence

Prompt diagnosis and emergency exploration of the scrotum increase the chances of saving the twisted testis, and 6 h is the time limit within which the testis is usually still viable, and orchiectomy can be avoided (Granados et al. 1998a, b; Della Negra et al. 2000; Shergill et al. 2002).

After 6 h from the onset of painful symptoms, irreversible infarction may result, and the need to perform orchiectomy is higher after 6 – 12 h. Within this lapse of time, orchiectomy becomes necessary in 17% of patients (Granados et al. 1998a, b). After 12 h, the chances of finding a viable testis decline dramatically, and testicular loss rate is up to 100% (Jefferson et al. 1997). After 24 h of torsion, the chances of finding a viable testis are very small, and do not exceed 5% in extensive case records (Nakajima et al. 1985; Hegarty et al. 2001). After 48 h, there is virtually no such possibility, and orchiectomy is necessary.

Anecdotally, cases of twisted testes being saved after longer periods of time – such as 7 days (Barbalias and Liatsikos 1999) or more – are reported in literature, but these are likely to be subtorsion episodes.

II.2.5.4 Undescended Testis

II.2.5.4.1 Summary

Early surgery has been proposed as a possibility to prevent spermatogenesis impairment. Poor fertility may occur not only following primary parenchymal degenerative change of the testis, but also as a consequence of gonadal blood flow disorder. Ischaemia – whether surgically induced, resulting from spermatic cord subtorsion, or due to altered tissue perfusion – will cause ipsilateral and contralateral oxidative stress.

II.2.5.4.2 Introduction

"Undescended testis" (UT) is found in 2 – 4% of boys born at term, and in approximately 1% of boys at the age of 1 year (Barthold and Gonzales 2003). As foetal development progresses, testes move from the first lumbar segment in a caudal direction together with the vas deferens, epididymis and spermatic vessels. From the 3rd to the 7th months, testes are situated by or in the proximity of the deep inguinal ring. Migration of testes into the scrotum occurs within the 8th month of intrauterine life. Possible causes of UT include: decreased intra-abdominal pressure, no or too long a gubernaculum testis, congenital defects of the testis, endocrine and environmental factors, anomalies of the genitofemoral nerve.

II.2.5.4.3 Consequences of Undescended Testes

Men with uni- or bi-lateral UT have a lower sperm count, poorer ejaculate quality and worse fertility rates than control groups (Kogan 1987; Yavetz et al. 1992). Eighty-nine percent of untreated patients with bilateral cryptorchidism develop azoospermia (Hadziselimovic 2002; Weidner et al. 2002). The histological hallmarks associated with UT become evident between the first and second years of life, and include tubules with a reduced diameter, a small germ cell population, defective germ cell maturation, polynuclear germ cells, peritubular fibrosis, seminiferous tubule sertolization, reduced number of Leydig cells, acrosomal deformity and Leydig cell vacuolization (Cortes et al. 1996; Huff et al. 2001; Rusnack et al. 2003). These changes can be detected in other pathological conditions, such as prolonged hyperthermia and experimental ischaemia, and are present in the spontaneously descended contralateral testis as well, albeit to a lesser extent.

II.2.5.4.4
Iatrogenic Ischaemia

Whatever the technique used for orchidopexy, adequate intratesticular blood flow needs to be preserved in order to maintain normal gonadal volume. Foetal testes are always supplied by at least two arteries – the testicular artery (primary) and the deferential artery (a branch of the inferior vesical artery) – and in 80% of cases by three or four arteries, including a possible repeat of the latter ones and the cremasteric artery (Sampayo et al. 1999). Testicular vessel dissection can cause testicular atrophy due to ischaemia. The incidence of this complication ranges from 8% for distally UT to as high as 25% for upper intra-abdominal testes, with higher risks for those techniques which involve high internal spermatic artery ligation (Docimo 1995). Poor blood supply to testes may accidentally result as a consequence of excessive spermatic cord dissection and cauterization, or spermatic vessel subtorsion following incorrect testis fixation inside the scrotum, or spermatic vessel ligation and division during Fowler-Stephens orchiopexy. Excessive axial tension of spermatic vessels and predominantly of the deferential artery, as a result of testicular traction following surgery, is an additional risk factor (Jarow 1991).

Experimentally, in prepubertal rats, spermatic artery and vein ligation causes an 18% reduction in blood flow to the testis (Pascual et al. 1990). Some authors observed that testicular artery ligation – still in rats – is accompanied by histological changes of the testis resulting in infertility (Kokoua et al. 2004). In men who underwent orchiopexy in childhood, anomalies of the testicular artery, as assessed by colour Doppler ultrasound, are found six times more frequently than for the artery of the spontaneously descended contralateral testis (Taskinen et al. 1996). Therefore, infertility in subjects with a history of UT could be ascribable not only to the well-known intrinsic damage of the dysgenetic gonad, but also to vascular injury during orchiopexy.

II.2.5.4.5
Ischaemia Due To Spermatic Cord Torsion

Previously some authors have reported that twisting of the spermatic cord is more frequent in UT than in testes that are regularly located in the scrotum (Schultz and Walker 1984). This event leads to acute ischaemia and, in UT, occurs more frequently in the intrauterine period. In newborn males with UT showing signs and symptoms of prenatal testicular torsion and undergoing exploratory emergency surgery, testicles are unviable and gangrenous in almost all cases, and orchiectomy is necessary (Herzog et al. 1987; Brandt et al. 1992).

Therefore, prenatal ischaemia results in testicular atrophy, a condition that is commonly referred to as absent testis. Whether monorchidism is the result of torsion, endocrinopathy, or other causes is an unrecognized fact, and only surgical exploration can help define its aetiology (Turek et al. 1994). Approximately 20% of undescended testes are not palpable, and the lack of a gonad is confirmed upon surgical exploration in about one-fifth of cases, in which, however, blind-ending cord structures such as vas, epididymis, fibrous/vascular tissue and small amounts of seminiferous tubules with germinal elements can be found up to 90% of the time (Lamesch 1994; Turek et al. 1994; Merry et al. 1997). The presence of Wolffian structures is evidence that the ipsilateral testis was present until at least the 16th week of gestation, vanishing at some point following induction of masculinization as a result of an intrauterine vascular accident or testicular torsion, more than twice as frequently as true testicular agenesis (Merry et al. 1997).

II.2.5.4.6
Ischaemia and Oxidative Stress

Experimental cryptorchidism in animal models shows that the UT is the site of changes that are typical of oxidative stress, which is attributable to absolute or relative tissue hypoxia as a consequence of the increased metabolic requirement of the hyperthermic gonad (Peltola et al 1995). In adult rat testes with surgically induced maldescent, there is an increase in lactic acid, hypoxanthines and the lipid peroxidation level that results from overproduction of free oxygen radicals secondary to ischaemia (Karnak et al. 1996a, b; Peltola et al. 1995). Moreover, a reduction in antioxidant enzyme levels, mainly Cu/Zn SOD, was documented; this is the expression of damage to the detoxifying ability of ROS (Ahotupa and Huhtaniemi 1992; Zini and Schlegel 1997).

In rats that were made unilaterally cryptorchid, clues of contralateral ischaemia such as an increase in lactic acid and hypoxanthines, besides a decrease in mean seminiferous tubular diameter, were observed – similarly to what happens in testicular torsion; however, this topic remains disputed (Karnak et al. 1996a, b). Unfortunately, the use of colour Doppler ultrasound to assess blood flow in UT is hampered by the small calibre of vessels and the relatively slow flows, in terms of both peak systolic velocity and end diastolic velocity. In these cases, impedance of the testicular artery, measured as the resistive index (RI), is the most reliable parameter. The testicular artery in UT has a significantly lower RI compared to the regularly located contralateral testis used as a control; histologically, this corresponds to a worse testicular biopsy score (Atilla et al. 1997).

References

Ahotupa M, Huhtaniemi I (1992) Impaired detoxification of reactive oxygen and consequent oxidative stress in experimental cryptorchid rat testis. Biol Reprod 46:1114–1118

Akgur FM, Kilinc K, Aktug T (1993) Reperfusion injury after detorsion of unilateral testicular torsion. Urol Res 21:395–399

Akgur FM, Kilinc K, Tanyel FC, Buyukpamukcu N, Hicsonmez A (1994) Ipsilateral and contralateral testicular biochemical acute changes after unilateral testicular torsion and detorsion. Urology 44:413–418

Atilla MK, Sargin H, Yilmaz Y, Odabas O, Keskin A, Aydin S (1997) Undescended testes in adults: clinical significance of resistive index values of the testicular artery measured by Doppler ultrasound as a predictor of testicular histology. J Urol 158:841–843

Barbalias GA, Liatsikos EN (1999) Testicular torsion: can the testicle be saved one week later? Int Urol Nephrol 31:247–251

Barrett-Connor E (2004) Cardiovascular risk stratification and cardiovascular risk factors associated with erectile dysfunction: assessing cardiovascular risk in men with erectile dysfunction. Clin Cardiol 27 (4 Suppl 1): I8–I13

Barthold JS, Gonzales R (2003) The epidemiology of congenital cryptorchidism, testicular ascent and orchiopexy. J Urol 170:2396–2401

Bocchio M, Desideri G, Scarpelli P, Necozione S, Properzi G, Spartera C, Francavilla F, Ferri C, Francavilla S (2004) Endothelial cell activation in men with erectile dysfunction without cardiovascular risk factors and overt vascular damage. J Urol 171:1601–1604

Bode-Boger SM, Boger RH, Alfke H, Heinzel D, Tsikas D, Creutzig A, Alexander K, Frolich JC (1996) L-Arginine induces nitric oxide dependent vasodilation in patients with critical limb ischemia. Circulation 93:85–90

Brandt MT, Sheldon CA, Wacksman J, Matthews P (1992) Prenatal testicular torsion: principles of management. J Urol 147:670–672

Camoglio FS, Zampieri N, Corroppolo M, Chironi C, Dipaola G, Giacomello L, Ottolenghi A (2004) Varicocele and retrograde adrenal metabolites flow. An experimental study on rats. Urol Int 73(4):337–342

Cavallini G, Caracciolo S, Vitali G, Modenini F, Biagiotti G (2004) Carnitine versus androgen administration in the treatment of sexual dysfunction, depressed mood, and fatigue associated with male aging. Urology 63:641–646

Chaki SP, Ghosh D, Misro MM (2003) Simultaneous increase in germ apoptosis and oxidative stress under acute unilateral testicular ischaemia in rats. Int J Androl 26:319–328

Chakraborty J, Hikim AP, Jhunjhunwala JS (1985) Stagnation of blood in the microcirculatory vessels in the testes of men with varicocele. J Androl 6(2):117–126

Chan PT, Goldstein M (2002) Medical backgrounder on varicocele. Drugs Today (Barc) 38:59–67

Ciftci AO, Muftuoğlu S, Cakar N, Tanyel FC (1997) Histological evidence of decreased contralateral testicular blood flow during ipsilateral testicular torsion. Br J Urol 80:783–786

Coolsaet BLRA (1980) The varicocele syndrome: venography determining the optimal level for surgical management. J Urol 124:833–839

Corona G, Mannucci E, Mansani R, Petrone L, Bartolini M, Giommi R, Mancini M, Forti G, Maggi M (2004) Aging and pathogenesis of erectile dysfunction. Int J Impot Res 16: 395–402

Cortes D, Thorup JM, Lindenberg S (1996) Fertility potential after unilateral orchiopexy: simultaneous testicular biopsy and orchiopexy in a cohort of 87 patients. J Urol 155:1061–1065

Dada R, Gupta NP, Kucheria K (2003) Spermatogenic arrest in men with testicular hyperthermia. Teratog Carcinog Mutagen Suppl 1:235–243

Della Negra E, Martin M, Bernardini S, Bittard H (2000) Spermatic cord torsion in adults. Prog Urol 10:265–270

Docimo SG (1995) The results of surgical therapy for cryptorchidism: a literature review and analysis. J Urol 154:1148–1152

El Sakka AI, Morsy AM, Fagih BI, Nassar AH (2004) Coronary artery risk factors in patients with erectile dysfunction. J Urol 172:251–254

Ferrini MG, Davila HH, Valente EG, Gonzalez-Cadavid NF, Rajfer J (2004) Aging-related induction of inducible nitric oxide synthase is vasculoprotective to the arterial media. Cardiovasc Res 61:796–805

Filho DW, Torres MA, Bordin AL, Crezcynski-Pasa TB, Boveris A (2004) Spermatic cord torsion and nitrogen species and ischemia-reperfusion injury. Mol Aspects Med 25:199–210

Foresta C, Caretta N, Rossato M, Garolla A, Ferlin A (2004) Role of androgens in erectile function. J Urol 171:2358–2362

Fung MM, Bettencourt R, Barrett-Connor E (2004) Heart disease risk factors predict erectile dysfunction 25 years later: the Rancho Bernardo Study. J Am Coll Cardiol 43:1405–1411

Gat Y, Bachar GN, Zukerman Z, Belenky A, Gornish M (2004) Varicocele: a bilateral disease. Fertil Steril 8:424–429

Gonzalez-Cadavid NF, Rajfer J (2000) Therapeutic stimulation of penile oxide synthase and related pathways. Drugs Today 36:163–174

Graif M, Hauser R, Hirshebein A, Botchan A, Kessler A, Yabetz H (2000) Varicocele and the testicular-renal venous route: hemodynamic Doppler sonographic investigation. J Ultrasound Med 19:627–631

Granados EA, Caicedo P, Garat JM (1998a) Testicular torsion between 6 and 12 hours. I. Arch Esp Urol 51:971–974

Granados EA, Caicedo P, Garat JM (1998b) Testicular torsion between 6 and 12 hours. II. Arch Esp Urol 51:975–977

Hadziselimovic F (2002) Cryptorchidism, its impact on male fertility. Eur Urology 41:121–123

Hagenas L, Ritzen EM, Svennson J, Hansson J, Hansson V, Purvis K (1978) Temperature dependence of Sertoli cell function. Int J Androl 2:449–453

Hamm B, Fobbe F, Sorensen R, Felsemberg D (1986) Varicoceles: combined sonography and thermography in diagnosis and posttherapeutic evaluation. Radiology 160:419–424

Hampl R, Lachman M, Novack Z (1992) Serum levels of steroid hormones in men with varicocele and oligospermia as compared to normozoospermic men. Exp Clin Endocrinol 100: 119

Hargreave TB (1993) Varicocele: a clinical enigma. Br J Urol 72:401–408

Hegarty PK, Walsh E, Corcoran MO (2001) Exploration of the acute scrotum: a retrospective analysis of 100 consecutive cases. Ir J Med Sci 170:181–182

Herzog B, Hadziselimovic F, Strebel C (1987) Primary and secondary testicular atrophy. Eur J Pediatr 146 (Suppl 2):S53–S55

Huff DS, Fenig DM, Canning DA, Carr MG, Zderic SA, Snyder HM 3rd (2001) Abnormal germ cell development in cryptorchidism. Horm Res 55:11–17

Intaglietta M, Johnson PC, Winslow RM (1996) Microvascular and tissue oxygen distribution. Cardiovasc Res 32:632–643

Jarow JP (1991) Clinical significance of intratesticular arterial anatomy. J Urol 145(4):777–779

Jefferson RH, Perez LM, Joseph DB (1997) Critical analysis of the clinical presentation of acute scrotum: a 9-year experience at a single institution. J Urol 158:1198–1200

Jevtich MJ, Khawand N, Vidic B (1990) Clinical significance of

ultrastructural findings in the corpus cavernosum of normal and impotent men. J Urol 143:289–293
Kanellis J, Kang DH (2005) Uric acid as a mediator of endothelial dysfunction, inflammation, and vascular disease. Semin Nephrol 25:39–42
Karaguzel G, Tanyel FC, Kilinc K, Buyukpamukcu N, Hicsonmez A (1994) The preventive role of chemical sympathectomy on contralateral testicular hypoxic parameters encountered during unilateral testicular torsion. Br J Urol 74:507–510
Karnak I, Gedikoglu G, Tanyel FC, Buyukpamukcu N, Hicsonmez A (1996a) The effects of chemical sympathectomy on contralateral histology, fertility and fecundity in unilateral abdominal testes. Br J Urol 77:580–584
Karnak I, Tanyel FC, Kilinc K, Buyukpamukcu N, Hicsonmez A (1996b) Tissue hypoxia in ipsilateral and contralateral testes undergoing surgically induced maldescent. Eur J Pediatr Surg 6:281–284
Kazama T (1995) Effect of experimental left varicocele on rat Leydig cell function. Nippon Hinyokika Gakkai Zasshi 86: 308–315
Kocakoc E, Kiris A, Orhan I, Bozgeyik Z, Kanbay M, Ogur E (2001) Incidence and importance of reflux in testicular veins of healthy men evaluated with color duplex sonography. Eur Urol 39:316–321
Kogan SJ (1987) Fertility in cryptorchidism. An overview in 1987. Eur J Pediatr 146 (Suppl 2):S21–S24
Kokoua A, Tre Yavo M, Santos KA, Homsy Y, Mobiot ML, Gnanazan Bi N'Guessan G (2004) Importance of the testicular artery: histo-functional approach and comparison between juvenile and adult rats. Morphologie 88:31–34
Kolettis PN, Stowe NT, Inman SR, Thomas AJ Jr. (1996) Acute spermatic cord torsion alters the microcirculation of the contralateral testis. J Urol 151:350–354
Lamesch AJ (1994) Monorchidism or unilateral anorchidism. Langenbecks Arch Chir 379:105–108
Li S, Hu L, Zhao J (2004) Effects of growth hormone on erectile function and number of nNOS-containing nerve fibers in internal iliac arterial ligation rats. Zhonghua Nan Ke Xue10:103–106
Little WC, Costantinescu M, Apllegate RJ, Kutcher MA, Burrows MT, Kahl FR et al (1988) Can coronary angiography predict the site of a subsequent myocardial infarction in patients with mild to moderate coronary artery disease? Circulation 78:1157–1166
Mancini M, Bartolini M, Maggi M, Innocenti P, Forti G (1996) The presence of arterial anatomical variations can affect the results of duplex sonographic evaluation of penile vessels in impotent patients. J Urol 155:1919–1923
Mancini M, Bartolini M, Maggi M, Innocenti P, Villari N, Forti G (2000a) Duplex ultrasound evaluation of cavernosal peak systolic velocity and waveform acceleration in the penile flaccid state: clinical significance in the assessment of the arterial supply in patients with erectile dysfunction. Int J Androl 23:199–204
Mancini M, Negri L, Maggi M, Nerva F, Forti G, Colpi GM (2000b) Doppler color ultrasonography in the diagnosis of erectile dysfunction of vascular origin. Arch Ital Urol Androl 72:361–365
Mancini M, Raina R, Agarwal A, Nerva F, Colpi GM (2004) Sildenafil citrate vs intracavernous alprostadil for patients with arteriogenic erectile dysfunction: a randomised placebo controlled study. Int J Impot Res 16:8–12
Mazzilli F, Rossi T, Marchesini M, Ronconi C, Dondero F (1994) Superoxide anion in human semen related to seminal parameters and clinical aspects. Fertil Steril 62:862–868
Merry C, Sweeney B, Puri P (1997) The vanishing testis: anatomical and histological findings. Eur Urol 31:65–67
Montorsi F, Briganti A, Salonia A, Rigatti P, Margonato A, Macchi A, Galli S, Ravagnani PM, Montorsi P (2003) Erectile dysfunction prevalence, time of onset and association with risk factors in 300 consecutive patients with acute chest pain and angiographically documented coronary artery disease. Eur Urol 44:360–365
Nakajima H, Yui Y, Hara M, Hasegawa J, Hirose H, Akimoto M (1985) Clinical examination of torsion of the spermatic cord – review of 177 cases reported in the recent Japanese literature including our present 7 cases. Hinyokika Kiyo 31:1371–1377
Nehra A, Goldstein I, Pabby A, Nugent M, Huang YH, de las Morenas A, Krane RJ, Udelson D, Saenz de Tejada I, Moreland RB (1996) Mechanisms of venous leakage: a prospective clinicopathological correlation of corporeal function and structure. J Urol 156:1320–1329
Nguyen L, Lievano G, Ghosh L, Radhakrishnan J, Fornell L, John E (1999) Effect of unilateral testicular torsion on blood flow and histology of contralateral testis. J Pediatr Surg 34:680–683
Pallwein L, Klauser A, Frauscher F, Pinggera GM, Studen M, Maneschg C, Helweg G, Bartsh G (2001) Adverse impact of nutcracker phenomenon on outcomes after varicocele repair. Color Doppler ultrasound demonstration. A.U.A. Annual meeting 2001; abstract 1602
Pascual JA, Villanueva-Mejer J, Rutgers JL, Lemni CA, Sikka SC, Ehrlich RM, Mena I, Rajfer J (1990) Long-term effects of prepubertal testicular vessel ligation on testicular function in the rat. J Urol 144:466–468
Peltola V, Huhtaniemi I, Ahotupa M (1995) Abdominal position of the rat testis is associated with high level of lipid peroxidation. Biol Reprod 53:1146–1150
Persson C, Diederichs W, Lue TF, Yen TS, Fishman IJ, McLin PH, Tanagho EA (1989) Correlation of altered penile ultrastructure with clinical arterial evaluation. J Urol 142: 1462–1468
Pritzker MR (1999) The penile stress test: a window to the hearts of men. Circulation 100 (Suppl 1):I711
Rodriguez-Rigau LJ, Weiss DB, Zuckerman Z, Grotyan HE, Smith KD (1978) A possible mechanism for the detrimental effect of varicocele on testicular function in men. Fertil Steril 30:577–585
Romeo C, Antonuccio P, Esposito M, Marini H, Impellizzeri P, Turiaco N, Altavilla D, Bitto A, Zuccarello B, Squadrito F (2004) Raxofelast, a hydrophilic vitamin E-like antioxidant, reduces testicular ischemia-reperfusion injury. Urol Res 32:367–371
Ruiz Rubio JL, Hernandez M, Rivera del los arcos L, Garcia-Sacristan A, Prieto D (2004) Mechanisms of prostaglandin E1-induced relaxation in penile resistance arteries. J Urol 171:968–973
Rusnack SL, Wu HY, Huff DS, Snyder HM 3rd, Carr MC, Bellah RD, Zderic SA, Canning DA (2003) Testis histopathology in boys with cryptorchidism correlates with future fertility potential. Urology 169:659–662
Salama N, Bergh A, Damber JE (2001) Microvascular testicular blood flow as evaluated by laser Doppler flowmetry after the surgical induction of varicocele. Arch Androl 46:197–204
Salama N, Bergh A, Damber JE (2003) The changes in testicular vascular permeability during progression of the experimental varicocele. Eur Urol 43:84–91
Saleh RA, Agarwal A, Sharma RK, Said TM, Sikka SC, Thomas AJ Jr (2003) Evaluation of nuclear DNA damage in spermatozoa from infertile men with varicocele. Fertil Steril 80: 1431–1436
Salman AB, Kilinc K, Tanyel FC (1997) Torsion of only spermatic cord in the absence of testis and/or epididymis results in contralateral testicular hypoxia. Urol Res 25:413–415

Salman AB, Mutlu S, Iskit AB, Guc MO, Mutlu M, Tanyel FC (1998) Haemodynamic monitoring of the contralateral testis during unilateral testicular torsion describes the mechanism of damage. Eur Urol 33:576–580

Saltzman EA, Guay AT, Jacobson J (2004) Improvement in erectile function in men with organic erectile dysfunction by correction of elevated cholesterol levels: a clinical observation. J Urol 172: 255–258

Sampayo FJ, Favorito LA, Freitas MA, Damiao R, Gouveia E (1999) Arterial supply of the human fetal testis during its migration. J Urol 161:1603–1605

Sarica K, Kupeli B, Budak M, Kosar A, Kavukcu M, Durac I, Gogus O (1997) Influence of experimental spermatic cord torsion on the contralateral testis in rats. Evaluation of tissue free oxygen radical scavenger enzyme levels. Urol Int 58:208–212

Sarteschi LM, Montorsi F, Fabris FM, Guazzoni G, Lencioni R, Rigatti P (1998) Cavernous arterial and arteriolar circulation in patients with erectile dysfunction: a power Doppler study. J Urol 159:428–432

Savas C, Ozogul C, Karaoz E, Bezir M (2002) Ischaemia, whether from ligation or torsion, causes ultrastructural changes on the contralateral testis. Scand J Urol Nephrol 36:302–306

Schultz KE, Walker J (1984) Testicular torsion in undescended testes. Ann Emerg Med 13:567–569

Shafik A (1991) The physiology of testicular thermoregulation in the light of new anatomical and pathological aspects. In: Zorgniotti AW (ed) Temperature and environmental effects on the testis. Plenum, New York, pp 153–172

Shergill IS, Foley Cl, Arya M, Bott SR, Mundy AR (2002) Testicular torsion unravelled. Hosp Med 63:456–459

Sigmund G, Gall H, Bahren W (1987) Stop-type and Shunt-type varicoceles: venographic findings. Radiology 163:105–110

Tarhan S, Gumus B, Gunduz I, Ayyildiz V, Goktan C (2003) Effect of varicocele on testicular artery blood flow in men – color Doppler investigation. Scand J Urol Nephrol 37:38–42

Tashi AI, Resim S, Caskurlu T, Dincel C, Bayraktar Z, Gurbuz G (2001) Color doppler ultrasonography and spectral analysis of venous flow in diagnosis of varicocele. Eur Urol 39: 316–321

Taskinen S, Lehtinen A, Hovatta O, Wikstrom S (1996) Ultrasonography and colour Doppler flow in the testes of adult patients after treatment of cryptorchidism. Br J Urol 78: 248–251

Tritto J, North MO, Dittmar A (2001) Micro-measurements of microcirculation perfusion and thermal parameters in human testis during microsurgery of varicocele. J Androl Suppl 114:P130

Tsai AG, Friesenecker B, Mazzoni MC (1998) Microvascular and tissue oxygen gradients in the rat mesentery. Proc Natl Acad Sci USA 95:6590–6595

Turek PJ, Ewalt DH, Snyder HM 3rd, Stamperfs D, Blyth B, Huff DS, Duckett JW (1994) The absent cryptorchid testis: surgical findings and their implications for diagnosis and aetiology. J Urol 151:718–720

Turner TT, Brown KJ (1993) Spermatic cord torsion: loss of spermatogenesis despite return of blood flow. Biol Reprod 49:401–407

Ushiyama M, Morita T, Kuramochi T, Yagi S, Katayama S (2004) Erectile dysfunction in hypertensive rats results from impairment of the relaxation evoked by neurogenic carbon monoxide and nitric oxide. Hypertens Res 27:253–261

Vignozzi L, Corona G, Petrone L, Filippi S, Morelli AM, Forti G, Maggi M (2005) Testosterone and sexual activity. J Endocrinol Invest 28:39–44

Vigueras RM, Reyes G, Rojas-Castaneda J, Rojas P, Hernandez R (2004) Testicular torsion and its effects on the spermatogenic cycle in the contralateral testis of the rat. Lab Anim 38: 313–320

Virag R, Floresco J, Richard C (2004) Impairment of shear-stress-mediated vasodilation of cavernous arteries in erectile dysfunction. Int J Impot Res 16:39–42

Weidner W, Colpi GM, Hargreave TB, Papp GK, Pomerol JM (2002) European guidelines on male infertility. Eur Urol 42:313–322

Wespes E, Goes PM, Schiffman S, Depierreux M, Vanderhaeghen JJ, Schulman CC (1991) Computerized analysis of smooth muscle fibers in potent and impotent patients. J Urol 146:1015–1017

Yavetz H, Harash B, Paz G, Yogev L, Jaffa AJ, Lessing JB, Homonnai ZT (1992) Cryptorchidism: incidence and sperm quality in infertile men. Andrologia 24:293–297

Yildiz O, Gul H, Ozgok Y, Onguru O, Kilciler M, Aydin A, Isimer A, Harmankaya AC (2003) Increased vasoconstrictor reactivity and decreased endothelial function in high grade varicocele; functional and morphological study. Urol Res 31: 323–328

Zini A, Schlegel PN (1997) Cu/Zn superoxide dismutase, catalase and glutathione peroxidase mRNA expression in the rat testis after surgical cryptorchidism and efferent duct ligation. J Urol 158:659–663

Zorgniotti AW (1980) Testis temperature, infertility and the varicocele paradox. Urology 16:7

II.2.6 Effects of Lifestyle and Toxicants

J. P. Bonde

Summary

A vast number of toxic chemicals encountered at the work place, in the environment or related to lifestyle have the potential to impair male reproductive health. The list of known male reproductive toxicants includes ionizing radiation, radiant heat exposure, inorganic lead and certain pesticides and organic solvents, but the number of chemicals that, according to experimental studies, have potential effects is much higher. Information on potential hazardous occupational and other toxic factors should be an important part of history taking among patients attending infertility clinics. The options for the disentanglement of occupational exposure in particular include:

- History taking about current occupational exposures
- Measurement of exposure levels in ambient air and tissues
- Observation of improvement in semen quality following temporary elimination of potential hazardous exposures – for instance by temporary referral to other work tasks.

II.2.6.1 Introduction

The aetiology of male infertility is unknown in the majority of cases in clinical practice. Deficits in knowledge fuels concern that is increasingly raised about the effect of occupational and environmental exposure on human semen quality and on what some interpret as genuine geographical differences and declining trends in sperm count. Although research methods in the field of reproductive epidemiology and male reproductive toxicology have improved substantially during past 20 years, the list of putative human male reproductive toxicants of relevance to the clinician remains limited. However, the vast number of exposures with limited evidence for male reproductive effects should be consulted by the clinician whenever suspicion is raised, because there are sound options for investigating the significance of toxic exposures in individual cases – in particular when toxic effects are not causing permanent damage to endocrine regulation or testicular tissues (Fig. II.2.5). For a scientific outline of the evidence on male reproductive toxicants in humans, the reader is referred to several reviews (Steeno and Pangkahila 1984; Schrag and Dixon 1985; Henderson et al. 1986; Baranski 1993; Bonde and Giwercman 1995; Lahdetie 1995; Tas et al. 1996; Giwercman and Bonde 1998; Figa-Talamanca et al. 2001; Bonde and Storgaard 2002; Sheiner et al. 2003). This chapter will briefly present the author's interpretation of present knowledge together with essential information on exposures that may help guide the clinician to identify cases of male infertility related to occupational factors in particular. Infertility caused by occupational exposure is not a prescribed occupational disease in any of the countries in the European Union, and this may partly explain why clinical cases of male occupation-related infertility are seldom diagnosed and reported. Clinical diagnoses in individual cases may have importance that reaches beyond worker compensation. Recognition of infertility caused by well-defined exposures in the workplace may enhance the improvement of working conditions to prevent additional cases. Moreover, the elimination of hazardous exposures and temporary referral to other work tasks might improve fecundity if the testicular damage is neither severe nor irreversible.

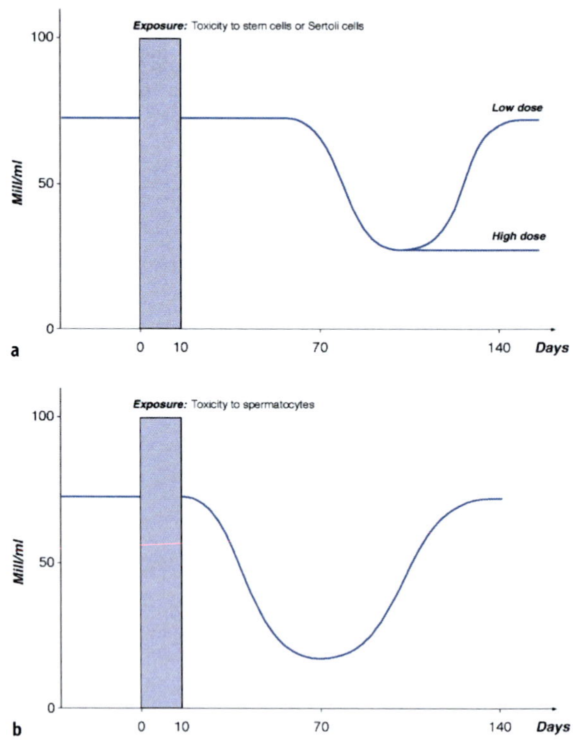

Fig. II.2.5a, b. Effects of reproductive toxicants on seminal characteristics according to site of action. Effects of stem cell and Sertoli cell toxicants are delayed and effects may be permanent if damage is severe (**a**) while the delay may be short and effects reversible following exposure to toxic substances acting at the later stages of spermatogenesis (**b**)

II.2

II.2.6.2 Lifestyle Factors

II.2.6.2.1 Tobacco Smoking

Considering the strong mutagenic, clastogenic<fn>A clastogen is a chemical agent that causes breaks in chromosomes</fn> and carcinogenic impacts of tobacco smoking, spermatogenesis and male fertility in *adult men* seem surprisingly resistant to tobacco smoke contaminants. While the probability of conception in a menstrual cycle (the fecundability) is reduced by some 30% if the woman is smoking, smoking in adult men seems not to have a strong impact on fecundability (Bolumar et al. 1996). This is consistent with a limited effect of smoking on sperm count. According to a meta-analysis of 20 different study populations worldwide, the sperm count is reduced by an average of 13 – 17% in adult male smokers (95% confidence interval, CI: 8 – 21%) (Vine et al. 1994).

Likewise, smoking seems not to have a major impact on semen volume, morphology, motility or chromatin integrity, although data linking smoking and these endpoints are more limited (Vine 1996; Vine et al. 1997; Spano et al. 1998). However, wives of smoking men have a lower chance of pregnancy with intrauterine insemination (IUI) and in vitro fertilization/intracytoplasmic sperm injection (IVF/ICSI) techniques, and several other more subtle effects of tobacco smoking have been demonstrated in recent studies. Thus several studies indicate that cigarette smoking is associated with oxidative DNA damage in human spermatozoa (Loft et al. 2003) and studies using fluorescence in situ hybridization have demonstrated an increased prevalence of aneuploidy of several chromosomes including 1, 7 and the sex chromosomes (Robbins et al. 1997; Rubes et al. 1998; Harkonen et al. 1999). Such findings raise concern as to the risk of cancer, birth defects and genetic diseases in the offspring, but so far there is only limited evidence for male-mediated developmental toxicity in male smokers. Moreover, smoking may have a major impact on male fertility through other exposure windows. Evidence is now accumulating that sons of mothers who smoked during their pregnancy have reduced sperm count (Jensen et al. 1998a, 2004; Storgaard et al. 2003), although findings are not entirely consistent (Ratcliffe et al. 1992). In one of these studies a 50% reduction of sperm count was observed in sons of heavily smoking mothers (Storgaard et al. 2003). Thus, at present the data seem to indicate that smoking by adult men has a minor impact on semen quality, while smoking by the mother during early pregnancy may have a major impact.

II.2.6.2.2 Alcoholic Beverages and Caffeine

Impaired testicular function in alcoholic addicts is well documented and may be caused by disturbed liver metabolism as well as toxic effects on the testis, including ethanol toxicity to Leydig cells (Gluud 1988), but fertility and conventional measures of semen quality seem not to be reduced in men with an intake of up to 15 – 20 alcoholic drinks a week (Gluud 1988; Jensen et al. 1998c; Juhl et al. 2001). There is limited evidence that coffee drinking (intake of caffeine) among women as well as men may be associated with reduced fertility, but only in non-smokers (Jensen et al. 1998b). Smoking may interfere with the metabolism of caffeine resulting in enhanced detoxification and elimination of caffeine metabolites.

II.2.6.2.3 Heat and Sedentary Body Posture

Social and economic development during the twentieth century dramatically changed everyday life for the majority of people in developed countries. One obvious consequence has been the shift from physically demanding work to sedentary work. A much larger fraction of the population sit in offices and transportation vehicles for a larger fraction of the time than previously. The question has been raised repeatedly of whether this shift in working and living conditions could influence male fertility through a disruption of testicular heat regulation (Mieusset and Bujan 1995). The testes are located outside the body to keep temperature of the germinal epithelium below the core temperature. It is well known that elevation of the testis temperature impairs and even inhibits spermatogenesis (Mieusset and Bujan 1995; Thonneau et al. 1998). External heating of the testis for a short period of time results in a dramatic but temporary decrease in sperm count after a delay of 6 – 8 weeks, and elevation of the core temperature by fever or extreme sauna bathing also reduces the sperm count (Procope 1965; Carlsen et al. 2003). Furthermore, work in a hot occupational environment and exposure to radiant heat among welders, foundry workers, ceramic workers and bakers may cause reduced sperm count (Bonde 1992; Figa-Talamanca et al. 1996; Thonneau et al. 1996, 1998), and disruption of testicular heat regulation may also be the cause of delayed conception in taxi drivers (Figa-Talamanca et al. 1996; Bujan et al. 2000). It is now well documented that the sedentary work position is associated with an increased scrotal temperature (Fig. II.2.6, Hjollund et al. 2000, 2002b).

Men sitting at work for 8 h a day have on average a 0.7 °C increased scrotal temperature during the day in comparison with employees spending fewer than 8 h in

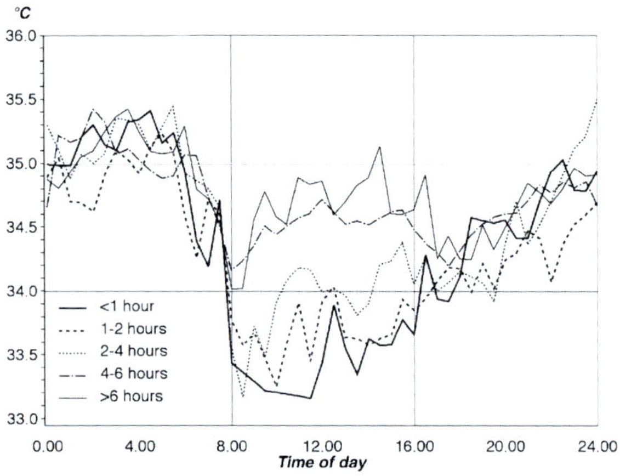

Fig. II.2.6. Scrotal temperature during night and day time according to the duration of sedentary body position during working hours. The natural decline of scrotal temperature during the day is partly inhibited by sitting at work (Hjollund et al. 2002b)

the sedentary body position. Although an increase of scrotal temperature of this order of magnitude might be sufficient to impair spermatogenesis, a reduced sperm count seems not to be related to sedentary work (Hjollund et al. 2002a; Stoy et al. 2004). Likewise it has been speculated whether tight underwear could act as a testicular suspensorium. Some studies on reduced sperm count related to the use of tight underwear and trousers have in fact been reported (Jung et al. 2005). In conclusion, it seems justified to pay attention to a possible temporary effect on sperm count in specific occupations with exposure to high levels of radiant heat and perhaps among professional drivers, while a sedentary work position in general and in office work seems unlikely to influence male fertility.

II.2.6.3 Workplace Factors

Exposure at the workplace is usually much higher than environmental exposures experienced by the general population. Although the number of people experiencing highly specific exposures is mostly low, individual risk may be high owing to high exposure levels. To date occupational studies of male fertility have contributed by far the most to current knowledge on toxic exposures and human male fertility. But as alert physicians pay attention to the possible impact of toxic and physical workplace exposures, much more can probably be learned about the impact of environmental exposures.

II.2.6.3.1 Ionizing Radiation

Health care and nuclear plant personnel, laboratory technicians, welding operators and radar technicians may be exposed to ionizing radiation at the workplace. The testis is one of the most radiosensitive tissues of the body. Spermatogonia are the most radiosensitive cells, spermatocytes are less vulnerable and spermatids are rather radio-resistant. A temporary reduction in sperm count occurs after a radiation dose of 0.15 Gy, while single exposures above 2 Gy may cause permanent azoospermia (Rowley et al. 1974; Littley et al. 1991; Ogilvy-Stuart and Shalet 1993). The decline in sperm count occurs with a delay of 50–60 days, consistent with the fact that the spermatogonia are the most radiosensitive. Workplace exposure to gamma-radiation is easy to monitor, while exposure to alpha- and beta-radiation by inhalation or ingestion of particles may easily escape recognition. However, according to the present occupational standards in industrial and research laboratories, exosure levels are far below background radiation. If the usual exposure threshold of 15 millisievert/year is not exceeded, testicular effects seem unlikely.

II.2.6.3.2 High-Frequency Electromagnetic Radiation (HHF, 300 kHz to 300 mHz, Short Waves or Microwaves)

High-frequency electromagnetic radiation is nonionizing radiation with a higher energy content than extremely low frequency electromagnetic radiation (see below). Exposure to HHF is increasing in society at large because of widespread use of cellular phones, among other devices. Occupational exposure occurs among military radar equipment operators and employees working with thermal plastic sealing, glue hardening, physiotherapy and telecommunication equipment. The apparent effect on semen quality of microwaves (100 mHz to 300,000 mHz) reported in an earlier East European study may result from the radiant heat associated with the exposure (Lancranjan et al. 1975a). The significance of reduced semen quality observed in military radar equipment operators in the USA and Denmark is uncertain (Lancranjan et al. 1975a, Weyandt et al. 1996, Hjollund et al. 1997). The effects observed in these small human populations are not corroborated by animal experimental evidence.

II.2.6.3.3 Extremely Low Frequency Electromagnetic Radiation

There has been a tremendous increase in the population's exposure to extremely low frequency electromagnetic radiation from household electrical equipment and power cables. Clues as to the possible significance for male reproductive health may be obtained from occupational studies. Metal welders are among the professionals with the greatest exposure because of their close proximity to power cables during electric arc welding. Comprehensive studies with full shift monitoring of electromagnetic fields provide no evidence that the endocrine profile or conventional semen characteristics are influenced by exposure to such fields (Hjollund et al. 1999). Moreover, there is a paucity of experimental evidence indicating that we should expect any effects.

II.2.6.3.4 Pesticides

Pesticides denote a large and heterogeneous group of chemicals sharing toxicity to living organisms. It has become evident from monitoring programmes of the general population over more than 20 years that several persistent organic pesticides are detectable in human tissues all over the globe, even including people living in the arctic regions. A United Nations working group has reported that 9 of the 12 most unwanted persistent organic pollutants are pesticides used on agricultural crops. Industrial workers engaged in the manufacture and formulation of pesticides may be exposed through multiple pathways, while the predominant route of exposure among applicators in greenhouses and agriculture seems to be through the skin. But spraying of pesticides may cause exposure through inhalation as well – unless the worker is adequately protected. Thousands of deaths are reported annually following acute intoxication in developing countries, and high-level exposure in the occupational setting as well as long-term low-level exposure of the general population continue to be of concern – not least from the point of view of male reproductive health. It is well known that the nematocide dibromochloropropane (DBCP) is detrimental to spermatogenesis in humans by as yet unknown mechanisms (Whorton et al. 1977; Potashnik et al. 1978; Whorton and Milby 1980; Whorton and Foliart 1983; Potashnik and Porath 1995). Azoospermia developed in some workers following low-level exposure for a short duration and in some cases seemed permanent, as an indication of severe stem cell or Sertoli cell toxicity. The severe reproductive effects of DBCP in humans were discovered in 1977, but their effects in rodent species had been known for decades. The substance has been prohibited in most countries for a long time, but during the past 20 years several other pesticides have been studied in occupational settings. Some agents seem to interfere with spermatogenesis although their effects are far less severe than DBCP (Whorton et al. 1979; Wong et al. 1979; Wyrobek et al. 1981; Ratcliffe et al. 1987). Examples include ethylene dibromide, which is structurally related to DBCP (Ratcliffe et al. 1987), carbaryl, which causes sperm morphology anomalies (Wyrobek et al. 1981), and 2,4-dichlorophenoxyacetic acid (Lerda and Rizzi 1991).

European studies of vineyard workers, organic and conventional farmers (Fig. II.2.7) and greenhouse workers with exposure to a wide range of different types of pesticides at low exposure levels have not revealed an effect on male fertility as measured by delayed time to conception, endocrine sex hormone profiles or semen characteristics (Larsen et al. 1998a, b, 1999; Thonneau et al. 1999); an exception is greenhouse workers, where results point to the impairment of several semen characteristics related to manual handling of cultures (Abell et al. 2000). Apparently inconsistent findings in occupational pesticide studies of male fertility may easily be explained by exposure to different chemicals at different levels (Rupa et al. 1991; de Cock et al. 1994; Curtis et al. 1999; Tielemans et al. 1999a, 1999b; Petrelli and Figa-Talamanca 2001; Greenlee et al. 2003; Hjollund et al. 2004; Sanchez-Pena et al. 2004). For the clinician, only limited specific information can be obtained from broad epidemiological studies with poorly characterized exposures. In the individual case emphasis must be on work history, exposure to specific chemicals and animal experimental evidence. Unfortunately, only a few pesticides can routinely be measured in blood, urine or semen.

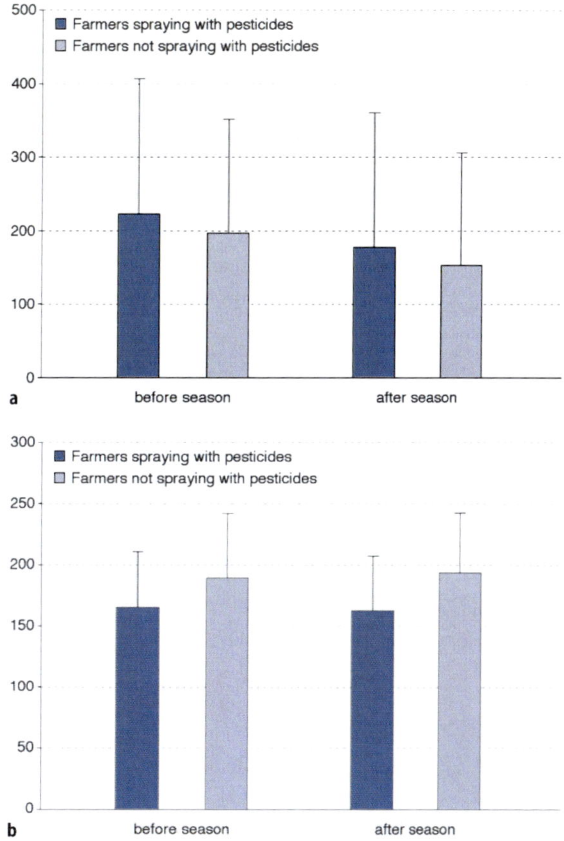

Fig. II.2.7a, b. Total sperm count (**a**) and serum inhibin B (**b**) throughout the season among Danish farmers using and not using pesticides for the crops. The controlled longitudinal design provides reliable evidence of limited effects, if any. Exposure levels are assumed to be low (Larsen et al. 1998a)

II.2

II.2.6.3.5 Inorganic Lead

Lead has widespread applications in industry. Workers in foundries, battery manufacturing plants, ceramic industries and pigment production may be exposed to high levels. But exposure to lead may occur – sometimes unexpectedly – in numerous other occupations, also including craftsmen. Previously, the general population has been heavily exposed to lead in gasoline, but population levels of blood lead declined dramatically after the introduction of non-leaded gasoline in many countries. Exposure levels in various European industries have also declined – according to one survey based upon some 45,000 blood samples from an average of 70 µg/dl in 1970 to 35 µg/dl in 1995 (Bonde et al. 1999).

In comparison with many other industrial chemicals, it is a great advantage that exposure to lead during the previous 30 days can be easily and reliably obtained by measuring lead levels in a blood sample. However, the relationship between lead in blood and target organs such as the testis is poorly characterized.

The toxicity of lead for male reproductivity in terms of impaired semen quality, hormonal imbalance and reduced fertility has been known for a long time, but the mechanisms involved and sites of action remain unclear. They may include a direct effect on the germinal epithelium or maturing spermatozoa, disruption of the endocrine regulation of spermatogenesis, or both (Apostoli et al. 1998). At very high exposure levels above 80–100 µg/dl blood, which may be associated with signs of clinical intoxication, lead exposure is associated with decreased libido and impotence – probably of central origin.

Several occupational surveys have linked exposure to inorganic lead in the exposure range above 50–60 µg/dl with a reduced sperm count in particular, but also with other semen characteristics and signs of male reproductive toxicity (Lancranjan et al. 1975b; Wildt et al. 1983; Assennato et al. 1986; Coste et al. 1991; Gennart et al. 1992; Lerda 1992; Alexander et al. 1996; Bonde and Kolstad 1997; Viskum et al. 1999; Bonde et al. 2002) although the literature is not entirely consistent (Bonde and Kolstad 1997; Robins et al. 1997; Joffe et al. 1999; Apostoli et al. 2000). The evidence in humans is supported by compelling evidence in mice, rabbits and some rat strains (Apostoli et al. 1998), but the question of the lowest level associated with an observed adverse effect remains open.

An international European study points to a threshold around 45 µg/dl below which effects on sperm count seem unlikely (Bonde et al. 2002). These findings are consistent with studies of delayed time to pregnancy not indicating effects in the lower exposure range below 50 µg/dl (Joffe et al. 1999). The lowest effect level of about 45 µg/dl of lead in blood is an average group threshold, which does not necessarily apply to all individual workers. It is likely that some workers are more susceptible to the actions of lead than others. The individual susceptibility could be influenced by genetic polymorphisms that modify the toxicokinetics of lead (Alexander et al. 1996). Variation in the distribution kinetics of lead across various tissues might also explain differences in individual susceptibility. A plot of the correlation between lead in blood and lead in spermatozoa reveals a large variation of sperm lead at a given blood lead level (Figs. II.2.8, II. 2.9). Since lead may be encountered in very diverse occupational settings, and is easily measured in blood, determination of this metal should probably be performed routinely when the suspicion is raised that occupational exposures might be of importance.

II.2.6.4.6 Cadmium

Exposure to cadmium fumes may be encountered in battery manufacture. In rodents cadmium produces

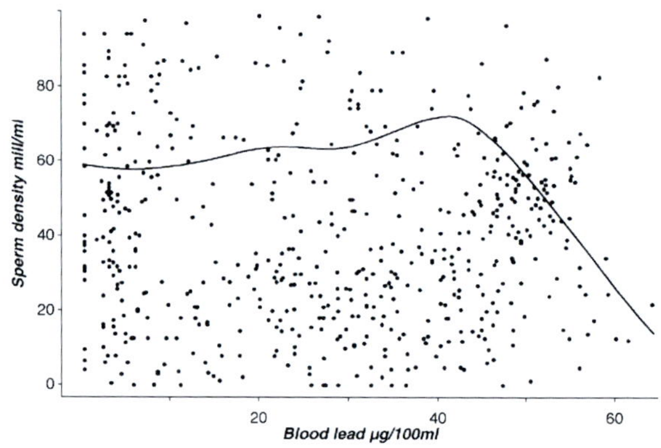

Fig. II.2.8. Concentration of sperm cells in fresh ejaculates in some 500 workers from UK, Belgium and Italy according to current blood lead level. No effects are observed below 45 µg lead per dl of blood (Bonde et al. 2002)

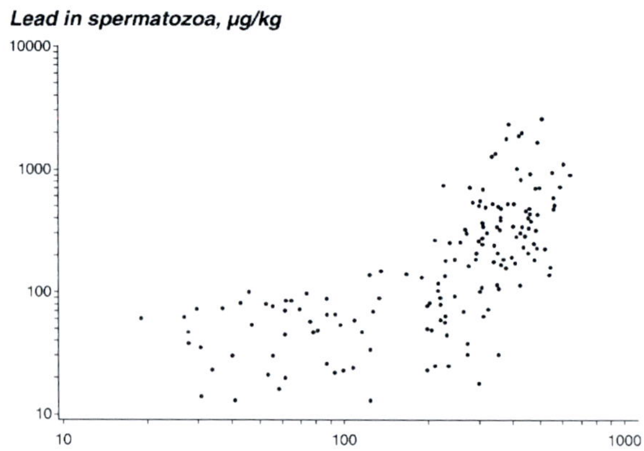

Fig. II.2.9. Relation between the concentration of lead in blood and spermatozoa (Bonde et al. 2002)

severe testicular damage even at low doses. The primary action involves damage to the testicular capillary epithelium. Despite remarkable findings in laboratory animals there is still inadequate data to assess the toxicity of cadmium to human male fertility.

II.2.6.4.7
Mercury

Both inorganic mercury and methyl mercury are taken up by the testis in mice (testicular half-life 3–4 and 56 days respectively) (Lee and Dixon 1975) and the early stages of spermatogenesis are particularly vulnerable to mercury at dose levels not producing systemic toxicity. Knowledge about the impact of mercury on human male reproductive function is limited, although the effects of mercury were implicated in a case study and a few epidemiological studies (Lee and Dixon 1975; Ernst and Bonde 1992a).

II.2.6.4.8
Manganese

Histopathological changes in testicular tissue have been shown to occur in different animal species following doses that were not otherwise toxic. It has been suggested that manganese inhibits succinic dehydrogenase in mitochondria, causing disruption of energy metabolism and cell death. An earlier epidemiological study revealed a decline in birth rate in workers exposed to high levels of manganese dust (Lauwerys et al. 1985), but the literature is inadequate to assess the toxicity of this metal in humans.

II.2.6.4.9
Hexavalent Chromium

Hexavalent chromium causes decreased epididymal sperm count and sperm motility in rats (Ernst 1990; Ernst and Bonde 1992b), but in welders with rather low exposure to airborne water-soluble hexavalent chromium no consistent effects on conventional semen characteristics or fertility rates have been found (Jelnes and Knudsen 1988; Bonde and Christensen 1991; Bonde and Ernst 1992). Welders using other welding methods and chromium platers may experience much higher exposure levels and may be at risk of effects on reproductive function.

II.2.6.4.10
Metal Welders

The prevalence of metal welding is about 5% in many countries throughout the world. The level and constituents of welding fume particulates is highly dependent on the type of metal and the welding technology. While electric rod welding (manual metal arc welding) and metal active gas welding are often associated with high exposure levels, far above 5 mg/m^3, tungsten inert gas welding confers much less exposure to welding fumes – often in the range below 1 mg/m^3. Several studies have demonstrated impaired semen quality, delayed time to conception and a reduced fertility rate in metal welders (Mortensen 1988; Bonde et al. 1990; Bonde 1990a, 1990b), but more recent studies have not corroborated earlier findings (Hjollund et al. 1998a, b). These apparent inconsistencies may be due to a recent reduction of exposure levels. The risk seems not to be related to welding on stainless steel, which may confer high exposure to hexavalent chromium. The mechanisms remain unclear. Exposure to extremely low frequency electromagnetic radiation is not a likely cause (Hjollund et al. 1999), and exposure to radiant heat is probably only important when preheated steel is welded (Bonde 1992). Suspicion should be raised if impaired semen quality with an unknown cause is revealed in a welder exposed to high levels of welding fume particulates (above 5–10 mg/m^3). This implies that only electric rod and metal active gas welding, but not tungsten inert gas welding, is relevant.

II.2.6.4.11
Organic Solvents

Among the widely used volatile, industrial, organic solvents, it seems that *carbon disulphide* carries a risk to the male reproductive system (Vanhoorne et al. 1994). This solvent is used in particular in the viscose-rayon industry. High-level exposure in the workplace may produce reduced sperm count, reduced sperm motility and increased frequency of abnormal sperm forms as well as endocrine effects, as suggested by reduced circulating levels of luteinizing and follicle stimulating hormone. *Styrene* is used in the manufacture of reinforced plastic products such as windmills and yachts. Manual laminating procedures often involve high exposure levels. There is limited evidence that inhalation of styrene may impair semen quality (Kolstad et al. 1999b) and an international study did not indicate that exposure of the male to styrene is related to delayed conception (Kolstad et al. 1999a). Animal as well as human data on the male reproductive effects of other widely used solvents, such as toluene, xylene, benzene, carbon tetrachloride and trichlorethylene, are limited.

Ethylene glycol ethyl or methyl ethers are solvents with low volatility, which increasingly have been used as substitutes for the highly volatile hydrocarbons in paints, adhesives, thinners, printing ink and anti-icing fluids. It has been estimated that two million workers are exposed to eight different glycol ethers in the USA. In experimental animals, these substances have revealed unequivocal evidence for male reproductive toxicity. Several studies in humans now document that these compounds impair human male reproductive health as well (Ratcliffe et al. 1989; Veulemans et al. 1993; Tielemans et al. 1999a).

The solvent 2-bromopropane has specific effects on rat spermatogonia (Omura et al. 1999; Son et al. 1999) and therefore it is interesting that six out of eight male workers at a Korean electronics company had a severely reduced sperm count (Kim et al. 1996). Clearly attention should be paid to this particular organic solvent for workers in the electronics industry.

II.2.6.4 Environmental Exposures

More than 10 years ago it was suggested that environmental toxicants with weak hormonal actions may interfere with the development of the gonads in prenatal life and during childhood, and cause impaired reproductive health in later life. While a large body of experimental and toxicological evidence addressing this hypothesis has emerged, knowledge on human exposure profiles and epidemiological evidence is limited (Sonnenschein and Soto 1998; Sharpe and Irvine 2004). A report from the European Commission identified 60 substances (29 chemical groups) from an initial list of 564 chemicals to be of high concern because of persistence, high volume and at least one study providing evidence of endocrine disruption in an intact organism. Polychlorinated biphenyls (PCBs) and dichlorodiphenyltrichloroethane (DDT) are of particular interest because these compounds are highly persistent in human tissues, with a half-life of 5–10 years, and exposure levels in the general population are well documented. The compounds have been released into the environment since the 1940s and accumulate in the aquatic environment in particular to reach high levels in predators at the top of the food chain. In addition to consumption of fatty fish the general population is exposed through diary products and meat. There is limited but accumulating epidemiological evidence that these compounds may reduce male fertility and result in subtle impairment of semen quality (Toft et al. 2004), but at present the evidence is far too crude to support the clinician in fertility workups or guidance of infertility patients. The same applies to several other potential compounds with weak hormone-like activity, such as phthalates (Duty et al. 2003; Hoppin 2003; Zhang et al. 2003). The issue of endocrine disrupting chemicals is dealt with more comprehensively elsewhere in this book. The general population is exposed to other chlorinated pesticides, see above, "Pesticides".

II.2.6.5 Male-Mediated Developmental Toxicity

Animal studies have demonstrated how mutagens and carcinogens are capable of introducing heritable genomic changes, which may result in reproductive failures such as miscarriage, congenital malformations and cancer in the offspring. Traslar et al. 1985 demonstrated how exposure of male rats to cyclophosphamide causes post implantation loss without interfering with fertility. Aneuploid sperm may not represent a hereditable risk if they are disadvantaged at fertilization with respect to normal sperm cells. However, in elegant studies Marchetti et al. (1999) demonstrated the absence of selection against aneuploid mouse sperm at fertilization. Thus the question about consequences of paternal exposures for pregnancy outcomes seems highly relevant, and since 1985 several synthetic chemicals have been found to induce genetic damage that is transmitted to the offspring. In humans, treatment with cytotoxic drugs and tobacco smoking have been associated with an increased frequency of aneuploidy in sperm cells (Rubes et al. 1998; Harkonen et al. 1999), but so far there is no clear evidence that developmental anomalies can be attributed to paternal smoking in spite of several findings suggesting such effects (Savitz 2003). Many epidemiologic studies indicate an association between certain paternal occupational exposures and adverse pregnancy outcomes (Savitz et al. 1994). However, in most cases positive findings obtained in one study have not been confirmed in other studies. Moreover, a study of ionizing irradiation, including about 70,000 children of atomic bombs survivors, did not demonstrate abnormal pregnancy outcomes related to paternal irradiation. Nevertheless, it is obvious that epidemiological research in this field has to overcome many difficulties and "no evidence" cannot be taken as "no effects". The question about paternal exposures in pregnancy outcomes is often raised in clinical practice, but so far no confirmative answers can be given.

II.2.6.6 Conclusion

The most obvious clinical consequence of male reproductive toxicity is delayed conception and infertility. For exposures acting after puberty the outcome will depend on the mechanisms involved. Thus the outcome is permanent sterility if the stock of stem cells is completely eradicated, whereas subfecundity may be rather temporary if post spermatogonial germ cells are affected. Only a few exposures, such as ionizing radiation, a high level of radiant heat, inorganic lead, certain pesticides and organic solvents, are well documented human male reproductive toxicants, but the list of potential reproductive toxicants is long. In clinical practice the clinician will have to take the vast body of experimental evidence into account when the suspicion is raised that some specific exposure is related to infertility. Data on occupational and lifestyle exposures should be an important part of history taking among patients attending infertility clinics.

References

Abell A, Ernst E, Bonde JP (2000) Semen quality and sexual hormones in greenhouse workers. Scand J Work Environ Health 26:492–500

Alexander BH, Checkoway H, van Netten C, Muller CH, Ewers TG, Kaufman JD, Mueller BA, Vaughan TL, Faustman EM (1996) Semen quality of men employed at a lead smelter. J Occup Med 53:411–416

Apostoli P, Kiss P, Porru S, Bonde JP, Vanhoorne M (1998) Male reproductive toxicity of lead in animals and humans. ASCLEPIOS Study Group. Occup Environ Med 55:364–374

Apostoli P, Bellini A, Porru S, Bisanti L (2000) The effect of lead on male fertility: a time to pregnancy (TTP) study. Am J Ind Med 38:310–315

Assennato G, Paci C, Baser ME, Molinini R, Candela RG, Altamura BM, Giorgino R (1986) Sperm count suppression without endocrine dysfunction in lead-exposed men. Arch Environ Health 41:387–390

Baranski B (1993) Effects of the workplace on fertility and related reproductive outcomes. Environ Health Perspect 101 [Suppl 2]:81–90

Bolumar F, Olsen J, Boldsen J (1996) Smoking reduces fecundity: a European multicenter study on infertility and subfecundity. The European Study Group on Infertility and Subfecundity. Am J Epidemiol 143:578–587

Bonde JP (1990a) Semen quality and sex hormones among mild steel and stainless steel welders: a cross sectional study. Br J Indust Med 47:508–514

Bonde JP (1990b) Subfertility in relation to welding. A case referent study among male welders. Dan Med Bull 37:105–108

Bonde JP (1992) Semen quality in welders exposed to radiant heat. Br J Indust Med 49:5–10

Bonde JP, Christensen JM (1991) Chromium in biological samples from low-level exposed stainless steel and mild steel welders. Arch Environ Health 46:225–229

Bonde JP, Ernst E (1992) Sex hormones and semen quality in welders exposed to hexavalent chromium. Hum Exp Toxicol 11:259–263

Bonde JP, Giwercman A (1995) Occupational hazards to male fecundity. Reprod Med Rev 4:59–73

Bonde JP, Kolstad H (1997) Fertility of Danish battery workers exposed to lead. Int J Epidemiol 26:1281–1288

Bonde JP, Storgaard L (2002) How work-place conditions, environmental toxicants and lifestyle affect male reproductive function. Int J Androl 25:262–268

Bonde JP, Hansen KS, Levine RJ (1990) Fertility among Danish male welders. Scand J Work Environ Health 16:315–322

Bonde JP, Joffe M, Danscher G, Apostoli P, Bisanti L, Giwercman A, Kolstad HA, Thonneau P, Roeleveld N, Vanhoorne M (1999) Objectives, designs and populations of the European Asclepios study on occupational hazards to male reproductive capability. Scand J Work Environ Health 25 [Suppl 1]:49–61

Bonde JP, Joffe M, Apostoli P, Dale A, Kiss P, Spano M, Caruso F, Giwercman A, Bisanti L, Porru S, Vanhoorne M, Comhaire F, Zschiesche W (2002) Sperm count and chromatin structure in men exposed to inorganic lead: lowest adverse effect levels. Occup Environ Med 59:234–242

Bujan L, Daudin M, Charlet JP, Thonneau P, Mieusset R (2000) Increase in scrotal temperature in car drivers. Hum Reprod 15:1355–1357

Carlsen E, Andersson AM, Petersen JH, Skakkebaek NE (2003) History of febrile illness and variation in semen quality. Hum Reprod 18:2089–2092

Coste J, Mandereau L, Pessione F, Bregu M, Faye C, Hemon D, Spira A (1991) Lead-exposed workmen and fertility: a cohort study on 354 subjects. Eur J Epidemiol 7:154–158

Curtis KM, Savitz DA, Weinberg CR, Arbuckle TE (1999) The effect of pesticide exposure on time to pregnancy. Epidemiology 10:112–117

de Cock J, Westveer K, Heederik D, te VE, van Kooij R (1994) Time to pregnancy and occupational exposure to pesticides in fruit growers in The Netherlands. Occup Environ Med 51:693–699

Duty SM, Silva MJ, Barr DB, Brock JW, Ryan L, Chen Z, Herrick RF, Christiani DC, Hauser R (2003) Phthalate exposure and human semen parameters. Epidemiology 14:269–277

Ernst E (1990) Testicular toxicity following short-term exposure to tri- and hexavalent chromium: an experimental study in the rat. Toxicol Lett 51:269–275

Ernst E, Bonde JP (1992a) Sex hormones and epididymal sperm parameters in rats following sub-chronic treatment with hexavalent chromium. Hum Exp Toxicol 11:255–258

Ernst E, Bonde JP (1992b) Sex hormones and epididymal sperm parameters in rats following subchronic treatment with hexavalent chromium. Hum Exp Toxicol 11:255–258

Figa-Talamanca I, Cini C, Varricchio GC, Dondero F, Gandini L, Lenzi A, Lombardo F, Angelucci L, Di Grezia R, Patacchioli FR (1996) Effects of prolonged autovehicle driving on male reproduction function: a study among taxi drivers. Am J Indust Med 30:750–758

Figa-Talamanca I, Traina ME, Urbani E (2001) Occupational exposures to metals, solvents and pesticides: recent evidence on male reproductive effects and biological markers. Occup Med (Lond) 51:174–188

Gennart JP, Buchet JP, Roels H, Ghyselen P, Ceulemans E, Lauwerys R (1992) Fertility of male workers exposed to cadmium, lead, or manganese 19. Am J Epidemiol 135:1208–1219

Giwercman A, Bonde JP (1998) Declining male fertility and environmental factors. Endocrinol Metab Clin North Am 27:807–830, viii

Gluud C (1988) Testosterone and alcoholic cirrhosis. Lægeforeningens, Copenhagen

Greenlee AR, Arbuckle TE, Chyou PH (2003) Risk factors for female infertility in an agricultural region. Epidemiology 14:429–436

Harkonen K, Viitanen T, Larsen SB, Bonde JP, Lahdetie J (1999) Aneuploidy in sperm and exposure to fungicides and lifestyle factors. ASCLEPIOS. A European Concerted Action on Occupational Hazards to Male Reproductive Capability. Environ Mol Mutagen 34:39–46

Henderson J, Baker HW, Hanna PJ (1986) Occupation-related male infertility: a review. Clin Reprod Fertil 4:87–106

Hjollund NH, Bonde JP, Skotte J (1997) Semen analysis of personnel operating military radar equipment. Reprod Toxicol 11:897

Hjollund NH, Bonde JP, Jensen TK, Ernst E, Henriksen TB, Kolstad HA, Giwercman A, Skakkebaek NE, Olsen J (1998a) Semen quality and sex hormones with reference to metal welding. Reprod Toxicol 12:91–95

Hjollund NH, Bonde JP, Jensen TK, Henriksen TB, Kolstad HA, Ernst E, Giwercman A, Pritzl G, Skakkebaek NE, Olsen J (1998b) A follow-up study of male exposure to welding and time to pregnancy. Reprod Toxicol 12:29–37

Hjollund NH, Skotte JH, Kolstad HA, Bonde JP (1999) Extremely low frequency magnetic fields and fertility: a follow up study of couples planning first pregnancies. The Danish First Pregnancy Planner Study Team. Occup Environ Med 56:253–255
Hjollund NH, Bonde JP, Jensen TK, Olsen J (2000) Diurnal scrotal skin temperature and semen quality. The Danish First Pregnancy Planner Study Team. Int J Androl 23:309–318
Hjollund NH, Storgaard L, Ernst E, Bonde JP, Olsen J (2002a) Impact of diurnal scrotal temperature on semen quality. Reprod Toxicol 16:215–221
Hjollund NH, Storgaard L, Ernst E, Bonde JP, Olsen J (2002b) The relation between daily activities and scrotal temperature. Reprod Toxicol 16:209–214
Hjollund NH, Bonde JP, Ernst E, Lindenberg S, Andersen AN, Olsen J (2004) Pesticide exposure in male farmers and survival of in vitro fertilized pregnancies. Hum Reprod 19: 1331–1337
Hoppin JA (2003) Male reproductive effects of phthalates: an emerging picture. Epidemiology 14:259–260
Jelnes JE, Knudsen L (1988) Stainless steel welding and semen quality. Reprod Toxicol 2:218–215
Jensen TK, Henriksen TB, Hjollund NH, Scheike T, Kolstad H, Giwercman A, Ernst E, Bonde JP, Skakkebaek NE, Olsen J (1998a) Adult and prenatal exposures to tobacco smoke as risk indicators of fertility among 430 Danish couples. Am J Epidemiol 148:992–997
Jensen TK, Henriksen TB, Hjollund NH, Scheike T, Kolstad H, Giwercman A, Ernst E, Bonde JP, Skakkebaek NE, Olsen J (1998b) Caffeine intake and fecundability: a follow-up study among 430 Danish couples planning their first pregnancy. Reprod Toxicol 12:289–295
Jensen TK, Hjollund NH, Henriksen TB, Scheike T, Kolstad H, Giwercman A, Ernst E, Bonde JP, Skakkebaek NE, Olsen J (1998c) Does moderate alcohol consumption affect fertility? Follow up study among couples planning first pregnancy. BMJ 317:505–510
Jensen TK, Jorgensen N, Punab M, Haugen TB, Suominen J, Zilaitiene B, Horte A, Andersen AG, Carlsen E, Magnus O, Matulevicius V, Nermoen I, Vierula M, Keiding N, Toppari J, Skakkebaek NE (2004) Association of in utero exposure to maternal smoking with reduced semen quality and testis size in adulthood: a cross-sectional study of 1,770 young men from the general population in five European countries. Am J Epidemiol 159:49–58
Joffe M, Bisanti L, Apostoli P, Shah N, Kiss P, Dale A, Roeleveld N, Lindbohm ML, Sallmen M, Bonde JP (1999) Time to pregnancy and occupational lead exposure. Asclepios. Scand J Work Environ Health 25 [Suppl 1]:64–65
Juhl M, Nyboe Andersen AM, Gronbaek M, Olsen J (2001) Moderate alcohol consumption and waiting time to pregnancy. Hum Reprod 16:2705–2709
Jung A, Leonhardt F, Schill WB, Schuppe HC (2005) Influence of the type of undertrousers and physical activity on scrotal temperature. Hum Reprod 1022–1027
Kim Y, Jung K, Hwang T, Jung G, Kim H, Park J, Kim J, Park J, Park D, Park S, Choi K, Moon Y (1996) Hematopoietic and reproductive hazards of Korean electronic workers exposed to solvents containing 2-bromopropane. Scand J Work Environ Health 22:387–391
Kolstad HA, Bisanti L, Roeleveld N, Bonde JP, Joffe M (1999a) Time to pregnancy for men occupationally exposed to styrene in several European reinforced plastics companies. Asclepios. Scand J Work Environ Health 25 [Suppl 1]:66–69
Kolstad HA, Bonde JP, Spano M, Giwercman A, Zschiesche W, Kaae D, Roeleveld N (1999b) Sperm chromatin structure and semen quality following occupational styrene exposure. Asclepios. Scand J Work Environ Health 25 [Suppl 1]:70–73
Lahdetie J (1995) Occupation- and exposure-related studies on human sperm. J Occup Environ Med 37:922–930
Lancranjan I, Maicanescu M, Rafaila E, Klepsch I, Popescu HI (1975a) Gonadic function in workmen with longterm exposure to microwaves. Health Physics 29:381–383
Lancranjan I, Popescu HI, Gavanescu O, Klepsch I, Serbanescu M (1975b) Reproductive ability of workmen occupationally exposed to lead. Arch Environ Health 30:396–401
Larsen SB, Giwercman A, Spano M, Bonde JP (1998a) A longitudinal study of semen quality in pesticide spraying Danish farmers. The ASCLEPIOS Study Group. Reprod Toxicol 12: 581–589
Larsen SB, Joffe M, Bonde JP (1998b) Time to pregnancy and exposure to pesticides in Danish farmers. ASCLEPIOS Study Group. Occup Environ Med 55:278–283
Larsen SB, Spano M, Giwercman A, Bonde JP (1999) Semen quality and sex hormones among organic and traditional Danish farmers. ASCLEPIOS Study Group. Occup Environ Med 56:139–144
Lauwerys R, Roels H, Genet P, Toussaint G, Bouckaert A, De Cooman S (1985) Fertility of male workers exposed to mercury vapor or to manganese dust: a questionnaire study. Am J Indust Med 7:171–176
Lee IP, Dixon RL (1975) Effects of mercury on spermatogenesis studied by velocity sedimentation cell separation and serial mating. J Pharmacol Exp Ther 194:171–181
Lerda D (1992) Study of sperm characteristics in persons occupationally exposed to lead. Am J Indust Med 22:567–571
Lerda D, Rizzi R (1991) Study of reproductive function in persons occupationally exposed to 2,4-dichlorophenoxyacetic acid (2,4-D). Mutat Res 262:47–50
Littley MD, Shalet SM, Morgenstern GR, Deakin DP (1991) Endocrine and reproductive dysfunction following fractionated total body irradiation in adults. Q J Med 78:265–274
Loft S, Kold-Jensen T, Hjollund NH, Giwercman A, Gyllemborg J, Ernst E, Olsen J, Scheike T, Poulsen HE, Bonde JP (2003) Oxidative DNA damage in human sperm influences time to pregnancy. Hum Reprod 18:1265–1272
Marchetti F, Lowe X, Bishop J, Wyrobek AJ (1999) Absence of selection against aneuploid mouse sperm at fertilization. Biol Reprod 61:948–954
Mieusset R, Bujan L (1995) Testicular heating and its possible contributions to male infertility: a review. Int J Androl 18: 169–184
Mortensen JT (1988) Risk for reduced sperm quality among metal workers, with special reference to welders. Scand J Work Environ Health 14:27–30
Ogilvy-Stuart AL, Shalet SM (1993) Effect of radiation on the human reproductive system. Environ Health Perspect 101 [Suppl 2]:109–116
Omura M, Romero Y, Zhao M, Inoue N (1999) Histopathological evidence that spermatogonia are the target cells of 2-bromopropane. Toxicol Lett 104:19–26
Petrelli G, Figa-Talamanca I (2001) Reduction in fertility in male greenhouse workers exposed to pesticides. Eur J Epidemiol 17:675–677
Potashnik G, Porath A (1995) Dibromochloropropane (DBCP): a 17-year reassessment of testicular function and reproductive performance. J Occup Environ Med 37:1287–1292
Potashnik G, Ben-Aderet N, Israeli R, Yanai-Inbar I, Sober I (1978) Suppressive effect of 1,2.dibromo-3-chloropropane on human spermatogenesis. Fertil Steril 30:444–447
Procope BJ (1965) Effect of repeated increase of body temperature on human sperm cells. Int J Fertil 10:333–339
Ratcliffe JM, Schrader SM, Steenland K, Clapp DE, Turner T, Hornung RW (1987) Semen quality in papaya workers with long term exposure to ethylene dibromide. Br J Ind Med 44:317–326

Ratcliffe JM, Schrader SM, Clapp DE, Halperin WE, Turner TW, Hornung RW (1989) Semen quality in workers exposed to 2-ethoxyethanol. Br J Ind Med 46:399–406
Ratcliffe JM, Gladen BC, Wilcox AJ, Herbst AL (1992) Does early exposure to maternal smoking affect future fertility in adult males? Reprod Toxicol 6:297–307
Robbins WA, Vine MF, Truong KY, Everson RB (1997) Use of fluorescence in situ hybridization (FISH) to assess effects of smoking, caffeine, and alcohol on aneuploidy load in sperm of healthy men. Environ Mol Mutagen 30:175–183
Robins TG, Bornman MS, Ehrlich RI, Cantrell AC, Pienaar E, Vallabh J, Miller S (1997) Semen quality and fertility of men employed in a South African lead acid battery plant. Am J Ind Med 32:369–376
Rowley MJ, Leach DR, Warner GA, Heller CG (1974) Effect of graded doses of ionizing radiation on the human testis. Radiat Res 59:665–678
Rubes J, Lowe X, Moore D, Perreault S, Slott V, Evenson D, Selevan SG, Wyrobek AJ (1998) Smoking cigarettes is associated with increased sperm disomy in teenage men. Fertil Steril 70:715–723
Rupa DS, Reddy PP, Reddi OS (1991) Reproductive performance in population exposed to pesticides in cotton fields in India. Environ Res 55:123–128
Sanchez-Pena LC, Reyes BE, Lopez-Carrillo L, Recio R, Moran-Martinez J, Cebrian ME, Quintanilla-Vega B (2004) Organophosphorous pesticide exposure alters sperm chromatin structure in Mexican agricultural workers. Toxicol Appl Pharmacol 196:108–113
Savitz DA (2003) Paternal exposure to known mutagens and health of the offspring: ionizing radiation and tobacco smoke. Adv Exp Med Biol 518:49–57
Savitz DA, Sonnenfeld NL, Olshan AF (1994) Review of epidemiologic studies of paternal occupational exposure and spontaneous abortion. Am J Ind Med 25:361–383
Schrag SD, Dixon RL (1985) Occupational exposures associated with male reproductive dysfunction. Annu Rev Pharmacol Toxicol 25:567–592
Sharpe RM, Irvine DS (2004) How strong is the evidence of a link between environmental chemicals and adverse effects on human reproductive health? BMJ 328:447–451
Sheiner EK, Sheiner E, Hammel RD, Potashnik G, Carel R (2003) Effect of occupational exposures on male fertility: literature review. Ind Health 41:55–62
Son HY, Kim YB, Kang BH, Cho SW, Ha CS, Roh JK (1999) Effects of 2-bromopropane on spermatogenesis in the Sprague-Dawley rat. Reprod Toxicol 13:179–187
Sonnenschein C, Soto AM (1998) An updated review of environmental estrogen and androgen mimics and antagonists. J Steroid Biochem Mol Biol 65:143–150
Spano M, Kolstad AH, Larsen SB, Cordelli E, Leter G, Giwercman A, Bonde JP (1998) The applicability of the flow cytometric sperm chromatin structure assay in epidemiological studies. Asclepios. Hum Reprod 13:2495–2505
Steeno OP, Pangkahila A (1984) Occupational influences on male fertility and sexuality. I. Andrologia 16:5–22
Storgaard L, Bonde JP, Ernst E, Spano M, Andersen CY, Frydenberg M, Olsen J (2003) Does smoking during pregnancy affect sons' sperm counts? Epidemiology 14:278–286
Stoy J, Hjollund NH, Mortensen JT, Burr H, Bonde JP (2004) Semen quality and sedentary work position. Int J Androl 27:5–11
Tas S, Lauwerys R, Lison D (1996) Occupational hazards for the male reproductive system. Crit Rev Toxicol 26:261–307
Thonneau P, Ducot B, Bujan L, Mieusset R, Spira A (1996) Heat exposure as a hazard to male fertility. Lancet 347:204–205
Thonneau P, Bujan L, Multigner L, Mieusset R (1998) Occupational heat exposure and male fertility: a review. Hum Reprod 13:2122–2125
Thonneau P, Abell A, Larsen SB, Bonde JP, Joffe M, Clavert A, Ducot B, Multigner L, Danscher G (1999) Effects of pesticide exposure on time to pregnancy: results of a multicenter study in France and Denmark. ASCLEPIOS Study Group. Am J Epidemiol 150:157–163
Tielemans E, Burdorf A, te Velde ER, Weber RF, van Kooij RJ, Veulemans H, Heederik DJ (1999a) Occupationally related exposures and reduced semen quality: a case-control study. Fertil Steril 71:690–696
Tielemans E, van Kooij R, te Velde ER, Burdorf A, Heederik D (1999b) Pesticide exposure and decreased fertilisation rates in vitro. Lancet 354:484–485
Toft G, Hagmar L, Giwercman A, Bonde JP (2004) Epidemiological evidence on reproductive effects of persistent organochlorines in humans. Reprod Toxicol 19:5–26
Trasler JM, Hales BF, Robaire B (1985) Paternal cyclophosphamide treatment of rats causes fetal loss and malformations without affecting male fertility. Nature 316:144–146
Vanhoorne M, Comhaire F, De Bacquer D (1994) Epidemiological study of the effects of carbon disulfide on male sexuality and reproduction. Arch Environ Health 49:273–278
Veulemans H, Steeno O, Masschelein R, Groeseneken D (1993) Exposure to ethylene glycol ethers and spermatogenic disorders in man: a case-control study. Br J Ind Med 50:71–78
Vine MF (1996) Smoking and male reproduction: a review. Int J Androl 19:323–337
Vine MF, Margolin BH, Morrison HI, Hulka BS (1994) Cigarette smoking and sperm density: a meta-analysis. Fertil Steril 61:35–43
Vine MF, Setzer RW Jr., Everson RB, Wyrobek AJ (1997) Human sperm morphometry and smoking, caffeine, and alcohol consumption. Reprod Toxicol 11:179–184
Viskum S, Rabjerg L, Jorgensen PJ, Grandjean P (1999) Improvement in semen quality associated with decreasing occupational lead exposure. Am J Indust Med 35:257–263
Weyandt TB, Schrader SM, Turner TW, Simon SD (1996) Semen analysis of military personnel associated with military duty assignments. Reprod Toxicol 10:521–528
Whorton MD, Foliart DE (1983) Mutagenicity, carcinogenicity and reproductive effects of dibromochloropropane (DBCP). Mutat Res 123:13–30
Whorton MD, Milby TH (1980) Recovery of testicular function among DBCP workers. J Occupat Med 22:177–179
Whorton MD, Krauss RM, Marshall S, Milby TH (1977) Infertility in male pesticide workers. Lancet 2:1259–1261
Whorton MD, Milby TH, Stubbs HA, Avashia BH, Hull EQ (1979) Testicular function among carbaryl-exposed employees. J Toxicol Environ Health 5:929–941
Wildt K, Eliasson R, Berlin M (1983) Effect of occupational exposure to lead on sperm and semen. Reprod Dev Toxicity Metals 279–300
Wong O, Utidjian MD, Karten VS (1979) Retrospective evaluation of reproductive performance of workers exposed to ethylene dibromide (EDB). J Occupat Med 21:98–102
Wyrobek AJ, Watchmaker G, Gordon L, Wong K, Moore HD, Whorton D (1981) Sperm shape abnormalities in carbaryl-exposed employees. Environ Health Perspect 40:255–265
Zhang YH, Chen BH, Zheng LX, Wu XY (2003) [Study on the level of phthalates in human biological samples]. Zhonghua Yu Fang Yi Xue Za Zhi 37:429–434

II.2.7 Influence of Systemic Diseases and Iatrogenic Factors on Sexual and Reproductive Functions

R. Bornman

Summary

Systemic diseases and ejaculatory dysfunction may be partly or entirely the cause of impaired male fertility. Certain medications may have a further negative effect on sperm function. If the physician is content to make a diagnosis on the semen analysis report without listening to the patient (history) or looking for specific signs (examination), very significant conditions may be overlooked. Unfortunately, this may lead not only to inappropriate management, but also to the loss of an opportunity to make a difference to the short- and long-term prognosis of both male reproductive and general health.

II.2.7.1 Introduction

A male factor is implicated in up to 50% of all infertile couples. The success of managing male factor infertility depends on both a clinical diagnosis and determination of the cause of the male factor infertility. There are many potential causes of male factor infertility and a systematic approach, therefore, is indispensable for directing the evaluation in order to make properly justifiable decisions about the diagnosis, aetiology and management.

As physicians we are all aware of the pitfalls of taking shortcuts in medicine – this is particularly true for andrology and male infertility. Only a detailed, complete medical history combined with a focused clinical examination will allow for appropriate laboratory and other studies. This requires that the managing physician has a definite understanding of the applied and integrative aspects of the genetics, anatomy and physiology of the male reproductive system. Without this, the evaluation may well become an incompetent exercise failing to elucidate the precise cause of infertility and resulting in the spider webs of inappropriate management.

II.2.7.2 Sexual and Reproductive Function

Male sexual dysfunction, observed by the absence of an erection, may be classified in the same way as female sexual dysfunction, according to DSM IV, into desire, arousal, orgasmic or pain disorders.

II.2.7.2.1 Libido

Testosterone is responsible for normal libido (sexual desire) and male psychosexual behaviour. In some cases, ejaculatory problems may occur in combination with loss of libido, and androgen deficiency (hypogonadism) starting as either pituitary or testicular dysfunction should be considered. Patients with hypogonadism may have decreased or absent ejaculation because the secretory function of the prostate and seminal vesicles is androgen dependent. If the seminal volume is normal, it seems unlikely that endocrine factors are responsible for loss of libido (Gerber and Brendler 2002).

The primary absence of sexual desire seems to be extremely rare. A decrease or complete loss of libido usually occurs secondarily. Organic causes such as dyspareunia (physical discomfort during intercourse), endocrine disturbances and chronic incapacitating disease, as well as iatrogenic causes such as anti-hypertensive drugs, sedatives and tranquilizers can change libido. A decrease in libido may also result from depression and a variety of medical illnesses that affect general health and well-being.

Erectile dysfunction, generally associated with reduced sexual desire and sometimes with orgasmic or ejaculatory dysfunction, is the major revealing symptom of hyperprolactinaemia in men, a condition that should not be neglected since many cases result from pituitary tumours, likely to result in serious complications (Buvat 2003). Prolactin (PRL) has a fundamental role in sexual activity and an elevated PRL level is associated with alterations in desire or libido. During chronic high levels of PRL in animals, Leydig cell sensitivity to luteinizing hormone (LH) stimulation changes and testosterone subsequently decreases (Huang et al. 2001). It also seems that PRL may be a feedback mechanism to central nervous system centres that control sexual arousal and behaviour. In both men and women plasma PRL concentrations are considerably increased for over 1 h following orgasm induced by either coitus or masturbation. Plasma PRL, however, remains unchanged following sexual arousal without orgasm (Exton et al. 2001; Kruger et al. 2002).

II.2.7.2.2 Emission and Ejaculation

The ejaculatory process consists of a well-timed sequence of neuromuscular events resulting in the expulsion of semen from the urethra. Subsequently the fertility potential will be affected by any neuromuscular involvement or anatomical/mechanical abnormalities.

Ejaculatory Dysfunction

Ejaculatory dysfunction is involved in < 2 % of causes of infertility (Wang et al. 1996). Congenital, pharmacological, metabolic, inflammatory and functional abnormalities are also potential causes, but some cases remain idiopathic.

Any process that interferes with the peristaltic contractions of the vas deferens and closure of the bladder neck may result in either failure of emission or retrograde ejaculation (Brugh et al. 2003). Ejaculatory dysfunction should be suspected in any patient with low-volume (< 1.0 ml) or absent ejaculate and should be distinguished from anorgasmia. In contrast, sperm will not be present in the urine of a patient with failure of emission, which must be diagnosed by clinical suspicion.

The causes of ejaculatory dysfunction are summarized in Table II.2.5.

Retrograde Ejaculation

Retrograde ejaculation is caused by incomplete closure of the bladder neck and subsequently sperm and seminal fluid are propelled backwards into the bladder through the bladder neck. The ejaculate volume is accordingly reduced or absent. Retrograde ejaculation is diagnosed by examining the post-ejaculate urine for sperm. Exact criteria have not been established for a positive post-ejaculate urinalysis, but the finding of > 10 sperm per high-power field confirms the presence of retrograde ejaculation.

Failure to Ejaculate (Anejaculation, Aspermia)

Patients who complain of absence of ejaculation should be questioned regarding loss of libido or other symptoms of androgen deficiency, present medications, diabetes and previous surgery. A careful history will usually determine the cause of this problem (Gerber and Brendler 2002).

Androgen deficiency results in decreased secretions from the prostate and seminal vesicles causing a reduction or loss of seminal volume. Sympathectomy or extensive retroperitoneal surgery, most particularly retroperitoneal lymphadenectomy for testicular cancer, may interfere with autonomic innervation of the prostate and seminal vesicles, resulting in the absence of smooth muscle contraction and absence of seminal emission at the time of orgasm. Pharmacologic agents, especially α-adrenergic antagonists, may interfere with bladder neck closure at the time of orgasm and subsequently result in retrograde ejaculation. Previous bladder neck or prostatic urethral surgery, most typically transurethral resection of the prostate, may interfere with bladder neck closure, resulting in retrograde ejaculation. Retrograde ejaculation may develop in diabetic men as part of the diabetic neuropathy.

Table II.2.5. Causes of ejaculatory dysfunction

Anejaculation	Retrograde ejaculation	Premature ejaculation
Traumatic Spinal cord injury Trauma to posterior urethra	**Traumatic** Spinal cord injury Trauma to posterior urethra	**Psychological**
Iatrogenic Retroperitoneal lymph node dissection Aortic aneurysm surgery Colorectal surgery Sympathectomy	**Iatrogenic** Retroperitoneal lymph node dissection Aortic aneurysm surgery Colorectal surgery Sympathectomy Prostatectomy Y-V plasty of bladder neck Posterior urethroplasty	**Systemic** Multiple sclerosis
Pharmacological Antihypertensives Antidepressants Antipsychotics Others including alcohol, etc.	**Congenital** Epispadias Exstrophy Posterior urethral valves	**Inflammatory** Prostatitis
Metabolic and systemic Diabetes mellitus Multiple sclerosis	**Pharmacological** Antihypertensives Antidepressants Antipsychotics Others including alcohol, etc.	**Other** Spinal cord tumour Benign prostatic hypertrophy
Psychological Delayed ejaculation *Idiopathic*	**Metabolic and systemic** Diabetes mellitus *Idiopathic*	

Premature Ejaculation

Premature ejaculation is characterized by the inability of the patient to control the time of ejaculation in a way that will allow his partner to reach an orgasm. Rapid (premature) ejaculation (RE) is a very common sexual disorder and may occur as a primary event or secondarily to underlying disease (Abdel-Hamid 2004). Premature ejaculation is clearly a very subjective symptom. It is common for men to ejaculate within 2 min after initiation of intercourse, and many men who complain of premature ejaculation in reality have normal sexual function with abnormal sexual expectations. Men with true premature ejaculation reach orgasm within less than 1 min after initiation of intercourse. This cause is almost always psychogenic and best treated by a clinical psychologist or psychiatrist who specializes in treating psychological aspects of male sexual dysfunction (Han et al. 2002).

Erectile dysfunction occurs in 3% to 5% of patients undergoing an open prostatectomy; it is more common in older men than in younger men.

Anorgasmia

Anorgasmia or the absence of orgasm is usually psychogenic or caused by certain medications used to treat psychiatric diseases. Sometimes, however, anorgasmia may be due to decreased penile sensation owing to impaired pudendal nerve function. Most commonly, this occurs in diabetics with peripheral neuropathy (Gerber and Brendler 2002).

Neurological

Diabetes mellitus causes peripheral nervous system injury resulting in possible retrograde ejaculation or anejaculation. Central nervous system lesions, such as spinal cord injury and myelodysplasia, can also cause ejaculatory dysfunction.

Failure of emission or ejaculation can also occur during retroperitoneal lymph node dissection for testicular cancer or other retroperitoneal abdominal or pelvic surgery when a portion of the sympathetic chain or pelvic nerves are also excised.

Drugs

Some medications will affect ejaculation, such as α-blockers (causing retrograde ejaculation), antidepressants, antipsychotics and some antihypertensives.

Anatomic causes of ejaculatory dysfunction include obstruction of the ejaculatory ducts and previous surgery on the bladder neck (Y-V plasty of the bladder neck, transurethral incision, or resection of the prostate). Retrograde ejaculation occurs in 80% to 90% of post-prostatectomy patients. The risk, however, can be reduced if the bladder neck is preserved at the time of surgery. Also, in 2% to 3% of patients a bladder neck contracture develops 6–12 weeks after an open prostatectomy, particularly in men who have a relatively small opening at the bladder neck at the end of the operation (Brugh et al. 2003).

II.2.7.2.3 Erectile Function

Male sexual dysfunction [*impotence* or *erectile dysfunction* (*ED*)] refers specifically to the persistent inability for at least 3 months to attain and maintain a penile erection sufficient for satisfactory sexual performance. ED is a symptom of disease and an important marker often of serious underlying pathology. ED is influenced by lifestyle factors (uncontrolled stress, lack of exercise, obesity, smoking, substance abuse) and lifestyle-associated diseases (hypertension, ischaemic heart disease, diabetes mellitus). These should be diagnosed as soon as possible, especially in younger men, when lifestyle changes may still be of benefit.

Studies show that blood testosterone concentrations are consistently lower among men with cardiovascular disease, suggesting a possible preventive role for testosterone therapy. Moreover, ED is frequently caused by pelvic arterial insufficiency due to atherosclerosis. This sentinel relationship to generalized atherosclerosis should not be overlooked in males complaining about infertility (Liu et al. 2003).

Systemic and iatrogenic causes of ED are summarized in Table II.2.6. Table II.2.7 lists the pharmacological causes of ED.

Table II.2.6. Medical conditions associated with erectile dysfunction

Factor	Conditions
Chronic medical illness	Diabetes mellitus, renal failure, anaemia
Medication and recreational drug use	Antihypertensives, antidepressants, alcohol, marijuana, cocaine
Atherosclerotic risk factors	Hypercholesterolaemia, hypertension, diabetes mellitus, family history
Pelvic, perineal, penile trauma	Pelvic fracture, cycling
Past surgery	Radical prostatectomy, laminectomy, vascular bypass surgery
Neurological disease	Multiple sclerosis, lumbosacral disc disease, spinal cord injury
Endocrinological disease	Hypogonadism, hyperprolactinaemia, thyroid disease
Psychiatric disease	Anxiety, depression
Sexually transmitted diseases	Retroviral disease, gonorrhoea, syphilis

Table II.2.7. Drugs often associated with erectile dysfunction

Antihypertensives	Thiazide diuretics, β-blockers, calcium channel blockers, angiotensin converting enzyme (ACE) inhibitors
Antidepressants	Tricyclic antidepressants, selective serotonin reuptake inhibitors (SSRIs)
Antiarrhythmics	Digoxin
Anti-androgens	Anti-androgens
H_2-blockers	Cimetidine
Recreational drugs	Alcohol, marijuana, cocaine, heroin

A careful history will often determine whether the problem is primarily psychogenic or organic. In men with psychogenic impotence, the condition frequently develops rather quickly secondary to a precipitating event such as marital stress or change or loss of a sexual partner. In men with organic impotence, the condition usually develops more insidiously and frequently can be linked to advancing age or other underlying risk factors.

In evaluating men with impotence, it is important to determine whether the problem exists in all situations. Many men who report impotence may not be able to have intercourse with one partner but will with another. Similarly, it is important to determine whether men are able to achieve normal erections with alternative forms of sexual stimulation (e.g. masturbation, erotic videos). Finally, the patient should be asked whether he ever notes nocturnal or early morning erections. In general, patients who are able to achieve adequate erections in some situations but not others have primarily psychogenic rather than organic impotence (Gerber and Brendler 2002).

Mechanical Causes of Sexual Dysfunction

Anatomical Penile Abnormalities

Congenital or acquired abnormalities of the penis may interfere with normal deposition of semen. The anatomical congenital variations include hypo-/epispadias and also Peyronie's disease. In hypospadias the urethra does not extend to the glans and the meatus is situated on the underside of the penis. In the majority of cases, glandular, coronal and distal hypospadias are observed, but penoscrotal or perineal hypospadias may occur.

In epispadias, the meatal opening is located on the dorsum of the penis and often forms an open urethral groove. In the majority of cases, epispadias will result in severe dorsal deviation of the penis, which may lead to disturbances in sperm deposition.

Phimosis is narrowing of the foreskin of the penis, either congenital or acquired. In secondary cases, diabetes mellitus, severe balanitis or lichen sclerosis et atrophicus may be responsible for infections and secondary phimosis. In individual cases, uncorrected phimosis may impair semen deposition and cause infertility (Gerber and Brendler 2002).

Table II.2.8. Systemic diseases and fertility

Disease	Possible cause of infertility
Diabetes	Neuropathy
Tuberculosis	Epididymitis, obstructive azoospermia
Chronic respiratory tract disease such as bronchiectasis, chronic sinusitis/bronchitis	Disorders of sperm cilia, complete asthenozoospermia, secretory disturbances in the epididymis resulting in obstructive azoospermia (Young syndrome)
Cystic fibrosis	Agenesis of vasa deferentia or seminal vesicles
Renal or hepatic dysfunction	Metabolic disorders
Fever > 38 °C	Suppression spermatogenesis (oligozoospermia)
Iatrogenic – chemotherapy, radiotherapy, medications such as nitrofurantoin, nitrodazole, sulphasalazine, spironolactone, colchicine	Teratozoo- or oligozoospermia
Surgery, anaesthesia, stress	Suppression hypothalamo-pituitary gonadal axis
STD such as syphilis, gonorrhoea, lymphogranulosum venereum, urethritis, *Chlamydia* infection	Granuloma and scarring with partial obstruction or antisperm antibodies
Mumps orchitis after puberty	Testicular ischaemia and fibrosis
Bilateral testicular trauma, torsion, undescended testis	Testicular damage
Occupational or environmental exposure to metals such as cadmium, mercury, lead; chemicals such as pesticides, phenol esters, ethylene, lifestyle related – excessive alcohol intake, heavy smoking, drug addiction	Testicular damage

II.2.7.3
Systemic Diseases and Fertility

Systemic conditions may contribute in various ways to impaired male fertility (Table II.2.8) (Comhaire 1996).

For a detailed discussion on lifestyle factors, the reader is also referred to Chap. II.2.6. Contaminants in tobacco smoke seem to have minor effects on adult males per se, but cigarette smoking may be associated with oxidative DNA damage in human spermatozoa and become clinically evident as male-mediated developmental toxicity in the offspring. Smokers are often heavy coffee drinkers, and caffeine itself may affect sperm parameters. Infertile men who smoke cigarettes have higher levels of seminal ROS than infertile nonsmokers. Given the potential adverse effects of smoking, physicians should advise infertile men who smoke cigarettes to quit.

Marinelli et al. (2004) reviewed the literature on alcohol use and semen quality, but studies on the effects of drinking habits on semen parameters seem insufficient to draw clear conclusions. In general, it seems that men with moderate alcohol consumption had fewer sperm defects than heavy drinkers (Auger et al. 2001).

References

Abdel-Hamid IA (2004) Phosphodiesterase 5 inhibitors in rapid ejaculation: potential use and possible mechanisms of action. Drugs 64:13 – 26

Auger J, Eustache F, Andersen AG, Irvine DS, Jorgensen N, Skakkebaek J, Suominen J, Toppari J, Vierula M, Jouannet P (2001) Sperm morphological defects related to environment, lifestyle and medical history of 1001 male partners of pregnant women from four European cities. Hum Reprod 16:2710 – 2717

Brugh VM III, Matschke HM, Lipshultz LI (2003) Male factor infertility. Endocrinol Metab Clin 32:689 – 707

Buvat J (2003) Hyperprolactinemia and sexual function in men: a short review. Int J Impotence Res 15:373 – 377

Comhaire FH (1996) Basic investigation of the infertile male and andrological aspects of erectile dysfunction. In: Comhaire FH (ed) Male infertility. Chapman and Hall, London, pp 134 – 142

Exton MS, Kruger TH, Bursch N et al (2001) Endocrine response to masturbation-induced orgasm in healthy men following a 3-week sexual abstinence. World J Urol 19:377 – 382

Gerber GS, Brendler CB (2002) Evaluation of the urologic patient: history, physical examination, and urinanalysis. In: Walsh PC (ed) Campbell's urology, 8th edn. Elsevier, Amsterdam, pp 83 – 110

Han M, Alfert HJ, Partin AW (2002) Retropubic and suprapubic open prostatectomy. In: Walsh PC (ed) Campbell's urology, 8th edn. Elsevier, Amsterdam, p 1433

Huang WJ, Yeh JY, Kan SF et al (2001) Effects of hyperprolactinemia on testosterone production in rat Leydig cells. J Cell Biochem 80:313 – 320

Kruger TH, Haake P, Hartmann U et al (2002) Orgasm-induced prolactin secretion: feedback control of sexual drive? Neurosci Biobehav Rev 26:31 – 44

Liu PY, Death AK, Handelsman DJ (2003) Androgens and cardiovascular disease. Endocr Rev 24:313 – 40

Marinelli D, Gaspari L, Pedotti P, Taioli E (2004) Minireviews of studies on the effects of smoking and drinking habits on semen parameters. Int J Hyg Environ Health 207:185 – 192

Wang R, Monga M, Helsstrom WJG (1996) Ejaculatory dysfunction. In: Comhaire FH (ed) Male infertility. Chapman and Hall, London, pp 134 – 142

II.2.8 Mechanisms of Pathogenesis of Uro-Genital Cancers

T. F. 'Aho, D. E. Neal

Summary

- Epidemiological studies have identified certain risk factors for uro-genital cancers.
- Defining the mechanisms by which these factors cause cancer remains ongoing.
- Carcinogenesis is usually a complex, multi-step process.
- Genetic and epigenetic mechanisms both play a role in carcinogenesis.
- An improved understanding of the mechanisms of carcinogenesis will translate into advancements in cancer prevention, detection and therapy.
- This chapter summarizes current opinion on mechanisms of carcinogenesis in general with specific comments on prostate, testis and penile cancer.

II.2

II.2.8.1
Pathogenesis of Cancer in General

II.2.8.1.1
Basic Principles of Carcinogenesis

Most cell populations in the adult human are differentiated and do not proliferate at a high rate. The rate of cell growth and division is tightly controlled. The basic underlying causes of cancer include the accumulation of many genetic and epigenetic alterations that result in independence from normal regulatory mechanisms.

Somatic Mutations

It is now generally accepted that carcinogenesis is a multi-step process that begins most commonly by somatic mutations in the DNA of a single cell (Fig. II.2.10). Mutations predisposing to cancer may occur in

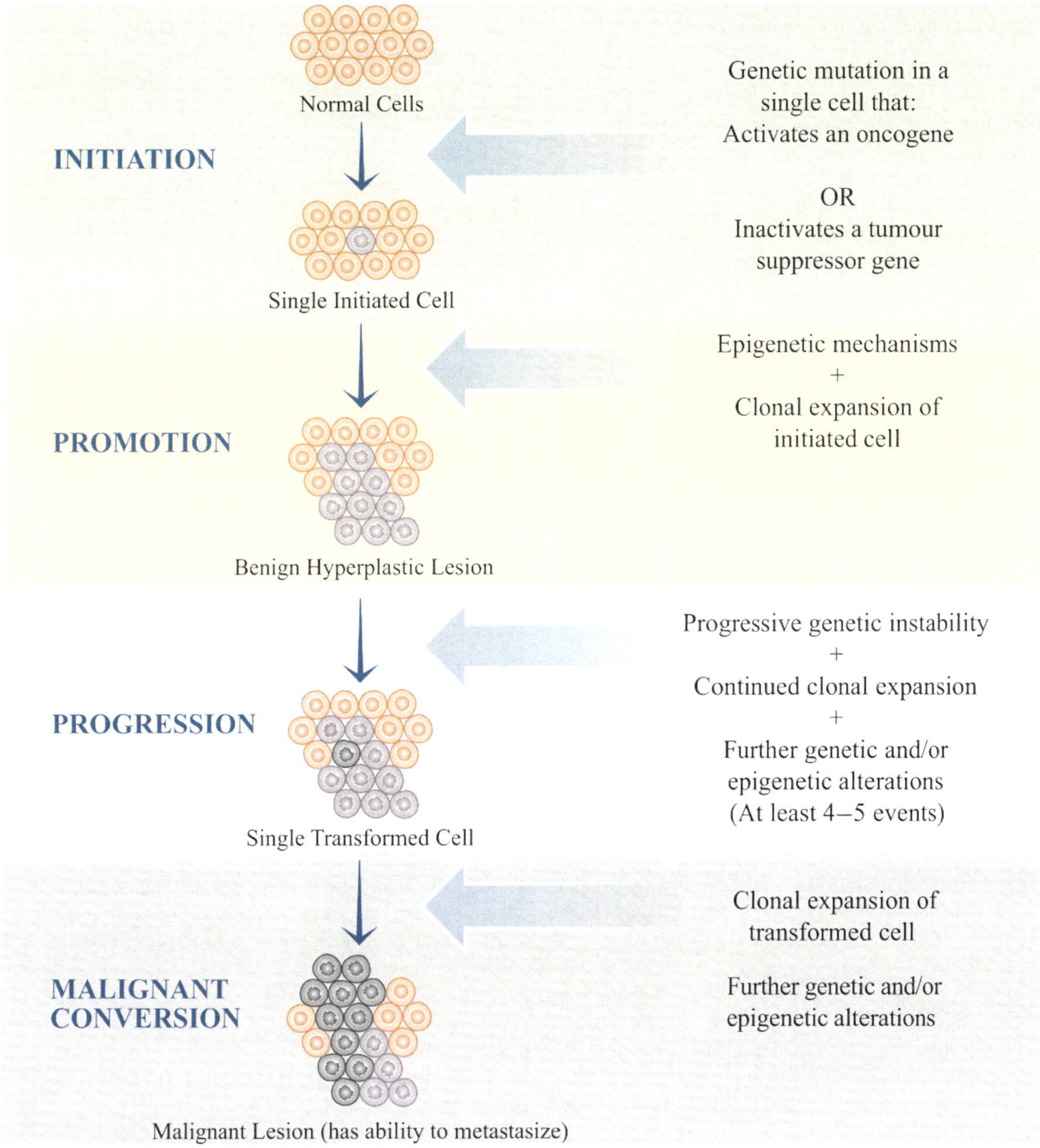

Fig. II.2.10. Stages of carcinogenesis

genes encoding proteins that affect a variety of regulatory processes including:

- Cell cycle regulation
- Apoptosis
- DNA repair
- Genetic stability
- Cell–cell and cell–matrix adhesion
- Transmembrane signalling
- Angiogenesis

The genes encoding these proteins can be divided into two functionally distinct groups: oncogenes and tumour suppressor genes.

Oncogenes

Of the approximately 25,000 genes in the human genome about 1% can be classified as proto-oncogenes. These are normal genes that code for proteins involved in diverse processes such as control of cell signalling and cell growth and angiogenesis. The proteins themselves can be classified into functional groups that include:

- Growth factors
- Receptor tyrosine kinases
- Membrane-associated non-receptor tyrosine kinases
- G-protein-coupled receptors
- Membrane-associated G-proteins
- Serine/threonine kinases
- Nuclear DNA-binding/transcription factors

When proto-oncogenes undergo a mutation or epigenetic alteration that confers a gain of function they become oncogenes, which predispose the individual to cancer. Oncogenes are dominant, therefore one abnormal allele increases the risk of cancer. The mechanisms include gene amplification, translocation and epigenetic mechanisms.

Tumour Suppressor Genes (TSGs)

TSGs, on the other hand, typically encode proteins involved in processes such as:

- Suppression of the cell cycle
- DNA repair in genetically abnormal cells
- Apoptosis if DNA damage is irreparable
- Cell–cell and cell-matrix adhesion
- Inhibition of metastasis

TSGs behave as recessives. Cells with one abnormal copy of the gene, which subsequently lose the normal copy [the process known as loss of heterogeneity (LOH)], are susceptible to cancer. Loss of function of both normal TSGs due to mutation, epigenetic change or deletion also increases the risk of cancer.

Epigenetic Alterations in Gene Expression

Whereas genetic mutations permanently alter the genome, epigenetic events modify gene expression without altering the genome sequence. There has been recent interest in the epigenetic silencing of TSGs by hypermethylation of gene regulatory DNA sequences (Garinis et al. 2002). This alters intra-nuclear protein–DNA interactions and the chromatin structure, affecting the rate of transcription and culminating in the under-expression of mRNA in cancers. Epigenetic mechanisms may also transform some proto-oncogenes. Unlike genetic mutations, epigenetic alterations are potentially reversible giving a degree of plasticity to the malignant phenotype.

Multi-Step Models of Carcinogenesis

Knudson's two-hit hypothesis noted that more than one genetic alteration in a cell is required for malignant transformation (Moolgavkar and Knudson 1981). Weinberg (1983) hypothesized that activation of at least two oncogenes in a specific order and context was necessary, and Barrett suggested that two different types of events were required (Boyd and Barrett 1990):

- Initiation: an irreversible mutational event arising from interaction with a carcinogen. Initiated cells must undergo further alteration by way of promotion and progression if they are to become malignant.
- Promotion, progression and malignant transformation: promoters, which may be endogenous (e.g. hormones, chronic inflammation) or exogenous (e.g. chemicals), act on initiated cells via reversible epigenetic mechanisms to form focal hyperplastic lesions. The resultant benign lesions may acquire progressively greater genetic instability and independent proliferative capacity until a clone of cells capable of autonomous cell division arises (progression). When this clone acquires the ability to metastasize, malignant transformation is complete.

Tumour kinetics imply that a series of four to five genetic and/or epigenetic events is required for a cancer to become clinically apparent.

Clonal Selection and Genetic Instability

Mutational events predisposing to cancer are rare, however once such an event has occurred carcinogenesis is accelerated by clonal selection and genetic instability. Clonal selection refers to the progressive outgrowth and eventual predominance of an initiated cell population that is less responsive to regulatory pathways than normal cells. As a less regulated clone predominates it becomes even more prone to mutation (genetic instability) which may render the clone even more independent of normal regulatory mechanisms. Hence there is serial amplification of clones that are progressively more predisposed to cancer.

II.2.8.1.2 Causes of Cancer

In vitro experiments, animal models and epidemiological studies suggest that most cancers are caused by the complex interaction of endogenous and exogenous factors which are modulated by the individual's age and genetic susceptibility to cancer.

Genetic Susceptibility

Some individuals are genetically more prone to cancer than others. Genetic polymorphisms affecting the following processes may render an individual more susceptible to oncogenic agents:

- Activation and detoxification of carcinogens
- DNA repair
- Cell cycle arrest coupled to DNA damage

The following are proposed mechanisms for some aetiological agents.

Hormones

Many endogenous and exogenous hormones provide a stimulus to cell proliferation, and mitogenesis increases the risk of accumulating random genetic mutations. If a series of random errors in the DNA of a cell enables it to escape normal regulatory mechanisms a cancer may develop. In contrast to chemical carcinogenesis where a specific initiator is required before carcinogenesis may proceed, none is required for hormonal carcinogenesis.

Viruses

It is estimated that around 15% of cancers worldwide may be caused by viruses. Tumour viruses are not usually complete carcinogens. The multi-step model of carcinogenesis applies, hence there may be a significant time delay between initial infection and emergence of a malignant phenotype, and most infected individuals do not develop cancer. There are two distinct groups of tumour viruses:

- DNA viruses (e.g. papilloma viruses) carry viral oncogenes that encode proteins essential for viral replication [the "large" T antigens (distinct from antigens on the surface of T cells)]. T antigen proteins may bind and inactivate host tumour suppressor proteins such as Rb and p53.
- Transforming retroviruses (e.g. human T cell lymphocytotrophic virus, HTLV) interact with host oncogenes in one of two ways:
  1. Transduction of a novel retroviral oncogene
     If insertion of the viral genome into an infected cell occurs near a host proto-oncogene, an excisional error could remove the proto-oncogene along with the viral genome. Subsequent alteration of the proto-oncogene by the virus may transform it into a viral oncogene.
  2. Retroviral integration-induced transformation
     Long terminal repeats (LTRs) are powerful transcriptional promoter sequences located at the end of retroviral genomes. If the random insertion of the viral genome into that of the host positions the LTRs close to a host proto-oncogene, it may be over-expressed.

Chronic Inflammation

Inflammatory cascades may generate oxidants and electrophiles that could damage DNA in a way that predisposes to cancer. Some chronic inflammatory lesions (e.g. proliferative inflammatory atrophy in the prostate) have been proposed as cancer precursors.

Chemicals

Chemical carcinogens are usually tissue specific. Indirect-acting carcinogens require activation by host enzymes in order to react with DNA whereas direct-acting carcinogens do not. Humans possess drug-metabolizing enzymes (xenobiotics) that may either detoxify or activate exogenous chemical carcinogens. The most important of these is the cytochrome P450 mono-oxygenase superfamily. Competition between activating and detoxifying pathways ultimately determines the effect of carcinogen exposure. Most direct carcinogens and activated indirect carcinogens react with DNA by transferring alkyl-, aryl- or aromatic amine groups. This results in fixation of nucleotide substitution or frameshift mutations.

Radiation

Ionizing radiation is a universal carcinogen with the potential to induce cancer in most tissues at any age. It can cause a range of seemingly random large-scale events resulting in DNA damage and mutations. As well as inducing cancer directly, radiation can render cells genetically unstable. Subsequent mutations in these unstable cells might then transform to a malignant phenotype.

Diet and Nutrition

It is estimated that dietary and nutritional factors contribute to around 35% of cancers. Two components have been implicated as causes of cancer:

- **Chemical carcinogens (micro-components)**
  The diet may contain potentially carcinogenic micro-components that are natural, synthetic or may result from cooking or contamination. Most occur at levels too low to cause a biological effect, but may interact with each other to predispose to cancer. Some react with DNA (e.g. heterocyclic aromatic amines produced by cooking proteinaceous food, and polycyclic aromatic hydrocarbons), whilst others do not (e.g. cadmium and arsenic). Compounds with anti-carcinogenic effects (e.g. vitamins A, C and E, folic acid, selenium and the isoflavones) may also be found in the diet.

- **Overnutrition (macro-components)**
  It is generally accepted that macro-components (e.g. animal fats rich in saturated fatty acids and excess calories) are greater contributors to cancer risk than micro-components. Epidemiological studies suggest that excess caloric intake and fat intake are independently associated with increased cancer incidence. Possible mechanisms include: increased cell proliferation, decreased cell death, hormonal imbalance and increased oxidative stress.

II.2.8.2 Pathogenesis of Prostate Cancer

II.2.8.2.1 Introduction

Prostate cancer is a heterogeneous disease with multifactorial aetiology involving genetic, epigenetic and environmental factors on a background of progressively increasing incidence with age (more so than for any other cancer). Prostate cancer may be sporadic, familial or hereditary; androgen receptor signalling plays a central role. Its pathogenesis remains poorly understood but the general principles of carcinogenesis apply (Fig. II.2.11). Multiple genes and variable phenotypic expression are likely involved (Visakorpi 2003; Deutsch et al. 2004).

II.2.8.2.2 Prostate Intraepithelial Neoplasia (PIN)

Whether a stepwise transition from low-grade to high-grade PIN (HGPIN) and then to prostate cancer exists remains controversial. A number of up-regulated and down-regulated genes have been identified in HGPIN and prostate cancer compared to normal prostate, and some of these may be involved in early prostate carcinogenesis (Ashida et al. 2004).

II.2.8.2.3 Proliferative Inflammatory Atrophy (PIA)

PIA arises when chronically inflamed prostate cells that have suffered oxidative damage attempt to regenerate.

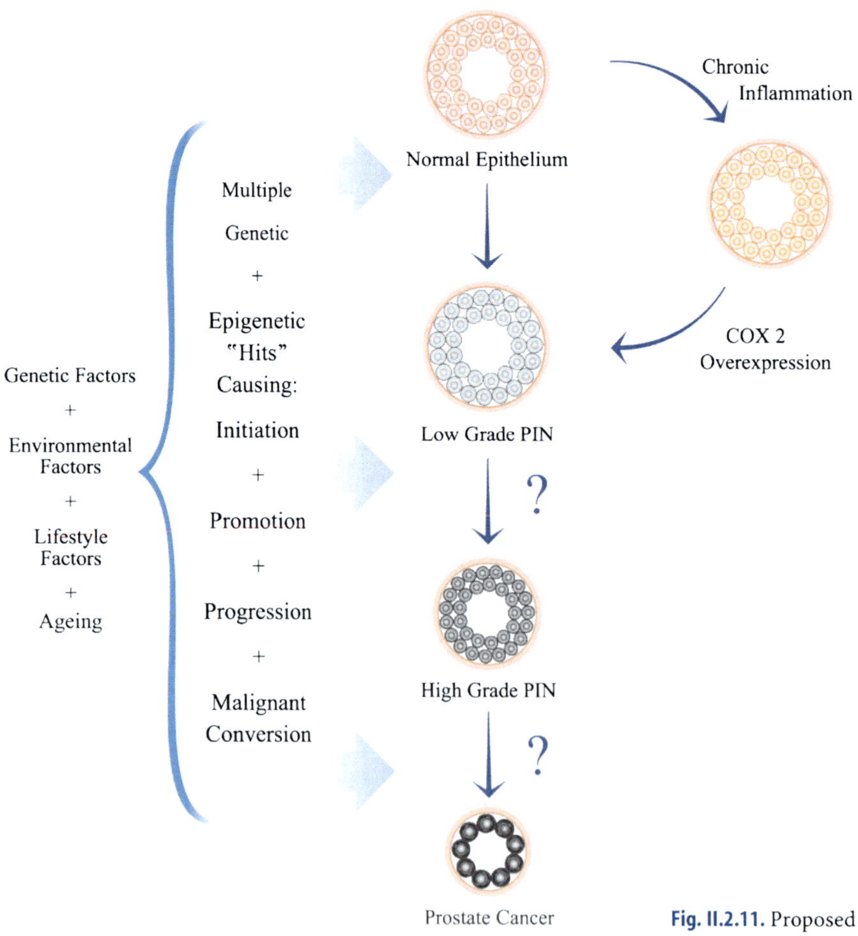

Fig. II.2.11. Proposed pathogenesis of prostate cancer

During this proliferative process there is usually increased expression of GSTP1 in an attempt to detoxify the inflammatory oxidants. If some cells are not able to increase GSTP1 expression (e.g. because of hypermethylation), they are potentially vulnerable to oxidative DNA damage. It has been suggested that PIA might be a precursor to PIN and prostate cancer.

II.2.8.2.4 Genetic and Epigenetic Factors

Although linkage analysis studies have identified multiple chromosomal loci for susceptibility to prostate cancer (e.g. HPC1, PCaP and CAPZB on chromosome 1; HPC2 or ELAC2 on chromosome 17; HPC20 on chromosome 20; and HPCX on the X chromosome), the linkages between these loci and prostate cancer are weak and no major predisposing genes have yet been found. The male relatives of females with BRCA2 mutations are at increased risk of prostate cancer and there is evidence of genetic linkage between breast cancer and prostate cancer outside these families. Some putative oncogenes and tumour suppressor genes have been identified as follows.

Oncogenes

The c-*myc* gene is located on chromosome 8q. Only 6% of primary cancers have increased 8q copy numbers compared to 89% of hormone refractory cancers, suggesting that c-*myc* may be involved in progression to androgen independence. Bcl-2 and ERBB-2 are also thought to be important in the progression to androgen independence. Insulin-like growth factor-1 (IGF-1) has growth-stimulating and anti-apoptotic effects on both androgen-dependent and -independent prostate cancer cell lines.

Tumour Suppressor Genes

The ribonuclease L gene (RNASEL) is the putative allele for the HPC-1 locus which has been found to predict prostate cancer risk in some families with a high prostate cancer frequency. It is pro-apoptotic and regulates cell proliferation. E-cadherin is a cell adhesion molecule that appears to suppress cancer invasion. Decreased E-cadherin expression occurs in around 50% of all prostate cancers. p53 helps regulate the cell cycle so that DNA damage can be repaired, or if irreparable the affected cells can undergo apoptosis. Mutations in p53 have been found in 3–79% of prostate cancers. p27 is involved in regulating the G1 phase of the cell cycle. Down-regulation of p27 has been associated with poorer prognosis in prostate cancer. Its association with HGPIN suggests that it may be an early event in prostate carcinogenesis. The PTEN gene is pro-apoptotic, regulates the cell cycle and inhibits angiogenesis. LOH at the PTEN location occurs in 15–49% of localized and greater than 50% of metastatic prostate cancer. Inactivation of both PTEN alleles occurs in less than 10% of localized and 30% of metastatic prostate cancer. Biallelic loss is associated with more aggressive disease than LOH.

Genetic Polymorphisms

Individuals carry two alleles for each gene. If many different alleles exist within the population, some combinations of alleles may predispose to cancer more than others. Examples of polymorphic genes that may be important in prostate cancer include genes coding for prostate specific antigen (PSA) and cytochrome-p450 isoforms; and genes involved in androgen metabolism [e.g. the androgen receptor (AR) and 5α-reductase (SRD5A2) genes].

Epigenetic Mechanisms

Epigenetic events are likely to be just as important as genetic mutations in prostate carcinogenesis. Examples include the hypermethylation of the GSTP1 gene promoter which has been detected in 70% of patients with HGPIN (suggesting that it may be an early event in prostate carcinogenesis) and greater than 90% of prostate cancers (the most common somatic alteration found so far in prostate cancer). GSTP1 codes for a detoxifying enzyme. Hypermethylation may render it ineffective, predisposing cells to genotoxic events.

II.2.8.2.5 Environmental Factors

The risk of prostate cancer in migrant populations tends to approach that of the society into which they assimilate, suggesting an important aetiological role for environmental factors. Phyto-oestrogens, selenium, lycopenes and vitamin D are associated with decreased prostate cancer incidence, whereas dietary fat and over-nutrition are associated with increased incidence. Further studies however are required to confirm these associations and to elucidate the underlying molecular mechanisms. Phyto-oestrogens (e.g. flavones, isoflavones and lignans) are naturally occurring plant compounds with oestrogen-like effects. Their cancer protective mechanisms might include: inhibition of 5α-reductase, decreasing dihydrotestosterone levels and inhibiting prostate cell growth and proliferation; induction of cell-cycle arrest and apoptosis; and inhibition of angiogenesis and metastasis. Soy beans are rich in isoflavones. Selenium is an essential trace element. A mounting body of evidence suggests it might be protective against prostate cancer. The molecular basis for this effect is starting to emerge and may involve effects on proliferation; carcinogen, androgen and fat metabolism; oxidative stress; inflammation; DNA repair; apoptosis; angiogenesis and immune function.

The mechanisms by which lycopenes (found in tomatoes) and vitamin D may decrease prostate cancer risk are poorly defined. The role of fatty acids is controversial but there is some evidence that omega-3 fatty acids decrease the risk of prostate cancer whilst omega-6 fatty acids increase it.

II.2.8.3 Pathogenesis of Testis Cancer

II.2.8.3.1 Introduction

Testicular cancers are a heterogeneous group consisting of germ cell (95%) and non-germ cell (5%) tumours. Testicular germ cell tumours (TGCT) are also heterogeneous. They often coexist with non-neoplastic lesions and consist of more than one histological type. Until the recent advent of micro-dissection techniques (capable of selecting specific cells for investigation) it had not been feasible to determine the molecular genetics of individual TGCT lesions. The origin and pathogenesis of TGCT remains obscure, however the multi-step model applies. Various stages of pathogenesis have been proposed (Fig. II.2.12) that incorporate the recent concept that TGCT is an uncommon manifestation of testicular dysgenesis syndrome (Skakkebaek et al. 2003).

II.2.8.3.2 Carcinoma In Situ

Carcinoma in situ (CIS) is recognized as a precursor lesion for most TGCT except infantile tumours and spermatocytic seminomas, implying that these may have a different pathogenesis. Up-regulation of C-KIT, ALPP, CCDN2 and ZNF354A genes and down-regulation of CDKN2D have been identified in CIS, therefore these alterations may occur early in testis carcinogenesis (von Eyben 2004).

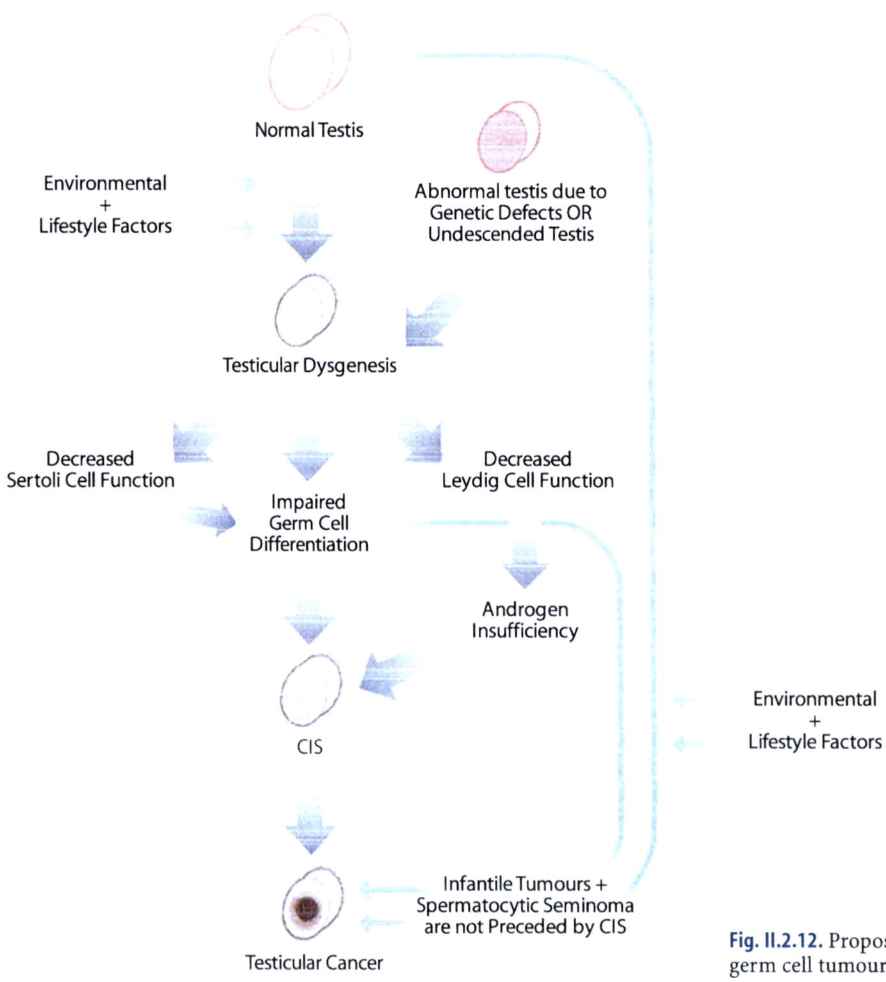

Fig. II.2.12. Proposed pathogenesis of testicular germ cell tumours

II.2.8.3.3
Genetic Factors

The increased familial risk in TGCT may be due to either heritable or environmental factors. Recent genome-wide screens suggest a locus of susceptibility on chromosome Xq27 that might also predispose to cryptorchidism (Holzik et al. 2004). The putative gene in this locus (TGCT-1) has yet to be identified.

It is well recognized that patients with intersex abnormalities (e.g. gonadal dysgenesis with Y chromosome abnormalities, and androgen insensitivity) are significantly at risk for TGCT. It has been proposed that Y chromosome deficiency in some cells (e.g. a low percentage of 45XO / 46XY aneuploidy), where the affected individual appears normal apart from unexplained infertility, might also predispose to TGCT.

TGCT characteristically show a gain of 12p-sequences, usually through isochromosome formation. A number of approaches are being used to identify the genes involved in testis carcinogenesis. Although a number of 12p genes are over-expressed in TGCT [e.g. BCAT1 (specific to non-seminomas), CCND2, GLU3, LRP6 and HPH1], their role awaits confirmation (Looijenga et al. 2003; Zafarana et al. 2003).

The testis is a unique environment where complex hormone-dependent interactions between Sertoli and germ cells regulate germ cell growth and differentiation. Various oncogenes and tumour suppressor genes coding for different classes of signalling molecules and pathways that are involved in these regulatory interactions have been proposed for TGCT (Devouassoux-Shisheboran et al. 2003), including the following.

Oncogenes

C-KIT encodes a tyrosine kinase receptor and is involved in germ cell proliferation during normal testicular development. C-KIT gain of function mutations have been identified in a minority of familial and sporadic TGCT. They appear more commonly in cases of bilateral TGCT and it has been suggested that they may occur early in embryogenesis in primordial germ cells that are subsequently distributed to both testes (Rapley et al. 2004). Activation or over-expression of genes encoding growth factors that stimulate proliferation (e.g. glial-derived neurotrophic factor, GDNF) and angiogenesis (e.g. vascular endothelial growth factor, VEGF) have also been identified in some TGCT compared with normal testicular germ cells.

Tumour Suppressor Genes

The Fas gene might be involved in the induction of apoptosis in testicular germ cells. Mutations that inactivate the Fas gene have been found in 28% of seminomas and 63% of embryonal carcinomas, but not in other histological types, suggesting a tumour suppressor role in the pathogenesis of at least some TGCT (Takayama et al. 2002). The transforming growth factor-β (TGF-β) family of growth factors regulates proliferation and differentiation. Loss of SMAD-4 expression (a component of the TGF-β signalling pathway) has been identified in some seminomas.

II.2.8.3.4
Intrauterine Environment

The hormonal milieu of the intrauterine environment might be a factor in testis carcinogenesis. Genetic disorders or exogenous factors that lead to a relative excess of oestrogens or a deficit of androgens in the first trimester might somehow cause primordial germ cells to transform into premalignant cells that are predisposed to CIS and TGCT.

II.2.8.3.5
Environmental Factors

The incidence of testicular cancer and poor semen quality have both increased significantly over the last two generations in different populations. It seems likely that environmental rather than genetic factors are responsible for this rapid change (Dieckmann and Pichlmeier 2004).

Hormone disrupters are environmental contaminants (natural and synthetic) that have oestrogenic or anti-androgenic effects. They have been increasingly identified over recent decades and include compounds found in pesticides, pharmaceuticals, plastics and detergents. By altering the hormonal milieu (especially during the vulnerable stage of embryonal sexual differentiation) they might predispose to TGCT. Certain dietary factors during childhood (e.g. a high dairy food intake) might also modify TGCT risk.

An association between smoking, maternal smoking during pregnancy and TGCT incidence has been suggested but the mechanisms have not yet been determined.

Non-seminomatous GCT are more common in some occupations (white-collar workers have 1.5–2× increased risk), implying that socioeconomic and/or lifestyle factors might be involved.

II.2.8.4
Pathogenesis of Penile Cancer

II.2.8.4.1
Introduction

Penile cancer is rare, therefore the mechanisms of its pathogenesis are not easily studied and remain poorly understood. A precursor condition (CIS, Bowen's disease or erythroplasia de Queyrat) is recognized, and associations with human papilloma virus (HPV), circumcision status and poor hygiene have been suggested by epidemiological studies (Dillner et al. 2000). It is likely that penile carcinogenesis is consistent with the multi-step model, and that a series of both genetic and epigenetic events is involved.

II.2.8.4.2 Genetic Factors

The HPV family are DNA viruses. Recognition of HPV-16 and -18 as aetiological agents in cervical cancer has stimulated investigation into whether they might have a similar role in penile cancer. HPV DNA has been detected in 10 – 100 % of penile cancers depending on the method used. Oncogenic HPV types (HPV-16 and -18) express the E6 and E7 oncoproteins, which bind to and inactivate the p53 and Rb suppressor gene products respectively. Other, non-viral methods of inactivating the Rb pathway might include: epigenetic methylation of the p16 promoter, and over-expression of the BMI-1 polycomb gene product (Ferreux et al. 2003). Cyclooxygenase-2 and microsomal prostaglandin E synthase-1, which are involved in the inflammatory cascade, have both been found to be over-expressed in CIS, invasive SCC and lymph node metastases (Golijanin et al. 2004). This supports the epidemiological association between chronic inflammation and penile cancer. The exact molecular mechanisms are as yet unknown.

II.2.8.4.3 Environmental Factors

Apart from lifestyles predisposing to HPV infection, the main environmental/lifestyle factors that have been associated with penile cancer are smoking, foreskin status and hygiene. Neonatal circumcision (but not circumcision later in life) seems protective against penile carcinoma, whereas phimosis and poor hygiene seem to predispose to it. The theory that these latter conditions allow unspecified carcinogens to accumulate in smegma and to subsequently initiate and promote carcinogenesis seems logical but is unproven at a molecular level. Also logical but unproven is the theory that smegma accumulation might result in chronic inflammation, the release of oxidative and electrophilic species, and subsequent DNA damage. Men exposed to psoralens and ultraviolet irradiation as treatment for psoriasis also seem at increased risk, presumably on the basis of genotoxic injury to oncogenes and/or tumour suppressor genes.

II.2.8.5 The Future

The recent availability of high throughput molecular technologies will allow the identification of many genes and proteins potentially relevant to the pathogenesis of various cancers. The challenge to the fields of genomics and proteomics will be to elucidate the molecular mechanisms and pathways responsible for carcinogenesis. Once these are understood there might be opportunities to accurately identify individuals at risk for cancer, and to modify their risk by lifestyle changes, gene therapy, chemoprevention or possibly prophylactic surgery. Such advancements will change the face of cancer management as we know it.

References

Ashida S et al (2004) Molecular features of the transition from PIN to prostate cancer: genome-wide gene-expression profiles of prostate cancers and PINs. Cancer Res 64:5963 – 5972

Boyd J, Barrett J (1990) Genetic and cellular basis of multistep carcinogenesis. Pharmaceut Ther 46:469 – 486

Deutsch E et al (2004) Environmental, genetic, and molecular features of prostate cancer. Lancet Oncol 5:303 – 313

Devouassoux-Shisheboran M et al (2003) Growth regulatory factors and signalling proteins in testicular germ cell tumours. APMIS 111:212 – 224

Dieckmann K, Pichlmeier U (2004) Clinical epidemiology of testicular germ cell tumors. World J Urol 22:2 – 14

Dillner J et al (2000) Etiology of squamous cell carcinoma of the penis. Scand J Urol Nephrol Suppl 205:189 – 193

Ferreux E et al (2003) Evidence for at least three alternative mechanisms targeting the p16/cyclin D/Rb pathway in penile carcinoma, one of which is mediated by high-risk human papillomavirus. J Pathol 201:109 – 118

Garinis G et al (2002) DNA hypermethylation: when tumour suppressor genes go silent. Hum Genet 111:115 – 127

Golijanin D et al (2004) Cyclooxygenase-2 and microsomal prostaglandin E synthase-1 are overexpressed in squamous cell carcinoma. Clin Cancer Res 10:1024 – 1031

Holzik M et al (2004) Genetic predisposition to testicular germ-cell tumours. Lancet Oncol 5:363 – 371

Looijenga L et al (2003) Role of gain of 12p in germ cell tumour development. APMIS 111:167 – 171

Moolgavkar S, Knudson A (1981) Mutation and cancer: a model for human carcinogenesis. J Natl Cancer Inst 66:1037 – 1052

Rapley E et al (2004) Somatic mutations of KIT in familial testicular germ cell tumours. Br J Cancer 90:2397 – 2401

Skakkebaek N et al (2003) Testicular cancer pathogenesis, diagnosis and endocrine aspects. In: McLachlan R (ed) Endocrinology of male reproduction. Endotext.com

Takayama H et al (2002) Frequent Fas gene mutations in testicular germ cell tumours. Am J Pathol 161:635 – 641

Visakorpi T (2003) The molecular genetics of prostate cancer. Urology 62 Suppl 5 A:3 – 10

von Eyben F (2004) Chromosomes, genes, and development of testicular germ cell tumours. Cancer Genet Cytogenet 151:93 – 138

Weinberg R (1983) Alteration of the genomes of tumour cells. Cancer 51:1971 – 1975

Zafarana G et al (2003) 12p-amplicon structure analysis in testicular germ cell tumours of adolescents and adults by array CGH. Oncogene 22:7695 – 7701

Diagnostic Tools II.3

II.3.1 History and Examination for Andrological Problems

T.B. Hargreave

Summary

- The most important first step in obtaining the clinical history is to take time to listen to what the man is complaining of.
- Careful clinical examination including full examination of the genitalia more often than not reassures the man that his problem is being assessed properly.
- Questionnaires and score sheets help with the assessment but do not replace the clinical assessment.
- Any younger man (under the age of 55) who complains of a testicular lump should have scrotal ultrasound unless the examining clinician is confident that the lesion is a benign one such as an epididymal cyst and can convey that confidence to the patient.
- It is easy to forget to note features during clinical examination, and the use of clinical examination checklists such as those in this chapter help prevent omissions.

II.3.1.1 History Taking

It is an old medical truth that the diagnosis is best made by careful history taking and clinical examination and that the most appropriate use of selected imaging and laboratory tests is to confirm the clinical diagnosis. The alternative methodology is to undertake a large number of screening blood tests, whole-body MRI scans, etc., but such an approach can result in spurious abnormal results which in turn can lead to costly, sometimes unpleasant, and possibly risky investigations that may not be necessary. Nevertheless, with increased understanding of molecular medicine there is likely to be an increasing role for blood tests both for diagnosis and screening, using newer molecular techniques such as gene array analysis and protein array analysis, particularly for selected at-risk groups. In this chapter the focus is on traditional history and clinical examination for common andrological problems.

Taking a medical history requires time and patience. The most important aspect is to listen to what the patient is saying before asking specific questions. It can be very helpful to ask the man to complete questionnaires prior to clinic attendance but even if this has been done it is best to start the consultation by giving the man time to tell you in his own words what the problem is. Do not be misled by preconceived ideas from a referral letter from another doctor.

II.3.1.2 Scheme for History Taking

History of main complaint – why has the man come to see you?
Problem-specific questions

- Infertility
- Sexual dysfunction and erectile problems
- Testicular pain
- Scrotal lumps
- Lower urinary tract symptoms
  - Prostate obstruction
  - Prostatitis
- Other andrological problems

II.3.1.2.1 General Medical History

Current or past significant medical problems. This should include details of any current or prior medication, whether prescribed or not. For men who may require surgery particular note should be made of any problems that may affect anaesthesia; for example, chest disease, allergies, impaired renal or liver function, cardiac or circulatory disease, etc.

II.3.1.2.2
Occupational History

A detailed occupational history may be directly relevant when dealing with male infertility (see Chap. II.2.6). Knowledge of the man's occupation is of general relevance to all andrological disorders when assessing the impact of the disorder on his work and life and for men who need surgery, in order to make arrangements for recovery time.

II.3.1.2.3
Lifestyle History

Use of tobacco, alcohol or "recreational drugs", weight, exercise and diet (see Chap. II.2.6).

II.3.1.2.4
Family and Social History

Note should be made of any family history of disease, for example a family history of prostate cancer in blood relatives is a good indication to start screening for prostate cancer at a younger age. Family history may also be relevant in genetic disorders. Social history includes taking a note of home circumstances.

II.3.1.2.5
Partner Involvement

In cases of male infertility it is best to see both partners. For men with testicular cancer sperm storage is a major consideration and the partner, if there is one, should be involved. For older men with prostate problems the partner is often able to give valuable information about the degree of disturbance from urinary symptoms. Also if the man wishes it is often very helpful for a partner to listen to the consultation as patients tend to forget what is said to them, particularly if they are stressed. Finally the partner may give insight into emotional disturbance and depression and this may be highly relevant in cases such as chronic testicular pain. However, there are situations where information is confidential and unknown to the partner and ideally clinical examination should be undertaken in a separate room so that the man has a chance to discuss any confidential aspects of medical history, for example prior children by another partner or previous sexually transmitted infection.

II.3.1.2.6
Communicating with the Patient after the Consultation

Patients are often stressed at the time of consultation because of worry about their condition and have poor recall of what has been said to them. It is almost always helpful to write to the patient after the consultation outlining the problem and what is proposed. In some clinics patients are given a tape recording of the consultation and this can be particularly helpful in the context of cancer care. My own practice is to copy all correspondence about a patient to the patient and in this correspondence I try to use ordinary language the patient will understand.

II.3.1.3
Problem-Specific Special History Taking

II.3.1.3.1
Special History: Male Partner of an Infertile Marriage

Different clinicians have their own approach to the initial assessment of the infertile couple. One way to ensure that complete information is obtained is to use a structured interview such as the World Health Organization simplified management scheme (WHO 1993). However, couples consulting about fertility problems are nearly always keen to provide information and during a 20-year period in Edinburgh we have used a comprehensive questionnaire and only 2 out of the first 2500 couples were unable or unwilling to answer all questions.

Check list for problem specific history for male infertility

- Duration of involuntary infertility
- Previous marriage, previous children, whether trying for children with another partner
- Previous investigation and treatment for infertility
- Episodes of high fever in the 3–4 months before any semen analysis
- History of any diseases which may impact on fertility (see Chap. II.2.7)
- Whether any medication is being taken with consideration of the impact of this on fertility (see Chap. II.2.7)
- History of any surgical procedure that may impact on fertility, e.g. urethral surgery, previous vasectomy (see Chap. I.5.1, vasectomy; Chap. II.2.7, influence of iatrogenic factors)
- History of any sexually transmitted infection (see Chap. I.1.6)
- History of any testicular injury, torsion, maldescent or malignancy (see Chaps. I.7.2, testicular trauma; I.3.10, congenital abnormality and infertility; I.7.1, torsion, I.8.2, testicular malignancy)
- Occupational history, exposure to heat, toxic chemicals, radiation, etc. (see Chap. II.2.6)
- Drugs of abuse (see Chap. II.2.6)
- Timing and frequency of sexual intercourse
- Difficulties with sexual and ejaculatory function (see Chap. I.4.3)
- Psychological problems (see Part I.4, "Problem: Sexual Dysfunction")

Both partners should be encouraged to attend during the initial interview but, if possible, physical examination of the man should be performed in a separate room as this gives each partner the opportunity to report any sensitive past history about which the other partner may be unaware; for example, previous sexually transmitted disease (STD) or pregnancies by a previous partner.

Duration of Involuntary Infertility

Sometimes also called the trying time, the duration of involuntary infertility is defined as the number of months the couple has been having sexual intercourse without the use of any contraceptive methods. The couple should be asked for how long unprotected intercourse has taken place. The duration of infertility is important as it gives prognostic information about the future chance for the couple (see Chap. II.3.2). If the duration of involuntary infertility is long then it is very likely that there is a severe biological problem, even if all the investigation results are within normal limits, however, the duration of involuntary infertility gives no information about whether there is a male or female problem.

Previous Marriage

In Scotland approximately one-third of marriages end in separation; in a Scottish clinic in 20% one or other or both partners have been previously married (in 8% the husband has had a previous marriage, in 7% the wife has had a previous marriage and 5% both partners). If there are any previous children or pregnancies this is strong evidence in favour of fertility in that partner, and previous unprotected intercourse without pregnancy with a prior partner is evidence for a fertility problem in that partner.

Previous Investigations and/or Treatment for Infertility

Knowledge of previous investigations or treatments is important as this may save the need for repeat investigations. Details of previous treatments should be noted with information on whether the treatment was prescribed and taken correctly and note of the results kept. However, it must also be remembered that fertility may change and the clinician should not rely too much on investigation results from a long time ago.

History of Diseases with Possible Adverse Effect on Fertility

Any serious illness may cause infertility because of generalized metabolic upset. This is usually but not always reversible with a return to health (see Chap. II.2.7). It is worth asking direct questions about respiratory disease, sense of smell, headaches and vision because men will not often volunteer these symptoms as they may not perceive any relevance to their fertility problem.

High Fever

A high fever exceeding 38 °C may suppress spermatogenesis over a period of up to 6 months. This may be particularly relevant after high fevers associated with tropical infectious diseases such as malaria, etc. If sperm analysis is poor, testicular size is normal, and there is history in the preceding 3 – 4 months of febrile illness such as influenza then sperm analysis should be repeated a month or two later, i.e. 4 – 5 months after the febrile illness; this should be done because the time for spermatogenesis and epididymal transit is approximately 3 months.

Medical Treatments

Treatment with medicines may cause temporary or permanent damage to spermatogenesis. Consideration needs to be given as to whether it is safe to stop the drug or whether there are any alternative preparations without deleterious effects on sexual function or semen quality [e.g. substitution of 5-aminosalicylic acid (5-ASA) instead of sulfasalazine in men with Crohn's disease] (Riley et al. 1987).

History of Surgery (see Chap. II.2.7)

There may be temporary depression of fertility after any surgical procedure, particularly where a general anaesthetic was administered. Also any surgery in the genital area may have caused damage.

Urinary Tract Infections

Urinary tract infections may occur in association with congenital abnormality or acquired abnormality such as post-gonococcal urethral stricture.

Reproductive Tract Infection, RTI (Sexually Transmitted Disease, STD) (see Chap. I.6.1)

It is often difficult to persuade men to give accurate information about sexually transmitted disease especially in the context of a joint consultation with their partner.

Epididymitis

Most men are unable to distinguish between epididymitis and orchitis and clinicians also may find this distinction difficult especially in the acute situation. The clinician should try to distinguish between acute generalized and severe scrotal pain suggestive of epididymo-orchitis and recurrent well-localized pain suggestive of chronic epididymitis. Epididymitis may result in obstruction.

Mumps Orchitis

Classical orchitis is associated with infectious parotitis (mumps) but may be caused by other virus infections, e.g. Coxsackie or herpes. Following an attack of mumps orchitis the recovery of fertility is variable; some men remain sterile but in other cases the time to recovery of sperm production may take as long as 2 years. Mumps before puberty and mumps not accompanied by orchitis do not interfere with fertility.

Testicular Injury: Bilateral Testicular Trauma

As a cause of infertility, this is rare (see Chap. I.7.2). A history of minor scrotal injury is common but it is doubtful if this is important in producing fertility problems. Injury should be recorded if accompanied by signs of tissue damage such as scrotal haematoma, haematospermia or haematuria. Subsequent testicular atrophy is a strong indication of the relevance of the traumatic incident. Unilateral injury may be important as it may cause extravasation of sperm or unilateral obstruction and antisperm antibody production.

Other Testicular Conditions

Testicular torsion (see Chap. I.7.1), varicocele (see Chap. I.3.12) and testicular maldescent (Chap. I.3.10).

An occupational history should be taken to identify exposure to toxic chemicals, heavy metals or excess heat or radiation (see Chap. II.2.6).

Drugs of abuse, excess cigarette smoking, and caffeine or alcohol consumption may affect male fertility (see Chaps. II.2.6, II.3.2) but there is controversy about their effects. It is particularly difficult to investigate the relationship with fertility because men who smoke also tend to drink alcohol, coffee, etc. Also it is difficult to persuade patients to give a truthful history because there is a general perception that doctors disapprove of these habits.

Timing of Sexual Intercourse

Sometimes either the man's or woman's work separates the couple or else shift work limits the opportunity for sexual intercourse. In most cases knowledge of the fertile period is not essential for fertility and indeed if the woman counts the days too avidly this can result in impotence on the man's part. In those cases where work causes separation it is important that the couple should be aware of the likely fertile time and the use of ovulation detection kits can help, provided the couple are properly instructed in their use. Some, usually younger, couples may experience infertility secondary to very frequent intercourse. This type of problem may be diagnosed if semen analysis is carried out:

1. after the couple's normal interval; and
2. after an interval of 2–3 days.

Intercourse has to occur several times a day or less than three times a month before there is likely to be any appreciable delay in fertility (Yaukey 1961). Some couples may concentrate on a recognized fertile period and understanding of the assessment of the timing of ovulation is consistent with fertility despite a low frequency of intercourse.

Difficulties with Sexual and Ejaculatory Function (Chap. I.3)

Difficulties with sexual intercourse causing infertility are identified in about 2% of couples. These difficulties may be associated with overt disorders such as paraplegia or other acquired neurological disorders or more rarely may be psychological. Therapeutic drugs are a rare cause of sexual problems in the age range of men attending infertility clinics. Sexual problems are not always evident from history taking and may only be detected during investigations because the man is unable or unwilling to provide a semen sample for analysis, or the wife is found to have an intact hymen, or there may be an unexplained lack of sperm in a post-coital test.

Premature Ejaculation

Ejaculation should occur intravaginally to be adequate. Anejaculation, ejaculation praecox (i.e. taking place before intromission), extravaginal ejaculation (e.g. associated with extreme hypospadias) and retrograde ejaculation should be noted. Premature ejaculation shortly after vaginal penetration is very common especially when a young man has a new partner, but this does not affect the chance of fertility. Persistent premature ejaculation prior to vaginal penetration is a rare cause of infertility and may be difficult to diagnose because the man may not volunteer this information and it is usually associated with psychological problems.

Psychological Problems

Psychosexual problems secondary to infertility are common if not universal but it is rare for infertility to occur as a result of psychosexual problems sufficiently severe to prevent intercourse (<1% in the clinic in Edinburgh). Psychological problems may be made worse if the fertility problem is prolonged and further aggravated by extended tests and treatments. An important aspect of management of the couple with a fertility problem is sympathetic and rapid investigation and counselling.

II.3.1.3.2
Special History: Sexual and Ejaculatory Dysfunction

In recent times male sexual dysfunction has been a taboo subject and men have not sought treatment. The advent of sildenafil (Viagra) and other effective therapy for erectile dysfunction has resulted in public discussion about men's sexual problems and increasingly men now seek advice. However, most men remain embarrassed about sexual dysfunction and inhibited from giving a history. The clinician should take time to listen to the problem and should avoid making any humorous or judgemental comments. It helps to put the man at ease if the clinician asks detailed questions without embarrassment; it often helps to put the man at ease if he is sent a detailed sexual function questionnaire prior to the consultation.

Bent Erections

If a man says that his erect penis is deformed this information is usually reliable and should not be dismissed. A simple problem such as a tight frenulum may be evident from examination and this is easily corrected by surgery; however, it may be more complicated such as the extreme angulation associated with a congenital short urethra. There may be confusion about the quality of erection perceived by the man to be adequate for sexual satisfaction and that necessary for fertility. For the latter it is sufficient only to achieve vaginal penetration.

Problems with Erectile Rigidity

In older men these are commonly secondary to vascular insufficiency. In younger men the problem is usually premature ejaculation or psychogenic. Careful history taking is needed to elicit that the loss of erection occurs after ejaculation, i.e. that the true problem is one of premature ejaculation rather than lack of rigidity. If a young man is unable to get an erection at all and there is no evidence of underlying congenital abnormality and if nocturnal penile tumescence testing shows nocturnal erections, then referral for expert psychosexual assessment is indicated as the problem is often complex and beyond the skill of andrology clinicians who do not have psychiatric expertise. For older men with vasculogenic erection it is helpful to use a scoring system such as the international index of erectile function.

Ejaculation Problems

Premature ejaculation is a common problem in younger men especially with a new partner. Lack of ejaculation may not be apparent if the man has never masturbated and may only be suspected if the man is unable to produce a semen sample. The usual first step in the diagnosis is to ask the man to collect a sample using a silicon condom. A history of a cloudy urine post orgasm indicates retrograde ejaculation and the need for microscopy of a post orgasm urine sample. Pain with ejaculation may indicate prostatitis but can also occur post incomplete lower spinal cord injury.

Problems with Penile Sensation

There is a general reduction in the sensitivity of the penis with ageing and an increase in the latent period. Isolated penile sensory disorders are seldom reported but can occur following nerve injury after radical prostate surgery. Penile anaesthesia is seen in the context of more general sensory loss in men with spinal injury, spinal cord tumour or multiple sclerosis. Urethral pain has a number of causes including bladder stone, urinary infection and urethritis from sexually transmitted infection. Urethral pain after sexual intercourse may be the result of prostatitis but may also occur as a result of allergy to the partner's secretions particularly if she has infection with *Candida* or *Trichomonas*. This problem can be suspected if the discomfort only occurs with unprotected sexual activity but not when using a condom.

II.3.1.3.3
Special History: Testicular Pain (see Chap. I.7.5)

History is directed to finding out possible causes of the pain such as varicocele, previous injury or inflammation. In men with longstanding pain it is important to distinguish those who have developed a chronic pain syndrome because further treatments to "cure" pain are risky and may make pain worse.

II.3.1.3.4
Special History: Scrotal Lumps (see Chap. I.8.1)

The main priority is to diagnose testicular cancer early and save the need for aggressive chemotherapy. Thus any younger man with a testicular lump should be assessed. History taking can be misleading as the man may give a history of minor injury to explain the lump. The most important part of the assessment is clinical examination and if there is any doubt at all then ultrasound examination. If clinical examination is normal but the man gives a history that one testicle feels different, heavier or in any way unusual, then ultrasound is warranted. It is worth remembering that the age range for testicular cancer is between 15 and 45 and that it is rare for men in their 60s to develop testicular cancer. Hydrocele is common in older men who often attend because they are concerned about possible cancer.

II.3.1.3.5 Special History: Lower Urinary Tract Symptoms, Prostate Obstruction and Prostatitis (see Chaps. I.9.1 and I.9.2)

In general it is daytime and nocturnal frequency of urination that causes the man to seek help but the andrologist must be wary of immediately ascribing these symptoms to prostatic disease as similar symptoms can be caused by other conditions such as transitional cell cancer of the bladder, or bladder overactivity (old terminology bladder instability). If the urine flow rate is poor then it is more likely that lower urinary tract symptoms relate to prostate disease. The most widely used validated instrument is the International Prostate Symptoms Score (IPPS) sheet.

II.3.1.3.6 Special History: Androgen Deficiency and Androgen Deficiency in Older Men

Androgen deficiency can be objectively diagnosed by serum androgen measurement in men who have lost both testicles, for example after bilateral testicular cancer. However, fortunately such a situation is rare and most men who believe they have androgen deficiency are much more difficult to assess. The diagnosis of androgen deficiency in older men is based on the finding of lower than normal testosterone levels in combination with symptoms indicative of androgen deficiency. However, these symptoms are nonspecific and can also be manifestation of other systemic disease, for example fatigue and tiredness may be associated with lack of androgen but may also relate to problems such as cardiac insufficiency, depression, etc. Because of the many confounding factors any man with potential androgen deficiency should be fully assessed for common diseases of ageing (see Chap. I.11). In the absence of any other systemic disorder the ageing male symptoms score can be used. In general the finding on clinical examination of normal-sized testicles with normal consistency makes the diagnosis of androgen deficiency unlikely. Also those men who are seeking androgens to enhance sexual performance usually have preserved libido and preservation of libido also makes the diagnosis of androgen deficiency less likely.

II.3.1.4 Clinical Examination for Andrological Conditions

The man should be examined in a warm room (20–24°C) in privacy. He should be examined both standing erect and lying on the examination couch. Clothing should be removed to enable general examination and also accurate assessment of the endocrine status and build. It is often convenient to apply simple objective tests at the time of physical examination, e.g. the testicular size can be measured with an orchiometer or ideally testicular size and venous return assessed by ultrasound and Doppler analysis.

II.3.1.4.1 General Examination

Observation is made of the body configuration and the degree of virilization, although the latter has only a very poor correlation with actual endocrine status. In Klinefelter syndrome the limbs may be disproportionately long in relation to the trunk but in many cases there are no obvious clinical features. In other chromosomal disorders there may be associated skeletal deformity (Chandley et al. 1980). A tall stature and immature physique may suggest an endocrinological factor resulting in delayed puberty. Other signs of hypoandrogenism include poor expression of secondary sex characteristics and scanty body hair. Often such patients have sought advice in adolescence because of delayed puberty and come to the infertility clinic with the diagnosis already made. Measurement of height and weight and blood pressure may give information about systemic disease. Being grossly overweight has been found to be associated with reduced testicular volume and impaired spermatogenesis (WHO 1987). Female fat distribution, with distribution of fat over the hips, and gynaecomastia may also indicate endocrinological abnormality. Any abnormality of secondary sexual development may be staged using Tanner's pubertal development scale.

II.3.1.4.2 Body Hair Distribution

Body hair is extremely variable, depending on racial, genetic and hormonal factors. In Caucasian but not Chinese men the distribution of body hair gives an indication of androgen production; this may be supplemented with questions about the frequency of shaving. Scanty body hair and infrequent shaving may indicate relatively low androgen production. Pubic hair is dihydrotestosterone dependent and axillary hair may be related to DHEA and the adrenarche.

II.3.1.4.3
Gynaecomastia (see Chap. I.10.1)

The breasts should be inspected and palpated for the presence or absence of glandular tissue. This is best done with the patient's hands placed behind his head to extend the pectoral muscles. Gynaecomastia is commonly seen in pubertal boys without any obvious hormonal abnormality. It is classically described as part of the Klinefelter syndrome. Gynaecomastia results from oestrogen androgen imbalance, either relative hyperoestrogenism or relative hypo-androgenism. It may be seen as a result of exposure to oestrogens, medication with digitalis, spironolactone, and also with antiandrogen treatment for prostate cancer (bicuclamide, etc.) An oestrogen-secreting tumour of the adrenal gland or testicle is another rare cause. Gynaecomastia may be seen in association with hyperprolactinaemia and in one-third of cases there is galactorrhoea (Thorner et al. 1974).

II.3.1.4.4
Inguinal Examination

Checklist for inguinal examination

Scars	Scars from orchidopexy in infancy may be very difficult to see under the pubic hair. The vas deference may have been injured during hernia repair in infancy Scars may indicate past or current infection with tuberculosis or lymphogranuloma venereum
Hernia and swelling	Once confidence has been gained it can help to examine the man standing up (be careful as young men are prone to syncope during testicular and inguinal examination)
Tenderness	Tenderness over the inguinal canal may indicate hernia If there is absence of the testicle within the scrotum, pressure over the inguinal canal may produce the sensation of testicular compression and indicate that the testicle is within the inguinal canal even if it cannot be clearly palpated. In this situation ultrasound confirms the position of the testicle
Glands	In men with penile inflammation or cancer it is important to carefully examine for lymph nodes in the inguinal and femoral area

II.3.1.4.5
Examination of the Penis

The penis should be inspected and palpated to detect hypospadias, surgical or traumatic scars, induration plaques or other pathology. The foreskin should always be retracted fully to detect problems such as meatal stricture or phimosis. Any ulceration or urethral discharge should be noted and, if present, further investigations should be performed to identify reproductive tract infection (RTI/STD) (see Chap. I.6.1). Penile deformity during erection may occur as a result of Peyronie's disease or because of inadequate surgical correction of chordee associated with hypospadias or in men with a congenital short urethra. The extent of the deformity will not be evident from clinical examination of the flaccid penis and it is wise in such cases to believe the patient and to use objective tests. The degree of penile deformity during erection can also be assessed either by asking the patient to take digital or Polaroid photos of his erect penis at home or by inducing an erection in the clinic with an injection into the corpora cavernosa of papaverine.

Checklist for examination of the penis and foreskin

Penis within normal size limits?	True micropenis is a rare problem (see Chaps. I.3.4)
Penile shaft skin normal?	Scars may indicate previous surgery for urethral stricture or chordee
Foreskin retracts fully?	Minor adhesions around the corona are a common problem Frenulum normal
Glans healthy?	Ulcers may indicate RTI/STD (see Chap. I.6.1) Premalignant lesions are more common in older men who do not retract their foreskin (see Chap.s I.8.3 and I.8.4)
Normal external urethral meatus?	Lips of meatus part easily and there is no stenosis? Position of the meatus normal? Hypospadias?
Man complains of bent or deformed erections	Are there any lumps or Peyronie's plaques palpable in the line of the corpora cavernosa? Examine man with an erect penis following an injection of prostaglandin or view digital or Polaroid photos of his erect penis

II.3.1.4.6
Examination of the Testis

The Position and Axis of the Testicle

Position and axis of the testicle is best determined with the man standing. The testes should both be palpable and low in the scrotum. Any abnormality in the site of the testes should be categorized as follows. High: in the scrotum, i.e. at the scrotal neck; inguinal: lying within the inguinal canal; ectopic: outside the normal pathway of descent, most commonly in the superficial inguinal pouch, but more rarely femoral or suprapubic. If the testes are impalpable they may be within the inguinal canal and atrophic or intra-abdominal or absent. Normally the testis lies in the scrotum vertically with the epididymis behind or medial. The testes may retract into the inguinal canal and this may be a problem particularly if it occurs during sexual intercourse and causes pain. However, this probably has no relevance to fertility. The horizontally lying testis is more liable to torsion. If such a patient gives a history of intermittent pain, and particularly if testicular volume is reduced or sperm concentration is low, testicular fixation should be considered.

Testicular Volume

Estimation of testicular volume is performed with the patient in recumbent position because of the risk of syncope. The scrotal skin is stretched over the testicle, the contours of which are isolated from the epididymis. The volume of each testis is compared with the corresponding ovoid of the modified Prader orchiometer. Alternatively callipers (Professor Stephen Seager, Fertility Research, Medlantic Research Foundation, George Hymen Memorial Research Building, Washington, USA) or hollow forms (Takihara et al. 1983) may be used. The modified Prader orchiometer has larger bead sizes to enable measurement of adult testes as the original instrument was designed to assess adolescents and children. The Takihara forms and Seager orchiometer are slightly more difficult to use but may give better inter-observer variation than the Prader orchiometer. The normal size may relate to ethnic group, but mostly depends on stature and is related to standardized body weight and body physique. In Orientals the mean testicular weight at autopsy of 100 individuals varying in age from late teens to seventies was: right testis 10 g (SE ± 0.3 g), left testis 9.4 g (SE ± 0.3 g) (Chang et al. 1960). Comparable data for 140 Caucasians gave the following measurements: right testis 21.6 g (SE ± 0.4 g), left testis 20.4 g (SE ± 0.5 g) (Olesen 1948). Most of the volume is accounted for by the seminiferous tubule mass. There is a strong correlation between the total testicular volume (the sum of the left and the right side added) and the sperm count per ejaculate (WHO 1987). For Caucasian men a size of less than 15 ml is indicative of damage to the seminiferous epithelium of that testis. Small firm testes, usually less than 3 ml in volume, are found in men with Klinefelter syndrome. Patients with hypogonadotrophic hypogonadism also have small testes, but the size is usually between 5 and 12 ml. A normal testicular volume in a man with azoospermia may indicate obstruction of sperm transport. An unduly large and asymmetrical testis may indicate testicular tumour. Symmetrical large testes, also called macro-orchia, are an occasional normal finding. False estimation of testicular volume may occur if there is hydrocele.

Testicular Consistency

This is normally estimated by gentle pressure. The normal consistency is rubbery. Soft testicles are nearly always associated with impaired spermatogenesis. Objective techniques using a tonometer have been tried and reduced testicular consistency has been shown to correlate with the presence of a varicocele (Lewis et al. 1985). At present few clinicians use objective techniques. Occasionally, patients are found with a hard testicle of normal or large volume and a testicular tumour may be present. If testes are hard and small, Klinefelter syndrome is suspected, whereas small and soft testes are commonly found in men with hypogonadotrophic hypogonadism.

Checklist for examination of the testicle

Both testicles in the scrotum?	Note should be made of any abnormality of descent including the testicle that lies at the scrotal neck
Testis axis	The normal axis is vertical with the epididymis lying behind or medial. Horizontal testes are more prone to torsion
Testis volume	When the problem is male infertility or suspected androgen deficiency the testicular volume should be measured using an objective method (Prader orchiometer, Takihara orchiometer, Seager orchiometer or ultrasound). The finding of normal-sized and normal consistency testis makes androgen deficiency an unlikely diagnosis
Testis consistency	This is based on experience as although there are objective methods they are not generally available. If the man indicates an area of his testis has changed in consistency then an ultrasound should be performed even if the clinician is unable to detect any abnormality
Testis contour	Care is taken to feel the testis for lumps. It is often helpful to ask the man to identify any lumps he can feel
Testis sensation and pain	Gentle squeezing of the testicle produces discomfort but this sensation is lost in conditions causing autonomic denervation (e.g. some men with diabetes) Pain in the testicle is usually poorly localized and felt as a general ache whereas epididymal pain is much better localized because of associated inflammation of the tunica and involvement of peripheral nerve pathways

Examination of the Epididymis

The normal epididymis is barely palpable, has a regular outline and soft consistency. Gentle palpation does not cause pain. Painful nodules may indicate epididymidis or sperm granulomata; those in the caput epididymidis suggest infection by *Chlamydia*. Painful swelling and/or nodularity of the caudal region may indicate gonococcal infection or inflammation or infection with urinary pathogens such as *Escherichia coli*. Sperm granulomata after previous vasectomy are also found in the caudal region. Cystic deformities may or may not be relevant to any obstruction. Painless craggy swelling of the epididymis may indicate tuberculous disease of the urinary tract.

Checklist for epididymal examination	
Is the anatomical relationship to the testicle normal?	The normal position of the epididymis is above, behind and below the testis
Any swellings, indurated areas or cysts expanding the head, body or tail of the epididymis	If yes, does the lesion involve the head, body or tail or all of the epididymis?
Any cysts adjacent to the epididymis	It is common to find small pedunculated cystic appendages in relation to the head of the epididymis (hydatid of Morgagni)
Any tenderness of the head, body or tail of the epididymis	The clinician should try to distinguish whether any discomfort is by pressure over a particular part of the epididymis or by pressure over the testicle or whether the pain is not well localized

Ultrasound examination may be useful to confirm major abnormalities in the epididymis, but does require the appropriate probe and is also dependent on skilled interpretation.

Examination of the Vasa Deferentia

Both vasa deferentia should be palpable and are felt as thin wire-like structures passing between the examining fingers. However, clinicians will sometimes miss bilateral absence of the vasa and it is worth re-examining all men with azoospermia, particularly if the testicular volume is normal and the ejaculate volume low. Bilateral absence is found in approximately 2% of men with obstructive azoospermia. Unilateral absence is much rarer and is often associated with an absence of the kidney on the same side. If the vas is present, note should be made of whether it is normal, thickened, nodular or painful upon pressure as this may indicate inflammation.

Checklist for the examination of the vas deferens	
Are both vasa palpable?	This can be difficult to determine especially if there has been previous orchidopexy and the cord is thickened. If the ejaculate volume is low in a man with azoospermia it is often worthwhile re-examining for absence of the vas deferens
Is the vas uniform?	If there are nodules palpable, this may indicate obstruction (e.g. previous vasectomy)
Is there a large gap between the cut ends of the vas deferens?	This is relevant in men who have had a previous vasectomy and who are seeking vasectomy reversal. If there is a very long gap this may make it impossible to undertake reversal surgery

Examination for Scrotal Swellings

The scheme for examination of scrotal swelling is shown in Fig. I.8.1 in Chap. I.8.1. If there is any doubt about the finding from clinical examination then scrotal ultrasound should be performed.

Checklist for the examination of scrotal lumps and swellings	
Where is the swelling in relation to the testicle?	Involving the testis – consider testicular malignancy Above – consider epididymal cyst, varicocele, hernia In front of – consider hydrocele Below – consider lesion of the tail of the epididymis
What is the consistency?	If the swelling is hard, consider testicular malignancy
Is the swelling painful to palpation?	If yes, consider epididymitis
Does the swelling disappear when lying down?	If yes, consider varicocele and indirect hernia

Examination of the Prostate Gland

Most men find prostate examination embarrassing and unpleasant and time should be taken to explain why the examination is needed and to obtain the man's agreement to this specific part of the clinical examination. Some men may decline prostate examination in which case an explanation should be given to the man of the risks he may run if prostate pathology is missed. Examination of the prostate gland is by rectal examination with the man in the lateral or knee elbow position.

Checklist for prostate examination	
Size	Although clinicians often write the size in grams this is not accurate and it is often best to restrict the size description to large, medium or small
Contour	Smooth or bumpy (irregular)
Median groove	Normally it is possible to feel a shallow groove separating the two prostate lobes although this feature may be lost when there is marked benign enlargement
Lateral grooves	The lateral margin of the prostate and the rectal wall form a groove which becomes more marked with prostate enlargement but may be lost if there is prostate cancer
Symmetry	Are the left and right lobes the same size
Consistency	With experience the clinician can categorize the consistency as normal, soft or boggy or hard or rock hard
The presence of any nodules	The size and location of any nodules should be recorded
Pain on palpation	The clinician should take care to distinguish abnormal pain and discomfort from a sense of urinary urgency which is normal during prostate palpation

It is often difficult to find out whether the man is experiencing true pain from prostate examination or just a more general discomfort and embarrassment. Use of the following words can help make this distinction: "I know that this is unpleasant and uncomfortable, but am I hurting you at all?"

Examination of the Seminal Vesicles

The seminal vesicles are not normally palpable. If they are palpable this usually indicates inflammation. Some men with characteristics of obstructive azoospermia have cystic deformities of the seminal vesicles, others may have agenesis. These abnormalities are best detected by ultrasound, preferably using a rectal probe.

List of Questionnaires and Score Sheets

WHO Structured Interview (Rowe et al. 2000)

The booklet has been extensively used in several countries and has been validated. The main disadvantage is the time needed for the interview.

Infertility Clinic Questionnaire (Edinburgh)

Designed to be sent to the couple prior to first appointment and to save the clinician time. Has been used by more than 2000 couples but not independently validated. High compliance rate. http://www.urologyedinburgh.co.uk/fertility_questionnaire.htm

Sexual Problems Questionnaire (Edinburgh)

Designed to be sent to the man prior to the first interview and to save the clinician time. Has been used by more than 500 men but not independently validated. Over 95% compliance rate. May help "break the ice" at the initial interview. http://www.urologyedinburgh.co.uk/sexual_function_questionnaire.htm

Vasectomy Reversal Questionnaire (Edinburgh)

Designed to help ensure completeness of information prior to giving advice about vasectomy reversal feasibility.

Testicular Pain Questionnaire (Edinburgh)

Designed to be used in the context of a structured interview to help distinguish neuropathic pain. Not validated. http://www.urologyedinburgh.co.uk/new_page_24.htm

International Index of Erectile Function (IIEF)

This is a validated instrument to assess the severity of impairment of stiffness of erections. This instrument does not assess ejaculatory and orgasmic dysfunction.

International Prostate Symptoms Score (IPSS)

This is a validated instrument to assess the severity of lower urinary tract symptoms in men with known prostatic obstruction.

Ageing Male Symptoms Score

This is a semi-validated scoring system to be used in conjunction with androgen measurement to establish the diagnosis of androgen deficiency in older men.

References

Chandley AC, Hargreave TB, Fletcher JM, Soos JM, Axworthy D, Price WH (1980) Trisomy 8. Report of a mosaic human male with near-normal phenotype and normal IQ, ascertained through infertility. Hum Genet 55:31–38

Hargreave TB (1990) Questionnaire for the infertile couple. In: Hargreave TB, Soon E (eds) Management of male infertility. PG Press, Singapore, p3

Lewis EL, Rasor MO, Overstreet JW (1985) Measurement of human testicular consistency by tonometry. Fertil Steril 43:911–916

Riley SA, Lecarpentier J, Mani V, Goodman Mi, Mandal BK Turnberg LA (1987) Sulphasalazine-induced seminal abnormalities in ulcerative colitis: results of mesalazine substitution. Gut 28:1008–1012

Rowe PJ, Comhaire FH, Hargreave TB, Mahmoud AMA (2000) WHO manual for the standardized investigation, diagnosis and management of the infertile male. Cambridge University Press, Cambridge

Takihara H, Sakatoku J, Fujii M, Nasu T, Cosentino IM, Cockett ATK (1983) Significance of testicular size measurement in andrology. I. A new orchiometer and its clinical application. Fertil Steril 39:836–840

Thorner MO, McNeilly AS, Hagan C, Besser GM (1974) Long-term treatment of galactorrhoea and hypogonadism with bromocriptine. Br Med J ii:419

WHO (1987) Towards more objectivity in diagnosis and management of male infertility. Int J Androl (Suppl 7)

Yaukey D (1961) Fertility differences in a modernising country: a survey of Lebanese couples. Princeton University Press, Princeton, N.J.

II.3.2 Semen Analysis and Sperm Function Tests

F. Comhaire, A. Mahmoud

Summary

- Conventional semen analysis, accurately measuring sperm concentration, motility and morphology, is the cornerstone of male fertility assessment.
- Both the technique of semen collection and the methods of laboratory analysis can influence the results dramatically.
- Semen analysis requires specific technical skills and training, as well as constant care for quality assurance.
- Each laboratory must define its own reference values, particularly for sperm motility and morphology.
- So-called advanced methods of semen analysis and functional tests are valuable instruments for research purposes, but do not contribute substantially to the management of the infertile couple.

II.3.2.1 Introduction

Semen analysis is the cornerstone of male infertility investigation. McLeod (1942), MacLeod and Gold (1953), Eliasson (1971) and Hellinga (1949, 1976) have created the scientific basis of conventional semen analysis, and the techniques recommended by them are still considered the reference for more advanced techniques. In order to perform correct semen analysis, the sample must be obtained and transported in agreement with strict guidelines (WHO 1999).

Conventional semen analysis includes measurements of particular aspects of spermatozoa and of seminal plasma. It is of the utmost importance to apply both internal and external quality control to the techniques of semen analysis, in order to reduce inter-observer errors and intra- and inter-assay variability, and to increase reproducibility.

II.3.2.2 Sample Collection and Delivery

Laboratory technicians should be informed that semen samples present a possible biohazard since they may contain harmful viruses, e.g. hepatitis viruses, human immunodeficiency viruses, herpes viruses, and should be handled with due care.

The subject should be provided with a clearly written instruction sheet concerning the collection and transport of semen.

1. The time interval between the last ejaculation and sample collection should be well defined and preferably constant in order to allow for reliable interpretation of the results, particularly of sperm concentration and motility. If, however, the period of sexual abstinence is outside of the suggested limits, the semen sample should still be analysed. If the result is normal, there is no need for a second analysis. When the duration of abstinence is in excess of 7 days, sperm motility, i.e. the proportion of spermatozoa with rapid progressive motility, may decline. If the duration of abstinence is less than 48 h, sperm concentration may be reduced, but motility will probably not be affected. Under particular circumstances, and when for example epididymal pathology is present, sperm characteristics may be better in samples collected after a short duration of abstinence (even only a few hours) than after longer periods.
2. Although repeat semen analysis is not mandatory if the result of the first analysis is completely normal, a second analysis may be recommended in cases with long-standing unexplained infertility, and provided complementary tests of sperm function can be performed.
3. Seminal plasma may exert an unfavourable effect on sperm motility that becomes more prominent as time elapses between ejaculation and analysis. Also, when semen is to be prepared for techniques of assisted reproduction, such as intra-uterine insemination or in vitro fertilization, processing of the sample should be performed immediately after liquefaction.
4. Special containers for semen analysis are available on the market. They have the advantage of allowing the estimation of sperm volume without the need for transferring the sample. In addition, the materials for manufacturing have been proven not to exert any negative effects on sperm motility or viability.
5. It has been shown that semen samples collected during intercourse using a special plastic condom tend to have a larger volume and higher concentration, with a resulting higher total count per ejaculate. Hence, the use of such condoms should be considered for the collection of a second semen sample if the first one shows a relatively low volume.

II.3.2.3 Initial Macroscopic Examination

II.3.2.3.1 Appearance

The semen sample is first evaluated by simple inspection. A normal sample has a grey-opalescent appearance, is homogeneous and liquefies within 60 min at room temperature under the influence of proteolytic enzymes of prostate origin. In some cases, complete liquefaction does not occur within 60 min and this fact should be recorded, as it suggests functional disturbance of the prostate.

The sample may appear clear if sperm concentration is too low. It may also appear brown when red blood cells are present in the ejaculate (haematospermia). The presence of mucous streaks may interfere with the counting procedure, and suggests inflammation or abnormal liquefaction. Normal semen samples may contain jelly-like grains which do not liquefy and are probably secreted by Cowper's' glands.

The sample should be examined immediately after liquefaction or within 1 h of ejaculation. Samples that do not liquefy need additional treatment such as exposure to bromelain or diluted trypsin, to make the sample amenable to analysis.

II.3.2.3.2 Volume

The volume of the ejaculate should be measured with either a graduated cylinder, or by aspirating the whole sample into a graduated syringe or pipette. If bioassays or semen culture are to be performed, sterile materials should be used in handling the semen samples. The bulk of the volume is secreted by the seminal vesicles, and between 0.5 and 1 ml originates from the prostate. A low ejaculate volume may suggest deficient secretion of the seminal vesicles whereas large volumes are sometimes found in association with varicocele.

II.3.2.3.3 Consistency

The consistency, also called viscosity, of the liquefied sample can be estimated by gently pushing the semen through a blunt injection needle (21G, internal diameter approximately 0.03 inches or 0.8 mm) and observing the length of the thread. A normal sample leaves the needle as small discrete drops, while in the case of abnormal consistency the drop will form a thread of more than 2 cm. Another method of estimating consistency does not use needles and is performed by introducing a glass rod into the sample and observing the length of the thread that forms on withdrawal of the rod. Again, the thread should not exceed 2 cm.

Increased viscosity has the same clinical meaning as abnormal liquefaction, and is related to prostate dysfunction.

II.3.2.3.4 pH

A drop of semen is spread evenly onto a pH paper (range pH 6.4–8.0) (Merck, Darmstadt, Art. 9557). After 30 s, the colour of the impregnated zone should be uniform and is compared with the calibration strip to read the pH. Whatever type of pH paper is used for this analysis, its accuracy should be checked against known standards before use in routine semen analysis.

The acidic secretions of the prostate and the alkaline secretions of the seminal vesicles determine the pH. It should normally be in the range of 7.2–7.8. A pH value exceeding 7.8 is related to decreased secretion of acidic products, such as citric acid, by the prostate. If the pH is less than 7.0 in a sample with small volume and azoospermia, congenital dysgenesis of the vas deferens, seminal vesicles and/or epididymides must be suspected.

II.3.2.4 Initial Microscopic Investigation

During the initial microscopic investigation, motility and concentration of spermatozoa are estimated and the presence of cells other than spermatozoa and of agglutination are determined.

II.3.2.4.1 Motility

A fixed volume of semen (10–15 µl) delivered with a micropipette is placed on a clean glass slide and covered with a coverslip sized between 20 mm × 20 mm or 24 mm × 24 mm. It is important that the volume of semen and the dimension of the coverslip are standardized, so that the analyses are always carried out on a preparation with fixed depth between 25 and 30 µm. This depth allows full expression of the rotating movement of normal spermatozoa. Alternatively, an aliquot of semen is placed in contact with the coverslip of a fixed depth disposable counting chamber (Fig. II.3.1).

The preparation is then examined at a magnification of 400–600×. An ordinary light microscope can be used for unstained preparations if the condenser is lowered to disperse the light, but a phase-contrast microscope is preferable.

The weight of the coverslip spreads the sample for optimal viewing, or this effect is obtained automatically when disposable counting chambers are used. The freshly made, wet preparation is left to stabilize for approximately 1 min. The examination can be performed

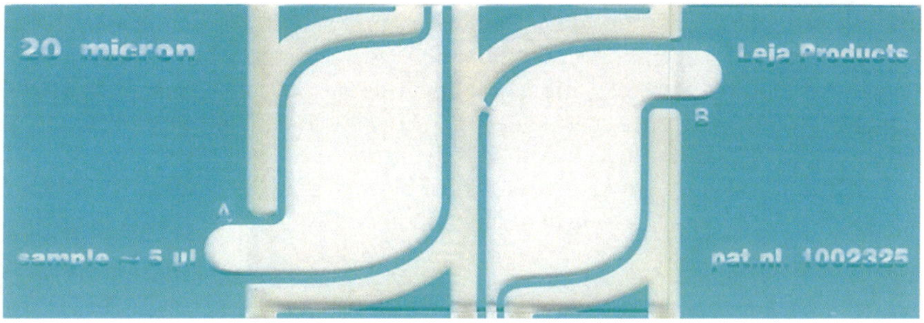

Fig. II.3.1. Disposable counting chamber

Table II.3.1. Grading of sperm motility

Grade (a):	if the spermatozoon has a rapid, linear, progressive motility (also referred to as excellent or good progression)
Grade (b):	if it has a slow or sluggish linear or nonlinear movement (also referred to as weak or moderate progression)
Grade (c):	if it has nonprogressive motility ("motile on the spot")
Grade (d):	if the spermatozoon is immotile

at room temperature, between 18 °C and 24 °C. Some laboratories may prefer assessing motility at 37 °C, using a heated microscope plate.

The microscopic field is scanned systematically and the motility of each spermatozoon encountered is classified. The categories for classifying sperm motility have been designated (a), (b), (c) and (d) (Table II.3.1). Usually, four to six fields are scanned to accumulate 100 successive spermatozoa, which are recorded by means of a laboratory counter, yielding a percentage of each motility category.

An alternative method consists of estimating the number of grade (a) spermatozoa in the entire visual field. Next the number of grade (b) cells is estimated, followed by the number of grade (c) and grade (d) cells. These numbers are added up, and the percentage of spermatozoa classified in each motility group is calculated.

It is recommended to repeat the procedure on a second drop of semen processed in the same way. For this reason, the disposable counting chamber contains at least two separate chambers and entries. Irrespective of the method used, the variability of results on the same sample should not exceed 10 %.

II.3.2.4.2 Estimation of Sperm Concentration

The concentration is estimated roughly during initial examination in order to determine the dilution factor to be used for the haemocytometer method, and to indicate whether centrifugation may be required to prepare an adequate smear for morphological analysis.

When using a preparation with a depth of 20 µm, and the diameter of the microscopic field is 250 µm, sperm concentration can be estimated from the mean number of spermatozoa per microscopic field under a 40× objective and multiplying this number by 10^6. For example, 40 spermatozoa per visual field can be considered roughly equivalent to 40 million spermatozoa per millilitre. In order to obtain a preparation with a standard depth of 20 µl, one drop of 11.5 µl of semen is placed on a microscope slide and covered with a coverslip of 24 mm × 24 mm. Alternatively, a disposable counting chamber with fixed depth of 20 µm can be used.

If the number of spermatozoa per visual field varies considerably, this indicates that the sample is not homogeneous, and that the sample should be mixed again thoroughly. The lack of homogeneity may also result from abnormal consistency or abnormal liquefaction, from aggregation of spermatozoa in mucus threads, or from sperm agglutination. These observations should be mentioned in the analysis report.

II.3.2.4.3 Cellular Elements other than Spermatozoa

The ejaculate usually contains cells other than spermatozoa. These include polygonal epithelial cells from the urethral tract. If many of these are present, and they are covered with bacteria, then it is probable that the sample is obtained by coitus interruptus, and the cells originate from the vagina. "Round cells" are present in almost every semen sample. They are spermatogenic cells and white blood cells. The concentration of these cells can be estimated per visual field in the wet preparation when the number of spermatozoa is estimated. Their concentration can be determined accurately using a haemocytometer or a disposable counting chamber.

If the concentration of round cells exceeds 10^6/ml or one per visual field using a 40× objective, a specific stain should be used to distinguish between the peroxidase-positive white blood cells and other cells. The staining procedure is performed on the fresh sample and is based on the fact that intact neutrophil polymorphonuclear granulocytes contain peroxidase

(Endtz 1972) (Leucoscreen, FertiPro, Beernem, Belgium). The peroxidase-negative cells include degranulated polymorphonuclear granulocytes, lymphocytes, and mainly immature germ cells, namely spermatids, spermatocytes and sometimes spermatogonia. Differentiation of peroxidase-negative round cells is often difficult and is usually not performed as part of basic semen analysis. If the concentration of peroxidase-positive cells exceeds 10^6/ml, further studies are required to establish if the man suffers from accessory gland infection.

A second method, described by Nahoum and Cardozo (1980), aims to count peroxidase-positive round cells in a haemocytometer. The following reagents are needed: saturated NH_4Cl solution (25 g per 100 ml); Na_2-EDTA 5% (vol/vol) in phosphate buffer (pH 6);

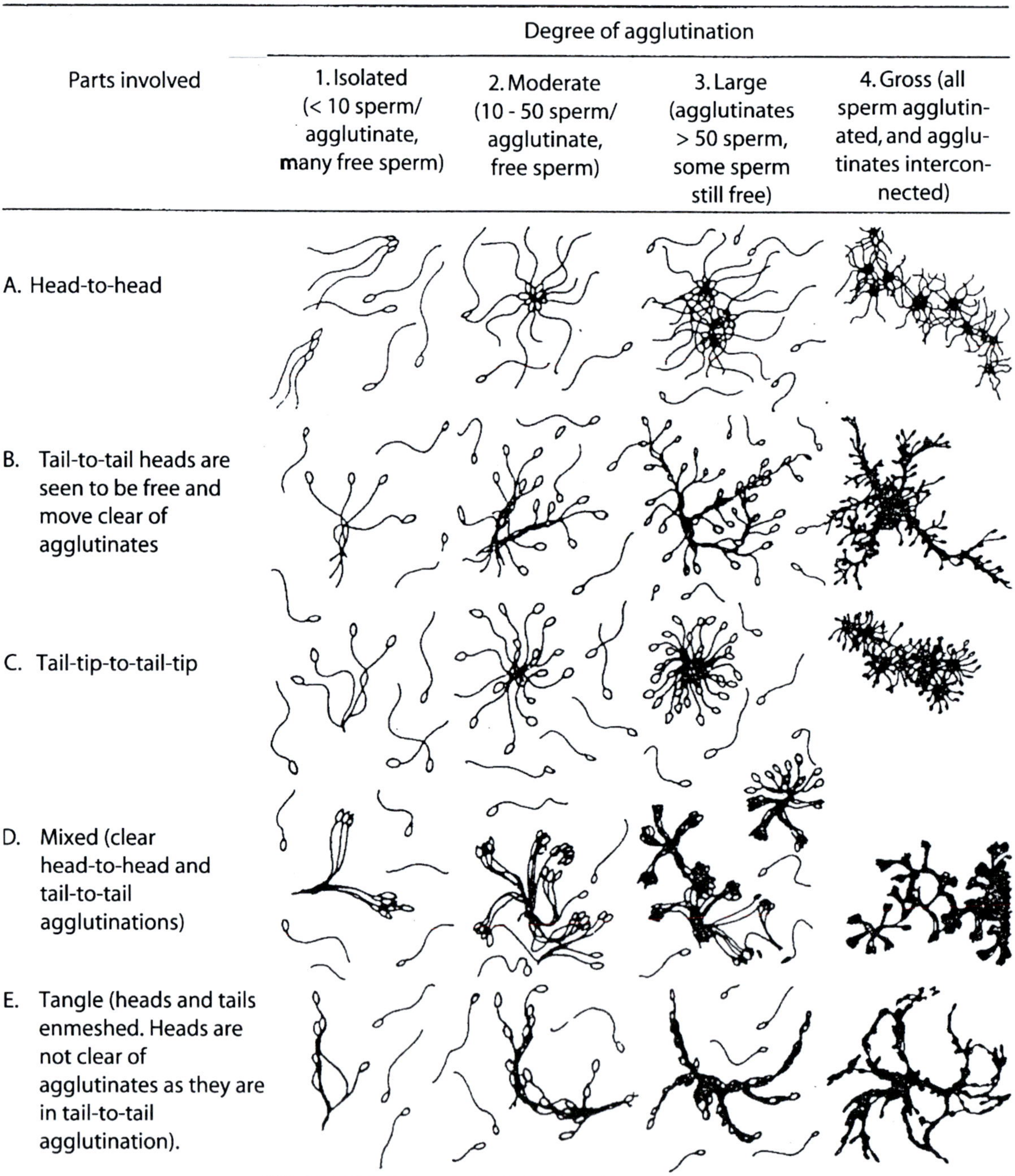

Fig. II.3.2. Standardized descriptions of type and degree of sperm agglutination. Descriptions are based on the type and degree of spermatozoa involved in the agglutination and the number of spermatozoa involved in the agglutination (Rose et al. 1976)

ortho-toluidine (0.025% vol/vol); and H_2O_2 (30% vol/vol in distilled water).

The working solution is prepared by adding 1 ml of saturated NH_4Cl solution, 1 ml of Na_2-EDTA 5% solution, 9 ml of ortho-toluidine solution and one drop of H_2O_2. This solution is mixed before use and can be conserved for 24 h after preparation.

The procedure consists of mixing 0.1 ml of semen with 0.9 ml of the working solution to achieve a total volume of 1 ml. This mixture is shaken for 2 min. It is then left for 20–30 min at room temperature and mixed again by shaking.

The mixture is now transferred onto a haemocytometer chamber for leukocytes (either Neubauer or Burker) and the number of peroxidase-positive cells that stain brown is counted. Peroxidase-negative cells remain unstained and are counted in the haemocytometer chamber. It is suggested to count 25 large squares in the improved Neubauer haemocytometer and to multiply the number of cells by 0.1 in order to obtain the concentration per millilitre.

II.3.2.4.4
Agglutination

Agglutination of spermatozoa means that motile spermatozoa stick to each other, head to head, mid-piece to mid-piece, tail to tail, or mixed, e.g. mid-piece to tail (Fig. II.3.2). The adherence of either immotile or motile spermatozoa to mucous threads, to cells other than spermatozoa, or to debris is not considered agglutination. The presence of agglutination is suggestive of, but not sufficient evidence to prove the existence of, an immunological factor of infertility.

The extent of agglutination may be important, but even the presence of only a few groups of small numbers of agglutinated spermatozoa should be recorded. In case of agglutination, sperm culture must be performed in order to exclude infection with *Escherichia coli*, and a direct mixed antiglobulin reaction (MAR) test or immunobead test is indicated to detect antisperm antibodies on the spermatozoa.

II.3.2.4.5
Sperm Viability

If the proportion of immotile spermatozoa exceeds 60–75%, a supra-vital staining technique is recommended. This staining is based on the principle that dead cells with damaged plasma membranes take up stain. Dead sperm cannot be used for in vitro fertilization (IVF), whereas living but immotile spermatozoa are suitable.

One drop of fresh sperm is mixed on a microscope slide with one drop of eosin 0.5%, and the mixture is examined using either bright light or phase-contrast microscopy. Using a laboratory counter, 100 spermatozoa are classified as either coloured orange-red, if the stain has passed through the membrane and therefore the cell is considered dead, or non-stained which are considered alive. Alternatively, 0.1 ml of fresh semen can be mixed with 0.1 ml of the 0.5% eosin solution in a test tube. After mixing, one drop of this solution is placed under a 20 mm × 20 mm or 24 mm × 24 mm coverslip.

The percentage of dead cells should not exceed the percentage of immotile (grade d) spermatozoa assessed at the same moment in time.

The result of the viability test correlates with that of the *hypo-osmotic swelling (HOS) test*, in so far as spermatozoa with a membrane that allows the dye to penetrate will not swell in the HOS test. Spermatozoa excluding the dye may either swell or die during the HOS test (van den Saffele et al. 1992).

The presence of a large proportion of viable but immotile cells may be indicative of structural defects of the flagellum, as part of immotile cilia syndrome. Such cells may still successfully fertilize oocytes during intracytoplasmic sperm injection (ICSI).

II.3.2.5
Evaluation of Morphological Characteristics

II.3.2.5.1
Slide Preparation and Staining

It is important to prepare a few smear slides from the fresh semen sample to be used for assessment of sperm morphology. The slide must be cleaned with detergent, washed in water and finally in alcohol, and dried before use. A drop of 7–10 µl semen is put onto one side of the slide. The sharp edge of another slide is placed in contact with the drop so that the drop spreads along the edge. The slide is then moved forward, dragging the drop of semen behind, to produce a feathered-edge smear. The smear is air-dried and fixed in a mixture of equal parts of ethanol and ether (Hellinga et al. 1973). Staining can be performed using the (simplified) Papanicolaou stain or a special stain for spermatozoa (Spermac).

II.3.2.5.2
Morphology Assessment

Various morphological abnormalities encountered are recorded by means of a tally form. It is preferable to use well-defined criteria for describing abnormal spermatozoa, and to consider all other cells, including those with borderline morphology, as normal (Comhaire et al. 1994b). This method results in a higher average of normal forms than the one applying "strict criteria" for normal sperm morphology, which classifies all the cells including borderline forms as abnormal (Menkveld et al. 1990).

Ideally shaped spermatozoa exhibit an oval-shaped head with regular outline and acrosomal cap covering more than one-third of the head surface. The head length is between 3 and 5 µm and the width must be between one-half and two-thirds of the length. When Papanicolaou-stained spermatozoa are observed under phase-contrast illumination, the acrosomal cap appears blue and the nuclear material of the head appears yellow. The mid-piece must be slender, less than one-third of the width of the head, straight and regular in outline. The mid-piece is aligned with the longitudinal axis of the head and is approximately 7 – 8 µm long. The tail is slender, uncoiled, and should present a regular outline. It is at least 45 µm in length. Size definitions of normal spermatozoa are sometimes different between authors, and may depend on the method of preparation of the smear (Hellinga et al. 1973). Increased or decreased head size occurs as the only abnormality in only 0.5% of spermatozoa with an oval head, normal mid-piece and tail. Hence, abnormalities of size are usually associated with other abnormalities.

Spermatozoa with a *tapering head* exhibit a diminished head width in relation to the head length, such that the width is less than half of the length. The head thus assumes a cigar-like shape which may or may not come to a point at the mid-piece.

Pyriform or pear-shaped head spermatozoa are those whose heads have an obvious or exaggerated tear-drop, tapered shape coming to a distinct point just above the mid-piece region.

Round head spermatozoa often have no acrosome and they may be present in large numbers in some semen samples.

Pin head: some spermatozoa, which are usually highly motile, do not present a clear head structure and seem to consist entirely of mid-piece and tail. They must be differentiated from spermatozoa with a small head.

Duplicate or double head spermatozoa have two distinct heads that may be of various shapes and sizes. The presence of a double head takes precedence over any other head type classification.

Amorphous head is the type of spermatozoon that has a bizarre shape of the head such that it cannot be put into any other category. The outline is always irregular.

Mid-piece Abnormalities

Mid-piece abnormalities include abnormal implantation of the mid-piece aside or angular to the longitudinal axis of the head, the presence of a cytoplasmic remnant, an abnormal width of the mid-piece, or broken mid-piece. The mid-piece may also be duplicated in cases with a double head.

Tail Abnormalities

Abnormalities of the tail include short tails, which are often excessively thick, broken tails, coiled tails, or tails that have an irregular outline as a result of disruption of the membrane. Sometimes the tail has a normal length but the extreme end is excessively thin.

II.3.2.6 Testing for Antibody-Coated Spermatozoa

The presence of sperm antibodies coating the spermatozoa is typical of, and is considered to be specific for, immunological infertility. Sperm antibodies in semen belong to the immunological classes IgG, IgA or, rarely, IgM. Some data suggest that IgA antibodies may have greater clinical importance than IgG antibodies as a cause of infertility (Kremer and Jager 1992). Testing for these antibodies is performed on fresh semen and uses the direct mixed antiglobulin reaction (MAR) test or the immunobead test.

II.3.2.6.1 Antibodies of the IgG Class

The *direct MAR test for IgG* is performed by mixing on a microscope slide one drop (approx. 10 µl) of fresh semen, one drop of latex particles coated with IgG, and one drop of antiserum from rabbit against human IgG. After 2 – 3 min the mixture is examined under the microscope. The percentage of motile spermatozoa with particles attached is counted using a laboratory counter. The SpermMar test is easier to perform, less cumbersome and more relevant than the *immunobead* test (Andreou et al. 1995). The diagnosis of immunological infertility is probable when 40% or more of the motile spermatozoa have particles adherent. Immunological infertility is suspected if 10 – 40% of the motile spermatozoa have adherent particles, when other tests are needed to confirm the diagnosis.

II.3.2.6.2 Antibodies of the IgA and IgM Classes

Direct MAR test for IgA or IgM is performed by mixing one drop of fresh semen containing motile spermatozoa with one drop of Latex particles that are coated with monoclonal antibodies against either human IgA or human IgM on a microscope slide. The preparation is covered with a large coverslip (24 mm × 32 mm) and observed immediately after mixing, as well as after 3 min. The percentage of motile spermatozoa with latex particles attached is calculated.

Additional tests such as the sperm-cervical mucus contact test, titration of sperm agglutinating antibodies in serum, and cytotoxicity tests will add weight and confirm or reject the diagnosis (Kremer and Jager 1992).

II.3.2.7 Counting of Spermatozoa

The reference method for sperm counting is the haemocytometer method, but disposable counting chambers may also be used with sufficient reliability (Mahmoud et al. 1997).

II.3.2.7.1 The Haemocytometer Method

Semen must be diluted whenever the haemocytometer method is used. The dilution medium consists of 50 g $NaHCO_3$, 10 ml of a 35% (vol/vol) formalin solution and distilled water to give a final volume of 1000 ml. Optionally, 5 ml of saturated aqueous gentian violet can be included. This stain need not be included if phase-contrast microscopy is used.

If the preliminary examination of the semen indicates that the concentration of spermatozoa present is either high ($>10 \times 10^7$/ml) or low ($<2 \times 10^6$/ml), then the dilution must be adjusted (see Fig. II.3.3). For samples with a sperm concentration estimated to be between 2×10^6 and 10×10^7/ml, a 1:20 dilution is used. This is obtained by mixing 50 µl of liquefied semen with 950 µl of diluent. For samples with low sperm count, a 1:10 dilution is made by mixing 100 µl of semen with 900 µl of diluent. Samples containing more than 10×10^7/ml spermatozoa are diluted 1:50 by adding 50 µl of semen to 2450 µl of diluent.

The specimens should be diluted in small clean glass tubes. The diluted specimen must be thoroughly mixed by hand and by vortex, after which a fixed volume is transferred to a haemocytometer and covered with a coverslip. The haemocytometer is allowed to stand for 1–5 min, preferably in a moist chamber to minimize drying. During this time the cells sediment. Counting is done under a light or phase-contrast microscope at a magnification of 100 or 400×. Only spermatozoa that are morphologically mature germinal cells with tails are counted.

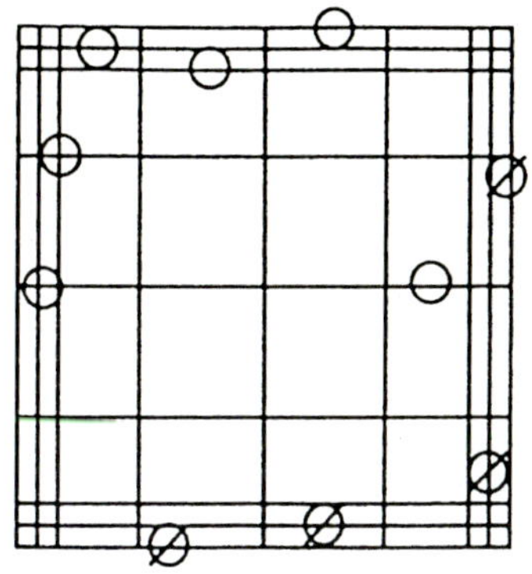

Fig. II.3.4. Cells on *top* and *left* touching middle line (O) are counted. Cells touching middle line at *bottom* and *right* are not counted (Ø)

The procedure for counting the spermatozoa in a haemocytometer chamber is as follows: the central square of the grid in an improved Neubauer haemocytometer contains 25 large squares, each with 16 smaller squares. For practical purposes it is recommended to count the number of spermatozoa that are present in 25 squares. If a spermatozoon lies on the line dividing two adjacent squares, it should be counted only if it is on the upper or the left side of the square being assessed (Fig. II.3.4). In order to determine the concentration of spermatozoa in the original semen sample in millions/ml, the number of spermatozoa counted in 25 large squares is multiplied by 0.1 if a dilution 1:10 has been applied, by 0.2 if a dilution of 1:20 is used, and by 0.5 a 1:50 dilution is used.

It is recommended to perform an in duplo count using a second aliquot of semen and the same dilution. Ideally, the result of both counts should not be more than 10% apart. In reality, the differences are often somewhat larger due to lack of homogeneity of the semen sample and errors during pipetting or dilution. Differences exceeding 10% indicate that the result is inadequate, and counting must be repeated.

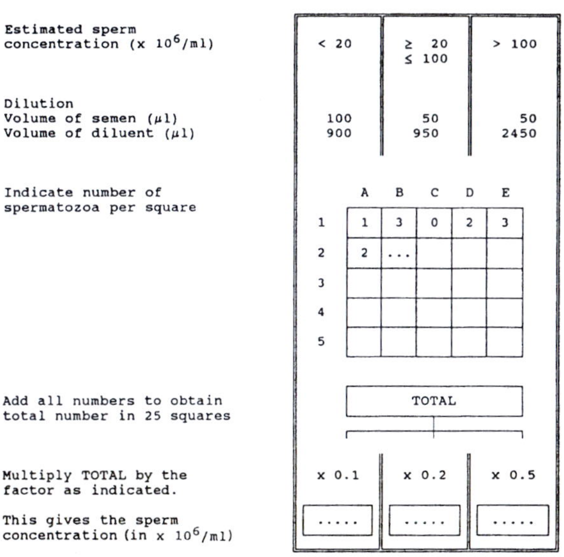

Fig. II.3.3. Practical record form for sperm concentration assessment

II.3.2.7.2 Disposable Fixed Depth Counting Chambers

An alternative procedure to determine sperm concentration is by employing special sperm counting chambers. Reusable counting chambers such as the one by Makler can be used without dilution of semen, but they may lack the accuracy of the haemocytometer technique (Mahmoud et al. 1997).

Another method uses disposable counting chambers (Fig. II.3.1). The counting chamber is filled with 5 μl semen. The semen flows into the counting chamber by making use of the physical properties of capillary flow. A special calibration grid must be introduced in the ocular, or disposable slides with a grid can be used. It is recommended to perform cell counting at the central part of the chamber, avoiding the inlet and outlet area.

The correlation between the result of sperm counting using the disposable slides and the haemocytometer is 0.95 and the coefficient of variation of the counting procedure is only slightly higher, namely 8% as compared to 6% with the haemocytometer (Mahmoud et al. 1997).

II.3.2.8 Semen Culture

Semen samples for bacteriological culture should be collected taking into account specific precautions to avoid contamination. Before obtaining the sample, the patient should pass urine. Next he should wash his hands and genital region with soap. He should rinse away the soap and dry with a fresh towel. The semen containers must be sterile. For a complete examination, the sample should be passed to a microbiology laboratory (Mobley 1975). Because seminal plasma has rather strong bacteriostatic capacity, it is recommended to dilute the semen specimen before inoculation. This can be done by adding 0.2 ml of sterile physiological saline to 0.2 ml of semen in a sterile glass or plastic test tube. Alternatively, the mixture may be aspirated directly in a sterile disposable syringe. After thorough mixing 50 μl of the mixture is homogeneously spread on a blood agar culture medium using an Ose. The blood agar is incubated overnight at 37°C. The number of colonies is counted and multiplied by 40 to give the number of colony forming units (CFUs) per ml.

If the number of CFUs is over 3000/ml, and culture is uniform, then further identification and an antibiogram are needed. Uniform growth of between 1000 and 3000 CFUs/ml is considered borderline, whereas the presence of fewer than 1000 CFUs/ml suggests contamination. Also, the nonuniform growth of more than 3000 CFUs of different species is considered to be contamination (Comhaire et al. 1980). Patients presenting a positive result on bacteriological culture of a first semen sample need to have the test repeated. It is only when culture is positive for the same bacterial species upon two semen analyses that bacterial infestation is considered of clinical importance.

The culture of seminal plasma may contribute to the diagnosis of male accessory gland infection, particularly of the prostate (Rowe et al. 2000). Semen culture must be performed on at least one semen sample from each patient, or when the subject has signs or symptoms of accessory gland infection, or the semen contains white blood cells exceeding 1×10^6/ml.

II.3.2.9 Summary of Basic Testing

When correctly performed, the techniques of basic semen analysis will give reliable and reproducible results on conventional sperm characteristics. Both internal and external quality control are mandatory, and strict standards for technical accuracy must be applied. In doing so, acceptable low levels of inter- and intraobserver variability can be obtained, and the results will have clinical relevance. Assessment of sperm characteristics gives important clues to the discrimination between infertile, subfertile and potentially fertile semen, and can to some extent predict the probability of occurrence of spontaneous conception, or help select the best method of treatment.

II.3.2.10 Advanced Assessment of Basic Sperm Characteristics

II.3.2.10.1 Sperm Concentration and Motility

Recent research and development permit the reliable measurement of patterns of sperm movement and the detailed assessment of sperm morphology through metric image analysis. There is some evidence supporting the superior capacity of objectively assessed sperm characteristics in discriminating between fertile and subfertile semen (Hinting et al. 1988a). Advanced techniques should not only permit more precise objective and reproducible analysis of conventional sperm characteristics, they should also allow for the measurement of complementary characteristics of, for example, sperm movement, such as curvilinear and linear velocity, cross beat frequency and lateral head displacement.

The first efforts to objectively assess sperm motility have been reported (Rothschild 1953), and several authors have described methods for the determination of motility characteristics.

Time exposure photography was introduced in the early 1950s (Rothschild 1953) and, after some modifications, it was made applicable to analysing human sperm motility (Overstreet et al. 1979). Spermatozoa are photographed under dark-field illumination for an exposure time of 1 s, during which images of both motile and immotile spermatozoa are recorded on film. The negatives are projected as a filmstrip and analysed on a specially designed console.

In order to overcome the blurriness and non-distinct images of motile spermatozoa, a *multiple exposure photography* method was developed (Makler 1978; Overstreet et al. 1979). An aliquot of undiluted semen is placed in a chamber with a depth of 10 μm, and spermatozoa are photographed for 1 s, while being exposed to six stroboscopic light pulses. As a result, motile spermatozoa appear on the photograph as a six-ringed chain. Immotile spermatozoa show a single image. This technique was simplified by using Polaroid photography and by modifying the stroboscopic apparatus.

With the *cinematographic technique* spermatozoa are filmed through the microscope by means of a movie camera and the tracks of the motile spermatozoa are analysed frame by frame.

The development of video cameras and software for image analysis has made assessment of sperm motility possible by fitting a video camera on the microscope (Katz et al. 1985). Quantitative measurements can be made directly from the video images, or the slow motion pictures can be analysed; alternatively there is computer analysis of the video images (computer assisted semen analysis or CASA) (Holt et al. 1985; Katz and Davis 1987; Ginsburg et al. 1988). Values are reported for sperm concentration, percent motility, velocity and linearity of sperm progression, maximum and mean amplitude of lateral head displacement and head beat cross frequency (Ginsburg et al. 1988).

A *simple semi-computerized method* has been developed for the objective assessment of sperm motility characteristics (Hinting et al. 1988b). By introducing a drawing tube between the objective and the oculars of a microscope, it is possible to observe motile spermatozoa and to track their movement manually with the help of a cursor on a digitizing tablet (Autosperm, Fertipro, Beernem, Belgium). This tablet generates data that can be analysed by a microcomputer programme (Hinting et al. 1988b).

The procedure yields optimal results in semen samples with sperm concentrations between 1×10^6 and 50×10^6/ml, and its reproducibility is excellent.

Two *major problems* have arisen with the CASA systems. The first resides in problems with the identification of spermatozoa against objects of similar size such as some round cells, cytoplasmic droplets or debris. In the older systems, particular characteristics of the head of the motile cells were defined first in order to identify all other spermatozoa. Estimation of the DNA content (Hamilton-Thorn) or of the presence of a sperm tail (Strömberg-Mika) has largely solved this problem. Errors are still induced by the arbitrary definition of minimal velocity criteria that may reduce the differences between study groups (Comhaire et al. 1992).

The second major problem is caused by the fact that the spatially average path of spermatozoa is computed by smoothing the periodical lateral wobble from the curvilinear trajectory using a fixed length running average. This induces errors that equally tend to reduce differences between specimens, particularly when analysing human sperm, because the motion characteristics of human spermatozoa are remarkably diverse. The introduction of adaptive smoothening and harmonic analysis (Davis et al. 1992) can only partially correct for these errors.

II.3.2.10.2 Morphology Analysis

Since Williams and Savage's statement: "in the microscopic study of spermatozoa, the morphology of the sperm head constitutes the greatest single source of information as to the fitness of these cells for reproduction" (Williams and Savage 1925), there has been a continuous debate on which criteria should be applied to define normal spermatozoa, and which classification of abnormal forms is most appropriate. Many authors (MacLeod and Gold 1951; Eliasson 1971; Hellinga 1976) advocate the use of strict criteria for sperm normality, while cells with borderline morphology must be considered abnormal (approach A). In contrast, Page and Houlding (1951) define the criteria of abnormal spermatozoa and consider all other cells normal (approach B). They do not claim any advantage of this approach, "except for a reduction in the errors of judgement between two observers". The controversy on morphology assessment has been revived through claims that the application of strict criteria for normality would give better results in terms of reproducibility, clinical accuracy and predictive power (Menkveld et al. 1990) than the more liberal criteria described by the World Health Organization (WHO 1987), for example. Fully automatic computer assisted systems for sperm morphology have been developed (CASA) (Katz et al. 1986; Wang et al. 1991; Davis et al. 1992).

In general, the reproducibility of results of approach B was found to be better than that of approach A (Comhaire et al. 1994b). Results of the two CASA systems matched closely in terms of reproducibility and correspondence with the average results of all centres, and they were intermediate between those of approaches A and B. The two CASA systems performed neither better nor worse than the human observer, confirming findings of Wang et al. (1991) and MacLeod et al. (1994).

II.3.2.11 Sperm Function Tests

After having been delivered into the vagina, spermatozoa need to "swim up" over a distance of about 8 cm, through the cervical channel, the uterus and part of the Fallopian tubes to reach the oocyte. Motility characteristics determine this process. During this passage the spermatozoa are capacitated. Next, a cohort of spermatozoa reaches the corona radiata which the hyaluronidase at the surface of the acrosomal cap assists in penetrating. When in contact with the zona pellucida, the sperm acquires hyperactivation, and the outer acrosome membrane fuses with the inner acrosome membrane. Proacrosin is activated to acrosin, and liberated to help the sperm head penetrate the zona by limited proteolysis. The spermatozoon then is immobilized and its head lays flat against the oolemma. Now the fusion of the sperm membrane and oolemma takes place, and the sperm is phagocytosed by the oocyte.

Several steps of this process can be assessed by means of in vitro tests. The interaction between semen and cervical mucus is assessed using a capillary (Kremer 1965; Kroeks and Kremer 1975) or on a microscope slide. Hyperactivation can be measured using CASA; the spontaneous and induced capacitation and acrosome reaction are evaluated using special staining methods (Henkel et al. 1993). The activity of acrosin of individual spermatozoa is measured by means of a proteolytic test (Henkel et al. 1995), or its total amount can be assessed with a biochemical test (AcroScreen). Sperm attachment to the zona pellucida is estimated using the hemizona test (Kruger et al. 1991; Oehninger et al. 1992) and binding to as well as passage through the oolemma followed by decondensation of the sperm head are assessed using the zona-free hamster oocyte test (Barros et al. 1978; Tyler et al. 1981).

These tests are difficult to standardize and they have largely lost significance for clinical practice and patient management in view of the availability of ICSI. They remain useful tools from the scientific point of view, more particularly in evaluating the positive or adverse effects of treatments.

II.3.2.12 Biological and Biochemical Tests on Semen

Attention has been directed to measurement of biochemical parameters of semen in an attempt to evaluate the fertilizing potential of men. Many of the biochemical markers related to seminal vesicles, prostate, epididymis, seminiferous tubules and spermatozoa have been investigated extensively, but few of these have proven clinically useful.

Biochemical tests on semen aim at evaluating the function of the accessory sex glands and testes, detecting causal factors of male infertility, and assessing the fertilizing potential of spermatozoa.

II.3.2.12.1 The Function of the Accessory Sex Glands

There are several biochemical markers of accessory gland function. Adequate secretion by the *seminal vesicles* is necessary to maintain optimal motility of spermatozoa (Okamura et al. 1986). The seminal vesicles produce and secrete reducing substances (fructose, ascorbic acid and ergothioneine), prostaglandins and bicarbonate. Reducing agents may be acting as physiologic antioxidants, preventing sperm agglutination and sperm membrane degeneration, whereas bicarbonate and prostaglandins act directly by stimulating motility through an effect on the adenylate cyclase system, increasing the production of cAMP (Gerozissis et al. 1982). Thus, the measurement of these compounds may be useful in the evaluation of semen quality.

Methods to determine seminal bicarbonate and prostaglandins are not available in most laboratories, but fructose is routinely assayed. Since seminal fructose is negatively correlated with sperm count and does not correlate with sperm motility, Gonzales et al. (1988) have used seminal fructose multiplied by the log of sperm count to obtain a value named "corrected fructose" which was lower in asthenozoospermic subjects, irrespective of the sperm count.

The secretion products of the *prostate* gland form about one-third of the seminal fluid, in which spermatozoa are suspended. The pH of expressed prostatic fluid is acidic with a mean of 6.7 in normal men, whereas it reaches a mean of 8.1 in men with chronic bacterial prostatitis. The markedly alkaline pH of prostatic secretion in chronic bacterial prostatitis is probably the cause of the ineffectiveness of cotrimoxazole and doxycycline treatment in this disease. The concentration of zinc in human seminal plasma and in sperm is extremely high compared with that of other body fluids and tissue (Halsted et al. 1974) and measurement of this substance may provide valuable information about the function of the prostate (Marmar et al. 1975).

The concentration of citric acid in semen gives a reliable measure of prostate gland secretion. Mann and Mann (1981) have speculated that citric acid may be important in maintaining the osmotic equilibrium of the semen, which will affect membrane function and morphology of the spermatozoa.

Gamma-glutamyl transpeptidase (GGT) in seminal fluid has been shown to be mainly prostatic in origin (Verhoeven and Steeno 1979). Delanghe et al. (1985) found a correlation between the glycosylation of seminal GGT on one hand, and acid phosphatase activity and the number of bacteria per millilitre of semen on the other. They suggested that inflammation of the accessory glands induces alteration in the glycosylation of GGT in seminal fluid and it appears that sialic acid plays a part in this process.

The diagnosis of an *epididymal pathological* condition or of an obstructive process at the deferent ducts level is of relevant importance. L-Carnitine, alpha-glucosidase and glycerylphosphoryl choline have been measured in human seminal plasma in this attempt. In patients with azoospermia, normal testicular volume and normal concentrations of testosterone and follicle-stimulating hormone (FSH), the determination of seminal alpha-glucosidase may be used to reliably identify the site of obstruction (Mahmoud et al. 1998; Comhaire et al. 2002). Alpha-glucosidase is secreted at the same site as the antioxidants by the epididymis. In cases of chronic epididymitis the secretion of both substances is decreased. This may enhance the possible imbalance between oxidative stress and antioxidants in semen.

II.3.2.12.2 Testicular Function

Transferrin is an essential factor secreted by Sertoli cells and the cycle of production of this protein seems to be linked to the cycle of the seminiferous epithelium (Mather et al. 1983). Transferrin is involved in the transport of iron to germ cells (Sylvester and Griswold 1984), and it acts as an antioxidant by binding iron in biological fluids. By comparing transferrin levels in seminal plasma from normal and vasectomized men, or men with congenital absence of the vas deferens, it has been found that about 80% of the transferrin in seminal plasma is derived from the testes. The concentration of seminal transferrin showed a strong positive correlation with the sperm count (Orlando et al. 1985; Liu et al. 1986), but there was no correlation with sperm motility or sperm morphology.

Transferrin does not seem to be useful in distinguishing between azoospermic patients with obstruction and those with failure of spermatogenesis. Hence, measurement of seminal plasma transferrin does not provide more information than sperm counting.

LDH-X is an isoenzyme of lactate dehydrogenase present in the human postpubertal testis and it is specific for germinal epithelium activity (Zinkham et al. 1964). LDH-X constitutes more than 80% of the total lactate dehydrogenase activity in mature spermatozoa (Montamat and Blanco 1976). In these cells, LDH-X is located in the cytosol as well as in the matrix of those mitochondria that form the mitochondrial sheath of the sperm mid-piece. Seminal LDH-X seems a more specific index of seminiferous tubular function because it comes entirely from the testis. The ratio of LDH-X over sperm concentration may serve as an indicator of the function of the seminiferous epithelium, and its assessment may provide a complementary instrument for the study of spermatogenesis (Eliasson and Virji 1985). On the other hand, seminal LDH-X does not correlate with sperm progressive motility, or with sperm viability and morphology.

Several *steroid hormones* have been identified in human seminal plasma. The most notable are testosterone and dihydrotestosterone. Purvis et al. (1975) found the levels of all steroids in seminal plasma to be significantly lower than the corresponding blood levels. Also, they found that the concentrations of dihydrotestosterone, pregnenolone and oestradiol were significantly lower in azoospermic subjects than in normals. The only pathological finding in seminal plasma of oligozoospermic subjects was a diminished level of dihydrotestosterone (Bain et al. 1979). Zalata et al. (1995) found testosterone and dihydrotestosterone in seminal plasma to be significantly lower in cases of azoospermia, and that there is a positive correlation between these androgens and the concentration of motile spermatozoa.

Studies relating seminal plasma *prolactin* concentration with sperm concentration and sperm motility give conflicting results (Aiman et al. 1988). The bulk of prolactin seems to originate from the seminal vesicles, and is related to the function of these glands, though the prostate may be another source of prolactin.

There are multiple forms of immunoreactive inhibin in seminal plasma. Measuring the concentration of inhibin B may help in the differential diagnosis of azoospermia (Garem et al. 2002).

Seminal plasma contains large amounts of other peptide factors such as beta-endorphin, calcitonin, epidermal growth factors, somatostatin and bombesin. The role of these peptides in seminal plasma is unknown.

Gamma interferon and the *tumour necrosis factor* (TNF) may affect the ability of human sperm to penetrate hamster eggs. Testicular *IL-1 alpha* seems to be produced by Sertoli cells and acts as a spermatogonial growth factor (Parvinen et al. 1991). *Interleukin-2* and its soluble receptor (IL-2 sR) increased at high concentration of polymorphonuclear neutrophil (PMN) elastase (Miska and Mahmoud 1993). The concentrations of *IL-6*, *its receptor*, and of *IL-1 beta* were unrelated to sperm concentration, motility and morphology and they were within normal limits in immunological cases. Both IL-6 and IL-6sR were higher in the first than in the second fraction of split ejaculates, and were within normal limits in vasectomized men, suggesting their mainly prostatic origin (Comhaire and Bosmans 1993). IL-6 concentration in seminal plasma was increased after testicular stimulation by means of injections of pure FSH, indicating its secretion by cells of Sertoli.

II.3.2.12.3 Markers of Infection or Inflammation

Infection of male accessory sex glands manifests itself by growth of a high number of aerobic pathogens upon semen culture and can affect the secretory functions of these organs. Furthermore, measurement of biochemical constituents in seminal plasma may help to confirm the diagnosis of male accessory gland infection, to identify the organs affected, and to differentiate against bacterial contamination (Comhaire et al. 1989). Using receiver-operating characteristic curves, it was established that estimation of ejaculate volume and measurement of the total output of citric acid, gamma-glutamyltranspeptidase or acid phosphatase are more relevant tests. Measurement of seminal fructose did not contribute to the diagnosis since its discriminating power is lower than that of the ejaculate volume, being also dependent on seminal vesicle function. The activity of alpha-glucosidase was decreased in patients with epididymitis.

Interleukin-6 and IL-1 beta are significantly higher in cases with accessory gland inflammation, and the former has a stronger power to discriminate between semen samples with a normal and those with an elevated concentration of white blood cells. The measurement of IL-6 in semen may contribute to the diagnosis of inflammatory disease of the accessory sex glands (Comhaire et al. 1994a).

II.3.2.12.4 Biochemical Markers of the Functional Capacity of Spermatozoa

The energy needed for motility is produced in the mitochondria of the mid-piece of the sperm. Approximately 90 % of the energy needed for motility is produced as *adenosine triphosphate (ATP)* and transported to the flagellum. In the flagellum, ATP is hydroxylated into adenosine diphosphate (ADP) and adenosine monophosphate (AMP) by the ATPase enzyme, which is present in the contractile protein of the dynein arms located in contact with the microtubular doublets (Comhaire et al. 1990). Assessment of ATP in semen is based on bioluminescence, a method that is rapid, simple and has high sensitivity, good recovery and good reproducibility (Fiorelli et al. 1982).

A significant correlation was found between ATP per millilitre of ejaculate and sperm concentration, number of motile spermatozoa per millilitre, capacity of spermatozoa to migrate against gravity and in vitro potential to penetrate zona-free hamster ova (Comhaire et al. 1983; Irvine and Aitken 1985; Mahmoud et al. 1994).

Reactive oxygen species (*ROS*), such as hydrogen peroxide, the superoxide anion and the hydroxyl radical, can be generated by living cells incubated under aerobic conditions. To counteract the effect of ROS, cells possess systems that scavenge ROS to prevent internal cellular damage. Human spermatozoa are especially sensitive to lipid peroxidation induced by oxygen reactive species because of their high content of polyunsaturated fatty acids (Aitken and Clarkson 1987), and it was suggested that ROS formation could play a pivotal role in the mechanism of idiopathic infertility and it has a detrimental effect on DNA fragmentation (Henkel et al. 2003, 2004).

II.3

Excessive generation of ROS leads to a diminished capacity for sperm–oocyte fusion because of changes in the fluidity and integrity of the plasma membrane following the initiation of lipid peroxidation (Zalata et al. 1998).

Glutathione tends to act against lipid peroxidation of the cell membrane. For this reason glutathione therapy has been proposed in various pathological situations in which ROS could create a pathogenetic effect. Glutathione therapy in infertile patients demonstrated a positive effect on sperm motility and morphology (Lenzi et al. 1993), and similar results were obtained with other antioxidants (Comhaire et al. 2000).

Acrosin is a sperm acrosomal serine proteinase that is involved in the acrosome reaction and binding of spermatozoa to the zona pellucida (Rogers and Bentwood 1982). Acrosin can be found on spermatozoa in both an active and inactive form, called pro-acrosin. The total acrosin activity of spermatozoa is defined as the amount of active (nonzymogen) acrosin associated with the spermatozoa plus the amount of active acrosin that is obtained by proacrosin activation. Spermatozoa from fertile men possess approximately three times as much acrosin as those from infertile men with at least one abnormal seminal parameter.

Low levels of acrosin are possibly associated with subfertility and infertility (Jeyendran et al. 1985), and acrosin activity of spermatozoa may be a useful complementary marker of semen quality.

Creatine phosphokinase (CK), the key enzyme in the synthesis and utilization of energy in sperm, has been found inversely correlated with sperm concentrations (Huszar et al. 1988). The CK activity differences in the swim up sperm fractions further suggested that the ejaculates are composed of biochemically different sperm subpopulations. However, there was no relationship between sperm CK activities and the values of sperm motility or morphology. An increased CK content is consistent with the increased retention of cytoplasm due to failure of spermatogenesis. As a consequence of the incomplete development, the biochemical maturity of the spermatozoa is retarded, leading to diminished sperm function including fertilizing potential (Huszar et al. 1990).

References

Aiman J, McAsey M, Harms L (1988) Serum and seminal plasma prolactin concentrations in men with normospermia, oligospermia, or azoospermia. Fertil Steril 49:133–137

Aitken RJ, Clarkson JS (1987) Cellular basis of defective sperm function and its association with the genesis of reactive oxygen species by human spermatozoa. J Reprod Fertil 81: 459–469

Andreou E, Mahmoud A, Vermeulen L, Schoonjans F, Comhaire F (1995) Comparison of different methods for the investigation of antisperm antibodies on spermatozoa, in seminal plasma and in serum. Hum Reprod 10:125–131

Bain J, Duthie M, Keene J (1979) Relationship of seminal plasma testosterone and dihydrotestosterone to sperm count and motility in man. Arch Androl 2:35–39

Barros C, Gonzelez J, Herrera E, Bustos-Obregon E (1978) Fertilizing capacity of human spermatozoa evaluated by actual penetration of foreign eggs. Contraception 17:87–92

Comhaire FH, Bosmans E (1993) Cytokines in semen of normal men and of patients with andrological diseases. The

American Fertility Society conjointly with the Canadian Fertility and Andrology Society, 11–14 October 1993, Montreal, Quebec, Canada. Fertil Steril Program Supplement:S44-S45
Comhaire F, Verschraegen G, Vermeulen L (1980) Diagnosis of accessory gland infection and its possible role in male infertility. Int J Androl 3:32–45
Comhaire F, Vermeulen L, Ghedira K, Mas J, Irvine S, Callipolitis G (1983) Adenosine triphosphate in human semen: a quantitative estimate of fertilizing potential. Fertil Steril 40:500–504
Comhaire FH, Vermeulen L, Pieters O (1989) Study of the accuracy of physical and biochemical markers in semen to detect infectious dysfunction of the accessory sex glands. J Androl 10:50–53
Comhaire FH, Vermeulen L, Fagla B (1990) Tests of spermatozoa function: ATP. In: Acosta AA, Swanson RJ, Ackerman SB, Kruger TF, van Zyl JA, Menkveld R (eds) Human spermatozoa in assisted reproduction. Williams and Wilkins, Baltimore, pp 102–105
Comhaire FH, Huysse S, Hinting A, Vermeulen L, Schoonjans F (1992) Objective semen analysis: has the target been reached? Hum Reprod 7:237–241
Comhaire F, Bosmans E, Ombelet W, Punjabi U, Schoonjans F (1994a) Cytokines in semen of normal men and of patients with andrological diseases. Am J Reprod Immunol 31: 99–103
Comhaire F, Schoonjans F, Vermeulen L, De Clercq N (1994b) Methodological aspects of sperm morphology evaluation: comparison between strict and liberal criteria. Fertil Steril 62:857–861
Comhaire FH, Christophe AB, Zalata AA, Dhooge WS, Mahmoud AM, Depuydt CE (2000) The effects of combined conventional treatment, oral antioxidants and essential fatty acids on sperm biology in subfertile men. Prostaglandins Leukot Essent Fatty Acids 63:159–165
Comhaire F, Mahmoud A, Schoonjans F, Kint J (2002) Why do we continue to determine α-glucosidase in human semen? Andrologia 34:8–10
Davis RO, Niswander PW, Katz DF (1992) New measures of sperm motion. I. Adaptive smoothing and harmonic analysis. J Androl 13:139–152
Delanghe J, Comhaire F, de Buyzere M, Vermeulen L (1985) Altered glycosylation of gamma-glutamyltranspeptidase (GGT) in seminal fluid from men with accessory gland infection. Int J Androl 8:186–192
Eliasson R (1971) Standards for investigation of human semen. Andrologie 3:49–64
Eliasson R, Virji N (1985) LDH-C4 in human seminal plasma and its relationship to testicular function. II. Clinical aspects. Int J Androl 8:201–214
Endtz AW (1972) Een methode om het vochtige urine sediment en het vochtige menselijk sperma rechtstreeks te kleuren. Ned Tijdschr Geneeskd 116:681–685
Fiorelli G, Orlando C, Caldini AL, Cuomo S, Serio M (1982) ATP and ADP measurement in human spermatozoa by luciferin-luciferase system. In: Serio M, Pazzagli M (eds) Luminescent assays: perspective in endocrinology and clinical chemistry. Raven, New York, pp 79–87
Garem YFE, Arini AFE, Beheiry AHE, Zeid SAA, Comhaire FH (2002) Possible relationship between seminal plasma inhibin B and spermatogenesis in patients with azoospermia. J Androl 23:825–829
Gerozissis K, Jouannet P, Soufir JC, Dray F (1982) Origin of prostaglandins in human semen. J Reprod Fertil 65:401–404
Ginsburg KA, Moghissi KS, Abel EL (1988) Computer-assisted human semen analysis. Sampling errors and reproducibility. J Androl 9:82–90
Gonzales GF, Garcia-Hjarles M, Napuri R (1988) Corrected seminal fructose levels: index of secretory activity of seminal vesicles. Arch Androl 21:135–142
Halsted JA, Smith JC Jr., Irwin MI (1974) A conspectus of research on zinc requirements of man. J Nutr 104:345–378
Hellinga G (1949) Het onderzoek bij stoornissen in de mannelijke vruchtbaarheid (The investigation in case of male subfertility). Academic Thesis, Amsterdam
Hellinga G (1976) Clinical andrology. William Heinmann, London
Hellinga G, Ruward R, Oppers VM (1973) The influence of fixation and staining on the morphology of spermatozoa. In: Fertility and sterility. Proceedings of the VII World Congress, Japan, Exerpta Medica, Amsterdam, pp 233–235
Henkel R, Müller C, Miska W, Gips H, Schill WB (1993) Determination of the acrosome reaction in human spermatozoa is predictive of fertilization in vitro. Hum Reprod 8:2128–2132
Henkel R, Müller C, Miska W, Schill WB, Kleinstein J, Gips H (1995) Acrosin activity of human spermatozoa by means of a simple gelatinolytic technique: a method useful for IVF. J Androl 16:272–277
Henkel R, Kierspel E, Hajimohammad M, Stalf T, Hoogendijk C, Mehnert C, Menkveld R, Schill WB, Kruger TF (2003) DNA fragmentation of spermatozoa and assisted reproduction technology. Reprod Biomed Online 7:477–484
Henkel R, Hajimohammad M, Stalf T, Hoogendijk C, Mehnert C, Menkveld R, Gips H, Schill WB, Kruger TF (2004) Influence of deoxyribonucleic acid damage on fertilization and pregnancy. Fertil Steril 81:965–972
Hinting A, Comhaire F, Schoonjans F (1988a) Capacity of objectively assessed sperm motility characteristics in differentiating between semen of fertile and subfertile men. Fertil Steril 50:635–639
Hinting A, Schoonjans F, Comhaire F (1988b) Validation of a single-step procedure for the objective assessment of sperm motility characteristics. Int J Androl 11:277–287
Holt WV, Moore HD, Hillier SG (1985) Computer-assisted measurement of sperm swimming speed in human semen: correlation of results with in vitro fertilization assays. Fertil Steril 44:112–119
Huszar G, Corrales M, Vigue L (1988) Correlation between sperm creatine phosphokinase activity and sperm concentrations in normospermic and oligospermic men. Gamete Res 19:67–75
Huszar G, Vigue L, Corrales M (1990) Sperm creatine kinase activity in fertile and infertile oligospermic men. J Androl 11:40–46
Irvine DS, Aitken RJ (1985) The value of adenosine triphosphate (ATP) measurements in assessing the fertilizing ability of human spermatozoa. Fertil Steril 44:806–813
Jeyendran RS, van der Ven HH, Kennedy WP, Heath E, Perez-Pelaez M, Sobrero AJ, Zaneveld LJ (1985) Acrosomeless sperm. A cause of primary male infertility. Andrologia 17:31–36
Katz DF, Davis RO (1987) Automatic analysis of human sperm motion. J Androl 8:170–181
Katz DF, Davis RO, Delandmeter BA, Overstreet JW (1985) Real-time analysis of sperm motion using automatic video image digitization. Comput Methods Programs Biomed 21:173–182
Katz DF, Overstreet JW, Samuels SJ, Niswander PW, Bloom TD, Lewis EL (1986) Morphometric analysis of spermatozoa in the assessment of human male fertility. J Androl 7:203–210
Kremer J (1965) A simple sperm penetration test. Int J Fertil 10:209–215
Kremer J, Jager S (1992) The significance of antisperm antibodies for sperm-cervical mucus interaction. Hum Reprod 7:781–784
Kroeks MV, Kremer J (1975) The fractional post-coital test performed in a square capillary tube. Acta Eur Fertil 6:371–375

Kruger TF, Oehninger S, Franken DR, Hodgen GD (1991) Hemizona assay: use of fresh versus salt-stored human oocytes to evaluate sperm binding potential to the zona pellucida. J In Vitro Fert Embryo Transf 8:154–156

Lenzi A, Culasso F, Gandini L, Lombardo F, Dondero F (1993) Placebo-controlled, double-blind, cross-over trial of glutathione therapy in male infertility. Hum Reprod 8:1657–1662

Liu DY, Cooper EJ, Baker HW (1986) Seminal transferrin, an index of Sertoli cell function: is it of clinical value? Clin Reprod Fertil 4:191–197

MacLeod IC, Irvine DS, Masterton A, Taylor A, Templeton AA (1994) Assessment of the conventional criteria of semen quality by computer-assisted image analysis: evaluation of the Hamilton-Thorn motility analyser in the context of a service andrology laboratory. Hum Reprod 9:310–319

MacLeod J (1942) An analysis in human semen of a staining method for differentiating live and dead spermatozoa. Anat Rec 83:573–578

MacLeod J, Gold RZ (1951) The male factor in fertility and infertility. IV. Sperm morphology in fertile and infertile marriage. Fertil Steril 2:394–414

MacLeod J, Gold RZ (1953) The male factor in fertility and infertility. VI. Semen quality and certain other factors in relation to ease of conception. Fertil Steril 4:10–33

Mahmoud AM, Comhaire FH, Vermeulen L, Andreou E (1994) Comparison of the resazurin test, adenosine triphosphate in semen, and various sperm parameters. Hum Reprod 9: 1688–1693

Mahmoud AM, Depoorter B, Piens N, Comhaire FH (1997) The performance of 10 different methods for the estimation of sperm concentration. Fertil Steril 68:340–345

Mahmoud AM, Geslevich J, Kint J, Depuydt C, Huysse L, Zalata A, Comhaire FH (1998) Seminal plasma alpha-glucosidase activity and male infertility. Hum Reprod 13:591–595

Makler A (1978) A new multiple exposure photography method for objective human spermatozoal motility determination. Fertil Steril 30:192–199

Mann T, Mann CL (eds) (1981) Male reproductive function and semen. Springer, Berlin Heidelberg New York, pp 171–174

Marmar JL, Katz S, Praiss DE, DeBenedictis TJ (1975) Semen zinc levels in infertile and postvasectomy patients and patients with prostatitis. Fertil Steril 26:1057–1063

Mather JP, Gunsalus GL, Musto NA, Cheng CY, Parvinen M, Wright W, Perez-Infante V, Margioris A, Liotta A, Becker R, Krieger DT, Bardin CW (1983) The hormonal and cellular control of Sertoli cell secretion. J Steroid Biochem 19:41–51

Menkveld R, Stander FS, Kotze TJ, Kruger TF, van Zyl JA (1990) The evaluation of morphological characteristics of human spermatozoa according to stricter criteria. Hum Reprod 5:586–592

Miska W, Mahmoud M (1993) Determination of soluble interleukin-2 receptor in human seminal plasma. Arch Androl 30:23–28

Mobley DF (1975) Semen cultures in the diagnosis of bacterial prostatitis. J Urol 114:83–85

Montamat EE, Blanco A (1976) Subcellular distribution of the lactate dehydrogenase isozyme specific for testis and sperm. Exp Cell Res 103:241–245

Nahoum CR, Cardozo D (1980) Staining for volumetric count of leukocytes in semen and prostate-vesicular fluid. Fertil Steril 34:68–69

Oehninger S, Franken D, Alexander N, Hodgen GD (1992) Hemizona assay and its impact on the identification and treatment of human sperm dysfunctions. Andrologia 24:307–321

Okamura N, Tajima Y, Ishikawa H, Yoshii S, Koiso K, Sugita Y (1986) Lowered levels of bicarbonate in seminal plasma cause the poor sperm motility in human infertile patients. Fertil Steril 45:265–272

Orlando C, Caldini AL, Barni T, Wood WG, Strasburger CJ, Natali A, Maver A, Forti G, Serio M (1985) Ceruloplasmin and transferrin in human seminal plasma: are they an index of seminiferous tubular function? Fertil Steril 43:290–294

Overstreet JW, Katz DF, Hanson FW, Fonseca JR (1979) A simple inexpensive method for objective assessment of human sperm movement characteristics. Fertil Steril 31:162–172

Page EW, Houlding F (1951) The clinical interpretation of 1000 semen analyses among applicants for sterility studies. Fertil Steril 2:140–151

Parvinen M, Soder O, Mali P, Froysa B, Ritzen EM (1991) In vitro stimulation of stage-specific deoxyribonucleic acid synthesis in rat seminiferous tubule segments by interleukin-1 alpha. Endocrinology 129:1614–1620

Purvis K, Landgren BM, Cekan Z, Diczfalusy E (1975) Indices of gonadal function in the human male. II. Seminal plasma levels of steroids in normal and pathological conditions. Clin Endocrinol (Oxf) 4:247–258

Rogers BJ, Bentwood B (1982) Capacitation, acrosome reaction and fertilization. In: Zaneveld LJD, Chatterton RT (eds) Biochemistry of mammalian reproduction. Wiley, New York, pp 203–230

Rose NR, Hjort T, Rumke P, Harper MJK, Vyazov O (1976) Techniques for detection of iso- and auto-antibodies to spermatozoa. Clin Exp Immunol 23:175–199

Rothschild (1953) A new method of measuring sperm speeds. Nature 171:512–513

Rowe PJ, Comhaire FH, Hargreave TB, Mahmoud AMA (2000) WHO manual for the standardized investigation, diagnosis and management of the infertile male. Cambridge University Press, Cambridge

Sylvester SR, Griswold MD (1984) Localization of transferrin and transferrin receptors in rat testes. Biol Reprod 31: 195–203

Tyler JP, Pryor JP, Collins WP (1981) Heterologous ovum penetration by human spermatozoa. J Reprod Fertil 63:499–508

van den Saffele J, Vermeulen L, Schoonjans F, Comhaire FH (1992) Evaluation of the hypo-osmotic swelling test in relation with advanced methods of semen analysis. Andrologia 24:213–217

Verhoeven G, Steeno O (1979) Evidence for the prostatic origin of gamma-glutamyltranspeptidase activity in human semen. Andrologia 11:163–167

Wang C, Leung A, Tsoi WL, Leung J, Ng V, Lee KF, Chan SY (1991) Computer-assisted assessment of human sperm morphology: usefulness in predicting fertilizing capacity of human spermatozoa. Fertil Steril 55:989–993

WHO (1987) WHO laboratory manual of the examination of human semen and sperm-cervical mucus interaction. Cambridge University Press, Cambridge

WHO (1999) WHO laboratory manual of the examination of human semen and sperm-cervical mucus interaction. Cambridge University Press, Cambridge

Williams WW, Savage A (1925) Observations on the seminal micropathology of bulls. Cornell Vet 15:353–375

Zalata A, Hafez T, Verdonck L, Vermeulen L, Comhaire F (1995) Androgens in seminal plasma: markers of the surface epithelium of the male reproductive tract. Int J Androl 18:271–277

Zalata AA, Christophe AB, Depuydt CE, Schoonjans F, Comhaire FH (1998) The fatty acid composition of phospholipids of spermatozoa from infertile patients. Mol Hum Reprod 4:111–118

Zinkham WH, Blanco A, Clowry LJ Jr. (1964) An unusual isozyme of lactate dehydrogenase in mature testes: localization, ontogeny, and kinetic properties. Ann NY Acad Sci 121: 571–588

II.3.3 Cytomorphological Semen Analysis

G. Haidl, H.-C. Schuppe

This chapter is dedicated to Professor Norbert Hofmann, Düsseldorf

Summary

Cytomorphological semen analysis is an essential part of the diagnostic work-up for male infertility. Apart from the assessment of sperm morphology, it should include the qualitative evaluation of cellular elements other than spermatozoa. Appropriate staining of routine semen smears allows one to differentiate "round cells" (which need to be differentiated with regard to their type and cytomorphological abnormalities) from the completely distinct population of leukocytes, such as neutrophils and macrophages. Moreover, erythrocytes, epithelial cells as well as agglutination of spermatozoa can be identified.

Classification of sperm morphology and its diagnostic and prognostic value are still a matter of debate. According to current WHO recommendations, strict criteria defining morphologically normal spermatozoa are widely used in andrology laboratories. Whereas official reference values are pending, recent studies suggest threshold values of 8–10% normal forms to distinguish between fertile and infertile men.

With regard to abnormal forms, head defects, neck and mid-piece defects, tail defects, and cytoplasmic droplets are considered as main categories and recorded for each spermatozoon. Beyond this descriptive approach, systematic analysis of the phenotype and degree of sperm pathology, e.g. by means of the Düsseldorf classification, may highlight underlying disorders of spermatogenesis and/or epididymal function. Ultrastructural evaluation allows further characterization of "systematic" defects affecting the majority of spermatozoa in a semen sample. Moreover, correlations between abnormal sperm morphology and chromosomal abnormalities should be taken into consideration when performing intracytoplasmic sperm injection (ICSI).

II.3.3.1 Introduction

Since Anton van Leeuwenhoek first described the existence of numerous animacula in the seminal fluid of animals and men, intensive research during the eighteenth and nineteenth centuries established the testicular origin and fundamental role of spermatozoa in fertilization. The introduction of modern morphological, biochemical and molecular techniques during the twentieth century resulted in characterization of various distinct sperm abnormalities in infertile males.

Standardized assessment of the conventional semen parameters, namely sperm concentration, motility and morphology, is mandatory for characterization of semen quality and an integral part of male infertility investigation (see Chap. II.3.2). However, the clinical significance of basic semen analysis is considered to be limited and no single test or even battery of tests definitely describes the fertilizing potential of spermatozoa in vitro or in vivo. In particular, evaluation of sperm morphology is hampered by methodological difficulties. However, there is substantial evidence that sperm morphology is the semen parameter with the best prognostic value concerning fertilization or pregnancy. With regard to identification of underlying causal factors and the degree of male fertility impairment, the diagnostic value of further cytomorphological semen analysis is often neglected.

II.3.3.2 Methodological Aspects

Appropriate cytomorphological semen analysis by means of light microscopy requires preparation of air-dried semen smears from fresh semen after complete liquefaction (see Chap. II.3.2; WHO 1999). It should be noted that the results largely depend on pretreatment of the glass slides, the quality of the smear, as well as fixation and staining methods used (Meschede et al. 1993; Menkveld et al. 1997). For optimal differential staining of spermatozoa, Papanicolaou or Shorr stain are recommended, alternative procedures include commercially available kits for rapid staining such as "Diff-Quik". Two hundred spermatozoa should be evaluated under oil-immersion at a magnification of 1000–1250×. In addition to the differentiation between morphologically normal and abnormal sperm, cytomorphological semen analysis should include the assessment of other cellular elements as well as noncellular abnormalities (Table II.3.2; see below).

A major problem in morphological assessment is the pleomorphism of human spermatozoa. Since the early 1950s, various classification systems have been published including both single and multiple entry systems (Ombelet et al. 1995). In the first WHO approach, a basic description of sperm morphology assessment was made, based on counting one abnormality per spermatozoon ("single entry"; ten different categories of abnormalities). During the following decades, recommendations concerning the classification method and respective reference values for the percentage of morphologically normal spermatozoa were changed (Ombelet et al. 1995; WHO 1992, 1999). In the fourth edition of the WHO manual (WHO 1999), a spermatozoon is considered normal if sperm head, neck, midpiece and tail adhere to the now widely used "strict criteria" (Table II.3.3; Fig. II.3.5a). These criteria are based on the morphology of postcoital spermatozoa found in the periovulatory cervical mucus at the level of the internal cervical os (Menkveld et al. 1990). However, in view of a controversial debate concerning quality control and clinical significance of the results, official reference values are pending (Comhaire et al. 1994; WHO 1999; Franken et al. 2000).

WHO guidelines consider it unnecessary to distinguish routinely between all variations in head shape and size, or between the various mid-piece and tail defects (WHO 1999). On the other hand, calculation of indices describing teratozoospermia has been suggested. After recording all abnormalities of each single sperm (head, neck and mid-piece, tail defects), the total number of defects can be divided by the number of spermatozoa with defects ("teratozoospermia index") or by the number of spermatozoa counted ("sperm deformity index"). As an alternative approach, the "Düsseldorf classification" introduced a systematic pattern analysis of sperm pathologies reflecting both the frequency and degree of specific defects (Table II.3.4; Hofmann and Haider 1985; Hofmann et al. 1995; Ombelet et al. 1995). Notably, the revised "Düsseldorf classification" also meets "strict criteria" for the definition of a normal spermatozoon.

Table II.3.2. Elements of cytomorphological semen analysis[a]

Morphologically normal spermatozoa[b]
Pathological phenotypes of spermatozoa and their differentiation[c]
Immature germ cells and their differentiation (i.e. spermatids, spermatocytes)
Leukocytes and their differentiation (i.e. neutrophils, macrophages)
Other cellular components (erythrocytes, epithelial cells)
Bacteria (nonadherent, adherent, intracellular)
Aggregation and agglutination of spermatozoa
Degree of "background" staining (seen with incomplete liquefaction, hyperviscosity)

[a] Requires high-quality semen smears and staining according to WHO recommendations (WHO 1999; see also Chap. II.3.2)
[b] See Table II.3.3
[c] See Table II.3.4

Table II.3.4. Düsseldorf classification of sperm morphology[a]

Morphologically normal spermatozoa[b]
Hyperelongation of sperm heads (I–III; including postacrosomal abnormalities)
Acrosome disorders (I–II; including vacuolated heads and round heads)
Combined defects (hyperelongation with acrosome disorders; I–II)
Amorphous forms
Pin heads
Duplicated/multiple forms
Size defects (small heads, large heads)
Mid-piece and/or flagellum disturbances (I–III)[c]

[a] Hofmann and Haider (1985); Hofmann et al. (1995); Ombelet et al. (1995)
[b] The revised classification meets strict criteria for the definition of normal spermatozoa
[c] Structural defects are differentiated from isolated staining abnormalities ("blue flagella")

Table II.3.3. Tygerberg strict criteria for morphologically normal spermatozoa[a]

Head	Smooth oval configuration Dimensions[b] Stain	 Length	 Width
	Papanicolaou Diff-Quik[c]	3.0–5.0 μm 5.0–6.0 μm	2.0–3.0 μm 2.5–3.5 μm
Acrosome	Acrosomal region should comprise 40–70% of the area of the head		
Borderline forms	Considered as abnormal		
Neck/mid-piece	No abaxial implantations; slender, approx. 1 μm in width and 6–7 μm in length Cytoplasmic droplets > 30% of head size are considered as abnormal		
Tail	Uniform, slightly thinner than the mid-piece, uncoiled with principal piece 45–50 μm and terminal segment 4–6 μm		

[a] Menkveld et al. (1990); Kruger and Franken (2004) [b] See also Eliasson (1971); WHO (1992, 1999)
[c] Comparable results obtained with Hemacolor stain

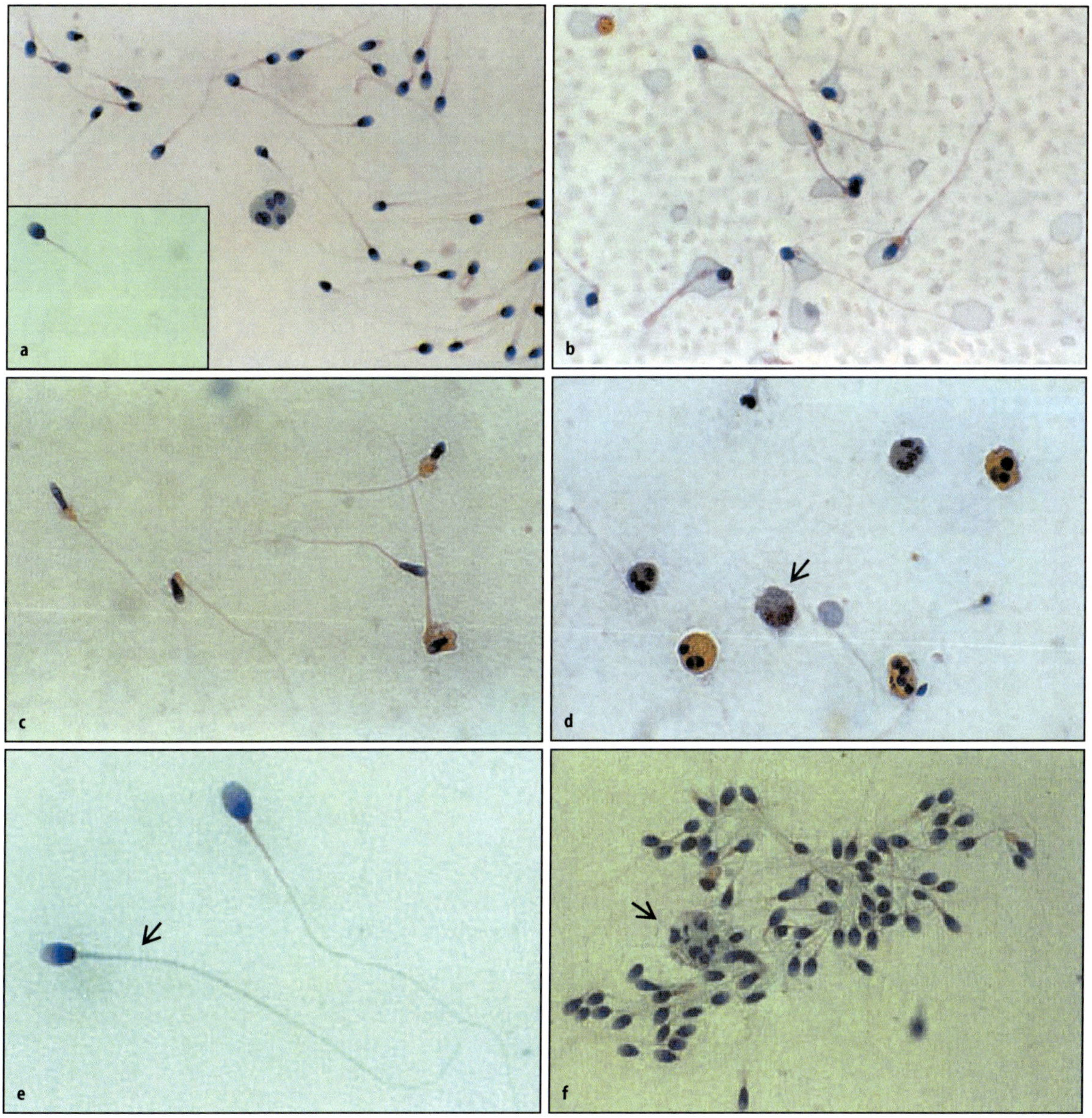

Fig. II.3.5a–f. Cytomorphological semen analysis. **a** Spermatozoa with morphologically normal heads (see *inset*) among others with minor deviations; note single neutrophil. **b** Spermatozoa with high-degree acrosomal deficiencies; note double head and additional defects of midpieces and flagella. **c** Hyperelongated sperm heads, some with concomitant acrosome disorders; note excessive cytoplasm and bend tails. **d** "Round cells" including multinuclear immature germ cells (spermatids) as well as neutrophils and a macrophage (→). **e** Abnormal staining of midpiece and flagellum ("blue flagellum";→). **f** Agglutination of spermatozoa (suggestive of surface-bound autoantibodies); note the macrophage phagocytosing spermatozoa (→). (Semen smears stained with modified Papanicolaou's; ×1000; see Hofmann et al. 1995; WHO 1999)

II.3.3.3 Predictive Value of Sperm Morphology In Vivo and In Vitro

Published literature using strict criteria for sperm morphology provides substantial evidence that the percentage of normally shaped spermatozoa in the ejaculate correlates with the results of conventional in vitro fertilization (Kruger et al. 1986, 1988; Hofmann et al. 1995; Coetzee et al. 1998). Fertilization rates above 80% were reported with semen samples containing >14% normal forms. A poor prognosis (fertilization rate 7.6%) was observed below a threshold of 5% normal forms. Values above or equal to this 5% strict-criteria threshold were also associated with significantly improved pregnancy rates following intrauterine insemination (IUI), whereas sperm morphology assessment according to WHO criteria did not reveal a comparable correlation (Van Waart et al. 2001). The predictive value of normal sperm morphology according to strict criteria for the outcome of IUI has been confirmed in further contributions (Hauser et al. 2001; Lee et al. 2002). A series of studies suggested threshold values of 8–12% for morphologically normal spermatozoa to distinguish between fertile and subfertile or infertile men with regard to natural conception (Ombelet et al. 1997; Bonde et al. 1998; Zinaman et al. 2000; Günalp et al. 2001; Guzick et al. 2001; Slama et al. 2002). There is, however, a considerable indeterminate range between results interpreted as fertile versus those associated with subfertility. Here, detailed analysis of the frequency and degree of sperm defects, i.e. the segment of minor aberrations, might improve the predictive value of sperm morphology. In contrast, fertilization and pregnancy rates following intracytoplasmic sperm injection (ICSI) have been considered as independent from sperm morphology (Nagy et al. 1995; Novero et al. 1997; Bonduelle et al. 2002; Check et al. 2003).

II.3.3.4 Clinical Relevance of Cytomorphological Semen Analysis

Cytomorphological analysis of sperm pathology represents an important step beyond mere counting of spermatozoa with a normal shape. Systematic assessment of morphological sperm defects and characterization of their severity give some insight into testicular pathologies, i.e. those affecting spermato- and/or spermiogenesis, as well as disturbances of epididymal function. This is emphasized by the "Düsseldorf classification", which reflects the principles of spermatid differentiation (chromatin condensation, acrosomal development, elongation, development of the terminal segment) (Hofmann and Haider 1985; Hofmann et al. 1995; Ombelet et al. 1995; Table II.3.4; Fig. II.3.5). Whereas hyperelongation of the postacrosomal region of sperm heads has been associated with Sertoli cell dysfunction and a more favourable prognosis, high-degree acrosome disorders and related combined defects are considered to be mostly of genetic origin and not reversible. Notably, spermatozoa with acrosome disorders have been shown to exhibit disturbances of chromatin condensation (Hofmann and Hilscher 1991; Chemes and Rawe 2003). With regard to sperm function, normal acrosomal morphology correlates with the inducibility of the acrosome reaction and sperm binding to the zona pellucida (Henkel et al. 2005).

Pattern analysis of sperm pathology is not restricted to head abnormalities, but includes mid-piece and tail (Tables II.3.4, II.3.5; Chemes and Rawe 2003). This approach allows one to distinguish between unfavourable structural defects of testicular origin and functional disturbances related to the epididymal passage and further transit through the genital tract as underlying causes of asthenozoospermia. The functional disturbances of the flagellar membrane are reflected by an atypical staining behaviour with Shorr or Papanicolaou staining. Whereas normal sperm tails stain red, disturbed epididymal maturation is indicated by bluish staining. Such spermatozoa, when retrieved from the epididymis, revealed a lack of membrane lipids associated with increased membrane rigidity and immotility without showing further structural defects (Haidl et al. 1993). Recording staining abnormalities of the flagella appears be a useful diagnostic tool as the underlying functional disturbances may respond to pharmacotherapy, i.e. in cases of chronic and mostly asymptomatic genital tract inflammation affecting the epididymis (Haidl 2002).

Although certain patterns of sperm pathology can be identified among infertile men, the combination of different abnormalities in individual patients is heterogeneous (Chemes and Rawe 2003). On the other hand, some patients reveal "systematic" defects such as globozoospermia affecting the majority of spermatozoa in a semen sample and resembling similar defects in other individuals (Table II.3.5). These anomalies tend to show family clustering and have proven or suspected genetic origin.

Poor sperm morphology, i.e. the presence of residual cytoplasmic droplets, also correlates with the sperm cell's own excessive production of reactive oxygen species and, thus, fertilizing potential (Gomez et al. 1996; Henkel et al. 2005). Spermatozoa with cytoplasmic residues have a higher quantity of cytoplasmic enzymes, such as creatine kinase or glucose-6-phosphate dehydrogenase, which are thought to stimulate the generation of reactive oxygen species.

Appropriate staining of routine semen smears allows the assessment of cellular elements other than spermatozoa. The detailed qualitative evaluation mainly concerns "round cells", i.e. type and cytomorphological abnormalities of spermatogenetic cells, which need to be distinguished from leukocytes such as neutrophils and macrophages (Johanisson et al. 2000). Definite quantification and differentiation of leukocyte subpopulations, however, require immunocytochemical techniques (Wolff 1995; WHO 1999; Villegas et al. 2002; see Chaps. I.3.13, II.2.4). Moreover, erythrocytes, epithelial cells, occurrence of crystalloid bodies as well as agglomeration and agglutination of spermatozoa can be identified. The latter phenomenon correlates with the detection of sperm autoantibodies in appropriate assays (see Chap. I.3.7).

Table II.3.5. Sperm pathology: examples of systematic defects[a]

	Disorder/Phenotype	Structural defect
Head defects	Globozoospermia	Lacking acrosome (loss of Golgi complex during spermiogenesis), associated with chromatin anomalies (failure of histone-protamine transition, increased DNA fragmentation)
	Acrosomal hypoplasia	Insufficient development of the acrosome (see above), often associated with abnormal chromatin maturation/condensation[b]
	"Crater defect"	Acrosomal malformation
Defects of head-neck attachment	Decapitated (acephalic) spermatozoa ("pin heads")	Failure of the connecting piece to attach to the spermatid nucleus
Mid-piece defects	"Thin mid-piece"	Deficiency or absence of mitochondria
Tail defects	Short ("stump") tail	Disorders of spermiogenesis, e.g. dysplasia of the fibrous sheath, associated with axonemal defects and mid-piece abnormalities
	Immotile cilia syndrome (primary ciliary dyskinesia)	Lack of dynein arms of microtubules and other axonemal defects
	"9+0" syndrome[c]	Missing central pair of microtubules of the axoneme

[a] For review see Chemes and Rawe (2003) [b] See also Table II.3.4 [c] Frequently associated with disorders of the fibrous sheath

II.3.3.5 Sperm Morphology and ICSI

There is increasing evidence that sperm morphology plays a significant role in ICSI outcome (Chemes and Rawe 2003). Although fertilization and pregnancy rates after ICSI were reported to be independent from the average percentage of normal forms in a semen sample, recent data suggest that pathomorphology of the individual sperm injected into the oocyte does influence ICSI results. Hence, a reduced implantation rate was observed when using abnormal spermatozoa for injection (De Vos et al. 2003). A significant sperm-related effect on blastomere cleavage has been demonstrated, which could be referred to sperm morphology according to strict criteria rather than sperm count or progressive motility (Salumets et al. 2002). Moreover, unexplained recurrent pregnancy loss is associated with sperm chromosome aneuploidy and sperm pathology (Carrell et al. 2003). The increased rate of chromosomal abnormalities found in spermatozoa with severe morphological abnormalities highlights the potential impact of sperm morphology on ICSI results (Martin et al. 2003; Vicari et al. 2003). Sperm chromatin anomalies were reported to exert a profound effect on fertilization failure in ICSI (Razavi et al. 2003). On the other hand, intracytoplasmic injection with morphologically selected sperm, i.e. those showing a normal nuclear shape, resulted in improved pregnancy rates (Berkovitz et al. 2004). In cases where no normal spermatozoa are available, it is suggested to select the less disturbed for injection, e.g. spermatozoa with hyperelongation of the postacrosomal region rather than those with acrosomal maldevelopment. In conclusion, sperm pathology and its pattern should not be neglected during both routine semen analysis and sperm selection prior to assisted fertilization.

References

Berkovitz A, Eltes F, Yaari S, Katz N, Barr I, Fishman A, Bartoov B (2004) The morphological normalcy of the sperm nucleus and pregnancy rate of intracytoplasmic injection with morphologically selected sperm. Hum Reprod 20:185–190

Bonde JP, Ernst E, Jensen TK, Hjollund NH, Kolstad H, Henriksen TB, Scheike T, Giwercman A, Olsen J, Skakkebaek NE (1998) Relation between semen quality and fertility: a population-based study of 430 first - pregnancy planners. Lancet 352:1172–1177

Bonduelle M, van Assche E, Joris H, Keymolen K, Devroey P, van Steirteghem A, Liebaers I (2002) Prenatal testing in ICSI pregnancies: incidence of chromosomal anomalies in 1586 karyotypes and relation to sperm parameters. Hum Reprod 17:2600–2614

Carrell DT, Wilcox AL, Lowy L, Peterson CM, Jones KP, Erickson L, Campbell B, Branch DW, Hatasaka HH (2003) Elevated sperm chromosome aneuploidy and apoptosis in patients with unexplained recurrent pregnancy loss. Obstet Gynecol 101:1229–1235

Check M, Check JK, Summers-Chase D, Swenson K, Yuan W (2003) An evaluation of the efficacy of in vitro fertilization with intracytoplasmic sperm injection for sperm with low hypoosmotic swelling test scores and poor morphology. J Assis Reprod Genet 20:182–185

Chemes HE, Rawe VY (2003) Sperm pathology: a step beyond descriptive morphology. Origin, characterization and fertility potential of abnormal sperm phenotypes in infertile men. Hum Reprod Update 9:405–428

Coetzee K, Kruger TF, Lombard CJ (1998) Predictive value of normal sperm morphology: a structured literature review. Hum Reprod Update 4:73–82

Comhaire F, Schoonjans F, Vermeulen L, De Clerq N (1994) Methodological aspects of sperm morphology evaluation: comparison between strict and liberal criteria. Fertil Steril 62:857–861

De Vos A, van de Velde H, Joris H, Verheyen G, Devroey P, van

II.3

Steirteghem A (2003) Influence of individual sperm morphology on fertilization, embryo morphology, and pregnancy outcome of intracytoplasmic sperm injection. Fertil Steril 79:42–48
Eliasson R (1971) Standards for investigation of human semen. Andrologia 3:49
Franken DR, Barendson R, Kruger TF (2000) A continuous quality control (CQC) program for strict sperm morphology. Fertil Steril 74:721–724
Gomez E, Buckingham D, Brindle J, Lanzafame F, Irvine DS, Aitken RJ (1996) Development of an image analysis system to monitor the retention of residual cytoplasm by human spermatozoa: correlation with biochemical markers of the cytoplasmic space, oxidative stress and sperm function. J Androl 17:276–287
Günalp S, Onculoglu C, Gurgan T Kruger TF, Lombard CJ (2001) A study of semen parameters with emphasis on sperm morphology in a fertile population: an attempt to develop clinical thresholds. Hum Reprod 16:110–114
Guzick DS, Overstreet JW, Factor-Litwack P, Brazil CK, Nakajima ST, Coutifaris C, Carson SA, Cisneros P, Steinkampf MP, Hill JA, Xu D, Vogel DL (2001) Sperm morphology, motility, and concentration in fertile and infertile men. N Engl J Med 345:1388–1393
Haidl (2002) Management strategies for male factor infertility. Drugs 62:1741–1753
Haidl G, Badura B, Hinsch KD, Ghyczy M, Gareiss J, Schill WB (1993) Disturbances of sperm flagella due to failure of epididymal maturation and their possible relationship to phospholipids. Hum Reprod 8:1070–1073
Hauser R, Yogev L, Botchan A, Lessing JB, Paz G, Yavetz H (2001) Intrauterine insemination in male factor subfertility: significance of sperm motility and morphology assessed by strict criteria. Andrologia 33:13–17
Henkel R, Maass G, Bödeker R-H, Scheibelhut C, Stalf T, Mehnert C, Schuppe HC, Jung A, Schill WB (2005) Sperm function and assisted reproduction technology. Reprod Med Biol 4:7–30
Hofmann N, Haider SG (1985) New results in the morphologic diagnosis of spermatogenesis disorders (German). Gynäkologe 18:70–80
Hofmann N, Hilscher B (1991) Use of aniline blue to assess chromatin condensation in morphologically normal spermatozoa in normal and infertile men. Hum Reprod 6:979–982
Hofmann N, Hilscher B, Möhrchen B, Schuppe HC, Bielfeld P (1995) Comparative studies on various modes of classification of morphology of sperm heads and results in in vitro fertilization – a preliminary report. Andrologia 27:19–23
Johanisson E, Campana A, Luthi R, de Agostini A (2000) Evaluation of "round cells" in semen analysis: a comparative study. Hum Reprod 6:404–412
Kruger TF, Franken DR (2004) Atlas of human sperm morphology evaluation. Taylor and Francis, London
Kruger TF, Menkveld R, Stander FSH, Lombard CJ, van der Merwe JP, van Zyl JA, Smith K (1986) Sperm morphologic features as a prognostic factor in in vitro fertilization. Fertil Steril 46:1118–1123
Kruger TF, Acosta AA, Simmons KF, Swanson RJ, Matta JF, Oehninger S (1988) Predictive value of abnormal sperm morphology in in vitro fertilization. Fertil Steril 49:112–117
Lee RK, Hou JW, Ho HY, Hwu YM, Lin MH, Tsai YC, Su JT (2002) Sperm morphology analysis using strict criteria as a prognostic factor in intrauterine insemination. Int J Androl 25:277–280
Martin RH, Greene C, Rademaker AW (2003) Sperm chromosome aneuploidy analysis in a man with globozoospermia. Fertil Steril 79 [Suppl 3]:1662–1664
Menkveld R, Stander F, Kotze T, Kruger TF, van Zyl JA (1990) The evaluation of morphological characteristics of human spermatozoa according to stricter criteria. Hum Reprod 5:586–592
Menkveld R, Laquet F, Kruger TF, Lombard CJ, Sanchez Sarmiento CA, de Villiers A (1997) Effects of different staining and washing procedures on the results of human sperm morphology evaluation by manual and computerised methods. Andrologia 29:1–7
Meschede D, Keck C, Zander M, Cooper TG, Yeung C, Nieschlag E (1993) Influence of three different preparation techniques on the results of human sperm morphology analysis. Int J Androl 16:362–369
Nagy ZP, Liu J, Joris H, Verheyen G, Tournaye H, Camus M, Derde MC, Devroey P, van Steirteghem AC (1995) The result of intracytoplasmic sperm injection is not related to any of the three basic sperm parameters. Hum Reprod 10:1123–1129
Novero V, Camus M, Tournaye H, Smitz J, Verheye G, Joris H, Derde MP, van Steirteghem A, Devroey (1997) Relationship between serum follicle stimulating hormone in the male and standard sperm parameters, and the results of intracytoplasmic sperm injection. Hum Reprod 12:59–63
Ombelet W, Menkveld R, Kruger TF, Steeno O (1995) Sperm morphology assessment: historical review in relation to fertility. Hum Reprod Update 1:543–557
Ombelet W, Bosmans E, Janssen M et al (1997) Semen parameters in a fertile versus subfertile population: a need for change in the interpretation of semen testing. Hum Reprod 12:987–993
Razavi S, Nasr-Esfahani MH, Mardani M, Mafi A, Moghdam A (2003) Effect of human sperm chromatin anomalies on fertilization outcome post-ICSI. Andrologia 35:238–243
Salumets A, Suikkari AM, Möls T, Söderström-Anttila V, Tuuri T (2002) Influence of oocytes and spermatozoa on early embryonic development. Fertil Steril 78:1082–1087
Slama R, Eustache F, Ducot B, Jensen TK, Joergensen N, Horte A, Irvine S, Suominen J, Andersen AG, Auger J, Vierula M, Toppari J, Andersen AN, Keiding N, Skakkebaek NE, Spira A, Jouannet P (2002) Time to pregnancy and semen parameters: a cross-sectional study among fertile couples from four European cities. Hum Reprod 17:503–515
Van Waart J, Kruger TF, Lombard CJ, Ombelet W (2001) Predictive value of normal sperm morphology in intrauterine insemination (IUI): a structured literature review. Hum Reprod Update 7:495–500
Vicari E, de Palma A, Burrello N, Longo G, Grazioso C, Barone N, Zahi M, D'Agata R, Calogero AE (2003) Absolute polymorphic teratozoospermia in patients with oligo-asthenozoospermia is associated with an elevated sperm aneuploidy rate. J Androl 24:598–603
Villegas J, Schulz M, Vallejos V, Henkel R, Miska W, Sanchez R (2002) Indirect immunofluorescence using monoclonal antibodies for the detection of leukocytospermia: comparison with peroxidase staining. Andrologia 34:69–73
Wolff H (1995) The biologic significance of white blood cells in semen. Fertil Steril 63:1143–1157
World Health Organization (1992) WHO laboratory manual for the examination of human semen and sperm-cervical mucus interaction, 3rd edn. Cambridge University Press, Cambridge
World Health Organization (1999) WHO laboratory manual for the examination of human semen and sperm-cervical mucus interaction, 4th edn. Cambridge University Press, Cambridge
Zinaman MJ, Brown CC, Selevan SG, Clegg ED (2000) Semen quality and human fertility. A prospective study with healthy couples. J Androl 21:145–153

II.3.4 Clinical Microbiology

H. G. Schiefer, A. von Graevenitz

Summary

Common pathogens and unconventional, fastidious bacteria, viruses, fungi and parasites are causative agents in male urogenital diseases. Uropathogens and sexually transmissible organisms must be considered. Diagnostic procedures and criteria for aetiological classification in cases of balanitis, urethritis, prostatitis, epididymitis, orchitis and male accessory gland infections are described and evaluated.

Of andrological importance are:

1. Infections of the male urogenital tract, frequently caused by sexually transmitted agents. Occasionally, they have deleterious consequences for fertility, e.g. azoospermia that follows epididymitis.
2. Agents (mostly viral) that cause systemic disease and are excreted in semen, e.g. human immunodeficiency virus (HIV), hepatitis B virus (HBV) and cytomegalovirus (CMV).

II.3.4.1 Normal Flora of the Male Urogenital Tract

With the exception of the external genitalia and the anterior third of the urethra, the male urogenital tract is devoid of microorganisms. The flora of the prepuce and anterior urethra is complex and inconsistent. Species and numbers depend on, among other things, age, personal hygiene, the patient's history (sexually transmitted diseases, urinary tract infections or manipulations), sexual activity (abstinence, monogamous or promiscuous relationships) and sexual practices (genital-genital, genital-anal, genital-oral). Beside microorganisms with low or no virulence for man one may encounter facultatively pathogenic ones, albeit mostly in small numbers.

Typical bacteria of the normal male urogenital tract (Bowie et al. 1977; Schiefer 1998) are coagulase-negative *Staphylococcus* spp., viridans streptococci, *Enterobacteriaceae* spp., *Acinetobacter* spp., *Corynebacterium* spp., *Neisseria* spp., *Mycobacterium smegmatis*, *Peptostreptococcus* spp., *Bacteroides* spp., *Fusobacterium* spp., *Mycoplasma* spp., and *Candida* spp. So far, there have been no data on possible viral or parasitic colonizers.

II.3.4.2 Diagnosis of Pathogens in the Male Urogenital Tract

Obligately pathogenic microorganisms in the male urogenital tract are *Mycobacterium (M.) tuberculosis*, *Neisseria (N.) gonorrhoeae*, *Chlamydia (C.) trachomatis*, *Treponema (T.) pallidum*, *Haemophilus (H.) ducreyi*, *Klebsiella (K.)* [*Calymmatobacterium (C.)*] *granulomatis*, herpes simplex virus 2 (HSV-2), human papilloma viruses (HPV), and *Trichomonas (T.) vaginalis*. In systemic disease human immunodeficiency viruses (HIV), hepatitis B virus (HBV), hepatitis C virus (HCV), hepatitis D virus (HDV), and cytomegalovirus (CMV) may be excreted with semen, often in high concentrations.

The interpretation of microbiological findings with regard to their relationship to clinical symptoms may be quite difficult in individual cases, particularly if no quantitative data are available. The finding of obligately pathogenic microorganisms or of a large number of facultatively pathogenic ones should be a sign of a pathological process, although there are asymptomatic carriers of *N. gonorrhoeae*, *C. trachomatis*, *T. vaginalis* and HSV-2.

The multitude of potential microorganisms and the difficulties in diagnosing some of them make it impossible to search every sample for all possible pathogens. Ambiguous results obtained by routine microbiology as well as scientific interest would call for a diagnostic armamentarium that exceeds that used in routine microbiology.

Depending on the clinical picture, the preliminary diagnosis and the organism(s) suspected, the following samples can be considered:

1. Samples from prepuce and urethra, on cotton-tipped fine wire, or on small plastic loops. Swabs or loops should be introduced 2–4 cm into the urethra in order to obtain mucosal cells.
2. Impression smears, e.g. from the prepuce in cases of balanitis, to be directly plated on media suitable for culture of potential pathogens.
3. Urogenital secretions, e.g. urethral discharge or prostatic fluid, obtained by means of a calibrated loop and placed into defined volumes (2 ml) of liquid transport media, e.g. trypticase soy broth with 0.5% bovine serum albumin.
4. Ejaculate. The patient should urinate first in order to eliminate part of the urethral flora. After cleansing prepuce and hands, the fluid is obtained by masturbation. Ejaculate culture is indicated after

$\geq 10^6$ peroxidase-positive leukocytes per ml have been detected by cytological analysis of semen. Attention: ejaculate may be contaminated by urethral flora (WHO 1999; Rowe et al. 2000).
5. Urine. For the diagnosis of extracellular microorganisms in urethritis and prostatitis, fractionated samples, e.g. those obtained by the "four-specimen-test" (Brunner et al. 1983; Weidner et al. 1987, 1994; Schiefer et al. 1993), should be obtained. For some nonculture tests, e.g. enzyme-linked immunosorbent assay (ELISA) or molecular biological techniques [ligase or polymerase chain reactions (LCR, PCR)], a portion of 20–30 ml, obtained approximately 2 h after the last voiding, may be used following centrifugation.
6. Immunological tests. A systemic immune response is tested in blood serum. Urogenital secreta may be used for testing the local immune response (Mestecky and Fultz 1999).
7. Biopsy, aspirated material, or scrapings. They can be used to detect intra- and extracellularly growing microorganisms by means of light or electron microscopy, culture or nucleic acid hybridization/amplification (Krieger et al. 1996b; Isenberg 1998; Tanner et al. 1999; Murray et al. 2003).

To ensure the survival of fastidious microorganisms that may be killed by drying or low temperatures, samples should be inoculated immediately on culture media or into special transport media, depending on the organisms to be cultured. Semen contains antibacterial factors, among them Zn-containing proteins, and proteases, and should be diluted before inoculation with the same or double volume of phosphate-buffered 0.145 M NaCl or of transport medium and should be homogenized on a vortex mixer. Prior to inoculation of cell cultures the homogenate should be centrifuged, and only the pellet should be used (Howell et al. 1986).

To obtain cell counts, defined volumes of secretions are used for culture so that the number of colonies, with the dilution factor taken into account, reflects the number of organisms per millilitre.

Various methods can be used to detect facultatively or obligately pathogenic microorganisms. Three levels of diagnostic workup will be distinguished, depending on the degree of diagnostic difficulty, personnel training, available instrumentation and reagents. For a critical analysis of the individual methods, we refer to Murray et al. (2003).

The standard diagnosis of urogenital infections (level II) for conventional bacteria and fungi involves culture of defined volumes of secretions, other samples in liquid transport media, or urine on the usual general/selective/indicator/fungal media, e.g. sheep blood, MacConkey, bromothymol blue-lactose-cystine (Sandys 1960), and Sabouraud plates. Incubation is for 24–48 h at 37 °C (72 h at 30 °C for fungal media). If obligately pathogenic and facultatively pathogenic microorganisms in significant numbers are found, they should be tested for antibiotic susceptibility (Isenberg 1998; Murray et al. 2003).

Level I:	Light microscopy, simple staining techniques, use of commercial media and simple identification techniques
Level II:	Culture and identification of microorganisms on various commercial and noncommercial media. Use of fluorescein- and peroxidase-labelled antibodies. ELISAs
Level III:	Special research techniques. Electron microscopy. Molecular techniques to detect and identify microorganisms: hybridization, nucleic acid amplification (PCR, LCR); amplification of the 16 S rRNA gene (rDNA) using specific or universal primers; sequencing (Krieger et al. 1996b; Isenberg 1998; Tanner et al. 1999; Murray et al. 2003).

II.3.4.2.1 *Neisseria* (*N.*) *gonorrhoeae*

The usual procedures are: microscopy of the material stained with Gram, methylene blue (I) or with fluorescein-labelled antibodies (II), and culture of fresh material (if possible, at body temperature) on modified Thayer–Martin selective medium (I) with subsequent colony identification (II) by patterns of acid production from glucose, maltose, lactose and fructose, or by coagglutination with antibody-labelled staphylococci (II). More recent and more sensitive procedures involve nucleic acid hybridization/amplification (III). The possible presence of β-lactamase should always be checked, e.g. by a nitrocefin test (important if no standardized test system for penicillin susceptibility is available) (Isenberg 1998; Murray et al. 2003).

II.3.4.2.2 *Treponema* (*T.*) *pallidum*

The serous fluid obtained from the primary lesion is examined by dark-field microscopy (I) or after staining with fluorescein-labelled antibodies (II). Later stages have to be diagnosed serologically (II) by means of treponema-specific tests [e.g., *Treponema pallidum* hemagglutination (TPHA) test, fluorescent treponemal antibody absorption (FTA-ABS) test] and treponema-nonspecific tests (e.g. VDRL or RPR card test). Antibodies develop slowly and can be detected at the earliest 2–3 weeks following infection. Approximately 12 weeks after infection, often in the secondary stage, almost all infected individuals will show a positive reaction (Isenberg 1998; Murray et al. 2003).

II.3.4.2.3
Mycobacterium (M.) tuberculosis

Since saprophytic mycobacteria (e.g. *M. smegmatis*) frequently occur on the prepuce, the finding of acid-fast bacteria (II) in urine, prostatic secretions and semen has to be interpreted with caution. The microbiological diagnosis is based on culture (II) or nucleic acid hybridization/amplification (III). Mycobacteria can also be stained in biopsy samples (Isenberg 1998; Murray et al. 2003).

II.3.4.2.4
Chlamydia (C.) trachomatis

The usual diagnostic tools are direct microscopy of elementary bodies using fluorescein-tagged antibodies (II), culture in cycloheximide-treated McCoy or BGMK cells (II), ELISA (II), and the more sensitive nucleic acid hybridization/amplification (III) (Isenberg 1998; Murray et al. 2003). The use of urine samples for the diagnosis of *C. trachomatis* infections is effective, but urine samples should be used in addition to conventional swabs instead of replacing them (Jensen et al. 2003). The microimmunofluorescence (MIF) test is valuable in the diagnosis of urogenital infections but is expensive and labour-intensive while the complement fixation (CF) test yields reliable results only for lymphogranuloma venereum. The value of *Chlamydia*-specific antibodies (IgM, IgG, IgA) in the diagnosis of urogenital infections using indirect immunofluorescence (IF) and immunoperoxidase (IPO) methods (II) is limited since these antibodies are genus-specific and thus will also be elevated in infections with *Chlamydophila pneumoniae* (Tuuminen et al. 2000). IgA levels in urogenital secretions may, in the future, be of more than academic interest (Mestecky and Fultz 1999).

II.3.4.2.5
Mycoplasma spp.

At least four mycoplasmas may colonize the urogenital tract: *Mycoplasma (M.) fermentans*, *M. hominis*, *M. genitalium* and *Ureaplasma (U.) urealyticum*. Only the latter three have pathogenic significance. Direct microscopy is unreliable. The usual diagnostic procedure (II) involves inoculation into solid media and in liquid enrichment and indicator media (Schiefer et al. 1993; Isenberg 1998; Schiefer 1998; Murray et al. 2003). Identification is based on the use of biochemical tests or fluorescein-labelled antibodies. Only semiquantitative analysis will lead to useful results. Serological tests are useless. *M. genitalium* can be detected by PCR or by primary culture on Vero cells, with subsequent culture in liquid and on solid media (Jensen et al. 1993, 1996; Taylor-Robinson 1996; Dupin et al. 2003).

II.3.4.2.6
Haemophilus (H.) ducreyi

The usual techniques are direct microscopy (I) of smears stained by Gram or Giemsa (I) and culture (II) on selective and enrichment media (Murray et al. 2003). A PCR (III) has been established as well (Murray et al. 2003).

II.3.4.2.7
Enterobacteriaceae spp.

Enterobacteriaceae spp. are cultured on selective media and identified according to biochemical reactions (Isenberg 1998; Murray et al. 2003). For the detection of *Klebsiella (K.)* [*Calymmatobacterium (C.)*] *granulomatis*, the most important technique is direct microscopy of Giemsa- or Wright-stained smears (I). Co-cultivation with monocytes and Hep-2 cells is possible (Kharsany et al 1996; Murray et al. 2003).

II.3.4.2.8
Streptococcus (S.) spp. and *Enterococcus (E.)* spp.

Streptococcus (S.) spp. and *Enterococcus (E.)* spp. are cultured on nonselective/selective media. Streptococci may be grouped by immunological techniques (II) (Murray et al. 2003).

II.3.4.2.9
Corynebacterium (C.) spp.

Corynebacterium (C.) spp. (e.g. *C. glucuronolyticum*, which is identical to *C. seminale*) are cultured on blood agar and speciated according to biochemical reactions (II) (Funke et al. 1995; Riegel et al. 1995; Murray et al. 2003).

II.3.4.2.10
Gardnerella (G.) vaginalis

The usual diagnostic tools are direct microscopy of Gram-stained smears and culture on selective media (II). Specific DNA probes have also been developed (Murray et al. 2003).

II.3.4.2.11
Anaerobes

Culture is performed by means of the usual anaerobic methods (II). Identification and quantification of the numerous anaerobes in the male urogenital tract are time- and labour-intensive and are rarely performed because of the questionable aetiological significance of these organisms (Eggert-Kruse et al. 1995; Isenberg 1998; Murray et al. 2003).

II.3.4.2.12
Herpes Simplex Virus 2 (HSV-2)

In smears of mucocutaneous lesions HSV antigen can be detected by ELISA (II). Cell culture allows for identification with fluorescein-labelled antibodies (III). HSV genome sequences can be amplified by type-specific PCR and detected by hybridization (III). Serology yields useful results only in primary infections and in older patients (Isenberg 1998; Murray et al. 2003).

II.3.4.2.13
Papilloma Viruses (HPV)

The diagnosis is a clinical one, to be confirmed by histopathology (III). Viruses are detected by nucleic acid hybridization or by PCR amplification of DNA obtained from biopsy samples (III) (Isenberg 1998; Murray et al. 2003).

II.3.4.2.14
Cytomegalovirus (CMV)

Cytomegalovirus (CMV) can be cultured in cell lines and detected with immunofluorescence techniques. The methods of choice, however, are detection by PCR (III) and by the presence of specific antibodies (Isenberg 1998; Murray et al. 2003).

II.3.4.2.15
Hepatitis Viruses

Important in this connection are HBV and, more rarely, HCV and HDV. Stage-specific diagnostic tests [antigens and antibodies, genome amplification by PCR (III)] are reviewed elsewhere (Isenberg 1998; Murray et al. 2003).

II.3.4.2.16
Human Immunodeficiency Viruses (HIV-1, HIV-2)

The usual method is serology for anti-HIV-antibodies by means of ELISA and immunoblot (III). These antibodies can be detected in most patients within 6–12 weeks and in >95% within 6 months following infection. Viral culture of lymphocytes and of various secretions is also possible, as is the detection of the HIV genome by PCR (III) (Isenberg 1998; Murray et al. 2003).

II.3.4.2.17
Yeasts

Standard methods are direct microscopy (I) and culture on selective media (II) (Isenberg 1998; Murray et al. 2003).

II.3.4.2.18
Trichomonas vaginalis

The method of choice is direct, if possible, dark-field microscopy (I) following suspension of the material in 0.145 M NaCl. The most sensitive detection method is culture, with subsequent microscopy of the (motile) trophozoites (II) (Isenberg 1998; Murray et al. 2003).

II.3.4.3 Microbiological Examinations in the Diagnosis of Male Urogenital Infections

II.3.4.3.1
Balanitis

Samples are swabbings or impression smears. The most frequent agents are *Enterobacteriaceae* spp., *Streptococcus* spp. (groups A, B), coagulase-positive *Staphylococcus* spp., *Gardnerella vaginalis*, HSV, *Candida* spp. and *Trichomonas vaginalis* (Schiefer 1998).

II.3.4.3.2
Urethritis

Evidence of ≥4 granulocytes per microscopic field (1000×) in the smear of urethral discharge, or of ≥15 granulocytes per microscopic field (400×) in the smear of the sediment of 3 ml of a first voided urine portion (VB1 = voided bladder urine 1) is indicative (Schiefer 1998).

Urethral discharge and the first voided portion of urine (VB1) are examined separately for common bacteria, gonococci, mycoplasmas, *C. trachomatis*, *T. vaginalis*, and *Candida* spp. Semiquantitative methods should be employed for common bacteria, mycoplasmas and yeasts.

Aetiological classification is based on the following criteria (Schiefer 1998):

1. (Quantitative) evidence of significantly high numbers of "conventional" bacteria, *Candida* spp. *Mycoplasma* spp., i.e. $\geq 10^4$ organisms per ml of urethral discharge, and $\geq 10^3$ organisms per ml of VB1.
2. (Qualitative) evidence of gonococci, *C. trachomatis*, *T. vaginalis*.

Patients suffering from chronic urethritis without discharge pose particular diagnostic problems. They should be examined for a possible "early morning urethral discharge" which can be observed prior to voiding morning urine. In addition, VB1 should be examined for granulocytes.

The most frequent agents of male urethritis are *N. gonorrhoeae*, *C. trachomatis*, *M. genitalium* and *U. urealyticum*. Mixed infections are common. Other microorganisms (*Enterobacteriaceae* spp., *Streptococcus* spp., *Staphylococcus aureus*, *Corynebacterium glucuronolyticum*, *Bacteroides ureolyticus*, *M. hominis*, *Candida* spp., HSV, *T. vaginalis*) are rare (Brunner et al. 1983; Hawkins et al. 1988; Jensen et al. 1993, 1996; Funke et al. 1995; Riegel et al. 1995; Schiefer 1998).

II.3.4.3.3 Prostatitis

This multifaceted syndrome has been classified by Drach et al. (1978) into acute bacterial, chronic bacterial and "abacterial" prostatitis, which have to be separated from prostatodynia in which prostatic secretions do not show signs of inflammation and do not yield infectious agents.

Difficulties in the separation of infectious, inflammatory, and noninflammatory forms have led to a new classification (Krieger et al. 1996a) based on symptomatology. It differentiates between:

1. Acute bacterial prostatitis, i.e. acute infection of the prostate.
2. Chronic bacterial prostatitis, i.e. recurrent prostatic infection.
3. Chronic prostatitis/chronic pelvic pain syndrome (no conventional microorganisms can be detected although symptoms are present) subdivided into:
   3a. Inflammatory subtype (elevated leukocyte numbers in ejaculate, prostatic secretions, or urine after prostatic massage).
   3b. Noninflammatory subtype (no leukocytes in the samples mentioned above).
4. Asymptomatic inflammatory prostatitis [no subjective symptoms but leukocytes in prostatic biopsy material and/or elevated leukocytes in ejaculate, prostatic secretions, or urine after prostatic massage, i.e. procedures performed after other pathologies, e.g., elevated prostate-specific antigen (PSA) levels, have been detected].

For the rare febrile acute bacterial prostatitis (category 1) microbiology of a urine sample should suffice. Prostatic massage is strictly contraindicated since it may induce sepsis.

Prostatitis (categories 2–4) is diagnosed according to the localization protocol of the "four-specimen-test" (Schiefer et al. 1993; Weidner et al. 1994; Schiefer 1998). The first voided urine portion (VB1) and the second voided (bladder) urine portion (VB2) are obtained separately. Following prostatic massage, expressed prostatic secretions (EPS) or, if the former are not available in sufficient amounts, urethral swabs are obtained. Then the patient urinates again and, as the fourth fraction, urine after prostatic massage (VB3) is obtained. Generally, ejaculate is also examined.

The diagnosis of prostatitis *sensu stricto* (categories 2, 3a and 4) is based on the detection of purulent prostatic secretions. If urethritis and urinary tract infections can be excluded, the presence of ≥ 10 granulocytes per microscopic field (1000×) in prostatic secretions is suggestive, while ≥ 20 granulocytes per microscopic field (1000×) is proof of prostatitis, as are ≥ 10 granulocytes per microscopic field (400×) in the cytocentrifugate of 3 ml of urine voided after prostatic massage (VB3) (Schiefer et al. 1993; Weidner et al. 1994; Schiefer 1998).

The optimal diagnostic strategy to differentiate between categories 3a (inflammatory) and 3b (noninflammatory) requires the evaluation of white blood cells in semen in addition to the traditional EPS examination. The presence of $\geq 10^6$ peroxidase-positive leukocytes per millilitre of ejaculate is considered representative of "significant leukocytospermia" indicating category 3a (Krieger et al. 2000).

Microbiological examination includes: (1) a semiquantitative analysis of Gram-positive and Gram-negative bacteria, mycoplasmas and yeasts in all fractions; (2) a qualitative examination for *C. trachomatis* and *N. gonorrhoeae* in the urethral swab after prostatic massage; and (3) microscopy for *T. vaginalis*. In case of clinical suspicion, morning urine and ejaculate are cultured for *M. tuberculosis*.

A shorter test comparing semiquantitatively urine cultures before and after prostatic massage would simplify the diagnosis (Nickel 1998).

The aetiological diagnosis of prostatitis requires either qualitative detection of gonococci, chlamydiae or trichomonads, or the presence of "conventional" bacteria, mycoplasmas, or yeasts at $\geq 10^4$/ml in EPS and $\geq 10^3$/ml in VB3, and $\leq 10^3$/ml in VB1 and VB2 ("prostatitis pattern") (Weidner et al. 1991, 1994; Schiefer et al. 1993).

The most important agents of acute and chronic bacterial prostatitis are Gram-negative bacteria (*Escherichia coli* in 80%, but also *Klebsiella* spp., *Enterobacter* spp., *Proteus* spp., *Pseudomonas* spp.), *Enterococcus* spp.; rarely, *Staphylococcus aureus*, *N. gonorrhoeae*, *Candida* spp., *T. vaginalis* (causing mostly urethroprostatitis) and *M. tuberculosis* (in chronic prostatitis). Yeast infections of the prostate, e.g. those due to *Cryptococcus neoformans* or *Candida* spp., are found in immunocompromised patients. The etiological role of *C. trachomatis*, *U. urealyticum* and viruses has not yet been elucidated (Weidner et al. 1991, 1994; Taylor-Robinson 1996; Schiefer 1998).

Inconsistent microbiological findings are frequent and are probably due to a focal localization of prostatitis (Weidner et al. 1991, 1994).

In the search for possible bacterial agents of chronic prostatitis/chronic pelvic pain syndrome (category 3) amplification of the 16 S rRNA gene (rDNA) has been tried using universal and bacteria-specific primers (Tanner et al. 1999; Krieger et al. 2000). This procedure is still in the research domain. However, preliminary data suggest that patients with the inflammatory subtype (category 3a) are significantly more likely to have bacterial DNA in their prostatic parenchyma than those with the noninflammatory subtype (category 3b) (Krieger et al. 1996b).

II.3.4.3.4 Epididymitis

Age and history of the patient are of particular importance in the diagnosis of epididymitis (Weidner et al. 1987). In younger patients with urethral discharge and no difficulty voiding, diagnostic procedures resemble those used in cases of urethritis. In patients without urethral discharge, diagnostic procedures follow the "four-specimen-test" (Weidner et al. 1987). In all other cases, particularly in patients over 35 years and in those with bladder outlet disturbances, a urinary tract infection should be suspected. In case of chronic epididymitis, morning urine (×3), ejaculate and urine voided after prostatic massage should be examined for *M. tuberculosis* (Weidner et al. 1987; Schiefer 1998).

In younger (<35 years), sexually active men without difficulty voiding, epididymitis is mostly caused by *N. gonorrhoeae* or *C. trachomatis*. Elderly men and those with bladder outlet disturbances have mostly urinary tract infections with bacteria identical to those causing epididymitis, i.e. *E. coli*, *Pseudomonas aeruginosa*, *Enterococcus* spp. and *M. tuberculosis* (Schiefer 1998).

II.3.4.3.5 Orchitis

Orchitis is a complication of many systemic bacterial infections, e.g. those due to *Salmonella typhi*, *Brucella* spp., *M. tuberculosis*, *M. leprae*, *Coxiella burnetii*, or of viral infections caused by the mumps virus, echo and arboviruses, the virus of lymphocytic choriomeningitis, and of *Plasmodium* spp. Clinical symptoms provide the clue (Schiefer 1998).

II.3.4.3.6 Male Accessory Gland Infections (MAGI)

Ejaculate originates from the testicles and epididymis (approx. 5%), the prostate (approx. 30%), the seminal vesicles (approx. 60%), and the bulbourethral and urethral glands (approx. 5%). The finding, on cytochemical and biochemical analysis of semen, of $\geq 10^6$ peroxidase-positive leukocytes/ml ("significant leukocytospermia"), ≥ 230 ng elastase/ml and ≥ 0.01 mg C3c complement/ml is indicative of an inflammation of the male accessory glands ("prostato-seminal vesiculitis", "male adnexitis", "epididymo-prostato-vesiculitis") as long as urethritis and urinary tract infections have been ruled out. Such findings call for microbiological analysis of the ejaculate (Ludwig et al. 1998; WHO 1999; Rowe et al. 2000), whereby growth of $\geq 10^3$/ml of potentially pathogenic bacteria, particularly of Gram-negative rods, is considered "significant bacteriospermia" (WHO 1999; Rowe et al. 2000). Localization of the inflammatory focus cannot be accomplished by culture of the ejaculate but rather requires a "four-specimen-test" (Schiefer et al. 1993; Weidner et al. 1994; Schiefer 1998). Analysis of various ejaculate fractions ("split ejaculate") – i.e. of the first fraction (approx. 0.6 ml) from the testicles and the epididymis, a second intermediate fraction (approx. 1.0 ml), and a third fraction from the seminal vesicles – allows, at best, an orientation.

II.3.4.3.7 Ejaculate as a Carrier of Microorganisms

Besides spermatozoa and cells of spermatogenesis ejaculate contains cells and secretions from epididymis, prostate, seminal vesicles and ejaculatory ducts. It is also mostly contaminated with organisms from the urethral residual flora. Localized or generalized infections can render ejaculate highly infectious. Obligate pathogens such as *N. gonorrhoeae*, *C. trachomatis*, *T. vaginalis* and facultatively pathogenic organisms such as *M. hominis*, *U. urealyticum*, group B streptococci and *Enterobacteriaceae* spp. can be detected in ejaculates. They attach to spermatozoa (Friberg et al. 1985) and can thus infect the female genital tract, particularly the endometrium and the tubal epithelium. Ejaculate may also transmit viruses, in particular HIV-1 and HIV-2, CMV, HBV and HPV (Craig et al. 1977; Mascola and Guinan 1986; Kashube et al. 1999).

Bacteria and viruses will not be killed by cryopreservation. Special precautionary measures are, therefore, necessary for semen used for artificial insemination. The donors are usually young, sexually active, unmarried men carrying a high risk of sexually transmitted disease(s). Men with histories of homosexual and prostitute encounters, frequently changing sexual partners, sexually transmitted diseases, drug abuse and blood transfusions to themselves or their partners should not be semen donors. Urogenital infection with HIV-1, HIV-2, CMV, HBV, HCV, HSV-2, HPV, *T. pallidum*, *C. trachomatis*, *N. gonorrhoeae*, *M. hominis*, *U. urealyticum*, group B streptococci and *T. vaginalis* are absolute or relative criteria for exclusion. Since the necessary tests cannot be completed on the day of semen donation, semen has to be cryopreserved and should only be used for insemination if tests on the donor have yielded negative findings 180 days later (Craig et al. 1977; Mascola and Guinan 1986; Liesnard 1998; British Andrology Society 1999).

References

Bowie WR, Pollock HM, Forsyth PS, Floyd JF, Alexander ER, Wang SP, Holmes KK (1977) Bacteriology of the urethra in normal men and men with nongonococcal urethritis. J Clin Microbiol 6:482–488

British Andrology Society (1999) British Andrology Society guidelines for the screening of semen donors for donor insemination. Hum Reprod 14:1823–1826

Brunner H, Weidner W, Schiefer HG (1983) Studies on the role of *Ureaplasma urealyticum* and *Mycoplasma hominis* in prostatitis. J Infect Dis 147:807–813

Craig JM, Barratt CLR, Kinghorn GR (1977) Semen donors and STD screening. Genitourin Med 73:280–283

Drach GW, Fair WR, Meares EM, Stamey TA (1978) Classification of benign diseases associated with prostatic pain: prostatitis or prostatodynia? J Urol 120:266

Dupin N, Bijaoui G, Schwarzinger M, Ernault P, Gerhardt P, Jdid R, Hilab S, Pantoja C, Buffet M, Escande JP, Costa JM (2003) Detection and quantification of *Mycoplasma genitalium* in male patients with urethritis. Clin Infect Dis 37:602–605

Eggert-Kruse W, Rohr G, Ströck W, Pohl S, Schwalbach B, Runnebaum B (1995) Anaerobes in ejaculates of subfertile men. Hum Reprod Update 1:462–478

Friberg J, Gleicher N, Suarez M, Confino E (1985) Chlamydia attached to spermatozoa. J Infect Dis 152:854

Funke G, Bernard KA, Bucher C, Pfyffer GE, Collins MD (1995) *Corynebacterium glucuronolyticum* sp. nov. isolated from male patients with genitourinary infections. Med Microbiol Lett 4:204–215

Hawkins DA, Fontaine EAR, Thomas BJ, Boustouller YL, Taylor-Robinson D (1988) The enigma of non-gonococcal urethritis: role for *Bacteroides ureolyticus*. Genitourin Med 64: 11–13

Howell CL, Miller MJ, Bruckner DA (1986) Elimination of toxicity and enhanced cytomegalovirus detection in cell cultures inoculated with semen from patients with acquired immunodeficiency syndrome. J Clin Microbiol 24:657–660

Isenberg HD (ed) (1998) Essential procedures for clinical microbiology. ASM Press, Washington DC

Jensen JS, Orsum R, Dohn B, Uldum S, Worm AW, Lind K (1993) *Mycoplasma genitalium*: a cause of male urethritis? Genitourin Med 69:265–269

Jensen JS, Hansen HT, Lind K (1996) Isolation of *Mycoplasma genitalium* strains from the male urethra. J Clin Microbiol 34:286–291

Jensen IP, Fogh H, Prag J (2003) Diagnosis of *Chlamydia trachomatis* infections in a sexually transmitted disease clinic: evaluation of a urine sample tested by enzyme immunoassay and polymerase chain reaction in comparison with a cervical and/or a urethral swab tested by culture and polymerase chain reaction. Clin Microbiol Infect 9:194–201

Kashube ADM, Dyer JR, Kramer LM, Raasch RH, Eron JJ, Cohen MS (1999) Antiretroviral-drug concentrations in semen: implications for sexual transmission of human immunodeficiency virus type 1. Antimicrob Agents Chemother 43:1817–1826

Kharsany ABM, Hoosen AA, Kiepiela P, Naicker T, Sturm AW (1996) Culture of *Calymmatobacterium granulomatis*. Clin Infect Dis 22:391

Krieger JN, Egan KJ, Ross SO, Jacobs R, Berger RE (1996a) Chronic pelvic pains represent the most prominent urogenital symptoms of chronic prostatitis. Urology 48:715–722

Krieger JN, Riley DE, Roberts MC, Berger RE (1996b) Prokaryotic DNA sequences in patients with chronic idiopathic prostatitis. J Clin Microbiol 34:3120–3128

Krieger JN, Jacobs RR, Ross SO (2000) Does the chronic prostatitis/pelvic pain syndrome differ from nonbacterial prostatitis and prostatodynia? J Urol 164:1554–1558

Liesnard CA (1998) Screening of semen donors for infectious diseases. Hum Reprod 13 [Suppl 2]:12–24

Ludwig M, Kümmel C, Schroeder-Printzen I, Ringert RH, Weidner W (1998) Evaluation of seminal plasma parameters in patients with chronic prostatitis or leukocytospermia. Andrologia 30 [Suppl. 1]:41–47

Mascola L, Guinan ME (1986) Screening to reduce transmission of sexually transmitted diseases in semen used for artificial insemination. New Engl J Med 314:1354–1359

Mestecky J, Fultz PN (1999) Mucosal immune system of the human genital tract. J Infect Dis 179 [Suppl 3]:S470–S474

Murray PR, Baron EJ, Jorgensen JH, Pfaller MA, Yolken RH (eds) (2003) Manual of clinical microbiology, 8th edn. ASM Press, Washington DC

Nickel JC (1998) Effective office management of chronic prostatitis. Urol Clin North Am 25:677–684

Riegel P, Ruimy R, de Briel D, Prévost G, Jehl F, Bimet F, Christen R, Monteil H (1995) *Corynebacterium seminale* sp. nov., a new species associated with genital infections in male patients. J Clin Microbiol 33:2244–2249

Rowe PJ, Comhaire FH, Hargreave TB, Mahmoud AMA (2000) WHO manual for the standardized investigation, diagnosis and management of the infertile male. Cambridge University Press, Cambridge

Sandys GH (1960) A new method of preventing swarming of *Proteus* sp. with a description of a new medium suitable for use in routine laboratory practice. J Med Lab Technol 17:224–233

Schiefer HG (1998) Microbiology of male urethroadnexitis: Diagnostic procedures and criteria for aetiologic classification. Andrologia 30 [Suppl 1]:7–13

Schiefer HG, Jantos C, Weidner W (1993) Prostatitis syndrome. Cytological and microbiological procedures for diagnosis and classification. Med Microbiol Lett 2:403–410

Tanner MA, Shoskes D, Shahed A, Pace NR (1999) Prevalence of corynebacterial 16 S rRNA sequences in patients with bacterial and "nonbacterial" prostatitis. J Clin Microbiol 37:1863–1870

Taylor-Robinson D (1996) Infections due to species of *Mycoplasma* and *Ureaplasma*: an update. Clin Infect Dis 23:671–684

Tuuminen T, Palomäki P, Paavonen J (2000) The use of serologic tests for the diagnosis of chlamydial infections. J Microbiol Methods 42:265–279

Weidner W, Schiefer HG, Garbe C (1987) Acute nongonococcal epididymitis. Aetiological and therapeutic aspects. Drugs 34 [Suppl. 1]:111–117

Weidner W, Schiefer HG, Krauss H, Jantos C, Friedrich HJ, Altmannsberger M (1991) Chronic prostatitis: a thorough search for etiologically involved microorganisms in 1461 patients. Infection 19 [Suppl. 3]:S119–S125

Weidner W, Madsen PO, Schiefer HG (eds) (1994) Prostatitis. Etiopathology, diagnosis and therapy. Springer, Berlin Heidelberg New York

World Health Organization (1999) WHO laboratory manual for the examination of human semen and sperm-cervical mucus interaction, 4th edn. Cambridge University Press, Cambridge

II.3.5 Hormonal Evaluation in Infertility and Sexual Dysfunction

D. Klingmüller, N. Bliesener, G. Haidl

Summary

Determinations of the serum concentrations of specific hormones are a prerequisite for the evaluation of infertility and sexual dysfunction. These are easy to perform and can shorten the diagnostic and therapeutic procedures. The most important hormones are FSH, LH and testosterone. Depending on the symptomatic findings, prolactin and thyroxine should also be determined. Knowledge of endocrine regulation and the variables affecting this is important for the interpretation of the hormone concentrations.

II.3.5.1 Introduction

Endocrine disorders are not the most frequent causes of male infertility and sexual dysfunction. Nevertheless, hormonal evaluation is a mandatory and initial component in the diagnosis of these disorders for several reasons. First, hormonal evaluations are easy to perform, results are mostly clear without ambiguity and the procedure is cost-effective. Second, if endocrine causes of male infertility and sexual dysfunction are not initially diagnosed, patients often undergo unnecessary diagnostic and therapeutic procedures. Third, treatment of infertility and sexual dysfunction of endocrine origin is mostly straightforward and very effective. Besides the hormonal evaluation, assessment of male patients suffering from infertility or sexual dysfunction includes a detailed history, a physical examination and a semen analysis. The analysis of diagnostic findings is based on knowledge of the endocrine regulation of the two main testicular functions, spermatogenesis and testosterone production.

Testicular dysfunction may result in reduced spermatogenesis with or without decreased testosterone production. The feedback relationships between hormones enable the physician to localize the endocrine dysfunction: in patients with a primary testicular dysfunction, serum concentrations of follicle-stimulating hormone (FSH) or FSH and luteinizing hormone (LH) are increased. In patients with a secondary dysfunction, such as a dysfunction of the pituitary or hypothalamus, FSH and LH concentrations are below normal or inappropriately normal. Additional routine determination of prolactin, thyroxin and inhibin B has been discussed. Depending on symptomatic findings, these hormones should be determined (see below).

Hormone determination is predominantly performed in serum. Hormone concentrations are very low, mostly in the nanomolar or even picomolar range. Highly sensitive assays such as radio, enzyme or fluorescence immunoassays (RIA, EIA, FIA) are able to measure substances at such low concentrations. The immunoassays of the various manufacturers often apply antibodies against different antigen determinants of the hormones. Thus their results often differ considerably, especially with peptide hormones. This must be taken into account when results of different assays are compared (Fig. II.3.6). Therefore, a normal range has to be determined for each method. The hormone concentrations are affected by several influential variables. Such variables are, for example, the patient's age, weight and the time of day of blood sampling. They are to be considered when blood samples are drawn or laboratory results are interpreted.

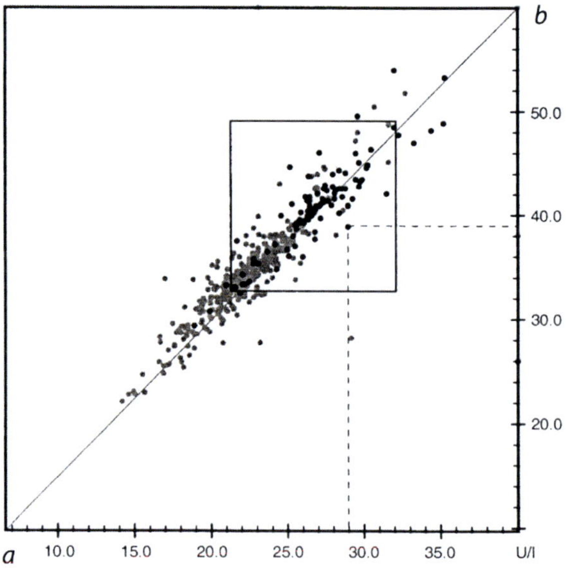

Fig. II.3.6a, b. Youden diagram of ring trials of Deutsche Gesellschaft für Klinische Chemie (DGKC, German Association of Clinical Chemistry). Luteinizing hormone (*LH*) concentrations in two samples (**a** and **b**) determined by 433 laboratories are shown. Own data (sample a: 29 U/l; sample b: 39.5 U/l) are indicated by *dotted lines*. The large scattering of all values, determined by testing methods from different manufacturers, is remarkable. Scattering of values measured with the same assay is less pronounced – indicated by *black dots*

II.3

II.3.5.2 Total Testosterone

Secretion of testosterone depends, among other things, on the patient's age and the time of day. It decreases with increasing age. Therefore, normal values are lower in elderly than in young men (Belanger et al. 1994). Testosterone secretion is regulated by a circadian rhythm with peak concentrations in the morning (Diver et al. 2003). In the evening, concentrations are up to 40% lower. Additionally, slight so-called ultradian fluctuations in testosterone concentrations may occur. Therefore, it is recommended to measure testosterone between 8:00 a.m. and 10:00 a.m. Since a single point plasma testosterone level is highly representative for the long-term hormonal milieu in men, pooled blood sampling is no longer recommended (Vermeulen and Verdonck 1992). In the case of subnormal or borderline low testosterone concentrations a second determination should be carried out.

In blood, testosterone is found free (approx. 2%) and bound to proteins (approx. 98%) (Bhasin et al. 1998). One fraction (approx. 40%) is firmly bound to sex hormone binding globulin (SHBG) with a binding constant of 1×10^9 l/mol (Hammond et al. 1980; Pardridge 1988). A large fraction (approx. 60%) is loosely bound to albumin with a binding constant of 3×10^4 l/mol. The combination of all testosterone fractions is termed total testosterone. The free as well as the albumin-bound testosterone are bioavailable.

Measurement of total testosterone provides an adequate assessment of Leydig cell function. Assessment of testosterone with a fluorescence or electrochemical luminescence analyser is widely used. A quantity of about 20 µl serum is sufficient. Analysis takes about 60 min. Both the precision and accuracy of these methods are very high, especially within the reference range. However, with low concentrations, the accuracy is considerably lower than with conventional radioimmunoassays (Taieb et al. 2002).

Measurement of free testosterone is advisable only when an alteration of the SHBG concentration is suspected. Numerous factors can influence the plasma concentration of SHBG (see below).

II.3.5.3 Free Testosterone

Several possibilities for determination or estimation of free testosterone exist. The most accurate method of determination is the equilibrium dialysis: serum is enriched with tracer amounts of the labelled hormone. The fraction of hormone passes through a semipermeable membrane and is then measured. Next, the absolute concentration of free hormone can be calculated as a product of the total hormone concentration and the fraction that is dialysable or the concentration of testosterone can be measured directly in the dialysate. This is a rather complicated and error-prone method performed in only a small number of specialist laboratories.

The "bioavailable" or non-SHBG-bound testosterone can be measured after separation by precipitating the SHBG-bound testosterone with 50% ammonium sulphate. Bioavailable testosterone corresponds with androgen-active testosterone. Its determination is also complex due to the precipitation step.

In the so-called analogue assay, a ^{125}I-labelled testosterone analogue with just a very slight affinity to SHBG and albumin is applied. Determinations performed with the presently commercially available analogue methods do not correlate with the results from equilibrium dialysis. Thus, these assays should not be used.

Free testosterone concentration can be calculated with the "testosterone calculator" using levels of total testosterone, SHBG and albumin (www.issam.ch). Vermeulen and co-workers showed a very high correlation between the calculated testosterone concentrations and those obtained by equilibrium dialysis. Generally, the free testosterone value (testosterone index), obtained by calculation from total testosterone and SHBG as determined by immunoassay, appears most suitable for clinical routine (Vermeulen et al. 1999).

Measurement of total testosterone with commercially available assays is sufficient for the differentiation between eugonadal and hypogonadal men. However, in many cases, these assays are not sensitive enough to measure low testosterone concentrations in prepubertal children and women (Taieb et al. 2003; Wang et al. 2004).

II.3.5.4 Luteinizing Hormone (LH) and Follicle-Stimulating Hormone (FSH)

Gonadotrophins LH and FSH are both produced by the pituitary. LH induces intratesticular testosterone synthesis. FSH mediates spermatozoa development in concert with testosterone. Since gonadotrophins are secreted in a pulsatile manner by the pituitary their reference range is very broad.

Highly sensitive detection systems for measurement of gonadotrophins applying two different monoclonal antibodies are commercially available. Of these, one is directed against the α-subunit and the other against the β-subunit of the hormones. Besides the immunoradioactive assays (IRMA), characterized by their high precision and high sensitivity, nonradioactive methods such as the immunofluorometric assay (IFMA) and the enzyme-linked immunosorbent assay (ELISA) have become more and more established. In these methods, fluorescent substances or enzymes are used instead of radioactive markers.

Measurements from assays of different manufacturers often vary considerably (Fig. II.3.6) and each assay has a different normal range. This fact has to be considered when comparing concentrations obtained by different methods.

Mutations of the LH-β-gene that cause structural changes of the binding site of the protein are rare. Due to such structural changes the antibodies of the assay can no longer bind the LH molecule and false low values are obtained. In these cases, examination of the bioactivity of LH via cell cultures is carried out, or an enzyme assay with antibodies of another specificity is applied.

The serum concentrations of FSH and LH provide important information on the cause of the testicular dysfunction. Subnormal or low normal testosterone concentrations accompanied by increased LH and FSH concentrations are characteristic of testicular hypogonadism. An increased FSH level with normal concentrations of serum testosterone and LH indicates impaired spermatogenesis with normal Leydig cell function. This combination is frequently found since spermatogenesis is more sensitive than Leydig cell function. A subnormal testosterone concentration and a low sperm count without an increase of gonadotrophins is indicative of a central dysfunction of the pituitary or the hypothalamus (hypogonadotrophic hypogonadism).

In adolescents with delayed puberty, it is often difficult to distinguish between constitutionally delayed puberty and other forms of hypogonadotrophic hypogonadism. Basal measurement of gonadotrophins and testosterone is mostly not sufficient to differentiate between these conditions. However, measuring LH levels stimulated by gonadotrophin releasing hormone (GnRH, 100 µg i.v.) is reported to enable the rapid and effective differential diagnosis of delayed puberty (Jungmann and Trautermann 1994). If there is a family history of constitutionally delayed puberty and the patient's bone age is delayed, constitutional delay in growth and puberty is most probable. When concurrent symptoms of pituitary insufficiency – especially diabetes insipidus – exist, magnetic resonance imaging (MRI) of the sella turcica has to be performed to detect central nervous system (CNS) tumours. In the case of Kallmann's syndrome – an innate form of hypogonadotrophic hypogonadism – the patient presents with anosmia and MRI reveals the absence of the olfactory bulb (Klingmüller et al. 1987).

II.3.5.5 Inhibin B

The glycoprotein inhibin B is produced by the Sertoli cells. Its production depends on the number of Sertoli cells, on germ cell factors and on gonadotrophins. In men, inhibin B is the major feedback regulator of FSH release. Unlike gonadotrophins, inhibin B can be detected in prepubertal males as it is produced in considerable amounts from birth. Its serum concentration displays a circadian rhythm with high concentrations in the morning and low concentrations in early evening (Brennemann et al. 1994).

The inhibin B-ELISA, developed by Groome, detects not only 31-kDa inhibin but also larger forms (Groome et al. 1996). This may explain why serum concentrations from oligo- and normozoospermic subjects overlap considerably (Winters and Plant 1999).

There is a weak positive correlation between inhibin B concentrations and sperm count. In patients with impaired spermatogenesis, inhibin B concentrations are lower compared to normal men. However, there are considerable overlaps between normal and oligozoospermic men. If spermatogenesis is severely impaired, e.g. following chemotherapy, inhibin B concentrations are severely reduced. Inhibin B is undetectable in patients suffering from Klinefelter syndrome or congenital anorchia. Measurements of inhibin B enable the physician to differentiate between these patients and patients with intra-abdominal testes (Kubini et al. 2000). In hypogonadotrophic hypogonadism inhibin B is also found to be subnormal.

The benefit of inhibin B in the diagnosis of male fertility is still ambiguous. Some studies reported inhibin B to be the most sensitive endocrine marker of spermatogenesis in infertile men (Klingmüller and Haidl 1997; Pierik et al. 1998). In contrast, Jensen et al. (1997) suggested that FSH is somewhat more appropriate for predicting impaired spermatogenesis. The positive prediction of impaired spermatogenesis was most reliable when the inhibin B/FSH ratio was applied (Jensen et al. 1997).

II.3.5.6 Anti-Müllerian Hormone

Anti-Müllerian hormone (AMH) is produced in Sertoli cells and it inhibits the Müllerian ducts during the male foetal period. In healthy boys, it is easily detected. During puberty, it decreases. Before the onset of puberty, it is used to determine the presence of gonads as it is non-existent in boys with congenital anorchia.

II.3.5.7 Oestradiol

In the male approximately 25% of oestradiol is produced by the testes and 75% is derived from extraglandular aromatization (Weinstein et al. 1974). Aromatase is found, inter alia, in Leydig cells, the adrenal cortex, fatty tissue and, to a lesser extent, in the brain (Steckelbroeck et al. 1999). In men, oestradiol is found free (2–3%) or loosely bound to albumin. About 30% is bound to SHBG with low affinity. Therefore the oestradiol concentration in men is not crucially influenced by changes of the SHBG level.

The classic detection methods for oestrogens are complex since interfering steroid metabolites must be chromatographically separated prior to quantification of oestrogens via an immunoassay. Unfortunately, the accuracy of the commercially available assays is very low at the low oestrogen levels we have to deal with in men. This applies in particular to automated multi-analyte systems (Taieb et al. 2002). Determination of oestradiol is of great importance in oestrogen-producing tumours, such as Leydig cell tumours. Due to the autonomous oestrogen production of such tumours, gonadotrophin and testosterone secretion can be reduced or suppressed.

In patients suffering from gynaecomastia caused by obesity, occasionally oestrogen levels are slightly elevated due to increased aromatase activity in fatty tissue.

II.3.5.8 Sex Hormone Binding Globulin (SHBG)

SHBG, a glycoprotein, binds testosterone and to a lesser extent other steroids, such as oestradiol, and thus increases their half-life in blood. In most cases, free testosterone correlates with total testosterone and determination of SHBG is not required.

The plasma concentration of SHBG can be influenced by several factors. A decrease of the SHBG level may be due to obesity or hyperinsulinaemia, but can also be due to a glucocorticoid excess, androgen excess, elevated progesterone levels, growth hormone excess and hypothyreosis. An increase in SHBG may be caused by ageing, but also by increased oestrogen levels, an androgen deficit, a growth hormone deficit, by hyperthyreosis or some anti-epileptics (Table II.3.6).

Table II.3.6. Variables influencing the SHBG level

Increased SHBG level	Decreased SHBG level
Hyperthyroidism	Obesity
Ageing	Hyperinsulinaemia
Growth hormone deficiency	Hypothyroidism
Chronic liver disease	Hypercortisolism
Oestrogen excess	Androgen excess
Androgen deficiency	

II.3.5.9 Prolactin

Hyperprolactinaemia inhibits GnRH secretion and thereby can cause a central hypogonadism. The higher the prolactin level the more the gonadal axis is suppressed and the more likely sexual dysfunction (impaired libido and/or erectile function) and infertility result. Breast symptoms such as galactorrhoea and gynaecomastia are rare signs of hyperprolactinaemia in men.

In men, the upper limit of the prolactin level is about 15 ng/ml. A prolactin concentration of more than 200 ng/ml is typical for a prolactinoma. In these cases, MRI of the pituitary is compelling.

Prolactin levels not exceeding 200 ng/ml are frequently detected in microprolactinoma (diameter less than 10 mm), but may also be caused by various drugs, especially dopamine antagonists such as metoclopramide, domperidone and almost every neuroleptic except the prolactin-sparing ones. The neuroleptics amisulpride, sulpiride and risperidone in particular are known to cause considerable prolactin elevations (Oseko et al. 1988; Schlosser et al. 2002; Kinon et al. 2003). Further causes of moderate prolactin elevations are hypothyreosis, chronic renal insufficiency and stress. One has to keep in mind that a rare cause of moderate prolactin elevation can be a mass lesion that compresses the pituitary stalk, and thereby disinhibits the dopamine-mediated blockade of prolactin secretion. Therefore, MRI should be performed if no other reason for a moderate hyperprolactinemia can be found (Molitch 1992).

If the prolactin concentration is very high (above 20,000 ng/ml), a high-dose hook effect may occur in the immunoassay due to the antigen excess, resulting in measurement of false low concentrations (St-Jean et al. 1996). If prolactin values are suspected to be very high, these false low measurements can be avoided by dilution of the serum sample.

II.3.5.10 Dihydrotestosterone

The serum concentration of dihydrotestosterone is approximately one-tenth of the concentration of testosterone. Prior to determination with an immunoassay, dihydrotestosterone should be chromatographically separated from testosterone to avoid cross-reaction of antibodies. Since serum concentrations from healthy and hypogonadal men overlap considerably, dihydrotestosterone is not suitable for the diagnosis of infertility and sexual dysfunction in men with normal genitalia. However, assessment of the basal and β-hCG-stimulated testosterone/dihydrotestosterone ratio is suitable for diagnosing 5α-reductase deficiency (Gad et al. 1997).

II.3.5.11 Hormonal Evaluation of Sexual Dysfunction

Sexual dysfunction is caused by numerous diseases. Endocrine causes include impairment of the hypothalamic–pituitary–testicular axis, hyperprolactinaemia, diabetes mellitus and, rarely, hyper- as well as hypothy-

Table II.3.7. Endocrine causes of sexual dysfunction

Primary or secondary testicular insufficiency
Thyroidal dysfunction
Hyperprolactinaemia
Diabetes mellitus
Cushing's disease

roidism and Cushing's disease (Table II.3.7). Testosterone deficiency can cause reduced sexual desire and impaired erectile function.

Endocrine disorders are rarely found to be the cause of sexual dysfunction, but they should be excluded in order to prevent the patients from undergoing unnecessary diagnostic and therapeutic procedures. In a study by Earle and Stuckey (2003), 1455 patients were screened for endocrine disorder as a cause of erectile dysfunction and the frequency was shown to be about 15%. They found abnormal values in testosterone (5.7%), prolactin (0.5%), thyroid function test (0.13%) and glucose (9.3%). The extent of hormone testing depends on the patient's medical condition. Altogether, the endocrine diagnosis of a sexual dysfunction is easy to perform, fast, effective and inexpensive (Fig. II.3.7, Table II.3.8).

Table II.3.8. Hormonal evaluation of sexual dysfunction. (*FSH* Follicle-stimulating hormone, *fT_4 free thyroxine, LH* luteinizing hormone, *SHBG* sex hormone binding globulin, *TSH* thyroid stimulating hormone)

Single measurement of total testosterone 8:00 – 10:00 a.m.
If low: check again
If low level is confirmed, assay:
LH, FSH
Prolactin
TSH, fT_4 (if thyroid dysfunction is suspected)
Glucose
In cases of conditions that might influence SHBG levels, check:
SHBG to calculate free testosterone

II.3.5.12 Human Chorionic Gonadotrophin (hCG) Stimulation Test

hCG, just as LH, stimulates testosterone production in Leydig cells. Before the onset of puberty, it is suitable for the determination of Leydig cell function. Various protocols exist for hCG stimulation testing. In general, 5000 IU hCG is applied intramuscularly (Knorr et al. 1979). Leydig cell function is assumed to be normal if the testosterone concentration increases by 1.5 – 2 ng/ml. Using this test, primary hypogonadism and disorders of testosterone synthesis can be detected. In boys with congenital anorchia, testosterone does not increase after stimulation by hCG. The diagnosis of congenital anorchia can be affirmed by measuring inhibin B and/or AMH (Kubini et al. 2000).

In adult men the hCG test is not required for analysing Leydig cell function, since basal measurement of testosterone and gonadotrophins provides sufficient information to make the diagnosis. In addition, the hCG test – in contrast to basal measurement of testosterone and gonadotrophins – is not suitable for differentiating between primary and central hypogonadism because in central hypogonadism, the testosterone increase after hCG is also subnormal as the testosterone-producing enzymes are downregulated.

II.3.5.13 Gonadotrophin Releasing-Hormone (GnRH) Stimulation Test

In adolescents the GnRH test seems to be useful to differentiate various forms of hypogonadotrophic (secondary) hypogonadism from more prevalent constitutional delay in puberty. This test differentiates patients

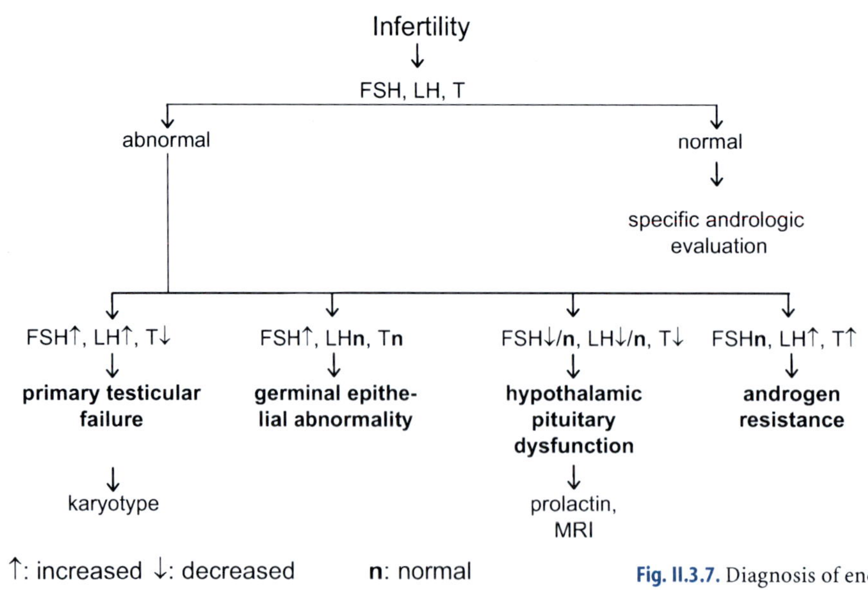

Fig. II.3.7. Diagnosis of endocrine causes of infertility

with hypogonadotrophic hypogonadism from constitutional delay in puberty with a sensitivity of 82% and a specificity of 98%. If LH is higher than 10 mU/ml 30 min after an acute i.v. dose of 100 μg GnRH, constitutional delay in puberty is most probable. Early diagnosis of this condition is of importance since late onset of sexual hormone replacement will worsen the outcome (Jungmann and Trautermann 1994).

In adult men, GnRH testing in the differential diagnosis of hypogonadotrophic hypogonadism seems to be of little practical value for several reasons (Vierhapper 1985; Pavord et al. 1992):

1. Basal measurement of testosterone (subnormal) and gonadotrophins (low or inappropriate normal) is almost always sufficient to make the diagnosis.
2. Individual fluctuations of the LH response in GnRH testing are known to be considerable.
3. GnRH testing has a low sensitivity since men with secondary testosterone deficiency frequently may have a normal response to an acute dose of GnRH.
4. GnRH testing does not differentiate between hypothalamic and pituitary disorder since a gonadotrophin response is reduced in both conditions.

In the late 1970s it was shown that measurement of the long-term GnRH responsiveness might be useful for localizing the disease (Snyder et al. 1979). In the light of steps made in imaging procedures, this test is not only to be regarded as expensive but even of limited clinical value. In a patient with pituitary adenoma, pituitary apoplexy following injection of GnRH was reported (Hiroi et al. 2001). In conclusion, we no longer recommend routine GnRH testing in adult men with hypogonadotrophic hypogonadism.

II.3.5.14 Stimulation Tests

II.3.5.14.1 hCG Stimulation Test

Indication

- Examination of Leydig cell function, anorchia and disorders of testosterone synthesis in children.

Method

- Measurement of testosterone between 8:00 and 10:00 a.m. before i.m. injection of 5000 IU hCG.
- Measurement of testosterone 72 h after i.m. injection of hCG.

Interpretation

- Testosterone increase of 1.5 – 2 ng/ml in prepubescent boys.

II.3.5.14.2 GnRH Stimulation Test

Indication

- Differential diagnosis of delayed puberty.
- Not indicated for routine testing of adult men suffering from secondary hypogonadism.

Method

- Measurement of LH before and 30 min after i.v. injection of 100 μg GnRH.

Interpretation

- Constitutional delay in puberty is most probable when LH is higher than 10 mU/ml 30 min after an acute i.v. dose of 100 μg GnRH (sensitivity: 82%, specificity: 98%) (Jungmann and Trautermann 1994).

Limitation in Adult Men

- Considerable variation of GnRH response.
- Low sensitivity.
- No differentiation of pituitary and hypothalamic disorders.

References

Belanger A, Candas B, Dupont A, Cusan L, Diamond P, Gomez JL, Labrie F (1994) Changes in serum concentrations of conjugated and unconjugated steroids in 40- to 80-year-old men. J Clin Endocrinol Metab 79:1086 – 1090

Bhasin S, Bagatell CJ, Bremner WJ, Plymate SR, Tenover JL, Korenman SG, Nieschlag E (1998) Issues in testosterone replacement in older men. J Clin Endocrinol Metab 83: 3435 – 3448

Brennemann W, Sommer L, Stoffel-Wagner B, Bidlingmaier F, Klingmüller D (1994) Secretion pattern of immunoreactive inhibin in men. Eur J Endocrinol 131:273 – 279

Diver MJ, Imtiaz KE, Ahmad AM, Vora JP, Fraser WD (2003) Diurnal rhythms of serum total, free and bioavailable testosterone and of SHBG in middle-aged men compared with those in young men. Clin Endocrinol (Oxf) 58:710 – 717

Earle CM, Stuckey BG (2003) Biochemical screening in the assessment of erectile dysfunction: what tests decide future therapy? Urology 62:727 – 731

Gad YZ, Nasr H, Mazen I, Salah N, el-Ridi R (1997) 5 Alpha-reductase deficiency in patients with micropenis. J Inherit Metab Dis 20:95 – 101

Groome NP, Illingworth PJ, O'Brien M, Pai R, Rodger FE, Mather JP, McNeilly AS (1996) Measurement of dimeric inhibin B throughout the human menstrual cycle. J Clin Endocrinol Metab 81:1401 – 1405

Hammond GL, Nisker JA, Jones LA, Siiteri PK (1980) Estimation of the percentage of free steroid in undiluted serum by centrifugal ultrafiltration-dialysis. J Biol Chem 255:5023 – 5026

Hiroi N, Ichijo T, Shimojo M, Ueshiba H, Tsuboi K, Miyachi Y (2001) Pituitary apoplexy caused by luteinizing hormone-

releasing hormone in prolactin-producing adenoma. Intern Med 40:747–750
Jensen TK, Andersson AM, Hjollund NH, Scheike T, Kolstad H, Giwercman A, Henriksen TB, Ernst E, Bonde JP, Olsen J, McNeilly A, Groome NP, Skakkebaek NE (1997) Inhibin B as a serum marker of spermatogenesis: correlation to differences in sperm concentration and follicle-stimulating hormone levels. A study of 349 Danish men. J Clin Endocrinol Metab 82:4059–4063
Jungmann E, Trautermann C (1994) [The status of the gonadotropin releasing hormone test in differential diagnosis of delayed puberty in adolescents over 14 years of age.] Med Klin (Munich) 89:529–533
Kinon BJ, Gilmore JA, Liu H, Halbreich UM (2003) Hyperprolactinemia in response to antipsychotic drugs: characterization across comparative clinical trials. Psychoneuroendocrinology 28 [Suppl 2]:69–82
Klingmüller D, Haidl G (1997) Inhibin B in men with normal and disturbed spermatogenesis. Hum Reprod 12:2376–2378
Klingmüller D, Dewes W, Krahe T, Brecht G, Schweikert HU (1987) Magnetic resonance imaging of the brain in patients with anosmia and hypothalamic hypogonadism (Kallmann's syndrome). J Clin Endocrinol Metab 65:581–584
Knorr D, Beckmann D, Bidlingmaier F, Helmig FJ, Sippell WG (1979) Plasma testosterone in male puberty. II. hCG stimulation test in boys with hypospadia. Acta Endocrinol (Copenh) 90:365–371
Kubini K, Zachmann M, Albers N, Hiort O, Bettendorf M, Wolfle J, Bidlingmaier F, Klingmüller D (2000) Basal inhibin B and the testosterone response to human chorionic gonadotropin correlate in prepubertal boys. J Clin Endocrinol Metab 85:134–138
Molitch ME (1992) Pathologic hyperprolactinemia. Endocrinol Metab Clin North Am 21:877–901
Oseko F, Oka N, Furuya H, Morikawa K (1988) Effects of chronic sulpiride-induced hyperprolactinemia on plasma testosterone and its responses to hCG in normal men. J Androl 9:231–233
Pardridge WM (1988) Selective delivery of sex steroid hormones to tissues by albumin and by sex hormone-binding globulin. Oxf Rev Reprod Biol 10:237–292
Pavord SR, Girach A, Price DE, Absalom SR, Falconer-Smith J, Howlett TA (1992) A retrospective audit of the combined pituitary function test, using the insulin stress test, TRH and GnRH in a district laboratory. Clin Endocrinol (Oxf) 36:135–139
Pierik FH, Vreeburg JT, Stijnen T, De Jong FH, Weber RF (1998) Serum inhibin B as a marker of spermatogenesis. J Clin Endocrinol Metab 83:3110–3114
Schlosser R, Grunder G, Anghelescu I, Hillert A, Ewald-Grunder S, Hiemke C, Benkert O (2002) Long-term effects of the substituted benzamide derivative amisulpride on baseline and stimulated prolactin levels. Neuropsychobiology 46:33–40
Snyder PJ, Rudenstein RS, Gardner DF, Rothman JG (1979) Repetitive infusion of gonadotropin-releasing hormone distinguishes hypothalamic from pituitary hypogonadism. J Clin Endocrinol Metab 48:864–868
Steckelbroeck S, Heidrich DD, Stoffel-Wagner B, Hans VH, Schramm J, Bidlingmaier F, Klingmüller D (1999) Characterization of aromatase cytochrome P450 activity in the human temporal lobe. J Clin Endocrinol Metab 84:2795–2801
St-Jean E, Blain F, Comtois R (1996) High prolactin levels may be missed by immunoradiometric assay in patients with macroprolactinomas. Clin Endocrinol (Oxf) 44:305–309
Taieb J, Benattar C, Birr AS, Lindenbaum A (2002) Limitations of steroid determination by direct immunoassay. Clin Chem 48:583–585
Taieb J, Mathian B, Millot F, Patricot MC, Mathieu E, Queyrel N, Lacroix I, Somma-Delpero C, Boudou P (2003) Testosterone measured by 10 immunoassays and by isotope-dilution gas chromatography-mass spectrometry in sera from 116 men, women, and children. Clin Chem 49:1381–1395
Vermeulen A, Verdonck G (1992) Representativeness of a single point plasma testosterone level for the long term hormonal milieu in men. J Clin Endocrinol Metab 74:939–942
Vermeulen A, Verdonck L, Kaufman JM (1999) A critical evaluation of simple methods for the estimation of free testosterone in serum. J Clin Endocrinol Metab 84:3666–3672
Vierhapper H (1985) LH-RH stimulated LH secretion in human endocrine disease. Acta Endocrinol Suppl (Copenh) 269:3–25
Wang C, Catlin DH, Demers LM, Starcevic B, Swerdloff RS (2004) Measurement of total serum testosterone in adult men: comparison of current laboratory methods versus liquid chromatography-tandem mass spectrometry. J Clin Endocrinol Metab 89:534–543
Weinstein RL, Kelch RP, Jenner MR, Kaplan SL, Grumbach MM (1974) Secretion of unconjugated androgens and estrogens by the normal and abnormal human testis before and after human chorionic gonadotropin. J Clin Invest 53:1–6
Winters SJ, Plant TM (1999) Partial characterization of circulating inhibin-B and pro-alphaC during development in the male rhesus monkey. Endocrinology 140:5497–5504

II.3.6 Tumour Markers in Andrology

M. E. BRACKE

Summary

Prostate specific antigen (PSA), α-fetoprotein (AFP) and human chorionic gonadotrophin (hCG) are important circulating tumour markers in the management of prostatic and testicular carcinomas. Their success is due to an attractive combination of sensitivity and specificity, ranking them among the best tools available in the clinical laboratory for the detection and therapeutic follow-up of these tumours. PSA, a member of the kallikrein superfamily with high specificity for the prostate, is probably the best circulating tumour marker available. Its performance is expected to be improved by introducing new methods into the clinical laboratory to assess PSA subfractions and other kallikreins, and by the application of artificial neural networks that integrate classic and new markers towards a powerful clinical output. While both AFP and hCG are useful for the follow-up of nonseminoma germ cell tumours of the testis, only hCG performs well in seminomas. New trends are set by technologies such as proteomics analysis of serum and polymerase chain reactions (PCR) to detect circulating cancer cells via their unique marker expression profiles.

II.3.6.1 Introduction

Compared to other fields of oncology, tumour markers in andrology are specific for certain types of tumours. Although this statement should not be taken too absolutely, markers such as prostate specific antigen (PSA), α-fetoprotein (AFP) and human chorionic gonadotrophin (hCG) for the management of prostatic and testicular carcinomas are among the best tools available in clinical laboratory oncology. In this chapter the main emphasis will be on those three markers, but attention will also be paid to other, often newly discovered, molecules.

II.3.6.2 Markers for Prostatic Carcinoma: Prostate Specific Antigen (PSA) and Others (Fig. II.3.8a)

II.3.6.2.1 History, Normal Function and Regulation

The history of tumour markers for prostatic carcinoma goes back to 1938 when prostatic acid phosphatase (PAP) was detected in serum of patients (Gutman and Gutman 1938). This marker dominated the field until PSA was discovered (Wang et al. 1979) and subsequently recognized as a circulating serum marker for prostatic carcinoma (Kuriyama et al. 1980). Since then PSA has proven to be the better tumour marker in terms of sensitivity and specificity for prostatic cancer, and has completely replaced PAP determinations. Recently, however, critical considerations concerning the value of PSA determinations have raised the need for new prostatic tumour markers with even better sensitivity and specificity profiles (Hernandez and Thompson 2004; Platz et al. 2004).

Furthermore, PSA has been shown to be a misnomer, because extraprostatic sources have been described, such as mammary carcinoma (Black and Diamandis 2000) and ileum (Olsson et al. 2005).

PSA is a secreted single-chain glycoprotein (molecular weight: 33 kDa), which is converted from its preproform into its pro-form upon secretion, and which becomes enzymatically active as a serine protease after cleavage of the inactive pro-form. PSA belongs to the kallikrein enzyme family, the largest group of serine proteases known, and is indeed identical to human kallikrein-3 (hK3) (McCormack et al. 1995; Rittenhouse et al. 1998). Secreted by the prostatic epithelium and the periurethral glands, enzymatically active PSA is present in seminal fluid, and is responsible for the liquefaction of the seminal coagulum. The enzyme is able to cleave multiple substrates, such as the seminal vesicle seminogelin proteins, fibronectin and insulin-like growth factor-binding protein-3 (Henttu and Vihko 1994), and new substrates are still being discovered using combinatorial substrate libraries (Matsumura et al. 2005).

The expression of PSA is sensitive to androgens, due to the presence of two androgen-responsive elements in the promoter of the PSA gene (Riegman et al. 1991; Cleutjens et al. 1996). This is also the case in females, where PSA is a serum marker for hyperandrogenic states, such as in some hirsute (Melegos et al. 1997) and in acromegalic (Manetti et al. 2004) women.

II.3.6.2.2 Application in Prostatic Cancer

In increasing order PSA determinations are powerful for screening, evaluation before treatment and follow-up of prostatic cancer. When a cut-off limit for serum PSA is set at 4.0 ng/ml, the marker shows a high sensitivity of 75 – 85 %, but a low specificity of 20 – 30 % to detect prostatic cancer (Waters 1999). This low specificity is due to the observation that elevated PSA con-

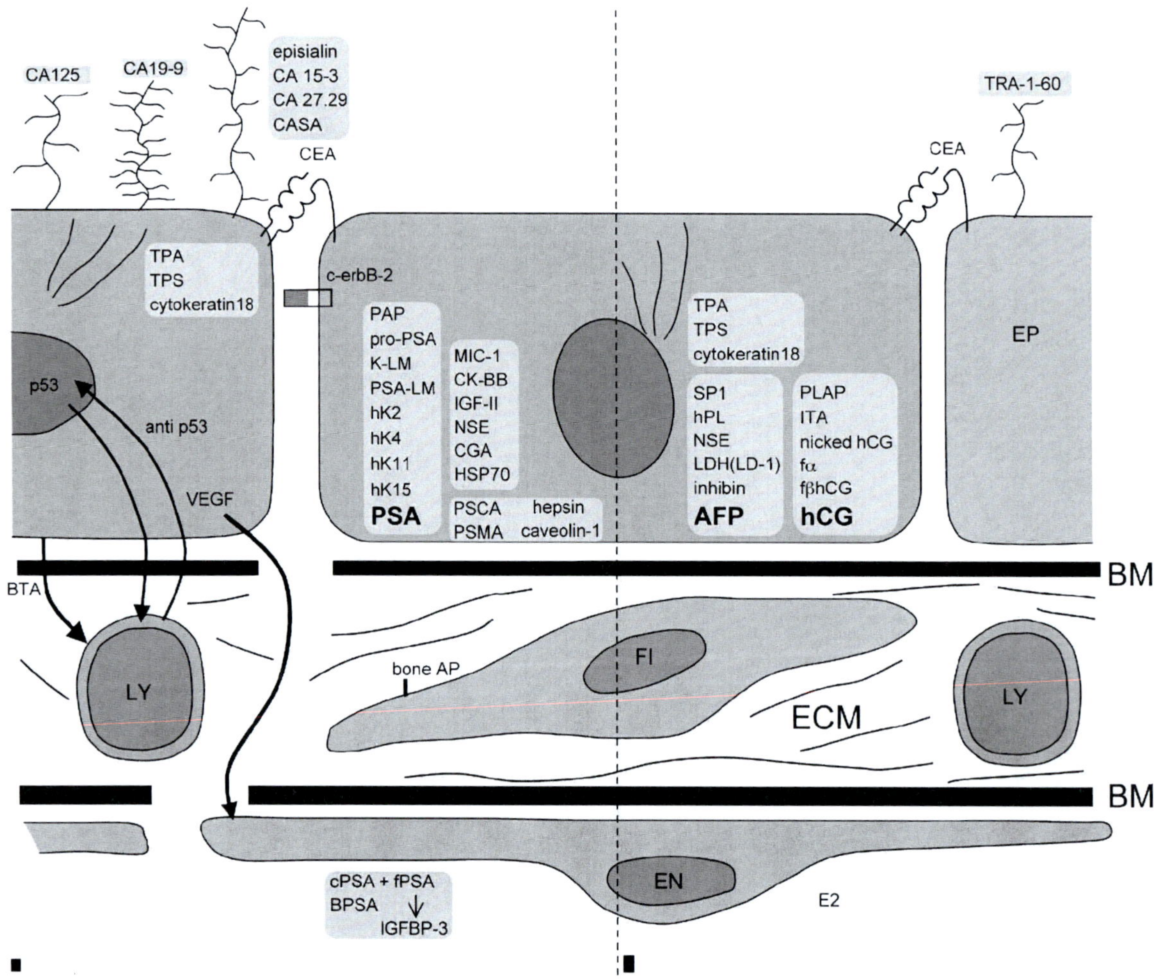

Fig. II.3.8a, b. Summary of circulating tumour markers of prostate (**a**) and testicular (**b**) cancer. Cancer is presented as a microecosystem consisting of epithelioid tumour cells (*EP*) interacting with stromal elements: fibroblasts and osteoblasts (*FI*), lymphocytes (*LY*) and extracellular matrix (*ECM*). Fragmented basement membranes (*BM*) separate the stroma from the EP and the vessel-lining endothelial cells (*EN*). The following molecules have been described as tumour markers. Mucins: CA125, CA 19–9, episialin (CA 15–3, CA 27.29 and CASA) and TRA-1–60. Cell-cell adhesion molecule: carcinoembryonic antigen (*CEA*). Soluble receptors: soluble c-erbB-2 (HER-2, neu). Intermediate filaments: tissue polypeptide antigen (*TPA*), TPA specific (*TPS*), cytokeratin 18. Cytoplasmic and secreted proteins: prostatic acid phosphatase (*PAP*), prostate specific antigen (*PSA*), pro-PSA, human kallikrein-2 linked molecule (*K-LM*), human PSA-linked molecule (*PSA-LM*), human kallikreins 2, 4, 11 and 15 (*hK2, hK4, hK11* and *hK15*), macrophage inhibitory cytokine 1 (*MIC-1*), creatine kinase BB (*CK-BB*), insulin-like growth factor II (*IGF-II*), neuron-specific enolase (*NSE*), chromogranin A (*CGA*), heat shock protein 70 (*HSP70*), pregnancy-specific beta 1-glycoprotein (*SP1*), human placental lactogen (*hPL*), lactate dehydrogenase (*LDH*) and its first isoenzyme (*LD1*), inhibin and alpha-fetoprotein (*AFP*), placental-like alkaline phosphatase (*PLAP*), human chorionic gonadotrophin (*hCG*), invasive trophoblast antigen (*ITA*), nicked hCG, free α-subunits (*fα*) and free β-hCG (*fβhCG*). Membrane-associated proteins: prostate stem cell antigen (*PSCA*), prostate-specific membrane antigen (*PSMA*), hepsin and caveolin-1. Immune surveillance-related molecules: anti p53 and bladder tumour antigen (*BTA*). Osteoblast-related marker: bone alkaline phosphatase (*bone AP*). Circulating markers: complexed PSA (*cPSA*), free PSA (*fPSA*), benign PSA (*BPSA*), IGF-binding protein-3 (*IGFBP-3*) and oestradiol (*E2*)

centrations are encountered not only in prostatic cancer, but also in other prostatic diseases such as benign prostatic hyperplasia (BPH) and prostatitis, although the concentration rarely exceeds 11.0 ng/ml in these noncancer conditions. For screening, use of PSA without digital rectal exam (DRE) is not recommended, because one-quarter of men with prostate cancer have PSA serum levels lower than 4.0 ng/ml. So, the most effective method for early detection of prostatic cancer is the combined use of DRE and PSA. If both are negative, the chance of cancer on biopsy varies from 4% to 9%, while if both are positive, the chance varies from 42% to 72% (Cooner et al. 1990; Hammerer and Huland 1994; Ellis et al. 1994; Catalona et al. 1994). It should not be overlooked, however, that high-grade prostatic cancer can occur in men screened with a PSA level below 4.0 ng/ml (Thompson et al. 2004).

In evaluation before treatment serum PSA has been

claimed to be useful for confirmation of the diagnosis, staging, differential diagnosis and prognosis of prostate cancer (Friedland et al. 2004; Shulman et al. 2004). Its main value, however, is associated with the search for a relevant tumour-associated antigen for treatment follow-up (Mann and Saller 1994a).

As for many other tumour markers, PSA finds an important application in the follow-up of prostatic cancer patients. If watchful waiting is the option, PSA doubling time and PSA slope can define a subgroup of patients with stable or decreasing levels with time (de Vries et al. 2004). In treated patients PSA evolution is used to monitor the treatment efficacy and to predict recurrence. PSA levels decrease during successful hormonal therapy, radiotherapy and surgical ablation of the prostate, and after radical prostatectomy PSA levels should fall down to undetectable levels within 4–6 weeks (Khan and Partin 2004). This period is in agreement with the biological PSA half-life of about 3 days on the one hand (Oesterling et al. 1988) and the high functional sensitivity of recent third-generation PSA assays on the other (Witherspoon and Lapeyrolerie 1997). The postoperative baseline PSA can predict disease relapse after radical prostatectomy, and a PSA nadir below 0.01 ng/ml appears critical to exclude residual disease (Doherty et al. 2000). Further follow-up of PSA levels is useful to anticipate recurrence, and the use of third-generation PSA assays can provide a mean additional lead time of 18 months over conventional assays (Ellis et al. 1997).

II.3.6.2.3 Increasing the Sensitivity and Specificity of PSA Determinations

As mentioned earlier, the introduction of second- and subsequently third-generation PSA assays (with functional sensitivities of 0.1 and 0.01 ng/ml respectively) were important steps to increase PSA sensitivity. Other variations have been developed to improve the sensitivity and specificity of PSA. Some PSA derivatives such as PSA velocity (the rate of change in PSA serum concentrations over time, PSA doubling time), PSA density (serum PSA over prostate volume), PSA transition zone density (serum PSA over the volume of the transition zone) and the use of age-specific reference values have proven to be useful in refining the clinical value of PSA results (Gustafsson et al. 1998). The measurement of free PSA (fPSA) in combination with total PSA (tPSA) in serum is an interesting tool for distinguishing between BPH and prostatic carcinoma. PSA circulates mainly as stable complexes with different enzyme inhibitors, among which α_1-antichymotrypsin (ACT) and α_2-macroglobulin (A2M) are quantitatively the most important ones (Christensson et al. 1990). The PSA–A2M complex cannot be detected by current immunoassays, because A2M shields all available epitopes on PSA, although recently new monoclonal antibodies were developed that could recognize this complex (Baumgart et al. 2004). From the tPSA currently measured in clinical laboratories 85–90% is complexed to ACT, while 10–15% is not complexed (fPSA). Because in PSA–ACT parts of the epitopes are shielded, it is possible to determine fPSA selectively, and compare the result with the one obtained for tPSA (provided the two measurements are equimolar). Due to the increased production of enzyme inhibitors in patients suffering from malignant tumours as compared to those with benign counterparts, the fraction of fPSA is generally lower in prostatic cancer than in BPH. This observation can be successfully exploited in the differential diagnosis, when tPSA concentrations are undecided (between 4 and 11 ng/ml) (Catalona 1996). So, the fPSA/tPSA ratio is now accepted as a diagnostic aid in selected cases, it can increase the specificity of PSA for cancer detection by about 20%, and it can reduce the number of unnecessary biopsies by about one-third (Reissigl et al. 1996). A "variant" of the fPSA assay is the complexed PSA (cPSA) assay, where the PSA–ACT complex is measured instead of the fPSA. This assay, which can be applied as a single determination without the need for tPSA, has also been reported to be useful in reducing the number of unnecessary biopsies (Parsons et al. 2004).

A new tool to improve the prostate cancer detection rate is the application of artificial neural networks. In a first stage these programmes learn to weigh different input data with back-propagated errors, and the output data are compared with the desired output step by step (training). In a later stage the trained network is tested for unknown data. The input data can vary among the different networks, but can include tPSA, fPSA, prostate volume, status of DRE, age and recently human kallikrein-2 (hK2) concentrations in serum (Djavan et al. 2002; Finne et al. 2002; Stephan et al. 2002a). In a multicentre evaluation of an artificial neural network to increase prostatic cancer detection and reduce unnecessary biopsies, the network data outperformed fPSA in specificity and sensitivity (Stephan et al. 2002b).

II.3.6.2.4 When and How to Take a Blood Sample for PSA

Serum PSA elevations occur as a result of disruption of the normal prostatic architecture, which allows access to the circulation. This takes place in prostatic disease (cancer, BPH and prostatitis) and after prostatic manipulation (prostate massage, biopsy) (Stamey et al. 1987). Prostatic trauma such as occurs after prostatic biopsy can result in a "leak" of PSA into the circulation that may require more than 4 weeks for return to baseline values (Yuan et al. 1992). DRE as performed in an office setting can lead to increases in serum PSA, but this does not appear to be clinically significant, because the change is within the error of the assay and rarely causes false-positive test results (Chybowski et al. 1992; Crawford et al. 1992). Flexible colonoscopy, however, affects serum PSA levels in certain patients (Barbatzas et al. 2004).

Once a blood sample is drawn, the PSA concentration is not stable due to enzymatic autolysis of the molecule. While tPSA and the complexes with enzyme inhibitors are relatively stable, fPSA is not. In practice this means that tPSA and cPSA are stable for 24 h at room temperature in samples without centrifugation, but that fPSA concentrations will drop by 25% under those conditions (Cartledge et al. 1999). It is recommended that samples meant for fPSA ratio or the percentage of tPSA are centrifuged as soon as possible and stored at 4 °C, provided the analysis can be done within 8 h after venepuncture. For delayed analyses the serum samples should be frozen at –20 °C (Sokoll et al. 2002) or –80 °C (Jung et al. 2000).

II.3.6.2.5
Alternative, Additional and New Markers for Prostatic Cancer

In the past several circulating tumour markers have been associated with prostatic carcinoma: circulating antibodies against p53 (anti-p53), bladder tumour antigen (BTA), MUC-1 or episialin (CA 27.29, CASA or CA 15–3), TPA (tissue polypeptide antigen), TPS (TPA specific), cytokeratin 18 (ck18), creatine kinase BB (CK-BB), CA 19–9, CA 125, carcinoembryonic antigen (CEA), insulin-like rowth factor II (IGF-II), vascular endothelial growth factor (VEGF), neuron-specific enolase (NSE) and c-erbB-2 ectodomains. None of these markers reaches the performance characteristics of PSA, but some of them may be useful as alternatives in the follow-up of PSA-negative prostatic cancers (Tricoli et al. 2004). Special attention has been paid in the recent literature to circulating prostate-specific membrane antigen (PSMA) (Douglas et al. 1997) as an alternative for PSA. Like prostate stem cell antigen (PSCA) this marker has not replaced PSA determinations in clinical practice (Bangma and Verhagen 2000). Promising results with BPSA, a variant of fPSA secreted excessively in BPH, indicate that this molecule can become useful for detecting and monitoring BPH (Canto et al. 2004).

Chromogranin A (CGA), like NSE, is a circulating marker for neuroendocrine differentiation of prostatic carcinomas, therapy resistance and bad prognosis (Isshiki et al. 2002).

Bone alkaline phosphatase (ostase) is present on the outer membrane of osteoblasts. There it forms tetramers, and it is released as dimers upon activation of the osteoblasts, such as in the case of metastases in the bone marrow. It belongs to the tissue nonspecific alkaline phosphatases (one of the four isoenzymes of the molecule), which are modified post-translationally into bone, liver or kidney variants. So, bone alkaline phosphatase is a sensitive metastasis marker in combination with PSA, although it should be emphasized that its elevation in blood is not specific for prostatic cancer (also elevated in, for example, advanced mammary carcinoma) nor for cancer in general (elevated in osteoporosis, renal osteodystrophy, bone fractures and Paget's disease). Mainly because of the close correlation with skeletal scans, bone alkaline phosphatase has found its clinical application in the follow-up of prostatic cancer (Cooper et al. 1994; Morote et al. 1996; Oremek et al. 1997; Wolff et al. 1998).

A number of candidates for new circulating markers have been launched. Two splice variants of PSA and human kallikrein-2, coined PSA-linked molecule (PSA-LM) and hK2-linked molecule (K-LM) (David et al. 2002), are currently under investigation. Pro-PSA was recently described as a better tool than fPSA to discriminate between prostatic cancer and BPH (Mikolajczyk et al. 2004). Some kallikreins, such as hK2, hK4, hK11 and hK15, are prostate-specific and can be expected to contribute as tumour markers in the future (Diamandis and Yousef 2002). Other interesting and potentially useful markers are hepsin (Klezovitch et al. 2004), caveolin-1 (Tahir et al. 2003), MIC-1 (Liu et al. 2003), insulin-like growth factor-binding protein-3 (Koistinen et al. 2002) and heat shock protein 70 (Abe et al. 2004). Last but not least, the introduction of new technologies such as proteomics (to assign protein profiles) (Ornstein et al. 2004) and real-time PCR (to detect circulating cancer cells) (Lintula et al. 2004) into the clinical laboratory will open new avenues for fine-tuning the detection and follow-up methods for prostatic cancer.

II.3.6.3
Markers for Testicular Carcinoma: α-Fetoprotein, Human Chorionic Gonadotrophin and Others (Fig. II.3.8b)

II.3.6.3.1
α-Fetoprotein (AFP)

AFP is an oncofoetal glycoprotein, which was first discovered in human foetal serum (Bergstrand and Czar 1956). In adult serum AFP concentrations are below 6 ng/ml (Masseyeff et al. 1974), and it is a sensitive tumour marker in cancer patients (Abelev et al. 1963; Tatarinov et al. 1963). The 70-kDa molecule is produced by the yolk sac and foetal liver, and it is the major circulating protein during foetal life. The AFP gene belongs to a multigene family to which albumin, afamin and vitamin D-binding globulin (Gc-globulin) also belong. In fact, AFP is considered the foetal counterpart of albumin (Ruoslahti and Terry 1976), and the switch from AFP to albumin (Tilghman and Belayew 1982) can be compared to the postnatal switch from haemoglobin F to haemoglobin A. The gene is flanked by a far upstream transcription control element with characteristics of an enhancer (Watanabe et al. 1987). As for albumin, transcription of AFP is downregulated by acute inflammation (negative acute phase protein), and theoretically this may act as a confounding element in the interpretation of serum AFP levels. Yet, this interference may practically be of little clinical relevance (Christiansen et al. 1995). The physiological role of AFP in the foetus is not entirely elucidated, but some consider it as an autocrine/paracrine growth factor acting on its own AFP receptor (Li et al. 2002), and AFP production is controlled by the extracellular matrix (Abelev and Eraiser 1999). Yet, AFP is not required for embryonic development, and AFP-null knock-out embryos develop normally, but AFP-null females are infertile due to a defect in the hypothalamic–pituitary system leading to anovulation (Gabant et al. 2002). AFP deficiency has been described in pregnant women (blood and amniotic fluid) and in their infants without phenotypic abnormalities (Greenberg et al. 1992). This appears to be a benign genetic trait analogous to analbuminaemia.

As a glycoprotein, AFP shows microheterogeneity largely due to variations in glycosylation. Based on affinity differences for several lectins, four patterns have been described: cord serum or liver type, hepatocellular carcinoma type, gastrointestinal tumour type and yolk sac tumour type (Taketa 1992).

AFP is the tumour marker of choice for nonseminoma germ cell tumours (NSGCT) (Smith 1970; Haije et al. 1976), whether they reside in the testis or in other organs (Ebi et al. 2003; Smith et al. 2004). Other cancers associated with elevated AFP serum levels are: hepatocellular carcinoma (often with levels exceeding 1000 ng/ml), choriocarcinoma, hepatoblastoma, yolk sac tumour, gastric and pancreatic carcinoma, cholangiocarcinoma, renal tumours, mammary carcinoma and leukaemia. Moderate elevations are found in other diseases, such as hepatitis, alcoholic liver steatosis and cirrhosis, haemochromatosis, mucoviscidosis and congenital nephrosis. Pregnancy is associated with elevated AFP concentrations in maternal blood and amniotic fluid: screening tests for neural tube defects and Down's syndrome are based on abnormally high and low maternal serum concentrations respectively. In hereditary persistence of AFP (HPAFP) the mean levels of serum AFP are 23-fold higher than in control individuals, and the trait can be confirmed by elevated AFP levels in family members (Schefer et al. 1998). In pure seminoma germ cell tumours (SGCT) serum AFP levels are not elevated, although "hidden" yolk sac elements can be present in histologically pure seminomas with detectable AFP mRNA in the tumours (Yuasa et al. 1999) and low serum AFP levels (< 16 ng/ml) (Nazeer et al. 1998). The correct classification of these tumours is important for the therapeutic strategy.

The list of circumstances associated with elevated serum AFP levels indicates that the specificity for NSGCTs is low, and the test cannot be advocated for screening purposes. It is, however, a useful marker for therapeutic follow-up and prognosis. A "half-life" shorter than 5 days, as determined by three measurements within 10 days after orchiectomy, indicates a favourable prognosis, as is a serum concentration below 1000 ng/ml before surgery. It should be noted on the one hand that increasing AFP serum concentrations do not necessarily indicate disease progression or recurrence, since concomitant liver dysfunction can be present (related to drug toxicity or viral hepatitis) (Germa et al. 1993). Persistent low and stable AFP levels on the other hand probably represent absence of active disease (Morris and Bosl 2000). Furthermore, the samples and the methods used for the follow-up of a patient should be standardized: determinations from serum give slightly higher results than those from plasma, and up to a 20 % bias error can exist between the different assay kits (Christiansen et al. 2001).

The analysis of the microheterogeneity in circulating AFP for differentiating between AFP variants from various sources has been claimed to add diagnostic information to plain AFP determinations. Concanavalin A could distinguish between AFP from NSGCT and liver disease (Saraswathi and Malati 1994; Mora et al. 1995), but additional lectins have been used as well (Yamamoto et al. 2003). In isoelectric focusing a band coined +III, mainly consisting of di- and asialo species, was associated with NSGCT (Johnson et al. 1995, 2000). Some authors have questioned the value of this assay (Vessella et al. 1984; de Takats et al. 1996), and technical sophistication has hampered its widespread introduction into the clinical laboratory. Finally, detection of germ-cell tumour cells in the peripheral blood by reverse transcription-PCR is a new marker seemingly with limited correlation with the AFP serum concentration, which deserves further clinical investigation (Hautkappe et al. 2000).

II.3.6.3.2 Human Chorionic Gonadotrophin (hCG)

hCG is a glycoprotein hormone with a molecular weight of 38 kDa and consists of a noncovalent dimer of an α- and a β-subunit. The α-subunit is common to other hormones such as human luteinizing hormone (hLH), follicle-stimulating hormone (hFSH) and thyroid-stimulating hormone (hTSH), while the β-subunit defines the endocrine function (Talmadge et al. 1983).

The hormone is not only heterogeneous in peptide structure but also in combination of subunits and in the structure of carbohydrate side chains. Common hCG-related molecules in serum samples include regular hCG, hyperglycosylated hCG (ITA), nicked hCG, nicked ITA, hCG missing the β-subunit C-terminal extension, free α-subunit, free β-subunit, free β-subunit missing the C-terminal extension, hyperglycosylated free β-subunit and nicked free β-subunit. The same molecules plus β-core fragment are present in urine samples (Cole and Sutton 2004). During pregnancy hCG is produced by the trophoblastic cells of the placenta, beginning at 12–14 days after conception. During the first trimester of pregnancy it stimulates the corpus luteum graviditatis to produce progesterone, which in turn maintains the secretory state of the endometrium. Other functions are induction of angiogenesis (during pregnancy and tumour development) (Zygmunt et al. 2002) and stimulation of growth (in bladder cancer cells) (Gillott et al. 1996). The production of hCG can be increased by cytokines (interleukin-1 and tumour necrosis factor).

Normally free βhCG concentrations in serum do not exceed 0.1 ng/ml. Together with AFP hCG is an independent marker of testicular NSGCT: in 40–50% of patients it is found at high serum concentrations and mainly circulates as an intact dimer. In embryonal carcinoma, teratocarcinoma and choriocarcinoma serum levels are typically elevated, but differentiated teratoma and yolk sac tumour do not produce hCG. In 20–40% of patients suffering from SGCT serum hCG concentrations are elevated, although usually to levels not as high as in NSGCT, and with a variable proportion of free β-subunits in addition to intact dimers (Saller et al. 1990). Non-Hodgkin lymphoma in the testis has been associated with elevated hCG levels as well (Moller 1996). The marker shows no specificity for testicular cancer, since moderately elevated serum concentrations are also found in malignancies from liver, pancreas, kidney, lung, breast, ovary, uterus, bladder, stomach, colon, oesophagus as well as in lymphoma and endocrine tumours. Yet, the marker has a place in the screening of patients at risk for developing testicular carcinoma: after orchiectomy for a tumour of the contralateral testis, in identical twins with testicular cancer and in intra-abdominal cryptorchid testes. Although hCG levels in serum correlate with the disease stage and with tumour burden, the main application of hCG is in the follow-up after orchiectomy (Perlin et al. 1976), and a serum "half-life" of more than 3 days, as calculated from weekly determinations (Seckl et al. 1990), indicates residual producing tumour and poor prognosis (Mazumdar et al. 2001). The lead time for tumour recurrence is about 2 months. Caution in the interpretation of follow-up levels, however, is needed in some instances. First, a transient increase shortly after chemotherapy ("marker surge") indicates tumour lysis rather than tumour progression (Horwich and Peckham 1986; Mohler et al. 1987; Beck et al. 2004). Second, circulating heterophilic antibodies have been described to generate false-positive hCG results (Trojan et al. 2004). Third, normalized hCG serum levels cannot exclude tumour persistence in every case. In about 20% of patients with mixed germ cell tumours, a transition of the histological tumour type from embryonal or teratocarcinoma to differentiated teratoma may occur, and this is accompanied by the disappearance of the marker (Mann and Saller 1994b).

hCG, especially the acidic variants produced by tumours, possess thyrotrophic activity (Mann et al. 1986). High levels of hCG (>20,000 IU/l) can stimulate the thyroid production of thyroxin and tri-iodothyronine, and provoke hyperthyroidism (Giralt et al. 1992; Derakhshani et al. 1999) or thyrotoxicosis (Goodarzi and Van Herle 2000). Moreover, hCG levels beyond 100 IU/l suppress pituitary hFSH production, and low serum levels in testicular cancer patients can be the result (Kovcin et al. 1997). The detection of germ-cell tumour cells in the peripheral blood by reverse transcription-PCR is a new technique that defines a patients group with poor prognosis (Hara et al. 2002). Finally, there is some debate concerning which type of assay to use for circulating hCG. Because hCG can circulate under many different variants, and some assays exclusively detect intact hCG dimers while others are designed to measure free β-subunits, it is not easy to predict which assays cover the right variants and are the most suitable ones for detection and follow-up of germ cell tumours. In the opinion of Cole and Sutton (2004) only two tests, the DPC Immulite (DPC, Los Angeles, Calif., USA) and UK RIA (radioimmunoassay) (used at Charing Cross Hospital, London, UK) appropriately detect all these hCG-related molecules.

II.3.6.3.3 Other Markers for Testicular Carcinoma

Placental-like alkaline phosphatase (PLAP) is an isoenzyme distinct from placental, intestinal and liver alkaline phosphatase, and is present in trace amounts in normal testes (Millan et al. 1982). The enzyme, also called Nagao or germ cell isoenzyme, shows enhanced expression in testicular germ cell tumours, especially in seminomas. Serum concentrations of PLAP are elevated in at least half of the seminoma patients (Tucker et al. 1985), and sensitivity can be enhanced to 82% by combining the marker with hCG and lactate dehydrogenase (Koshida et al. 1996). The marker is not specific for several reasons: immunoassays cannot distinguish between placental and germ cell alkaline phosphatases, half of smokers show elevated serum levels (Koshida et al. 1990) and colonic adenocarcinomas can also provoke increased serum concentrations of PLAP (Harmenberg et al. 1991).

Inhibin B is a dimer belonging to the transforming growth factor β superfamily of ligands that have roles in reproduction and development (Brown et al. 2000). The hormone is secreted by Sertoli cells in the testis, and it inhibits hFSH secretion by the pituitary gland. In this way serum concentrations of inhibin reflect the Sertoli cell function (Bergh and Cajander 1990; Peters et al. 2000). Because in the rare Sertoli cell tumours serum inhibin levels are elevated, and return to normal after orchiectomy, inhibin is propagated as a useful marker in the management of these testicular tumours (Toppari et al. 1998). In the interpretation of inhibin levels in serum, it should be noted that testicular enlargement with elevated serum inhibin concentrations also occurs in patients with pituitary macroadenomas secreting hFSH (Heseltine et al. 1989).

Lactate dehydrogenase (LDH) and more specifically its first isoenzyme (LD-1) is a useful marker for seminoma and for testicular germ cell tumours in general (Lippert et al. 1981; von Eyben 1983; von Eyben and Skude 1984), and serum levels reflect the tumour burden (Lippert and Javadpour 1981). The specificity of LDH is low, as a variety of nonmalignant diseases and minimal tissue damage can also lead to pathologic serum levels. Nevertheless, LDH is of some value in the follow-up of marker-negative patients and can indicate a persistent tumour or a recurrence.

In the past several other circulating tumour markers have been associated with testicular carcinoma: TPA (tissue polypeptide antigen), TPS (TPA specific), cytokeratin 18 (ck18), NSE (neuron-specific enolase), free α-subunits, CEA (carcinoembryonic antigen), hPL (human placental lactogen), SP1 (pregnancy-specific beta 1-glycoprotein) and oestradiol. Finally, the clinical value of the mucin-like TRA-1–60 antigen awaits further evaluation (Gels et al. 1997; Lajer et al. 2002).

References

Abe M, Manola JB, Oh WK, Parslow DL, George DJ, Austin CL, Kantoff PW (2004) Plasma levels of heat shock protein 70 in patients with prostate cancer: a potential biomarker for prostate cancer. Clin Prostate Cancer 3:49–53

Abelev GI, Eraiser TL (1999) Cellular aspects of alpha-fetoprotein reexpression in tumors. Semin Cancer Biol 9:95–107

Abelev GI, Perova SD, Khramkova NI, Postnikova ZA, Irlin IS (1963) Production of embryonal alpha-globulin by transplantable mouse hepatomas. Transplantation 1:174–180

Bangma CH, Verhagen PC (2000) Blood and serum substances for markers of prostate cancer. Microsc Res Tech 51:430–435

Barbatzas C, Dellis A, Grivas I, Trakas N, Ekonomou A, Kostakopoulos A (2004) Colonoscopy effects on serum prostate specific antigen levels. Int Urol Nephrol 36:203–206

Baumgart Y, Otto A, Schafer A, Usbeck E, Cott C, Schott A, Tornack M, Wenzel A, Mossie A, Birkenmeier G (2004) Characterization of novel monoclonal antibodies for prostate-specific antigen (PSA) with potency to recognize PSA bound to alpha2-macroglobulin. Clin Chem 51:84–92

Beck SD, Patel MI, Sheinfeld J (2004) Tumor marker levels in post-chemotherapy cystic masses: clinical implications for patients with germ cell tumors. J Urol 171:168–171

Bergh A, Cajander S (1990) Immunohistochemical localization of inhibin-alpha in the testes of normal men and in men with testicular disorders. Int J Androl 13:463–469

Bergstrand CG, Czar B (1956) Demonstration of a new protein fraction in serum from the human fetus. Scand J Clin Lab Invest 8:174

Black MH, Diamandis EP (2000) The diagnostic and prognostic utility of prostate-specific antigen for diseases of the breast. Breast Cancer Res Treat 59:1–14

Brown CW, Houston-Hawkins DE, Woodruff TK, Matzuk MM (2000) Insertion of Inhbb into the Inhba locus rescues the Inhba-null phenotype and reveals new activin functions. Nat Genet 25:453–457

Canto EI, Singh H, Shariat SF, Lamb DJ, Mikolajczyk SD, Linton HJ, Rittenhouse HG, Kadmon D, Miles BJ, Slawin KM (2004) Serum BPSA outperforms both total PSA and free PSA as a predictor of prostatic enlargement in men without prostate cancer. Urology 63:905–910

Cartledge JJ, Thompson D, Verril H, Clarkson P, Eardley I (1999) The stability of free and bound prostate-specific antigen. BJU Int 84:810–814

Catalona WJ (1996) Clinical utility of measurements of free and total prostate-specific antigen (PSA): a review. Prostate Suppl 7:64–69

Catalona WJ, Richie JP, Ahmann FR, Hudson MA, Scardino PT, Flanigan RC, deKernion JB, Ratliff TL, Kavoussi LR, Dalkin BL et al (1994) Comparison of digital rectal examination and serum prostate specific antigen in the early detection of prostate cancer: results of a multicenter clinical trial of 6,630 men. J Urol 151:1283–1290

Christensson A, Laurell CB, Lilja H (1990) Enzymatic activity of prostate-specific antigen and its reactions with extracellular serine proteinase inhibitors. Eur J Biochem 194:755–763

Christiansen M, Hogdall CK, Brihmer C (1995) Alpha-fetoprotein and the acute phase response. A study using acute pelvic inflammatory disease as a model system. Clin Chim Acta 235:71–79

Christiansen M, Hogdall CK, Andersen JR, Norgaard-Pedersen B (2001) Alpha-fetoprotein in plasma and serum of healthy adults: preanalytical, analytical and biological sources of variation and construction of age-dependent reference intervals. Scand J Clin Lab Invest 61:205–215

Chybowski FM, Bergstralh EJ, Oesterling JE (1992) The effect of digital rectal examination on the serum prostate specific antigen concentration: results of a randomized study. J Urol 148:83–86

Cleutjens KB, van Eekelen CC, van der Korput HA, Brinkmann AO, Trapman J (1996) Two androgen response regions cooperate in steroid hormone regulated activity of the prostate-specific antigen promoter. J Biol Chem 271:6379–6388

Cole LA, Sutton JM (2004) Selecting an appropriate hCG test for managing gestational trophoblastic disease and cancer. J Reprod Med 49:545–553

Cooner WH, Mosley BR, Rutherford CL Jr, Beard JH, Pond HS, Terry WJ, Igel TC, Kidd DD (1990) Prostate cancer detection in a clinical urological practice by ultrasonography, digital rectal examination and prostate specific antigen. J Urol 143:1146–1152

Cooper EH, Whelan P, Purves D (1994) Bone alkaline phosphatase and prostate-specific antigen in the monitoring of prostate cancer. Prostate 25:236–242

Crawford ED, Schutz MJ, Clejan S, Drago J, Resnick MI, Chodak GW, Gomella LG, Austenfeld M, Stone NN, Miles BJ et al (1992) The effect of digital rectal examination on prostate-specific antigen levels. J Am Med Assoc 267:2227–2228

David A, Mabjeesh N, Azar I, Biton S, Engel S, Bernstein J, Romano J, Avidor Y, Waks T, Eshhar Z, Langer SZ, Lifschitz-Mercer B, Matzkin H, Rotman G, Toporik A, Savitsky K, Mintz L (2002) Unusual alternative splicing within the human kallikrein genes KLK2 and KLK3 gives rise to novel prostate-specific proteins. J Biol Chem 277:18084–18090

de Takats PG, Jones SR, Penn R, Cullen MH (1996) Alpha-foetoprotein heterogeneity: what is its value in managing patients with germ cell tumours?. Clin Oncol (R Coll Radiol) 8:323–326

de Vries SH, Raaijmakers R, Kranse R, Blijenberg BG, Schroder FH (2004) Prostate cancer characteristics and prostate specific antigen changes in screening detected patients initially treated with a watchful waiting policy. J Urol 172:2193–2196

Derakhshani P, Klotz T, Heidenreich A, Engelmann U (1999) Diffuse metastasized testicular teratoma and paraneoplastic thyreotoxicosis. Case report and literature review. Urol Int 63:265–267

Diamandis EP, Yousef GM (2002) Human tissue kallikreins: a family of new cancer biomarkers. Clin Chem 48:1198–1205

Djavan B, Remzi M, Zlotta A, Seitz C, Snow P, Marberger M (2002) Novel artificial neural network for early detection of prostate cancer. J Clin Oncol 20:921–929

Doherty AP, Bower M, Smith GL, Miano R, Mannion EM, Mitchell H, Christmas TJ (2000) Undetectable ultrasensitive PSA after radical prostatectomy for prostate cancer predicts relapse-free survival. Br J Cancer 83:1432–1436

Douglas TH, Morgan TO, McLeod DG, Moul JW, Murphy GP, Barren R 3rd, Sesterhenn IA, Mostofi FK (1997) Comparison of serum prostate specific membrane antigen, prostate specific antigen, and free prostate specific antigen levels in radical prostatectomy patients. Cancer 80:107–114

Ebi H, Nakata M, Tahara M, Igarashi T, Kawada K, Itoh K, Ueda R, Minami H (2003) Extragonadal germ cell tumors in Japan. Cancer Sci 94:1107–1111

Ellis WJ, Chetner MP, Preston SD, Brawer MK (1994) Diagnosis of prostatic carcinoma: the yield of serum prostate specific antigen, digital rectal examination and transrectal ultrasonography. J Urol 152:1520–1525

Ellis WJ, Vessella RL, Noteboom JL, Lange PH, Wolfert RL, Rittenhouse HG (1997) Early detection of recurrent prostate cancer with an ultrasensitive chemiluminescent prostate-specific antigen assay. Urology 50:573–579

Finne P, Auvinen A, Aro J, Juusela H, Maattanen L, Rannikko S, Hakama M, Tammela TL, Stenman UH (2002) Estimation of prostate cancer risk on the basis of total and free prostate-specific antigen, prostate volume and digital rectal examination. Eur Urol 41:619–626

Friedland SJ, Aronson WJ, Kane CJ, Terris MK, Presti JC Jr, Trock B, Amling CL (2004) Biochemical outcome after radical prostatectomy among men with normal preoperative serum prostate-specific antigen levels. Cancer 101:748–753

Gabant P, Forrester L, Nichols J, Van Reeth T, De Mees C, Pajack B, Watt A, Smitz J, Alexandre H, Szpirer C, Szpirer J (2002) Alpha-fetoprotein, the major fetal serum protein, is not essential for embryonic development but is required for female fertility. Proc Natl Acad Sci USA 99:12865–12870

Gels ME, Marrink J, Visser P, Sleijfer DT, Droste JH, Hoekstra HJ, Andrews PW, Schraffordt Koops H (1997) Importance of a new tumor marker TRA-1-60 in the follow-up of patients with clinical stage I nonseminomatous testicular germ cell tumors. Ann Surg Oncol 4:321–327

Germa JR, Llanos M, Tabernero JM, Mora J (1993) False elevations of alpha-fetoprotein associated with liver dysfunction in germ cell tumors. Cancer 72:2491–2494

Gillott DJ, Iles RK, Chard T (1996) The effects of beta-human chorionic gonadotrophin on the in vitro growth of bladder cancer cell lines. Br J Cancer 73:323–326

Giralt SA, Dexeus F, Amato R, Sella A, Logothetis C (1992) Hyperthyroidism in men with germ cell tumors and high levels of beta-human chorionic gonadotropin. Cancer 69:1286–1290

Goodarzi MO, Van Herle AJ (2000) Thyrotoxicosis in a male patient associated with excess human chorionic gonadotropin production by germ cell tumor. Thyroid 10:611–619

Greenberg F, Faucett A, Rose E, Bancalari L, Kardon NB, Mizejewski G, Haddow JE, Alpert E (1992) Congenital deficiency of alpha-fetoprotein. Am J Obstet Gynecol 167:509–511

Gustafsson O, Mansour E, Norming U, Carlsson A, Tornblom M, Nyman CR (1998) Prostate-specific antigen (PSA), PSA density and age-adjusted PSA reference values in screening for prostate cancer – a study of a randomly selected population of 2,400 men. Scand J Urol Nephrol 32:373–377

Gutman AB, Gutman EE (1938) An "acid" phosphatase occurring in the serum of patients with metastasising carcinoma of the prostate gland. J Clin Invest 17:473–478

Haije WG, Talerman A, Boekestein-Tjahjadien HM, Baggerman L (1976) Alpha fetoprotein (AFP) in the serum of patients with germ cell tumors. The value of AFP determination for diagnosis and follow-up. Ned Tijdschr Geneeskd 120:855–859

Hammerer P, Huland H (1994) Systematic sextant biopsies in 651 patients referred for prostate evaluation. J Urol 151:99–102

Hara I, Yamada Y, Miyake H, Hara S, Gotoh A, Fujisawa M, Okada H, Arakawa S, Kamidono S (2002) Detection of beta-human chorionic gonadotropin expressing cells by nested reverse transcriptase-polymerase chain reaction in the peripheral blood stem cells of patients with advanced germ cell tumor. J Urol 167:1487–1491

Harmenberg U, Koha M, Makiya R, Koshida K, Brismar B, Stigbrand T, Wahren B (1991) Identification and characterization of alkaline phosphatase isozymes in human colorectal adenocarcinomas. Tumour Biol 12:237–248

Hautkappe AL, Lu M, Mueller H, Bex A, Harstrick A, Roggendorf M, Ruebben H (2000) Detection of germ-cell tumor cells in the peripheral blood by nested reverse transcription-polymerase chain reaction for alpha-fetoprotein-messenger RNA and beta human chorionic gonadotropin-messenger RNA. Cancer Res 60:3170–3174

Henttu P, Vihko P (1994) Prostate-specific antigen and human glandular kallikrein: two kallikreins of the human prostate. Ann Med 26:157–164

Hernandez J, Thompson IM (2004) Prostate-specific antigen: a review of the validation of the most commonly used cancer biomarker. Cancer 101:894–904

Heseltine D, White MC, Kendall-Taylor P, De Kretser DM, Kelly W (1989) Testicular enlargement and elevated serum inhibin concentrations occur in patients with pituitary macroadenomas secreting follicle stimulating hormone. Clin Endocrinol (Oxf) 31:411–423

Horwich A, Peckham MJ (1986) Transient tumor marker elevation following chemotherapy for germ cell tumors of the testis. Cancer Treat Rep 70:1329–1331

Isshiki S, Akakura K, Komiya A, Suzuki H, Kamiya N, Ito H (2002) Chromogranin a concentration as a serum marker to predict prognosis after endocrine therapy for prostate cancer. J Urol 167:512–515

Johnson PJ, Ho S, Cheng P, Chan A, Leung T, Yuen J (1995) Germ cell tumors express a specific alpha-fetoprotein variant detectable by isoelectric focusing. Cancer 75:1663–1668

Johnson PJ, Poon TC, Hjelm NM, Ho CS, Blake C, Ho SK (2000) Structures of disease-specific serum alpha-fetoprotein isoforms. Br J Cancer 83:1330–1337

Jung K, Lein M, Brux B, Sinha P, Schnorr D, Loening SA (2000) Different stability of free and complexed prostate-specific

antigen in serum in relation to specimen handling and storage conditions. Clin Chem Lab Med 38:1271–1275
Khan MA, Partin AW (2004) Management of patients with an increasing prostate-specific antigen after radical prostatectomy. Curr Urol Rep 5:179–187
Klezovitch O, Chevillet J, Mirosevich J, Roberts RL, Matusik RJ, Vasioukhin V (2004) Hepsin promotes prostate cancer progression and metastasis. Cancer Cell 6:185–195
Koistinen H, Paju A, Koistinen R, Finne P, Lovgren J, Wu P, Seppala M, Stenman UH (2002) Prostate-specific antigen and other prostate-derived proteases cleave IGFBP-3, but prostate cancer is not associated with proteolytically cleaved circulating IGFBP-3. Prostate 50:112–118
Koshida K, Stigbrand T, Munck-Wikland E, Hisazumi H, Wahren B (1990) Analysis of serum placental alkaline phosphatase activity in testicular cancer and cigarette smokers. Urol Res 18:169–173
Koshida K, Uchibayashi T, Yamamoto H, Hirano K (1996) Significance of placental alkaline phosphatase (PLAP) in the monitoring of patients with seminoma. Br J Urol 77:138–142
Kovcin VN, Jelic SB, Ivanovic SM, Babovic NL (1997) Serum gonadotropin levels in patients with germ-cell tumors of the testis: interrelations, possible cross-reactions and interpretation of beta-HCG level. Int J Biol Markers 12:55–60
Kuriyama M, Wang MC, Papsidero LD, Killian CS, Shimano T, Valenzuela L, Nishiura T, Murphy GP, Chu TM (1980) Quantitation of prostate-specific antigen in serum by a sensitive enzyme immunoassay. Cancer Res 40:4658–4662
Lajer H, Daugaard G, Andersson AM, Skakkebaek NE (2002) Clinical use of serum TRA-1–60 as tumor marker in patients with germ cell cancer. Int J Cancer 100:244–246
Li MS, Li PF, Yang FY, He SP, Du GG, Li G (2002) The intracellular mechanism of alpha-fetoprotein promoting the proliferation of NIH 3T3 cells. Cell Res 12:151–156
Lintula S, Vesalainen S, Rannikko A, Zhang WM, Finne P, Stenman J, Stenman UH (2004) Quantification of prostate specific antigen mRNA levels in circulation after prostatic surgery and endocrine treatment by quantitative reverse transcription-polymerase chain reaction. Scand J Clin Lab Invest 64:93–100
Lippert MC, Javadpour N (1981) Lactic dehydrogenase in the monitoring and prognosis of testicular cancer. Cancer 48:2274–2278
Lippert M, Papadopoulos N, Javadpour N (1981) Role of lactate dehydrogenase isoenzymes in testicular cancer. Urology 18:50–53
Liu T, Bauskin AR, Zaunders J, Brown DA, Pankhurst S, Russell PJ, Breit SN, Panhurst S (2003) Macrophage inhibitory cytokine 1 reduces cell adhesion and induces apoptosis in prostate cancer cells. Cancer Res 63:5034–5040
Manetti L, Lupi I, Genovesi M, Morselli L, Grasso L, Nencetti C, Gasperi M, Bogazzi F, Bartalena L, Martino E (2004) Serum prostate-specific antigen concentration is increased in acromegalic women. J Endocrinol Invest 27:643–647
Mann K, Saller B (1994a) Tumours of the prostate gland. In: Klapdor R (ed) Tumour markers in clinical oncology: an overview. Sorin Biomedica, Turin, pp 145–150
Mann K, Saller B (1994b) Tumours of the testis. In: Klapdor R (ed) Tumour markers in clinical oncology: an overview. Sorin Biomedica, Turin, pp 151–156
Mann K, Schneider N, Hoermann R (1986) Thyrotropic activity of acidic isoelectric variants of human chorionic gonadotropin from trophoblastic tumors. Endocrinology 118:1558–1566
Masseyeff R, Bonet C, Drouet J, Sudaka P, Lalanne C (1974) Radioimmunoassay of alpha-fetoprotein. I. Technique and serum levels in the normal adult. Digestion 10:17–28
Matsumura M, Bhatt AS, Andress D, Clegg N, Takayama TK, Craik CS, Nelson PS (2005) Substrates of the prostate-specific serine protease prostase/KLK4 defined by positional-scanning peptide libraries. Prostate 62:1–13
Mazumdar M, Bajorin DF, Bacik J, Higgins G, Motzer RJ, Bosl GJ (2001) Predicting outcome to chemotherapy in patients with germ cell tumors: the value of the rate of decline of human chorionic gonadotrophin and alpha-fetoprotein during therapy. J Clin Oncol 19:2534–2541
McCormack RT, Rittenhouse HG, Finlay JA, Sokoloff RL, Wang TJ, Wolfert RL, Lilja H, Oesterling JE (1995) Molecular forms of prostate-specific antigen and the human kallikrein gene family: a new era. Urology 45:729–744
Melegos DN, Yu H, Ashok M, Wang C, Stanczyk F, Diamandis EP (1997) Prostate-specific antigen in female serum, a potential new marker of androgen excess. J Clin Endocrinol Metab 82:777–780
Mikolajczyk SD, Catalona WJ, Evans CL, Linton HJ, Millar LS, Marker KM, Katir D, Amirkhan A, Rittenhouse HG (2004) Proenzyme forms of prostate-specific antigen in serum improve the detection of prostate cancer. Clin Chem 50:1017–1025
Millan JL, Eriksson A, Stigbrand T (1982) A possible new locus of alkaline phosphatase expressed in human testis. Hum Genet 62:293–295
Mohler JL, Siami PF, Flanigan RC (1987) False positive beta-human chorionic gonadotropin in testicular cancer. Urology 30:252–254
Moller MB (1996) Association of testicular non-Hodgkin's lymphomas with elevated serum levels of human chorionic gonadotropin-like material. Oncology 53:94–98
Mora J, Gascon N, Tabernero JM, Germa JR, Gonzalez F (1995) Alpha-fetoprotein-concanavalin A binding as a marker to discriminate between germ cell tumours and liver diseases. Eur J Cancer 31A:2239–2242
Morote J, Lorente JA, Encabo G (1996) Prostate carcinoma staging. Clinical utility of bone alkaline phosphatase in addition to prostate specific antigen. Cancer 78:2374–2378
Morris MJ, Bosl GJ (2000) Recognizing abnormal marker results that do not reflect disease in patients with germ cell tumors. J Urol 163:796–801
Nazeer T, Ro JY, Amato RJ, Park YW, Ordonez NG, Ayala AG (1998) Histologically pure seminoma with elevated alpha-fetoprotein: a clinicopathologic study of ten cases. Oncol Rep 5:1425–1429
Oesterling JE, Chan DW, Epstein JI, Kimball AW Jr., Bruzek DJ, Rock RC, Brendler CB, Walsh PC (1988) Prostate specific antigen in the preoperative and postoperative evaluation of localized prostatic cancer treated with radical prostatectomy. J Urol 139:766–772
Olsson AY, Bjartell A, Lilja H, Lundwall A (2005) Expression of prostate-specific antigen (PSA) and human glandular kallikrein 2 (hK2) in ileum and other extraprostatic tissues. Int J Cancer 113:290–297
Oremek GM, Kramer W, Seiffert UB, Jonas D (1997) Diagnostic value of skeletal AP and PSA with respect to skeletal scintigram in patients with prostatic disease. Anticancer Res 17:3035–3036
Ornstein DK, Rayford W, Fusaro VA, Conrads TP, Ross SJ, Hitt BA, Wiggins WW, Veenstra TD, Liotta LA, Petricoin EF 3rd (2004) Serum proteomic profiling can discriminate prostate cancer from benign prostates in men with total prostate specific antigen levels between 2.5 and 15.0 ng/ml. J Urol 172:1302–1305
Parsons JK, Brawer MK, Cheli CD, Partin AW, Djavan R (2004) Complexed prostate specific antigen (PSA) reduces unnecessary prostate biopsies in the 2.6–4.0 ng/mL range of total PSA. BJU Int 94:47–50
Perlin E, Engeler JE Jr., Edson M, Karp D, McIntire KR, Wald-

mann TA (1976) The value of serial measurement of both human chorionic gonadotropin and alpha-fetoprotein for monitoring germinal cell tumors. Cancer 37:215–219
Peters MA, de Jong FH, Teerds KJ, de Rooij DG, Dieleman SJ, van Sluijs FJ (2000) Ageing, testicular tumours and the pituitary-testis axis in dogs. J Endocrinol 166:153–161
Platz EA, De Marzo AM, Giovannucci E (2004) Prostate cancer association studies: pitfalls and solutions to cancer misclassification in the PSA era. J Cell Biochem 91:553–557
Reissigl A, Klocker H, Pointner J, Fink K, Horninger W, Ennemoser O, Strasser H, Colleselli K, Holtl L, Bartsch G (1996) Usefulness of the ratio free/total prostate-specific antigen in addition to total PSA levels in prostate cancer screening. Urology Suppl 48:62–66
Riegman PH, Vlietstra RJ, van der Korput JA, Brinkmann AO, Trapman J (1991) The promoter of the prostate-specific antigen gene contains a functional androgen responsive element. Mol Endocrinol 5:1921–1930
Rittenhouse HG, Finlay JA, Mikolajczyk SD, Partin AW (1998) Human kallikrein 2 (hK2) and prostate-specific antigen (PSA): two closely related, but distinct, kallikreins in the prostate. Crit Rev Clin Lab Sci 35:275–368
Ruoslahti E, Terry WD (1976) Alpha foetoprotein and serum albumin show sequence homology. Nature 260:804–805
Saller B, Clara R, Spottl G, Siddle K, Mann K (1990) Testicular cancer secretes intact human choriogonadotropin (hCG) and its free beta-subunit: evidence that hCG (+hCG-beta) assays are the most reliable in diagnosis and follow-up. Clin Chem 36:234–239
Saraswathi A, Malati T (1994) Clinical relevance of alphafetoprotein microheterogeneity in alphafetoprotein-secreting tumors. Cancer Detect Prev 18:447–454
Schefer H, Mattmann S, Joss RA (1998) Hereditary persistence of alpha-fetoprotein. Case report and review of the literature. Ann Oncol 9:667–672
Seckl MJ, Rustin GJ, Bagshawe KD (1990) Frequency of serum tumour marker monitoring in patients with non-seminomatous germ cell tumours. Br J Cancer 61:916–918
Shulman MJ, Karam JA, Benaim EA (2004) Prostate-specific antigen doubling time predicts response to deferred antiandrogen therapy in men with androgen-independent prostate cancer. Urology 63:732–736
Smith AA, Weng E, Handler M, Foreman NK (2004) Intracranial germ cell tumors: a single institution experience and review of the literature. J Neurooncol 68:153–159
Smith JB (1970) Alpha-fetoprotein: occurrence in certain malignant diseases and review of clinical applications. Med Clin North Am 54:797–803
Sokoll LJ, Bruzek DJ, Dua R, Dunn W, Mohr P, Wallerson G, Eisenberger M, Partin AW, Chan DW (2002) Short-term stability of the molecular forms of prostate-specific antigen and effect on percent complexed prostate-specific antigen and percent free prostate-specific antigen. Urology 60:24–30
Stamey TA, Yang N, Hay AR, McNeal JE, Freiha FS, Redwine E (1987) Prostate-specific antigen as a serum marker for adenocarcinoma of the prostate. N Engl J Med 317:909–916
Stephan C, Cammann H, Semjonow A, Diamandis EP, Wymenga LF, Lein M, Sinha P, Loening SA, Jung K (2002a) Multicenter evaluation of an artificial neural network to increase the prostate cancer detection rate and reduce unnecessary biopsies. Clin Chem 48:1279–1287
Stephan C, Jung K, Cammann H, Vogel B, Brux B, Kristiansen G, Rudolph B, Hauptmann S, Lein M, Schnorr D, Sinha P, Loening SA (2002b) An artificial neural network considerably improves the diagnostic power of percent free prostate-specific antigen in prostate cancer diagnosis: results of a 5-year investigation. Int J Cancer 99:466–473
Tahir SA, Ren C, Timme TL, Gdor Y, Hoogeveen R, Morrisett JD, Frolov A, Ayala G, Wheeler TM, Thompson TC (2003) Development of an immunoassay for serum caveolin-1: a novel biomarker for prostate cancer. Clin Cancer Res 9: 3653–3659
Taketa K (1992) Alpha-fetoprotein in the 1990s. In: Sell S (ed) Serological cancer markers. Humana, Totowa, New Jersey, pp 31–46
Talmadge K, Boorstein WR, Fiddes JC (1983) The human genome contains seven genes for the beta-subunit of chorionic gonadotropin but only one gene for the beta-subunit of luteinizing hormone. DNA 2:281–289
Tatarinov IS, Afanas'eva AV, Parfenova LF (1963) On the development of the serum proteins in human ontogenesis. Vopr Med Khim 37:403–410
Thompson IM, Pauler DK, Goodman PJ, Tangen CM, Lucia MS, Parnes HL, Minasian LM, Ford LG, Lippman SM, Crawford ED, Crowley JJ, Coltman CA Jr. (2004) Prevalence of prostate cancer among men with a prostate-specific antigen level ≤4.0 ng per milliliter. N Engl J Med 350:2239–2246
Tilghman SM, Belayew A (1982) Transcriptional control of the murine albumin/alpha-fetoprotein locus during development. Proc Natl Acad Sci USA 79:5254–5257
Toppari J, Kaipia A, Kaleva M, Laato M, de Kretser DM, Krummen LA, Mather JP, Salmi TT (1998) Inhibin gene expression in a large cell calcifying Sertoli cell tumour and serum inhibin and activin levels. APMIS 106:101–112
Tricoli JV, Schoenfeldt M, Conley BA (2004) Detection of prostate cancer and predicting progression: current and future diagnostic markers. Clin Cancer Res 10:3943–3953
Trojan A, Joller-Jemelka H, Stahel RA, Jacky E, Hersberger M (2004) False-positive human serum chorionic gonadotropin in a patient with a history of germ cell cancer. Oncology 66:336–338
Tucker DF, Oliver RT, Travers P, Bodmer WF (1985) Serum marker potential of placental alkaline phosphatase-like activity in testicular germ cell tumours evaluated by H17E2 monoclonal antibody assay. Br J Cancer 51:631–639
Vessella RL, Santrach MA, Bronson D, Smith CJ, Klicka MJ, Lange PH (1984) Evaluation of AFP glycosylation heterogeneity in cancer patients with AFP-producing tumors. Int J Cancer 34:309–314
von Eyben FE (1983) Lactate dehydrogenase and its isoenzymes in testicular germ cell tumors: an overview. Oncodev Biol Med 4:395–414
von Eyben FE, Skude G (1984) Lactate dehydrogenase and its isoenzyme, LDH-1, in serum are markers of testicular germ cell tumors. Clin Chem 30:340–341
Wang MC, Valenzuela LA, Murphy GP, Chu TM (1979) Purification of a human prostate specific antigen. Invest Urol 17: 159–163
Watanabe K, Saito A, Tamaoki T (1987) Cell-specific enhancer activity in a far upstream region of the human alpha-fetoprotein gene. J Biol Chem 262:4812–4818
Waters WB (1999) Rational uses of PSA testing. In: AACC Proceedings. Tumor markers: successful laboratory practice for today and tomorrow.
Witherspoon LR, Lapeyrolerie T (1997) Sensitive prostate specific antigen measurements identify men with long disease-free intervals and differentiate aggressive from indolent cancer recurrences within 2 years after radical prostatectomy. J Urol 157:1322–1328
Wolff JM, Ittel T, Borchers H, Brauers A, Jakse G (1998) Efficacy of skeletal alkaline phosphatase and prostate-specific antigen in the diagnosis of bone metastasis in cancer of the prostate. Urol Int 61:12–16
Yamamoto R, Ohkouchi T, Wakui Y, Minobe S, Watari H, Shimizu K, Satomura S, Sakuragi N (2003) A study on the microheterogeneity of alpha-fetoproteins produced by yolk sac

and germ cell tumors. Acta Obstet Gynecol Scand 82: 876–882
Yuan JJ, Coplen DE, Petros JA, Figenshau RS, Ratliff TL, Smith DS, Catalona WJ (1992) Effects of rectal examination, prostatic massage, ultrasonography and needle biopsy on serum prostate specific antigen levels. J Urol 147:810–814
Yuasa T, Yoshiki T, Ogawa O, Tanaka T, Isono T, Mishina M, Higuchi K, Okada Y, Yoshida O (1999) Detection of alpha-fetoprotein mRNA in seminoma. J Androl 20:336–340
Zygmunt M, Herr F, Keller-Schoenwetter S, Kunzi-Rapp K, Munstedt K, Rao CV, Lang U, Preissner KT (2002) Characterization of human chorionic gonadotropin as a novel angiogenic factor. J Clin Endocrinol Metab 87:5290–5296

II.3.7 Technical Investigations Including Imaging Procedures: Doppler, MRI, PET, Echo for Tumours

E.L.F. Nijs, R.H. Oyen

Summary

Scrotal ultrasonography (US) and transrectal ultrasonography (TRUS) are the imaging techniques of choice in the evaluation of male infertility. Both US and TRUS are diagnostic tools to assess for the presence of congenital abnormalities or acquired causes.

In selected cases ultrasonography can also be used for guidance for several procedures. US with Doppler can be used to select the appropriate site for sperm retrieval and TRUS can be utilized to guide for seminal vesicle puncture for seminal vesiculography.

Percutaneous or surgical vasography (or deferentography) has now been replaced by magnetic resonance imaging (MRI) and occasionally by TRUS-guided seminal vesiculography in combination with aspiration. This technique may be of importance at the time of microsurgical correction of obstruction of the vas deferens (vasovasostomy or vasoepididymostomy).

MRI is the first examination technique in evaluation of the hypothalamic–pituitary axis and is an adjunctive tool after US and TRUS in selected cases of persistent or complex diagnostic problems or equivocal results.

At present, positron emission tomography (PET) is indicated in urologic oncology (mainly testicular cancer), but PET has no indications in the evaluation of infertile men.

For all emergencies in andrology, including testicular torsion, testicular trauma, priapism and penile fracture, the imaging technique of choice is US in combination with Doppler. MR only serves as a problem-solving technique in these patients.

II.3.7.1 Ultrasound (US)

II.3.7.1.1 Technique

Ultrasonography is a noninvasive imaging technique based on high-frequency sound waves. The frequency of sound waves for imaging purposes ranges typically between 2 and 15 MHz and thus is much higher than 20 kHz, which is the upper limit of human hearing.

An essential part of an ultrasound machine is the transducer that is placed on the skin or intracavitarily. Transducers are equipped with piezoelectric crystals with the ability to change electric energy into sound waves and vice versa. The transducer sends out high-frequency sound waves into the patient (transmitter function). When the sound waves hit a boundary between tissues (e.g. between fluid and soft tissue, soft tissue and bone) some of the sound waves are reflected back and the remainder penetrate further until they reach another boundary and are reflected back. The crystals convert these reflected sound waves or echoes into electrical waves (receiver function) which are then transferred to the computer that converts and displays them as a 2-D grey-scale image on the screen.

For appropriate scrotal and prostate imaging dedicated linear transducers of at least 7.5 MHz are required.

II.3.7.1.2 Clinical Indications

US in combination with Doppler will be the first and only imaging technique in many diseases of the penis and the scrotal contents, including congenital and acquired diseases such as trauma, tumours, infection/inflammation and vascular disorders.

MRI is mainly indicated as a problem-solving modality in selected cases.

Peyronie's Disease (Induratio Penis Plastica) (Fig. II.3.9a–l)

Chronic inflammation of the tunica albuginea, enveloping the corpora cavernosa, leads to fibrosis and focal or diffuse thickening, called penile plaques. These plaques may or may not calcify and cause painful penile deformity during erection. In severe cases this may interfere with sexual intercourse. The diagnosis can be made by palpation of the penis. Ultrasound is used to evaluate the plaque size and consistency (ranging from hypoechoic to hyperechoic with retro-acoustic shadow) and is able to monitor therapy effectiveness (Fornara and Gerbershagen 2004). In these patients there is a higher incidence of arterial, venous and mixed vascular impotence (see Sect II.3.7.2.2, subsection "Erectile Dysfunction").

Testicular Volume and Testicular Echogenicity

Ultrasound is not indicated for the evaluation of testicular volume (Schiff et al. 2004) except in patients where the physical examination raises difficulties such as in patients with a large hydrocele.

The normal testis has a homogeneous fine granular appearance. In infertile men abnormal testicular echo

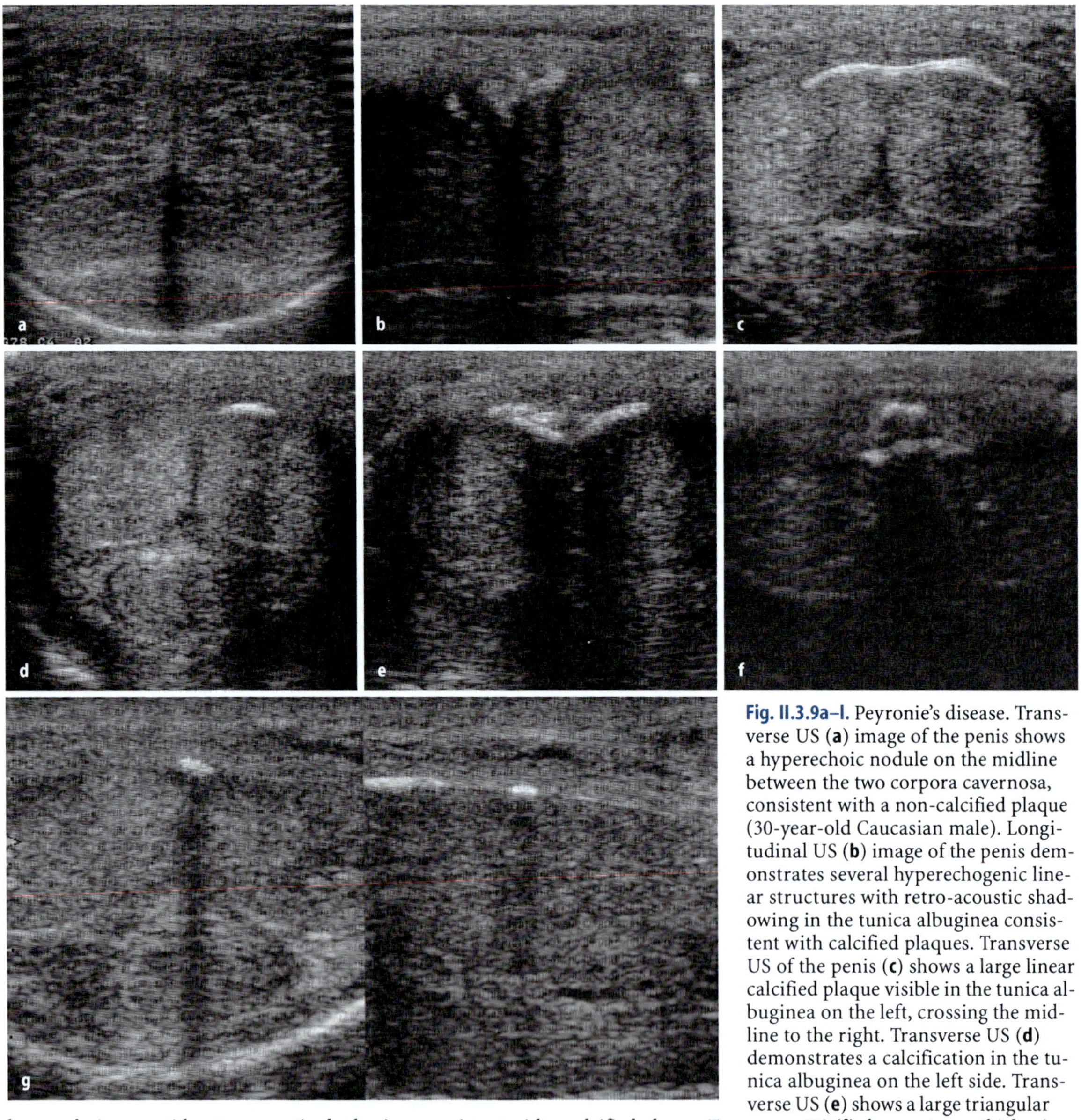

Fig. II.3.9a–l. Peyronie's disease. Transverse US (**a**) image of the penis shows a hyperechoic nodule on the midline between the two corpora cavernosa, consistent with a non-calcified plaque (30-year-old Caucasian male). Longitudinal US (**b**) image of the penis demonstrates several hyperechogenic linear structures with retro-acoustic shadowing in the tunica albuginea consistent with calcified plaques. Transverse US of the penis (**c**) shows a large linear calcified plaque visible in the tunica albuginea on the left, crossing the midline to the right. Transverse US (**d**) demonstrates a calcification in the tunica albuginea on the left side. Transverse US (**e**) shows a large triangular hyperechoic area with retro-acoustic shadowing, consistent with a calcified plaque. Transverse US (**f**) demonstrates thickening of the tunica albuginea, seen as a slightly hypoechoic band crossing the midline, with two linear calcifications in the centre: partially calcified plaque. Transverse (*left image*) and longitudinal (*right image*) (**g**) in the same patient. Transverse US shows a small calcification at the midline in the tunica albuginea, but on the longitudinal image several larger calcifications can be seen

Fig. II.3.9. (Cont.) Transverse (*left image*) (**h**) demonstrates a large calcified plaque in the tunica albuginea on the right side. Longitudinal US confirms these findings. Longitudinal US (**i**) shows multiple large calcifications in the tunica albuginea. Longitudinal US of the penis (**j**) demonstrates multiple hyperechoic rounded areas in the tunica albuginea, consistent with calcified plaques. Transverse US (**k**) shows a wedge-shaped hyperechoic structure at the midline in the tunica albuginea: calcified plaque. Transverse US (**l**) demonstrates several calcifications between the corpora cavernosa

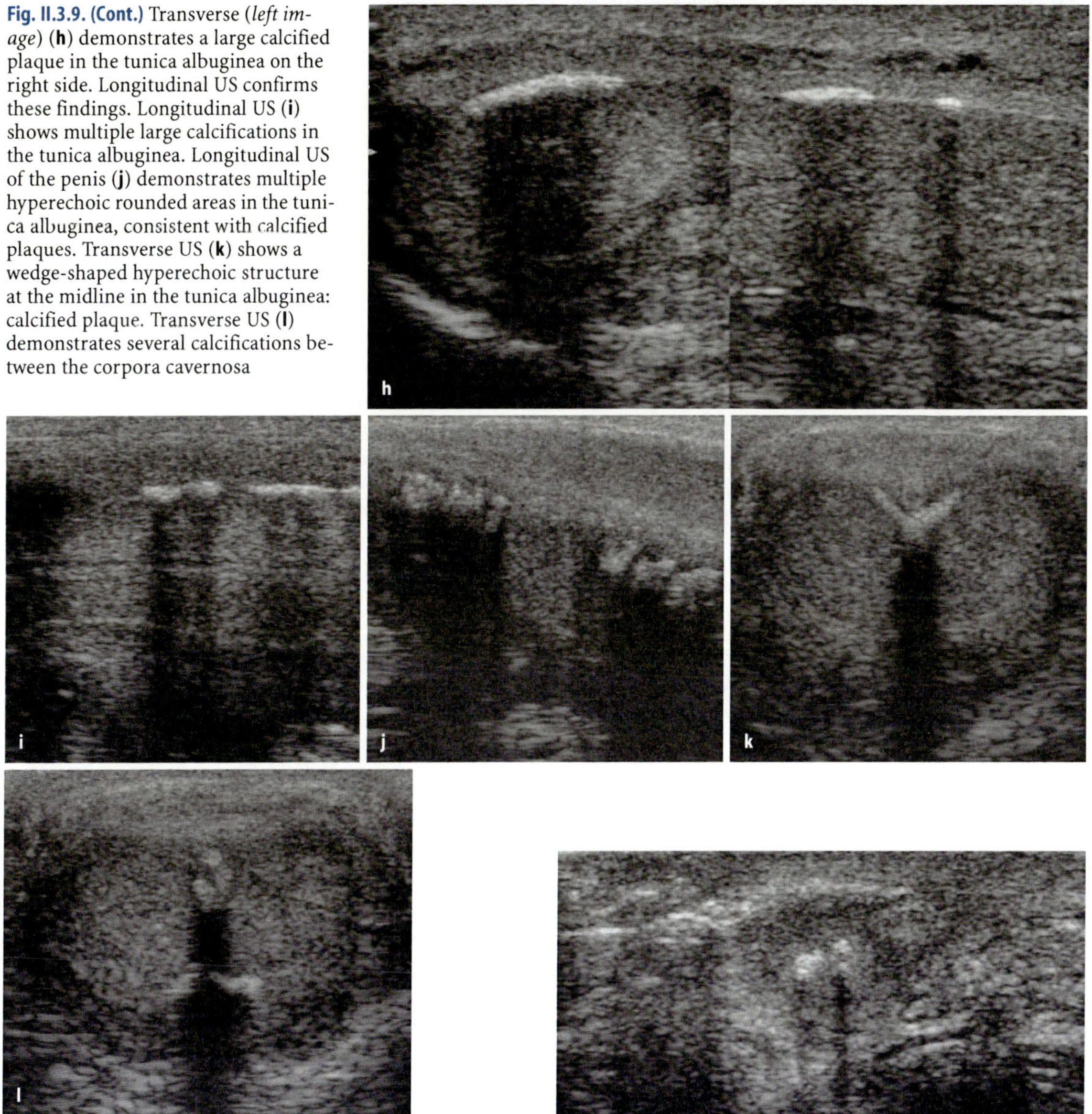

patterns can be expected such as patchy heterogeneity, hypoechoic lesions or echogenic foci. Such findings have been associated with a reduced testicular biopsy score and sperm count (Lenz et al. 1994).

Cryptorchidism (Figs. II.3.10, II.3.11)

One of the causes of hypofertility is undescended testis or a history of undescended testis. An undescended testis is abnormal in many ways (small volume, altered morphology, decreased echogenicity and presence of microlithiasis) and there is a definite increase in the incidence of testicular tumours. In general, testicular tumours are also predominately hypoechoic and this might jeopardize the US diagnosis of these lesions in

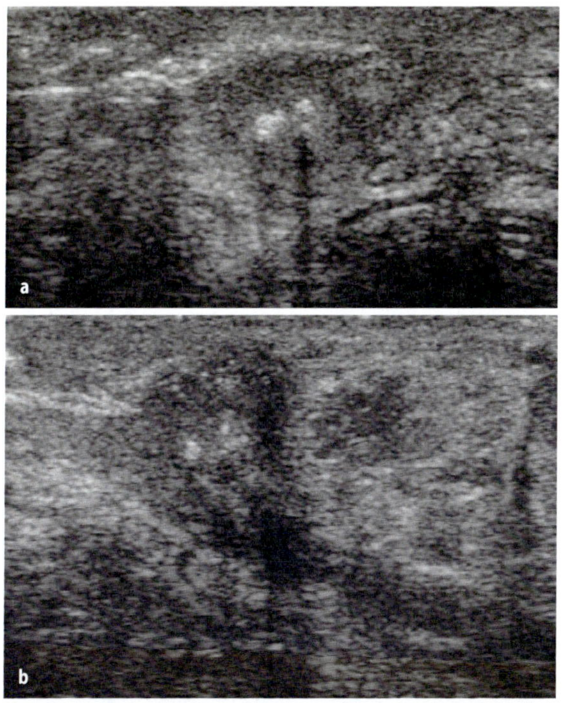

Fig. II.3.10a, b. Cryptorchidism. Transverse (**a**) and longitudinal (**b**) US demonstrates an atrophic/hypoplastic testicle in the inguinal canal with a hypoechoic appearance and several hyperechogenic spots centrally, consistent with calcifications

II.3

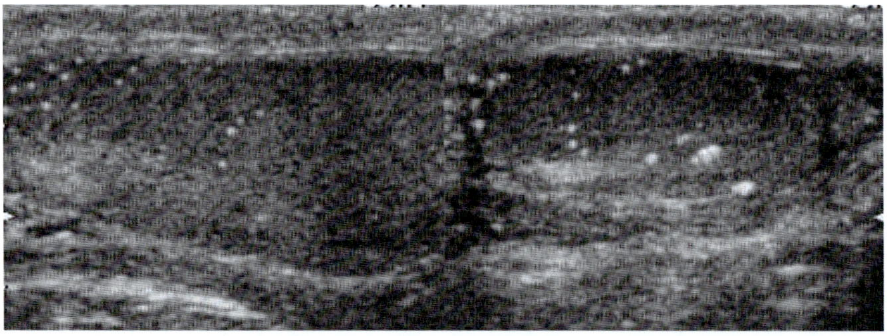

Fig. II.3.11. Testicular microlithiasis. Corrected cryptorchidism. Longitudinal US shows multiple tiny hyperechogenic spots in both hypoplastic testes, consistent with testicular microlithiasis

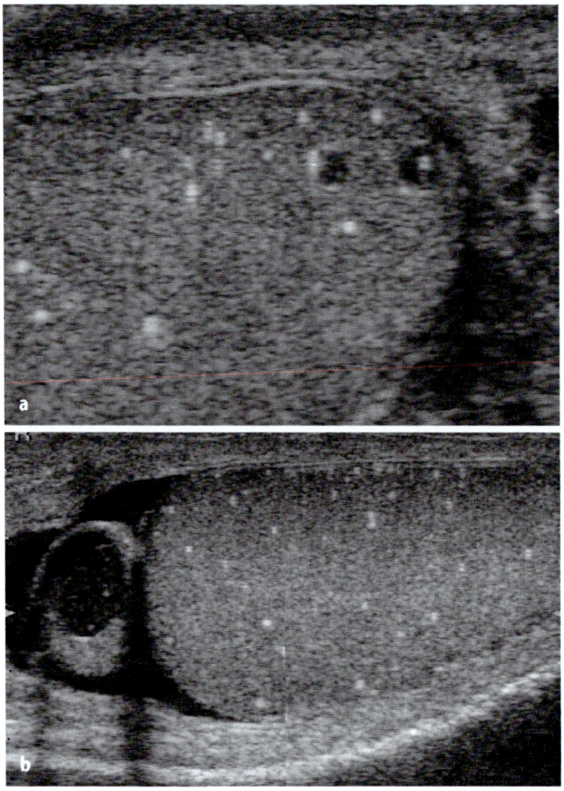

Fig. II.3.12a, b. Testicular microlithiasis. Longitudinal US (**a**) shows multiple tiny echogenic spots throughout the testicle, consistent with testicular microlithiasis. Near the lower pole, some of the calcifications seem to be located in or at the border of a subtle hypoechoic lesion. Longitudinal US (**b**) demonstrates multiple small calcifications in the testicle. There is a cyst in the epididymal head

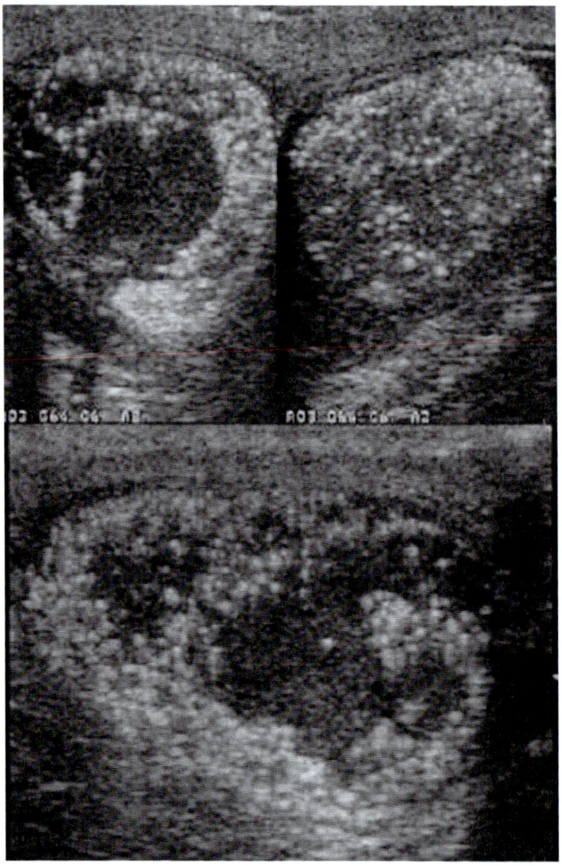

Fig. II.3.13. Testicular microlithiasis and seminoma. The *upper right* image shows a transverse view of the left testicle with the typical "snowstorm image", indicating testicular microlithiasis. The *upper left* image demonstrates a comparable transverse view of the right testicle where a large hypoechoic lesion can be seen "disrupting" the homogeneous snowstorm pattern. The *lower image* is a longitudinal view of the right testicle with a very large hypoechoic lesion centrally

the hypoechoic testis. Scrotal US is definitely indicated in these patients to detect testicular neoplasms at an early stage.

Testicular Microlithiasis (Figs. II.3.11–II.3.13)

Testicular microlithiasis is a rare condition with a reported incidence ranging from 0.6% to 9% in the general population (Thomas et al. 2000). It is more frequently seen in patients with cryptorchidism. Some authors also report an association with infertility (Aizenstein et al. 1998; Thomas et al. 2000) although there is no definite proof.

On US, single or multiple tiny hyperechoic spots are seen in the seminiferous tubules of the testis. Based on the number of calcifications, a classification system (grades I–III) may be used.

Caution is necessary since testicular microlithiasis seems to be associated with a higher risk of developing germ cell tumours (Miller et al. 1996; Thomas et al. 2000). Regular (6–12 months) US follow-up is recommended (Miller et al. 1996), especially in high-grade microlithiasis.

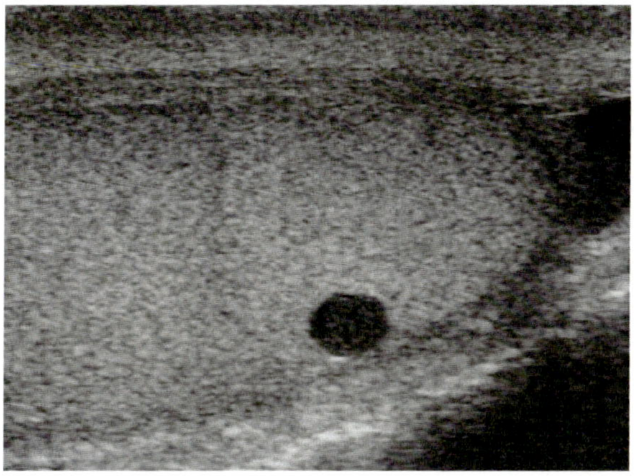

Fig. II.3.14. Testicular cyst. Longitudinal US shows a well-circumscribed rounded lesion near the lower pole of the testicle which appears very hypoechoic with some internal reflections

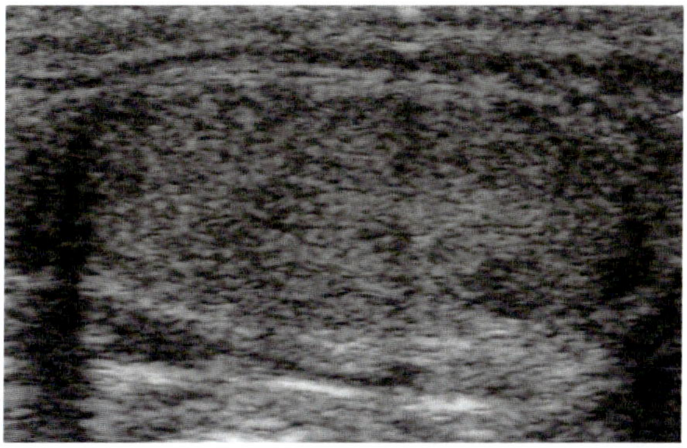

Fig. II.3.15. Leydig cell hyperplasia. Longitudinal US of the testicle demonstrates a heterogeneous appearance of the testicular parenchyma with multiple ill-marginated hypoechoic lesions. The patient was referred for infertility

Testicular Neoplasms (Figs. II.3.14–II.3.22)

The incidence of testicular cancer has been on the increase worldwide since the late twentieth century and there seems to be a higher incidence of testicular cancer in infertile men compared to the general population. Several reports state that a palpable lesion is present only in some patients (Pierik et al. 1999; Carmignani et al. 2004). In practice some authors have suggested that a routine scrotal US is indicated in all infertile men to detect testicular malignancies at early stages (impalpable) (Thomas 2004).

Most tumours have mixed echogenicity on US, with a predominately hypoechoic background and with or without calcifications or cystic areas. There are no typi-

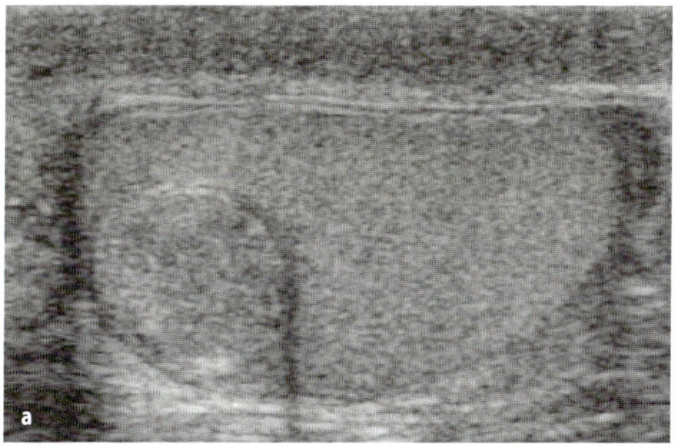

Fig. II.3.17a–c. Epidermoid cyst in a 27-year-old male with infertility. Longitudinal (**a**) US of the left testicle shows a rounded lesion in the upper pole of the testicle with a hyperechoic rim and a slightly hypoechoic centre. Near the centre of the lesion however are some hyperechoic spots. Transverse (**b**, **c**) scans of the left testicle demonstrate the same lesion which is well delineated and with mixed echogenicity. The testis was removed and the diagnosis of this benign tumour (teratoma here presenting as an epidermoid cyst) was obtained. However, there was tubular fibrosis, diffuse extensive intratubular germ cell dysplasia (*ITGCNU*), and a microfocus of invasive seminoma

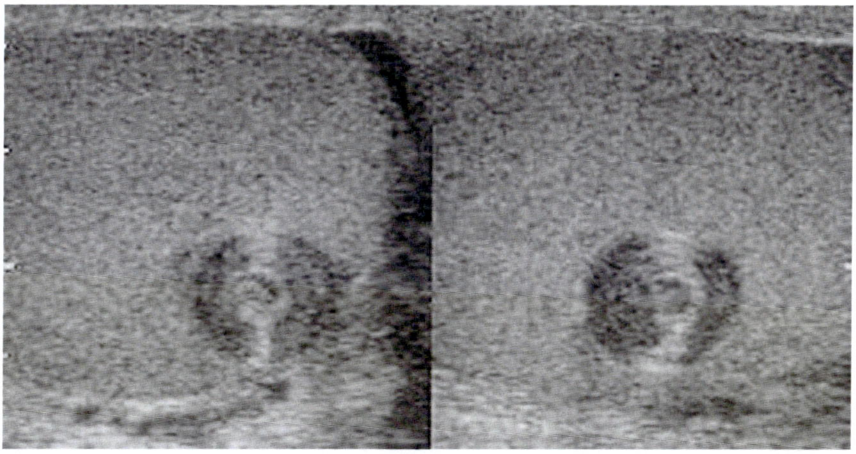

Fig. II.3.16. Epidermoid cyst. Transverse and longitudinal testicular US shows a well-delineated rounded hypoechoic lesion with concentric layering. This appearance is typical of an epidermoid cyst; yet not all epidermoid cysts have this appearance on US

II.3

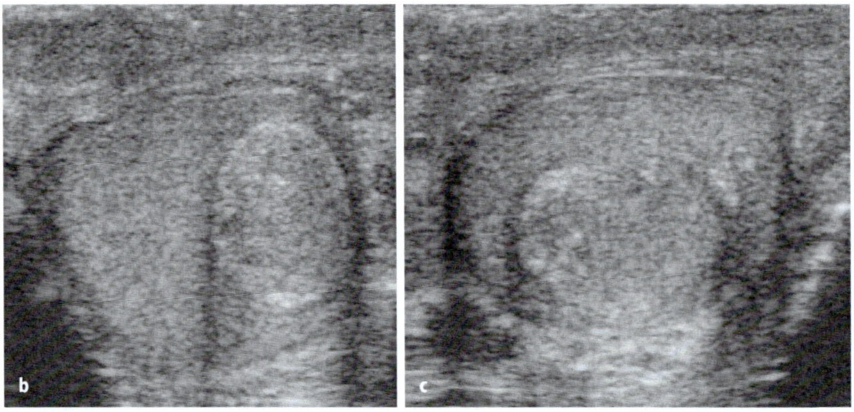

Fig. II.3.17 (Cont.)

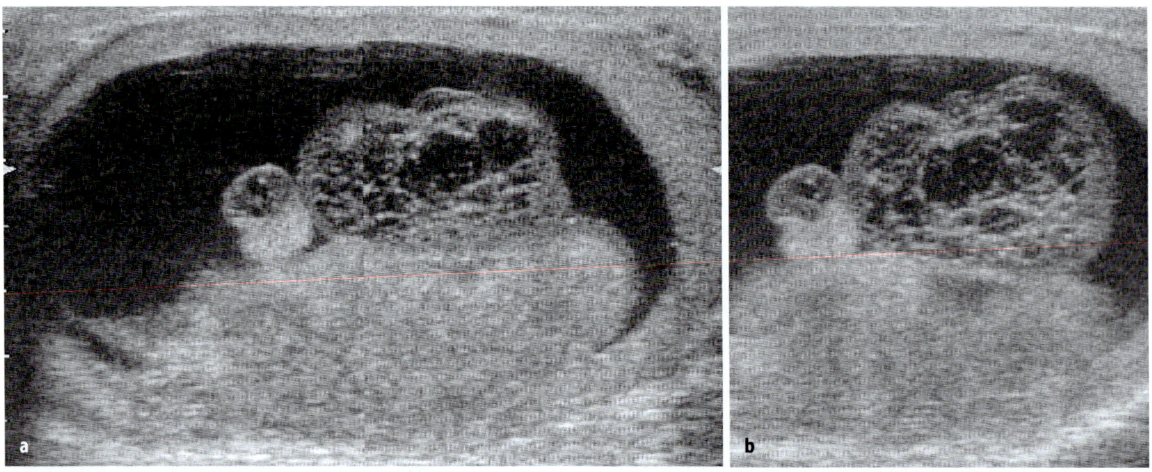

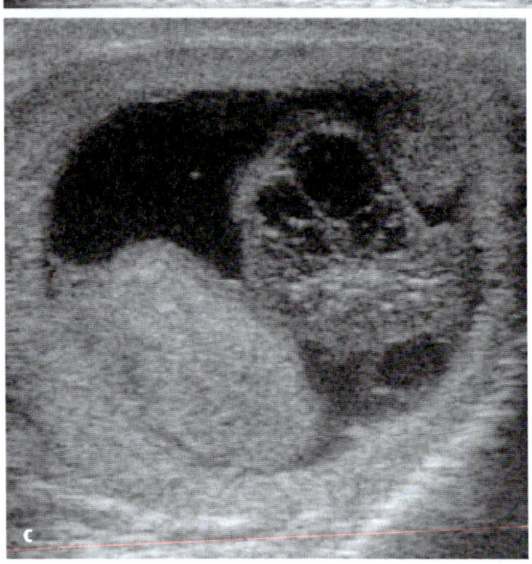

Fig. II.3.18a–c. Teratoma. Longitudinal US (**a**) of a testicle infiltrated completely by a large mass lesion consisting of different components: there is a large anechoic area (fluid) and there are several soft-tissue components with varying appearance; some appear hyperechogenic, others contain hypoechoic areas. Detailed view of the different soft-tissue components (**b**). Transverse US (**c**) illustrates the large cystic component and at least three different soft-tissue components (hyperechoic, mixed echo pattern with cystic areas and a hypoechoic component)

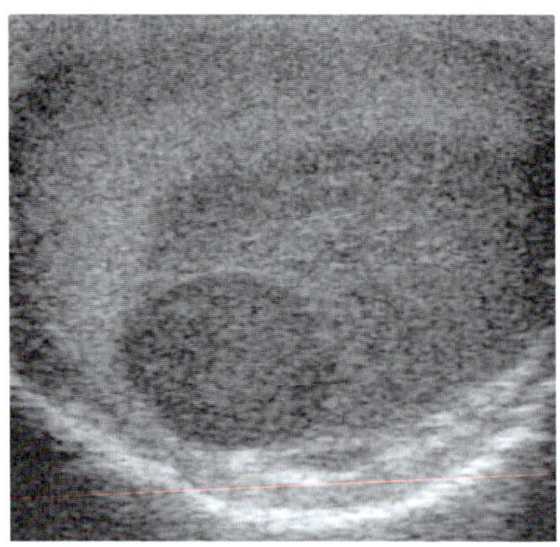

Fig. II.3.19. Seminoma. Transverse US of the testis demonstrates a rounded bilobar hypoechoic lesion in the periphery of the testicular parenchyma. Multinodular hypoechoic testicular masses are more frequently seen in seminoma

▷
Fig. II.3.20a, b. Seminoma. Longitudinal (**a**) and transverse (**b**) US of the testicle shows a small homogeneous hypoechoic lesion near the lower pole of the testicle. There is nothing specific about this lesion

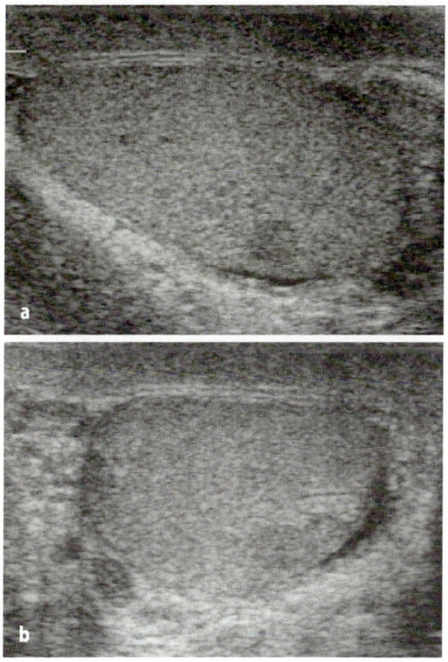

▷▷
Fig. II.3.21a, b. Mixed germ cell tumour. Firm testis at palpation. Longitudinal US (**a**) shows at least two hypoechoic lesions in the centre of the testicle and a third almost isoechoic lesion with an anechoic rim in the periphery of the testis. Spot view of the lesions (**b**). Mixed germ cell tumour consisting predominantly of embryonic carcinoma, and microscopic foci of yolk sac tumour and teratoma

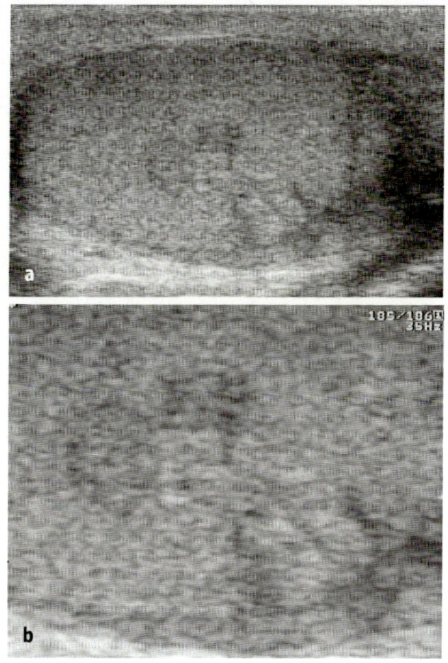

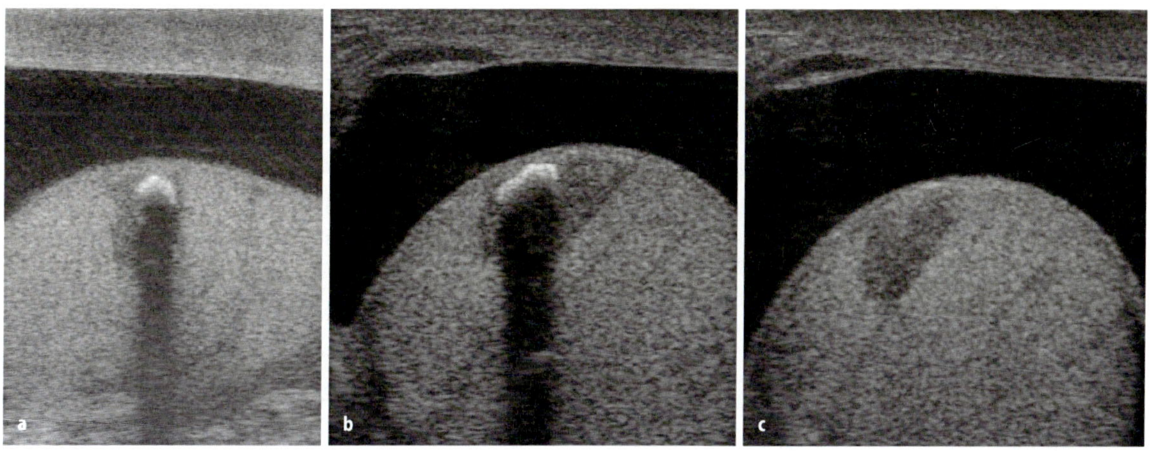

Fig. II.3.22a–c. Testicular scar and calcification. Longitudinal US (**a**) demonstrates a wedge-shaped hypoechoic area harbouring a hyperechoic curvilinear structure with a retro-acoustic shadow, consistent with calcification. The fluid surrounding the testicle represents a hydrocele. Transverse US (**b**) shows the calcification and the hypoechoic area which is now better appreciated. On this transverse view (**c**), the calcification is not visible. The well-circumscribed triangular hypoechoic area however is well seen

cal or reliable imaging characteristics for histological characterization of testicular tumours (Oyen et al. 1999; Oyen 2002; Woodward et al. 2002).

Evaluation of Obstructive Azoospermia (Cornud et al. 1997)

For a quick overview, see also Table II.3.9.

Azoospermia or Severe Oligozoospermia with a Normal Volume Ejaculate: Proximal Obstruction (*Figs. II.3.23, II.3.24*)

Scrotal US has no significant role in these patients since the enlargement of the epididymis is also palpable. US, however, has a much more important role when the obstruction is proximal to the junction of the head and body of the epididymis. In this case biochemical epididymal markers will be normal as will be the physical examination. Only US can demonstrate the obstruction by isolated dilation of the rete testis.

Table II.3.9. Evaluation of obstructive azoospermia

	Proximal obstruction	Proximal obstruction at the level of the epididymis	Distal obstruction CBAVD	Distal obstruction with palpable vas deferens
Semen analysis	Azoospermia or severe oligozoospermia Normal volume ejaculate Normal fructose Alkaline pH>7 Normal biochemical epididymal markers	Azoospermia or severe oligozoospermia Normal volume ejaculate Normal fructose Alkaline pH>7 Low biochemical epididymal markers	Azoospermia or severe oligozoospermia Low-volume ejaculate Low fructose Acid pH<7	Azoospermia or severe oligozoospermia Low-volume ejaculate Low fructose Acid pH<7
Scrotal US	Isolated dilation of rete testis	Enlargement of epididymis Hypoechoic epididymis Dilation of epididymal tube	Dilation of the efferent ducts Abrupt stop at the body of the epididymis	Obstructive epididymis
TRUS	Normal or signs of chronic prostatitis	Normal or signs of chronic prostatitis	Absence of vasal ampullae 90% abnormalities seminal vesicle (ranging from uni- or bilateral absence to hypoplasia, cysts, calcifications, hyperechoic appearance)	Median cyst (Mullerian/utricular or Wollfian) Dilation of seminal vesicles Seminal vesicle cyst Lithiasis in ejaculatory ducts or vasal ampulla Chronic prostatitis (patchy pattern of peripheral zone) Prostate cancer

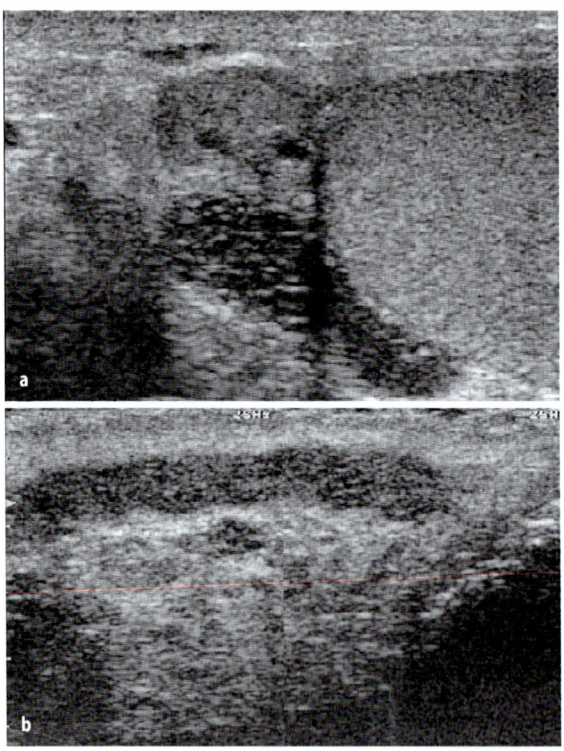

Fig. II.3.23a, b. Agenesis of the epididymal tail. Longitudinal scrotal US (**a**) demonstrates an enlarged epididymal head and body which appear hypoechoic (dilated), indicating an obstruction more distally. The epididymal tail is absent. The testicle appears normal. Longitudinal US (**b**) in the same patient again shows the cystically enlarged epididymis over its full length, including head and body, and confirms the absence of the epididymal tail

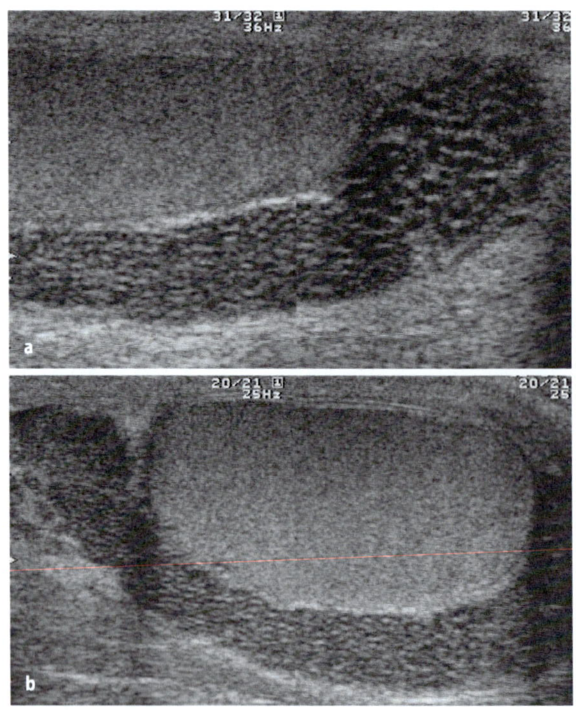

Fig. II.3.24a, b. Obstruction of the epididymis after vasectomy. Longitudinal US (**a**) demonstrates the dilated epididymal body and tail with a hypoechoic (cystic) appearance, indicating an obstruction more proximally. Longitudinal US (**b**) in the same patient again shows the cystically dilated epididymis (head and body)

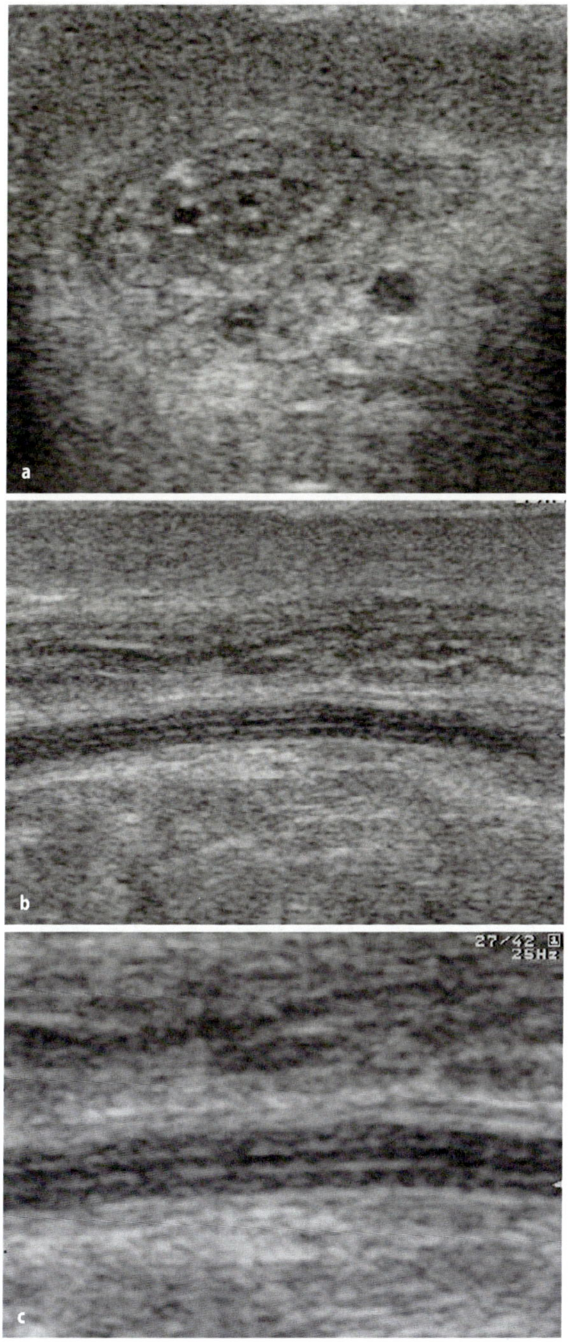

Fig. II.3.25a–c. Normal deferent duct. Transverse US (**a**) demonstrates a small rounded hypoechoic area with two linear hyperechogenic structures in the centre. This is the normal deferent duct in transverse section. Longitudinal US (**b**) shows a long tubular hypoechoic structure with two hyperechoic lines centrally: normal deferent duct. Spot view longitudinal US (**c**) again demonstrating the normal deferent duct. The appearance is explained by the thick smooth muscle wall enveloping the lumen of the deferent duct

Azoospermia or Severe Oligozoospermia with Low Volume Ejaculate (<2 ml): Distal Obstruction *(Figs. II.3.25–II.3.35)*

Since normal fructose levels in semen indicate normal function of the seminal vesicles, low fructose levels strongly suggest vasal aplasia or distal obstruction at the level of the distal vas, vasal ampulla, seminal vesicles, ejaculatory ducts or periurethral prostate (Kuligowska and Fenlon 1998).

The two vasa deferentia cannot be felt. Congenital bilateral absence of vas deferens (CBAVD) is strongly suspected when there is total azoospermia, semen volume is below 1 ml, fructose level is below the detection limit and pH<7 as prostatic secretions mainly contribute to the semen volume. The agenesis starts at the junction of the body and tail of the epididymis. Clinically the dilation of the epididymal head and body can be palpated. Additional renal US is recommended in these patients since 43% of patients will have renal anomalies ranging from unilateral renal agenesis, crossed fused ectopia or ectopic pelvic kidney. CBAVD is observed in 98% of men with cystic fibrosis. It is

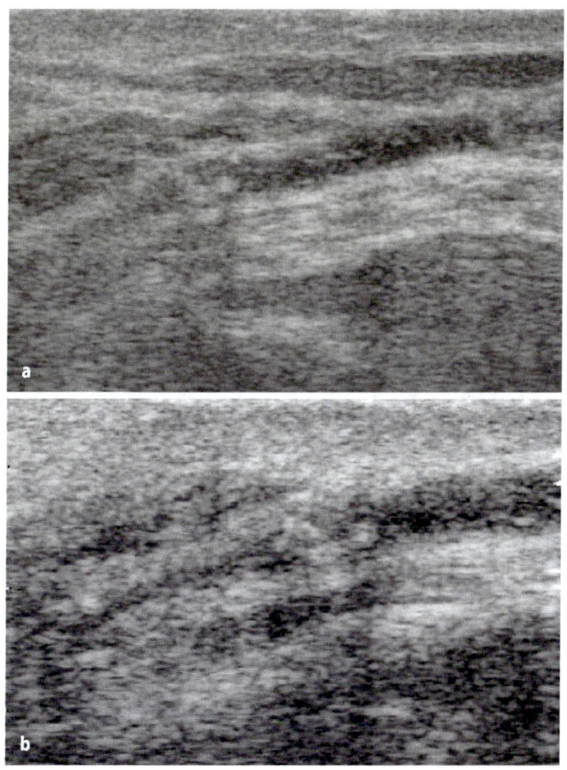

Fig. II.3.26a, b. Obstruction at the level of the deferent duct. Longitudinal US (**a**) demonstrates a normal appearance of the deferent duct on the *right side* of the image, followed by an abrupt stop seen as a hyperechoic structure in the centre of the deferent duct. Spot view longitudinal US (**b**). There is some retro-acoustic shadowing behind the hyperechoic structure in the deferent duct, consistent with calcification. Another calcification can be seen just distal to it

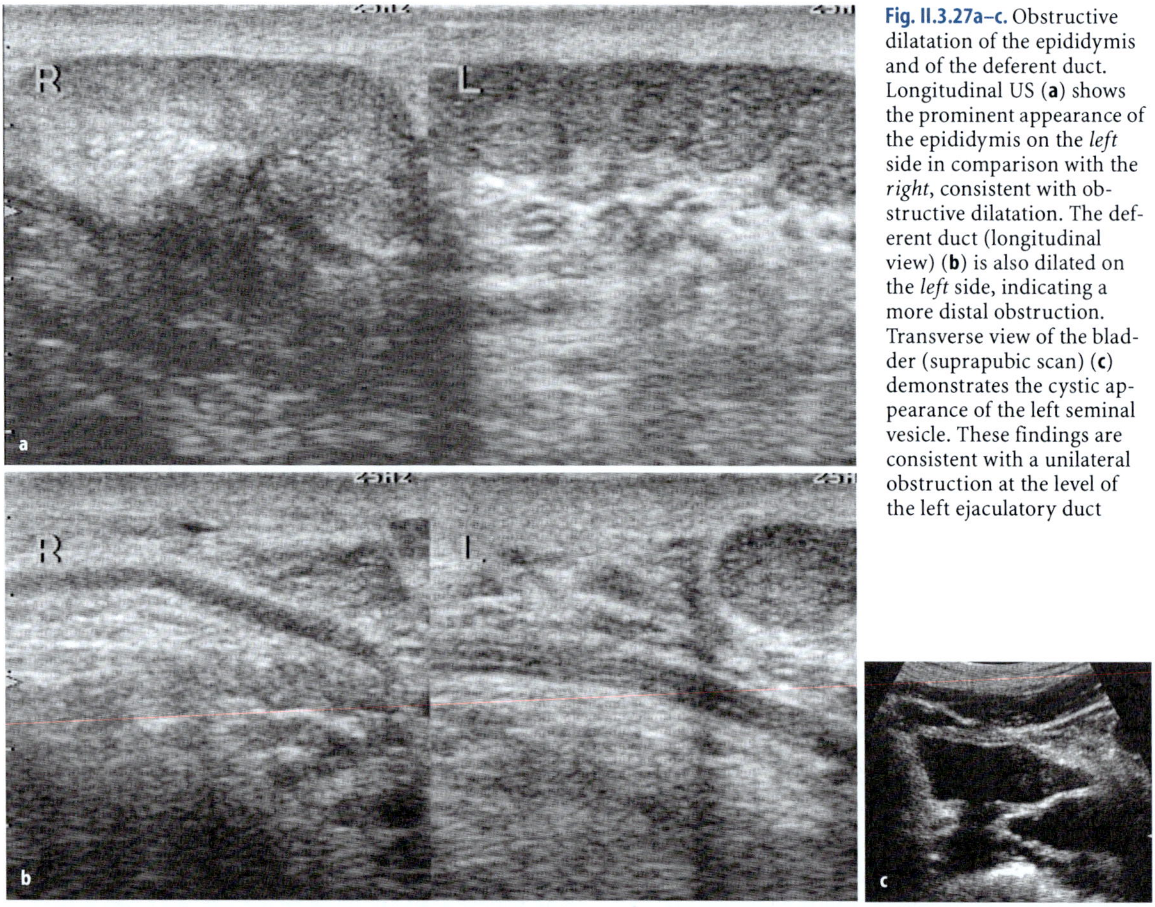

Fig. II.3.27a–c. Obstructive dilatation of the epididymis and of the deferent duct. Longitudinal US (**a**) shows the prominent appearance of the epididymis on the *left* side in comparison with the *right*, consistent with obstructive dilatation. The deferent duct (longitudinal view) (**b**) is also dilated on the *left* side, indicating a more distal obstruction. Transverse view of the bladder (suprapubic scan) (**c**) demonstrates the cystic appearance of the left seminal vesicle. These findings are consistent with a unilateral obstruction at the level of the left ejaculatory duct

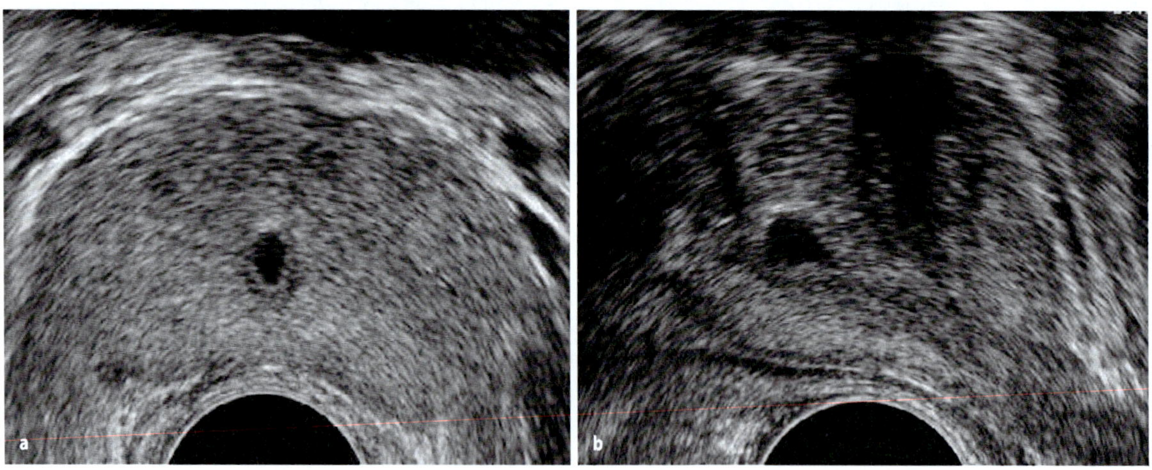

Fig. II.3.28a, b. Utricular cyst. Transverse US (**a**) at the base of the prostate shows a small hypoechoic "cyst" in the centre: small midline cyst. Longitudinal US (**b**) at the midline confirms the presence of a small cystic lesion posterior to the prostatic urethra

now thought to be an acquired lesion, which also explains incomplete forms with variable presentation (normal volume ejaculate, moderately reduced fructose and pH>7).

Two Vasa Deferentia are Palpable

The obstruction can be complete (1 ml) or partial (1.5–2 ml volume ejaculate), congenital (compression by median cyst) or acquired (distal inflammatory or traumatic stenosis).

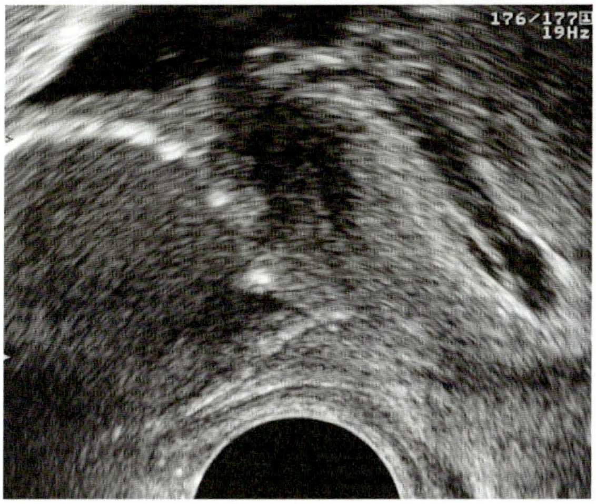

Fig. II.3.29. Midline cyst. Sagittal transrectal ultrasonography (*TRUS*) shows a large hypoechoic lesion at the midline at the base of the prostate, consistent with a midline cyst. In the periphery of this cyst, several hyperechoic foci are seen, indicating calcifications of its wall

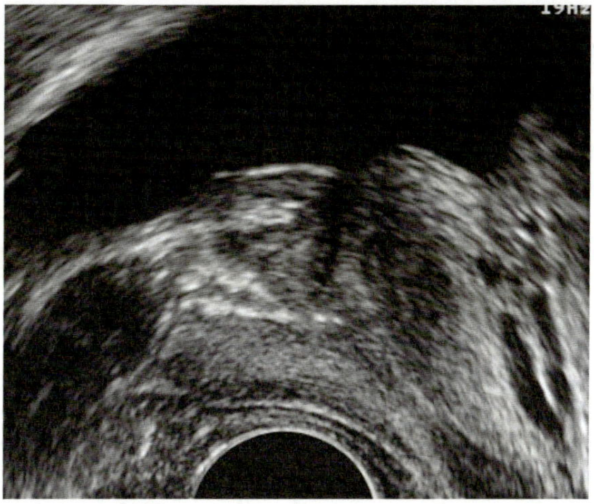

Fig. II.3.31. Calcifications of the ejaculatory duct complex. Sagittal TRUS shows multiple hyperechogenic foci in or around the ejaculatory duct, consistent with multiple calcifications. The seminal vesicle appears enlarged, indicating obstruction of the ejaculatory duct

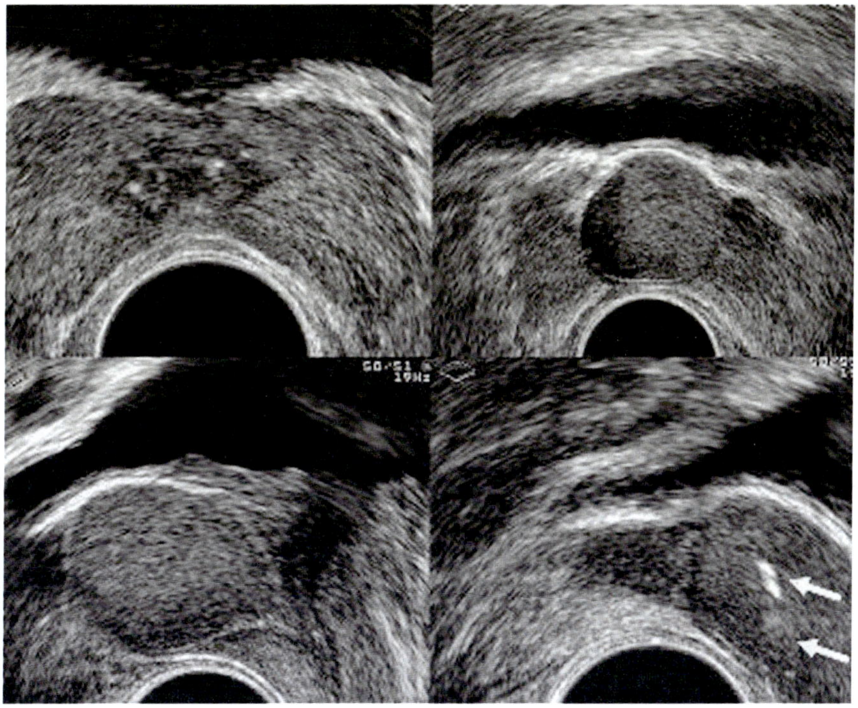

Fig. II.3.30. Aspiration of complicated midline cyst. *Left upper image*: transverse TRUS at the base of the prostate demonstrates a slightly hypoechoic structure at the midline. *Right upper image*: transverse TRUS in the same patient, slightly cephalad to the previous image. A well-defined rounded structure is visible at the midline, consistent with a midline cyst. The cyst contains a fluid level with multiple small internal reflections in the lower part, consistent with debris, e.g. after haemorrhage and/or infection. *Left lower image*: sagittal TRUS through the lower part of the lesion again shows the rounded hypoechoic midline cyst at the base of the prostate. *Right lower image*: sagittal TRUS guiding transrectal aspiration of the cyst (*arrows* indicating the needle)

Median cysts are subdivided into two categories: Müllerian or utricular cysts (contain no semen) and Wolffian cysts (contain semen). When the ejaculatory ducts are compressed by these cysts, they become obstructive. However, on US dilation of the seminal vesicles or vasal ampullae may be absent and mild dilation of the seminal vesicles may be physiological.

Stones are mainly located at the vasal ampulla, the ejaculatory duct or the verumontanum (periurethral prostate). Distal ejaculatory duct stenosis may also be acquired by inflammation, which can sometimes be suggested by associated features of (chronic) prostatitis revealed by US.

Multifocal obstruction cannot be diagnosed with US. Vasography has been the gold standard for years, but has been replaced by MRI or puncture of the

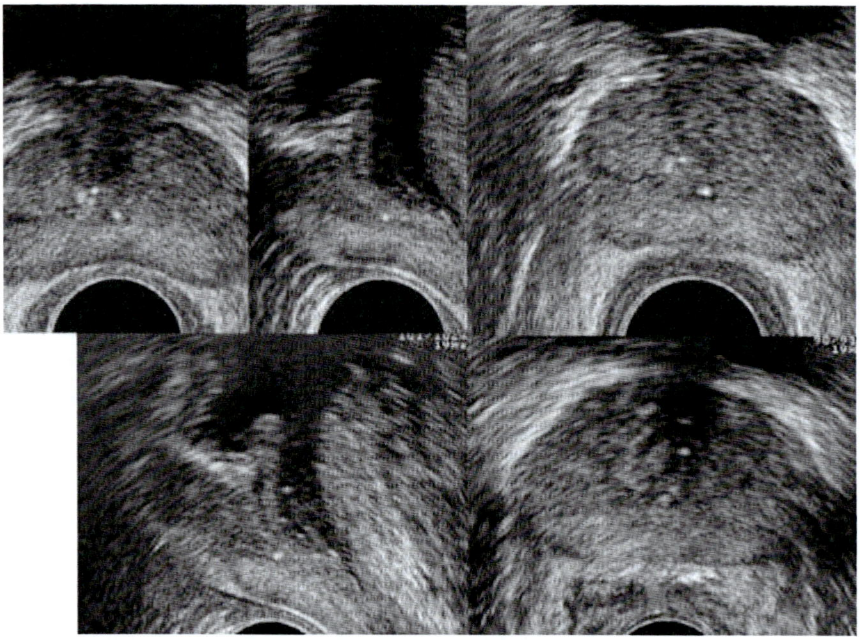

Fig. II.3.32. Calcifications of the ejaculatory duct complex. Transverse TRUS (*left upper, right upper, right lower image*) demonstrates several small punctiform hyperechogenic foci in the vicinity of the ejaculatory duct near the colliculus seminalis. Sagittal US (*middle upper image, left lower image*) again shows the small calcifications along the course of the ejaculatory duct

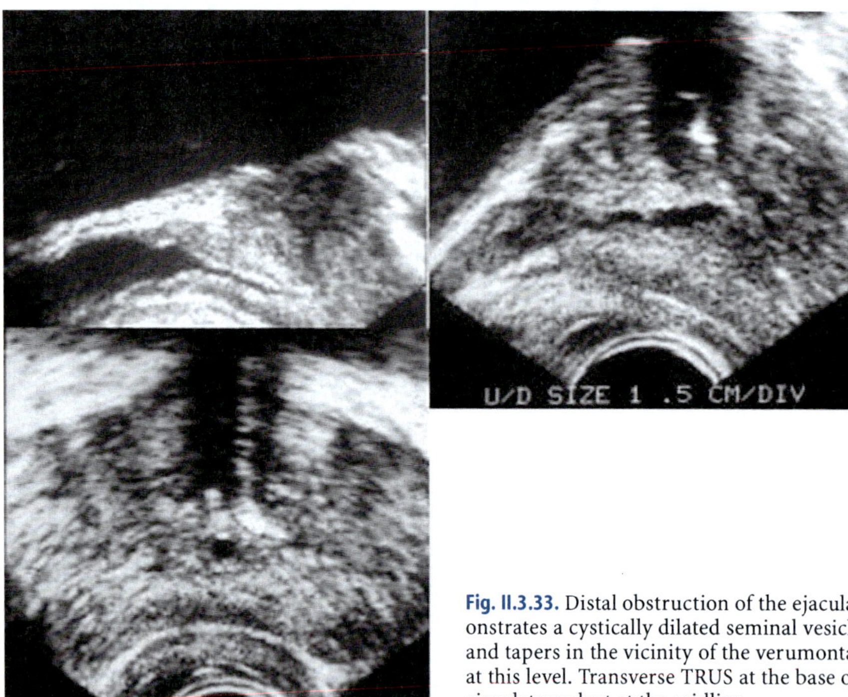

Fig. II.3.33. Distal obstruction of the ejaculatory ducts. Sagittal TRUS demonstrates a cystically dilated seminal vesicle. The ejaculatory duct is dilated and tapers in the vicinity of the verumontanum, indicating an obstruction at this level. Transverse TRUS at the base of the prostate shows the dilated ejaculatory duct at the midline

seminal vesicles under TRUS guidance with or without vesiculography. If motile sperm can be demonstrated, this indicates the absence of a proximal obstruction. Likewise if no motile sperm can be found, then the azoospermia is not due to a distal obstruction.

Partial obstruction cannot be documented by any imaging modality (Jones et al. 1997).

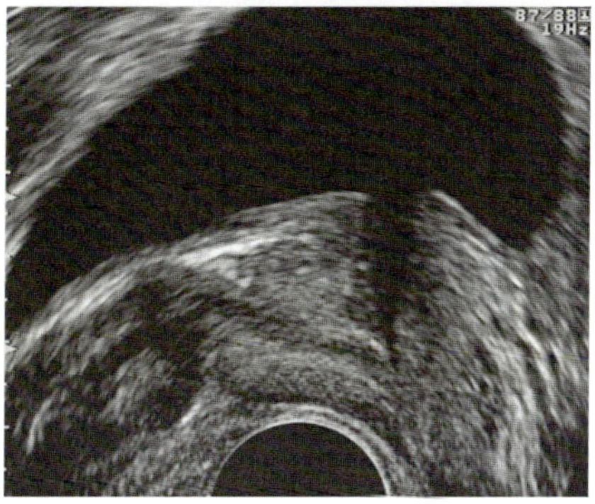

▷
Fig. II.3.34. Distal obstruction of the ejaculatory duct. Sagittal TRUS demonstrates cystic dilatation of the seminal vesicle and an enlarged ejaculatory duct, consistent with a distal obstruction (at the verumontanum)

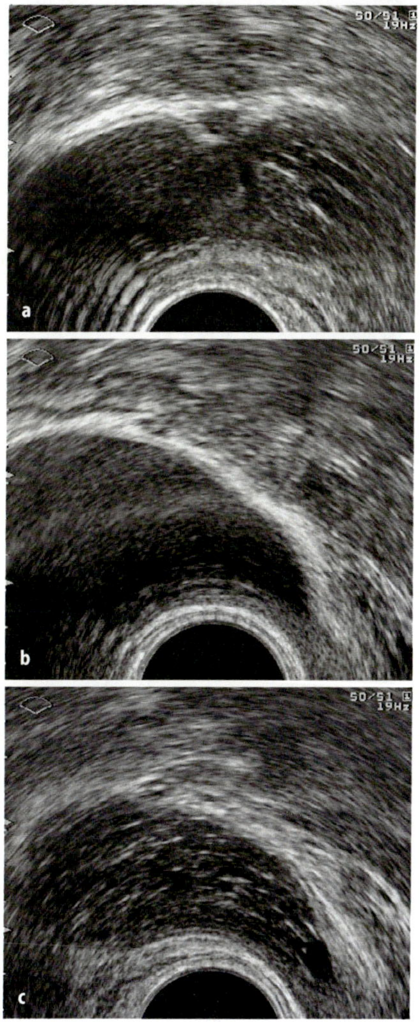

▷▷
Fig. II.3.35a–c. Cystically dilated seminal vesicles. Patient with autosomal dominant polycystic kidney disease (*ADPKD*). Transverse (**a**) and parasagittal (**b**, **c**) TRUS at the level of the seminal vesicles shows that both seminal vesicles are enlarged and have a cystic appearance. These are mega seminal vesicles in patients with ADPKD not likely to be explained by obstruction

II.3.7.2 Doppler

II.3.7.2.1 Technique

Doppler is a noninvasive US-based imaging technique that measures movement or flow. The scanning can be done continuously (continuous wave Doppler, CW) or pulsed (pulsed Doppler, PW).

Continuous wave instruments have a transducer with separate piezoelectric crystals: one to continuously produce the sound waves and one to receive the reflected echoes. The main disadvantage is that the depth information is lost; this technique works well for superficial vessels and is very sensitive to weak signals.

Pulsed wave instruments use the same transducer as on a regular ultrasound machine. A burst of sound waves is transmitted and then the returning signal is received. This process is repeated in a very short timeframe. By comparing the information from the consecutive cycles flow calculation can be obtained. In colour Doppler mode the direction and the velocity of the flow can be shown, while in power Doppler mode only the velocity can be determined, yet with greater sensitivity.

In both colour and power Doppler mode a small area can be selected for spectral analysis. Spectral Doppler mode plots this information in a velocity versus time graph with negative velocity indicating opposite flow direction. From the spectral waveform, additional quantitative parameters can be derived.

Since colour and power Doppler provide a limited amount of information over a large region, and spectral Doppler provides more detailed information about a specific area, these modes are complementary and, in practice, are used as such.

II.3.7.2.2 Clinical Indications

Erectile Dysfunction

Vasculogenic impotence is one of the major causes of erectile dysfunction. The more invasive techniques such as arteriography, cavernosometry and cavernosography have been replaced by colour or power Doppler US in combination with the intracavernosal injection of vasoactive drugs (such as prostaglandin E_1, alprostadil, papaverine). Certain authors use oral intake of sildenafil, a combination of oral drugs and intracavernosal injection or a transurethral injection (e.g. transurethral alprostadil: less effective and less reliable in comparison with intracavernous alprostadil; Ahn et al. 2004). The most often used drug is prostaglandin E_1 intracavernosally.

After pharmacological induction of erection, the cavernosal artery (right and/or left) will be interrogated. The diameter of this artery is no longer routinely used by several authors as the correlation with the peak systolic velocity (PSV) or with the clinical grading of the erection is weak. Spectral waveforms are obtained from the cavernosal artery which will show typical features in a certain time course. Early in tumescence there will be an increase of the systolic and diastolic flow which will then decrease and eventually there will be reversal of the diastolic flow as veno-occlusion occurs. A PSV of 35 cm/s or greater is diagnostic of a sufficient arterial inflow, while a PSV of 25 cm/s or less indicates arterial insufficiency. A venous leak or venogenic impotence is diagnosed if the end diastolic velocity (EDV) is greater than 5 cm/s, provided that the arterial inflow is sufficient. Abnormal draining veins may be present but are not necessary for the diagnosis (Wilkins et al. 2003).

The intermediate values are not specific. Research however has shown that the cavernosal arteries give rise to the capillary arteries (nutrient vessels for the corpus cavernosum) and the helicine arteries, which connect directly to the cavernous sinusoids. Power Doppler is needed to visualize these small arteries and the same haemodynamic variables have been studied in different patient groups (Sakamoto et al. 2002). Three-dimensional representation of the arterial supply has been described by some authors but the benefit for diagnosis and therapy remains questionable.

Varicocele (Figs. II.3.36, II.3.37)

Varicocele is a very common finding and can be seen in 20–40% of infertile men. Colour Doppler US is a very reliable test for detecting nonpalpable reflux (probably the only significant subclinical varicocele) or for confirming questionable reflux at clinical examination. This will be further discussed in the next chapter.

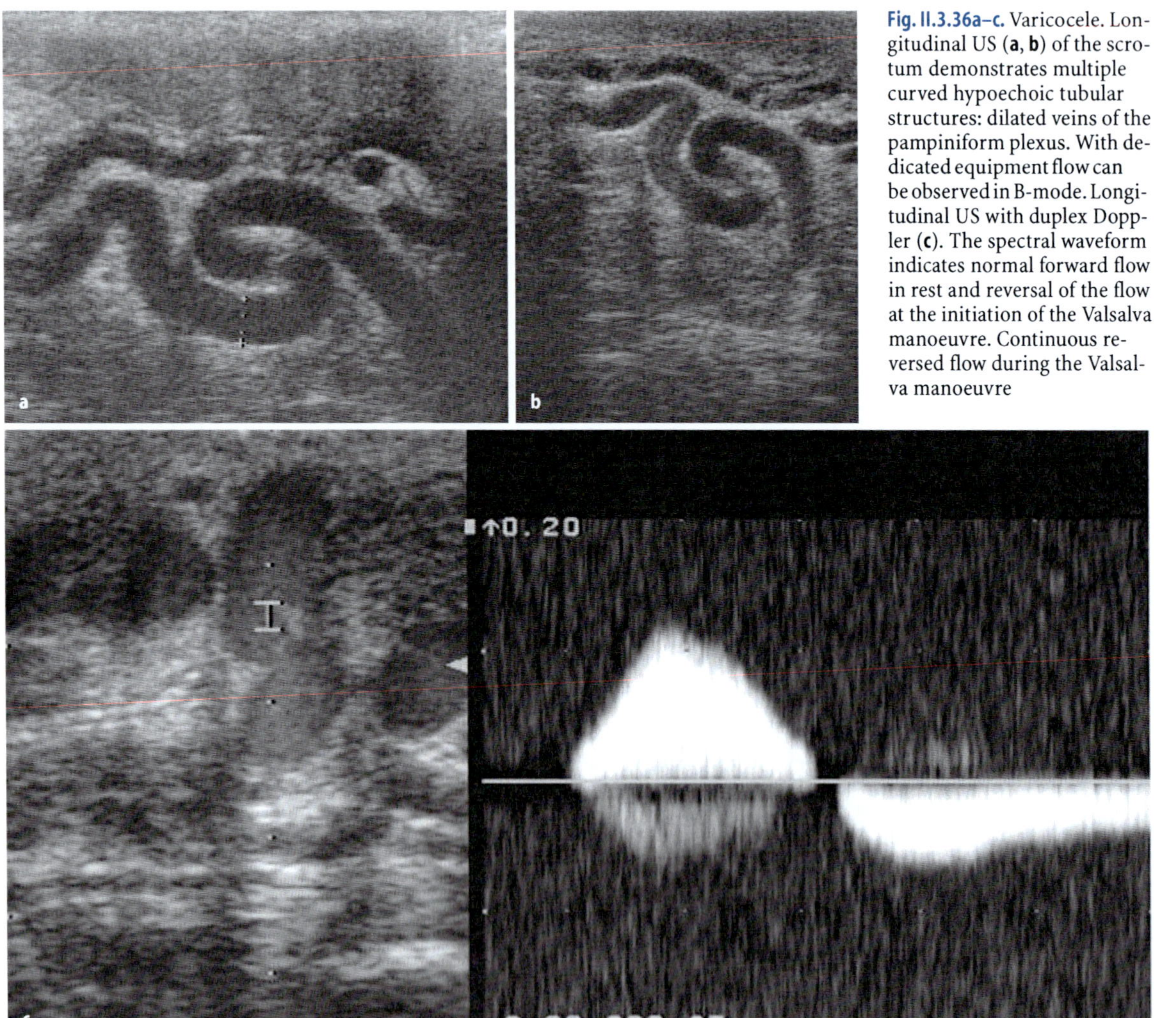

Fig. II.3.36a–c. Varicocele. Longitudinal US (**a**, **b**) of the scrotum demonstrates multiple curved hypoechoic tubular structures: dilated veins of the pampiniform plexus. With dedicated equipment flow can be observed in B-mode. Longitudinal US with duplex Doppler (**c**). The spectral waveform indicates normal forward flow in rest and reversal of the flow at the initiation of the Valsalva manoeuvre. Continuous reversed flow during the Valsalva manoeuvre

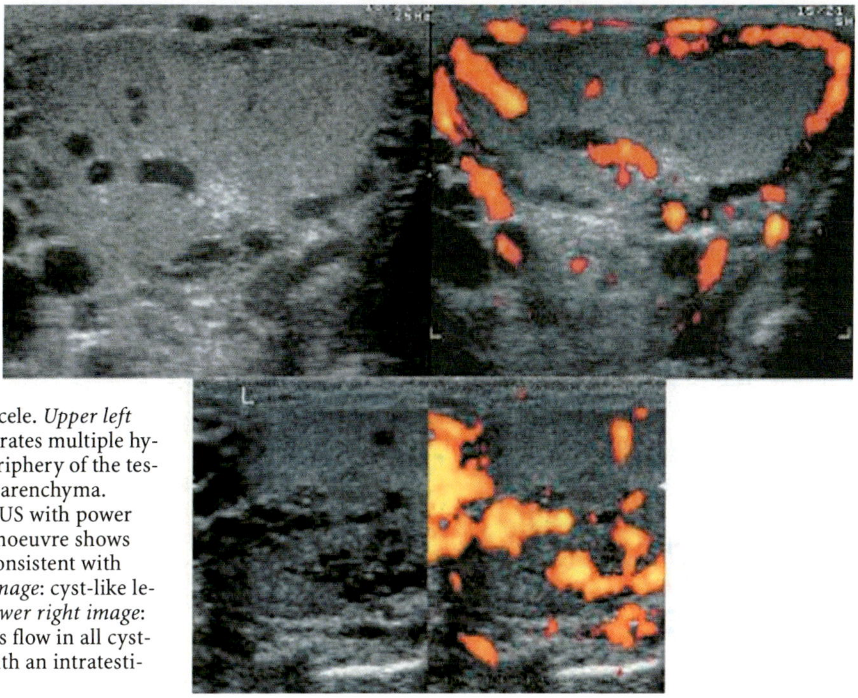

Fig. II.3.37. Intratesticular varicocele. *Upper left image*: longitudinal US demonstrates multiple hypoechoic ovoid lesions in the periphery of the testicle as well as in the testicular parenchyma. *Upper right image*: longitudinal US with power Doppler during the Valsalva manoeuvre shows that all these ovoid lesions are consistent with vascular structures. *Lower left image*: cyst-like lesions throughout the testicle. *Lower right image*: US with power Doppler confirms flow in all cyst-like lesions. This is consistent with an intratesticular varicocele

Tumours

Doppler will be used in the evaluation of tumours of the male genital tract, mainly to differentiate between a nontumorous mass lesion (such as a haematoma) and a tumour, by demonstrating the presence of vessels in a tumour. Such sophisticated techniques will not help to differentiate between a benign and a malignant tumour, to further differentiate between the different types of tumours and nor will they help to indicate the grade of malignancy of a tumour.

Guidance for Sperm Retrieval

Instead of performing random biopsy samples for testicular sperm extraction (TESE) in preparation for assisted reproduction, some authors have suggested that sperm quality and quantity depend on tissue perfusion within the testicle. Therefore, they propose that testicular biopsy samples should be taken from areas with high perfusion, which can be demonstrated by using power Doppler (with or without 3D mapping) (Har-Toov et al. 2004) or contrast-enhanced US with a laser Doppler scanner (Herwig et al. 2004). These techniques may reduce the number of biopsies, improve the outcome and have the potential to reduce testicular damage (Har-Toov et al. 2004).

II.3.7.3 MRI (Magnetic Resonance Imaging)

II.3.7.3.1 Technique

An MRI system is basically a large magnet in which the patient is installed. The human body consists largely of water molecules (two atoms of hydrogen joined to one atom of oxygen – H_2O). Hydrogen atoms consist of outer shells of one negatively charged particle (electron) buzzing around and a nucleus with a positive charge. These nuclei behave like small magnets and when placed in the powerful magnetic field of the MR system, about half line up in the direction of the magnetic field and about half line up in the opposite direction. After sending in a radio wave, the orientation of these tiny magnets can be changed, to resonate absorbing energy at a resonance frequency that depends directly on the strength of the magnetic field. The resulting magnetic signal can be detected and decoded by the computer into a 2D image. MRI enables scanning of the body or parts of it noninvasively in any spatial plane.

Pacemakers and certain metals are incompatible with MR.

II.3.7.3.2 Clinical Indications

Hypothalamo–Pituitary Axis

The method of choice for visualizing the hypothalamo-pituitary axis is MRI (Rhoden et al. 2003).

Penis and Scrotal Contents

Imaging of the penis can be done with or without the intracavernosal administration of prostaglandin E_1. MRI of the penis and scrotal contents is in almost all instances performed after an initial inconclusive evaluation using US with or without Doppler. Intravenous administration of contrast may be indicated to further evaluate the scrotal and penile abnormalities. The MR indications are listed in Table II.3.10.

Obstructive Azoospermia (Figs. II.3.38, II.3.39)

Endorectal MRI of the prostate and ejaculatory complex can be performed and provides high-resolution images. Again MRI is indicated as a problem-solving technique only.

Table II.3.10. MR indications

	Malignant tumour	Benign mass	Trauma	Vascular disorders	Follow-up after treatment
Penis (Pretorius,2001)	Squamous cell carcinoma Sarcoma - Epitheloid sarcoma - Kaposi sarcoma - Leiomyosarcoma - Rhabdomyosarcoma Penile metastases - Primary malignancies genitourinary tract - Colon - Stomach - Esophagus - Pancreas	Cowper duct Syringocele Periurethral abscess Partial cavernosal thrombosis Peyronie's disease	- Penile fracture - Tears of tunica albuginea - Posterior urethral injury	Arteriogenic impotence (large vessels)	After partial or total penectomy - Tumor recurrence - Postsurgical findings - Complications of surgery - Penile prostheses
Testicle	Germ cell tumors - Seminomas - Nonseminomatous tumors - Embryonal carcinoma - Yolk sac tumor - Choriocarcinoma - Teratoma Mixed germ cell tumor	Sertoli cell tumor Leydig cell tumor 90% benign Intratesticular cyst Epidermoid cyst Congenital adrenal hyperplasia Sarcoidosis	Testicular fracture	(segmental) testicular infarction	

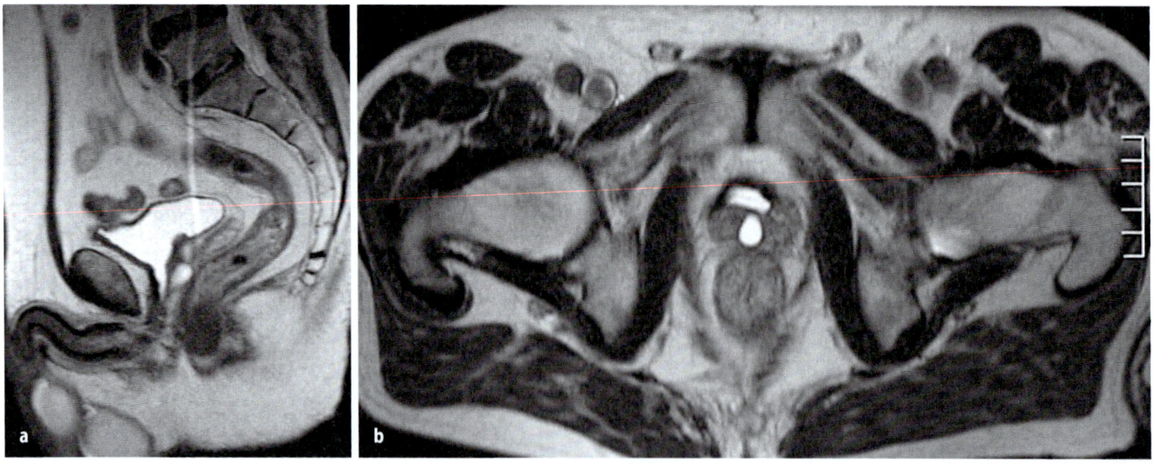

Fig. II.3.38a, b. Utricular cyst – MRI. Sagittal T2-weighted image (**a**) demonstrates a well-defined hyperintense lesion at the midline, just posterior to the prostatic urethra. Axial T2-weighted MR (**b**) shows a rounded hyperintense lesion at the midline near the base of the prostate

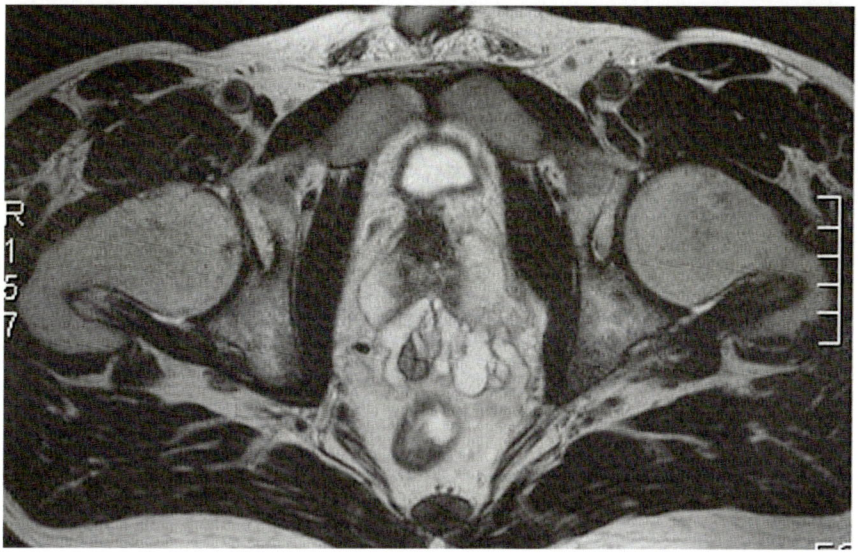

Fig. II.3.39. Cystic seminal vesicles – MRI. Axial T2-weighted image shows cystically dilated seminal vesicles and dilatation of the ejaculatory duct bilaterally, indicating a more distal obstruction

II.3.7.4 PET (Positron Emission Tomography)

II.3.7.4.1 Technique

PET is a functional imaging modality that studies specific biochemical processes noninvasively (e.g. glucose metabolism). Many types of malignant tumours have an accelerated rate of glycolysis when compared to normal tissue and, therefore, today PET is mainly used in the field of oncology. The most commonly used radiotracer is the glucose analogue 2-deoxy-2 [^{18}F]fluoro-D-glucose (FDG). FDG is preferentially taken up by tumour cells after intravenous injection and phosphorylated by hexokinase to FDG-6-PO_4. FDG-6-PO_4 cannot be further metabolized in the glycolytic pathway, in contrast to glucose-6-PO_4, and remains trapped intracellularly. Larger amounts of FDG-6-PO_4 are stored in malignant cells in comparison to the normal surrounding tissues and this can be displayed as increased activity that delineates the hypermetabolic tumour.

II.3.7.4.2 Clinical Indications

Testicular Cancer

In urologic oncology FDG PET has been most widely studied for the staging and follow-up of seminomatous and nonseminomatous germ cell tumours of the testicle. For staging purposes, there is still some disagreement, in that some studies will indicate a higher sensitivity and specificity for PET in comparison to CT, whereas others cannot demonstrate a significant difference between these two imaging modalities. The two main disadvantages are that PET is unable to detect metastatic lesions less than 5 mm in diameter (whereas CT is able to) and that PET has a low sensitivity to detect mature teratoma (Shvarts et al. 2002; Spermon et al. 2002). Further studies are required to evaluate the possible utility in this area.

On the other hand, PET has proven its value in the assessment of residual mass after chemotherapy. This is the only imaging modality that enables differentiation between viable tumour and fibrosis (De Santis et al. 2004). PET needs to be done 2 weeks after chemotherapy however, because of false-negative findings due to early suppression of metabolic activity immediately after chemotherapy and false-positive findings due to increased macrophage activity in absorption of necrotic tissue, respectively (Shvarts et al. 2002). PET also has the ability to predict the response to chemotherapy in patients with metastatic germ cell tumours after their induction chemotherapy and before the start of salvage chemotherapy. PET may also be possibly beneficial in monitoring therapy response, with a positive response indicated by a decrease in FDG uptake. When tumour markers increase, PET is able to identify the place of tumour recurrence sooner in comparison to CT.

Prostate Cancer

Overall the results are much less promising for FDG PET in the evaluation of prostate cancer because of the significant overlap between prostate cancer and benign prostate hypertrophy and the inability of FDG PET to differentiate between postoperative scar and local tumour recurrence (Shvarts et al. 2002; Hain and Maisey 2003). Also there seems to be no correlation between FDG uptake and tumour grading (Gleason grade) in contrast to other tumours. FDG PET is also less sensitive than a conventional bone scan in the evaluation of bone metastases (Hain and Maisey 2003).

More recent studies focus on using other tracers such as [^{11}C]methionine, [^{11}C]choline, [^{18}F]-labelled choline and [^{11}C]acetate to improve the results of PET and they seem to be more promising.

II.3.7.5 Emergencies in Andrology

II.3.7.5.1 Testicular Torsion (Figs. II.3.40, II.3.41)

US in combination with Doppler is the modality of choice for evaluating testicular torsion (Pavlica and Barozzi 2001). Grey-scale US can vary from a normal appearance to a very oedematous and heterogenic appearance consistent with a recent onset versus a more advanced stage. The absence of flow demonstrated by colour and/or power Doppler is the key criterion for this diagnosis. The diagnosis can be more challenging in cases of partial or incomplete torsion. In these patients arterial flow can still be detected and even reactive hyperaemia may be seen, but the resistive index will show an increase and there may be inversion of the diastolic flow (Pavlica and Barozzi 2001).

II.3.7.5.2 Priapism (Fig. II.3.42)

In priapism Colour Doppler is indicated to differentiate between high-flow and low-flow priapism.

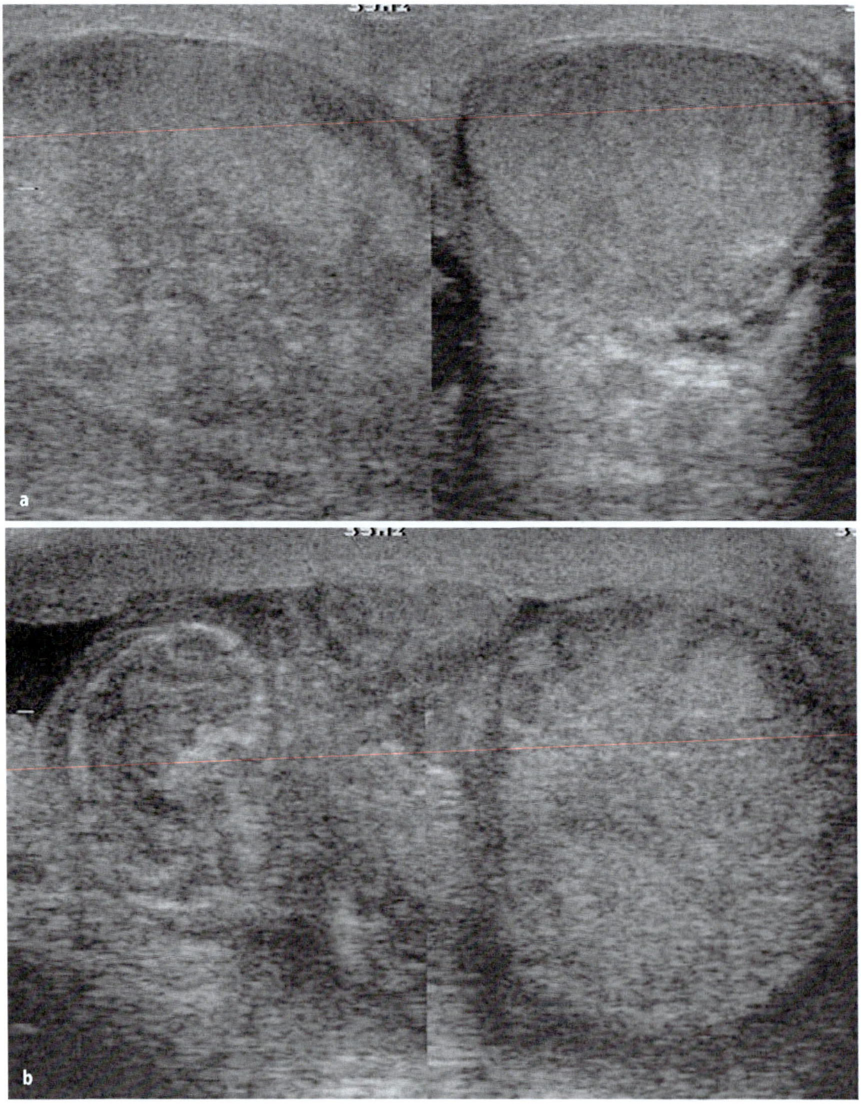

Fig. II.3.40a–c. Testicular torsion. Transverse US (**a**) demonstrates the normal left testicle with a homogeneous appearance. The right testicle is enlarged and is heterogeneous. Longitudinal US (**b**) showing the enlarged heterogeneously right testicle and the thickening of the adjacent portion of the spermatic cord

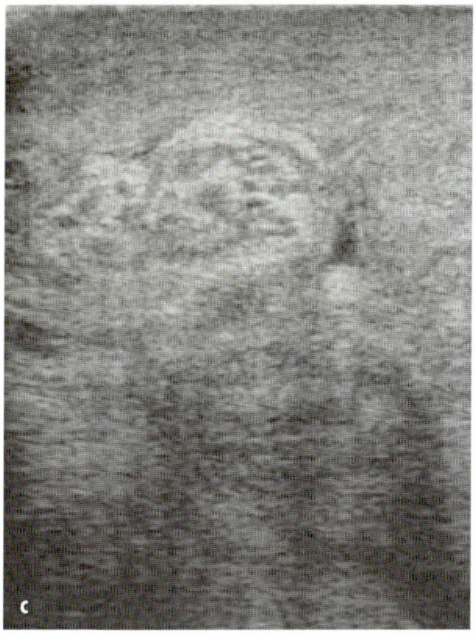

Fig. II.3.40. (Cont.) Transverse US view (**c**) of the proximal portion of the spermatic cord which is oedematous (swollen and hyperechoic fat) and twisted

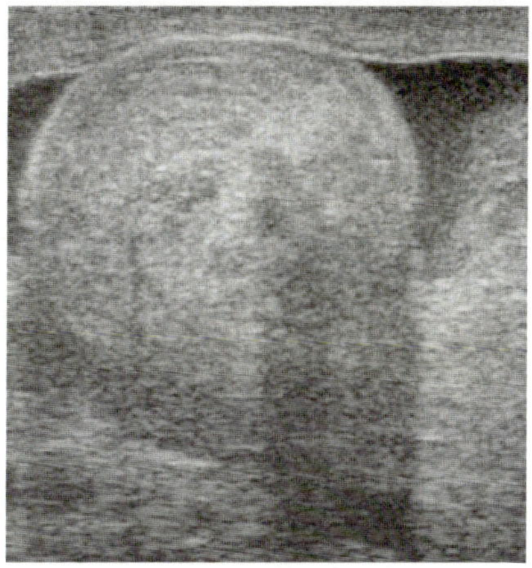

Fig. II.3.41. Testicular torsion. "Swirling sign" of the spermatic cord: typical of intravaginal testicular torsion

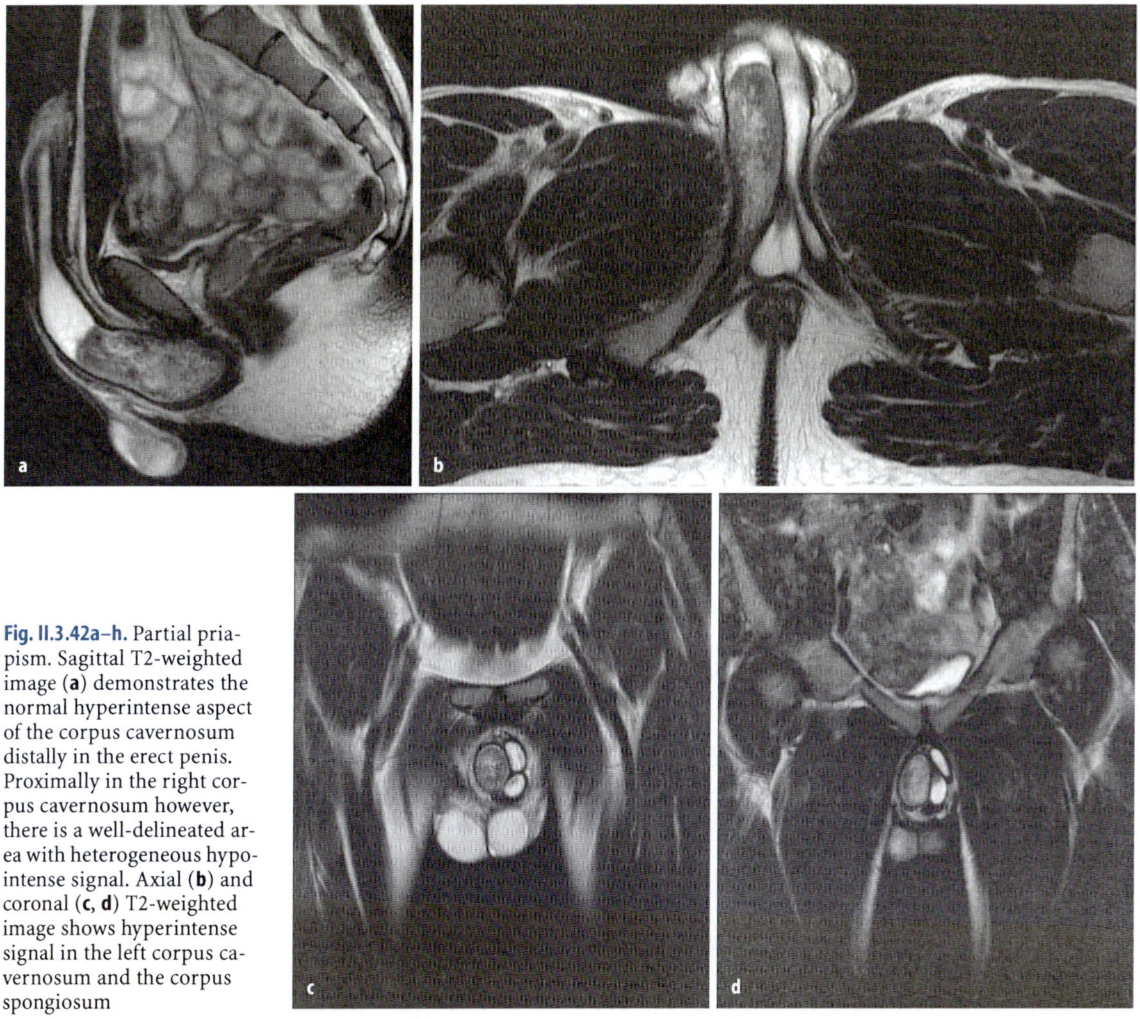

Fig. II.3.42a–h. Partial priapism. Sagittal T2-weighted image (**a**) demonstrates the normal hyperintense aspect of the corpus cavernosum distally in the erect penis. Proximally in the right corpus cavernosum however, there is a well-delineated area with heterogeneous hypointense signal. Axial (**b**) and coronal (**c, d**) T2-weighted image shows hyperintense signal in the left corpus cavernosum and the corpus spongiosum

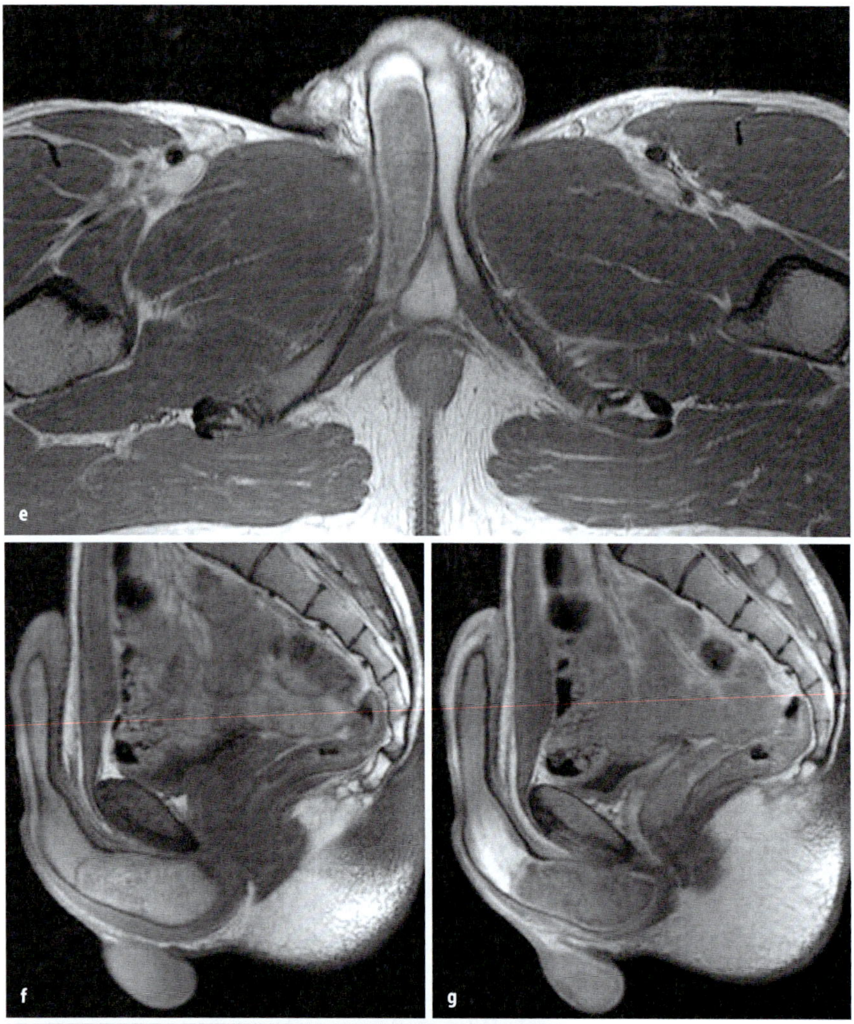

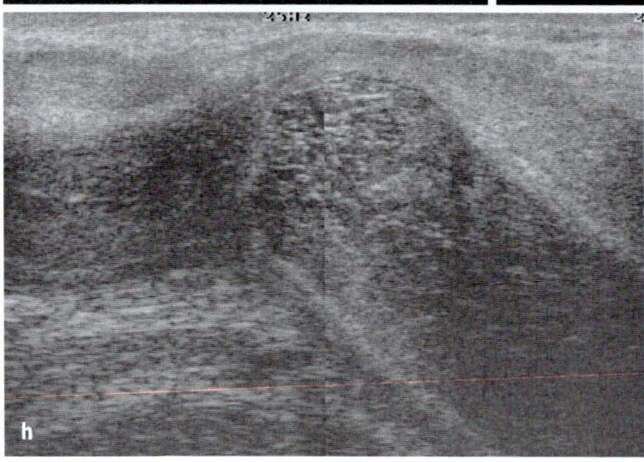

Fig. II.3.42. (Cont.) The right corpus cavernosum has a heterogeneous hypointense signal near the base and is widened compared to the normal left side. Axial (**e**) and sagittal (**f**, **g**) T1-weighted image shows the prominent aspect of the corpus cavernosum at the base; this area also demonstrates a slightly heterogeneous appearance in comparison with the normal hyperintense signal distally. With US (**h**), the swelling and mass in the base of the corpus cavernosum is well appreciated

II.3.7.5.3
Testicular Trauma (Figs. II.3.43, II.3.44)

Testicular US is the imaging technique of choice and is able to discern between scrotal hematoma, haematocele, testicular haematoma and testicular rupture (discontinuation of the tunica albuginea) (Pavlica and Barozzi 2001). In the acute phase a haematoma will appear hyperechogenic, but the echogenicity changes rapidly as a function of the organization and liquefaction of the blood clot.

II.3.7.5.4
Penile Fracture

Penile fracture is most often the result of vigorous sexual intercourse. Patients will present with acute pain, swelling and sudden loss of erection. US can demonstrate a haematoma (due to rupture of a superficial vessel or due to a tunica albuginea defect) and document the tunica albuginea defect itself. The tunica albuginea is visible as a hyperechogenic line on US and the defect presents as an interruption of this line.

The same findings (haematoma and defect in the tunica albuginea) can be visualized on MR.

II.3

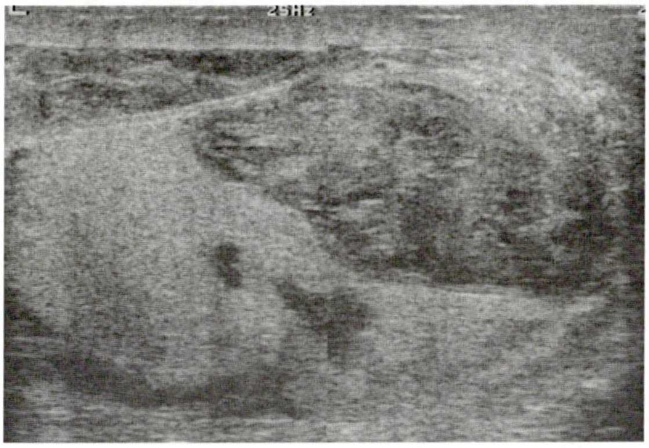

Fig. II.3.43. Testicular trauma. Motorcycle accident. Longitudinal US shows a well-delineated heterogeneous area in the left testicle, consistent with a haematoma. The tunica albuginea is ruptured. Haematocele

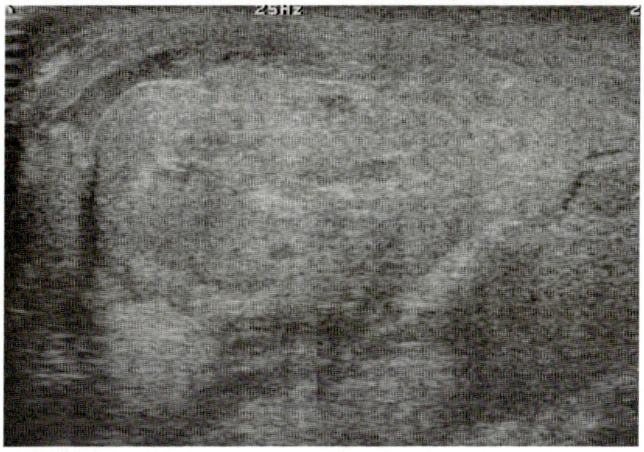

Fig. II.3.44. Testicular trauma. Football trauma. Longitudinal US. The right testicle is no longer well delineated by a hyperechogenic line (tunica albuginea) and appears very heterogenic consistent with laceration of the testicle and disruption of the tunica albuginea, and with intra- and peritesticular haematoma

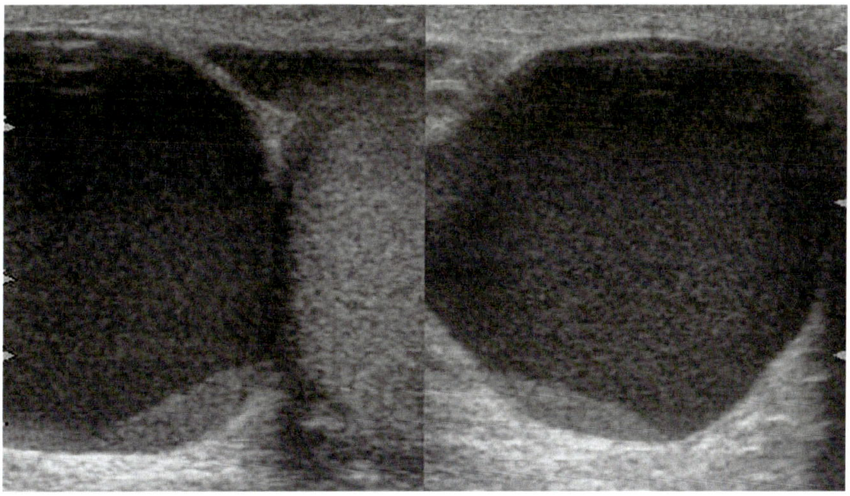

Fig. II.3.45. Spermatocele. Longitudinal and transverse US shows a sharply demarcated, rounded structure adjacent to the upper pole of the testicle. This structure is hypoechoic with multiple internal reflections and a fluid level: this sediment has settled at the depending portion of the spermatocele

II.3.7.6 Tumours

II.3.7.6.1 Epididymal Cysts (Fig. II.3.45)

Epididymal cysts are very common lesions and have been reported in as many as 70% of men who undergo US (Oyen 2002). They are most often found in the head and appear as asonant well-defined lesions. They can be single or multiple and vary from very small to large.

II.3.7.6.2 Epididymal Tumours

In contrast to the epididymal cyst, solid lesions of the epididymis are rare. The most common tumour is the adenomatoid tumour, which is benign and originates most often in the tail. A sperm granuloma can be seen in patients after vasectomy.

II.3.7.6.3 Testicular Cancer

See "Testicular Microlithiasis".

II.3.7.6.4 Penile Cancer

Most primary malignant tumours of the penis are squamous cell carcinoma. Physical examination cannot always determine the presence or absence of cavernosal invasion. In these instances US and/or MRI with or without artificial erection and/or intravenous contrast administration can be done. MRI is the most sensitive method (Scardino et al. 2004), but will have some false-positive results (Lont et al. 2003).

References

Ahn HS, Lee SW, Yoon SJ, Hann HJ, Hong JM (2004) A comparison of colour duplex sonography after transurethral alprostadil and intracavernous alprostadil in the assessment of erectile dysfunction. J Int Med Res 32:317–323
Aizenstein RI, DiDomenico D, Wilbur AC, O'Neil HK (1998) Testicular microlithiasis: association with male infertility. J Clin Ultrasound 26:195–198
Carmignani L, Gadda F, Mancini M et al (2004) Detection of ultrasonographic lesions in severe male infertility. J Urol 172:1045–1047
Cornud F, Belin X, Delafontaine D, Amar T, Hélénon O, Moreau JF (1997) Imaging of obstructive azoospermia. Eur Radiol 7:1079–1085
De Santis M, Becherer A, Bokemeyer C et al (2004) 2-^{18}Fluorodeoxy-D-glucose positron emission tomography is a reliable predictor for viable tumor in postchemotherapy seminoma: an update of the prospective multicentric SEMPET trial. J Clin Oncol 22:1034–1039
Fornara P, Gerbershagen HP (2004) Ultrasound in patients affected with Peyronie's disease. World J Urol 22:365–367
Hain SF, Maisey MN (2003) Positron emission tomography for urological tumours. BJU Int 92:159–164
Har-Toov J, Eytan O, Hauser R, Yavetz H, Elad D, Jaffa AJ (2004) A new power doppler ultrasound guiding technique for improved testicular sperm extraction. Fertil Steril 81:430–434
Herwig R, Tosun K, Pinggera GM et al (2004) Tissue perfusion essential for spermatogenesis and outcome of testicular sperm extraction (TESE) for assisted reproduction. J Assist Reprod Genet 21:175–180
Jones TR, Zagoria RJ, Jarow JP (1997) Transrectal US-guided seminal vesiculography. Radiology 205:276–278
Kuligowska E, Fenlon HM (1998) Transrectal US in male infertility: spectrum of findings and role in patient care. Radiology 207:173–181
Lenz S, Thomsen JK, Giwercman A, Hertel NT, Herts J, Skakkebaek NE (1994) Ultrasonic texture and volume of testicles in infertile men. Hum Reprod 9:878–881
Lont AP, Besnard APE, Gallee MPW, Van Tinteren H, Horenblas S (2003) A comparison of physical examination and imaging in determining the extent of primary penile carcinoma. BJU Int 91:493–495
Miller RL, Wissman R, White S, Ragosin R (1996) Testicular microlithiasis: a benign condition with a malignant association. J Clin Ultrasound 24:197–202
Oyen R, Verbist B, Verswijvel G (1999) Imaging of testicular neoplasms. In: Petrovich Z, Baert L, Brady LW (eds) Carcinoma of the kidney and testis, and rare urologic malignancies. Springer, Berlin Heidelberg New York
Oyen RH (2002) Scrotal ultrasound. Eur Radiol 12:19–34
Pavlica P, Barozzi L (2001) Imaging of the acute scrotum. Eur Radiol 11:220–228
Pierik FH, Dohle GR, van Muiswinkel JM, Vreeburg JT, Weber RF (1999) Is routine scrotal ultrasound advantageous in infertile men? J Urol 162:1618–1620
Pretorius ES, Siegelman ES, Ramchandani P, Banner MP (2001) MR imaging of the penis. Radiographics 21:S283–S298
Rhoden EL, Estrada C, Levine L, Morgentaler A (2003) The value of pituitary magnetic resonance imaging in men with hypogonadism. J Urol 170:795–798
Sakamoto H, Shimada M, Yoshida H (2002) Hemodynamic evaluation of the penile arterial system in patients with erectile dysfunction using power Doppler imaging. Urology 60:480–484
Scardino E, Villa G, Bonomo G et al (2004) Magnetic resonance imaging combined with artificial erection for local staging of penile cancer. Urology 63:1158–1162
Schiff JD, Li PS, Goldstein M (2004) Correlation of ultrasonographic and orchidometer measurements of testis volume in adults. BJU Int 93:1015–1017
Shvarts O, Han K, Seltzer M, Pantuck AJ, Belldegrun AS (2002) Positron emission tomography in urologic oncology. Cancer Control 9:335–342
Spermon JR, De Geus-Oei LF, Kiemeney LALM, Witjes JA, Oyen WJG (2002) The role of ^{18}fluoro-2-deoxyglucose positron emission tomography in initial staging and re-staging after chemotherapy for testicular germ cell tumours. BJU Int 89:549–556
Thomas AJ (2004) Should testicular ultrasound be considered a medically necessary test for the spermatogenically impaired male? J Urol 172:829–830
Thomas K, Wood SJ, Thompson AJM, Pilling D, Lewis-Jones DI (2000) The incidence and significance of testicular microlithiasis in a subfertile population. Br J Radiol 73:494–497
Wilkins CJ, Sriprasad S, Sidhu P (2003) Colour doppler ultrasound of the penis. Radiology 58:514–523
Woodward PJ, Sohaey R, O'Donoghue MJ, Green DE (2002) From the archives of the AFIP Tumors and tumorlike lesions of the testis: radiologic-pathologic correlation. Radiographics 22:189–216

II.3.8 Technical Investigations Including Imaging Procedures: Colour Flow Doppler and Thermography for the Detection of Reflux in Varicocele

Y. Gat, M. Gornish

Summary

Based on our recent findings and on flow mechanics analysis of the impaired testicular venous drainage system, the following statements can be made:

1. Varicocele is predominantly a bilateral venous disease.
2. Internal spermatic veins with incompetent valves are associated with retroperitoneal collaterals and small bypasses.
3. Right varicocele exists in 86% of infertile men with varicocele.
4. In 92% of these patients it is impossible to produce back flow even by the Valsalva manoeuvre, since the right ISV inserts directly into the inferior vena cava.
5. Fluid mechanics analysis, supported by venographies, clearly proves that ISV back flow cannot be evoked on the right side, so right varicocele cannot be detected by palpation.
6. Only in 8% of patients, whose right ISV inserts into the right renal vein (a mirror image of the left side), can reflux be produced by the Valsalva manoeuvre. In these cases only, right varicocele can be detected by palpation.
7. Thermography, based on conductivity of the heat and not on blood flow, is an effective screening tool for detecting right varicocele and, combined with ultrasonography, yields the best results.
8. Small and impalpable veins have the same detrimental effect as large veins since the elevated hydrostatic pressure, which causes hypoxia in the testicular microcirculation, depends on the height of the blood column and not on its diameter.
9. Left high ligation is incomplete treatment since it ignores right-side involvement and venous collaterals and bypasses.
10. Adequate treatment is achieved by transvenous embolization or by microsurgery, both of which successfully occlude the ISV, including the associated network of bypasses. These treatments allow the return of normal, oxygenated blood flow to the testicular microcirculation, seminiferous tubules, Sertoli cells and Leydig cells and in significant numbers restore fertility.

II.3.8.1 Introduction on the Bilaterality of the Disease

Varicocele is a bilateral vascular disease involving a network of collaterals and small, retroperitoneal bypasses. The right and the left testicular venous drainage systems are complex and not identical to each other. In order to detect varicocele in the right side, one needs more than simple physical examination. It is important to understand the hydraulic systems involved in the testicular blood supply and drainage system, using the tools of physics, hydraulics, flow mechanics and material strength.

Recent data have demonstrated that varicocele is a bilateral disease (Gat et al. 2004a). Studies have shown that physical examination may miss the diagnosis of bilateral varicocele in 92% of cases (Gat et al. 2004b).

There is a misunderstanding among clinicians that varicocele is a left-sided disease and this has led to misdiagnosis and partial treatment (of the left side only and ignoring hidden venous bypasses), which is not adequate to correct the problem.

The reason why right varicocele cannot be diagnosed by palpation lies in the anatomy of the right internal spermatic vein (ISV), which is different from that of the left ISV. On the left, when the Valsalva manoeuvre is performed the elevated pressure results in increasing pressure in the renal vein. Since the pressures of the left renal vein and the left spermatic vein are close, the pressure in the left renal vein then exceeds the pressure in the left ISV. As blood flows from high to low pressures, the venous blood in the left renal vein now flows in two directions: in the usual one to the inferior vena cava (IVC) and back flow to the left ISV. The clinician can feel the retrograde flow by palpation, while the reflux of blood dilates the ISV and the pampiniform plexus.

On the right, the hydraulic mechanism is completely different. The pressure in the right ISV is around 10 mmHg. The pressure in the IVC is on average 0 mmHg (from –5 to +5 mmHg). The patient cannot raise the hydrostatic pressure in the IVC above the pressure in the right ISV, a fact that can be clearly seen on venography.

Since the flow is always from high to low pressure, blood cannot flow back from the inferior vena cava to the right ISV (as needed to produce back flow). If elevated pressures were maintained in the IVC, it would cause the patient to faint.

Thus, back flow cannot be produced in the right ISV even with the use of the Valsalva manoeuvre. Therefore, palpation of the right testis is not a reliable diagnostic test. Only in 5–8% of cases (where the right ISV inserts into the right renal vein, the mirror image of the left side) will the Valsalva manoeuvre yield back flow and palpation of the spermatic veins be used to diagnose right varicocele. In our recent study we demonstrated that palpation misses 92% of right varicocele cases. For this reason varicocele was diagnosed primarily as a left-sided disease for many decades in the medical literature.

Physical examination may have high sensitivity for varicocele on the left, but not on the right. Additional modalities should be applied for patients in whom varicocele is suspected clinically.

An effective, noninvasive method is thermography (Varicoscreen®) of the scrotum. This diagnostic tool for varicocele was first developed and evaluated by Comhaire et al. (1976).

From a physics point of view this tool demonstrates transfer of the heat within fluid (blood), and it does not depend on back flow of the fluid. When the one-way valves in the right ISV have been damaged or malfunction and there is stagnation of the blood, the high temperature of the blood in the abdominal portion of the ISV (at 37°C) is transferred downstream towards the right testis by convection of fluid particles. Therefore, thermography is able to detect varicocele without back flow since the incompetent valves in the ISV enable the free transfer of heat by conductivity.

The discussion of these methods is based on studies showing a significant elevation in intratesticular and scrotal skin surface temperatures in patients with varicocele, and a temperature difference of 0.5°C to 3.0°C between hyperthermal hemiscrotums and the healthy contralateral side (Goldstein and Eid 1989).

Hamm et al. (1986) reported a sensitivity of 98.3%, a specificity of 100% and an accuracy of 98.4% for thermography. They suggested that thermography is the most sensitive and reliable method for detecting varicocele, and that it permits rapid, simple and noninvasive diagnosis of even subclinical varicocele. Trum et al. (1996) noted a 97% sensitivity for Varicoscreen thermography in 63 patients (95% confidence interval, CI, 0.83–1.0). Another study (Pochaczevsky et al. 1986) reported agreement between thermography and spermatic venography findings in 15 out of 17 cases. These rates correspond to our thermography results of 98.9% sensitivity, 98.5% accuracy and 100% positive predictive value (PPV) for left-sided varicocele, and 95.6%, 94.9% and 98%, respectively, for right-sided varicocele (Gat et al. 2004b). On the left side, there were two false-negatives and one false positive; on the right side, there were seven false-negatives and three false-positives. In our recent study (Gat et al. 2004c), contact scrotal thermography had the highest sensitivity and accuracy of the noninvasive methods for detecting varicocele.

II.3.8.2 How to Use Contact Scrotal Thermograph

Contact thermography is performed with the patient upright and undressed, after remaining for 5 min at room temperature of not less than 22°C, as described by Comhaire et al. (1976). The penis is taped to the abdominal wall and the genital region is exposed. The investigator then brings the scrotum forward with both hands to apply the Varicoscreen, a flexible liquid crystal thermostrip film. The screen scale ranges from 31.3°C to 35.3°C, with a colour change every 0.8°C. In the healthy male, the temperature of the scrotal skin is symmetrically distributed and does not exceed 32.5°C, corresponding to a brown or reddish colour.

In men with varicocele or retrograde flow, the temperature is higher than in controls and the colour changes to dark green, violet or blue; the last two are diagnostic. We also compared scrotal temperature distribution patterns of the two sides, and the intensity and extension of the hyperthermia in the standing position and during the Valsalva manoeuvre. A temperature differential of 0.8°C or more, encompassing at least 25% of the area of one hemiscrotum, is considered indicative of varicocele. Bilateral varicocele can be suspected if the entire scrotum is warmer than the anterior thigh. Using this method, the accuracy and sensitivity of contact scrotal thermography as a diagnostic screening tool of varicocele is extremely high and actually the best noninvasive modality in comparison with the "gold standard" invasive tool of venography, as demonstrated by Comhaire et al. (1981) and further supported by studies with adolescent patients (Gat et al. 2003) and adults (Gat et al. 2004a).

II.3.8.2.1 Colour Flow Doppler Ultrasonography

Doppler ultrasound has also been shown to be accurate for the diagnosis of clinical and subclinical varicocele (McClure and Hricak 1986; Petros et al. 1991; Eskew et al. 1993; Hoekstra and Witt 1995; Chiou et al. 1997). Not only does it measure the diameter of the ISV and pampiniform plexus, it also detects the presence of retrograde venous flow, which is the apparent mechanism by which varicocele produces a pathological effect on spermatogenesis. Moreover, ultrasound has the advantage of detecting the presence of testicular abnormalities such as testicular masses, torsion, spermatocele, epididymal lesions and hydrocele. However, its diagnostic criteria for varicocele are poorly defined and vary among different investigators. We used those recommended by Chiou et al. (1997); namely, detection of

2 to 3 venous channels of more than 3 mm in diameter and reflux during the Valsalva manoeuvre for 1 s or more. Eskew et al. (1993) reported a sensitivity of 85% for scrotal ultrasound detection of subclinical varicocele. One study (Petros et al. 1991) reported a 93% detection rate of subclinical varicocele using venography as the gold standard, and another (Chiou et al. 1997) found a sensitivity of 93% and a specificity of 85% compared to physical examination. These findings correspond to our results (Gat et al. 2004c) for colour Doppler ultrasound: for left varicocele, 98% sensitivity, 97.9% accuracy and 98.4% PPV; for right varicocele, 77.3% sensitivity, 71.8% accuracy and 86.6% PPV. On the left side, there were 2 false-negatives and 2 false-positives, and on the right side, there were 36 false-negatives and 19 false-positives when venography was used as the standard. We noted a good correlation between colour Doppler ultrasound and thermography and venography, with ultrasound being a more objective assessment than physical examination. When the results of ultrasound Doppler and thermography were equivocal, venography was used as the reference standard. The anatomical differences between the right and the left side can explain the low sensitivity, accuracy and PPV on the right side compared to the left. Therefore, the preferred strategy is to evaluate all patients with infertility by ultrasound Doppler and thermography in order to detect bilateral varicocele.

II.3.8.2.2 How to Use Ultrasound Doppler

Ultrasound Doppler is performed with an up-to-date imager, such as ATL HDI 3000 or 5000 unit, using a 10 MHz multifrequency linear transducer. Machine settings are adjusted to optimize the detection of blood flow.

The examination is done with the patient in the supine position with his scrotum supported by a towel placed over his upper thighs. The penis is placed on the abdomen and covered with a drape for minimal exposure of the patient and maximal access for the physician. Since the detrimental effects of varicocele exist only in upright or sitting position and there is no adverse effect in horizontal position, there is no use in examining the patient horizontally. The best way to detect and evaluate varicocele – which yields the highest accuracy and sensitivity compared to venography, especially on the right side – is while standing (Gat et al. 2004b).

Each side of the scrotum is scanned from the level of the testicular hilus to the neck of the scrotum in longitudinal and transverse sections, and the scrotal septum is examined in the transverse plane. Vascular channels in the spermatic cord are noted, and vessel diameters are measured by electronic callipers. The presence of testicular abnormalities, spermatocele, epididymal lesions and hydrocele is recorded. The patient is then asked to stand upright for 5 min, and the examination is repeated. The Valsalva manoeuvre is used in the supine and upright positions. The maximum diameter of the scrotal veins is recorded, and the appearance of the venous pampiniform plexus is noted. The flow velocity of the main vein is measured before and after the Valsalva manoeuvre.

The sonographic diagnosis of varicocele is based on the detection of two to three venous channels, one of which measures >3 mm in diameter, and reflux during the Valsalva manoeuvre. Patients without reflux or with Valsalva-induced reflux for <1 s are considered normal; patients with reflux for >1 s are considered to have varicocele.

II.3.8.2.3 Contact Scrotal Thermography Combined with Colour Doppler Ultrasonography

When contact scrotal thermography is combined with colour Doppler ultrasound, the sensitivity, specificity, accuracy and PPV for left varicocele are 100%, 33.3%, 99.0% and 98.9%, respectively; for right varicocele, 97.4%, 58.3%, 90.3% and 91.1%, respectively (Gat et al. 2004c). These results support the claim that combined thermography and colour Doppler ultrasound is the most sensitive strategy for the diagnosis of varicocele (Netto et al. 1984; Hamm et al. 1986). However, based on the presented sensitivities and specificities and accuracy of each diagnostic modality, compared to the standard of venography, it appears that thermography is the best single test.

II.3.8.3 Medical Importance of the Complete and Accurate Diagnosis of Varicocele

Recent editorial comments by Nagler (2004) are in conflict with our anatomic and physical findings. However, three major issues need to be addressed in confronting Nagler's comments. First, is there a relationship between varicocele and male infertility? Second, is subclinical varicocele relevant to male infertility, and does it requires treatment? Third, what is the best diagnostic test for varicocele if there is an indication to treat?

These issues have serious implications in the treatment of infertile males and since the missed diagnosis of right varicocele by palpation has led to these questions and doubts, they demand proper explanation in this chapter.

II.3.8.4 Is There a Relationship Between Varicocele and Male Infertility?

The assertion that varicocele does not relate to male infertility is supported by the comprehensive meta-analysis of seven prospective randomized studies conducted in the last two decades, which concluded that "varicocele repair does not seem to be an effective treatment for male subfertility" (Evers and Collins 2003). This is further supported by a comprehensive analysis presented in *Cochrane Database Systems Review* 2004 (Evers and Collins 2004), where the reviewers concluded that the result of eight controlled prospective randomized studies indicated "no benefit of varicocele treatment over expectant management in subfertile couples in whom varicocele in the man is the only abnormal finding".

The results of these multicentre data analyses are not surprising since, according to the usual practice, the vast majority of patients in these studies were treated on the left side only. Until now, the bilaterality of varicocele has gone largely unrecognized and the network of venous bypasses and collaterals is undetected at high ligation. Thus, they were either not treated, or only partially treated. We have estimated that only some 20 % of the patients in these studies on which those conclusions are based were adequately treated. These include patients who did not have right varicocele; those whose varicocele was not associated with collaterals and venous bypasses or those who did not have significant inter-testicular venous connections. The remaining 80 % were only partially treated and showed either no improvement or merely transient improvement in fertility. When partial treatment (left high ligation - occlusion of the main ISV) alone is performed, the remaining collateral veins will enlarge to accept a greater volume of blood, in accordance with a simple law of flow mechanics regarding hydrodynamic equilibrium in the drainage system of elastic vessels. That eventually results in what we call "survived", or "secondary" varicocele (mistakenly called "recurrent varicocele" in the medical literature).

Another aspect that raises doubts about the meta-analysis is that it included studies concluding that treatment of varicocele or consultation only yielded the same results. This absurd statement can exist only when you treat the patient and you think that you treat, but actually you do not, because the medical procedure is not adequate. Extensive studies on patients suffering from azoospermia or extremely severe oligoasthenoteratozoospermia (OAT) (concentration less than 1.0 million/ml), treated mainly bilaterally with microsurgery or embolization, showed significant improvement in spermatogenesis (60 %) and achievement of pregnancies (30 %) (Matthews et al. 1998; Pasqualotto et al. 2004; Gat et al. 2005a). It is clear that patients with azoospermia or extremely severe OAT, per definition, cannot achieve spontaneous pregnancy without treatment. It means that the patients selected for the studies in the meta-analysis did not include severe cases, which are about 30 – 40 % in the population of male infertility, and/or the treatment was not complete as mentioned above. To state that treatment of a disease and no treatment have the same results means that either there is "no disease" or the "treatment" is not the required complete treatment.

Our conclusion is that the proper interpretation of these two comprehensive meta-analyses should state that inadequate treatment techniques carried out in these studies for varicocele repair indeed do not improve fertility in affected males. The fundamental error in this approach to varicocele treatment stems from ignoring the pathophysiologic role of hydrostatic pressure, and its effects on both sides.

II.3.8.5 Is Subclinical Varicocele Relevant to Male Infertility and Does it Require Treatment?

We maintain that varicocele is indeed the main cause of male infertility. The poor results of inadequate treatment have led those working in the field to ignore the pathophysiologic connection between the cause of varicocele (hydrostatic pressure and hypoxia) and its ultimate effect on sperm production.

As we have stated above it is the small veins that do significantly contribute to the problem of high hydrostatic pressure that causes hypoxia (Gat et al 2005b) in the microcirculatory system of the testes, which make its proper treatment more complex than the solution provided by the simple traditional surgical techniques.

The hydrostatic pressures can be estimated according to Eq. 1, which determines pressure as a function of the fluid column height derived from Pascal's law (Streeter 1971, p 31):

$$P = h * \varphi$$

Where P is hydrostatic pressure, h is height of the fluid column and φ is density.

Each 1.0 cm of blood column contributes 0.77 mm Hg to the total pressure (Ganong 1999).

According to Eq. 1, the hydrostatic pressure, created by destruction of the one-way valves in the testicular venous drainage system, depends primarily on the height of the vessels and the density of the blood. The pressure transmitted through the ISV does not depend on the diameter or geometry of the veins. Small veins, which may not be palpable by the fingers of the best clinician, can be as effective in transmitting these elevated pressures to the pampiniform plexus. Regardless of whether the vessels are palpable or not, the very existence of blood vessels without competent one-way valves that produce 40 cm of blood column causes elevated hydrostatic pressure (Streeter 1971). This pressure leads to stagnation of blood flow in the microcirculatory system and hypoxia in the testicular tissues (Chakraborty et al. 1985). Hypoxia will cause tissue damage and progressive deterioration of sperm production resulting in infertility (Matthews et al. 1998; Cozzolino and Lipshultz 2001; Gat et al. 2005a).

II.3.8.6 Is Ultrasonography a Better Diagnostic Tool Because Venography is Subject to Technical Variations?

Venography shows, in real time, the direction of blood flow in the spermatic veins and, when performed using manual injections with a tilt-table apparatus, one can demonstrate the residual traces of incompetent or damaged valves, partially or intermittently competent valves, and the collaterals and venous bypasses associated with varicocele. The imaging achieved with ultrasonography may provide certain additional information about blood flow in the testis, but cannot address the anatomy of the retroperitoneal ISV system. More important to our discussion of right-sided reflux, since the flow in the IVC cannot be reversed from the IVC into the right ISV (study to be published), ultrasonography cannot detect reflux easily on the right side. Imaging using colour flow Doppler has a minimal resolution threshold of flow. It is difficult to detect small amounts of reflux in the right system, even for an experienced ultrasonographer.

A simple, sensitive and easy to use detector for screening right varicocele is contact thermography (Comhaire et al. 1976; Kunnen and Comhaire 1992; Gat et al. 2004b). Contact thermography is based on the conductivity of the heat transferred from the abdominal level of the right spermatic vein downstream to the level of the pampiniform plexus where the patient is being examined. It does not depend on blood flow. Since it is impossible to produce back flow in the right side (reflux) by venography, higher sensitivity and accuracy are achieved by thermography.

II.3.8.7 Why Right Varicocele Could Not be Detected

On the left side, retrograde flow in ISV is obtained during a Valsalva maneuver-induced compression of the renal vein. The slight reduction in volume then results in a pressure rise in the renal vein, which is sufficient to cause back-flow in the left ISV.

On the right side, it is impossible to detect varicocele effectively on physical examination, since it is impossible to produce back-flow by Valsalva manoeuvre in 92% of the cases where the internal spermatic veins (ISV) are inserted to the inferior vena cava (IVC). This can be explained at three levels:

A. From the *physiologic flow* point of view: (1) All interconnected veins to the IVC must flow to the IVC in order to maintain continuous flow to the heart. That is why the pressure in the IVC is the lowest in the venous system. (2) If the patient could produce back-flow by Valsalva manoeuvre in the right ISV, the blood flow in the IVC would have to be reversed, resulting in syncope.

B. From the *hydrodynamic* point of view: The pressure difference between IVC (–5 to +5 mm Hg) and the ISV (10 – 12 mm Hg) is too high to allow reversal of the pressure gradient in order to produce back-flow for the detection of right varicocele.

C. From the *observational* point of view: While performing venographies, patients fail to produce back-flow by Valsalva manoeuvre except in those cases where the right ISV is inserted to the right renal vein (8%).

As explained, in 92% of patients (in whom the ISV enters the IVC) back-flow cannot be elicited. As a result, the diagnosis of the right side was missed and therefore the right side was not treated (Gat 2005b).

II.3.8.8 Goren-Gat Technique for Detection and Treatment of Right and Left Varicocele

The goal of treatment is the identification and occlusion of the abnormal ISV (right and left) and all of its associated collateral veins. These retroperitoneal collaterals, if not treated, will allow the backflow of blood to continue by way of venous bypasses, and perpetuate the detrimental effects of the varicocele (Fig. II.3.46.1).

Access is gained to the inferior vena cava by way of the right common femoral vein, with a protective 6.5F (3 mm) sheath placed at the entry site until the procedure is completed. The guiding catheter is positioned in the left renal vein, over the vertebral bodies. The left side is usually treated first. For the right ISV, the original guiding catheter is replaced by a "shepherd's hook"-shaped catheter which is positioned in the inferior vena cava, above the orifice of the right renal vein. On both sides, a 3F superselective catheter with hydrophilic tip is advanced through the guiding catheter and will either enter the orifice of the ISV directly, or, if there is a competent upper valve, will lodge in the valve. If this occurs (in ~20% of the cases), the patient is placed in 10-15 deg Trendelenburg and, using a series of deep inspirations following Valsalva manoeuvre, the valve can usually be passed. In most cases, after passing the upper valve, the catheter will advance retrograde in

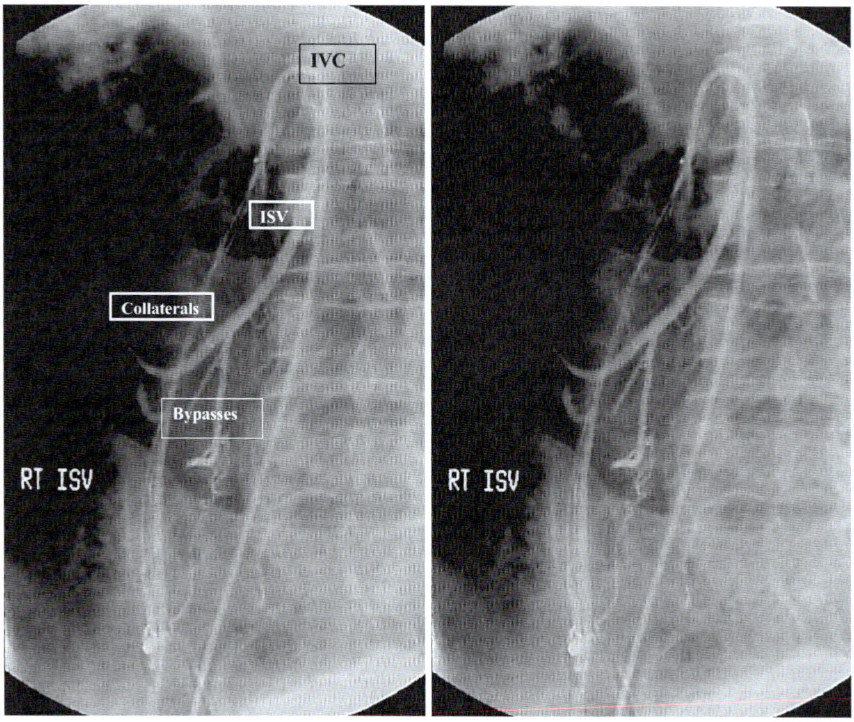

Fig. II.3.46. Right varicocele with associated network of bypasses and retroperitoneal collaterals. The right internal spermatic vein (ISV) inserts into the inferior vena cava (*IVC*). One-way valves are absent. The venous bypasses lack valves. Back-flow (reflux) is seen during fluoroscopy as contrast material flows freely downstream from point (IVC) towards the testes. The vertical height of the blood column from point (IVC) to the pampiniform plexus is about 35 cm. It exerts a hydrostatic pressure of 27 mm Hg, which exceeds the pressure of the arteriolar system (about 18 mm Hg) in the testicular microcirculation

the ISV down to the inguinal ligament, since the lower valves tend to be incompetent in most cases even when the upper, orificial valve is competent. Occasionally, the catheter will encounter additional ostensibly competent or semi-competent valves in the lower abdomen or pelvis. If so, these are passed with additional manoeuvres as above. The catheter will sometimes enter smaller collateral veins and then cannot be advanced further. Invariably, injection of radioopaque contrast material will show downward filling of the vessel (reflux) and communication with the major ISV. This explains the "paradox" of competent ISV orificial valves in the face of clear evidence of pathologic reflux. Our experience is the basis of our assertion that the direction of venous valvular destruction progresses upward as a result of the persistent hydrodynamic overload over time.

II.3.8.9 'Recurrent' Varicocele After Left High Ligation is Actually 'Survived' Varicocele

Associated bypasses are produced in varicocele; they are of very small diameter, 0.1 – 0.2 mm, and without one-way valves. They assist the impaired drainage system in draining the blood by 'capillary force' (P), which depend on the surface tension (σ) and on the diameter d) of the vessel:

$$P = \sigma / d$$

After performing left high ligation that occludes the main draining vessel (ISV) only, the small bypasses have to include a higher volume of blood and their diameters enlarge. When the diameter enlarges, the phenomenon of 'capillary force' does not exist any more and these bypasses, which at the first stage assist in elevating the venous blood upwards against the gravity, turn after a short time into 'secondary' or 'survived' varicocele as seen in our venographies, performed after failed left high ligation, mistakenly called 'recurrent varicocele' in the medical literature.

This means that most of the studies on varicocele treatment based on left high ligation reflect partial or transient treatment or no treatment at all.

These findings suggest that for decades most varicocele patients have been treated only partially (since right varicocele was not detected and ignored). It further suggests that most of the statistics that raised doubts about the connection between varicocele and male infertility may not reflect clinical reality, since the diagnostic and the treatment modality were not appropriate. Since right varicocele could not be diagnosed by palpation, the treatment was incomplete (left high ligation), which led to poor and inconsistent results, which in turn led to misleading conclusions in the medical literature disconnecting varicocele from male infertility. Varicocele should be diagnosed as a bilateral disease associated with a network of bypasses and treated accordingly.

References

Chakraborty J, Hikim AP, Jhunjhunwala JS (1985) Stagnation of blood in the microcirculatory vessels in the testes of men with varicocele. J Androl 6:117 - 126

Chiou KR, Anderson JC, Wobig RK, Rosinsky DE, Matamoros A, Chen WS, Taylor RJ (1997) Color Doppler ultrasound criteria to diagnose varicoceles: correlation of a new scoring system with physical examination. Urology 50:953 - 956

Comhaire F, Monteyne R, Kunnen M (1976) The value of scrotal thermography as compared with selective retrograde venography of the internal spermatic vein for the diagnosis of subclinical varicocele. Fertil Steril 27:694 - 698

Comhaire F, Kunnen M, Nahum C (1981) Radiological anatomy of the internal spermatic veins in 200 retrograde venograms. Int J Androl 4:379 - 387

Cozzolino DJ, Lipshultz LI (2001) Varicocele as a progressive lesion: positive effect of varicocele repair. Hum Reprod Update 7:55 - 58

Eskew A, Watson N, Wolfman R, Bechtold R, Scharling E, Jarow J (1993) The accuracy of ultrasonographic diagnosis of varicoceles. Fertil Steril 60:693 - 697

Evers J, Collins A (2003) Assessment of efficacy of varicocele repair for male subfertility: a systematic review. Lancet 361: 1849 - 1852

Evers JL, Collins JA (2004) Surgery or embolization for varicocele in subfertile men. Cochrane Database Syst Rev: CD000479

Ganong WF (1999) Medical physiology, 19th edn. Lange Medical Books/McGraw-Hill, New York, pp 550 - 567

Gat Y, Zukerman Z, Bachar GN, Feldberg DO, Gornish M (2003) Adolescent varicocele: is it a unilateral disease? Urology 62:742 - 746; Editorial comment p 746; Reply by authors pp 746 - 747

Gat Y, Bachar GN, Zukerman Z, Belenky A, Gornish M (2004a) Varicocele: a bilateral disease. Fertil Steril 81:424 - 429; Editorial comments in J Urol 2004; 172:790 - 791

Gat Y, Bachar GN, Zuckerman Z, Belenky A, Gornish M (2004b) Physical examination may miss the diagnosis of bilateral varicocele: a comparative study of 4 diagnostic modalities. J Urol 172 (4 Pt 1):1414 - 1417; Editorial commentary and authors' reply in J Urol 2005; 173:2208 - 2209

Gat Y, Gornish M, Belenky A, Bachar GN (2004c) Elevation of serum testosterone and free testosterone after embolization of the internal spermatic vein for the treatment of varicocele in infertile men. Hum Reprod 19:2303 - 2306; Editorial comments in J Urol 2005; 173:2079

Gat Y, Bachar GN, Everaert K, Levinger U, Gornish M (2005a) Induction of spermatogenesis in azoospermic men after internal spermatic veins embolization for the treatment of varicocele. Hum Reprod 20:1013 - 1017

Gat Y, Chakraborty J, Zukerman Z, Gornish M (2005b) Varicocele, hypoxia, and male infertility. Fluid mechanics analysis of the impaired testicular venous drainage system. Hum Reprod 20:2614 - 2619

Goldstein M, Eid JF (1989) Elevation of intratesticular and scrotal skin surface temperature in men with varicocele. J Urol 142:743 - 745

Hamm B, Fobbe F, Sorensen R, Felsenberg D (1986) Varicoceles: combined sonography and thermography in diagnosis and posttherapeutic evaluation. Radiology 160:419

Hoekstra T, Witt MA (1995) The correlation of internal spermatic vein palpability with ultrasonographic diameter and reversal of venous flow. J Urol 153:82 - 84

Kunnen M, Comhaire F (1992) Nonsurgical cure of the varicocele by transcatheter embolization of the internal spermatic veins with tissue adhesive (histoacryl transparent). In: Castaneda-Zuniga WR, Tadavarthy SM (eds) Interventional radiology, 2nd edn, part 2.Williams and Wilkinson, Baltimore, Md., pp 73 - 100

Matthews GJ, Matthews ED, Goldstein M (1998) Induction of spermatogenesis and achievement of pregnancy after microsurgical varicolectomy in men with azoospermia and severe oligoasthenospermia. Fertil Steril 70:71 - 75

McClure DR, Hricak H (1986) Scrotal ultrasound in infertile man: detection of subclinical unilateral and bilateral varicoceles. J Urol 135:711 - 715

Nagler HM (2004) Varicocele. Where, why and, if so, how? J Urol 172 (4Pt1):1239 - 1240

Netto NR, Lemos GC, Barbosa EM (1984) The value of thermography and of the Doppler ultrasound in varicocele diagnosis. Int J Fertil 29:176 - 179

Pasqualotto FF, Lucon AM, Hallak J, Goes PM, Saldanha LB, Arap S (2003) Induction of spermatogenesis in azoospermic men after varicocele repair. Hum Reprod 18:108 - 112

Petros JA, Andriola GL, Middletoon WD, Picus DA (1991) Correlation of testicular color Doppler ultrasonography, physical examination and venography in the detection of left varicocele in men with infertility. J Urol 145:785 - 788

Pochaczevsky R, Lee WJ, Mallett E (1986) Management of male infertility: roles of contact thermography, spermatic venography, and embolization. AJR 147:97

Streeter VL (1971) Fluid mechanics, 5th edn. McGraw-Hill, New York, p 77

Trum JW, Gubler FM, Laan RL, Van der Veen F (1996) The value of palpation, varicoscreen contact thermography and colour Doppler ultrasound in the diagnosis of varicocele. Hum Reprod 11:1232 - 1235

II.3.9 Evaluation of Testicular Biopsy Samples from the Clinical Perspective

M. Bergmann

Summary

Testicular biopsy is indicated therapeutically in cases of obstructive azoospermia, and also in cases of hypergonadotrophic testicular azoospermia to recover testicular spermatozoa (testicular sperm extraction = TESE) for assisted reproduction by intracytoplasmic sperm injection (ICSI). A diagnostic biopsy is indicated in cases of refertilization after vasectomy, and also to exclude a testicular tumour. According to European Association of Urology (EAU) guidelines, several testicular samples from three different locations should be taken because of regional differences in spermatogenesis. Histological evaluation is recommended instead of testicular fine needle aspiration (TEFNA). Specimens should be fixed in Bouin's solution to ensure good preservation of tissue structure and to allow the application of modern histological techniques such as in situ hybridization and immunohistochemistry for evaluating gene expression at the mRNA and protein levels. Diagnosis of pre-invasive carcinoma in situ (CIS, synonym: testicular intraepithelial neoplasia = TIN) is based on the immunohistochemical demonstration of placenta-like alkaline phosphatase (PLAP), which is exclusively expressed in CIS cells. Histological evaluation should be performed using a "score count" system, determining at least the percentage of seminiferous tubules containing elongated spermatids, which is the most important parameter for TESE/ICSI, together with a cytological analysis, which gives further causal evidence for the observed spermatogenic impairment. Testicular biopsy is an invasive surgical operation with a high impact on patients with severe spermatogenic impairment, and should therefore be performed only by considering strict criteria of indication, surgical procedure and histological evaluation in qualified centres that are **certified**, i.e. recommended by the European Academy of Andrology (EAA).

II.3.9.1 Indication

Testicular biopsy is an invasive diagnostic tool to evaluate spermatogenesis and has to be performed only following strict criteria. It completes history taking, physical examination, scrotal ultrasonography, ejaculate and hormonal analysis. It is indicated in cases of azoospermia, when obstruction of the genital tract is suspected because of normal testicular volume, normal follicle-stimulating hormone (FSH) levels (≤7 IU/l), and low levels of epididymal (α-glucosidase, L-carnitine) or seminal vesicle (fructose) markers. It should also be performed in the case of refertilization (vaso-vasostomy) after vasectomy or micro-surgical-epididymal sperm aspiration (MESA) to exclude impairment of the seminiferous epithelium. In both cases, cryopreservation of at least part of the biopsy sample offers the opportunity for testicular sperm extraction (TESE) in combination with intracytoplasmic sperm injection (ICSI), if chirurgical refertilization techniques fail. It is also indicated in cases of testicular hypergonadotrophic azoospermia suggested by high levels of FSH (≥7 IU/l) indicating focal or total Sertoli cell only syndrome (SCO) (Bergmann et al. 1994). In these cases, TESE from remaining focal areas of spermatogenesis within the testis and ICSI form the only rational therapy for assisted reproduction. A diagnostic biopsy is indicated in cases of inhomogeneous testicular ultrasonography to exclude pre-invasive carcinoma in situ (CIS, synonym: testicular intraepithelial neoplasia: TIN) (von Eckardstein et al. 2001). Biopsy of the contralateral testis is indicated when a testicular tumour is clinically evident, because contralateral CIS is reported to have a prevalence of about 5–6%, and of about 2–4% in cases of adult cryptorchidism (Rørth et al. 2000). Testicular biopsy may also be indicated in azoospermic Klinefelter patients, because spermatogenesis, even at a very low rate, might occur allowing TESE and ICSI (Lanfranco et al. 2004). Indications for performing a testicular biopsy are summarized in Table II.3.11.

Table II.3.11. Indications for testicular biopsy

In the case of
Obstructive azoospermia including refertilization after vasectomy (vaso-vasostomy) for TESE/ICSI
Hypergonadotrophic azoospermia for TESE/ICSI
To exclude testicular tumour
In the case of
Contralateral testis in the case of unilateral testicular tumour
Sonographic testicular microlithiasis
Adult cryptorchidism

II.3

II.3.9.2 Preparation

Different surgical techniques for obtaining testicular tissue are used. Percutaneous testicular fine needle aspiration (TEFNA) has been recommended for both the assessment of spermatogenesis (Craft et al. 1997) and sperm retrieval in nonobstructive azoospermia (Lewin et al. 1999) assuming a less traumatic nature compared to the main approach of open TESE (Silber et al. 1995). However, it was shown in a controlled animal model system that TEFNA may also produce widespread architectural distortion of seminiferous tubules, especially after repeated punctures, leaving only Sertoli cells (SCO) as well as focal chronic inflammation and necrosis. The latter was also shown to occur after TESE (Shufaro et al. 2002).

A technique combining cryopreservation, TESE and histology was first developed by Jezek et al. (1998). It was later improved and published as "EAU Guidelines on Male Infertility" by Weidner et al. (2002). This technique includes histological evaluation using a scoring system of three biopsies per testis, which are taken from different locations taking account of the testicular vascularization pattern (Fig. II.3.47). Two parts of the biopsy sample are cryopreserved to recover spermatozoa for ICSI, and to be stored. The third part is fixed and embedded for histological evaluation, because it offers the opportunity for a causal histological evaluation of spermatogenesis. Formalin fixation of specimens as regularly used in pathology cannot be recommended because of severe shrinkage artefacts, making a detailed histological evaluation impossible (Fig. II.3.48a). Fixation in glutaraldehyde, and subsequent embedding in Epon does provide optimal preservation of the structure, allowing semi-thin and ultra-thin electron microscopy (see Holstein et al. 1988). This technique allows clear identification of atypical germ cells in the case of testicular intraepithelial neoplasia (CIS/TIN), because of their nuclear structure and large amounts of intracytoplasmic glycogen granules (Fig. II.3.48b). However, this material is not suitable for the application of modern histological techniques such as immunohistochemistry or in situ hybridization, which provide evidence of gene expression at the protein and mRNA levels. Therefore, fixation in Bouin's solution and embedding in paraffin wax is recommended (Figs. II.3.48c, II.3.49a–c).

For histological evaluation, the biopsy sample should be about the size of a rice grain, showing about 25–30 tubular cross-sections that are shown to be representative of the whole organ (Holstein et al. 1988). However, taking three biopsy samples on each side, our own data of score analysis revealed that there are regional differences within the same testis in respect of spermatogenesis, indicating focal impairment in about 12% of testis specimens (Fig. II.3.52b). In addition, the diagnostic safety in the detection of CIS is significantly increased by taking multiple testicular biopsy samples (Kliesch et al. 2003).

II.3.9.3 Evaluation

Histological evaluation has first to detect and/or to exclude the presence of atypical germ cells (CIS/TIN), which are known to be the precursors of most seminomatous and nonseminomatous germ cell tumours, with the exception of spermatocytic seminoma (Dieckmann and Huland 2001). On paraffin sections these cells can be detected by immunohistochemistry using

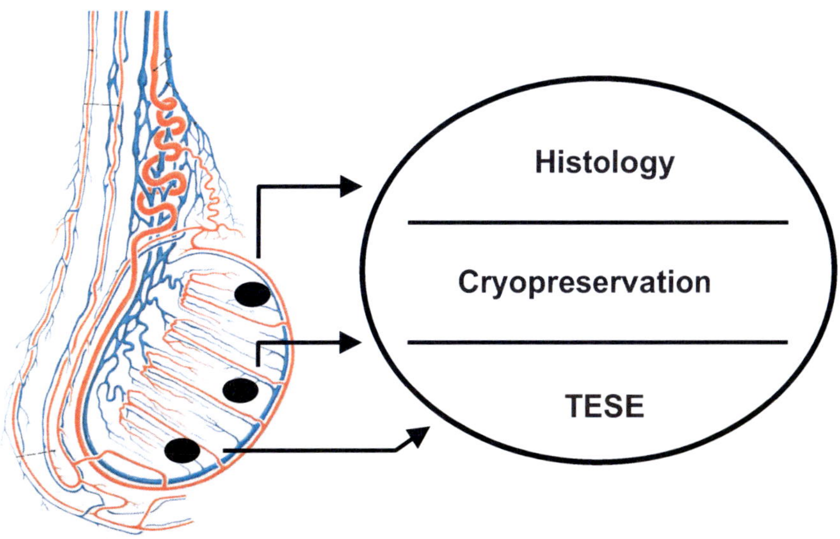

Fig. II.3.47. Scheme of testicular biopsy from three different locations per testis (modified according to Weidner et al. 2002)

II.3

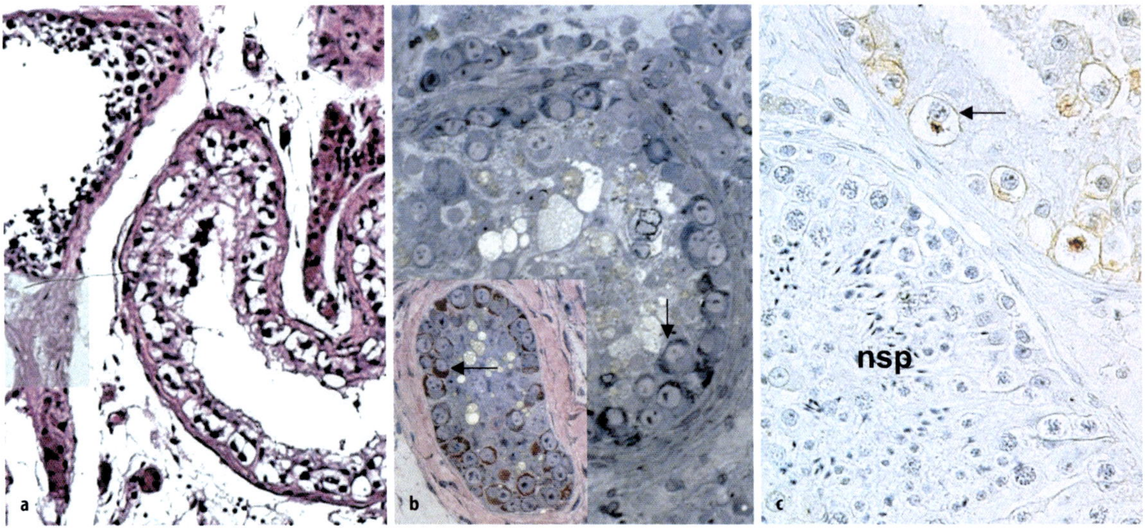

Fig. II.3.48a–c. Seminiferous tubules containing carcinoma in situ (*CIS*). **a** Formalin-fixed, paraffin section; haematoxylin and eosin staining. Note severe shrinkage artefacts of the tissue. **b** Glutaraldehyde fixation, semi-thin section; methylene blue staining. Note typical large nuclei including numerous nucleoli, and dark cytoplasmic glycogen (*arrow*) which can be selectively stained by PAS (*arrow*) (*inset*). **c** Bouin fixation, paraffin section, immunohistochemical staining against placenta-like alkaline phosphatase (*PLAP*). Note membrane-bound immunoreaction of CIS cells (*arrow*). (*nsp* Seminiferous epithelium showing intact spermatogenesis.) Primary magnification: **a** × 20; **b–c** × 40

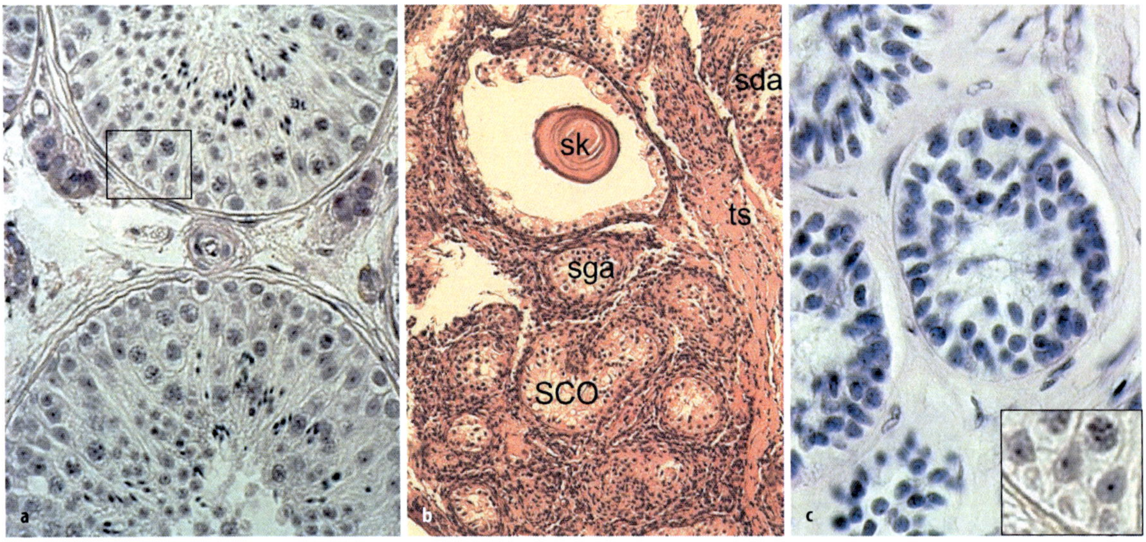

Fig. II.3.49a–c. Testicular histology. **a** Seminiferous tubules showing intact spermatogenesis. **b** Mixed atrophy showing maturation arrest at the level of early round spermatids (*sda*) or spermatogonia (*sga*), only Sertoli cells (*SCO*) or only lamina propria (tubular shadows = *ts*) in adjacent tubules. Note intratubular concentric spherical concrements derived from basal lamina (*sk*). **c** Prepubertal seminiferous cord within an adult testis showing undifferentiated Sertoli cells indicated by round to oval nuclear appearance compared to nuclei of normal Sertoli cells (*inset* = magnification of rectangle a). **a–c** Paraffin sections, haematoxylin and eosin staining; primary magnification: **a** × 40, **b** × 20, **c** × 40

different markers, and most commonly by the presence of placenta-like alkaline phosphatase (PLAP) (Fig. II.3.48c) (Beckstead 1983).

Histological evaluation of any testicular tissue showing impaired spermatogenesis often provides so-called mixed atrophy (Sigg 1979), i.e. the simultaneous occurrence of seminiferous tubules showing at least qualitatively intact spermatogenesis, spermatogenic arrest at different levels of spermatogenesis including tubules with just Sertoli cells (Sertoli cell only = SCO) or even just lamina propria (tubular shadows) in adjacent tubules within the same testis (Fig. II.3.49a–c). Therefore, a semi-quantitative "score count " evaluation, i.e. according to Johnson (1970) or Bergmann and Kliesch

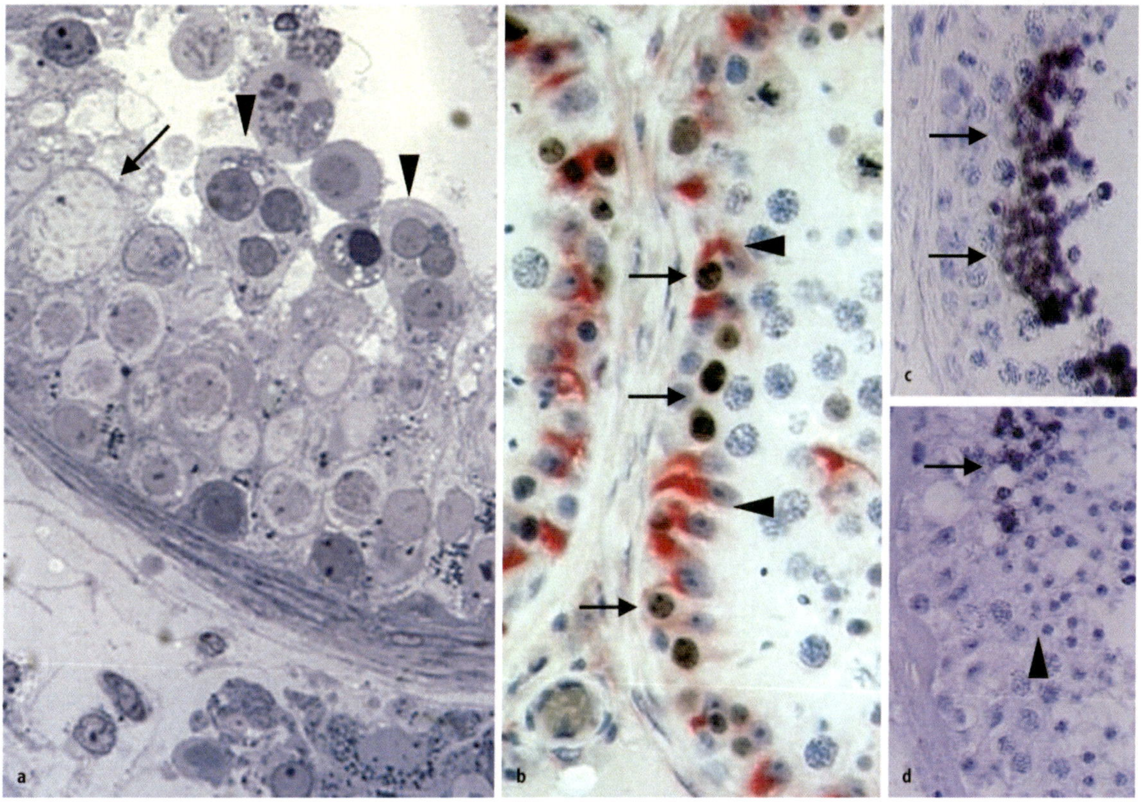

Fig. II.3.50a–d. Histological evaluation using different methodological approaches. **a** Meiotic arrest as indicated by megalospermatocytes (*arrow*) and defects in spermiogenesis indicated by multinucleated spermatids (*arrowheads*). Semi-thin section, methylene blue, primary magnification: ×40. **b** Double immunohistochemistry against s-phase-related Ki-67 protein staining spermatogonial nuclei (*arrows*), and vimentin intermediate filaments staining Sertoli cell cytoplasm (*arrowheads*). Paraffin section, haematoxylin counterstaining; primary magnification: × 40. **c, d** In situ hybridization against protamine mRNA expression in early round spermatids (*arrows*); **c** normal spermatogenesis; **d** hypospermatogenesis. Note the reduced number of labelled spermatids in the case of hypospermatogenesis despite normal histological appearance (*arrowhead*). Paraffin section, haematoxylin counterstaining; primary magnification: × 40

(1998), is necessary. The Johnson score provides a scoring of every tubule within a given histological section, and is highly recommended for oligozoospermic patients, because a high correlation between testicular biopsy score and sperm count is found. However, oligozoospermia is not a current indication for testicular biopsy. In contrast, the score according to Bergmann and Kliesch (1998) (Fig. II.3.50a, b) is based only on the percentage of tubules within the biopsy section showing elongated spermatids, because the occurrence of these spermatids is of main interest in most cases when TESE and ICSI are performed.

Histological evaluation additionally has to include a consideration of cytological alterations. Meiotic defects resulting in so-called megalospermatocytes (Holstein and Eckmann 1986; Johannisson et al. 2003) or multinucleated spermatids representing defects in spermiogenesis (see Holstein et al. 1988) can be recognized on semi-thin sections without any gene or protein expression analysis (Fig. II.3.51a). Estimation of spermatogonial mitotic activity, which is known to be reduced together with spermatogenic impairment, requires an immunohistochemical approach using antibodies against s-phase-related proteins such as K-67 or PCNA (Fig. II.3.51b) (Steger et al. 1998). In biopsy samples showing hypospermatogenesis, in situ hybridization revealed a reduced number of spermatids showing protamine gene expression (Fig. II.3.51c, d) (Steger et al. 2001) which was later confirmed by quantitative polymerase chain reaction (PCR) analysis (Steger et al. 2003). These data gave evidence that "hypospermatogenesis" results from different defects and impairments in germ cell development and differentiation.

Alterations of somatic Sertoli cells are regularly found as signs of differentiation deficiency. This is suggested on routine paraffin sections by round to oval nuclei in Sertoli cells within immature seminiferous cords compared to the normal irregular shape with large and numerous clefts of Sertoli cells within normal seminiferous epithelium (Fig. II.3.49c), and was first proved by Bruning et al. (1993) using computer-assisted three-

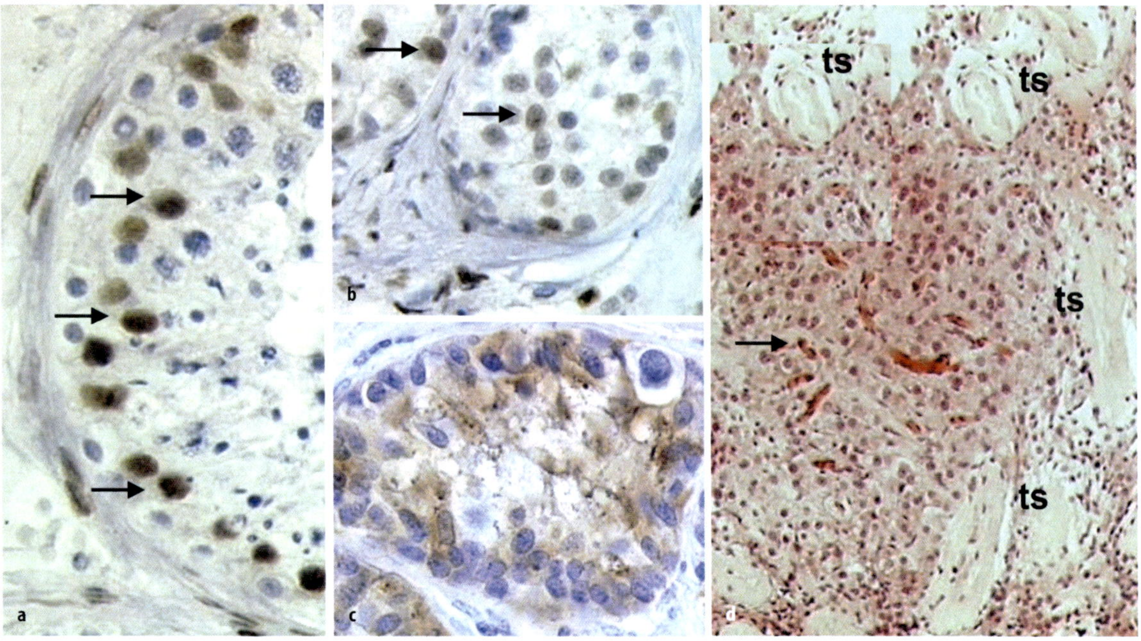

Fig. II.3.51a–d. Immunohistochemistry of Sertoli cell differentiation. **a, b** Androgen receptor expression in Sertoli cell nuclei of normal seminiferous epithelium (**a**) and in prepubertal seminiferous cords (*arrows*). Note only weak expression in some Sertoli cell nuclei in prepubertal seminiferous cords. **c** Persistence of anti-Müllerian hormone expression in Sertoli cells in prepubertal seminiferous cords. **a–c** Paraffin sections, haematoxylin counterstaining; primary magnification: ×40. **d** Typical testicular histology of a Klinefelter patient showing focal Leydig cell hyperplasia (*arrow*), and total atrophy of the seminiferous epithelium resulting in "tubular shadows" (*ts* = only lamina propria). Paraffin section, haematoxylin and eosin staining; primary magnification: **a** ×10

dimensional reconstruction. Sertoli cell differentiation deficiency shown by different markers is now widely accepted to be associated with spermatogenic impairment, and was reviewed by Sharpe et al. (2003).

Sertoli cells are the only cells within the seminiferous epithelium expressing androgen (Fig. II.3.51) as well as FSH receptors. In cryptorchidism, this androgen receptor expression is significantly reduced, as shown by Regadera et al. (2001) using quantitative immunohistochemistry. This is also true for Sertoli cells within premature seminiferous cords found in infertile men (Fig. II.3.51b), which additionally show the persistence of anti-Müllerian hormone expression (Fig. II.3.51c) (Steger et al. 1996). Leydig cells regularly show hyperplasia, which is typically found associated with Sertoli cell only syndrome, i.e. in Klinefelter patients (Fig. II.3.51c).

Taken together, score count evaluation together with a cytological analysis (Fig. II.3.52a, b) provide the opportunity for causal histological evaluation, giving rise to retrospective studies considering histological evaluation and successful TESE/ICSI. Such studies have the potential to facilitate successful assisted reproduction.

Testicular biopsy is an invasive surgical operation with a high impact on patients with severe spermatogenic impairment, and should therefore be performed only after considering strict criteria of indication, surgical procedure and histological evaluation in qualified centres that are certified, i.e. by the European Academy of Andrology (EAA).

Evaluation of testicular biopsy

Name, prename: Date of birth:

Date of biopsy:

Clinic:

Clinical diagnosis:

Criteria	biopsy right			biopsy left		
Semiquantitative	number of tubules			number of tubules		
spermatogenesis up to	1	2	3	1	2	3
- elongating spermatids						
- round spermatids						
- primary spermatocytes						
- spermatogonia						
Sertoli-cell-only						
tubular shadows						
total						
score						
Morphological evaluation						
tubules containing						
- multinuclear spermatids						
- multinuclear spermatocytes						
- multinuclear spermatogonia						
- megalospermatocytes						
- megalospermatogonia						
- degenerating germ cells						
tubular diverticle						
thickening of lamina propria						
morphology of Sertoli cells						
morphology of Leydig cells						
interstitium						
peculiar features						
Diagnosis						

Fig. II.3.52.a Form for evaluation

Evaluation of testicular biopsy

Name, prename: NN　　　　Date of birth: x x

Date of biopsy: x x

Clinic: x x

Clinical diagnosis: hypergonadotropic azoospermia

Criteria	biopsy right			biopsy left		
Semiquantitative	number of tubules			number of tubules		
spermatogenesis up to	1	2	3	1	2	3
- elongating spermatids				11		11
- round spermatids						6
- primary spermatocytes						13
- spermatogonia						
Sertoli-cell-only	42	23	10	18	37	35
tubular shadows		20				
total			95			132
score	0	0	0	4	0	2
Morphological evaluation						
tubules containing						
- multinuclear spermatids				8		6
- multinuclear spermatocytes						
- multinuclear spermatogonia						
- megalospermatocytes						
- megalospermatogonia						
- degenerating germ cells						
tubular diverticle						
thickening of lamina propria	partly					
morphology of Sertoli cells						
morphology of Leydig cells						
interstitium						
peculiar features						
Diagnosis	-SCO - focal total atrophy			- SCO - focal spermatogenesis		

Fig. II.3.52.b Example of biopsy evaluation of a hypergonadotrophic azoospermic patient showing total Sertoli cell only syndrome within the right and left testis, and additional focal areas of spermatogenesis within the upper and lower pole of the left testis. Cytoplasmic analysis also revealed an impairment of spermiogenesis (multinuclear spermatids)

References

Beckstead JH (1983) Alkaline phosphatase histochemistry in human germ cell neoplasms. Am J Surg Pathol 7:341–349

Bergmann M, Kliesch S (1998) Hodenbiopsie. In: Krause W, Weidner W (eds) Andrologie. Enke, Stuttgart, pp 66–71

Bergmann M, Behre HM, Nieschlag E (1994) Serum FSH and testicular morphology in male infertility. Clin Endocrinol 40:133–136

Bruning G, Dierichs R, Stümpel C, Bergmann M (1993) Sertoli cell nuclear changes in human testicular biopsies as revealed by three dimensional reconstruction. Andrologia 25:311–316

Craft I, Tsirigotis M, Courtald E, Farrer-Brown G (1997) Testicular needle aspiration as an alternative to biopsy for the assessment of spermatogenesis. Hum Reprod 10:1483–1487

Dieckmann KP, Huland H (2001) Hodentumoren. In: Hautmann RE, Huland H (eds) Andrologie. Springer, Berlin Heidelberg New York, pp 223–236

Holstein AF, Eckmann C (1986) Megalospermatocytes: indicators of disturbed meiosis in man. Andrologia 18:601–609

Holstein AF, Schirren C, Roosen-Runge EC (1988) Illustrated pathology of human spermatogenesis. Grosse, Berlin

Jezek D, Knuth UA, Schulze W (1998) Successful testicular sperm extraction (TESE) in spite of high serum follicle stimulating hormone and azoospermia: correlation between testicular morphology, TESE results, semen analysis and serum hormone values in 103 infertile men. Hum Reprod 13:1230–1234

Johannisson R, Schulze W, Holstein AF (2003) Megalospermatocytes in the human testis exhibit asynapsis of chromosomes. Andrologia 35:146–151

Johnson SG (1970) Testicular biopsy score count – a method for registration of spermatogenesis in human testis: normal values and results in 335 hypogonadal males. Hormone 1:2

Kliesch S, Thomaidis T, Schütte B, Pühse G, Kater B, Roth S, Bergmann M (2003) Update on the diagnostic safety for detection of testicular intraepithelial neoplasia (TIN). APMIS 111:70–75

Lanfranco F, Kamischke A, Zitzmann M, Nieschlag E (2004) Klinefelter's syndrome. Lancet 364:273–284

Lewin A, Reubinoff B, Porat-Kratz A (1999) Testicular needle aspiration: the alternative method for sperm retrieval in non-obstructive azoospermia. Hum Reprod 14:1785–1790

Regadera J, Martinez-Garcia F, Gonzalez-Peramato P, Serrano A, Nistal M, Suarez-Quian C (2001) Androgen receptor expression in Sertoli cells as a function of seminiferous tubule maturation in the human cryptorchid testis. J Clin Endocrinol Metab 86:431–421

Rørth M, Raijpert-De Meyts E, Andersson L, Diekmann K-P, Fossa SD, Grigor KM, Hendry WF, Herr HW, Looijenga LH, Oosterhuis JW, Skakkebaek NE (2000) Carcinoma in situ of the testis. Scand J Urol Nephrol Suppl 205:166–186

Sharpe RM, McKinnell C, Kivlin C, Fisher S (2003) Proliferation and functional maturation of Sertoli cells, and their relevance to disorders of testis function in adulthood. Reproduction 125:769–784

Shufaro Y, Prus D, Laufer N, Simon A (2002) Impact of repeated testicular fine needle aspirations (TEFNA) and testicular sperm extraction (TESE) on the microscopic morphology of the testis: an animal model. Hum Reprod 17:1795–1799

Sigg C (1979) Klassifizierung tubulärer Hodenatrophien bei Sterilitätsabklärungen. Bedeutung der sogenannten bunten Atrophie. Schweiz Med Wschr 109:1284–1293

Silber SJ, Van Steirteghem AC, Liu J, Nagy Z, Tournaye H, Devreoey P (1995) High fertilization and pregnancy rate after intracytoplasmic sperm injection with spermatozoa obtained from testicular biopsy. Hum Reprod 10:148–152

Steger K, Rey R, Kliesch S, Louis F, Schleicher G, Bergmann M (1996) Immunohistochemical detection of immature Sertoli cell markers in testicular tissue of infertile adult men: a preliminary study. Int J Androl 19:122–128

Steger K, Aleithe I, Behre H-M, Bergmann M (1998) The proliferation of spermatogonia in normal and pathologic human seminiferous epithelium: an immunohistochemical study using monoclonal antibodies against Ki-67 protein and proliferating cell nuclear antigen PCNA). Mol Hum Reprod 4: 227–233

Steger K, Failing K, Klonisch T, Behre HM, Manning M, Weidner W, Hertle L, Bergmann M, Kliesch S (2001) Round spermatids from infertile men exhibit decreased levels of protamine-1 and protamine2 mRNA. Hum Reprod 16:709–716

Steger K, Fink L, Failing K, Bohle RM, Kliesch S, Weidner W, Bergmann M (2003) Decreased protamine-1 transcript levels in testes from infertile men. Mol Hum Reprod 9:331–336

von Eckardstein S, Tsakmakidis G, Kamischke A, Rolf C, Nieschlag E (2001) Sonographic testicular microlithiasis as an indicator of premalignant conditions in normal and infertile men. J Androl 22:818–824

Weidner W, Colpi GM, Hargreave TB, Papp GK, Pomerol JM, The EAU Working Group on Male Infertility (2002) EAU guidelines on male infertility. Eur Urol 42:313–322

II.3.10 Genetics and Male Infertility

T.B. Hargreave, D.J. Elliott

Summary

- Karyotype analysis should be undertaken for all men with low sperm concentration who are seeking fertility treatments.
- Chromosomes are relatively sticky and fragile, and translocation of genetic material from one chromosome to another occurs in approximately 1 in 500 people. People with balanced translocations are normal but will produce some sperm or eggs with extra or missing genetic material and this will result in a foetus with an imbalanced translocation.
- Klinefelter syndrome 47XXY is the most frequent sex chromosome abnormality.
- Partners of men with congenital bilateral absence of the vas deferens should also be tested for cystic fibrosis transmembrane conductance regulator (CFTR) mutations prior to any fertility treatment so that the couple can be given an accurate risk assessment of having a child with cystic fibrosis.
- Y microdeletions will be passed to sons and it can be predicted that some of these in their turn may have fertility problems.

II.3.10.1 Introduction

The advent of in vitro fertilization (IVF) and intracytoplasmic sperm injection (ICSI) has opened the door to fertility for many couples for whom there had been no reasonable prospect of conception. IVF was introduced to overcome the problem of bilateral Fallopian tube occlusion, however it soon became apparent that this technology could enable fatherhood for men with very low sperm counts and severely impaired spermatogenesis. It has been known for a long time that there is a higher rate of chromosomal and genetic abnormalities detected in peripheral blood leukocytes from such men and it is now known that some men with a normal constitutional genetic make-up have genetic abnormalities confined to the germ-cell line and in whom abnormalities can only be detected by the examination of sperm. Before the advent of IVF and ICSI, this was mainly of academic interest but now there is the potential for these defects to be passed on to the next generation. Thus, there is a need for infertility clinicians to have a good understanding of the genetics of male as well as female infertility.

II.3.10.2 Basic Information about the Human Genetic Code

The normal human cell has 46 chromosomes arranged as 22 pairs of autosomes and either two X chromosomes in the female or an X and Y in the male. On these chromosomes are arranged approximately 30,000 genes that encode proteins (Lander et al. 2001). The chromosomes package six to seven billion base pairs of deoxyribonucleic acid (DNA). The DNA is arranged as sequences of the four DNA nucleotides adenosine, cytosine, thymine and guanine (ACTG) and it is this sequence that spells out the sequence of amino acids in proteins. The sequences of the nucleotides are arranged into protein-describing areas called EXONS and non-protein-describing areas called INTRONS and also special sequences to indicate the beginning and end of genes. Usually the sequence of amino acids in a protein is derived from information from several EXONS joined or "spliced" together in the nucleus before the proteins are made in the cytoplasm. Splicing is under the control of proteins and RNAs in a complex called the spliceosome. Splicing allows mixing and matching of exons to enable the formation of different proteins with shared common sequences and thus maximizes the efficiency of the genetic information. Only 2% of the human genome encodes proteins. The function of the remaining 98% of the genetic material is largely unknown although some of it may be to do with regulating genes. The preservation over 400 million years of some non-protein-coding sequences between men, mice and fugu fish indicates a likely vital role for some of these sequences. Some chromosomes are much richer in gene coding sequences than others; for example, chromosome 19 has sequences for at least 1461 genes including those that code for cardiovascular disease, insulin-dependent diabetes and migraines, whereas by contrast chromosome 5 is nearly 3 times the size of chromosome 19 and yet it only contains some 923 protein-encoding genes and has vast regions known as gene deserts.

Genes can be classified into functional classes; for example, oncogenes, check point genes, genes regulating apoptosis, etc. Genes may be arranged in functional clusters. The male sex-determining gene SRY is located on the short arm of the Y and there are several genes involved with spermatogenesis on the long arm of the Y chromosome.

Humans share common genes with all living creatures. We differ from our closest relatives, the chimpanzees, by approximately 1.6% of our DNA and diverged from a common ancestor about 7 million years ago. Gorillas differ in approximately 2.3% of their DNA from chimpanzees and us and diverged from our (humans and chimpanzees) common ancestor about 10 million years ago. All the above species diverged from monkeys about 32 million years ago and there is a DNA difference of only 7.5% (Sibley et al. 1990). Our kinship with primates and mammals allows appropriate animal models to be used to study human genetic mechanisms both generally and with respect to male fertility.

Spermatozoa and oocytes are different from other cells in the body because the DNA content is half that of other cells. This reduction in DNA content occurs when the spermatocytes undergo meiotic division to form haploid round spermatids. The round spermatids elongate in a process called spermiogenesis and during this process the DNA becomes compacted in the sperm head. These changes are under genetic control but we are only now beginning to understand the mechanisms. It is estimated that 2000 genes are involved in the regulation of spermatogenesis and that of these 20–30 genes are located on the long arm of the Y chromosome (Hackstein et al. 2000). In general, autosomal genes that regulate spermatogenesis are concerned with the regulation of metabolic processes in other cells in the body as well as in the cells of spermatogenesis, whereas Y genes are not essential for vital functions other than male reproduction. Our new understanding of the genetics of spermatogenesis holds promise for the development of new treatments for male infertility and novel non-hormonal methods of male contraception.

II.3.10.3 Chromosomal Abnormalities and Male Fertility

There are various different types of chromosomal abnormality including the absence of chromosomes or the presence of supernumerary chromosomes or translocation of sections of chromosome or abnormal shaped chromosome such as ring forms.

Peripheral blood chromosomal abnormalities are more common in infertile men and in infertile male partners in couples seeking ICSI than in the general population (Van Assche et al. 1996). In a survey of pooled data from 11 publications reporting on 9766 infertile men (Johnson 1998), there was an incidence of chromosomal abnormalities of 5.8%. Of these, sex chromosome abnormalities accounted for 4.2% and autosomal abnormalities for 1.5%. For comparison, the incidence of chromosome abnormalities in pooled data from three series including a total of 94,465 newborn male infants was 0.38%, and of these 131 (0.14%) were sex chromosome abnormalities and 232 (0.25%) were autosomal abnormalities (Van Assche et al. 1996).

In a population of 781 male partners in couples undergoing ICSI, 30 men (3.8%) had chromosomal abnormalities. Of these there were 10 (1.2%) sex chromosome aberrations and 20 (2.6%) autosomal aberrations (Peschka et al. 1999).

Chromosomes are relatively sticky and fragile and translocation of genetic material from one chromosome to another occurs in approximately 1 in 500 people. A balanced reciprocal translocation is when there is exchange between two different chromosomes but there is no loss or gain of genetic material. People with balanced translocations are normal but will produce some sperm or eggs with extra or missing genetic material and this will result in a foetus with an imbalanced translocation. One of the more common examples is translocation of genetic material between chromosome 21 and 14 and whilst the carrying parent is normal some gametes contain extra material from chromosome 21 and this can result in a baby with Down's syndrome. This particular scenario accounts for approximately 4% of cases of Down's syndrome. Another type of translocation is where chromosomes join around their centre to form one long chromosome. This is called a Robertsonian translocation. It occurs among chromosomes 13, 14, 15, 21 and 22 (most commonly between chromosomes 13, 14 and 14, 21) and is present in 1 in 1000 in the general population. A person with a Robertsonian translocation only has 45 chromosomes but is normal provided there is no missing material (balanced Robertsonian translocation). However, gametes may contain a whole extra chromosome and, for example, this is another cause of trisomy 21 (Down's syndrome).

II.3.10.3.1 Sex Chromosomal Abnormalities

The effect of sex chromosome abnormalities depends on whether the problem affects the X or the Y chromosome. In general, the Y chromosome does not carry genes essential for life, which is not surprising as half of humanity does not have one!

Klinefelter Syndrome and Variants (47XXY, 46XY; 47XXY Mosaicism)

Klinefelter syndrome is the most frequent sex chromosome abnormality, which occurred in 66 (0.07%) phenotypically newborn males in pooled data from cytogenetic analysis of 94,465 newborn infants (Van Assche et al. 1996). In azoospermic men the prevalence of Klinefelter syndrome has been found to be approximately 10% in Western countries (De Braekeleer and Dao 1991) and approximately 7.5% in Japanese men (Okada et al. 1999). Adult males with Klinefelter's have firm small testicles with very few or no germ cells; this is to be distinguished from men with other causes of damage to spermatogenesis who usually have soft small testicles. The phenotype can vary from a normally virilized man to one with stigmata of androgen deficiency including female hair distribution and scanty body hair. Classically a man with Klinefelter syndrome has long legs and, if eunuchoid, long arms as well because of late epiphyseal closure. A longitudinal study of children with sex chromosome abnormalities has been reported (Ratcliffe 1999).

Leydig Cell Function is Commonly Impaired in Men with Klinefelter Syndrome (Wang et al. 1975)

Testosterone levels may be normal or low, oestradiol levels normal or increased and follicle-stimulating hormone (FSH) levels increased. Surprisingly, libido is often normal despite low testosterone levels but with ageing there is often a need for androgen replacement; thus men with Klinefelter syndrome should be offered longer-term supervision in addition to the management of their fertility problems. Reduced Leydig cell function is also relevant in the context of sperm retrieval for ICSI as there may be long-term post biopsy lower testosterone levels (Okada et al. 2004). Also adequate levels of androgens are being implicated in the development of behaviour and language and this is relevant as ICSI may increase the chances of birth of babies with Klinefelter syndrome (Simpson et al. 2003). In a series of 147 men with complete Klinefelter syndrome 47XXY, as determined by peripheral blood karyotype (Okada et al. 1999), spermatozoa were detected in the ejaculate in only one man, and in his case repeat peripheral blood karyotype still failed to detect any mosaicism. If this experience is typical, men with complete Klinefelter syndrome may be advised that the prospects of sperm recovery from the ejaculate are poor. Mature spermatozoa can be recovered from testicular tissue from men with apparent complete Klinefelter syndrome (Foresta et al. 1999) and in many centres this is being done (Ulug et al. 2003; Komori et al. 2004). At present there are no reliable prebiopsy criteria to indicate the chance of success (Vernaeve et al. 2004) all the more since the chances of finding sperm may decrease with age (Lin et al. 2004). There is a risk of offspring with Klinefelter, and preimplantation genetic diagnosis (PGD) is now being offered in some centres (Kahraman et al. 2003; Staessen et al. 2003).

When advising a man with Klinefelter syndrome about the chances of sperm recovery from testicular tissue, the andrologist should consider the chances of obtaining sperm and the risk of subsequent testosterone deficiency as it has been shown that even minimal biopsy is associated with long-term testosterone deficit (Okada et al. 2004). If the man has absolute azoospermia verified by examination of centrifuged deposits of at least three ejaculate samples and if karyotype shows no evidence of mosaicism, then the chance of recovering sperm is approximately 50% (Vernaeve et al. 2004) and may involve extensive testicular dissection with a significant risk of reduction of Leydig cell mass. Arrangements should be made for the long-term endocrine follow-up of all men with Klinefelter syndrome who undergo testicular biopsy to recover sperm.

Men with Klinefelter mosaicism 46XY/47XXY have variable germ-cell presence and variable sperm production. Until the advent of IVF and ICSI this was academic, but it is now important to diagnose mosaicism because some sperm retrieved may be expected to be normal and can be used for fertilization. Preimplantation fluorescent in situ hybridization (FISH) analysis of cells from embryos can be used to confirm normality (Tournaye et al. 1996). The production of 24XY sperm has been reported in 0.9% (Chevret et al. 1996) and 2.1% (Martini et al. 1996) of men with Klinefelter mosaicism, and in 1.36–25% of men with somatic karyotype 47XXY (Cozzi et al. 1994; Guttenbach et al. 1997; Estop et al. 1998; Foresta et al. 1998; Hennebicq et al. 1999). It is not known whether haploid sperm in Klinefelter syndrome is always the result of a clone of normal cells in a mosaic population or whether in certain circumstances some 47XXY male germ cells are viable and capable of producing haploid sperm.

Sex Chromosome Abnormalities in Babies Conceived Through Intracytoplasmic Sperm Injection

There are a number of reports that indicate a higher than normal frequency of sex chromosome abnormalities in children conceived through ICSI compared with that in the normal population. The underlying mechanism is not yet known, but there are several possibilities discussed in the literature. These include Klinefelter's mosaicism with an aneuploid cell line confined to the germ cells and thus not detectable by peripheral blood karyotyping (Persson et al. 1996) or the production of 47XY diploid sperm; this has been reported in sperm from severely oligozoospermic men with a normal karyotype (Foresta et al. 1996). It has been suggested that mutations confined to the germ cells may arise when the primordial germ cells are in the extra-embryonic cell mass before these cells migrate back into the embryo (Persson 1999). A third possibility is that low levels of mosaicism may be missed during routine karyotype analysis.

47 XYY a Rarer Abnormality and Often Associated with an Apparently Normal Sperm Analysis

Males with 47 XYY are seen more frequently in the infertile population and FISH analysis of spermatozoa indicates that although the majority of sperm are normal (Martini et al. 1996), there is an increase in disomy (Chevret et al. 1997; Martin et al. 1999).

II.3.10.3.2
Autosomal Abnormalities in Men with Azoospermia and Severe Oligozoospermia

In addition to an increase in sex chromosome abnormalities there is also an increase in autosomal abnormalities in populations of men with non-obstructive azoospermia or severe oligozoospermia (Chandley et al. 1975; Moog et al. 1996). Usually autosomal disorders do not cause infertility in isolation but reduced spermatogenesis is the consequence of a more general disturbance in phenotype and patients with these problems are often known to doctors because of other developmental abnormalities and do not present de novo with infertility. It is worthwhile performing karyotype analysis for any man with infertility who has clinical stigmata such as facial asymmetry or other congenital abnormality. In view of the known excess of autosomal abnormalities in men with severe oligozoospermia it is appropriate to perform karyotyping for all such men where it is proposed to use ICSI to enable fertility and to offer genetic counselling when abnormalities are discovered. Karyotype analysis may be normal but this does not exclude genetic defects and patients and infertility clinicians need to understand the limitations of karyotype analysis. From time to time, men may ask for ICSI who are known to have an autosomal defect. In these cases genetic counselling is required, and should address the concerns of the man for his genetic condition as well as any reproductive implications.

II.3.10.4
Genetic Defects and Male Fertility

Changes in the sequence of DNA are called mutations and while mutations may occasionally be beneficial and become preserved in evolution often they result in defective genetic function. It has been postulated that many mutations occur in the testis during spermatogenesis and that the testicle is "the engine of evolution" and that the external position of the testes is because a cooler temperature damps down the mutation rate (Short 1997). Mutations may involve relatively large chunks of the gene but there are also many examples of where the alteration of a single base pair on the original DNA (point mutation) can have a profound effect on phenotype. Genetic defects may be single or multiple and may be inherited or the result of new mutation. They may be inherited in a dominant pattern as in Huntington's chorea or a recessive pattern as in cystic fibrosis and may have variable penetrance.

When mutations are in exons there is an alteration in the protein produced and in many cases a marked resulting alteration in phenotype. Mutations of non coding areas (introns) are less well understood but can affect the amount of protein produced by making the reading of protein-encoding RNA from the original DNA less efficient; for the andrologist one of the best known examples of this is the 5 T intron abnormality that occurs in the cystic fibrosis transmembrane gene complex (CFTR) and which is found either alone or with exon mutations in men with congenital absence of the vas deferens (see below).

Most if not all genes on the Y chromosome are to do with the regulation of male differentiation and defects will be manifested as phenotypic abnormality except sometimes where there are autosomal replacement homologues of the gene, e.g. the Y-linked DAZ gene has an autosomal homologue called DAZL which might provide some overlapping gene function. X-linked genes may be dominant (e.g. hypophosphatemic rickets) or recessive (e.g. Duchenne's muscular dystrophy). X-linked dominant genes will alter the phenotype in both sexes but X-linked recessive genes will only be manifest in the male.

II.3.10.4.1
X-Linked Genetic Disorders and Male Fertility

Each man has only one X chromosome and therefore an X-linked recessive disorder will be manifest in males and the defect will be transmitted through his daughters to his grandsons (Fig. II.3.53). In addition there is a suggestion that the X chromosome may contain a preponderance of genes involved in spermatogenesis (Wang et al. 2001).

Kallman's Syndrome

The commonest X-linked disorder in infertility practice is Kallman's syndrome and the most common form of this is X-linked recessive caused by a mutation in the KALIG-1 gene on Xp22.3 (Franco et al. 1991). This gene is involved with the regulation of cell adhesion and axonal path finding. Patients with Kallman's syndrome

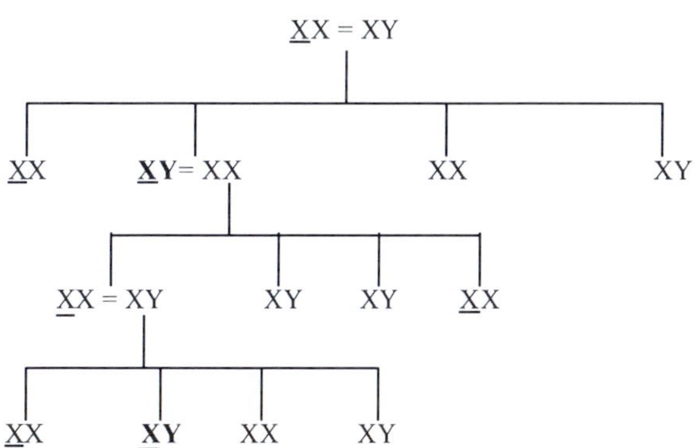

Fig. II.3.53. Diagram of X-linked recessive inheritance, showing transmission through daughters to grandsons. Sons are not affected, and therefore phenotypic disorders will skip generations and may be hard to detect

have hypogonadotrophic hypogonadism and may have other clinical features including anosmia, facial asymmetry, cleft palate, colour blindness, deafness, maldescended testes and renal abnormalities. Other rare forms of Kallman's syndrome have been described, including an autosomal dominant (Sauten and Paulsen 1973) and an autosomal recessive form. It is important for the andrologist to note that some men with Kallman's syndrome have an isolated gonadotrophin deficiency without any other phenotypic abnormalities and that these men may sometimes present de novo with infertility, which can be treated successfully by hormone replacement therapy.

Androgen Insensitivity – Reifenstein Syndrome, Morris Syndrome, Hairless Women

The rare disorder of androgen insensitivity may sometimes first present with infertility. The condition has an X-linked recessive inheritance and is caused by one or more defects in the androgen receptor gene, which is located on Xq 11–12. The phenotype may range from complete testicular feminization with an immature female phenotype, to an apparently normal male with infertility, although the latter is rare. In our clinic we conducted a structured genetic search for androgen receptor deficiency among those men with normal phenotype but with high normal testosterone levels and low sperm counts; however, we failed to find any cases using base-pair mismatch analysis technology (Tincello et al. 1997). In the course of our study we reported several de novo mutations of the androgen receptor, but in all cases these were associated with obvious genital abnormalities, such as hypospadias. We concluded that androgen insensitivity in the infertile male in the absence of any genital abnormality is rare.

Excessive amplification of trinucleotide repeats (CAG) in the translated part of the androgen receptor gene is associated with various neurodegenerative diseases such as Huntington's disease. There has been debate about whether sons of infertile men conceived through ICSI may be with an increased number of CAG repeats in exon 1 compared with their fathers and whether these sons may be at risk of neurodegenerative disease but this is thought to be unlikely (Vogt 1999).

The number of CAG repeats may also be of relevance to prostate cancer. Men with fewer than 22 repeats may be at more risk of developing prostate cancer than those with more repeats (Nelson and Witte 2002) but this association has not been found in a Japanese population (Li et al. 2003).

Other X Disorders

There is a case report (Gonialves et al. 1996) of an azoospermic man with biopsy-proven spermatogenetic arrest who was found to have a submicroscopic interstitial deletion on the Xp pseudoautosomal region in peripheral blood and skin fibroblast samples. Other genetic and chromosome studies were entirely normal, including probing of the Yq region. It is also worth noting a report of two men with azoospermia and X pseudoautosomal deletions (Gabriel-Robez et al. 1990). So far there have been no other reported examples of X-linked disorders affecting male fertility, and if such disorders exist and are not associated with azoospermia, these would skip generations of males and will be very difficult to define.

X-Linked Disorders that are not Associated with Male Infertility

There are many rare X-linked disorders not associated with infertility. For example, Menkes disease is an X-linked recessive disturbance of copper metabolism associated with progressive neurological symptoms (Horn et al. 1992). Family history is important as it is very difficult to recognize such disorders, especially if there have been several generations of female births and where a recessive X-linked gene has been carried through these generations without any clinical stigmata. Management is in the normal way by giving the couple choices after appropriate genetic counselling including consideration about the severity of any disorder that may result. It may be appropriate to offer the couple pre-implantation sex determination and only to replace female embryos or in some situations not to embark on fertility treatment at all.

II.3.10.4.2 Y Genes and Male Infertility

Y chromosome genes are subject to different evolutionary pressure compared with all other genes. Spermatogenesis is lifelong and is the result of rapid cell division, and in principle there is much lifetime chance for production of sperm with mutant genes compared with oogenesis, which involves much small numbers of cells, occurs early in life and is followed by a long inert period, and this is despite the fact that, cell for cell, oogenesis is actually more error prone (Hunt and Hassold 2002).

Normally autosomal genes can undergo DNA repair when they pair with their opposite number during mitotic division but for Y genes this pairing cannot happen since most of the Y chromosome excluding the pseudoautosomal region is different from the X. Instead there are multiple copies of genes arranged in mirror images (palindromes) which might act to repair themselves by gene conversion and because of this when genetic material is deleted there is a variable phenotype depending on the number of gene copies deleted (Rozen et al. 2003; Skaletsky et al. 2003).

Y Microdeletions

In 1992 we reported three men with severe damage to spermatogenesis and an apparently normal chromosome analysis but where molecular probes revealed microdeletions on the long arm of the Y chromosome (Ma et al. 1992; Vogt et al. 1992). We were stimulated to probe the long arm of the Y because of a report (Tiepolo and Zuffardi 1976) of men with azoospermia and deletions of the long arm of the Y transecting interval 6 with the loss of all distal genetic material and also by our own finding of an infertile man with a short arm dicentric Y (Chandley et al. 1986). Following our 1992 report there have been a large number of publications of case series and it is clear that while microdeletions may occur in the fertile population (Pryor et al. 1997) they are more prevalent in the infertile populations (Table II.3.12).

To date the microdeletions detected have been rather large but there are reports of much smaller deletions encompassing single genes (Foresta et al. 2000). Microdeletions have been found in three non-overlapping regions of the Y chromosome, AZF a-b-c (Vogt et al. 1996). The proximal part of the AZFc microdeletion is sometimes designated AZFd. These microdeletions are thought to occur between the palindromic and direct repeats (Repping et al. 2002). Involvement of several genes has been described, and these include RBM (Ma et al. 1993), DAZ (Reijo et al. 1995), DFFRY (Brown et al. 1998), DBY and CDY (Fig. II.3.54). The abnormalities most commonly reported in the literature are microdeletions in the AZFc region encompassing copies of the DAZ gene. However, there is no exact correlation between DAZ deletion and the degree of spermatogenesis, perhaps because there are four DAZ copies on the Y and also a very similar autosomal homologue called DAZL. There is a report of a man with severely damaged spermatogenesis who has normal peripheral blood leukocyte DAZ expression, but with an absence of testicular DAZ expression (Ferlin et al. 1999). The same explanations may be postulated as discussed above for 47XY sperm (i.e. low levels of mosaicism or perhaps mutations in the extra-embryonic cell mass).

DAZ and RBM Genes

The first candidate gene for spermatogenesis was identified from our unit and is now called RBM (RNA binding motif). There is a family of up to 50 RBM genes

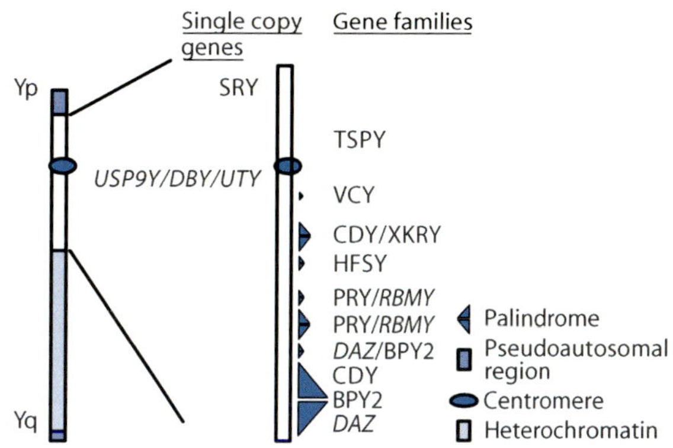

Fig. II.3.54. The human Y chromosome has a long and a short arm separated by the centromere. At the tips of each arm are the pseudoautosomal regions, which are homologous to the X chromosome. The male-specific part of the Y chromosome is composed of heterochromatin and euchromatin (not shaded and shown enlarged on the *right-hand side* of the figure). The euchromatin has now been sequenced and is composed of a mixture of single copy genes (including SRY, the sex determining gene) and large inverted repeats (palindromes) containing gene families. Deletion of the genes and gene families shown in *bold italics* has been implicated in male infertility. Not all Y chromosome genes are shown. For a full catalogue, see *Nature* 423: 825–837

(Cooke et al. 1996), and while most copies are probably inactive, deletions of the AZFb region cause functional inactivation of RBM. Sequencing of the human Y chromosome has identified six potentially active RBM genes, all of which are deleted in the AZFb region (Skaletsky et al. 2003). The DAZ gene (formerly known as SPGY) was the second candidate gene to be described and is also a member of a family of similar genes (Saxena et al. 1996).

Both DAZ and the RBM gene families encode proteins with a conserved protein domain called an RNA recognition motif (RRM), which means they are probably involved in the metabolism of RNA. RBM is a nuclear protein, whereas DAZ protein is cytoplasmic, but expression of both is restricted to the male germ line. RBM protein is most closely related in sequence to hnRNPG, a member of a group of nuclear proteins called hnRNPs (heterogeneous nuclear RNA ribonucleoproteins). hnRNPs are involved in many aspects of RNA metabolism, including packaging of RNA, transport to the cytoplasm and splicing. However, hnRNPG is ubiquitously expressed, indicating a function that is required for all cell types (Soulard et al. 1993; Caceres et al. 1994; Delbridge et al. 1998). RBM probably regulates splicing events essential for spermatogenesis (Elliot et al. 1998), whereas DAZ is important for gametogenesis in both sexes and, because of its cytoplasmic location, may be involved in the male in regulating protein translation during spermatogenesis.

The X and the Y chromosomes were originally a pair of autosomes that became specialized as sex chromo-

Table II.3.12. Men with microdeletions. Presented are published case series data. (*astheno* Asthenozoospermia, *azoo* azoospermia, *oligo* oligozoospermia, *STS* sequence tagged site.)

Reference	Observation	No. of men	No. with deletion	%
Ma et al. (1992)	Various all Yq	Various	3 Azoo-oligo	
Mallidis et al. (1996)	1 AZFc	186	5	3%
Kent-First et al. (1999)	Multiplex STS all Yq	239	24	(18–22%)
Kupker et al. (1996)	6 all Yq	80 Oligo 40 Azoo	0 3	 7.5% Azoo
Kobayashi et al. (1994)		53	10	16%
Najmabadi et al. (1996)	26 interval 6	16 Fertile men 7 Fertile women 50 Azoo 10 Oligo 15 X-linked	0 0 10 1 0	 20% Azoo 10% Oligo
Reijo et al. (1996)	83 all Yq	89 Azoo	12	13%
Qureshi et al. (1996)	23 all Yq	51 Azoo 38; $<5.0\times10^6$ sperm per ml; oligo 11; $>5.0\times10^6$ sperm per ml 80 Fertile	4 4 0 0	8% Azoo 11%; $<5.0\times10^6$ sperm per ml
Reijo et al. (1996)	118 probes all Yq	35 Severe oligo	2	5.7%
Foresta et al. (1996		16 Azoo 23; $<5.0\times10^6$ sperm per ml	5 6	31% 26%
Stuppia et al. (1996)	13 probes interval 6	33 Azoo-oligo; 10 normal		8%
Vogt et al. (1996)	76 probes al Yq	370 Azoo-oligo 200		3.2%
Pryor et al. (1997)	85 probes all Yq	200 Infertile 200 Normal	14 4	7% 2%
Foresta et al. (1997)	15 probes all Yq	38 Azoo-oligo 10 Normal		37.5% Azoo 22.7% Oligo 0% Normal
Simoni et al. (1997)	4 probes AZF a-b-c	168 Azoo-oligo 86 Normal		3%
Girardi et al. (1997)	36 all Yq	160 Infertile 6 Fertile		5%
Stuppia et al. (1998)	27 interval 6	50 Azoo-oligo 10 Normal		14%
Krausz et al. (1999)		22 Azoo 42; $<1\times10^6$ sperm per ml 53 Oligozoo 13 Astheno $>20\times10^6$ sperm per ml 4 Normal	1 2 0 0 0	4.5% 4.7%
Kleiman et al. (1999)		133 Oligo/azoo	8	6.01%

somes. The gene encoding hnRNPG is found on the X chromosome (Delbridge et al. 1999). This means that RBMX and RBM were original members of the pair of autosomes that gave rise to the X and Y chromosomes and so are very ancient (and probably important) genes. Consistent with this, RBM is a highly conserved gene and has been found on the Y chromosomes of all mammalian species so far tested (Schempp et al. 1995) including marsupials (Delbridge et al. 1997). In addition to these copies on the sex chromosomes, there are a number of autosomal genes which encode proteins almost identical to hnRNPG. One of these autosomal genes on chromosome 11 is only expressed during meiosis, and is called HNRNPGT (Elliott et al. 2000). Because of its restricted expression in male germ cell development, HNRNPGT is a candidate infertility gene, and a variant allele of this gene is associated with male infertility (Westerveld et al. 2004).

DAZ is found only in humans and old world primates, but an autosomal homologue (DAZL) is present in mammals and is found in mice on chromosome 17. This autosomal homologue is also present in humans on chromosome 3p24 (Dorfman et al. 1999), and may account for the varied spermatogenesis in men with AZFc deletions. DAZL is essential for male and female fertility in mice: homozygous knockout DAZL males do not progress past meiosis, while female mice without the DAZL gene have a failure of proper development of the female genital tract (Saunders et al. 2003). It is also possible that defects in autosomal DAZL genes could be the explanation for some cases of female infertility associated with primary amenorrhoea. Both DAZ and DAZL are expressed in early primordial germ cells and spermatogonia, and then later in meiotic cells. In contrast a third member of this gene family, BOULE, is only expressed in meiosis (Xu et al. 2001). BOULE is thought to be the ancestral member of the DAZ family since it is also found in flies, where it regulates translation of the transcript encoding the CDC25 phosphatase twine. Both Boule and twine are needed for meiotic entry in flies (Maines and Wasserman 1999), and a human BOULE transgene can rescue a fly boule mutation! Consistent with an equally important role in human fertility, BOULE and CDC25A proteins are absent in some infertile men who are arrested in meiosis (Luetjens et al. 2004).

Other Y Genes

Several other genes on the long arm of the Y have been described (Fig. II.3.53) but in general microdeletions in regions other than AZFc are less frequent. In the AZFa region, deletion of the DBY gene, which encodes a protein that unwinds RNA, causes infertility (Foresta et al. 2000) and single gene deletions and point mutations of the USP9Y gene, which is involved in controlling protein stability, cause infertility (Sun et al. 1999). In addition to removing RBM, deletions of the AZFb region of the Y chromosome remove other genes, including HSFY (Tessari et al. 2004).

Clinical Implications of Y Microdeletions

There are no reports that men with microdeletions have any phenotypic abnormalities other than abnormal spermatogenesis and men with microdeletions appear to be in perfect health in every other respect (Mallidis et al. 1996; Najmabadi et al. 1996).

As there is only one Y chromosome we may predict that Y microdeletions will be transmitted to their sons; although this is likely to be infrequent in the normal population, because without ICSI treatment men with

Table II.3.13. Transmission of Y chromosome deletion from father to son. (Adapted from the Table presented by Dr K McElreavey, Institute Pasteur Paris and presented at the Y Gene conference Royal College of Physicians Edinburgh 1998.) (*ICSI* Intracytoplasmic sperm injection, *TESA* testicular sperm aspiration)

Authors	Y deletion son	Y deletion father	Method of conception and semen concentration (millions per ml)
Kobayashi et al. (1994)	AZFc	AZFc	?
Vogt et al. (1996)	AZFc	AZFc	$<0.1\times10^6$
Kent-First et al. (1996)	Small near AZFc Small near AZFc Large AZFc -AZFb	Small near AZFc Not detected Not detected	ICSI Normal
Pryor et al. (1997)	sY153-sY267 sY207-sY272	sY153-sY267	0.3×10^6
Stuppia et al. (1997)	AZFc	AZFc (smaller)	$<2\times10^6$
Mulhall et al. (1997)	Ongoing twin pregnancy	AZFc	ICSI
Silber et al. (1998)	Two ongoing pregnancies Two ongoing one twin AZFc	AZFc Azoospermic AZFc Oligospermic	TESE-ICSI ICSI
Kamischke et al. (1999)	AZFc	AZFc	ICSI Normal
Kleiman et al. (1999)	AZFc	AZFc (sY153,sY254,sY255, DAZ,sY158)	TESE-ICSI
Page et al. (1999)	Twin both AZFc AZFc AZFc	AZFc Azoospermic AZFc Azoospermic AZFc Azoospermic	ICSI ICSI ICSI

very low sperm counts are less likely to father children. However, some cases have been reported in the literature (Table II.3.13). It may be important that in two of the cases the microdeletion appears to be larger in the son than the father. More information is needed from father/son pairs where the son has a very low sperm count and also about the outcome of ICSI attempts where sperm have been used from men with microdeletions and there is a need for long term follow-up of any male children. However, although it may be desirable to obtain information about the genetic status of ICSI babies there are ethical questions about whether young babies should be tested and, if so, whether the test results should be identifiable.

Testing for Y Microdeletions

Testing for microdeletions is now widespread in IVF and ICSI units, but there is no standardized methodology and it is therefore difficult to make direct comparisons between reported results (Table II.3.12). Several centres have developed screening methodologies (Henegariu et al. 1994; Qureshi et al. 1996; Vogt et al. 1996; Kent-First et al. 1999). As there is no correlation between histopathology and deletion of DAZ, it is premature to rely on specific gene probes because these will fail to detect a significant proportion of men with microdeletions. In a study to compare results from 28 different European laboratories (Simoni et al. 1998) it was concluded that the use of a high number of primers did not improve the accuracy of results, and recommendations are being produced for standardization. A commercial testing kit is now available (www.promega.com/moldx/). In general, deletions affecting the AZFa and AZFb regions are associated with more profound derangement of spermatogenesis and poorer prognosis for sperm recovery and ICSI (Hopps et al. 2003) and the larger the AZFc microdeletion the more likely it is that the phenotype is azoospermia (Fernandes et al. 2004). However, testing using peripheral blood may not be reliable. Lack of DAZ messenger RNA in testicular cells has been reported in a man with apparently normal DAZ gene constitution on DNA extraction from leukocytes (Repping et al. 2002). There may also be very small deletions encompassing active copies of DAZ, mosaicism, or abnormalities in DAZ transcription.

Advice to Couples Where the Man has a Y Microdeletion

What advice can we give our patients? It is probably unnecessary to test for microdeletions in men where ICSI is being used to overcome obstructive azoospermia, as in these men spermatogenesis should be normal. For other men with severely damaged spermatogenesis testing for microdeletions before ICSI is desirable, but as these men and their male children are unlikely to have any phenotypic abnormality other than damaged spermatogenesis it is reasonable to take into account the availability, cost and limitations of present methods of testing and to discuss this with the couple. If a man with Y chromosome microdeletions and his partner wish to proceed with ICSI they can be advised that microdeletions will be passed to sons but not to daughters, but that it is unknown to what extent a son who inherits a microdeletion will in turn have a fertility problem. The couple may be told that there is no evidence of any other health consequences of microdeletions. In a study of the actual decisions taken by couples in the situation in the Netherlands and Belgium it was found that most chose to proceed with ICSI but that 21% refrained from treatment or chose donor insemination but that this was strongly influenced by the opinion of the counsellor (Nap et al. 1999).

II.3.10.4.3 Cystic Fibrosis Mutations and Male Infertility

Cystic fibrosis, a fatal autosomal recessive disorder, is the most common genetic disease of Caucasians; 1 in 25 are carriers of recessive gene mutations involving the cystic fibrosis transmembrane conductance regulator (CFTR) gene. This gene, located on the short arm of chromosome 7, encodes a membrane protein that functions as an ion channel and also influences the formation of the ejaculatory duct, seminal vesicle, vas deferens and distal two-thirds of the epididymis. Congenital bilateral absence of the vas deferens (CBAVD) is associated with mutations in the CFTR gene, and is found in approximately 2% of men with obstructive azoospermia attending our clinic in Edinburgh, Scotland (Donat et al. 1997). However, the incidence in men with obstructive azoospermia will vary in different countries, depending on the prevalence of cystic fibrosis mutations in the population (Wu et al. 2004) and the prevalence of other causes of obstruction. In those countries with a high prevalence of sexually transmitted infection, CBAVD as a cause of azoospermia will be relatively infrequent compared with azoospermia associated with postgonococcal epididymitis. The clinical finding of absent vas deferens is easy to miss and all men with azoospermia should be very carefully examined, particularly if semen analysis reveals azoospermia in association with a semen volume of less than 1.0 ml and with acidic pH (<7.0).

More than 400 mutations of the CFTR gene have been characterized (Dean and Santis 1994). In published series of men with CBAVD who have been tested for varying numbers of mutations, the more mutations tested for, the higher the percentage of men found to have mutations. In more recent publications (Oates and Amos 1994; Tournaye et al. 1994; Mercier et al. 1995) detection rates have been higher (75%, 70%, 81%, 76% respectively) whereas in older publications detection rates have been around 40%. In a review of published series of 449 men with CBAVD the ΔF508 mutation was detected in 244 men, the R117H mutation in 54 men and the W1282X mutation in 37. Sixty-three other mutations were detected in between one and nine men but not all mutations were tested for in all case series (De-Braekeleer and Ferec 1996). It seems likely that as more and more mutations are defined and tested for that, approaching 100% of men with CBAVD will be found to have mutations. At present it is not practical to test for all known mutations, as many have a very low prevalence in a particular population and in most places testing is restricted to the 20–30 mutations that occur most commonly in that community.

Mutations may be found in both copies of the CFTR gene but in most men with CBAVD they are found in only one copy. In some of these supposedly heterozygous cases there may be an unknown second mutation but there is also another interesting mechanism. In up to 63% of these a DNA variant called the 5 T allele can be detected in one of the introns of the other allele of the CFTR gene (Chillon et al. 1995), and we have confirmed these observations in our own patients. The 5 T allele causes the CFTR transcript to be inefficiently spliced in the nucleus, decreasing the amount of functional CFTR protein (Chu et al. 1993; Hefferon et al. 2004).

Further work is needed to fully understand the genetics of CBAVD. It is noteworthy that the heterozygous men with CBAVD whom we see in our clinic often have mild clinical stigmata of cystic fibrosis, e.g. history of chest infections. It will therefore be important to follow up children born after ICSI and where the father has CBAVD and is either hetero- or homozygous. Men with mild clinical stigmata should be advised to avoid smoking as their respiratory reserve will be reduced compared with normal.

There have been reports of CFTR mutations in men with severe oligozoospermia but without absence of the vas deferens and it has been postulated that the CFTR complex may also relate to spermatogenesis (van der Ven 1996). While the relationship between absence of the vas deferens and CFTR mutations is becoming well established the role of these mutations in spermatogenetic defects is as yet unclear.

Advice for Couples Where the Man has Congenital Bilateral Absence of the Vas Deferens

CFTR mutations have implications for clinical infertility practice. When the male partner has CBAVD it is important to test the female partner for cystic fibrosis mutations as well as the male partner. If she is also found to be a carrier then there must be very careful consideration about whether the couple wish to proceed with ICSI using the husband's sperm as the chance of a baby with cystic fibrosis will be 25% if he is heterozygous or 50% if he is homozygous. If the female partner is negative for known mutations her chance of being a carrier of unknown mutations is about 0.4% and in these circumstances the chance of her heterozygous partner fathering a child with cystic fibrosis is approximately 1:410. These figures are estimates calculated using the known mutation frequency in Caucasian populations but will vary depending on the frequency of the different mutations in different populations. In the context of ICSI preimplantation diagnosis of CFTR status can be used to avoid a CFTR homozygous baby (Moutou et al. 2004).

Unilateral (and Bilateral) Absence/Abnormality of the Vas and Renal Abnormalities

Unilateral absence of the vas deferens is usually associated with ipsilateral absence of the kidney (Drake and Quinn 1996) and probably has a different genetic causation. Men with unilateral absence of the vas deferens are usually fertile and the condition is most commonly encountered as an incidental finding in the vasectomy clinic. Nevertheless, there have been recent reports that some men with unilateral absence have cystic fibrosis mutations, and these may represent incomplete CBAVD rather than true unilateral agenesis. Also it has been reported that some men with bilateral absence of vas deferens and renal abnormalities do not have CFTR abnormalities (Augarten et al. 1994). There is a need for reports of further case series of men with bilateral and unilateral absence of vas deferens, with accurate documentation of cystic fibrosis mutations and renal status.

When a man is found to have a unilateral absence of the vas and with normal kidneys, or bilateral absence or bilateral abnormality, then tests for cystic fibrosis mutations should be undertaken. However, if the results are negative and if the renal anatomy has not been defined, then it is worthwhile obtaining an abdominal ultrasound to define urinary tract anatomy. Findings may range from unilateral absence of the vas with ipsilateral absence of the kidney, to bilateral vasal abnormalities and renal abnormalities, such as pelvic kidney.

II.3.10.4.4 Autosomal Gene Defects with Severe Phenotypic Abnormalities as well as Infertility

There are a number of inherited disorders with severe or considerable generalized abnormalities as well as infertility (Table II.3.14). Such patients will be well known to doctors, often from childhood, and any fertility problem should be managed in the context of the care of the man as a whole, and with consideration of

Disorder	Phenotype	Genetic basis
Prader-Willi syndrome	Obesity, mental retardation	Deletion of 15q12 on paternally inherited chromosome
Bardet-Biedl syndrome	Obesity, mental retardation, retinitis pigmentosa, polydactyly	Autosomal-recessive 16q21
Cerebellar ataxia and hypogonadotrophic hypogonadism	Eunuchoidism and disturbances of gait and speech	Autosomal-recessive
Noonan's syndrome	Short stature, webbed neck, cardiac and pulmonary abnormality, cryptorchidism	Autosomal-dominant
Myotonic dystrophy	Muscle wasting, cataract testicular atrophy	Autosomal-dominant 19q13.3
Dominant polycystic kidney disease	Renal cysts, obstruction from epididymal cysts	Autosomal-dominant 16p13.3 and 4q
5α-reductase deficiency	Perineal or scrotal hypospadias, vaginal pouch, immature female phenotype	Autosomal-recessive

Table II.3.14. Less common inherited disorders associated with infertility and other alterations to phenotype

his and his partner's ability to care for a child should treatment be successful. Cryptorchidism is associated with both infertility and testicular cancer, and occurs in 3–4% of newborn boys. Mutations in the genes encoding insulin-like 3 (INSL3) and its receptor GREAT/Lgr8 are found in some patients with undescended testes, and in animal models these genes affect testicular descent in mice (Bogatcheva and Agoulnik 2005).

II.3.10.4.5 Autosomal Gene Defects and Male Fertility, but in the Absence of Overt Phenotypic Abnormality

Lillford et al. (1994) reported an epidemiological study which indicated that reduced male fertility may run in some families, and there is some molecular evidence that there may be autosomal defects that could account for this. It is difficult to know how many autosomal genes are specific for fertility, but estimates from the number of genes required in model organisms suggest that it may be in the order of 1500 (Hackstein et al. 2000). Because of the large number of potential genes which might be affected in infertile men, any indication of genes or an array of genes which might be more frequently disrupted would be useful diagnostically.

Homozygous disruption of a number of genes causes infertility in mice; for example, those encoding the ubiquitin conjugating enzymes hHR6A and hHR6B (Roest et al. 1996). These enzymes are implicated in post replication repair. Heterozygous male mice and knockout female mice are completely normal and able to transmit the defect, which, however, caused deranged spermatogenesis in homozygous mice. It is possible that similar hHR6B mutations may cause male infertility in man. If this is the case then there may be an enhanced chance of passing such a defect by ICSI as the male partner will be more likely than normal to carry such a defect and will thus pass the defect to half of his offspring. The chance of the offspring being affected will depend on the prevalence rate of these mutations in the general community. This may be quite low as there will have been a tendency to select against such mutations because of their anti fertility effect. Another gene potentially involved in ubiquitinylation is the Y-encoded USP9Y, which encodes a ubiquitin C-terminal hydrolase and which is mutated in some infertile men (Sun et al. 1999).

II.3.10.4.6 Unknown Genetic Disorders and Male Fertility

The search for genes on the long arm of the Y chromosome has given opportunities to find similar genes on the autosomes. In the mouse, the autosomal version of DAZ, DAZLA, has been found on mouse chromosome 17, and the human homologue of DAZLA has been mapped to chromosome 3p. Disruption of a number of autosomal loci in transgenic mice results in infertility, suggesting that defects in a number of genes might cause idiopathic infertility in humans (Venables and Cooke 2000). For example, it has been reported that male *Drosophila mojavensis* made sterile by having its Y chromosome replaced with that of the sibling species *Drosophila arizonae* has fertility restored by material from the fourth chromosome of *D. arizonae* (Pantazidis et al. 1993). These various observations raise the possibility of human autosomal-recessive disorders with homozygosity affecting spermatogenesis. This theoretical mechanism could account for a proportion of the men with unexplained deranged spermatogenesis. It has been postulated that follicle-stimulating hormone receptor mutations may account for some cases of male infertility, but, although allelic variants are present, these are detected in equal frequency in fertile and infertile men and do not seem to be relevant to fertility (Simoni et al. 1999).

II.3.10.5 DNA Methylation and Gene Imprinting and Ageing Changes

Methylation of the DNA base cytosine contributes to silencing and condensation of DNA, so the corresponding genes tend to be inactivated. Cytosine methylation and inactivation of genes occur as part of the ageing process and also as an important part of the mechanism of sex differentiation by silencing genes on the inactive X chromosome. DNA remodelling also has a very important role in spermatogenesis, since the DNA of the haploid round spermatids has to be condensed into the much smaller volume present in sperm. This occurs during spermiogenesis, and may involve the CDY gene which is deleted in some infertile men (Lahn et al. 2003).

II.3.10.5.1 Genetic Imprinting Disorders in Male Infertility

There is evidence that there is an increase in the human overgrowth condition called the Beckwith-Wiedemann syndrome in babies born by ICSI (DeBaun et al. 2003) and this condition is associated with failure of imprinting. Beckwith-Wiedemann syndrome is a growth disorder characterized by some or all of the following clinical features: macroglossia, omphalocele, umbilical hernia, diastasis recti, above average birth weight and length, visceromegaly, hemihypertrophy of part or all of the body, and finally typical facial features including earlobe creases, prominent occiput and naevus flammeus (strawberry mark on the forehead and eyelids). The prevalence of Beckwith-Wiedemann syndrome is difficult to establish because of underreporting of cases with minimal stigmata.

There are attempts to overcome maturation arrest by altering tissue culture characteristics (Tesarik 2004) and in the context of this line of treatment it will be important to evaluate the effect on normal imprinting mechanisms.

II.3.10.5.2 Ageing and Male Infertility

Sperm from older men have an increased incidence of XY, YY and XX disomy (Gazvani et al. 2000). Also, children born of older men may have an increased chance of genetic defects; for example, an increased incidence of the rare congenital disorder Apert syndrome (Tolarova et al. 1997). Apert syndrome is characterized by craniosynostosis, syndactyly and other malformations, and is caused by a paternal mutation in which cytosine is substituted by guanine in the fibroblast receptor-2 gene (Moloney et al. 1996; Tolarova et al. 1997). Based on this evidence, there are concerns about the genetic integrity of sperm from older men and this has led to recommendations for an upper age limit for men who wish to donate sperm to a sperm bank. In the USA (Linden and Centola 1997), UK (British Andrology Society 1999) and France (Lansac et al. 1997), there is now a recommended or required upper age limit of 35–45 years. More research is needed to define the exact risk according to age.

II.3.10.6 Mitochondrial Abnormalities

In addition to the nuclear genome, mitochondria contain their own genetic material. Very few if any mitochondria make a paternal contribution to the embryo, and therefore these are unlikely to be a significant factor in inherited male infertility. However, clearly defective mitochondrial function in sperm may, by way of poor sperm motility, be a cause of infertility. There is concern that the ICSI process may allow transmission of paternal mitochondria between generations, but in a study of nine children conceived by ICSI no paternal mitochondria were detected (Danan et al. 1999).

Human mitochondrial DNA is replicated by a DNA polymerase encoded by the nuclear genome called POLG, which contains a polyglutamine tract of typically ten amino acids. In men with sperm quality defects, the number of glutamines in this tract has been reported to vary (Rovio et al. 2001). Sperm from men homozygous for POLG alleles without the common ten glutamine repeat are less able to achieve fertilization, but this could be successfully treated by ICSI (Jensen et al. 2004).

II.3.10.7 Inherited Cytoplasmic Disorders and Male Fertility

In humans the cytoskeleton is a paternal contribution and thus in theory there is the possibility of non-DNA transmitted cytoskeleton abnormalities when very defective spermatozoa are used (Simmerly et al. 1995). Whether this actually occurs is not known.

II.3.10.8 Chromosomal and DNA Abnormalities in Sperm

There is less information about the incidence of genetic abnormalities in sperm. In general, tests on peripheral blood leukocytes may indicate that the man has abnormal chromosomal or genetic make-up, and this may be reflected in his sperm. However, another mechanism for the introduction of genetic abnormality in gametes is derangement of mitosis in the testis, and in this situation tests on peripheral blood leukocytes will all be normal and only by studying the sperm will abnormalities become apparent (Martin et al. 2003). In particular, men with meiotic arrest have been shown to have increased frequency of mutations in germ cells, suggesting that the DNA repair machinery may be compromised in these cells, and this is obviously important regarding the health of any children they might have as a result of assisted reproduction therapy (Nudell et al. 2000).

II.3.10.9 Chromosomal Abnormalities in Sperm

Large numbers of sperm can be tested using multicolour FISH analysis, whereas previously sperm karyotyping was by hamster penetration assay, a method that was both laborious and insensitive. Several studies of spermatozoa using FISH (Martin 1996; Finkelstein et al. 1998; Zhang 2004) have shown an increased frequency of both autosomal and sex chromosome aneuploidy. Typically, a standard karyotype analysis is performed on 20–30 cells. However, in a study in which 1000 cells were analysed using FISH (Gazvani et al. 2000) the median incidence of sex chromosome aneuploidy was found to be 1.5% in ten oligozoospermic men compared with 0.3% in ten fertile men. Also, it was postulated that mitotic instability in infertile men could be the result of failure of the mitotic checkpoint gene MAD2L1.

II.3.10.9.1 DNA Strand Breakages in Sperm

A Japanese group (Kuroki et al. 1999) have used polymerase chain reaction (PCR) to assess DNA differences in the Y chromosome [PCR single-strand confirmation polymorphism, PCR restriction fragment length polymorphism and PCR for three polymorphic loci: SRY, DXYS5Y(47z/stu 1) and DYS287 (YAP)]. They used their results to classify the Y chromosome into four haplotypes: I, II, III and IV. The frequency of occurrence of these haplotypes was studied in a population of 198 fertile men and 106 azoospermic men (azoospermic men with Y microdeletions were excluded). It was found that men with haplotype II had a lower sperm concentration than men with the haplotypes III and IV, and that the frequency of haplotype II is more common in the azoospermic men than in normal men. This work indicates a significant genetic contribution to male fertility potential.

Men with infertility have an increase in damage to sperm DNA compared with fertile men (Irvine et al. 2000) and this increased DNA fragmentation is associated with poorer IVF pregnancy rates (Henkel et al. 2004). One of the mechanisms of damage to DNA is oxidation (Bjelland and Seeberg 2003) and this is particular relevant in men with damaged spermatogenesis and leukospermia where free oxygen radical levels are high. Sperm from older men have increased DNA damage compared to those from younger men and this may be one of the mechanisms contributing to the slight increase in risks to children born of older fathers.

There is increasing evidence that sperm abnormalities may be common, and further investigations are needed of sperm from men in well-defined clinical categories (Table II.3.15). Also, when considering such studies, it is relevant to investigate the population of sperm that would normally be used in an ICSI procedure. In a study of sperm in a swim up preparation, the frequency of DNA breaks was reduced by one-third in motile sperm (Van Kooij et al. 2004).

Table II.3.15. Suggested male risk categories for the follow-up of children born by intracytoplasmic sperm injection. The male diagnostic categories descend in order of genetic and diagnostic precision. (*CBAVD* Congenital bilateral absence of the vas deferens)

Men with sex chromosome abnormality on peripheral blood karyotyping
Men with autosomal chromosome abnormality on peripheral blood karyotyping
Men with obstructive azoospermia secondary to CBAVD
Men with damaged spermatogenesis and Y microdeletions
Men with other defined genetic disorders
Men with normal spermatogenesis and obstructive azoospermia; for example, after failed vasectomy reversal but where karyotyping and genetic tests have not been undertaken or if they have been performed are normal. In this category there is no reason to predict any genetic abnormality different from that in the general population
Men with normal karyotype and normal genetic tests but where spermatids have been used. In cases where karyotype or genetic tests are abnormal then the followed-up category should probably be considered under one of the above groups
Men with testicular maldescent
Men with impaired spermatogenesis secondary to cancer chemotherapy
Men with impaired spermatogenesis secondary to known mitogen (e.g. occupational hazard)
Men with damaged spermatogenesis of unknown aetiology

Paternal RNA

Paternal RNAs are delivered to the egg at fertilization but it is not known whether these have a role in the early molecular events after fertilization but it is hypothesized that the defect could account for some cases of unexplained male factor infertility (Ostermeier et al. 2004).

II.3.10.10 Risks of Intracytoplasmic Sperm Injection

Intracytoplasmic sperm injection (ICSI) is now used to enable men with severe damage to spermatogenesis to father children in situations formerly considered hopeless and where only a very few spermatozoa can be obtained. This has led to worries that children may be born with foetal abnormality, because by bypassing the selective processes of the female genital tract and coverings of the egg the process could enable defective sperm to fertilize, or that eggs may be fertilized that would otherwise not do so. It is reassuring that the collected statistics of foetal abnormality from ICSI centres show similar rates of congenital malformations compared with the general population (Bonduelle et al. 2002; Pinborg et al. 2004) but despite this some concern remains because the indications for ICSI are constantly being extended to include fertilization with immature sperm forms and potentially damaged sperm. It will be particularly important to continue to monitor foetal abnormality rates with detailed subgroup analysis according to the clinical and molecular diagnosis of the father (see Table II.3.14). ICSI has meant that some men with Klinefelter syndrome can become fathers. One of the most common aneuploidies in humans is trisomy 21 (Down's syndrome) and there is evidence that men with Klinefelter syndrome also produce sperm with high levels of disomy of chromosome 21 (Hennebicq et al. 2001). Hence any embryos from Klinefelter fathers derived by ICSI should be carefully screened.

II.3.10.11 Ethical Considerations, Genetic Counselling and Intracytoplasmic Sperm Injection

The main difficulties will occur where there is a conflict of interest between the wishes of the couple and the interests of a future child.

The best initial management is to give the couple full information about the risks to the child and then for the couple to decide whether to proceed or not. However, in the situation where both partners are known to carry defects (for example cystic fibrosis mutations), there can be up to a 50% chance of the birth of a child who will develop clinical cystic fibrosis and die young after a number of years of morbidity. In this situation, many clinicians and infertility clinic personnel may feel that their duty of care to the future child and the interests of society as a whole outweigh the wishes of the individual couple, and that it is not ethical to proceed and that ICSI should not be offered to the couple.

Table II.3.16. Problems faced by germline therapy

Uncertainty and risk
The commonly perceived slippery slope, particularly regarding genetic enhancement
Lack of consent by future generations
Inappropriate allocation of health care resources
Intrinsic immorality

Data from Hefferon et al. (2004)

In some countries law may govern these matters and then there is no choice, but in the absence of law this type of conflict makes the doctors' role very difficult. Each case has to be judged on its merits and in the context of what is available and affordable in the local health care system. When there is a conflict that cannot be resolved by agreement the interests of a future child probably take precedence over the interests of a couple. If the decision is taken to proceed, it is important for the couple to appreciate fully what may be in store for a future child, and it is often appropriate for arrangements to be made for the couple to visit another family where there is a teenager or older person suffering from the condition. Also, the couple will need to give consideration to preimplantation diagnosis and replacement only of normal embryos or, if this is not available, amniocentesis and genetic diagnosis and the possibility of termination.

ICSI is new technology, but perhaps the greatest potential application is the window of opportunity for germline therapy. At present this is considered unethical and sometimes illegal. Nevertheless, the following hypothetical situation may help focus debate. Suppose a couple decide to go ahead with ICSI in a situation in which both partners are known to have cystic fibrosis mutations, but after successful pregnancy would not contemplate amniocentesis and abortion. If in this situation it was possible to correct the mutation before embryo replacement, which would be less harmful – to repair the defect and enable the birth of a child without cystic fibrosis, or not to repair the defect and for a child to be born with cystic fibrosis? These arguments can be extended to correction of oncogenes and other defects. The risks of germline therapy (Table II.3.16) have been summarized by Fiddler and Pergament (1996) in a review article, which gives powerful argument in favour of germline therapy.

II.3.10.12 Conclusion

We are beginning to understand the genetic basis of infertility, and the advent of ICSI makes this of practical relevance. This is because couples need to be given information about potential risks to children, and for some there may be opportunities to select genetically healthy IVF embryos for replacement. This necessitates good understanding of genetics by clinical staff and the public at large. In the present review, the emphasis is on the description of the more common genetic disorders that are likely to be encountered by the infertility clinicians, such as Klinefelter syndrome, CBAVD and Y microdeletions. Our understanding of the genetics of male fertility is increasing exponentially and it is likely that genetic treatments will become available. Infertility clinicians will need to keep up to date with fast moving scientific advances to best advise infertile couples. It will be increasingly important that infertility clinicians keep in mind the fundamental ethical principles of beneficence, autonomy and justice, and to have the knowledge to advise and be able to manage situations when there are conflicts of interest or principle.

References

Augarten A, Yahav Y, Kerem BS, Halle D, Laufer J, Szeinberg A, Dor J et al (1994) Congenital bilateral absence of the vas deferens in the absence of cystic fibrosis. Lancet 344:1473–1474

Bjelland S, Seeberg E (2003) Mutagenicity, toxicity and repair of DNA base damage induced by oxidation. Mutat Res 531:37–80

Bogatcheva NV, Agoulnik AI (2005) INSL3/LGR8 role in testicular descent and cryptorchidism. Reprod Biomed Online 10:49–54

Bonduelle M, Liebaers I, Deketelaere V, Derde MP, Camus M, Devroey P, Van Steirteghem A (2002) Neonatal data on a cohort of 2889 infants born after ICSI (1991–1999) and of 2995 infants born after IVF (1983–1999). Hum Reprod 17: 671–94

British Andrology Society (1999) British Andrology Society guidelines for the screening of semen donors for donor insemination. Hum Reprod 14:1823–1826

Brown GM, Furlong RA, Sargent CA, Erickson RP, Longepied G, Mitchaeli M et al (1998) Characterisation of the coding sequence and fine mapping of the human DFFRY gene and comparative expression analysis and mapping to the Sxr^b interval of the mouse Y chromosome of the Dffry gene. Hum Mol Genet 7:97–107

Caceres C, Ribes E, Muller S, Cornudella L, Chiva M (1994) Characterization of chromatin-condensing proteins during spermatogenesis in a neogastropod mollusc (*Murex brandaris*). Mol Reprod Dev 38:440–452

Chandley AC, Edmond PE, Christie S, Gowans I, Fletcher J, Frackiewicz A, Newton M (1975) Cytogenetics and infertility in man. Results of a five year study of men attending a subfertility clinic. Ann Hum Genet 39:231–254

Chandley AC, Ambros P, McBeath S, Hargreave TB, Kilanowski F, Spowart G (1986) Short arm dicentric Y chromosome with associated structural defects in a sterile man. Hum Genet 73:350–353

Chevret E, Rousseaux S, Monteil M (1996) Increased incidence of hyperhaploid 24 XY spermatozoa detected by three-colour FISH in a 46XY/47XXY male. Hum Genet 97:171–175

Chevret ERS, Monteil M, Usson Y, Cozzi J, Pelletier R, Sele B (1997) Meiotic behaviour of sex chromosomes investigated by three-colour FISH on 35142 sperm nuclei from two 47,XYY males. Hum Genet 99:407–412

Chillon M, Casals T, Mercier B, Bassas L, Lissens W, Silber S, Romey MC et al (1995) Mutations in cystic fibrosis gene in patients with congenital absence of the vas deferens. N Engl J Med 332:1475–1480

Chu CS, Trapnell BC, Curristin S, Cutting GR, Crystal RG (1993) Genetic basis of variable exon 9 skipping in cystic fibrosis transmembrane conductance regulator mRNA. Nat Genet 3:151–156

Cooke HJ, Lee M, Kerr S, Ruggiu M (1996) A murine homologue of the human DAZ gene is autosomal and expressed only in male and female gonads. Hum Mol Genet 5:513–516

Cozzi J, Chevret E, Rousseaux S (1994) Achievement of meiosis in XXY germ cells: study of 543 sperm karyotypes from an XY/XXY mosaic patient. Hum Genet 93:32–34

Danan C, Sterberg D, Steirteghem AV, Cazeneuve C, Duquesnoy P, Besmond C et al (1999) Evaluation of parental mitochondrial inheritance in neonates born after intracytoplasmic sperm injection. Am J Hum Genet 65:463–473

This paper confirms that paternal mitochondria are not relevant

De Braekeleer M, Dao TN (1991) Cytogenetic studies in male infertility: a review. Hum Reprod 6:245–250

De Braekeleer M, Ferec C (1996) Mutations in the cystic fibrosis gene in men with congenital bilateral absence of the vas deferens. Mol Hum Reprod 2:669–677

Dean M, Santis G (1994) Heterogenicity in the severity of cystic fibrosis and the role of the CFTR gene mutations. Hum Genet 93:364–368

DeBaun MR, Niemitz EL, Feinberg AP (2003) Association of in vitro fertilization with Beckwith-Wiedemann syndrome and epigenetic alterations of LIT1 and H19. Am J Hum Genet 72:156–160

Delbridge ML, Harry JL, Toder R, Waugh O'Neill RJ, Kun Ma, Chandley AC, Marshall Graves JA (1997) A human candidate spermatogenesis gene, RBMI, is conserved and amplified on the marsupial Y chromosome. Nature Genet 15:131–136

Delbridge ML, Ma K, Subbarao MN, Cooke HJ, Bhasin S, Graves JAM (1998) Evolution of mammalian HNRPG and its relationship with the putative azoospermia factor RBM. Mammalian Genome 9:168–170

Delbridge ML, Lingenfelter PA, Disteche CM, Graves JA (1999) The candidate spermatogenesis gene RBMY has a homologue on the human X chromosome. Nat Genet 22:223–224

Donat R, McNeill AS, Fitzpatrick DR, Hargreave TB (1997) The incidence of cystic fibrosis gene mutation in patients with congenital bilateral absence of the vas deferens in Scotland. Br J Urol 79:74–77

Dorfman DM, Genest DR, Reijo-Pera RA (1999) Human DAZL1 encodes candidate fertility factor in women that localizes to the prenatal and postnatal germ cells. Hum Reprod 14:2531–2536

Drake MJ, Quinn FM (1996) Absent vas deferens and ipsilateral multicystic dysplastic kidney in a child. Br J Urol 77:756–757

Elliot DJ, Oghene K, Makarova O, Hargreave TB, Chandley AC, Eperon IC, Cooke HJ (1998) Dynamic changes in the subnuclear organisation of pre-mRNA splicing proteins and RBM during human germ cell development. J Cell Sci 111:1255–1265

Elliott DJ, Venables JP, Newton CS, Lawson D, Boyle S, Eperon IC, Cooke HJ (2000) An evolutionarily conserved germ cell-specific hnRNP is encoded by a retrotransposed gene. Hum Mol Genet 9:2117–2124

Estop AM, Munne S, Cieply KM, Vandermark KK, Lamb AN, Fisch H (1998) Meiotic products of a Klinefelter 47,XXY male as determined by sperm fluorescence in-situ hybridization analysis. Hum Reprod 13:124–127

Ferlin A, Moro E, Onisto M, Toscano E, Brettelia A, Foresta C (1999) Absence of testicular DAZ gene expression in idiopathic severe testiculopathies. Hum Reprod 14:2286–2292

Fernandes S, Paracchini S, Meyer LH, Floridia G, Tyler M, Smith C, Vogt PH (2004) A large AZFc deletion removes

DAZ3/DAZ4 and nearby genes from men in Y haplogroup N. Am J Hum Genet 74:180–187
Fiddler M, Pergament E (1996) Germline gene therapy: its time is near. Mol Hum Reprod 2:75–76
Finkelstein S, Mukamel E, Yavetz H, Paz G, Avivi L (1998) Increased rate of nondisjunction in sex cells derived from low quality semen. Hum Genet 102:129–137
Foresta C, Rassato M, Garolla A et al (1996) Male infertility and ICSI: are there any limits? Hum Reprod 11:2347–2348
Foresta C, Ferlin A, Garolla A et al (1997) Y-Chromosome deletions in idiopathic severe testiculopathies. J Clin Endocrinol Metab 82:1075–1080
Foresta C, Galeazzi C, Bettella A, Stella M, Scandellari C (1998) High incidence of sperm sex chromosomes aneuploidies in two patients with Klinefelter's syndrome. J Clin Endocrinol Metab 83:203–205
Foresta C, Galeazzi C, Bettella A, Marin P, Rossato M, Garolla A, Ferlin A (1999) Analysis of meiosis in intratesticular germ cells from subjects affected by classic Klinefelter's syndrome. J Clin Endocrinol Metab 84:3807–3810
This paper provides good insight into the debate about whether men with complete (nonmosaic) Klinefelter's syndrome can produce sex chromosome haploid gametes
Foresta C, Ferlin A, Moro E (2000) Deletion and expression analysis of AZFa genes on the human Y chromosome revealed a major role for DBY in male infertility. Hum Mol Genet 9:1161–1169
Franco B, Guioli S, Pragliola A, Incerti B, Bardoni B, Tonlorenzi R, Carrozzo R et al (1991) A gene deleted in Kallmann's syndrome shares homology with neural cell adhesion and axonal path-finding molecules. Nature 353:529–536
Gabriel-Robez O, Rumpler Y, Ratomponirina C, Petit C, Levilliers J, Croquette MF, Couturier J (1990) Deletion of the pseudoautosomal region and lack of sex chromosome pairing at pachytene in two infertile men carrying an X-Y translocation. Cytogenet Cell Genet 54:38–42
Gazvani MR, Wilson EDA, Richmond DH, Howard PJ, Kingsland CR, Lewis-Jones DI (2000) Evaluation of the role of mitotic instability in karyotypically normal men with oligozoospermia. Fertil Steril 73:51–55
Girardi SK, Mielnik A, Schlegel PN (1997) Submicroscopic deletions in the Y chromosome of infertile men. Hum Reprod 12:1635–1641
Gonialves J, McElreavey K, Carreiro H, Vale F, Marques R, Simao L et al (1996) An azoospermic man with a submicroscopic interstitial deletion on the Xp pseudoautosomal region [abstract]. In: Human Reproduction, Vol 11, Abstract book, 1 June 1996, 12th Annual Meeting, Maastricht, 30 June to 3 July 1996. European Society of Human Reproduction and Embryology, ISSN 0268–1161 Coden HUREEE, Oxford University Press
Guttenbach M, Michelmann HW, Hinney B, Engel W, Schmid M (1997) Segregation of sex chromosomes into sperm nuclei in a man with 47,XXY Klinefelter's karyotype: a FISH analysis. Hum Genet 99:474–477
Hackstein JH Hochstenbach R Pearson PL (2000) Towards an understanding of the genetics of human male infertility: lessons from flies. Trends Genet 16:565–572
Hefferon TW, Groman JD, Yurk CE, Cutting GR (2004) A variable dinucleotide repeat in the CFTR gene contributes to phenotype diversity by forming RNA secondary structures that alter splicing. Proc Natl Acad Sci USA 101:3504–3509
Henegariu O, Hirschmann P, Killian K, Kirsch S, Lengauer C, Maiwald R et al (1994) Rapid screening of the Y chromosome in idiopathic sterile men, diagnostic for deletions in AZF, a genetic Y factor expressed during spermatogenesis. Andrologia 26:97–106
Henkel NDI, Hajimohammad M, Stalf T, Hoogendijk C, Mehnert C, Menkveld R, Gips H, Schill WB, Kruger TF (2004) Influence of deoxyribonucleic acid damage on fertilization and pregnancy. Fertil Steril 81:965–972
Hennebicq S, Pelletier R, Rousseaux S, Sele B (1999) Segregation of sex chromosomes in a Klinefelter patient (47,XXY) [abstract]. In: Human Reproduction, Vol 14, Abstract book, 1 June 1999, 15th Annual Meeting, Tours, 26–30 June 1999. European Society of Human Reproduction and Embryology, ISSN 0268–1161 Coden HUREEE, Oxford University Press
Hennebicq S, Pelletier R, Bergues U, Rousseaux S (2001) Risk of trisomy 21 in offspring of patients with Klinefelter's syndrome. Lancet 357:2104–2105
Hopps CV, Mielnik A, Goldstein M, Palermo GD, Rosenwaks Z, Schlegel PN (2003) Detection of sperm in men with Y chromosome microdeletions of the AZFa, AZFb and AZFc regions. Hum Reprod 18:1660–1665
Horn N, Tonnesen T, Tumer Z (1992) Menkes disease :an X-linked neurological disorder of copper metabolism. Brain Pathol 2:351–362
Hunt PA, Hassold TJ (2002) Sex matters in meiosis. Science 296:2181–2183
Irvine DS, Twigg JP, Gordon EL, Fulton N, Milne PA, Aitken RJ (2000) DNA integrity in human spermatozoa: relationships with semen quality. J Androl 21:33–44
This is one of the first papers to look at DNA in sperm in a large number of men with infertility and to pose the question about mitotic abnormalities in the germ-cell line. It is likely that many more similar studies will be published
Jensen M, Leffers H, Petersen JH, Nyboe Andersen A, Jorgensen N, Carlsen E, Jensen TK, Skakkebaek NE, Rajpert-De Meyts E (2004) Frequent polymorphism of the mitochondrial DNA polymerase gamma gene (POLG) in patients with normal spermiograms and unexplained subfertility. Hum Reprod 19:65–70
Johnson MD (1998) Genetic risks of intracytoplasmic sperm injection in the treatment of male infertility: recommendations for genetic counseling and screening. Fertil Steril 70:397–411
Kahraman S, Findikli N, Berkil H, Bakircioglu E, Donmez E, Sertyel S, Biricik A (2003) Results of preimplantation genetic diagnosis in patients with Klinefelter's syndrome. Reprod Biomed Online 7:346–352
Kamischke A, Gromoll J, Simoni M, Behre HM, Nieschlag E (1999) Transmission of a Y chromosomal deletion involving the deleted in azoospermia (DAZ) and chromodomain (CDYI) genes from father to son through intracytoplasmic sperm injection. Hum Reprod 14:2320–2322
Kent-First MG, Kol S, Maullem A, Blazer S, Itskovitz-Eldor J (1996) Infertility in intracytoplasmic sperm injection-derived sons. Lancet 348:332
Kent-First M, Muallem A, Shultz J Pryor J, Roberts K, Nolten W, Meisner L, Chandley A, Gouchy G, Jorgensen L, Havighurst T, Grosch J (1999) Defining regions of the Y-chromosome responsible for male infertility and identification of a fourth AZF region (AZFD) by Y-chromosome microdeletion detection. Mol Reprod Dev 53:27–41
Kleiman SE, Yogev L, Gamzu R, Hauser R, Botchan A, Lessing JB et al (1999) Genetic evaluation of infertile men. Hum Reprod 14:33–38
Kobayashi K, Mizuno K, Hida A et al (1994) PCR analysis of the Y chromosome long arm in azoospermic patients – evidence for a second locus required for spermatogenesis. Hum Mol Genet 3:1965–1967
Komori S, Horiuchi I, Hamada Y, Hasegawa A, Kasumi H, Kondoh N, Sawai H, Toji H, Shigeta M, Shima H, Koyama K (2004) Birth of healthy neonates after intracytoplasmic injection of ejaculated or testicular spermatozoa from men

with nonmosaic Klinefelter's syndrome: a report of 2 cases. J Reprod Med 49:126–130

Krausz C, Bussani-Mastellone C, Granchi S, McElreavey K, Scarselli G, Forti G (1999) Screening for microdeletions of Y chromosome genes in patients undergoing intracytoplasmic sperm injection. Hum Reprod 14:1717–1721

Kupker W, Ludwig M, Hahn K et al (1996) Prevalence of microdeletions in the azoospermia factor region of the Y chromosome in cases of azoospermia and severe oligoasthenoteratozoospermia. 12th Annual Meeting of the EHSRE, Maastricht 1996. Hum Reprod 11:57

Kuroki Y, Iwamoto T, Lee J, Yoshiike M, Nozawa S, Nishida T et al (1999) Spermatogenic ability is different among males in different Y chromosome lineage. Hum Genet 44:289–292

This is potentially a landmark paper. These authors found that sperm with different Y chromosome DNA lineages may have different fertility potential. We still know relatively little about the Y chromosome, and this paper opens up new avenues of enquiry

Lahn BT, Tang ZL, Zhou J, Barndt RJ, Parvinen M, Allis CD, Page DC (2003) Previously uncharacterized histone acetyltransferases implicated in mammalian spermatogenesis. EMBO Rep 4:877–82 [Epub 2003 August 08. Related Articles, Links Cdyl: a new transcriptional co-repressor. Proc Natl Acad Sci USA 2002 99:8707–8712. Epub 2002 June 18]

Lander ES, Linton LM, Birren B, Nusbaum C, Zody MC, Baldwin J, Devon K, Dewar K, Doyle M, FitzHugh W et al (2001) Initial sequencing and analysis of the human genome. Nature 409:860–921

Lansac J, Thepot F, Mayuax MJ (1997) Pregnancy outcome after artificial insemination or IVF with frozen semen donor: a collaborative study of the French CECOS Federation on 21,597 pregnancies. Eur J Obstet Gynecol Reprod Biol 74: 223–228

Li C, Gronberg H, Matsuyama H, Weber G, Nordenskjold M, Naito K, Bergh A Bergerheim U, Damber JE, Larsson C, Ekman P (2003) Difference between Swedish and Japanese men in the association between AR CAG repeats and prostate cancer suggesting a susceptibility-modifying locus overlapping the androgen receptor gene. Int J Mol Med 11:529–533

Lillford R, Jones AM, Bishop DT, Thronton J, Mueller R (1994) Case control study of whether subfertility in men is familial. Br Med J 309:507–573

Lin YM, Huang WJ, Lin JS, Kuo PL (2004) Progressive depletion of germ cells in a man with nonmosaic Klinefelter's syndrome: optimal time for sperm recovery. Urology 63: 380–381

Linden JV, Centola G (1997) New American Association of Tissue Banks standards for semen banking. Fertil Steril 68: 597–600

Luetjens CM, Xu EY, Rejo Pera RA, Kamischke A, Nieschlag E, Gromoll J (2004) Association of meiotic arrest with lack of BOULE protein expression in infertile men. J Clin Endocrinol Metab 89:1926–1933

Ma K, Sharkey A, Kirsch S, Vogt P, Keil R, Hargreave TB et al (1992) Towards the molecular localisation of the AZF locus: mapping of microdeletions in azoospermic men within 14 subintervals of interval 6 of the human Y chromosome. Hum Mol Genet 1:29–33

Ma K, Inglis JD, Sharkey A, Bickmore WA, Hill RE, Prosser EJ et al (1993) A Y chromosome gene family with RNA-binding protein homology: candidates for the azoospermia factor AZF controlling human spermatogenesis. Cell 75:1–20

Maines JZ, Wasserman SA (1999) Post-transcriptional regulation of the meiotic Cdc25 protein Twine by the Dazl orthologue Boule. Nat Cell Biol 1:171–174

Mallidis C, Loveland K, Najmabadi H, McLaughlin R, Baker G, Bhasin S, de Kretser DM (1996) The incidence of the deleted in azoospermia gene in infertile men. In: Human Reproduction, Vol 11, Abstract book, 1 June 1996, 12th Annual Meeting, Maastricht, 30 June to 3 July 3 1996, European Society of Human Reproduction and Embryology, ISSN 0268–1161 Coden HUREEE, Oxford University Press

Martin RH (1996) The risk of chromosomal abnormalities following ICSI. Hum Reprod 11:924–925

Martin RH, McInnes B, Rademaker AW (1999) Analysis of aneuploidy for chromosomes 13, 21, X and Y by multicolour fluorescence in situ hybridisation (FISH) in a 47,XYY male. Zygote 7:131–134

Martin RH, Rademaker AW, Greene C, Ko E, Hoang T, Barclay L, Chernos J (2003) A comparison of the frequency of sperm chromosome abnormalities in men with mild, moderate, and severe oligozoospermia. Biol Reprod 69:535–539

Martini E, Geraedts JPM, Liebaers I, Land JA, Capitanio GL, Ramaekers FCS, Hopman AHN (1996) Constitution of semen samples from XYY and XXY males as analysed by in-situ hybridization. Hum Reprod 11:1638–1643

Mercier B, Verlingue C, Lissens W, Silber SJ, Noveli G, Bonduelle M et al (1995) Is congenital bilateral absence of vas deferens primary form of cystic fibrosis ? Analysis of the CFTR gene in 67 patients. Am J Hum Genet 56:272–277

Moloney DM, Slaney SF, Oldridge M, Wall SA, Sahlin P, Stenman G, Wilkie AO (1996) Exclusive paternal origin of new mutations in Apert syndrome. Nature Genet 13:48–53

Moog U, Coonen E, Dumoulin JCM, Engelen JJM (1996) Karyotypes of men involved in ICSI programmes: the Maastricht experience, April 1994 to date [abstract]. In: Human Reproduction, Vol 11, Abstract book, 1 June 1996, 12th Annual Meeting, Maastricht, 30 June to 3 July 1996. European Society of Human Reproduction and Embryology, ISSN 0268–1161 Coden HUREEE, Oxford University Press

Moutou C, Gardes N, Viville S (2004) Duplex, triplex and quadruplex PCR for the preimplantation genetic diagnosis (PGD) of cystic fibrosis (CF), an exhaustive approach. Prenat Diagn 24:562–569

Mulhall JP, Reijo R, Alagappan R, Brown L, Page D, Carson R, Oates RD (1997) Azoospermic men with deletion of the DAZ gene cluster are capable of completing spermatogenesis: fertilization, normal embryonic development and pregnancy occur when retrieved testicular spermatozoa are used for intracytoplasmic sperm injection. Hum Reprod 12:503–508

Najmabadi H, Huang V, Yen P, Subbarao MN, Bhasin D, Banaag L et al (1996) Substantial prevalence of microdeletions of the Y chromosome in infertile men with idiopathic azoospermia and oligozoospermia detected using a sequence-tagged site-based mapping strategy. J Clin Endocrinol Metab 81: 1347–1352

Nap AW, Van Golde RJ, Tuerlings JH, De Sutter P, Pieters MH, Giltay JC, Kastrop PM, Braat DD, Kremer JA (1999) Reproductive decisions of men with microdeletions of the Y chromosome: the role of genetic counselling. Hum Reprod 14: 2166–2169

Nelson KA, Witte JS (2002) Androgen receptor CAG repeats and prostate cancer. Am J Epidemiol 155:883–890

Nudell D, Castillo M, Turek PJ, Pera RR (2000) Increased frequency of mutations in DNA from infertile men with meiotic arrest. Hum Reprod 15:1289–1294

Oates RD, Amos JA (1994) The genetic basis of congenital bilateral absence of the vas deferens and cystic fibrosis. J Androl 15:1–8

Okada H, Fujioka H, Tatsumi N, Kanzaki M, Okuda Y, Fujisawa M et al (1999) Klinefelter's syndrome in the male infertility clinic. Hum Reprod 14:946–952

Okada H, Shirakawa T, Ishikawa T, Goda K, Fujisawa M, Kamidono S (2004) Serum testosterone levels in patients with nonmosaic Klinefelter syndrome after testicular sperm extraction for intracytoplasmic sperm injection. Fertil Steril 82:237–238

Ostermeier GC, Miller D, Huntriss JD, Diamond MP, Krawetz SA (2004) Reproductive biology: delivery spermatozoan RNA to the oocyte. Nature 429:154

Page DC, Silber S, Brown LG (1999) Men with infertility caused by AZFc deletion can produce sons by intracytoplasmic sperm injection, but are likely to transmit the deletion and infertility. Hum Reprod. 14:1722–1726

Pantazidis AC, Galanopoulos VK, Zouros E (1993) An autosomal factor from *Drosophila mojavensis* restores normal spermatogenesis in Drosophila males carrying the *D. arizonae* Y chromosome. Genetics 134:309–318

Persson JW (1999) A hypothesis on the origin of germ cell mutation and evolutionary role of extraembryonic mutation. Hum Reprod 14:1840–1841

In this paper we are reminded that germ cells migrate into the embryo from the extra-embryonic cell mass, and this may explain how it is possible to have mutations that are unique to the germ cell line. There is increasing realization that we may need to do cytogenetic studies on the sperm rather than on peripheral blood cells

Persson JW, Peter GB, Saunders DM (1996) Is ICSI associated with risks of genetic disease ? Implications for counselling, practice and research. Hum Reprod 11:921–924

Peschka B, Leygraaf J, van der Ven K, Montag M, Schartmann B, Schubert R et al (1999) Type and frequency of chromosome aberrations in 781 couple undergoing intracytoplasmic sperm injection. Hum Reprod 14:2257–2263

Pinborg A, Loft A, Rasmussen S, Schmidt L, Langhoff-Roos J, Greisen G Andersen AN (2004) Neonatal outcome in a Danish national cohort of 3438 IVF/ICSI and 10,362 non-IVF/ICSI twins born between 1995 and 2000. Hum Reprod 19:435–441

Pryor JL, Kent First M, Muallem A et al (1997) Microdeletions in the Y chromosome of infertile men. N Engl J Med 336:534–539

Qureshi SJ, Ross AR, Ma K, Cooke HJ, McIntyre MA, Hargreave TB (1996) Polymerase chain reaction screening for Y chromosome microdeletions: a first step towards the diagnosis of genetically determined spermatogenetic failure in men. Mol Hum Reprod 2:775–779

Ratcliffe S (1999) Long term outcome in children of sex chromosome abnormalities. Arch Dis Child 80:192–195

Reijo R, Lee TY, Salo P, Alagappan R, Brown LG, Rosenberg M, Rozen S et al (1995) Diverse spermatogenic defects in humans caused by Y chromosome deletions encompassing a novel RNA-binding protein gene. Nature Genet 10:383–393

Reijo R, Alagappan PK, Patrizio P et al (1996) Severe oligozoospermia resulting from deletions of azoospermia factor gene on Y chromosome. Lancet 347:1290–1293

Repping S, Skaletsky H, Lange J, Silber S, Van Der Veen F, Oates RD, Page DC, Rozen S (2002) Recombination between palindromes P5 and P1 on the human Y chromosome causes massive deletions and spermatogenic failure. Am J Hum Genet 71:906–922

Roest HP, Van Klaveran J, de Wit J, van Gurp CG, Koken MHM, Vermy M (1996) Inactivation of the HR6B ubiquitin conjugating DNA repair enzyme in mice causes male sterility associated with chromatin modification. Cell 86:799–810

Rovio AT, Marchington DR, Donat S, Schuppe HC, Abel J, Fritsche E, Elliott DJ, Laippala P, Ahola AL, McNay D, Harrison RF, Hughes B, Barrett T, Bailey DM, Mehmet D, Jequier AM, Hargreave TB, Kao SH, Cummins JM, Barton DE, Cooke HJ, Wei YH, Wichmann L, Poulton J, Jacobs HT (2001) Mutations at the mitochondrial DNA polymerase (POLG) locus associated with male infertility. Nat Genet 29:261–262

Rozen S, Skaletsky H, Marszalek JD, Minx PJ, Cordum HS, Waterston RH, Wilson RK, Page DC (2003) Abundant gene conversion between arms of palindromes in human and ape Y chromosomes. Nature 423:873–876

Saunders PT, Turner JM, Ruggiu M, Taggart M, Burgoyne PS, Elliott D, Cooke HJ (2003) Absence of mDazl produces a final block on germ cell development at meiosis. Reproduction 126:589–597

Sauten RJ, Paulsen CA (1973) Hypogonadotrophic eunuchoidism. I. Clinical study of the mode of inheritance. J Clin Endocrinol Metab 36:47–54

Saxena R, Brown LG, Hawkins T, Alagappan RK, Skaletsky H, Reeve MP, Reijo R, Rozen S, Dinulos MB, Disteche CM, Page DC (1996) The DAZ gene cluster on the human Y chromosome arose from an autosomal gene that was transposed, repeatedly amplified and pruned. Nat Genet 14:292–299

Schempp W, Binkele A, Arnemann J, Glaser B, Ma K, Taylor K et al (1995) Comparative mapping of YRRM and TSPY related cosmids in man and homonoid apes. Chromosome Res 3:227–237

Short RV (1997) The testis, the witness of the mating system, the site of mutation and the engine of desire. Acta Paediatr (Suppl) 422:3–7

Sibley CG, Comstock JA, Ahlquist JE (1990) DNA hybridization evidence of hominoid phylogeny : a re-analysis of the data. J Mol Evol 30:202–236

Silber SJ, Alagappan R, Brown LG, Page DC (1998) Y chromosome deletions in azoospermic and severely oligozoospermic men undergoing intracytoplasmic sperm injection after testicular sperm extraction. Hum Reprod 13:3332–3337

Simmerly C, Wu GJ, Zoran S et al (1995) The paternal inheritance of the centrosome, the cells microtubular organizing center in humans and the implications for infertility. Nature Med 1:47–52

Simoni M, Gromoll J, Dwoniczak B et al (1997) Screening for deletions of the Y chromosome involving the DAZ (deleted in Azoospermia) gene in azoospermia and severe oligozoospermia. Fertil Steril 67:542–547

Simoni M, Kamischke A, Nieschlag E (1998) Current status of the molecular diagnosis of Y-chromosomal microdeletions in the work-up of male infertility. Initiative for international quality control. Hum Reprod 13:1764–1768

This paper represents welcome step towards laboratory quality control of Y microdeletion analysis. It is still very difficult to compare results from different centres, because all use different sequence tagged sites in their analyses

Simoni M, Gromoll J, Hoppner W, Kamischke A, Krafft T, Stahle D, Nieschlag E (1999) Mutational analysis of the follicle-stimulating hormone (FSH) receptor in normal and infertile men: identification and characterization of two discrete FSH receptor isoforms. J Clin Endocrinol Metab 84:751–755

Simpson JL, de la Cruz F, Swerdloff RS, Samango-Sprouse C, Skakkebaek NE, Graham JM, Hassold T, Aylstock M, Meyer-Bahlburg HF, Willard HF, Hall JG, Salameh W, Boone K, Staessen C, Geschwind D, Giedd J, Dobs AS, Rogol A, Brinton B, Paulsen CA (2003) Klinefelter syndrome: expanding the phenotype and identifying new research directions. Genet Med 5:460–468

Skaletsky H, Kuroda-Kawaguchi T, Minx PJ, Cordum HS, Hillier L, Brown LG, Repping S, Pyntikova T, Ali J, Bieri T, Chinwalla A, Delehaunty A, Delehaunty K, Du H, Fewell G, Fulton L, Fulton R, Graves T, Hou SF, Latrielle P, Leonard S, Mardis E, Maupin R, McPherson J, Miner T, Nash W, Nguyen C, Ozersky P, Pepin K, Rock S, Rohlfing T, Scott K, Schultz B, Strong C, Tin-Wollam A, Yang SP, Waterston RH, Wilson RK, Rozen S, Page DC (2003) Related articles, links [Abstract]. The male-specific region of the human Y chromosome is a mosaic of discrete sequence classes. Nature 423:825–837

Soulard M, Della Valle V, Siomi MC, Pinol-Roma S, Codogno P, Bauvy C et al (1993) hnRNP G: sequence and characterization of a glycosylated RNA-binding protein. Nucleic Acids Res 21:4210–4217

Staessen C, Tournaye H, Van Assche E, Michiels A, Van Landuyt L, Devroey P, Liebaers I, Van Steirteghem A (2003) PGD in 47,XXY Klinefelter's syndrome patients. Hum Reprod Update 9:319–330

Stuppia L, Mastroprimiano G, Calabrese G et al (1996) Microdeletions in interval 6 of the Y chromosome detected by STS-PCR in 6 of 33 patients with idiopathic oligo- or azoospermia. Cytogenet Cell Genet 72:155–158

Stuppia L, Gatta V, Mastroprimiano G (1997) Clustering of Y chromosome deletions in subinterval E of interval 6 supports the existence of an oligozoospermia critical region outside the DAZ gene. J Med Genet 34:881–883

Sun C, Skaletsky H, Birren B, Devon K, Tang Z, Silber S, Oates R, Page DC (1999) An azoospermic man with a de novo point mutation in the Y-chromosomal gene USP9Y. Nat Genet 23:429–432

Tesarik J (2004) Overcoming maturation arrest by in vitro spermatogenesis: search for the optimal culture system. Fertil Steril 81:1417–1419

Tessari A, Salata E, Ferlin A, Bartoloni L, Slongo ML, Foresta C (2004) Characterisation of HSFY, a novel AZFb gene on the Y chromosome with a possible role in spermatogenesis. Mol Hum Reprod 10:253–258

Tiepolo L, Zuffardi O (1976) Location of factors controlling spermatogenesis in the nonfluorescent portion of the human Y chromosome long arm. Hum Genet 34:119–124

Tincello DG, Saunders PTK, Hargreave TB (1997) Preliminary investigations on androgen receptor gene mutations in infertile men. Mol Hum Reprod 3:941–943

Tolarova MM, Harris JA, Ordway DE, Vargervik K (1997) Birth prevalence, mutation rate, sex ratio, parent's age and ethnicity in Apert syndrome. Am J Med Genet 72:394–398

Tournaye H, Devroey P, Liu J, Nagy Z, Lissens W, Van Steirteghem A (1994) Microsurgical epididymal sperm aspiration and intracytoplasmic sperm injection: a new effective approach to infertility as a result of congenital bilateral absence of the vas deferens. Fertil Steril 61:1045–1051

Tournaye H, Staessen C, Liebaers I, Van Assche EV, Devroey P Bonduelle M Steirteghem AV (1996) Testicular sperm recovery in nine 47 XXY Klinefelter patients. Hum Reprod 11: 1644–1649

Ulug U, Bener F, Akman MA, Bahceci M (2003) Partners of men with Klinefelter syndrome can benefit from assisted reproductive technologies. Fertil Steril 80:903–906

Van Assche E, Bonduelle M, Tournaye H, Joris H, Verheyen G, Devroey P et al (1996) Cytogenetics of infertile men. Hum Reprod 11 [Suppl 4]:1–24

van der Ven K, Messer L, van der Ven H, Jeyendran RS, Ober C (1996) Cystic fibrosis mutation screening in healthy men with reduced sperm quality. Hum Reprod 11:513–517

Van Kooij RJ, de Boer P, De Vreedenb-Elbertse JM, Ganga NA, Singh N, Te Velde (2004) The neutral comet assay detects double strand DNA damage in selected and unselected human spermatozoa of normospermic donors. Int J Androl 27:140–146

Venables JP, Cooke HJ (2000) Lessons from knockout and transgenic mice for infertility in men. J Endocrinol Invest 23:584–591

Vernaeve V, Staessen C, Verheyen G, Van Steirteghem A, Devroey P, Tournaye H (2004) Can biological or clinical parameters predict testicular sperm recovery in 47,XXY Klinefelter's syndrome patients? Hum Reprod 19:1135–1139

Vogt PH (1999) Risk of neurodegenerative diseases in children by intracytoplasmic sperm injection? Lancet 354:611–612

Vogt is best known for his work on Y microdeletions in the fruit fly and in humans, and he has made significant contributions to our knowledge. In this erudite review, he examines the possibility that genetic anticipation may make children who are conceived through ICSI more likely to have neurodegenerative disease, but concludes that it is unlikely

Vogt P, Chandley AC, Hargreave TB, Keil R, Ma K, Sharkey A (1992) Microdeletions in interval 6 of the Y chromosome of males with idiopathic sterility point to disruption of AZF, a human spermatogenesis gene. Hum Genet 89:491–496

Vogt P, Edelmann A, Kirsch S (1996) Human Y chromosome azoospermic factors AZF mapped to different regions in Ya11. Hum Mol Genet 5:933–943

Wang C, Baker HWG, Burger HG et al (1975) Hormonal studies in men with Klinefelters syndrome. Clin Endocrinol 4: 399–414

Wang PJ, McCarrey JR, Yang F, Page DC (2001) An abundance of X-linked genes expressed in spermatogonia. Nat Genet 27:422–426

Westerveld GH, Gianotten J, Leschot NJ, van der Veen F, Repping S, Lombardi MP (2004) Heterogeneous nuclear ribonucleoprotein G-T (HNRNP G-T) mutations in men with impaired spermatogenesis. Mol Hum Reprod 10:265–269

Wu CC, Hsieh-Li HM, Lin YM, Chiang HS (2004) Cystic fibrosis transmembrane conductance regulator gene screening and clinical correlation in Taiwanese males with congenital bilateral absence of the vas deferens. Hum Reprod 19:250–253

Xu EY, Moore FL, Pera RA (2001) A gene family required for human germ cell development evolved from an ancient meiotic gene conserved in metazoans. Proc Natl Acad Sci USA 98:7414–7419

Zhang LU (2004) Investigation of the frequency of chromosomal aneuploidy using triple fluorescence in situ hybridization in 12 Chinese infertile men. Chinese Med J 117: 503–506

II.3.11 Tumour Genetics (Prostate/Testis/Penis)

O. Tatarov, D. Kirk

Summary

- Family history is a major risk factor for prostate cancer
- Prostate cancer developing before age 55 is frequently inherited
- Brothers of men with testis cancer have an eight- to tenfold risk themselves of testis cancer
- Bilateral testis cancer may carry a higher genetic risk
- The rarity of penile cancer makes hereditary risks difficult to define

II.3.11.1 Genetic Aspects of Prostate Cancer

In addition to age and race, several large case–control and cohort studies have confirmed that family history is a major risk factor in prostate cancer (Cannon et al. 1982; Steinberg et al. 1990; Carter et al. 1992; Gronberg et al. 1996). From twin registries of Denmark, Sweden and Finland, 42% of prostate cancers were attributed to inheritance (Lichtenstein et al. 2000). The number of affected relatives and their age at diagnosis affect the risk. A brother or father with prostate cancer increases the risk by twofold to threefold, greater the younger the affected relative (Cannon et al. 1982; Ghadirian et al. 1997; Matikaine et al. 2001). A large proportion of prostate cancer in men under 55 years old is thought to be inherited (Zeegers et al. 2003).

"Hereditary prostate cancer", which simulates a Mendelian dominant trait, is suggested when prostate cancer occurs in three or more first-degree relatives; in each of three generations in the paternal or maternal lineage; or in two or more first- or second-degree relatives under the age of 55 (Damber 2001; Nieder et al. 2003). However, as few as one or two affected relatives ("familial prostate cancer") may indicate an increased risk (Steinberg et al. 1990).

Affected brothers confer a greater risk than affected fathers. This may be due to X-linked or recessive inheritance, although the reason for the difference is unknown. Detailed information regarding risk ratios related to family history of prostate cancer was presented in a meta-analysis of 33 epidemiological studies (Table II.3.17).

Clinical presentation, response to treatment and survival do not appear to be different in patients with inherited and sporadic forms of disease, with no statistical differences in symptoms, pathologic stage, Gleason scores, margins or in prostate specific antigen (PSA) recurrence (Gronberg et al. 1998; Valeri et al. 2000; Bratt et al. 2002). Thus, the arguments about PSA testing and screening are in theory no different than those in sporadic disease, but clearly in practice those with close relatives, particularly where the disease was fatal, will have a greater anxiety creating a desire for screening. However, counselling before PSA testing is no less important.

There have been recent reports that men with a positive family history of prostate cancer may be at risk for other malignancies. In the Li–Fraumeni dominantly inherited cancer syndrome, caused by constitutional mutations in the TP53 or CHK2 genes, affected family members develop, apart from prostatic adenocarcinoma, at an early age rhabdomyosarcomas, soft tissue sarcomas, breast cancer, brain tumours, osteosarcoma, leukaemia and pancreatic carcinoma. Individuals with inherited mutations of BRCA1 and BRCA2 (breast cancer genes) are also thought to be at higher risk for prostate cancer. A possible increased risk for colon cancer, non-Hodgkin's lymphoma, rectal cancer and brain cancer in first-degree relatives of patients with prostate cancer (Goldgar et al. 1994; Gronberg et al. 2000) might be due to genetic predisposition resulting in a family cancer syndrome, but the alternative explanation of a common environmental exposure has not been excluded.

II.3.11.2 Genetics of Testicular Cancer

Testicular germ-cell tumours (TGCT) are the most common type of malignancy in men aged 15–45 years. The important risk factors for TGCT are family history

Table II.3.17. Relative risk related to family history of prostate cancer. (*CI* Confidence interval.) Adapted from Zeegers et al. (2003)

Risk group	Relative risk for prostate cancer
Brother with prostate cancer diagnosed at any age	3.4 (95% CI = 3.0–3.8)
Father with prostate cancer diagnosed at any age	2.2 (95% CI = 1.9–2.5)
One affected first-degree relative diagnosed at any age	2.6 (95% CI = 2.3–2.8)
One affected second-degree relative diagnosed at any age	1.7 (95% CI = 1.1–2.6)
Affected first-degree relative(s) diagnosed age <65 years	3.3 (95% CI = 2.6–4.2)
Affected first-degree relative(s) diagnosed age >65 years	2.4 (95% CI = 1.7–3.6)
Two or more affected first-degree relatives diagnosed at any age	5.1 (95% CI = 3.3–7.8)

(UK Testicular Cancer Study Group 1994), cryptorchidism (Swerdlow et al.1997) and previously diagnosed TGCT (Osterlind et al. 1991; Wanderas et al.1997).

Twenty-five different hereditary disorders or constitutional chromosomal anomalies have been reported in patients with TGCT. In some there are also defects in urogenital differentiation suggesting a correlation with testicular dysgenesis syndrome, of which testicular cancer is thought to be part (Lutke Holzik et al. 2003). Patients with Klinefelter syndrome (47 XXY) and XY gonadal dysgenesis have a substantial risk of developing germ-cell tumours. Approximately 8% of cases of mediastinal (extragonadal) GCT have Klinefelter syndrome, although tumours in their testes are rare, probably because of lack of testicular germ cells.

Familial cases account for 1.0–5.5% of testicular cancers (Forman et al. 1992; Heimdal et al. 1996; Dieckman and Pichlmeier 1997; Sonneveld et al. 1999). Some 1–3% of men with TGCT have an affected first-degree relative. Brothers of those with the disease have a relative risk of TGCT of 8–10 whereas for the sons the relative risk is 4–6 (Heimdal et al. 1996; Dieckman and Pichlmeier 1997; Sonneveld et al. 1999). This high relative risk is unlikely to be due to a shared environmental factor (Lutke Holzik et al. 2004).

Bilateral involvement of paired organs is considered to be an important sign of hereditary cancer. Early somatic mutation of tyrosine kinase receptor gene (KIT) is believed to predispose patients to the bilateral TGCT (Looijenga et al. 2003). Several association studies have also linked the risk of TGCT to HLA genes that might play a role in the immune response to various carcinogenic factors (Birkeland et al. 1995; Bateman and Howell 1999; Spano et al. 2002). Finally, there is circumstantial evidence that patients with TGCT and their relatives might be at risk for developing tumours at other sites such as colon, kidney, pancreas, bladder, thyroid and lung (Goss and Bulbul 1990; Dong et al. 2001).

In both prostate cancer and TGCT, several putative susceptibility genes are thought to confer an increased risk. However, no definitive genetic tests are available for these conditions. Progress in bioinformatics and molecular biology is expected to facilitate further advance in exploration of genetic predisposition to prostatic and testicular carcinomas as well as improve our understanding of non-hereditary cancers.

II.3.11.3 Genetics of Penile Cancer

Penile squamous cell carcinoma is a rare disease and there is a relatively small amount of information regarding hereditary aspects. Data are usually limited to case reports, with no statistically sound publications (Raney and Jhaveri 1981).

II.3.11.4 Genetic Testing

A statement from the American Society of Clinical Oncology provides indications for genetic testing (American Society of Clinical Oncology 2003):

1. The individual has personal or family history features suggestive of a genetic cancer susceptibility condition
2. The test can be adequately interpreted
3. The results will aid in diagnosis or influence the medical or surgical management of the patient or family members at hereditary risk of cancer.

Individuals undergo genetic screening to determine whether a gene predisposing to certain type of cancer has been inherited. The process involves constructing and evaluating a pedigree, eliciting a personal and family medical history, and providing information about genetic risk. Where a genetic test is not available, an age-related risk estimate can be provided from the pedigree analysis in order to decide when clinical screening should be offered. Those thought to be at increased risk for inherited cancer should be encouraged to participate in established research programmes. Candidates for genetic testing should first receive counselling on the various medical uncertainties and psychosocial risks and benefits involved in genetic testing (Petersen 2000; American Society of Clinical Oncology 2003).

Family history information must be summarized in the form of a pedigree or family tree. This is a standardized graphic representation of family relationships in which patterns of disease transmission are tracked (Bennett et al. 1995). This facilitates identification of patterns of transmission, recognition of specific hereditary cancer syndromes and assists in determining the best methods for risk assessment.

Factors suggesting inherited cancer risk include the following:

- Clustering of the same type of cancer in close relatives
- Unusually early age of cancer onset
- Two or more primary cancers in a single relative
- Evidence of autosomal dominant inheritance
- Bilaterality in paired organs
- Patterns of cancer in the family that are associated with a known cancer syndrome.

References

American Society of Clinical Oncology (2003) American Society of Clinical Oncology policy statement update: genetic testing for cancer susceptibility. J Clin Oncol 21:2397–2406

Bateman AC, Howell WM (1999) Human leukocyte antigens and cancer: is it in our genes? J Pathol 188:231–236

Bennett RL, Steinhaus KA, Uhrich SB et al (1995) Recommendations for standardized human pedigree nomenclature. J Genet Couns 4:267–279
Birkeland SA, Storm HH, Lamm LU et al (1995) Cancer risk after renal transplantation in the Nordic countries, 1964–1986. Int J Cancer 60:183–189
Bratt O, Dumber JE, Emanuelsson M, Gronberg H (2002) Hereditary prostate cancer:clinical characteristics and survival. J Urol 167:2423–2426
Cannon L, Bishop DT, Skolnick M et al (1982) Genetic epidemiology of prostate cancer in the Utah Mormon genealogy. Cancer Surv 1:47–69
Carter BS, Beaty TH, Steinberg GD et al (1992) Mendelian inheritance of familial prostate cancer. Proc Natl Acad Sci USA 89:3367–3371
Damber JE (2001) Familial aggregation of prostate cancer management while waiting for the identification of hereditary prostate cancer genes. Eur Urol 39 [Suppl. 4]:19–21
Dieckman KP, Pichlmeier U (1997) The prevalence of familial testicular cancer: an analysis of two patient populations and a review of the literature. Cancer 80:1954–1960
Dong C, Lonnstedt I, K. Hemminki (2001) Familial testicular cancer and second primary cancers in testicular cancer patients by histological type. Eur J Cancer 37:1878–1885
Forman D, Oliver RT, Brett AR et al (1992) Familial testicular cancer: a report of the UK family register, estimation of risk and an HLA class 1 sib-pair analysis. Br J Cancer 65:255–262
Ghadirian P, Howe GR, Hislop TG et al (1997) Family history of prostate cancer: a multi-center case-control study in Canada. Int J Cancer 70:679–681
Goldgar DE, Easton DF, Cannon-Albright LA, Skolnick MH (1994) Systematic population-based assessment of cancer risk in first-degree relatives of cancer probands. J Natl Cancer Inst 86:1600–1608
Goss PE, Bulbul MA (1990) Familial testicular cancer in five members of a cancer-prone kindred. Cancer 66:2044–2046
Gronberg H, Damber L, Damber JE (1996) Familial prostate cancer in Sweden. A nationwide register cohort study. Cancer 77:138–143
Gronberg H, Damber L, Tavelin B, Damber JE (1998) No difference in survival between sporadic, familial and hereditary prostate cancer. Br J Urol 82:564–567
Gronberg H, Bergh A, Damber JE, Emanuelsson M (2000) Cancer risk in families with hereditary prostate carcinoma. Cancer 89:1315–1321
Heimdal K, Olsson H, Trestly S et al (1996) Familial testicular cancer in Norway and Southern Sweden. Br J Cancer 73:964–969
Lichtenstein P, Holm NV, Verkasalo PK et al (2000) Environmental and heritable factors in the causation of cancer – analyses of cohorts of twins from Sweden, Denmark, and Finland. N Engl J Med 343:78–85
Looijenga LH, de Leeuw H, van Oorschot M et al (2003) Stem cell factor receptor (c-KIT) codon 816 mutations predict development of bilateral testicular germ-cell tumours. Cancer Res 63:7674–7678
Lutke Holzik MF, Sijmons RH, Sleijfer DT et al (2003) Syndromic aspects of testicular carcinoma. Cancer 97:984–992
Lutke Holzik MF, Rapley EA, Hoekstra HJ et al (2004) Genetic predisposition to testicular germ-cell tumours. Lancet Oncol 5:363–371
Matikaine MP, Pukkala E, Schleutker J et al (2001) Relatives of prostate cancer patients have an increased risk of prostate and stomach cancers: a population-based, cancer registry study in Finland. Cancer Causes Control 12:223–230
Nieder AM, Taneja SS, Zeegers MPA, Ostrer H (2003) Genetic counselling for prostate cancer risk. Clin Genet 63:169–176
Osterlind A, Berthelsen JG, Abildgaard N et al (1991) Risk of bilateral testicular germ cell cancer in Denmark 1960–1984. J Natl Cancer Inst 83:1391–1395
Petersen GM (2000) Genetic testing. Hematol Oncol Clin North Am 14:939–952
Raney AM, Jhaveri KK (1981) Familial carcinoma of penis. NY State J Med 81:1786–1787
Sonneveld DJ, Sleijfer DT, Schraffordt Koops H et al (1999) Familial testicular cancer in a single-centre population. Eur J Cancer 35:1368–1373
Spano JP, Atlan D, Breau JL, Farge D (2002) AIDS and non-AIDS-related malignancies: a new vexing challenge in HIV-positive patients: part II, cervical and anal squamous epithelial lesions, lung cancer, testicular germ cell cancers, and skin cancers. Eur J Intern Med 13:227–232
Steinberg GD, Carter BS, Beaty TH et al (1990) Family history and the risk of prostate cancer. Prostate 17:337–347
Swerdlow AJ, Higgins CD, Pike MC (1997) Risk of testicular cancer in cohort of boys with cryptorchidism. BMJ 314: 1507–1511
UK Testicular Cancer Study Group (1994) Aetiology of testicular cancer: association with congenital abnormalities, age at puberty, infertility, and exercise. BMJ 308:1393–1399
Valeri A, Azzouzi R, Drelon E et al (2000) Early-onset hereditary prostate cancer is not associated with specific clinical and biological features. Prostate 45:66–71
Wanderas EH, Fossa SD, Tretli S (1997) Risk of a second germ cell cancer after treatment of a primary germ cell cancer in 2201 Norwegian male patients. Eur J Cancer 33:244–252
Zeegers MP, Jellema A, Ostrer H (2003) Empiric risk of prostate carcinoma for relatives of patients with prostate carcinoma: a meta-analysis. Cancer 97:1894–1903

II.4 Therapeutic Options

II.4.1 Introduction to Surgical Section

In this section there are descriptions of the operative technique for some commonly performed operations on the male genitalia. Often such operation are delegated to inexperienced doctors, and unfortunately this can result in lifelong disability; for example care needs to be taken with adult circumcision not to remove too much skin from the shaft of the penis. The authors all have considerable personal experience of performing the techniques described and also have all been involved in teaching technique. There are many alternative operations to those described but the techniques in this section work well and are safe. The reader will find description of the following operations: circumcision, penile prosthesis, penile straightening, orchiopexy, removal of an epididymal cyst, hydrocele, vasectomy and vasectomy reversal. In Chap. II.4.17 the reader will find description of sperm recovery. The repertoire of operations is limited to those most commonly performed and the reader is referred to a dedicated surgical manual such as Campbell's Urology for other surgical procedures.

II.4.2 Surgical Procedures in Andrology

Christine Evans

II.4.2.1 Scrotal Surgery

The advantage of operating on the scrotum is that it is extremely accessible and the anatomy is easy to see and to learn; the drawback is that, if not done with attention to detail, the surgery can lead to bleeding (very vascular area) and post operative infertility and at worst ischaemic problems of the testis.

In order to open the scrotum knowledge of scrotal layers is needed, as is anatomy of the testis (Fig. II.4.1). The testis is oval in shape and measures about 4 cm by 2 cm by 2.5 cm. The dense covering is called the tunica albuginea as it is whitish in colour. The epididymis lies posterior along the length of the testis and has a head, body and tail, and the tail becomes the vas deferens which runs proximally to form the spermatic cord with the testicular vessels. The testis and epididymis are covered by the tunica vaginalis derived from the peritoneum with a parietal layer, and a visceral layer with a potential space which contains a small amount of fluid. Covering the testis is the internal spermatic fascia, cremasteric muscle, the external spermatic fascia and then skin.

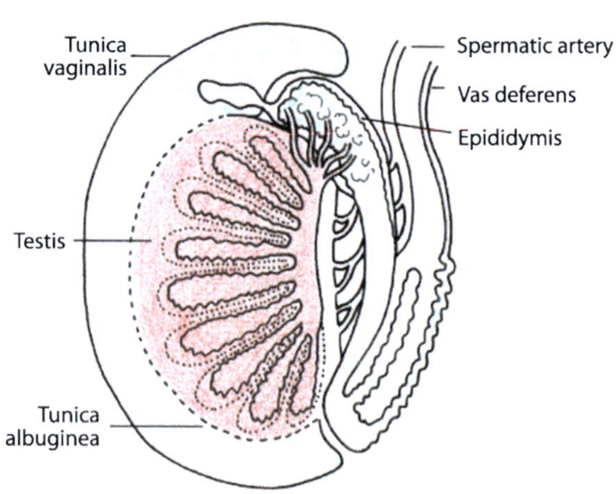

Fig. II.4.1. Sagittal section of the testis

II.4.2.1.1
Scrotal Incisions

If unilateral surgery is to be performed, a single incision on that side may be made either longitudinally or in the transverse direction. If both sides require surgery a single midline or transverse incision can be made; the latter usually has a less obvious scar but due to the rugose nature of the skin the scars are not usually obvious. If the operation requires exposure to get up to the external ring, bilateral operations are best done through two longitudinal incisions of adequate size. Certain scrotal operations are best performed through a groin incision, especially those for orchiectomy for testicular tumours, so the cord can be occluded prior to mobilization of the whole testis from the scrotum. Also for orchiopexy where access to above the internal ring is required, adequate exposure in the groin is needed, to allow maximal mobilization to get the testis fixed in the scrotum comfortably.

Scrotal incisions nearly always heal well with minimal scarring. Subcutaneous tissue can be approximated by several interrupted absorbable sutures such as 3.0 vicryl and the skin can be closed with a subcuticular absorbable suture such as undyed Vicryl or Monocryl. There is no need to use nonabsorbable sutures that need to be removed; men do not like having stitches removed from the genital area, nurses do not like to have to do this and often the stitches are difficult to find once the scrotal skin has contracted. Generally scrotal skin incisions heal in 3 – 5 days.

II.4.2.2
Anaesthesia for Scrotal, Inguinoscrotal and Penile Surgery

Scrotal procedures can be undertaken with general, spinal or field block anaesthesia. Effective testicular anaesthesia can be obtained by injecting 2 – 5 ml of 0.5% levobupivacaine into the cord at the level of the external inguinal ring with an additional 2 – 5 ml into the scrotal skin at the scrotal neck and in the area of the incision. It is important to wait for sufficient time for the anaesthetic to take effect (10 – 15 min) and to test for effective anaesthesia before commencing surgery. A useful variation in technique is to use a mixture of lignocaine and levobupivacaine because lignocaine acts more speedily than levobupivacaine but does not last the 4 – 6 h that is obtained after levobupivacaine.

Inguinoscrotal surgery can be undertaken using a field block. However, most surgeons prefer the use of general anaesthesia because of unfamiliarity with the surgical and field block techniques and because of the time taken to achieve effective regional anaesthesia. A larger volume of local anaesthetic is needed. A long needle is used (e.g. a spinal needle) and three of injections of 5 ml anaesthetic are made above the inguinal ligament in a vertical line above a point one-third from the lateral end of the ligament. The needle is passed through the skin and subcutaneous tissue and through the fascia overlying the abdominal wall muscles before the injection is made. With practice the passage of the needle through the fascia can be felt. The objective is to block the segmental nerves as they run from lateral to medial. In addition, an injection is made into the cord within the inguinal canal and also over the incision. Once the injections have been given 10 – 15 min should be allowed before testing for effective anaesthesia, especially if the local anaesthetic has been diluted.

Most penile surgery can be undertaken with penile block anaesthesia. An injection is made into the skin about 1 cm above the superior border of the base of the penis over the pubic bone. Using a long needle the injection is deepened until the needle abuts the pubic bone. The angle of the injection is then altered so that the needle passes just under the underside of the pubic symphysis between the symphysis and the penis. At this point the needle is slightly angulated to one side of the midline and then the other and approximately 5 ml of anaesthetic solution injected on each side. After a wait of 5 – 10 min the penis is tested for anaesthesia and if not complete a further injection can be given.

It is important not to exceed local anaesthetic safe doses within a 4-h period total. The total safe dose of bupivacaine or levobupivacaine is 2 mg/kg and for lignocaine it is 3 mg/kg (without adrenaline) or 7 mg/kg (with adrenaline). When using mixtures of local anaesthetics, remember that toxic doses are additive. In order to have sufficient volume and also not to exceed toxic doses, local anaesthetic solutions can be further diluted to make 0.25% or 0.125% solutions.

II.4.2.2.1
Adjuvant Local Anaesthetic

It is kind to patients and may help prevent chronic pain to give local anaesthetic with levobupivacaine as an adjunct in all general anaesthetic scrotal and penile procedures.

II.4.2.3
Surgical Procedures on the Scrotum

- Orchiopexy for imperfect descent of the testes
- Exploration and fixation for torsion of the testes
- Exploration for infective conditions
- Orchiectomy for malignant and benign disease
- Subcapsular orchiectomy
- Excision of epididymal cysts/spermatocele
- Operations for hydrocele
- Epididymectomy

- Ligation of varicocele
- Vasectomy
- Reversal of vasectomy (vasovasostomy)
- Vasoepididymostomy for epididymal obstruction
- Exploratory scrototomy/vasography

II.4.2.4 Surgery for Adult Hydrocele

A hydrocele is a collection of usually clear yellow fluid between the two layers of tunica vaginalis and can get to a very large size (Fig. II.4.2). Most hydroceles occur spontaneously and no underlying cause can be identified. Sometimes hydroceles occur in older men with heart failure because of altered scrotal circulatory dynamics. More rarely hydroceles occur as a reaction to inflammation or testicular tumour. Small hydroceles can be left alone. In younger men the underlying testicle should be visualized by ultrasound or the hydrocele can be aspirated and the testicle palpated. However, aspiration is not curative as the fluid quickly recollects and each aspiration risks the introduction of infection. Injection with sclerosing agent is not recommended.

II.4.2.4.1 Hydrocele of Testis

Lord's Procedure

The operation described by Lord (1964) is done through a scrotal incision (Figs. II.4.3, II.4.4). The procedure can be done under general spinal or local anaesthesia; if the latter, a good cord block with additional local anaesthesia to the skin is required. Holding the hydrocele firmly in the left hand (if right handed) the anterior scrotal skin is stretched. An incision

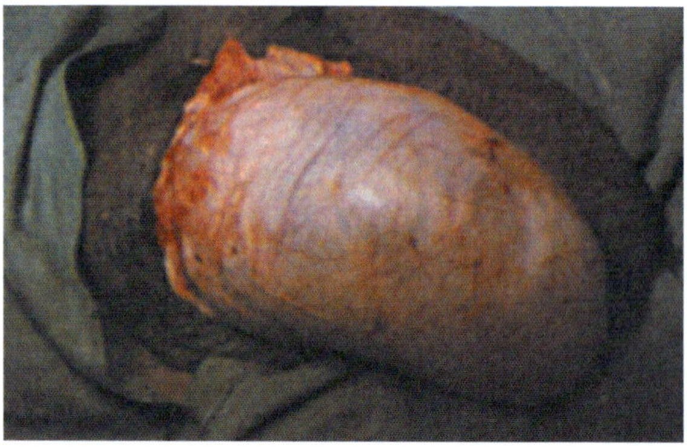

Fig. II.4.2. Hydrocele

3–4 cm in length is made through skin and subcutaneous tissues until the tunica vaginalis reached. It is best to coagulate with diathermy any blood vessels as you go because they are easy to see when the tissues are stretched but less so afterwards when the skin is not stretched. The tunica vaginalis is incised and the fluid drained off; there is no need to mobilize further. The testis is lifted up, inspected and then five to six gathering sutures are made into the tunica, which has been everted backwards away from the testis itself, and the tunica now forms a collar behind the testis. Before closing the skin and dartos together careful haemostasis is essential. If there is doubt about haemostasis a scrotal drain can be used, but usually haemostasis is adequate. A firm scrotal support should be used postoperatively. The advantage of the Lord's procedure is that there is minimal tissue dissection and this reduces the occurrence of postoperative bleeding. A disadvantage of the procedure is that the gathering up and pleating of the hydrocele sac can result in a rather lumpy testicle, particularly if the hydrocele wall is thickened.

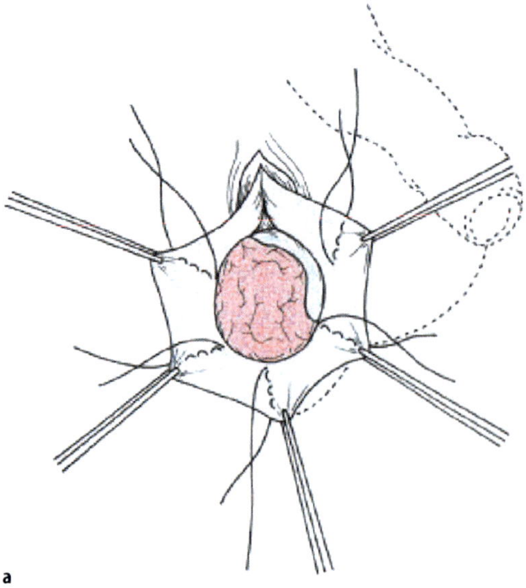

a

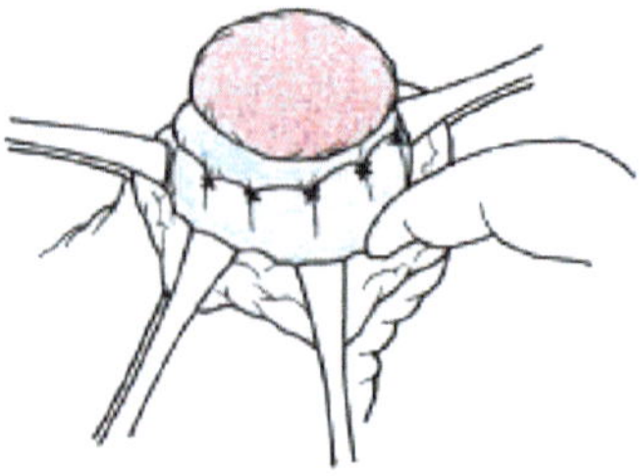

b

Fig. II.4.3. Drawing of Lord's procedure

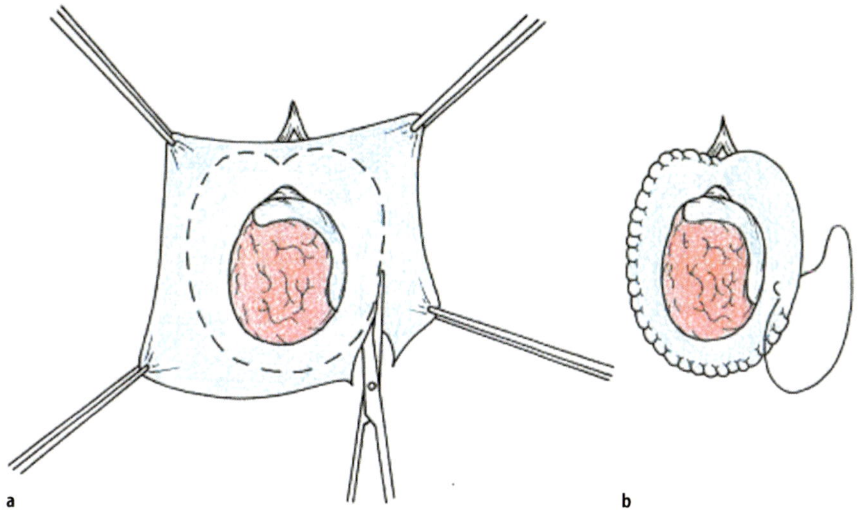

Fig. II.4.4. Excision of hydrocele with oversewn edge

Repair of Hydrocele by Excision of the Tunica Vaginalis

An alternative operation is to excise the tunica vaginalis and this is usually the best technique if the hydrocele is very large or if the tunica is thickened. Once the tunica is excised close to the testis, bleeding points must be dealt with by diathermy and a running stitch before returning the testis to the scrotum. Bleeding can be a particular problem after hydrocele excision and although it is always more bothersome for patient and surgeon it is often best to use a drain, and provided all is well remove it the next day. This is especially so if large areas of hydrocele wall have been excised.

Postoperatively the scrotal swelling may take up to 4 weeks to settle. There is nearly always some residual thickening, and the man should be warned that a minor degree of thickening and lumpiness is likely to remain after surgery especially after an operation for a longstanding hydrocele.

II.4.2.5 Excision of Epididymal Cyst/Spermatocele

II.4.2.5.1 Epididymal Cyst

An epididymal cyst is a retention cyst in the epididymis that can be single or multiple, and the fluid is clear (Fig. II.4.5). A spermatocele contains sperm and the fluid is cloudy.

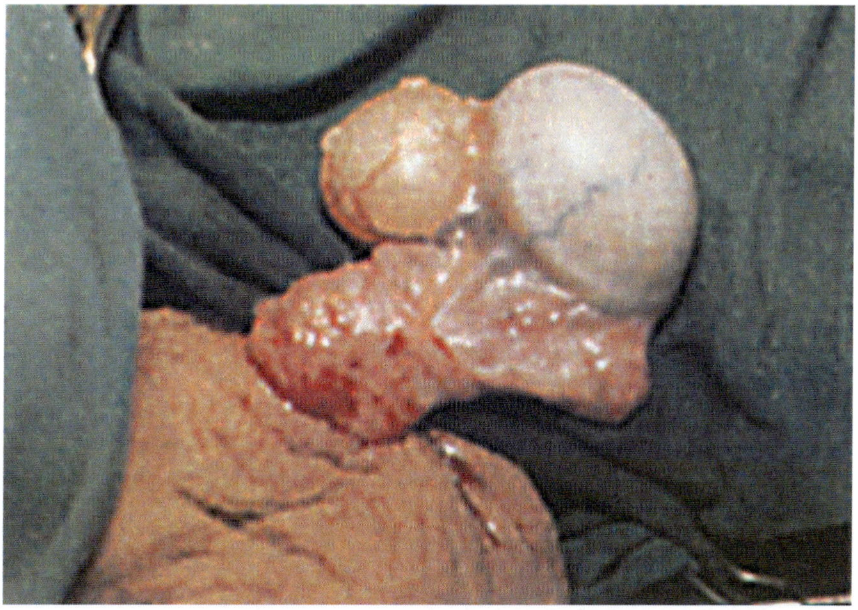

Fig. II.4.5. Epididymal cyst

Epididymal Cyst with Normal Testis

Through a scrotal incision the tunica is opened and the testis plus cyst is delivered into the wound. The cyst is excised off the testis and the plane is usually easy to find and dissect off (Fig. II.4.6). Be careful to cauterize vessels going to the cyst by diathermy. These cysts tend to recur and if they do or are multiple then epididymectomy is advised. All epididymal surgery, including removal of a solitary epididymal cyst, carries the risk of blockage to the epididymal duct and obstruction to sperm on that side. Therefore, all men considering epididymal surgery should be advised about possible risks to fertility. In the case of a small cyst in a younger man it is often best to reassure the man that there is no danger of cancer but not to operate. Care should be taken to ensure adequate haemostasis but not to use excessive diathermy because this may damage the epididymal duct or the blood supply to the testicle. In selected cases (e.g. only one testicle) the operating microscope can be used to help identify anatomy and reduce the chance of damage.

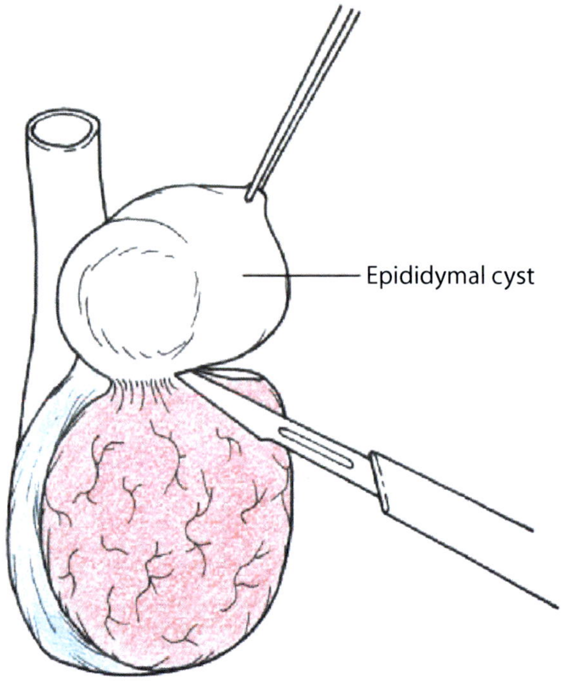

Fig. II.4.6. Excision of epididymal cyst

Epididymectomy

Through the scrotal incision the tunica albuginea is opened and the testis and epididymis delivered. Separation of the epididymis is commenced at the lower pole, with great care taken of the vessels entering behind into the middle part of the testis at the mesorchium. The vas can be divided anywhere in the scrotum but it is best done as near to the external ring as possible. The man should be warned about the rare possibility of damage to the blood vessels supplying the testicle and postoperative testicular atrophy.

II.4.2.6 Undescended Testis in the Adult

Postpubertal boys and even adults may present with undescended testes, although this condition is usually picked up in infancy. There are three indications for operative surgery: one is to maximize the chances of fer-

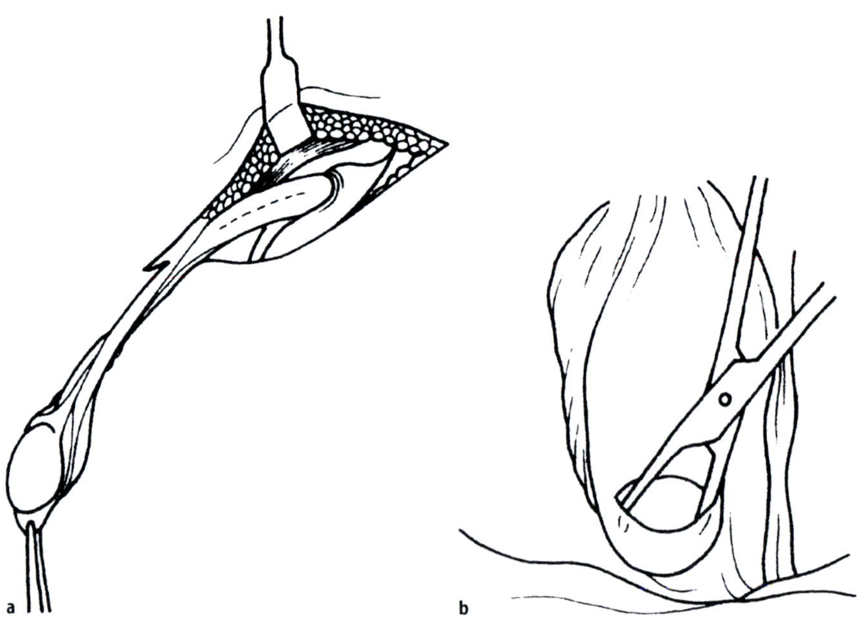

Fig. II.4.7. Surgery for undescended testis. **a** Mobilisation of the testis and spermatic cord for orchidopexy. **b** Formation of pouch

tility, although if the other testis is normally descended it will make little difference; the second is to place the testicle in the scrotum so that any abnormality can be more easily detected (this is important as there is an increased risk of testicular malignancy in men with testicular maldescent, see Chap. I.8.2); the third indication is for cosmetic reasons.

II.4.2.6.1
Orchiopexy (Fig. II.4.7)

An incision is made above and parallel to the medial half of the inguinal ligament. The testis may be in the inguinal canal or in a pouch superficial to the external ring. In the latter case the testicular blood vessels emerge from the external inguinal ring and turn upwards to run to the testicle so that as the testicle lies in the superficial inguinal pouch the vessels lie inferiomedial to the testicle. Care has to be taken with the dissection as this anatomical relationship of testicle and blood vessels is exactly opposite to the normal situation. The inguinal canal is opened by incising the external oblique parallel to the ligament. The cord is mobilized and the tissues of the cord gently cleared of the vessels and the vas up to and above the internal ring. A hernial sac and/or pad of fat is often present, usually lying anterior to the vas deferens and testicular blood vessels. Care must be taken not to injure the vas deferens or testicular blood vessels as the posterior wall of the hernia sac is dissected. If there is a sac it should be dissected, twisted to expel any contents back into the abdominal cavity and tied with a transfixion suture at the level of the internal inguinal ring. If at this stage the testis can be placed within the scrotum no further dissection is needed; however, if not, the dissection of the testicular blood vessels and vas deferens can be extended above the internal ring to the retroperitoneal tissues with care taken to divide all bands of fibrous tissue and strands of muscle. After this has been done it is nearly always possible to place the testicle into the scrotum without tension on the cord. If the patient has proved his fertility and has consented, and if the testis is small or cannot be placed in the scrotum, orchiectomy can be considered, as long as the other testicle is normal.

Once the testicle has been mobilized the length of the mobilization is tested by holding the testicle over the scrotum. Provided the length is adequate to avoid tension, a tract has to be made into the scrotum. The tissues from the inguinal wound to the inside of the scrotum are broken down by finger dissection to create a tract from the external inguinal ring into the scrotum. Stretching the skin of the most dependent point of the hemiscrotum over the finger, an incision is made transversely and a pouch big enough for the testis is dissected between the skin and the dartos muscle. A small puncture is then made through the dartos muscle with long-handled artery forceps and the tips are then manipulated though the previously created tract to the inguinal canal and the testis picked up and pulled through into the pouch. Care must be taken not to twist the vessels and a check made that the testis is lying comfortably and is not pulling back into the groin. All wounds are closed, the inguinal wound in layers. Usually the puncture through the dartos muscle is sufficient to keep the testicle in place, but if there is any tendency for the testicle to slip back upwards it should be fixed in position with one or two interrupted absorbable sutures.

II.4.2.7
Circumcision in Adults

The need for circumcision in adults is usually for phimosis, paraphimosis if the prepuce remains tight after reduction, and a premalignancy or actual malignancy affecting the prepuce alone.

This operation is frequently performed by trainee surgeons early in their training and sometimes the results are not as good as they should be. Circumcision should be carefully taught and performed by competent surgeons as a bad cosmetic result can seriously affect the patient both sexually and psychologically.

II.4.2.7.1
Sleeve Technique for Retractable Foreskins

The foreskin is retracted and the skin marked 0.5 – 1 cm proximal to the corona and incised with a knife to make a clean straight incision circumferentially; on the ventral surface the frenulum is incised and the vessels ligated. Care must be taken with diathermy as there have been instances of loss of the penis secondary to coagulation of the whole of the penis. Bipolar diathermy is generally advised; if this is not available and monopolar diathermy is used, then fine diathermy forceps should be used and great care taken to pick up vessels very accurately and use only short bursts of current and to observe that diathermy is working instantly. The foreskin is then pulled back over the glans and the site of the second incision is made just at the level of the corona; the skin is incised and the tissues between the two incisions removed (Fig. II.4.8). Do not put too much tension on the skin when pulling the foreskin back over the glans prior to marking the skin for the second incision. This is to avoid removing too much skin from the penile shaft. Careful haemostasis is needed with diathermy and ties for larger vessels. The skin should be closed with fine absorbable sutures (e.g. 4.0 Vicryl).

A dressing is optional. It is advised to avoid sexual intercourse for 4 weeks and it often helps to advise the man to use a condom for the first few occasions to protect the suture line.

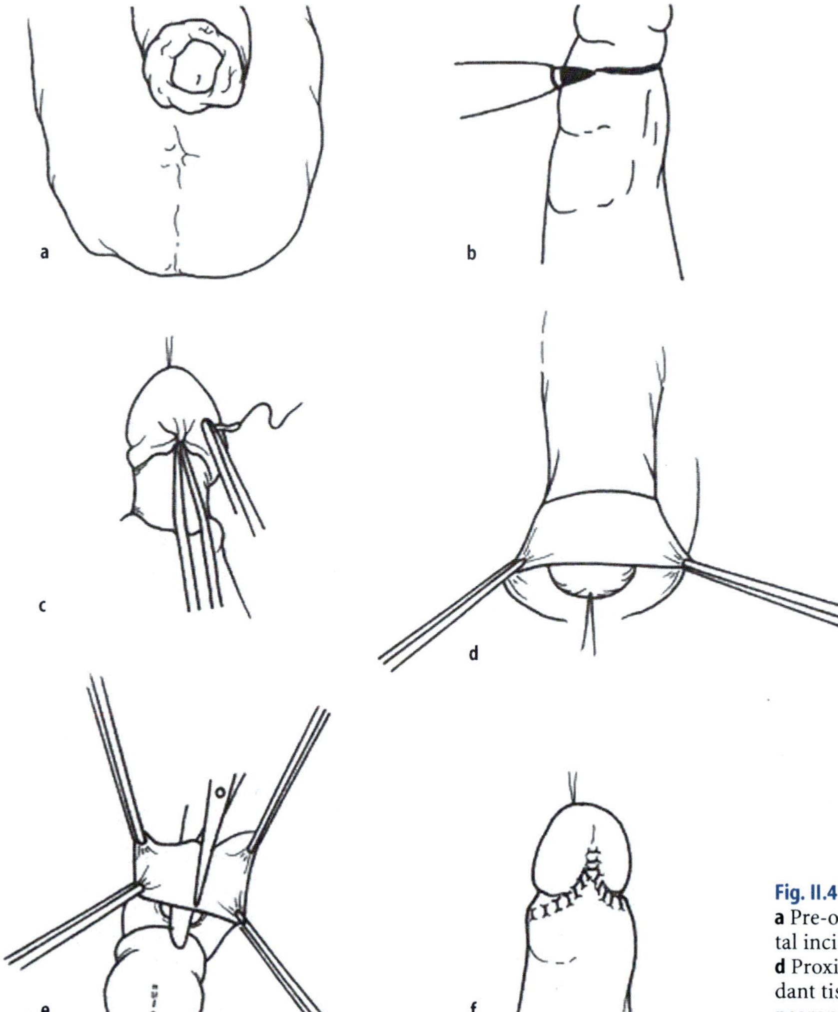

Fig. II.4.8. Circumcision sleeve technique. **a** Pre-operative. **b** Foreskin retracted distal incision marked. **c** Frenuloplasty. **d** Proximal incision marked. **e** Redundant tissue excised. **f** Post-operative appearance ventral surface

II.4.2.7.2 Technique for Phimosis

In this technique the skin is marked with the foreskin a bit stretched just distal to the corona. Then a dorsal slit is performed through both layers of the foreskin to the level of the skin mark at the corona (Fig. II.4.9). The mark on the skin is the mark for excision through both layers, either with scissors or knife – the latter has a neater cut for cosmesis. Careful haemostasis is needed and the skin edges closed with absorbable interrupted fine sutures. Dressing is optional. Histology is advised if the prepuce not entirely normal.

Postoperative complications include bleeding, infection, complaints about cosmetic appearance, complaints about pain and skin tension during erection and oversensitivity of the glans.

Bleeding is an inherent risk of the procedure but can be minimized by careful technique. Infection may be reduced by administering a single dose of broad-spectrum antibiotics just prior to surgery. Antibiotics should be given if phimosis is severe, especially if there is balanitis. If a day case procedure is undertaken the man should be instructed to remain off work for the first three to four postoperative days, to avoid contact sports and any activity that increases intra-abdominal pressure. The commonest postoperative problem is haematoma. Patients dislike it when too much skin is excised which is why care must be made to mark the skin pre incision without pulling on the prepuce too much. The glans, not used to being exposed, will be hypersensitive initially and to protect the meatus from rubbing on underpants, and causing meatal stenosis, some lubricant may be applied to this site only. The man should be advised to use a condom during sexual intercourse for 6–8 weeks postoperatively until the wound has completely healed.

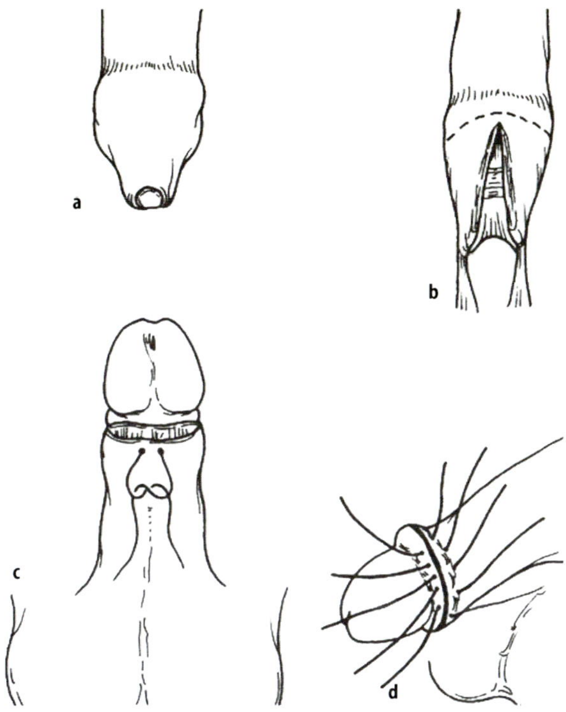

Fig. II.4.9. Circumcision with dorsal slit. **a** Pre-operative phimosis. **b** Dorsal slit. **c** Frenular suture. **d** Sutures in place

II.4.2.8 Insertion of Penile Prosthesis

II.4.2.8.1 Who Gets Penile Prostheses?

Penile prostheses are inserted in those patients who have erectile dysfunction and have failed to respond to all other medical treatments, are willing to undergo surgery and will use the prosthesis. Those patients with organic causes of impotence are more often considered and it is especially useful in Peyronie's disease with associated impotence, as moulding and the prosthesis itself will straighten the angulated penis as well as improve rigidity.

The main types are malleable semi-rigid rods. These are simple to put in and less expensive but stick out all the time and so are not suitable for single men, those who attend swimming pools or gyms, teachers or those dealing or living with children. The inflatable prostheses are more expensive, more difficult to insert and need manual dexterity for either the patient or partner to work it but they are much more satisfactory as they deflate. The satisfaction rate is 90% and the main complications are sepsis (particularly in men with diabetes), mechanical breakdown, glans droop and auto-inflation; these occur on average in 5% of patients. Also sepsis is more common in re-operations. These problems need to be discussed with the patient and partner preoperatively, whose expectations must not be too high as the penis will never be as good as when the patient was in his youth; however, they should manage to have penetrative intercourse with ejaculation as long as ejaculation was present preoperatively.

II.4.2.8.2 Preoperative Preparation

Urinary flow rate measurement is advised especially in the neuropathic patient, after pelvic surgery and in the older patient. Lower bowel clearance is needed in difficult cases or if the lithotomy position is used. Antibiotics are essential, and they should cover Gram-positive cocci and Gram-negative bacilli and start preoperatively (e.g. rectal metronidazole, intravenous cephalosporin or gentamicin and ampicillin). The first dose is given at induction and continued for 48 h and then oral ciprofloxacin for a further 5 days. Pubic shaving is recommended in theatre with an exaggerated skin preparation. A catheter is not usually needed and is only another added source of infection. The urethra is easy to identify at operation. A solution of dilute gentamicin and ampicillin is instilled prior to insertion of the components after dilatation of the corpora and dissection of the scrotum and extravesicular space as well as after closure.

II.4.2.8.3 Surgical Approaches

The choice of surgical approach depends on the prosthesis.

A subcoronal incision can be used for semi-rigid prostheses, if a circumcision is needed it should be carried out initially; if not, the posterior part of the prepuce is incised. This can be achieved with either two longitudinal incisions either side of the urethra onto the tunica albuginea or an inverted "V" incision at the apex of the frenulum and extending laterally close to the corona for 2–3 cm. The tissues are then dissected off the tunica albuginea. A vertical incision about 3 cm is made longitudinally into the tunica (easiest between stay sutures) about 2 cm from the corona either side of the urethra, which is avoided. The corpora are then dilated with Hegar dilators (size 7 to 13) straight down to the proximal end; the dilator can be felt tapping the ischium proximally. The corpora, which is distal to the incision, is 2–3 cm and should also be dilated into the glans, but not through the tunica. Remember the tunical covering goes to the mid glans level, so be gentle, as ham-fistedness means disruption of the tunica and a much greater chance of erosion, especially with a semi-rigid prosthesis which is rigid and not anchored (Fig. II.4.10). The size to be implanted is selected by a measuring tool; there are two diameters and the largest diameter will fit if the 13 dilator has been used. It is important not to implant a prosthesis that is too long, and

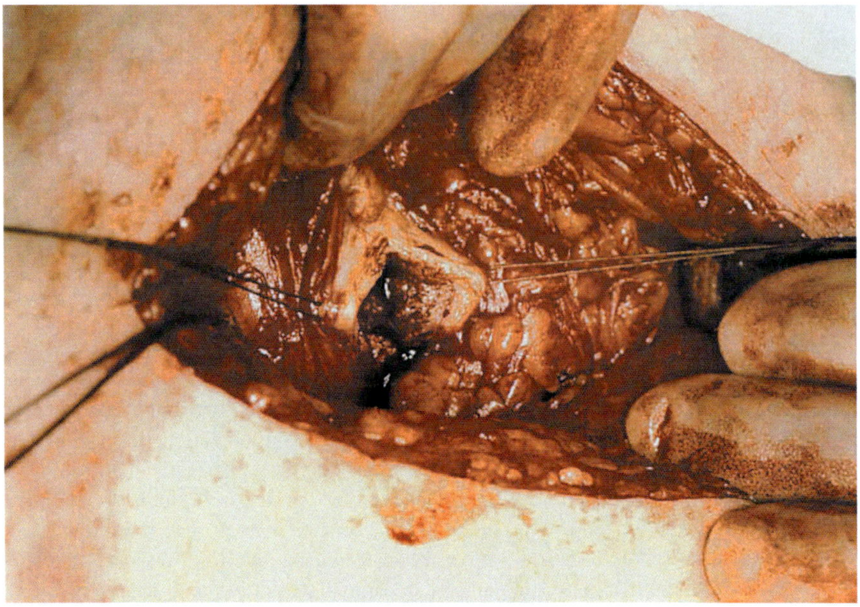

Fig. II.4.10. The tunica opened and the erectile tissue inside

rear tip extenders (RTE) can be used to shorten or lengthen the prosthesis as needed. If the corpora are not the same length then cross dilation has occurred, which can be assessed by inserting Hegar dilators on each side at the same time. Care should be taken to ensure that the tip of the prosthesis supports the glans to avoid the complication of glans droop. Insert the antibiotic solution here. Close the corpora using 4/0 or 3/0 absorbable sutures and then close the skin. Avoid a dressing on completion, and compression is not advisable as it can compromise the glandular blood supply.

II.4.2.8.4 Penoscrotal Approach

This approach is used for inflatable cylinders, two-part inflatable cylinders, for difficult fibrotic corpora and for re-operations (with the patient in the lithotomy position).

The incision is made in the junction of the scrotum and penis on the dorsal surface; a transverse incision allows for better access to proximal corpora. Avoid the urethra if difficult to see or feel and insert a catheter for the duration of the operation. The corpora are incised in the middle on either side of the urethra for 2–3 cm, and the incision must be long enough to accept the prosthesis both distally and proximally. The distal end of the inflatable cylinder can be inserted using a Furlow tool (already threaded with the suture in the tip of the prosthesis), passed carefully on a needle inside the corpora and pulled out of the glans tip (Fig. II.4.11). The corpora are closed with 3/0 or 4/0 absorbable sutures. These closing sutures can either be placed before insertion of the cylinder, left long and then tied once the cylinders are in position, or a special needle guard tool can be used to protect the cylinder whilst suturing. An unrecognized hole in the cylinders is an expensive disaster. Even though the cylinders are inflated while the patient is on the table (Fig. II.4.12), the hole may not be recognized for a further 6 weeks when the cylinders are regularly inflated. The pump is placed in the scrotum and the reservoir under the abdominal muscles. This can be done by a separate incision in the groin, or by a blind technique using an incision at the external ring and a finger to create a space behind the pubic bone extraperitoneally to hold the reservoir, which is then filled with 60 ml saline. This latter technique is less safe than the former.

II.4.2.8.5 Infrapubic Approach

This single incision is easier for multipart inflatables. Also the scar is placed within the pubic hair and is less noticeable. The incision is made 10 cm transversely across the pubic symphysis giving easy access to the corpora, as they appear below the pubic bone. The neurovascular bundle should be noted and avoided. The corporal incision is made longitudinally on either side of the neurovascular bundle and long enough to take a size 14 Hegar dilator. Dilatation of the corpora from size 7 to 14 Hegar is performed both distally into the glans, but not perforating the tunica, and proximally. The distinctive feeling of tapping on the bone is felt proximally and care should be taken to avoid disrupting the proximal tunica. It is important to dilate to Hegar size 14 to fit in the cylinders and the cylinder tubing into the proximal corpora. The length of corpora is de-

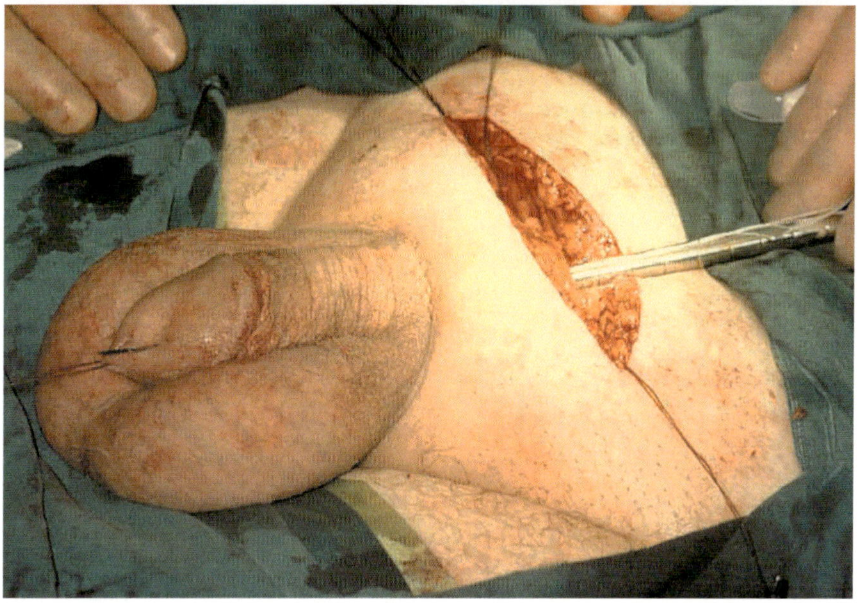

Fig. II.4.11. The Furlow tool passing up the corpus with the cylinder threaded on the needle issuing from the glans

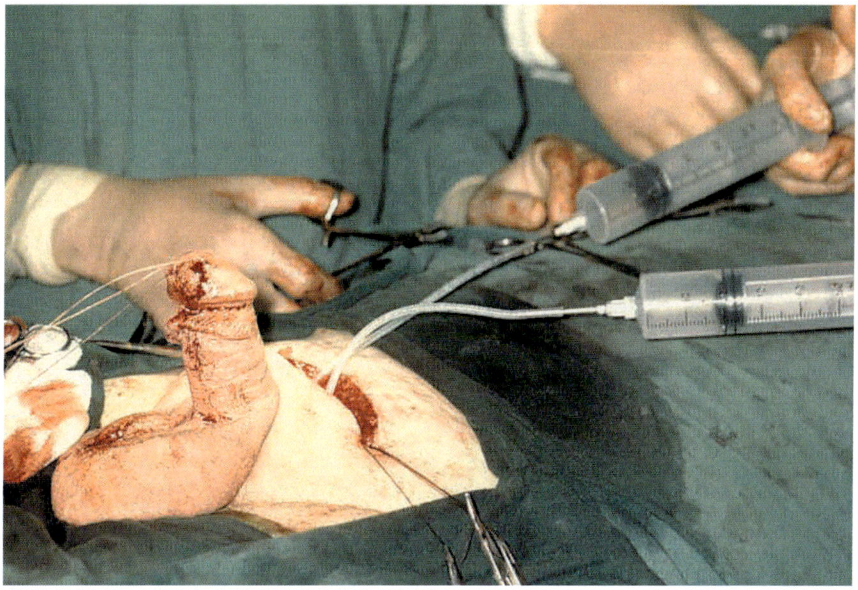

Fig. II.4.12. The cylinders inserted in both corpora and being filled with fluid

termined using a Furlow tool to measure distally and proximally. The selected cylinder size can be lengthened by RTEs; the cylinder should fit closely but not be too long. The suture at the end of the cylinder is threaded on a straight needle and passed with the needle protected in the Furlow tool to the distal corpora and brought through the glans tip on each side. The proximal part of the cylinder with the tubing and RTE is pushed down onto the ischium on each side. Inflating and deflating the cylinders at this stage straightens the cylinders inside the corpora, which are then closed with 3/0 or 4/0 absorbable sutures. There is a special closing tool to prevent puncturing the cylinders. Using the same incision the rectus muscle is separated in the midline and a space made extraperitoneally, by the bladder, to insert the 60-ml or 100-ml reservoir, depending on the cylinder size. The reservoir is filled with saline and the contrast medium is no longer needed. The pump is then placed in the most dependent part of the scrotum in a dartos pouch. All areas are irrigated with antibiotic solution. The two tubes from the pump to the cylinders are joined with connectors, as is the reinforced tubing from the pump to the reservoir. Special connecters are available with a "quick-connect" closing tool, which are easy to use and almost impossible to pull apart. The whole prosthesis is then checked for function and satisfactory fit, left deflated and the wound closed in layers.

A few problems that can occur at operation are now described. Cross dilation can be corrected by re-dilating the corpora, leaving a dilator first in one side and then the other. Tunical disruption, which is important particularly with semi-rigid prostheses, needs either direct closure or closing using a Dacron sleeve in the proximal end. Disruption of the urethra, which usually occurs at the meatus when the dilation has been difficult or the operator is heavy handed. It is advisable to abandon the procedure and re-operate a few weeks later when the breach has healed. Poor fit, which is caused by difficult or inadequate dilation. Most corpora are of similar size, and a difference in size of less than 1 cm will not be noticed by the patient; anything more than this will be unsightly. Cylinders that do not enter the glans may occur because of individual anatomical differences, but will lead to a floppy glans or "droop". These problems may be corrected by additional dilation. When there is difficulty closing the corpora, or a slim or fibrotic penis, it is advisable to avoid using synthetic material to close, as it is an added source of infection.

II.4.2.8.6 Re-exploration of Prosthesis

This is usually for mechanical breakdown or sepsis (Fig. II.4.13). If one of the components is not working it may be possible to replace that one component. The surgery is not necessarily difficult but care must be taken not to damage surrounding structures and, in order not to damage the prosthetic component that is still working, use a cutting diathermy to cut down onto the prosthesis as it will not damage the silicone. If the prosthesis has been in for more than 3 years it is better to replace all components and these are now provided free by the manufacturers. The difficult part of this is replacing the cylinders, and the corpora will need resizing as they will have become more capacious to accommodate the previous implant.

If overt pus is present it is advised to remove all components and wait 6 months before replacement. The repeat operation may well be extremely difficult due to fibrosis and shortening of the corpora. If there is erosion or sepsis without culture, then the technique is to remove the components, and wash the sites with hydrogen peroxide, dilute betadine and antibiotics thoroughly for 5 min before implanting a new prosthesis. This will have an 80% salvage rate and the corporeal size is maintained (Mulcahy 1991).

Penile prostheses give very acceptable and satisfactory results in patients with impotence, and while the surgery should not be embarked upon lightly, many marriages and partnerships are saved, especially in younger patients.

Suggested Reading

Campbell M, Retik AB, Vaughan ED, Wein AJ, Walsh PC (eds) (1998) Campbell's urology, 7th edn. Saunders, Philadelphia

References

Evans C (1998) The use of penile prostheses in the treatment of impotence. Br J Urol 81:591–598
Lord PH (1964) A bloodless operation for the radical cure of idiopathic hydrocele. Br J Surg 51:914–916
Mulcahy JJ (1991) The management of complications of penile implants. Prob Urol 5:608–627

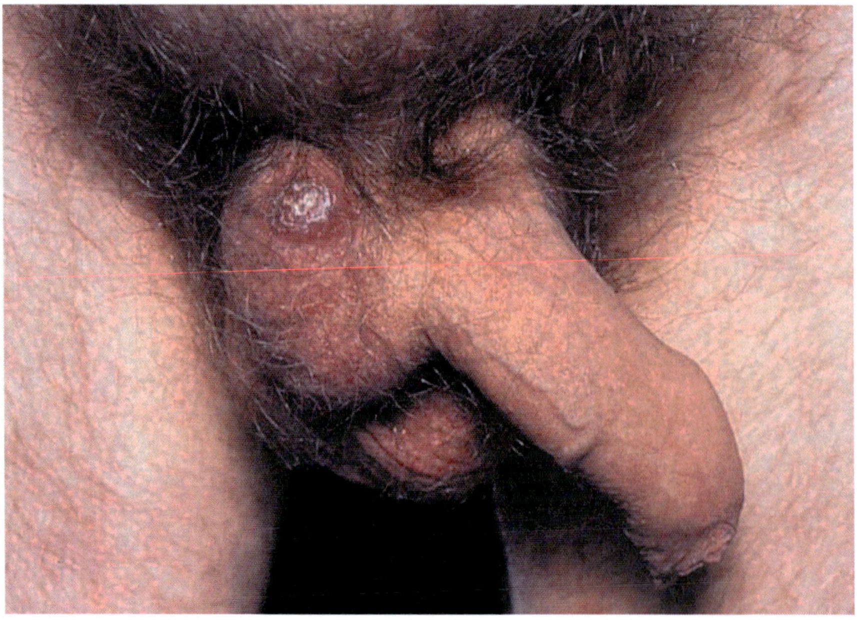

Fig. II.4.13. Erosion of the pump in the scrotum secondary to low grade infection, the pump was replaced and resited on other side

II.4.3 Vasectomy Technique

T.B. Hargreave

There are numerous ways to perform the operation of vasectomy but few have been subject to proper assessment by rigorous audit or clinical trial.

The ideal vasectomy would be easy to do, have no complications and be 100% reversible. No technique fulfils all these objectives.

Prior to operation the man should be given appropriate information and it helps if he is given written information as well (Appendix 1). Consent for the operation should be given by the man and it helps if this is documented. It is also appropriate to notify his partner as she must understand the need to continue contraceptive precautions until post vasectomy semen analysis shows no sperm and the man can be given the "all clear". The form in Appendix 2 documents both consent by the man and partner notification.

It is important to ensure and test for adequate anaesthesia. If the vas can be felt and manipulated to near the surface of the skin then local anaesthetic is usually the safest and cheapest option. If, however, the cord is thickened, for example after previous orchiopexy, or the scrotum is very tight then general anaesthesia may be needed depending on the skill of the surgeon. This author has seen two men with severe disabling chronic pain syndromes following vasectomy and in both cases the men gave a history of the surgeon continuing to proceed with the operation despite the man complaining of severe pain.

The techniques described below each have merits. There is no longer a role for the old fashioned "wrecking technique", which involved removal of a long length of vas and doubling back the ends, because simpler techniques are equally or more effective, less invasive and have lower complication rates. The vas can be occluded with vicryl ties, metal clips or cautery but silk ties should not be used as they can be a cause of a chronic discharging scrotal sinus.

There are two main parts of the vasectomy operation.

Step one is location and dissection of the vas from its fascial sheath. The best technique depends on the experience and case load of the surgeon.

1. Needle fixation technique of location and dissection (Fig. II.4.14). This technique is good for the occasional vasectomist because once the vas has been fixed by the needle it is difficult for the vas to get "lost" by dropping back into the wound. The main disadvantage is that because a scalpel is used to make the incision it cannot be called a no scalpel technique and thus has a less appealing name, although in reality the size of the scalpel incision is nearly the same as the puncture wound made by the "no scalpel forceps". Once the vas has been fixed by the needle a second injection of local anaesthetic is given, using a longer needle, into the sheath and tissue adjacent to the vas approximately 2 cm above the point where the vas will be occluded near the scrotal neck. This has the effect of creating a mini-field block but does not compromise the operation because any swelling caused by the

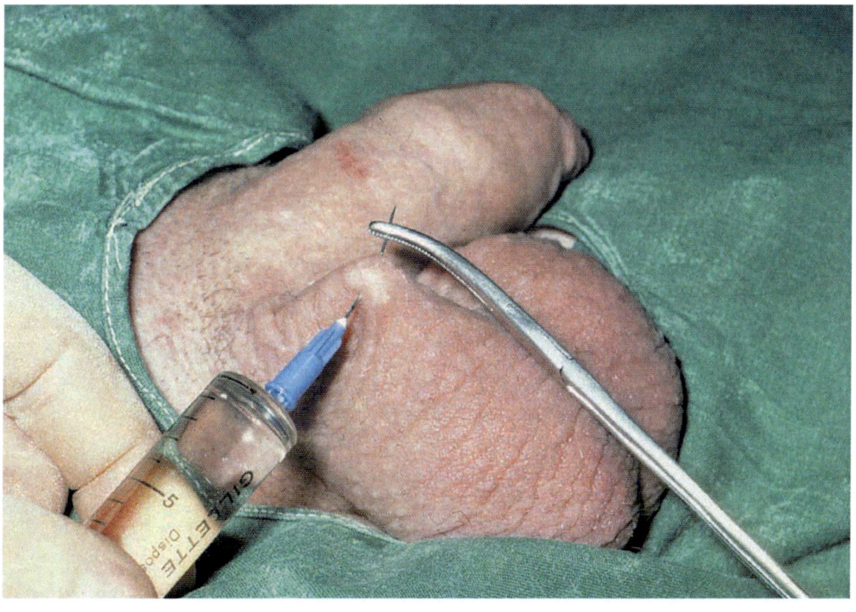

Fig. II.4.14. Needle fixation technique. The vas is manipulated close to the skin and then local anaesthetic is injected into the skin and around the vas as the needle is passed under the vas and out through the skin. An artery forceps is then clamped to the needle thus fixing the vas under the skin. Using a second needle further local anaesthetic is then given around the vas and in the direction of the vas proximally towards the scrotal neck

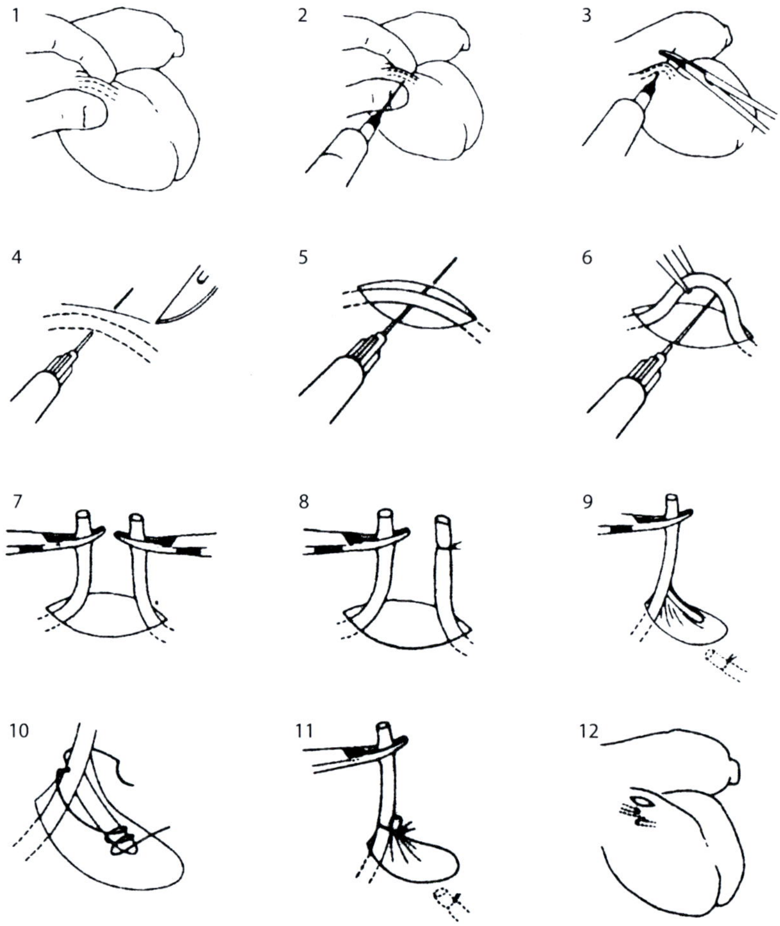

Fig. II.4.15. Step by step diagram of the needle fixation technique and separation of the vas ends by a tissue plane

local anaesthetic injection is a centimetre or two proximal to the site of the vasectomy. Once the vas has been cleanly separated from it sheath and surrounding tissues vas occlusion can be undertaken in a number of different ways (see below). In Fig. II.4.15 the needle fixation and dissection technique is shown including vas occlusion with the tissue plane technique (see below).

2. The no scalpel technique of fixation and dissection was invented by Professor Li in Sichuan and is probably the most widely used technique in the world. There is general agreement that this approach has fewer side-effects and lower complications than an incisional approach (Aradhya et al. 2005). The technique requires special instruments (Fig. II.4.16) and depends on picking up the vas accurately and the surgeon holding it between the fingers. This can be difficult if the man has thick scrotal skin. The exact technique can be learnt from a short film "No scalpel vasectomy" made by WHO but is illustrated in the figure (Fig. II.4.17). It is a technique that is best used by vasectomy surgeons who undertake regular vasectomy operating sessions because the vas can be more easily lost after injection of the local anaesthetic and before it is fixed with the ring clamp and it takes practice to acquire the trick of fixing the vas with the surgeon's fingers. Once the vas has been divided then step two is to use an effective method of occlusion.

Techniques that are widely used include the tissue plane technique, cautery and the use of ligaclips.

1. The tissue plane technique. The vas is covered by a fascial sheath and this sheath is used to separate the cut vas ends. The most usual technique is to identify and clamp and tie both ends as shown in Fig. II.4.15 step 7 and step 8 and then to allow one end of the vas to return to the inside of the sheath (Fig. II.4.15 step 9) and to close the hole in the sheath in such a way as to keep the other end of the vas outside the sheath (Fig. II.4.15 step 10 and step 11). The tissue plane technique has been shown to reduce failure by about half when compared to a technique of simple ligation and excision of a length of vas (Sokal et al. 2004a) and the latter should no longer be used. However, the tissue plane technique may not be appropriate in all cir-

cumstances because it is important to fix the fascial sheath in such a way as to prevent the outside sheath vas end pulling back through the buttonhole in the fascia. If the fixing stitch used to do this is pulled too tightly (Fig. II.4.15 step 11) then it can cheese wire through the vas with the result that both vas ends are in close proximity again and the vasectomy may fail. The tissue plane technique requires a degree of surgical precision and delicate technique and may not be suitable in all clinic settings.

2. Use of ligaclips. The advantage of ligaclips is that the vas is occluded but does not necrose. The disadvantages are that some men can feel a lump and the cost of the clips. There has been no formal clinical trial to compare ligaclips with either fascial inter-

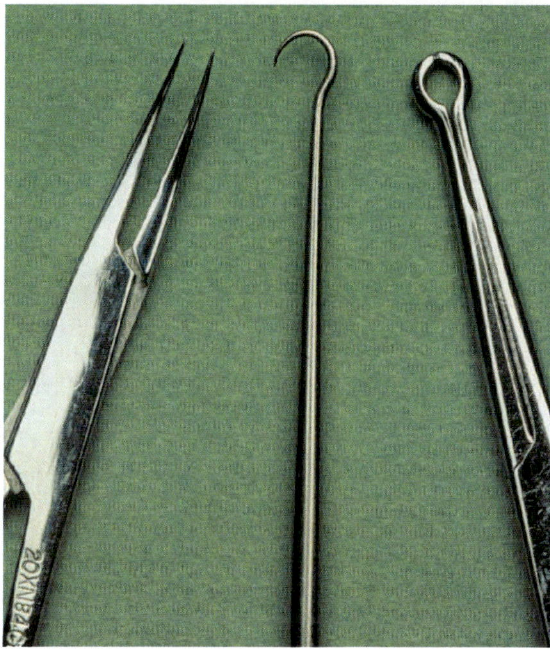

Fig. II.4.16. No scalpel vasectomy instruments. Sharp artery forceps for making the puncture and ring forceps for grasping the vas. If an ordinary artery forceps is used to grasp the vas it is rather easy to crush right through the vas and then for each end to drop back into the wound; if this happens it can be very difficult to find the lost end

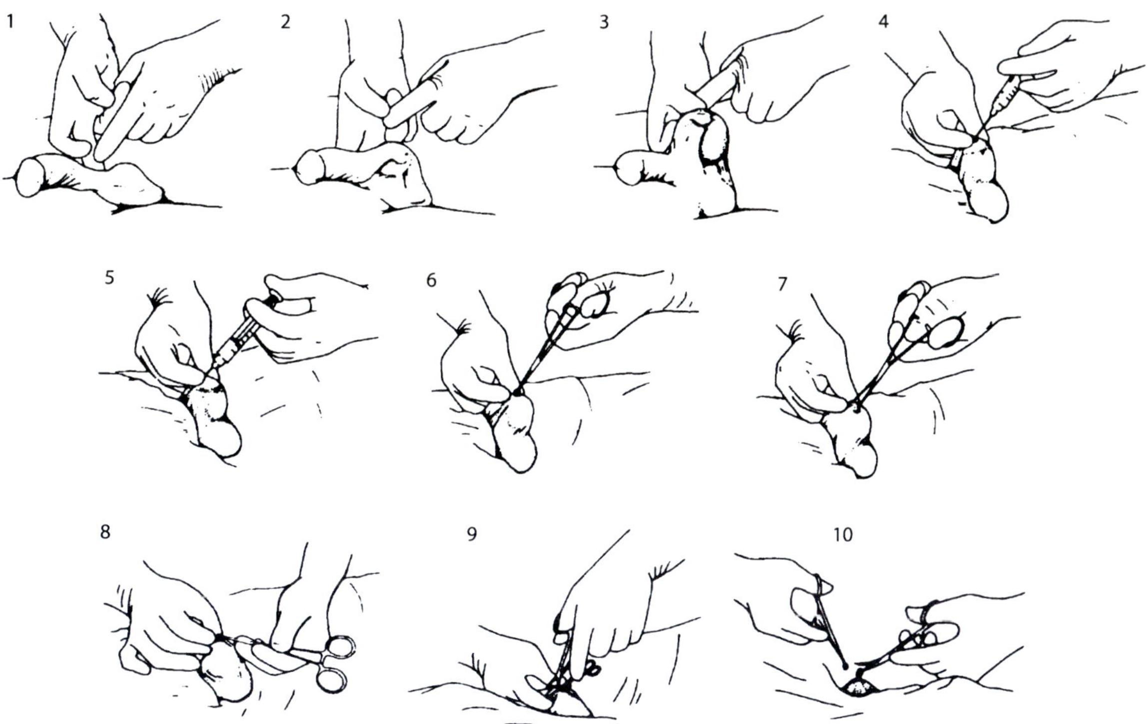

Fig. II.4.17. No scalpel technique step by step. *1–3* The vas is hooked towards the surface of the skin by the operator's middle finger and positioned just under the surface of the skin. *4* About 0.25 ml of local anaesthetic is injected into the skin at the site of the future puncture. *5* The vas is held taut and the anaesthetic needle is then advanced along the line of the vas and approximately 2 ml of local anaesthetic is injected. This anaesthetic is proximal and well away from the site of the vasectomy puncture, does not interfere with the operation site and causes a mini-field block of the vas distal to the site of the injection. *6, 7* The vas is grasped with the ring forceps (see Fig. II.4.16). It is best to push on the vas with the forceps closed and then to open the forceps while pushing on the vas and then to close them around the vas. This minimizes the amount of redundant skin that may be picked up with the vas. *8* The ring is flipped downwards to cause a loop of vas to stand out. *9* The puncture forceps (see Fig. II.4.16) is opened and using one of the blades a puncture is made through the skin and into the vas. The puncture wound is then enlarged by inserting the closed puncture forceps and gently opening them several times. *10* Using one blade of the puncture forceps the vas is skewered and with a rotating movement brought to the outside. The rest of the vasectomy may then proceed as in Fig. II.4.15

position or cautery probably because such trials tend to be conducted in developing countries where men are willing to join studies in exchange for cost-free surgery and because it is too costly to supply the clips in resource-poor settings. However, despite the lack of clinical evidence the technique of using clips is widely used and this indicates efficacy. Formal clinical trail data are needed.

3. Cautery of the vas end. The technique is to insert the cautery probe into the vas lumen to a depth of 0.5 mm (and no more) and to cauterize each end. Clips or sutures should not be used as well as cautery as their use causes the vas ends to necrose and may render the occlusion ineffective. In an analysis of data from two different studies (Sokal et al. 2004b), one a large multicentre case series of cautery and the other a randomized study of fascial interposition (WHO film, "No scalpel vasectomy"), it was concluded that cautery was superior to fascial interposition in terms of efficacy. The studies analysed in this comparison were undertaken by Family Health International (FHI) in a variety of clinics in different countries, some of them developing countries. This context is important because the overall failure rates were higher than those normally reported in case series studies in developed countries, probably because the FHI studies included a wide variety of resource settings and surgeons with different levels of experience. As stated above the fascial interposition technique is very technique dependent, difficult to standardize and because of all these factors the results of the FHI studies must be interpreted with caution.
4. Combination of cautery and fascial interposition. This technique was first described by Schmidt (1987) where 0.5 mm of vas was cauterized and fascial interposition undertaken, and the present evidence suggests that this combination of cautery and fascial interposition may be the most efficacious technique (Labrecque et al. 2004).

Appendix 1

Information sheet that can be given to men to remind them of points discussed during vasectomy counselling

Information About Vasectomy

Vasectomy is the surest method of family planning available apart from complete abstinence! However, no doctor can guarantee vasectomy as a method of contraception. The failure rate is approximately 1 in 1000; for comparison, the failure rate after female Fallopian tube tying is approximately 1 in 100. There are two times when failure may occur.

Early failure occurs within the first 3 months of operation and is usually because of technical difficulties with the operation or the very rare condition of an extra vas deferens on one or other side. Sperm count performed approximately 3 months after operation detects this type of failure.

Late failure is a more difficult problem. The cut ends of the vas occasionally heal up again and sometimes years after the original operation. The exact frequency with which this occurs is difficult to know but is probably about 1 in 2000. Unfortunately there is no way to guarantee against this happening. It is worth noting that vasectomy is the surest method of sterilization now and that the failure rate after female sterilization is much higher. The only sure method of avoiding pregnancy is complete abstinence!

Vasectomy should be regarded as an irreversible procedure. You should regard vasectomy as a permament procedure because although it is often possible to try vasectomy reversal there is no guarantee that it can be obtained in any individual case. This point is particularly important to consider when children are very young. What would happen if disaster struck and a child of yours dies? When children are very young can you be sure that there will be no change of mind about wanting more of a family in a year or two.

After vasectomy you remain fertile until you have ejaculated about 30 times (usually 3–4 months). This is because there are storage areas for sperm (the seminal vesicles) inside the body. It takes about 20–30 ejaculations before all the sperm are cleared away and therefore you and your partner should use your usual methods of contraception until sperm samples have been tested and the "all clear" given. Normal practice is to have two semen samples tested 3–4 months after the operation. At this time 7 out of 10 men will be found to be "all clear", but for the remaining 3 out of 10 men it takes longer. By 6 months the "all clear" can be expected in 17 out of every 20 men and by 12 months, 99 out of every 100 men. Once you have been told there are no sperm in the ejaculate then you can reasonably stop using other methods of contraception. As stated above, in approximately 3 out of 10 men the 4-months samples come back showing some sperm. If in fact the sample shows very small numbers of non-moving sperm then the risk of pregnancy is very low and is 5 pregnancies in every 10,000 couples. This low risk is not significantly different from the risk if the sample is completely free of sperm. Therefore, in the situation where the 4-months sample shows very small numbers of non-moving sperm, many men and their partners will choose to stop other methods of contraception. However, the traditional advice has always been to wait until two samples are completely clear.

Serious Complications are Very Rare

Two particular immediate complications of vasectomy are bleeding and wound infection. If either of these occurs then the period off work will be longer than normal. The reason these complications sometimes occur is because the scrotum (bag for the testicles) is made of soft stretchy skin and is situated in an area of the body where contamination from the bowel can occur. The chance of these complications is reduced if plans are made to spend the first day after operation lying down for as much time as possible with the scrotum as the highest point of the body, i.e. lying flat. Also hard manual work, heavy lifting or straining should be avoided for 2 weeks after the operation. It is best not to have sex for about 2 weeks after the operation.

Later Complications

A bothersome later complication that occurs in about 1 in 100 men is discomfort in the epididymis. This is the soft tissue next to the testicle and it is in this area that the sperm dissolve away. Continuing minor discomfort can occur if there is leakage of sperm from this area causing a localized inflammation. If this occurs it usually settles down after a few months but very occasionally it may be more troublesome so that further treatment for the pain is needed and very, very rarely (1 in 20,000) this can be completely incapacitating, causing an inability to work and the need for continuing treatments and operations.

Other late complications that have been reported in the medical literature include an increased risk of testicular and prostate cancer, increased risk of kidney stone formation and an increased risk of heart disease. These reports have been taken very seriously by a number of organizations including some of the large medical insurance companies in the USA and the World Health Organization. It is true to say that so far in large studies there is no evidence of any increased risk of testicular cancer, heart disease or kidney stone formation and it is unlikely that vasectomy causes an increase in the risk of prostate cancer. It is worth noting that in one of the larger USA studies the men who have had a vasectomy are living a little longer than a comparison group of men who have not had a vasectomy!

Also, it is worth noting that risks of *complications after female sterilization* are greater than the risks of vasectomy and that the risks of having another baby are greater than the risks from either male or female sterilization.

May I Store Sperm Before Vasectomy?

It is certainly possible to store sperm in liquid nitrogen and for sperm samples to be kept for many years. This facility is available for young men with cancer who are about to undergo treatment, which may cause sterility. Sperm storage is subject to the 1990 Human Fertilisation and Embryology Act of Parliament and can only be undertaken in a licensed centre. If you wish to arrange storage you may contact one of the HFEA licensed sperm storage facilities.

A Final Word About Risks

In recent years there have been several court cases about vasectomy and it is now generally accepted that people need to know about rare risks when making a decision about non essential "quality of life" surgery. I have therefore given you information about lots of possible risks of vasectomy but it is important to keep these risks in perspective and to bear in mind the risks of alternative solutions. Female sterilization by tying the Fallopian tubes has a higher failure rate than vasectomy and more complications because it is necessary to enter the abdominal cavity and to use a general anaesthetic. Taking all these factors into account compared with other solutions vasectomy is more sure and less risky.

Appendix 2

Document suitable for recording the man's consent to vasectomy and notification of his partner about the need to continue contraception until the "all clear" has been given

Consent Form For Vasectomy

Name and Address

I have read the information sheet about vasectomy and wish to proceed with the operation of vasectomy.

Signed

Date

The consent signed above is sufficient to allow the operation to proceed but please also ask your wife/ partner to read the information about vasectomy. It is helpful but not essential if she signs the statement below to indicate that she has had the opportunity to read the information.

Partner Notification

Please note the information about the need to continue contraception after the operation of vasectomy and until the "all clear" has been given. Please note that once the operation of vasectomy has been done it should be regarded as permament.

I am aware that my husband/partner plans to have the operation of vasectomy for contraceptive purposes and I have noted the need to continue contraceptive precautions after the operation of vasectomy and until the "all clear" has been given.

Signed by spouse/partner

Date

Vasectomy Surgeon's Statement

I have explained to this patient that vasectomy should be regarded as a permanent method of contraception and that there is no guarantee that vasectomy can be reversed. I have also explained that there is a failure rate and that very rarely (1 in 2000) sperm may appear in the ejaculate years later and very occasionally this may result in pregnancy. I have explained that vasectomy is the surest method of either male or female contraception. I have also discussed early complications of bleeding and infection and later complications of testicular discomfort and the very rare late complication of severe incapacitating testicular pain.

Vasectomy Surgeon

Date

References

Aradhya KW, Best K, Sokal DC (2005) Recent developments in vasectomy. Br Med J 330:296–2999

Labrecque M, Dufresne C, Barone MA, St-Hilaire K (2004) Vasectomy surgical techniques: a systematic review. BMC Med 2:21

Schmidt SS (1987) Vasectomy. Urol Clin North Am 14:149–154

Sokal DC, Irsula B, Hays M, Chen-Mok M, Barone M (2004a) Vasectomy by ligation and excision, with or without fascial interposition: a randomized controlled trial. BMC Med 2:6

Sokal D, Irsula B, Chen-Mok M, Labrecque M, Barone MA (2004b) A comparison of vas occlusion techniques: cautery more effective than ligation and excision with fascial interposition. BMC Urol 4:12

II.4.4 Vasovasostomy and Vasoepididymostomy

A.M. Belker

Summary

Vasovasostomy almost always is performed for the reversal of an elective vasectomy. Vasoepididymostomy, which involves anastomosis of the vas deferens to the epididymal tubule, is required to bypass an obstruction in the epididymis that may result from congenital conditions, infection or from obstruction within the epididymis after a vasectomy. Patients who consider these procedures should be counselled about the possibility of undergoing surgical or percutaneous needle aspiration to obtain spermatozoa for in vitro fertilization (IVF) with intracytoplasmic sperm injection (ICSI) as an alternative to surgical reconstruction.

During a vasectomy reversal, the surgeon's decision to perform vasovasostomy or vasoepididymostomy is influenced by the sperm quality in the intraoperative vas fluid and the gross appearance of that fluid. If spermatozoa are absent from the vas fluid, the cause could be a back-pressure-induced rupture of the epididymal tubule with subsequent obstruction to the passage of spermatozoa. In such cases, vasoepididymostomy is required. The results of both vasovasostomy and vasoepididymostomy are significantly better when these procedures are performed with microsurgery than when microsurgery is not used. Comparable results of vasovasostomy are obtained with microsurgical modified one-layer and two-layer anastomoses, although the author prefers the two-layer method for reasons explained in the text.

When vasoepididymostomy is required, it may be difficult to determine the location within the epididymis at which the obstruction is present. If the point of obstruction is unclear, the surgeon should sample the epididymal tubular fluid at the lowest accessible level in the epididymis and subsequently at progressively higher epididymal levels until a level is reached at which spermatozoa are present in the tubule. The anastomosis is performed at the lowest level at which spermatozoa are found to be present in the epididymal tubular fluid. The microsurgical method of vasoepididymostomy creates a direct connection of the mucosa of the vas deferens to the edges of the epididymal tubule. A modified microsurgical method of vasoepididymostomy creates an end-to-side intussusception of the epididymal tubule into the lumen of the vas. The latter method is simpler to perform and seems to obtain results that are comparable to those of the more tedious alternative, microsurgical end-to-side anastomotic method.

The results of vasovasostomy become progressively poorer as the time from the vasectomy until its reversal lengthens. Spermatozoa should appear in the semen within 2 months after vasovasostomy, but may not appear until as long as 12–18 months after vasoepididymostomy. The average postoperative interval until a pregnancy occurs after vasovasostomy is 12 months. There are few reports of the average interval until a pregnancy occurs after vasoepididymostomy.

II.4.4.1
Indications

Either vasovasostomy or vasoepididymostomy, which sometimes is referred to as epididymovasostomy, may be required for vasectomy reversal (see Chap. I.5.2) or for the treatment of congenital or acquired obstructions of the vas deferens or the epididymis that result in azoospermia (see Part I). The latter conditions usually are discovered during the evaluation of a couple's infertility. Either procedure also may be required for the relief of postvasectomy pain, which fortunately occurs infrequently after vasectomy. Both procedures may be performed with local, regional or general anaesthesia and commonly are performed on an outpatient basis.

II.4.4.2
Contraindications

The contraindications to these procedures are the same as the contraindications mentioned in Chap. I.5.2.

II.4.4.3
Alternative Procedures

When advising patients about the chances of a pregnancy occurring after vasovasostomy and vasoepididymostomy, surgeons should be familiar with the pregnancy rates and comparative expenses associated with retrieval of spermatozoa for in vitro fertilization (IVF) with intracytoplasmic sperm injection (ICSI) (Kolettis and Thomas 1997) and should discuss these alternatives with patients. A consideration of which procedures may be paid by the couple's health insurance coverage will influence the couple's choice in countries in which such a consideration applies.

In some centres, intraoperative retrieval of sperm from the vas, epididymis or testis is performed to cryopreserve sperm for possible later use for IVF/ICSI in case the vasovasostomy or vasoepididymostomy fails. In my centre, the additional expense for intraoperative sperm cryopreservation is over US$1000 due to the requirement of the cryobank for the man to be tested for HIV, hepatitis B and C and syphilis before sperm may be cryopreserved, in addition to the costs for freeze/thaw testing and the first year of sperm storage. The performance of percutaneous testicular sperm aspiration in the office to obtain sperm for IVF/ICSI in case the surgical anastomosis fails costs much less than the amount needed for intraoperative sperm cryopreservation in my centre. Such a discrepancy in costs does not exist in all centres. **If the surgeon elects to perform intraoperative sperm harvesting for cryopreservation, it is necessary for the surgeon to alert the cryobank laboratory personnel that the sperm should be frozen in aliquots suitable for IVF/ICSI, because the relatively small numbers of sperm harvested would not be useful for intrauterine insemination or for IVF without ICSI.**

II.4.4.4
Factors That Influence Choice of Vasovasostomy or Vasoepididymostomy

A surgical incision is made at the level of vasal obstruction. After the upper and lower ends of the vas deferens (subsequently referred to as the vas) have been isolated surgically, the scarred ends are resected. The surgeon must be certain that all of the scar tissue is removed from each end of the vas. This is ascertained by observing that the remaining severed end of the vas bleeds freely. After the scarred ends of the vas have been resected, patency of the abdominal end of the vas is assured by instilling 5 ml of Ringer's solution through a 24-gauge blunt tip needle inserted into the abdominal end. Patency is assured if the fluid flows freely. If the fluid does not flow freely, an operative vasogram is performed to determine if an obstruction also exists at a higher level.

After the scarred testicular end of the vas has been resected, fluid that exudes from this end is inspected with a laboratory microscope to determine if spermatozoa are present in the fluid (Fig. II.4.18). If intact

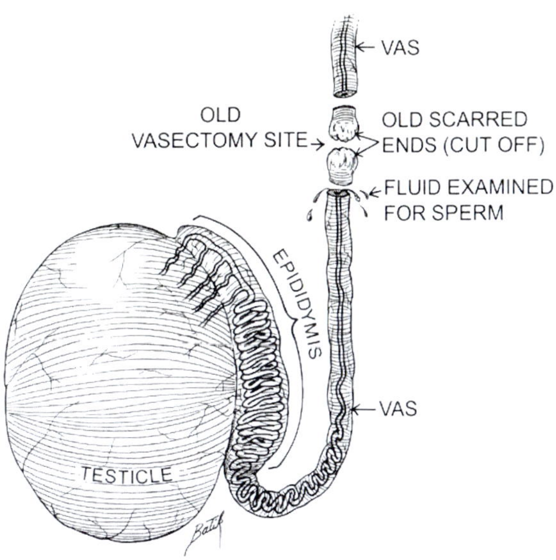

Fig. II.4.18. The scarred ends of the vas are resected. Fluid from the testicular end is examined with a laboratory microscope to determine if spermatozoa are present in the fluid. Patency of the abdominal end of the vas then is assured by instilling Ringer's solution into the abdominal end (not shown in figure). [Reproduced with permission from Belker AM (1985) Vasectomy and its reversal. *Primary Care* 12:703–717]

Table II.4.1. Postoperative patency and pregnancy rates according to intraoperative quality of spermatozoa in vas fluid when that quality was identical bilaterally (Belker et al. 1991)

Intraoperative vas fluid sperm quality	Sperm in semen Number[a]	(%)	Pregnancy Number[a]	(%)
Grade 1 – mainly normal motile sperm	116/123	(94)	62/98	(63)
Grade 2 – mainly normal non-motile sperm	199/220	(91)	89/165	(54)
Grade 3 – mainly sperm heads (no tails)	67/70	(96)	36/72	(50)
Grade 4 – only sperm heads	55/73	(75)	31/70	(44)
Grade 5 – no sperm	50/83	(60)	20/65	(31)

[a] Numerator indicates number of patients achieving postoperative patency or pregnancy and denominator indicates number of patients in each group

spermatozoa are present, vasovasostomy is performed. The results of vasovasostomy vary according to the grade of quality of spermatozoa in the fluid obtained intraoperatively from the testicular end of the vas (Table II.4.1) (Belker et al. 1991). If the fluid contains only sperm heads (without attached tails) or no spermatozoa are present, the surgeon should inspect the epididymis to determine if a clearly defined level of obstruction exists. This determination is made by the observation of dilation of the epididymal tubule above and collapse of the tubule below the point of obstruction. If a clearly defined point of epididymal obstruction is identified, then vasoepididymostomy, rather than vasovasostomy, will be required to reverse a vasectomy (Silber 1979).

When grade 3 sperm (Table II.4.1) quality is present in the intraoperative vas fluid, most surgeons perform vasovasostomy. When spermatozoa are absent from the intraoperative vas fluid, the surgeon may be guided by the gross appearance of the vas fluid (Belker et al. 1991). Generally, when spermatozoa are absent from the intraoperative vas fluid, watery (clear, colourless and transparent) vas fluid indicates that success will occur with vasovasostomy even though spermatozoa may be absent from the intraoperative fluid. However, the presence of thick, creamy fluid generally indicates that vasoepididymostomy is required (Belker et al. 1991). When grade 4 (Table II.4.1) sperm quality is present, some surgeons recommend vasovasostomy, while others recommend vasoepididymostomy. Unfortunately, there still is not universal agreement on the choice between vasovasostomy and vasoepididymostomy when grade 4 or 5 sperm quality is present in the intraoperative vas fluid, with the exception of the observation of an obvious point of epididymal obstruction, which clearly indicates the performance of vasoepididymostomy. The decision about which procedure should be performed is made independently on each side.

When the testicular biopsy of an azoospermic man who has a normal semen volume and no history of previous surgery reveals normal spermatogenesis, the obstruction is almost always in the epididymis. Using a scrotal incision, a microsurgical hemitransection of the vas is made in the lowermost portion of the vas. If spermatozoa are present in the fluid obtained from the opening in the vas, the obstruction is above that level and an operative vasogram is performed. If spermatozoa are absent from the vas fluid, the obstruction is in the epididymis. In this situation, the surgeon completes the transection of the vas, ligates the testicular end of the vas and passes the abdominal end through a surgically created opening in the parietal tunica vaginalis to prepare for the performance of vasoepididymostomy.

II.4.4.5 Surgical Techniques

II.4.4.5.1 Placement of Incisions

In order to perform vasovasostomy, it usually is necessary to create only very short (3–5 cm long) vertical scrotal incisions, and it is not necessary to extrude the testicle and epididymis from the scrotum. In situations in which the previous vasectomy was performed very high in the scrotum or an unusually long length of the vas was resected at the time of the vasectomy, an infrapubic incision (Belker 1988), or preferably modified infrapubic incisions lateral to each side of the base of the penis (Fig. II.4.19) (Belker 1995), may be useful to mobilize a sufficiently long segment of the abdominal end of the vas to perform either vasovasostomy or vasoepididymostomy without tension on the anastomosis. When vasoepididymostomy is required while using modified infrapubic incisions, it is possible to displace the scrotal contents upward through these incisions to perform the anastomosis (Belker 1988).

When obstruction of the vas results from an injury to the vas during bilateral inguinal hernia repair, an inguinal incision obviously is needed. A useful "trick of the trade" in such situations is to perform laparoscopic mobilization of the abdominal end of the vas, with passage of the abdominal end through a surgically created puncture in the external inguinal ring.

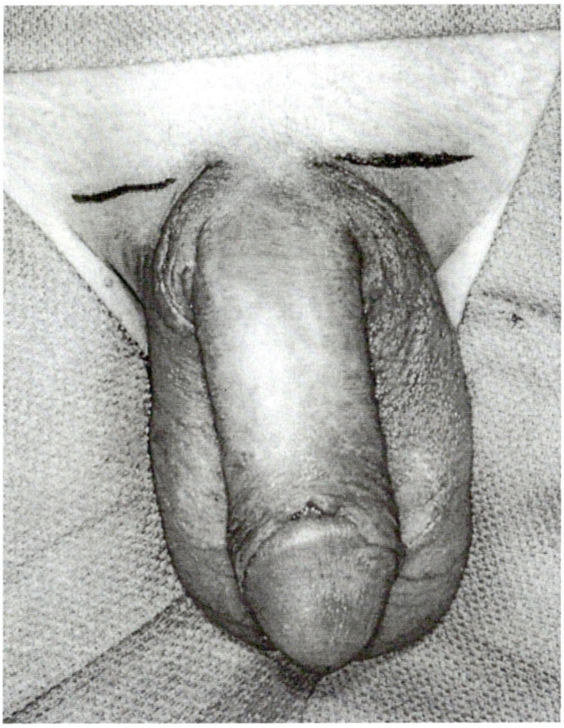

Fig. II.4.19. The locations of modified infrapubic incisions, which are useful for isolating the ends of the vas when the vasectomy was performed at a very high level or when an unusually long segment of the vas was removed during the vasectomy, are indicated by markings on the skin lateral to each side of the base of the penis. [Reproduced with permission from Belker AM (1995) Microsurgical vasovasostomy: two-layer technique. In: Goldstein M (ed) *Surgery of male infertility.* Saunders, Philadelphia, pp 61–66]

II.4.4.5.2 Vasovasostomy

During mobilization of the ends of the vas, it is important to remove completely the scarred ends of the vas, which assures that viable tissue will be present on each side of the anastomosis. It also is important to avoid devascularization of the ends of the vas. This is accomplished by leaving enough tissue surrounding each end to be able to observe that each end bleeds freely. Bipolar, rather than monopolar, cautery is recommended when cauterizing bleeding vessels in the adventitia of the vas. It is important to avoid cautery of the transected surface of each end of the vas in order to prevent the creation of scar tissue in that location. A sufficient length of each end of the vas must be mobilized to prevent tension on the anastomosis.

There now is virtually universal agreement that the results of microsurgical vasovasostomy are superior to the results of vasovasostomy performed without optical magnification. Microsurgical anastomoses are more successful than anastomoses performed without the aid of microsurgery because microsurgery affords

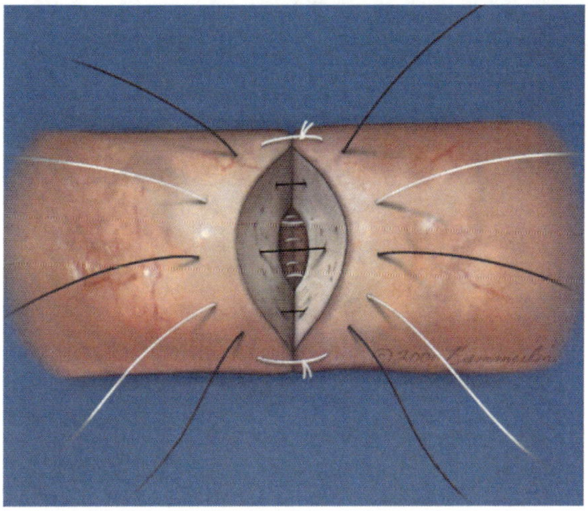

Fig. II.4.20. Schmidt's modified one-layer method of microsurgical vasovasostomy. Full thickness sutures are shown in white and outer muscular layer sutures are shown in black. (Reproduced with permission; ©2001 Bammerlin, Louisville, Kentucky, USA.)

precise approximation of the mucosal edges of the vas, thus creating a leak-proof anastomosis. The adverse effects of an anastomotic leak of spermatozoa with the resulting anastomotic sperm granuloma were shown clearly in a study of the results of various types of anastomoses in laboratory animals (Hagan and Coffey 1977).

The microsurgical anastomosis may be performed with either a modified one-layer or a two-layer technique. The modified one-layer anastomosis (Schmidt 1978) is performed using six to eight interrupted full thickness sutures of 9–0 nylon placed equidistantly around the circumference of each end of the vas, followed by the placement of more superficial outer muscular layer sutures of 9–0 nylon between adjacent full thickness sutures (Fig. II.4.20).

The two-layer end-to-side microsurgical anastomosis (Belker 1997) is performed by placing six to eight interrupted sutures of 10–0 nylon through the mucosa of each end of the vas, followed by the placement of approximately eight interrupted sutures of 9–0 nylon through the outer muscular layer of the vas (Fig. II.4.21). A folding vas approximating clamp is useful to perform this anastomosis (Belker 1980, 1995).

II.4.4.5.3 Vasoepididymostomy

This procedure is performed by creating vertical scrotal incisions that are adequately long to extrude the scrotal contents. The parietal tunica vaginalis is opened and the abdominal end of the vas is passed through a surgical puncture in the parietal tunica vaginalis. Perivasal tissue is attached to the parietal tunica vaginalis

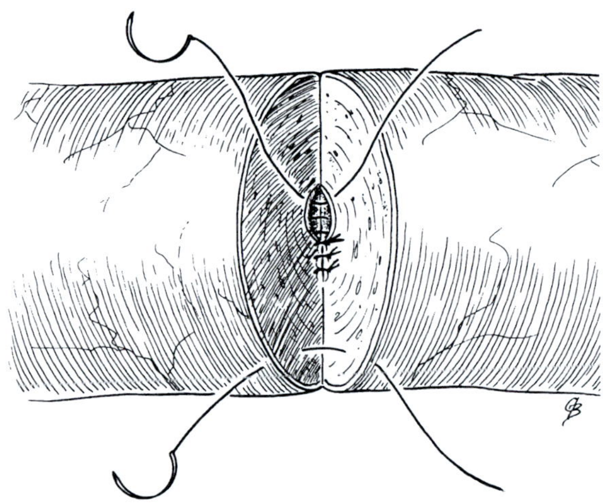

Fig. II.4.21. The two-layer method of microsurgical vasovasostomy. Inner mucosal edges are approximated with interrupted 10–0 nylon sutures and outer muscular edges are approximated with interrupted 9–0 nylon sutures. [Reproduced with permission from Belker AM (1985) Vasectomy and its reversal. *Primary Care* 12:703–717]

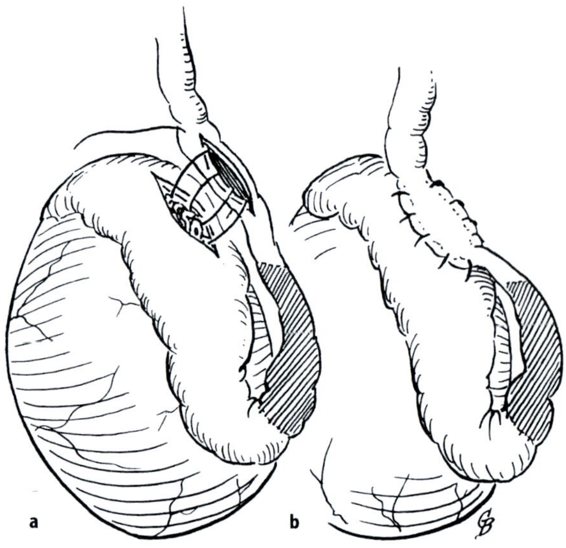

Fig. II.4.22a, b. The older nonmicrosurgical method of vasoepididymostomy relied upon creation of a fistula between several openings in the epididymal tubule and the lumen of the vas. [Reproduced with permission from Belker AM (1981) Vasovasostomy. In Resnick MI (ed) *Current trends in urology*, vol 1. Williams and Wilkins, Baltimore, Md., pp 20–41]

at two to four intervals along the portion of the vas that now is inside the tunica vaginalis. This manoeuvre prevents tension on the anastomosis.

If the level of epididymal obstruction is evident by inspection of the epididymis, the epididymal tubule is isolated just above that level. If a clear point of obstruction is not evident, the epididymal tubule is isolated at its lowest accessible level and fluid obtained from the opening in the tubule is inspected with a laboratory microscope to determine if intact spermatozoa are present. If intact spermatozoa are not present, the surgeon then opens the epididymal tubule at progressively higher levels until spermatozoa are found to be present in the tubular fluid.

Although pregnancies have been reported to result from anastomosis of the vas to the caput epididymidis (Silber 1989) and to the vasa efferentia (Silber 1988; Weiske 1994), the results of vasoepididymostomy are increasingly successful the lower the anastomosis is performed in the epididymis (Schoysman and Bedford 1986; Schoysman 1993; Jarow et al. 1997). While it is important to perform the anastomosis at the lowest possible epididymal level, the level must be at a point in the epididymis at which spermatozoa are present in the epididymal tubular fluid, which assures that the anastomosis will be performed above the obstruction in the epididymis. Although vasovasostomy may have a successful result despite the intraoperative absence of spermatozoa from the vas fluid, vasoepididymostomy never will be successful when performed at an epididymal level at which spermatozoa are absent from the epididymal tubular fluid (Niederberger and Ross 1993).

Before the introduction of a microsurgical method of vasoepididymostomy, the anastomosis was accomplished by connecting the edges of the opened epididymal tunic to the edges of the end of the vas, thus creating a fistula between the underlying openings in the epididymal tubule and the vas (Fig. II.4.22). The method now preferred is a microsurgical end-to-side anastomosis. This type of anastomosis results in approximation of the edges of the epididymal tubule to the mucosa of the vas. The end-to-side anastomosis may be performed either by connecting the edges of the opened epididymal tubule to the mucosa of the vas and then connecting the edges of the epididymal tunic to the outer muscular layer of the vas (Fig. II.4.23) (Thomas 1987) or by the "triangulation intussusception" method (Figs. II.4.24, II.4.25) (Berger 1998; McCallum et al. 2002). Both of these methods accomplish end-to-side anastomosis of a specific portion of the epididymal tubule to the mucosa of the vas. However, the "triangulation intussusception" method is technically simpler and therefore requires less time than the alternative end-to-side method (Thomas 1987).

In order to isolate the epididymal tubule, it is necessary to open the epididymal tunic first. This is achieved either by microsurgically incising the overlying epididymal tunic or by microsurgically resecting an oval of the tunic. After the tunic has been opened, a microsurgical scalpel is used to gently incise repeatedly the tissue that overlies the tubule. When most of the overlying tissue has been incised and the outline of the tubule becomes evident, a microsurgical Vannas scissors, which has blunt tips, may be used to incise the remaining tissue that overlies the epididymal tubule. An aid to isola-

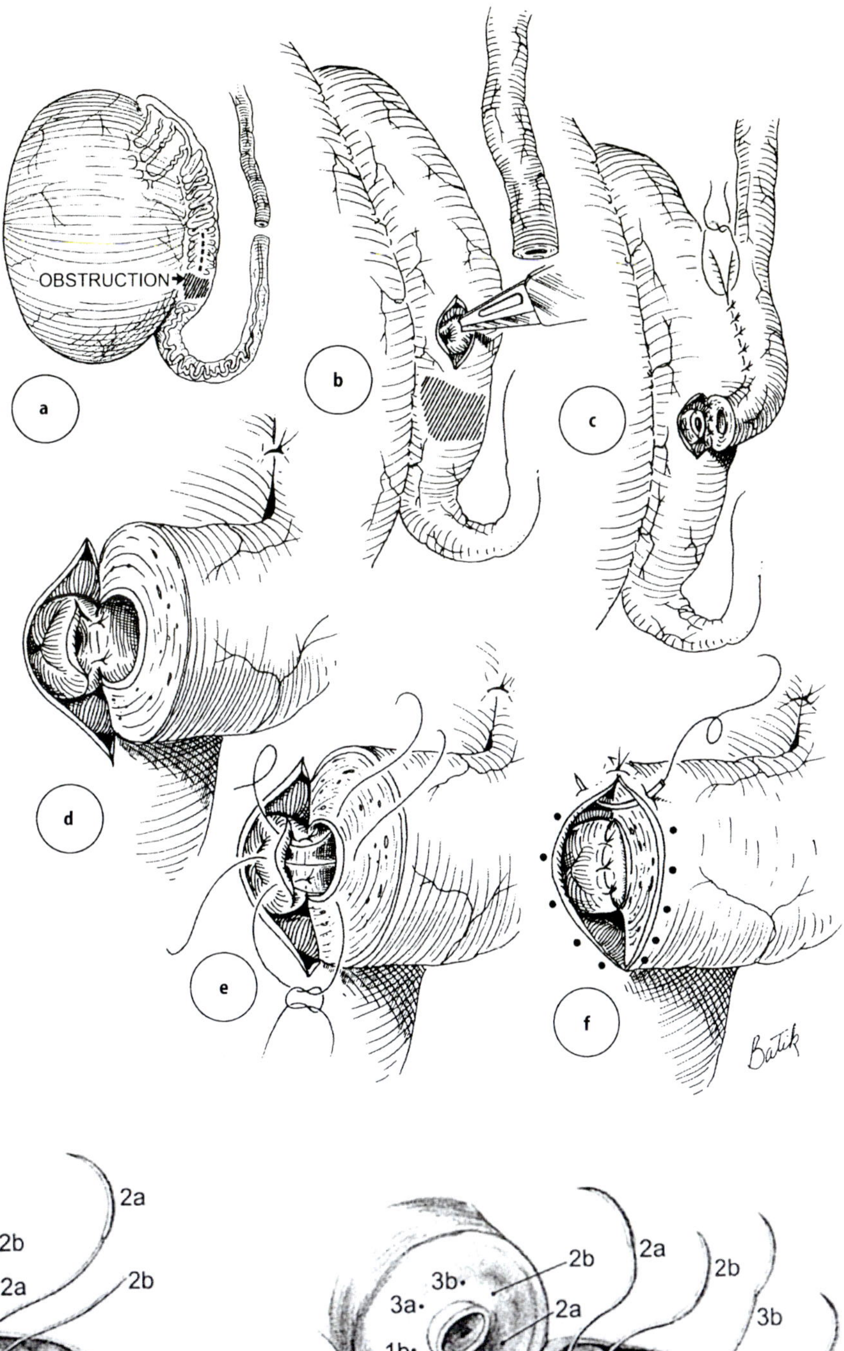

Fig. II.4.23a–f. Thomas' microsurgical end-to-side method of vasoepididymostomy. **b** Incision into epididymal tubule. **d, e** Edges of opened epididymal tubule approximated to edges of vas mucosa. **c, f** Edges of epididymal tunic approximated to edges of outer muscular layer of vas. [Reproduced with permission from Crais TF Jr (1983) Reproductive and urogenital microsurgery. *Clinics in Plastic Surgery.* Saunders, Philadelphia, 10:155–171]

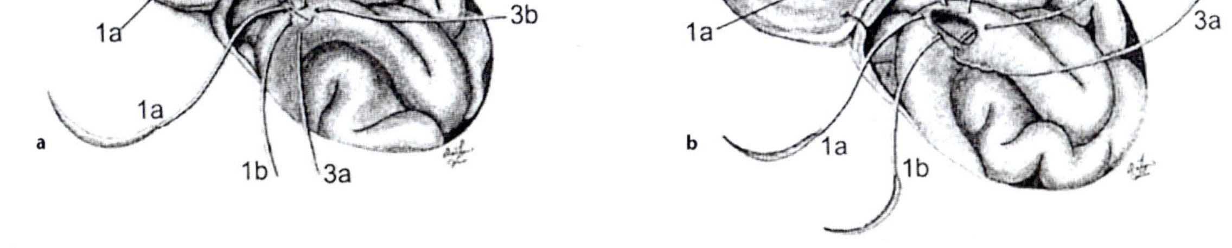

Fig. II.4.24a–d. Berger's triangulation intussusception method of microsurgical vasoepididymostomy. **a** Placement of the three triangulating sutures into the epididymal tubule. Diagram does not show that the needle of one end of each suture should be placed into the tubule before any of those needles are pulled through the tubule (see text and Fig. II.4.25)

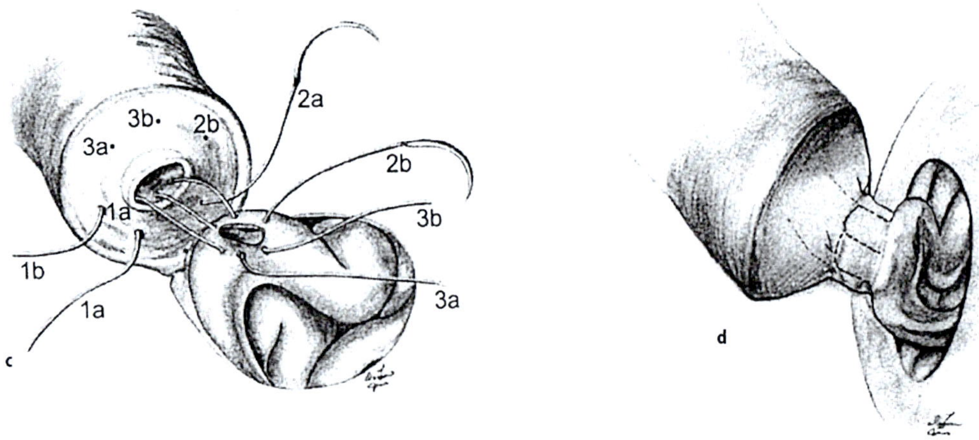

Fig. II.4.24. (Cont.) After the tubule is opened, "*a*" and "*b*" ends of each suture are placed through corresponding locations in vas, thus intussuscepting the tubule into the lumen of the vas. After inner layer sutures are tied, edges of epididymal tunic are approximated to edges of the outer muscular layer of the vas (not shown in diagram). (©2004 Urology Surgical Associates, PSC, Louisville, Kentucky, USA)

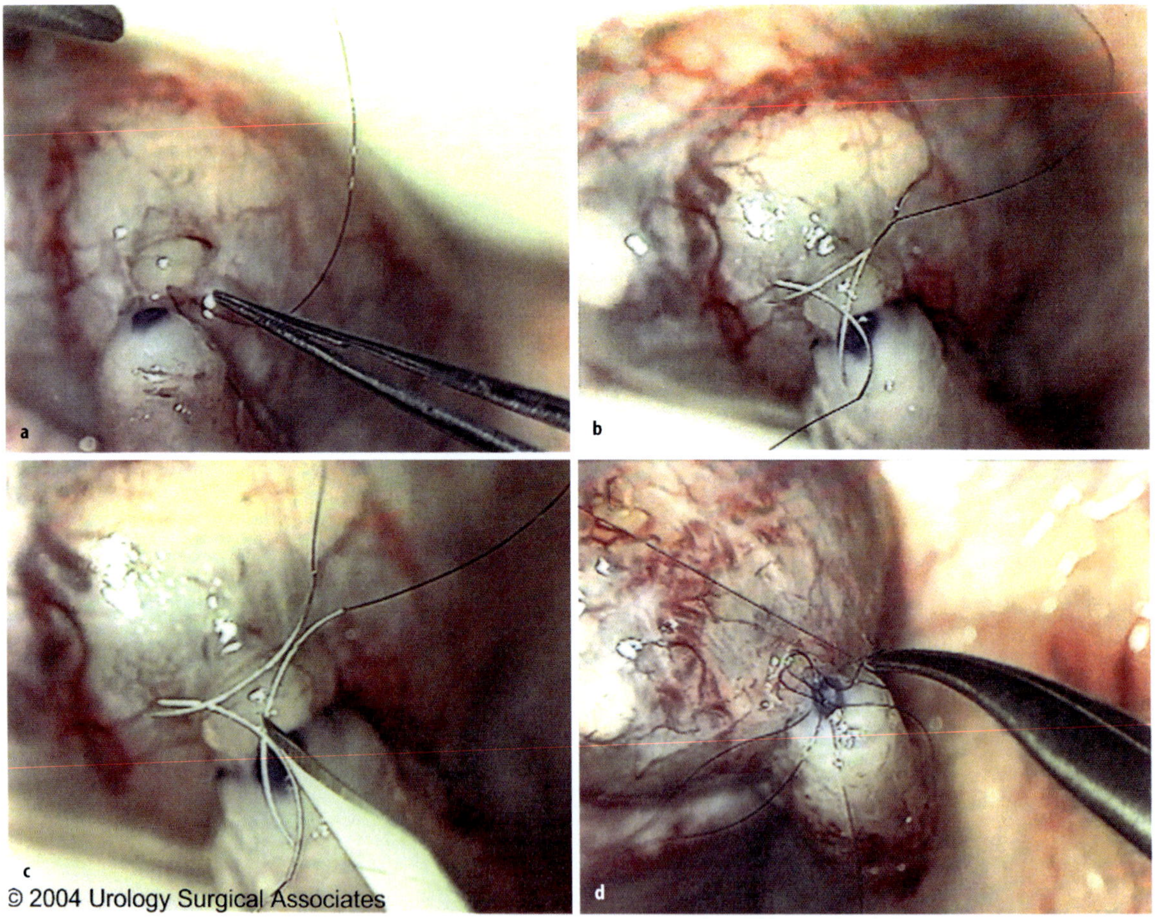

Fig. II.4.25. Operative photograph of Berger's triangulation intussusception method of microsurgical vasoepididymostomy. Vas at *bottom* and epididymal tubule *above* in all photos. Mucosa of vas stained with blue dye. **a** Posterior muscular layer of vas approximated to edge of epididymal tunic. **b** All three triangulating needles are placed into epididymal tubule before any needle is pulled through the tubule. Apex of triangle points toward the vas. **c** Incision of tubule between triangulating needles made with microsurgical scalpel blade. **d** First double armed inner layer suture being tied (©2004 Urology Surgical Associates, PSC, Louisville, Kentucky, USA)

II.4

tion of the epididymal tubule is the use of compression of the epididymis between the surgeon's index finger and thumb. Such compression results in displacement of the tubule to a superficial level just below the epididymal tunic and allows the surgeon to dissect the tubule from the surrounding tissue easier than when compression is not used.

Both methods of microsurgical end-to-side anastomosis are simpler to perform when double armed sutures of 10–0 nylon having a length of 2.5 cm are used for the inner layer suturing. The use of such short sutures helps prevent tangling that may occur when longer sutures are used. If the end-to-side anastomotic technique shown in Fig. II.4.23 is used, the tubule may be opened either by incising it or by excising an oval of the superficial portion of the tubule with microsurgical scissors. The latter option may result in the removal of too large a part of the tubule. It therefore seems more expedient simply to incise the superficial portion of the tubule in order to open it.

When the microsurgical "triangulation intussusception" method (Fig. II.4.24) is performed, it is useful to place the needles of one end of each of the three double armed triangulating sutures of 10–0 nylon into the unopened epididymal tubule and then incise the tubule between the triangulating needles before any needle is withdrawn from the tubule (Fig. II.4.25). If each needle is withdrawn from the tubule immediately after it has been placed into the tubule, the leakage of tubular fluid around the trailing suture may result in collapse of the tubule and thus create difficulty in placing the remaining triangulating sutures. After all three needles have been placed into the tubule, the tubule has been opened and microscopic examination of the tubular fluid verifies the presence of spermatozoa, the needles are withdrawn from the tubule and the needles on each end of each suture are placed through corresponding points in the vas (Fig. II.4.24). These sutures in the vas should include the mucosa and the inner portion of muscular layer. After these inner layer sutures have all been tied, the anastomosis is completed by connecting the outer muscular layer of the vas to the incised edges of the epididymal tunic identical to the method of performing the outer layer suture placement when the more tedious end-to-side method shown in Fig. II.4.23 is used.

After the anastomosis has been completed, the scrotal contents are replaced within the scrotum, parietal tunica vaginalis is closed, Dartos layer edges are approximated and skin is closed. A dressing and scrotal support then are applied.

II.4.4.6 Postoperative Care

Patients are advised to remain at home for 7 days postoperatively. They also are advised to wear a scrotal support and to avoid heavy physical activity for 4 weeks postoperatively. The observation of disrupted anastomoses at the time of exploration of failed vasovasostomy procedures prompted such advice. Sexual intercourse is restricted to a minimum of 2 weeks postoperatively. The latter restriction is based upon the observation in canine vasovasostomy procedures that 2 weeks was required for the anastomotic healing process to be sufficiently advanced that a leak of spermatozoa would be unlikely at the time of an ejaculation (Schmidt 1966). Because an anastomotic leak of spermatozoa and the resulting anastomotic sperm granuloma decrease patency rates after vasovasostomy (Hagan and Coffey 1977), this 2-week restriction from intercourse is emphasized to patients. Semen analyses are obtained every 2–3 months until either pregnancy or stable semen parameters occur.

If the concentration of spermatozoa becomes normal after vasovasostomy but motility is absent, the cause usually is the development of cicatricial obstruction of the anastomoses, and the subsequent development of azoospermia may be expected. Reduced, but not absent, sperm motility may result from the presence of antisperm antibodies, epididymal dysfunction or the beginning of anastomotic scar formation that eventually may lead to permanent anastomotic obliteration. Although epididymal dysfunction is believed to be a reason for some instances of reduced sperm motility after vasectomy reversal, there unfortunately is no available test to measure epididymal function or dysfunction. Whether or not reduced sperm motility is due to beginning anastomotic scar tissue formation will become apparent with the results of sequential semen analyses over ensuing months. If sperm motility is progressively lower and eventually absent, the surgeon may confidently conclude that the reason for such a sequence of events is anastomotic scarring that eventually results in permanent anastomotic occlusion.

Reduced sperm motility is not necessarily an indication of the presence of antisperm antibodies. However, when a patient has reduced sperm motility after a vasectomy reversal, it seems prudent to obtain a test to determine if such antibodies may be present. Antisperm antibodies are present in the serum of about 70% of vasectomized men (Linnet 1983). Linnet (1983) demonstrated that men with the highest serum titres of agglutinating antisperm antibodies were the men most likely to have such antibodies appear in the semen after vasectomy reversal, and that such antibodies in the semen seemed to impair fertility after a reversal procedure. Unfortunately, few laboratories currently perform antisperm antibody testing using the older agglutination method. Most laboratories now test for anti-immunoglobulins A and G (IgA and IgG) (see Chap. I.3.7). There is no clinical study to suggest that measurement of a man's *serum* immunoglobulin level before a vasectomy reversal can predict if his fertility may be impaired after the reversal procedure. If sperm motility is reduced or if there is no apparent reason for infertility after a vasectomy reversal, then measurement of IgG and/or IgA on the surface of sperm in the semen using either a direct immunobead or SpermMAR test (see Chap. I.3.7) may indicate that antisperm antibodies are causing the problem. If infertility after a vasectomy reversal is suspected to result from antisperm antibodies or epididymal dysfunction, most authorities now agree that intracytoplasmic sperm injection (ICSI) with in vitro fertilization (IVF) (see Chap. II.4.16) is the best therapy.

II.4.4.7 Complications

Postoperative bleeding and infection fortunately occur rarely after either vasovasostomy or vasoepididymostomy. Late anastomotic scarring that results in azoospermia after the previous return of spermatozoa to the semen has been reported to occur in from 3% (Belker et al. 1985) to 12% (Matthews et al. 1995) of men after vasovasostomy. The rate of either late azoospermia or the appearance of only non-motile spermatozoa in the semen after the initial appearance of motile spermatozoa has been reported to be as high as 21% after vasoepididymostomy (Matthews et al. 1995).

II.4.4.8 Results

The influence of the obstructive interval, which is the duration of time from the vasectomy until its reversal, on postoperative patency and pregnancy rates is shown in Table II.4.2. The obstructive interval is the most important preoperative factor that can be used to guide a couple to understand the chances for both the return of spermatozoa to the semen and of pregnancy. The overall rates of the return of spermatozoa to the semen and of pregnancy, respectively, are 86% and 52% for initial vasovasostomy procedures, and 75% and 43% for repeat procedures (Belker et al. 1991).

After microsurgical vasoepididymostomy, spermatozoa return to the semen of from 60% to 85% of men, and pregnancy occurs in 20% to 44% of their partners (Matthews et al. 1995; Kolettis and Thomas 1997; Kim et al. 1998). The "triangulation intussusception" method appears to achieve results comparable to those obtained with the alternative microsurgical end-to-side method (Berger 1998; McCallum et al. 2002). The results of vasoepididymostomy may depend on the aetiology of epididymal obstruction (Kim et al. 1998).

If spermatozoa do not return to the semen within 2 months or certainly by 4 months postoperatively, it can be assumed that vasovasostomy has failed. However, there may be a delay in the appearance of spermatozoa in the semen after vasoepididymostomy for reasons that are not clearly understood (Schoysman 1990). Jarow et al. (1995) reported that 18 of 44 (41%) patients who were azoospermic at the time of the first postoperative semen analysis had delayed appearance of spermatozoa in the semen, with a mean delay of 6 months and a range of 3–15 months.

Patients are informed that the average interval until a pregnancy occurs after microsurgical vasovasostomy is 12 months and that most pregnancies do not occur until 24 months postoperatively (Belker et al. 1991). An average interval to pregnancy after vasoepididymostomy is not known. However, the time interval for pregnancy to occur has been reported to be as long as 24 months postoperatively in the female partners of 117 patients (Schoysman 1993). If the female partner does not become pregnant within 1 year after stable semen parameters have been attained, she should undergo a fertility evaluation.

The resolution of post-vasectomy pain can be expected in the majority of patients who undergo vasectomy reversal for the purpose of pain relief. Myers et al. (1997) reported relief of post-vasectomy pain in 24 of 32 men following vasectomy reversal, and in 3 of 6 men who underwent a second reversal because of persistent pain after the first reversal. Thus, 27 of the 32 men (84%) reported by Myers et al. (1997) had relief of pain after vasectomy reversal. Nangia et al. (2000) reported relief of post-vasectomy pain in 9 of 13 (69%) men following vasectomy reversal. Patients who enquire about post-vasectomy pain relief by undergoing vasectomy reversal should be informed that a reversal will relieve such pain in the majority of patients, but that pain relief cannot be guaranteed if a reversal is performed.

Table II.4.2. Effect of the duration of the obstructive interval on the result of vasovasostomy (Belker et al. 1991)

Duration of obstructive interval (years)	Sperm in semen Number[a]	(%)	Pregnancy Number[a]	(%)
<3	86/89	(97)	56/74	(76)
3–8	525/600	(88)	253/478	(53)
9–14	205/261	(79)	92/209	(44)
≥15	32/45	(71)	11/37	(30)

[a] Numerator indicates number of patients achieving postoperative patency or pregnancy and denominator indicates number of patients in each group

II.4

II.4.4.9 Conclusions

Microsurgical methods of vasovasostomy and vasoepididymostomy have improved the success rates of both procedures. Surgeons must obtain formal microsurgical laboratory training and subsequently practise microsurgical anastomotic procedures before attempting to perform them clinically. The mere use of an operating microscope and microsurgical instruments will lead to suboptimal results without such training and practice. Patients who are considering undergoing either procedure should verify the training, experience and results of the particular surgeon who will perform the procedure.

Before patients consider either of these reconstructive microsurgical procedures, they should be informed about the comparative expense and success rates of sperm retrieval with IVF and ICSI. This allows patients to reach their own conclusions about which method to achieve a pregnancy is best suited to their needs and financial resources.

References

Belker AM (1980) Microsurgical two-layer vasovasostomy: simplified technique using hinged, folding-approximating clamp. Urology 16:376 – 381

Belker AM (1988) Infrapubic incisions for specific vasectomy reversal situations. Urology 32:413 – 415

Belker AM (1995) Microsurgical vasovasostomy: two-layer technique. In: Goldstein M (ed) Surgery of male infertility. Saunders, Philadelphia, pp 61 – 66

Belker AM (1997) Vasovasostomy. In: Hellstrom WJG (ed) Male infertility and sexual dysfunction. Springer, Berlin Heidelberg New York, pp 230 – 243

Belker AM, Thomas AJ Jr, Fuchs EF, Konnak JW, Sharlip ID, Thomas AJ Jr (1985) Transient fertility after vasovasostomy in 892 patients. J Urol 134:75 – 76

Belker AM, Thomas AJ Jr, Fuchs EF, Konnak JW, Sharlip ID, Thomas AJ Jr (1991) Results of 1,469 microsurgical vasectomy reversals by the Vasovasostomy Study Group. J Urol 145:505 – 511

Berger RE (1998) Triangulation end-to-side vasoepididymostomy. J Urol 159:1951 – 1953

Hagan KF, Coffey DS (1977) The adverse effects of sperm during vasovasostomy. J Urol 118:269 – 273

Jarow JP, Sigman M, Buch JP, Oates RD (1995) Delayed appearance of sperm after end-to-side vasoepididymostomy. J Urol 153:1156 – 1158

Jarow JP, Oates RD, Buch JP, Shaban SF, Sigman M (1997) Epididymovasostomy outcomes based upon level of anastomosis and intraepididymal sperm quality. Assisted Reprod Reviews 7:179 – 183

Kim ED, Winkel E, Orejuela F, Lipshultz LI (1998) Pathological epididymal obstruction unrelated to vasectomy: results with microsurgical reconstruction. J Urol 160:2078 – 2080

Kolettis PN, Thomas AJ Jr (1997) Vasoepididymostomy for vasectomy reversal: a critical assessment in the era of intracytoplasmic sperm injection. J Urol 158:467 – 470

Linnet L (1983) Clinical immunology of vasectomy and vasovasostomy. Urology 22:101 – 114

Matthews GJ, Schlegel PN, Goldstein M (1995) Patency following microsurgical vasoepididymostomy and vasovasostomy: temporal considerations. J Urol 154:2070 – 2073

McCallum S, Li PS, Shenykin Y, Su L-M, Chan P, Goldstein M (2002) Comparison of intussusception pull-through and conventional end-to-side microsurgical vasoepididymostomy: prospective randomized controlled study in male Wistar rats. J Urol 167:2284 – 2288

Myers SA, Mershon CE, Fuchs EF (1997) Vasectomy reversal for treatment of the post-vasectomy pain syndrome. J Urol 157:518 – 520

Nangia AK, Myles JL, Thomas AJ Jr (2000) Vasectomy reversal for the post-vasectomy pain syndrome: a clinical and histological evaluation. J Urol 164:1939 – 1942

Niederberger C, Ross LS (1993) Microsurgical epididymovasostomy: predictors of success. J Urol 149:1364 – 1367

Schmidt SS (1966) Anastomosis of the vas deferens: an experimental study. I. J Urol 75:300 – 303

Schmidt SS (1978) Vasovasostomy. Urol Clin North Am 5: 585 – 592

Schoysman R (1990) Vaso-epididymostomy – a survey of techniques and results with considerations of delay of appearance of spermatozoa after surgery. ACTA Eur Fertil 21:239 – 245

Schoysman R (1993) Clinical situations challenging the established concept of epididymal physiology in the human. ACTA Eur Fertil 24:55 – 60

Schoysman RJ, Bedford JM (1986) The role of the human epididymis in sperm maturation and sperm storage as reflected in the consequences of epididymovasostomy. Fertil Steril 46:293 – 299

Silber SJ (1979) Epididymal extravasation following vasectomy as a cause for failure of vasectomy reversal. Fertil Steril 31:309 – 315

Silber SJ (1988) Pregnancy caused by sperm from vasa efferentia. Fertil Steril 49:373 – 375

Silber SJ (1989) Apparent fertility of human spermatozoa from the caput epididymis. J Androl 10:263 – 269

Thomas AJ Jr (1987) Vasoepididymostomy. Urol Clin North Am 14:527 – 538

Weiske W-H (1994) Pregnancy caused by sperm from vasa efferentia. Fertil Steril 62:642 – 643

II.4.5 Nonsurgical Cure of Varicocele by Transcatheter Embolization of the Internal Spermatic Vein(s) with a Tissue Adhesive

J. Kunnen, M. Kunnen

Summary

Transcatheter treatment of varicoceles by means of embolization with a tissue adhesive is performed under local anaesthesia, on an outpatient basis, and has a low technical failure (< 1 %), a low recurrence (2 %) and only 0.3 % complication rate.

Considering these advantages, together with the favourable results in terms of repair of fertility, embolization of the internal spermatic vein(s) with a tissue adhesive is to be considered the treatment of first choice for varicocele-associated infertility; furthermore early diagnosis and nonsurgical treatment of varicocele(s) at school age is indicated. Also local scrotal discomfort and even sexual inadequacy may react favourably to this therapy.

II.4.5.1 Introduction

Varicocele is the most common detectable cause of male infertility. It is caused by a disturbance of the efflux of venous blood from the testicle(s) due to the inversion of blood flow in the internal spermatic vein(s).

Impairment of testicular and epididymal function probably results from the countercurrent exchange of noradrenaline from the refluxing venous blood into the testicular arterial blood, at the level of the pampiniform plexus.

The latter causes chronic vasoconstriction of the intratesticular arterioles and decreased tissue perfusion with degeneration of Sertoli cells and, finally, decreased production of spermatozoa. Varicoceles may cause local discomfort and are associated with prostatovesiculitis as well as sexual inadequacy.

II.4.5.2 Diagnostic Venography

In 1976 one of the authors (M.K.) worked out a method for selective venography of the internal spermatic vein(s), which he claimed to be safe and suitable for routine use (Comhaire and Kunnen 1976). At present this method is put into practice all over the world.

Using this technique one succeeds in visualizing not only those varicoceles that were already detected by clinical examination, but also the ones we have called subclinical, and which are detected by means of contact thermography using Varicoscreen®, developed by Comhaire, or Doppler flow measurement.

During venography right-sided varicoceles should be searched for systematically since we have found varicoceles to be bilateral in up to 24 % of patients. In these cases we could show that the right internal spermatic vein nearly always connects with the renal vein or with the renal or perirenal venous plexus.

II.4.5.3 Treatment by Embolization

In the presence of a varicocele, diagnostic venography is immediately followed by nonsurgical treatment by means of transcatheter superselective embolization with a tissue adhesive (Kunnen 1980, 1982; Kunnen and Comhaire 1991). This method is relatively simple, safe and indeed successful.

According to our technique 99 % of all varicoceles, including both those on the right side and those on the left, may be treated under local anaesthesia and on an outpatient basis. More than 3400 patients have been treated in the 25 years of experience. The method is safe, as it has no side-effects; its complication rate is only 0.3 %, which is much lower than that of surgery. The same is true for the rate of varicocele persistence or recurrence, which is 2 % at the left side and less than 1 % at the right side.

II.4.5.4 General Information

The catheterization is performed from the right groin under local anaesthesia and according to a strict protocol, exclusively using coaxial catheters. A left and a right Kunnen spermatic set are manufactured by Cook (Denmark). The left one contains a 6Fr cobra-shaped outer catheter and a suitable 0.038" flexible guidewire, and a straight 3Fr inner catheter provided with an opaque marker at the tip, also with a suitable 0.021" guidewire. The right set contains a 6Fr hooked outer catheter and a straight 3Fr inner catheter. The guidewires of the left set are also used on the right side.

Diagnostic venography should always precede the therapeutic procedure. One starts with the hooked catheter, which is the outer part of the *right* spermatic set. First the *right* renal and internal spermatic veins are examined. The right renal vein is catheterized,

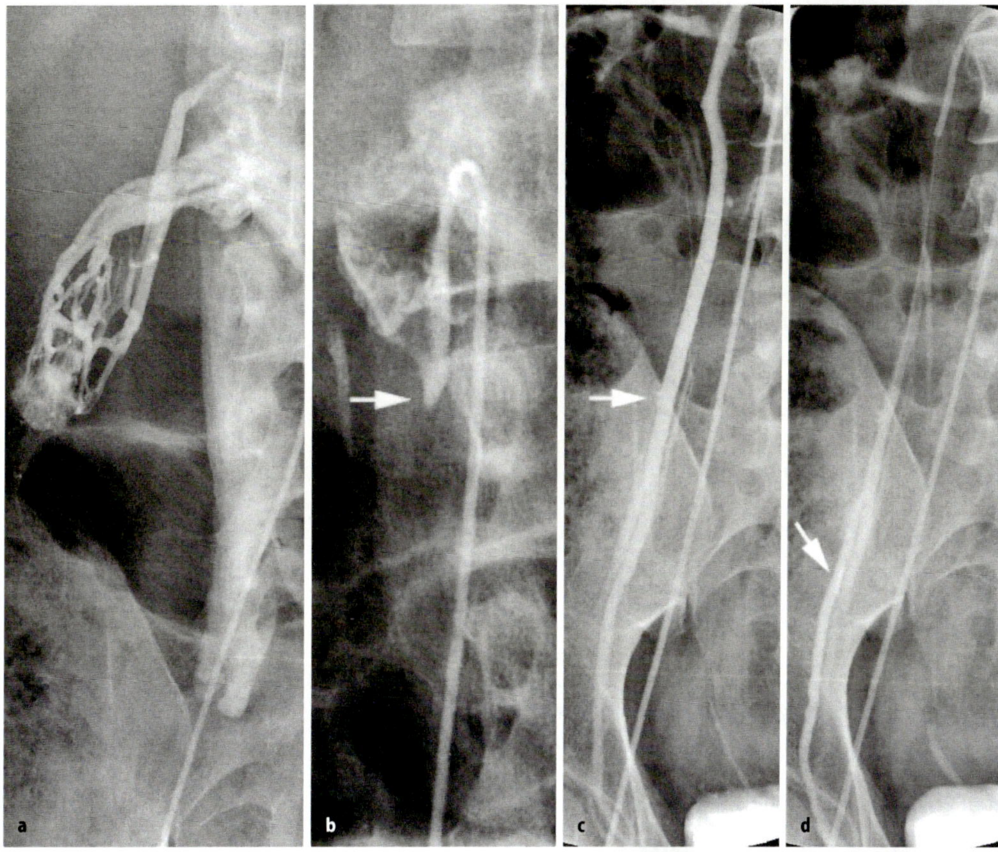

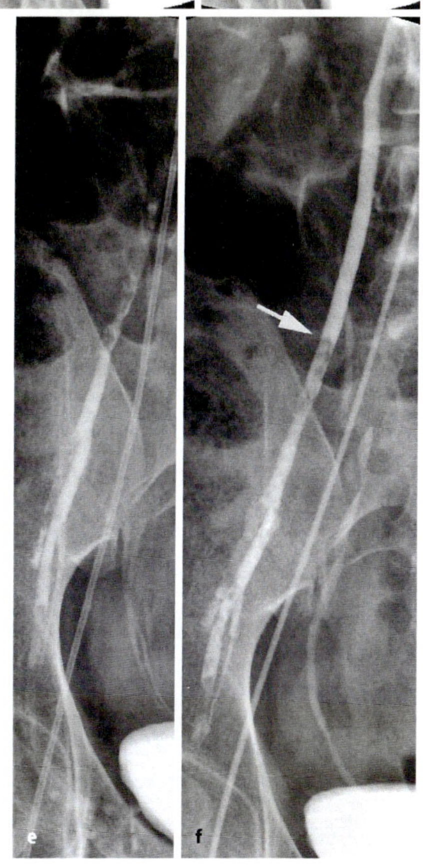

Fig. II.4.26a–f. A 26-year-old man presents with primary infertility; on clinical examination a grade III varicocele is found on the left side. No right varicocele is detected clinically. Phlebography and treatment of a subclinical right varicocele is presented. **a** Selective venography of the right renal vein: nice opacification of all the intrarenal veins, showing a normal aspect; no renospermatic reflux. **b** Selective venography of the outlet of the right internal spermatic vein: competent valve (*arrow*). **c** Superselective venography of the right internal spermatic vein after passing the outlet valve: clear reflux and presence of the outlet of a renospermatic bypass (*arrow*). **d** Superselective internal spermatic venography: the embolization catheter is placed in the lateral branch of the bifurcated distal spermatic vein (*arrow*). **e** Plain X-ray after embolization: the embolus, Histoacryl Transparent®, opacified with Lipiodol Ultrafluid® is clearly shown in the internal spermatic branches. **f** Selective control venography of the right internal spermatic vein: total occlusion at the level of L5 (*arrow*). Successful treatment of the right subclinical varicocele

II.4

probing the segmentary veins with the flexible 0.038" guidewire (Fig. II.4.26a). The venogram has to show the segmentary veins clearly. It is mandatory to use a tilting examination table and to bring the patient into a semi-erect position; he has to perform a Valsalva manoeuvre. Then 10 – 15 ml of contrast medium is injected by hand. We use non-ionic Iohexol (Omnipaque® 240, Amersham Health, Norway), which yields practically no side-effects.

Collaterals connecting to the spermatic vein or a direct connection between the renal and the spermatic vein have to be sought. In the presence of a competent valve at the outlet of the right internal spermatic vein (Fig. II.4.26b) we try to pass this valve by means of the straight 3Fr inner catheter, with the 0.021" guidewire. This increases the percentage of positive tests impressively, especially at the right side (Gat et al. 2004). When this is unsuccessful or in the presence of a second competent valve, the venography of the right side is regarded as negative.

If this right venography is positive, i.e. if retrograde opacification of the right spermatic vein is visualized (Fig. II.4.26c), this vein should be catheterized coaxially, angiographed superselectively (Fig. II.4.26d) and embolized with a tissue adhesive (Fig. II.4.26e). The occlusion should be monitored by means of selective venography 10 min later (Fig. II.4.26f). The venography of the *right* side is positive in 25 % of our patients presenting with a varicocele.

Then we have to proceed with the *left*-sided diagnostic venography using the 6Fr cobra-shaped catheter of the left spermatic set. This catheter is pushed into the segmentary renal veins, probing them with the flexible tip of the 0.038" guidewire. This venography has to show the segmentary veins clearly and should disclose insufficiency of the valve at the outlet of the left internal spermatic vein, yielding reflux into it (Fig. II.4.27a). In cases with a competent outlet valve, reflux via perirenal collaterals may bypass the valve to drain into caudal, insufficient parts of the spermatic vein: we call these vessels perirenal collaterals or renospermatic bypasses. Even in the case of a competent valve without apparent renospermatic bypasses, this valve must be passed coaxially in search of more distal bypasses.

If the left venography is positive the internal spermatic vein should be catheterized selectively (Fig. II.4.27b), angiographed superselectively by coaxial catheter (Fig. II.4.27c) and embolized with a tissue adhesive (Fig. II.4.27d). The occlusion should be monitored by means of venography 10 min later, selectively in the internal spermatic vein (Fig. II.4.27e) and in the left renal vein (Fig. II.4.27f).

II.4.5.5 Specific Information on Superselective, Coaxial Catheterization and Embolization

The outer catheter is placed in the outlet of the internal spermatic vein. A selective spermatic venogram is carried out.

The thin (3Fr) inner catheter, fitted with the small guidewire (0.021") included in the left spermatic set, is pushed through the outer catheter to enter the spermatic vein. During this procedure the tip of the guidewire extends slightly beyond the tip of the thin catheter, which presents an opaque marker. The catheters are slightly moistened with glucose 5 % through a T-adaptor or a haemostatic valve. The thin inner catheter moves more easily when the patient coughs, or performs a Valsalva manoeuvre; this is especially of interest in order to pass competent valves. The exact localization of the catheter is monitored by injections of small quantities of contrast medium. The exact site for the embolization is selected inferior to the lowest anastomosis between the spermatic vein and the (peri)renal venous plexus and, preferentially, superior to possible bifurcations. At this stage superselective venograms may be of great value.

The patient is examined on a remote-controlled tilting table, which is brought into the near-horizontal position – in fact 2 to 30° – in order to stop blood flow in the internal spermatic vein. Injecting a small bolus of contrast medium also controls the latter. *This procedure is extremely important as it excludes accidental embolization of the renal vein as well as injection into the pampiniform plexus.*

First a tuberculin *syringe* is filled with 1 ml 10 % glucose and connected to the plastic 3-way stopcock of the embolization catheter, which itself is filled with 5 % glucose. The glucose solution slows down the polymerization of the tissue adhesive.

In a *second syringe*, the following substances are aspirated in sequence: first 0.4 – 0.5 ml Lipiodol Ultrafluid® (Guerbet, France) and next 0.5 ml *n*-butyl-cyanoacrylate (Histoacryl Transparent®, Braun, Melsungen, Germany). Rarely more than one ampule, i.e. 0.6 ml of tissue adhesive, is necessary. The contrast medium – the Lipiodol Ultrafluid® – is used not only to delineate the non-opaque embolus of tissue adhesive on the TV screen and the X-ray images, but also to slow down the polymerization.

The *second syringe* is connected to the 3-way stopcock, and its contents are injected into the embolization catheter and pushed into the spermatic vein by means of the contents of the *first syringe*. 0.7 ml of 10 % glucose from the first syringe is injected in order to push the embolus completely into the spermatic vein. The coaxial embolization catheter is immediately pulled back by 2 or 3 cm and the remaining 0.3 ml 10 %

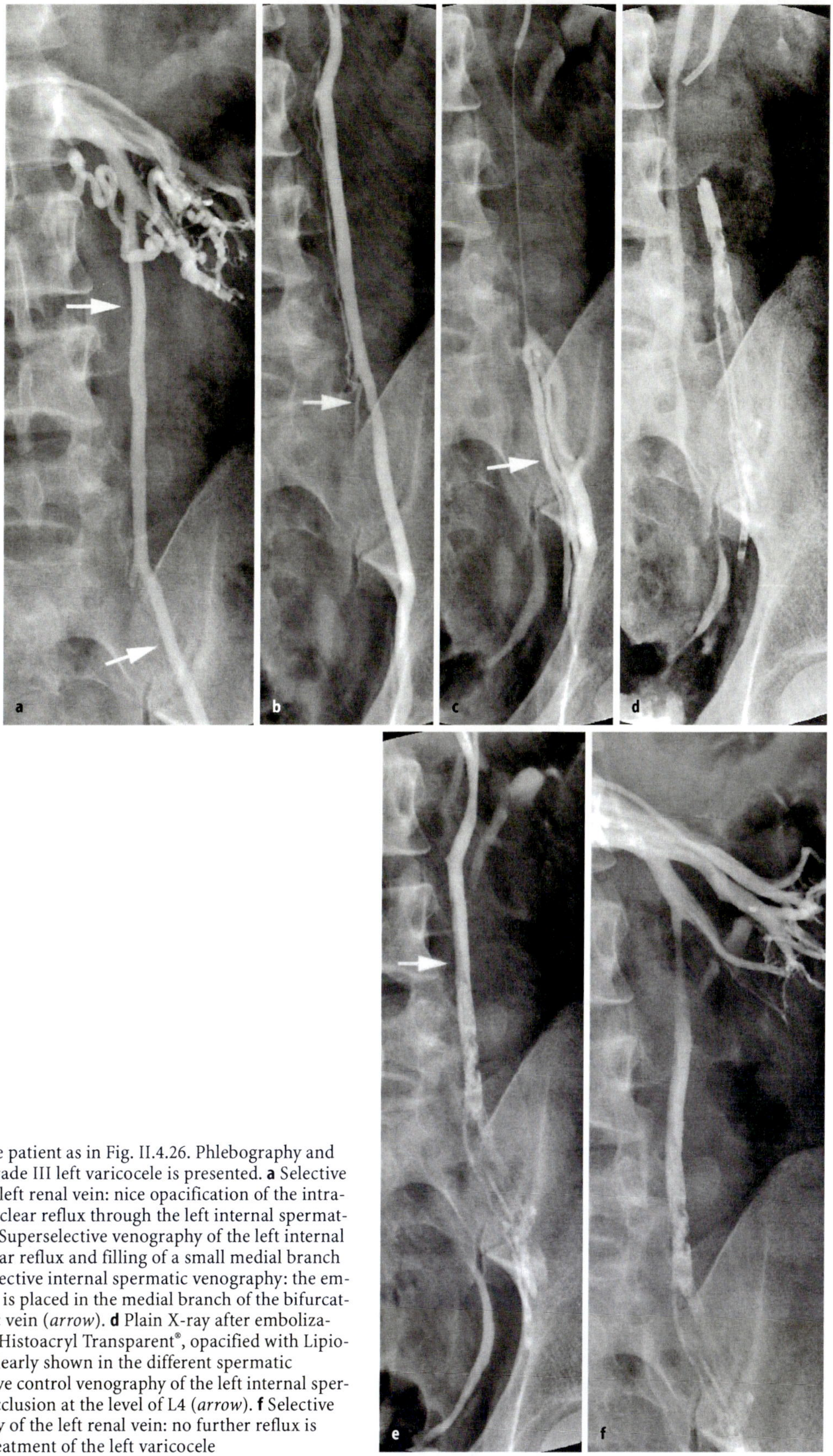

Fig. II.4.27a–f. Same patient as in Fig. II.4.26. Phlebography and treatment of the grade III left varicocele is presented. **a** Selective venography of the left renal vein: nice opacification of the intrarenal veins, with a clear reflux through the left internal spermatic vein (*arrows*). **b** Superselective venography of the left internal spermatic vein: clear reflux and filling of a small medial branch (*arrow*). **c** Superselective internal spermatic venography: the embolization catheter is placed in the medial branch of the bifurcated distal spermatic vein (*arrow*). **d** Plain X-ray after embolization: the embolus, Histoacryl Transparent®, opacified with Lipiodol Ultrafluid® is clearly shown in the different spermatic branches. **e** Selective control venography of the left internal spermatic vein: total occlusion at the level of L4 (*arrow*). **f** Selective control venography of the left renal vein: no further reflux is seen. Successful treatment of the left varicocele

glucose from the *first* syringe is injected in order to completely remove all tissue adhesive from this catheter. After that, the inner catheter is completely withdrawn from the outer one, which itself is pulled back into the caval vein where blood is aspirated. If it is not possible to aspirate blood, the caval vein wall may adhere to the tip of the catheter; this can be avoided by placing the tip of the catheter in the left common iliac vein. Whenever aspiration of blood remains impossible, occlusion of the outer catheter by a residue of tissue adhesive should be suspected and the outer catheter should also be withdrawn. It is replaced by a new outer catheter (all catheters can be obtained separately, i.e. not only in sets). In these rare cases one can cut the external part of the occluded catheter obliquely, introduce a 6Fr sheath over it, withdraw the catheter and replace it with the new one, fitted with the 0.038" flexible guidewire.

As soon as the tissue adhesive comes in contact with blood it polymerizes to form a permanent occlusion. The embolus is seen on the X-ray images.

A venography is performed about 10 min later through the outer catheter, replaced in the segmentary veins. First the renal vein is injected without a Valsalva manoeuvre in order to check its integrity. The renal vein is then injected during a Valsalva manoeuvre, showing incomplete filling of the spermatic vein. Finally the embolized spermatic vein is selectively visualized, confirming the occlusion to be complete.

Our method is also perfectly suited to the treatment of large veins. It usually allows the embolization of veins presenting complex anatomic conditions. Generally such patients can be treated with one single embolus, provided the ideal site for occlusion is carefully searched for and reached by the embolization catheter. In 12% of cases a second embolization during the same session is necessary to occlude all spermatic branches.

In more than 30% of cases, the internal spermatic vein presents a competent outlet valve, but reflux occurs through one or even several renospermatic bypasses. With our technique these competent valves may be passed using the coaxial catheter in 99% of those cases and the patients can be treated successfully by embolizing the insufficient caudal part of the spermatic vein.

II.4.5.6 Data on Tissue Adhesives and Sclerosing Agents

In the first 6 years use was made of the tissue adhesive isobutyl 2-cyanoacrylate, registered name Bucrylate®, manufactured by Ethicon (Somerville, USA). Primarily it was designed for wound closure.

At the end of 1985, Ethicon suddenly decided to withdraw Bucrylate® from the market; to the best of our knowledge, no clear explanation has been given.

For 19 years we have successfully used *n*-butyl 2-cyanoacrylate (Histoacryl® from Braun, Melsungen, Germany). One should *not use* the classical Histoacryl *Blue®*, as it polymerizes too rapidly. We use Histoacryl *Transparent®* very successfully. By enhancing the concentration of the inhibitor P_2O_5 the polymerization is delayed. It seems worthwhile mentioning that Histoacryl® is authorized by Canadian but not by American authorities.

Recently a new European tissue adhesive, co-monomer *n*-butyl cyanoacrylate (Glubran®2/Viareggio, Italy), got a CE label, and the use for intravascular embolization is clearly mentioned by the company; perhaps this drug will be authorized by the FDA.

We were also very successful with another group of 282 patients, treating their varicoceles by superselective sclerotherapy with 5 ml of 3% sodium tetradecyl sulphate solution (Thrombovar® from Lepetit, France; Sotradecol®, Elkins-Sinn, N.J., USA). Provided the blood flow is arrested by tilting the examination table, and adopting the same coaxial technique, the authors seldom observed pain or scrotal swelling. We do consider the fact that one has to postpone the post-embolization venography for at least 30 min after injecting the sclerosing agent, a clear drawback. In 35% of cases a second dose of Thrombovar® had to be given, as the occlusion was incomplete; this means another 30-min wait, and performing a second control venography. Nevertheless, superselective sclerotherapy is a good alternative in countries where tissue adhesives are not available.

In contrast, metallic coils are not suitable for spermatic vein occlusion because they leave the accompanying veins and renospermatic bypasses open. Moreover, coil-treated vessels may also remain open or become partly patent later. Finally, the presence of coils may render distal coaxial catheterization of the spermatic vein and correct embolization with tissue adhesive impossible.

II.4.5.7 Results in 3043 Consecutive Patients

In total, 3450 patients have been examined for a clinical problem of varicocele, 2718 between 1979 and 2000 by M.K. et al. at the University Hospital of Ghent and 732 between 1993 and 2004 by J.K. at the ZNA Middelheim Hospital in Antwerp (Belgium).

Here we report on 3043 consecutive patients from 1985 to 2004. The age of these patients ranged 4–72 years (mean 24.5; 1171 patients were under 20).

Twenty-nine men (1.0%) had unilateral right varicoceles, 2228 (73.2%) unilateral left varicoceles and 736 (24.2%) bilateral varicoceles, of which 22 had already been unsuccessfully treated by surgical ligation on the left side.

Almost 41,7% of patients presented with primary infertility, 8.0% with secondary infertility, 7.7% with local discomfort, 1.1% with sexual inadequacy and 41.5% were treated preventively.

Our results revealed that 2906 of 2928 (99.2%) left varicoceles and 757 of 764 (99.1%) right varicoceles were successfully treated.

Persistent varicocele was detected in 5 of 757 (0.66%) on the right side and re-embolized successfully. Out of the 59/2906 (2.03%) persistent left varicoceles, 53 could be treated by re-embolization and 6 by surgical ligation.

In three patients (0.09%) the inner catheter was glued in the spermatic vein; they were operated uneventfully.

Thanks to coaxial catheterization tissue adhesive never migrated. In two patients an inguinal haematoma was treated conservatively. Rarely, patients developed some pain or scrotal swelling requiring symptomatic antiphlogistic therapy. Hydrocele never occurred.

The irradiation dose was negligible, as the scrotum was always X-ray shielded. Since 2002 the use of pulsed fluoroscopy has further reduced irradiation.

II.4.5.8 Effect on Semen and Pregnancies

Two-thirds of patients improved their semen quality after varicocele treatment and, overall, half of them were successful in achieving pregnancy. The probability was 3.9% per cycle. This is significantly better than the expected treatment-independent pregnancy rate, which is estimated to be 1.5% per cycle (Comhaire and Kunnen 1985).

The duration of infertility does not influence the probability of post-treatment pregnancy. The coincidence of additional pathology interfering with the fertility of the male or the female partner decreases the probability of success, as do the findings of an elevated pre-treatment serum concentration of follicle-stimulating hormone, a small total testicular volume (i.e. less than 28 ml) and very poor semen quality (Kunnen and Comhaire 1986).

Depending on the latter the probability of conception varies between 8% and 80%. Patients with azoospermia or circulating sperm antibodies stand such poor chances of success that treatment should probably not be offered to them.

II.4.5.9 Conclusion

Varicocele is a bilateral disease and the possible right varicocele must always be sought by phlebography. In cases presenting with a competent outlet valve an effort should be made to pass it, in order to find clinically significant renospermatic bypasses by superselective phlebography in the internal spermatic vein.

Superselective transfemoral spermatic vein(s) embolization with tissue adhesive is highly effective (99% successful) and safe (0.3%, mostly minor, complications). A good control phlebography at the end of the session should exclude spermatic branches that remain permeable.

References

Comhaire F, Kunnen M (1976) Selective retrograde venography of the internal spermatic vein: a conclusive approach to the diagnosis of varicocele. Andrologia 8:11–24

Comhaire F, Kunnen M (1985) Factors affecting the probability of conception after treatment of subfertile men with varicocele by transcatheter embolization with Bucrylate. Fertil Steril 43:781–786

Gat Y, Bachar GN, Zukerman Z, Belenky A, Gornish M (2004) Varicocele: a bilateral disease. Fertil Steril 81:424–429

Kunnen M (1980) Neue Technik zur Embolisation der Vena spermatica interna: intravenöser Gewebekleber. Fortschr Röntgenstr 133:625–629

Kunnen M (1982) Non-surgical cure of varicocele by transcatheter embolization of the internal spermatic vein with bucrylate. In: Zeitler E, Jecht E (eds) Varicocele and male infertility (Recent Advances in Radiodiagnostic and Therapy). Springer, Berlin Heidelberg New York, pp 153–161

Kunnen M, Comhaire F (1986) Fertility after varicocele embolization with bucrylate. Ann Radiol 29:169–171

Kunnen M, Comhaire F (1991) Non-surgical cure of varicocele by transcatheter embolization of the internal spermatic vein(s) with a tissue adhesive (Histoacryl Transparent). In: Castaneda-Zuniga W (ed) Interventional radiology (Golden Series). Williams and Wilkins, Baltimore, Md., pp 73–101

II.4.6 Hormonal Treatment of Infertility

F. Comhaire, A. Mahmoud

Summary

- Treatment of patients with hypogonadotrophic hypogonadism by means of purified urinary or recombinant gonadotrophins induces or restores complete spermatogenesis, though sperm concentration may remain relatively low necessitating complementary intra-uterine insemination or in vitro fertilization (IVF) for successful conception.
- The use of gonadotrophins or luteinizing hormone releasing hormone (LHRH) does not improve the fertility of men with idiopathic oligozoospermia.
- Treatment with tamoxifen (20 mg/day), with or without testosterone undecanoate, results in a threefold increase of spontaneous pregnancies, within 6 months.
- Tamoxifen is the treatment of first choice in patients with idiopathic oligozoospermia and sperm concentrations between 2 and 10–12 million/ml, a percentage of spermatozoa with normal morphology better than 4%, and serum gonadotrophin levels that are not elevated.

II.4.6.1 Introduction

Normal spermatogenesis requires adequate testicular stimulation. Pulsatile secretion of luteinizing hormone releasing hormone (LHRH) by the hypothalamus induces pulsatile release of luteinizing hormone (LH) by the pituitary, causing pulsatile secretion of testosterone by the Leydig cells. The latter is released in the interstitial fluid surrounding the seminiferous tubules, which are exposed to extremely high concentrations of testosterone. Stimulation of Sertoli cells by follicle stimulating hormone (FSH) is required for optimal spermatogenesis, although some degree of spermatogenesis can be maintained through the effect of testosterone alone (Sharpe et al. 1993). Hypogonadotrophic hypogonadism results from inadequate testicular exposure to endogenous gonadotrophins, usually both LH and FSH. The isolated deficiency of LH secretion has been described as "fertile eunuch syndrome", where spermatogenesis seems to proceed normally but virilization is inadequate as a result of insufficient exposure to androgens. The opposite situation, with normal LH and testosterone secretion but deficient FSH secretion, may also occur. It has been suggested that inadequate bioactivity of gonadotrophins, the concentration of which is identified as normal by radioimmunoassay, may play a role in impaired sperm production (Rowe 1988). This hypothesis has been questioned since more adequate enzyme-linked immunosorbent assay (ELISA) methods have been introduced for gonadotrophin assessment.

Abnormalities of the biosynthesis of testosterone by Leydig cells have been reported in certain men with poor sperm production, but these findings are probably due to artefacts of the in vitro testing systems. Androgen receptor inadequacy may, perhaps, occur in some infertile men (Ochsenkuhn and de Kretser 2003).

The Sertoli cells play a major role in the "nutrition" of spermatogenic cells. Inadequate stimulation of these cells, or defects of their biosynthetic and/or enzymatic activity because of "immaturity" have been suggested as a possible cause of deficient spermatogenesis.

Attention has focused on the role of endogenous and exogenous oestrogens in the pathogenesis of idiopathic oligozoospermia. These patients present with oligozoospermia, normal or slightly decreased testicular volume, testosterone in the low-normal range, and serum concentrations of LH and FSH that are not elevated.

Since approximately one-quarter of men do not show any demonstrable cause of their deficient sperm production (idiopathic oligozoospermia), hormones have been prescribed to them. We will discuss the effects of androgens, gonadotrophins, aromatase inhibitors and anti-oestrogens.

II.4.6.2 Androgens

II.4.6.2.1 Testosterone

Testosterone is poorly taken up after oral administration. It is given parentally as either short-acting testosterone phenylpropionate, or long-acting testosterone enanthate, or a mixture of several esters. After injection, such esters increase the concentration of testosterone in peripheral blood in excess of the normal physiological concentration during at least the first 3–5 days. Testosterone is aromatized in the liver, in fat tissue and by hypothalamic cells, resulting in an increased oestradiol concentration which suppresses the secretion of LHRH and of LH and FSH, and inhibits spermatogenesis. Hence, high-dose androgen therapy has a suppressive rather than stimulating effect on spermatogenesis, and it has been applied for contraceptive purposes (Swerdloff et al. 1979).

II.4.6.2.2 Androgen Derivatives

Testosterone derivatives have been developed adapting the molecular structure such that the substance is taken up after oral administration and that aromatization to oestrogens is decreased. A number of publications have suggested a potential benefit of mesterolone (Schering, Berlin, Germany) (Schellen and Beek 1972; Von Mauss 1974; Barwin 1982). However, no beneficial effect on semen characteristics or on the occurrence of pregnancies was observed when the usual dose of 75 mg/day of mesterolone was given (WHO 1989). Neither was treatment with a high mesterolone dose of 150 mg/day effective in a double-blind trial that extended over a 12-month period (Gerris et al. 1991).

Testosterone-undecanoate (Andriol, Organon, The Netherlands) is a non-toxic testosterone derivative that is absorbed after oral administration (Horst et al. 1976) and increases the concentration of mainly 5-alpha-dihydrotestosterone in peripheral blood (Skakkebaek et al. 1981). Testosterone-undecanoate exerts little suppressive effect on hypothalamo–pituitary function when given in the recommended dose of 120 mg/day (Luisi et al. 1978). Because spermatogenesis and epididymal function largely depend on high local concentrations of both testosterone and dihydrotestosterone, trials were undertaken on the effect of 120 or 240 mg/day testosterone-undecanoate for the treatment of patients with idiopathic oligozoospermia. The favourable effect observed with the first dose (Pusch 1989) was not confirmed when the high dose of 240 mg/day was given (Comhaire 1990). The only positive effect on sperm characteristics was a moderate increase of the percentage of live spermatozoa, but no effect was observed on sperm concentration, proportion motility, linear velocity or sperm morphology.

II.4.6.3 Gonadotrophins

II.4.6.3.1 Urinary Gonadotrophins

Whereas treatment with human menopausal gonadotropin (hMG, a source of both FSH and LH), or with purified urinary FSH together with human chorionic gonadotrophin (hCG) is of great benefit to patients with hypogonadotrophic hypogonadism (Liu et al. 1999), its possible usefulness in men with normo-gonadotrophic idiopathic oligozoospermia has not been proven. Meta-analysis of published data indicates an average success rate of 3.8 conceptions per cycle, but most studies refer to short periods of treatment (Winters and Troen 1982).

Patients who do not present an increase of testosterone concentration during treatment with tamoxifen may benefit from gonadotrophin treatment, since it can be hypothesized that their hypothalamo pituitary function is impaired or suppressed.

II.4.6.3.2 Recombinant Gonadotrophins

The advent of recombinant pure FSH may open new avenues for gonadotrophin treatment. Indeed, pure FSH will probably not suppress the pulsatile release of LHRH and LH, maintaining the pulsatile exposure of the seminiferous tubules to highly variable and elevated testosterone concentrations. In uncontrolled trials, a satisfactory success rate of pure FSH treatment was reported in patients with idiopathic oligozoospermia (Foresta et al. 2002; Caroppo et al. 2003), but this was not confirmed in a placebo-controlled trial (Kamischke et al. 1998). Recombinant FSH treatment has also been recommended for patients with failed IVF due to poor semen quality (Acosta et al. 1992), though this approach has become obsolete since the introduction of intracytoplasmic sperm injection (ICSI).

II.4.6.4 Luteinizing Hormone Releasing Hormone (LHRH)

Pulsatile LHRH can be delivered by means of a portable computerized pump, resulting in a physiological stimulation of pituitary gonadotrophin secretion. This treatment may offer new prospects for the management of patients with hypogonadotrophic hypogonadism of hypothalamic origin. Preliminary trials of treating patients with normo- or hyper-gonadotrophic idiopathic testicular failure with pulsatile LHRH have given inconclusive or negative results (Comhaire 1992).

Nasal or subcutaneous application of high doses of LHRH agonists results in downregulation of pituitary gonadotrophin secretion and suppression of testicular function, both hormonogenesis and spermatogenesis.

II.4.6.5 Treatments Interfering with Oestradiol

Treatment may aim at interfering with the biological effect of oestradiol, either through inhibiting its synthesis by means of aromatase inhibitors, or through blocking its effect on target cells by anti-oestrogens.

II.4.6.5.1 Testolacton

Experience with testolacton, a potent aromatase inhibitor, has been moderately positive in an open study on a small number of patients (Vigersky and Glass 1981), but no significant effect was observed in controlled double-blind trials (Dony et al. 1985; Clark and Sherins 1989). Newer aromatase inhibitors (anastrozole, exemestan, letrozol) have not been tested for the treatment of idiopathic oligozoospermia.

II.4.6.5.2 Anti-oestrogens

Anti-oestrogens have largely been used in the treatment of patients with oligozoospermia. Clomiphene citrate is a racemic mixture of two isomers, and it exerts a significant intrinsic oestrogenic activity in addition to its dominant anti-oestrogenic effect (Heller et al. 1969). No beneficial effect of clomiphene citrate was evidenced for the treatment of patients with idiopathic oligozoospermia in a double-blind trial organized by World Health Organization (WHO 1992).

Tamoxifen is a specific anti-oestrogen and is devoid of intrinsic oestrogenic activity when applied at the dose of 20 mg/day in men (Comhaire 1976). This substance stimulates the hypothalamic release of LHRH by setting the threshold of feedback at a higher level. As a result, the secretion of LH, FSH and testosterone is increased by between 60% and 100% (Fig. II.4.28). A more than twofold increase of sperm concentration occurs after 4–6 months of treatment (Vermeulen and Comhaire 1978), with significant increase of sperm motility and linear velocity (Fig. II.4.29). Sperm morphology is barely influenced. In a meta-analysis of 6 studies involving 402 patients followed during a total of 2025 months, the overall success rate was 29% with a monthly conception rate of 4.6%.

The effective cumulative pregnancy rate during tamoxifen intake evidences a clear-cut increase in the 4th, 5th and 6th months of treatment, whereas no such effect seems to be present during the initial 2 months (Fig. II.4.30). This is probably related to the fact that several months of treatment is needed before the full effect on spermatogenesis occurs. Tamoxifen treatment was found to result in a stronger positive effect on pregnancy rates in cases with low pre-treatment sperm concentration (Comhaire 2000).

Adamopoulos et al. (2003) published the outcome of a prospective double-blind, placebo-controlled trial

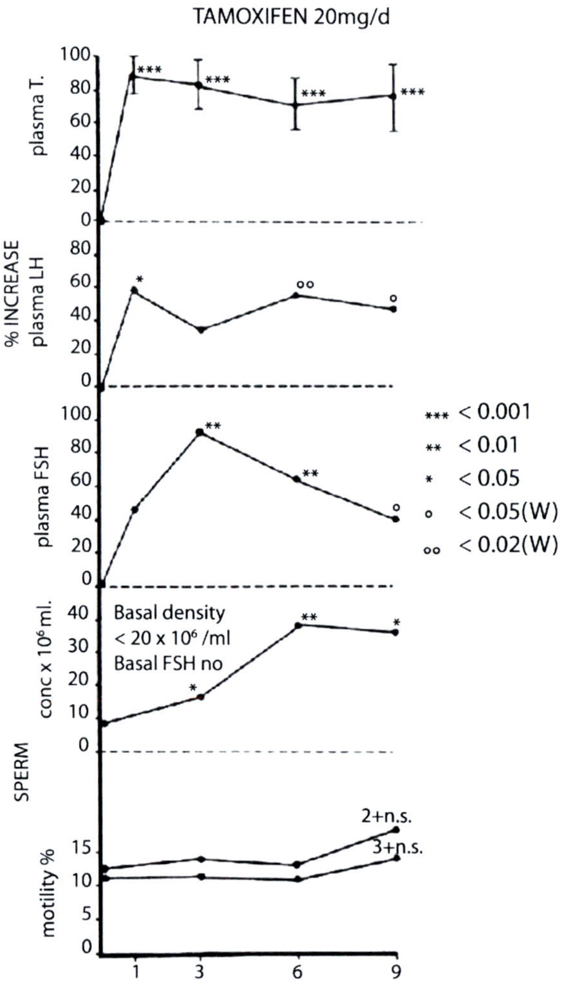

Fig. II.4.28. Effects of treatment with 20 mg per day of tamoxifen for 9 months, given to patients with idiopathic oligozoospermia, on the plasma concentrations of testosterone (ng/dl), LH and FSH (% increase over basal value), sperm concentration (million/ml) and motility [% spermatozoa with motility 2 = grade (b) motility; 3 = grade (a) motility]. (From Vermeulen and Comhaire 1978)

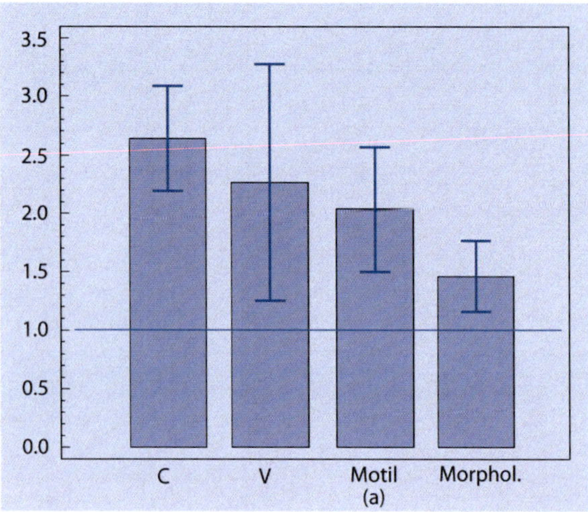

▷ **Fig. II.4.29.** Ratio of sperm concentration (*C*), linear velocity (*V*), grade (a) motility [*Motil (a)*] and morphology (*Morphol.*) after 6 months of treatment with tamoxifen 20 mg per day orally divided by the values before treatment

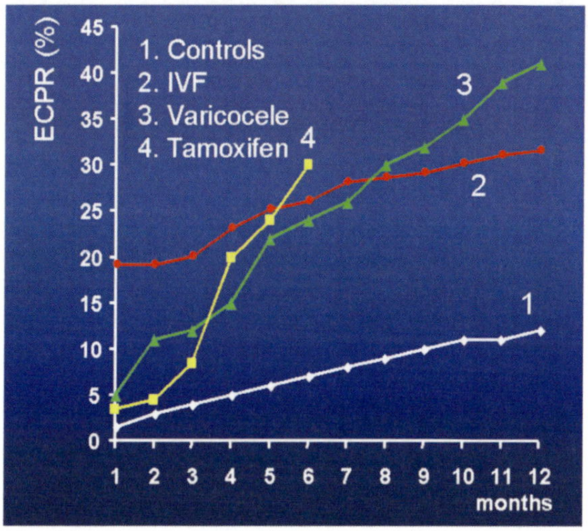

Fig. II.4.30. Effective cumulative pregnancy rate (in %, including only pregnancies resulting in successful delivery) during a follow-up period of 12 months, among couples with infertility of at least 12 months duration, no demonstrable abnormalities in the female partner, and a male factor. [*1* Controls are couples receiving counselling ("tender loving care"), *2* treatment by means of in vitro fertilization (with or without ICSI), *3* treatment of varicocele, *4* treatment with tamoxifen 20 mg/day orally)

treating patients suffering from idiopathic oligozoospermia with a combination of tamoxifen and testosterone-undecanoate. They reported a significant favourable effect of this treatment with the spontaneous pregnancy rate being 3.2 times higher in the treated cases than in the placebo controls.

II.4.6.6 Conclusion

New insights into the physiology of testicular regulation and better understanding of the pathogenesis of idiopathic male infertility hold out hope for the future possibilities of hormonal treatment. At present, the hormonal therapeutic arsenal remains limited. Antioestrogen treatment with tamoxifen is indicated, particularly in cases with low sperm concentration (ideally between 2 and 10–12 million/ml) and moderately disturbed sperm morphology. Tamoxifen treatment has little effect when sperm morphology is severely abnormal with less than 4% normal spermatozoa. Also, treatment with tamoxifen seems pointless in cases with elevated serum gonadotrophin levels and/or very small testicular volume.

References

Acosta AA, Khalifa E, Oehninger S (1992) Pure human follicle stimulating hormone has a role in the treatment of severe male infertility by assisted reproduction: Norfolk's total experience. Hum Reprod 7:1067–1072

Adamopoulos DA, Pappa A, Billa E, Nicopoulou S, Koukkou E, Michopoulos J (2003) Effectiveness of combined tamoxifen citrate and testosterone undecanoate treatment in men with idiopathic oligozoospermia. Fertil Steril 80:914–920

Barwin BH (1982) Mesterolone: a new androgen for the treatment of male infertility. In: Bain J, Schill WB, Schwarzstein L (eds) Treatment of male infertility. Springer, Berlin Heidelberg New York, pp 117–123

Caroppo E, Niederberger C, Vizziello GM, D'Amato G (2003) Recombinant human follicle-stimulating hormone as a pretreatment for idiopathic oligoasthenoteratozoospermic patients undergoing intracytoplasmic sperm injection. Fertil Steril 80:1398–1403

Clark RV, Sherins RJ (1989) Treatment of men with idiopathic oligozoospermic infertility using the aromatase inhibitor, testolactone. Results of a double-blinded, randomized, placebo-controlled trial with crossover. J Androl 10:240–247

Comhaire F (1976) Treatment of oligospermia with tamoxifen. Int J Fertil 21:232–238

Comhaire F (1990) Treatment of idiopathic testicular failure with high-dose testosterone undecanoate: a double-blind pilot study. Fertil Steril 54:689–693

Comhaire FH (1992) Conventional treatment of oligo-asthenoteratozoospermia. In: Frick J (ed) Die Anwendung von GnRH und GnRH-Analoga in der Urologie. Blackwell, Vienna, pp 115–123

Comhaire F (2000) Clinical andrology: from evidence-base to ethics. The 'E' quintet in clinical andrology. Hum Reprod 15:2067-2071

Dony JM, Smals AG, Rolland R, Fauser BC, Thomas CM (1985) Effect of lower versus higher doses of tamoxifen on pituitary-gonadal function and sperm indices in oligozoospermic men. Andrologia 17:369–378

Foresta C, Bettella A, Merico M, Garolla A, Ferlin A, Rossato M (2002) Use of recombinant human follicle-stimulating hormone in the treatment of male factor infertility. Fertil Steril 77:238–244

Gerris J, Comhaire F, Hellemans P, Peeters K, Schoonjans F (1991) Placebo-controlled trial of high-dose mesterolone treatment of idiopathic male infertility. Fertil Steril 55: 603–607

Heller CG, Rowley MJ, Heller GV (1969) Clomiphene citrate: a correlation of its effect on sperm concentration and morphology, total gonadotropins, ICSH, estrogen and testosterone excretion, and testicular cytology in normal men. J Clin Endocrinol Metab 29:638–649

Horst HJ, Holtje WJ, Dennis M, Coert A, Geelen J, Voigt KD (1976) Lymphatic absorption and metabolism of orally administered testosterone undecanoate in man. Klin Wochenschr 54:875–879

Kamischke A, Behre HM, Bergmann M, Simoni M, Schafer T, Nieschlag E (1998) Recombinant human follicle stimulating hormone for treatment of male idiopathic infertility: a randomized, double-blind, placebo-controlled, clinical trial. Hum Reprod 13:596–603

Liu PY, Turner L, Rushford D, McDonald J, Baker HW, Conway AJ, Handelsman DJ (1999) Efficacy and safety of recombinant human follicle stimulating hormone (Gonal-F) with urinary human chorionic gonadotrophin for induction of spermatogenesis and fertility in gonadotrophin-deficient men. Hum Reprod 14:1540–1545

Luisi M, Eliasson R, Kicovic PM, Franchi F, Alicicco E (1978) Hypothalamic-pituitary responsiveness to clomiphene stimulation during a placebo controlled study of testosterone undecanoate therapy in normal men. In: Fabbrini A, Steinberger E (eds) Recent progress in andrology. Academic, London, pp 469–475

Ochsenkuhn R, de Kretser DM (2003) The contributions of de-

ficient androgen action in spermatogenic disorders. Int J Androl 26:195–201
Pusch HH (1989) Oral treatment of oligozoospermia with testosterone-undecanoate: results of a double-blind-placebo-controlled trial. Andrologia 21:76–82
Rowe PJ (1988) WHO's approach to the management of the infertile couple. In: Neglo-Vilar A, Isidori A, Paulson J, Abdelmassih R, de Castro MPP (eds) Andrology and human reproduction. Raven, New York, pp 291–309
Schellen TM, Beek JM (1972) The influence of high doses of mesterolone on the spermiogram. Fertil Steril 23:712–714
Sharpe RM, Millar M, McKinnell C (1993) Relative roles of testosterone and the germ cell complement in determining stage-dependent changes in protein secretion by isolated rat seminiferous tubules. Int J Androl 16:71–81
Skakkebaek NE, Bancroft J, Davidson DW, Warner P (1981) Androgen replacement with oral testosterone undecanoate in hypogonadal men: a double blind controlled study. Clin Endocrinol (Oxf) 14:49–61
Swerdloff RS, Campfield LA, Palacios A, McClure RD (1979) Suppression of human spermatogenesis by depot androgen: potential for male contraception. J Steroid Biochem 11: 663–670
Vermeulen A, Comhaire F (1978) Hormonal effects of an anti-estrogen, tamoxifen, in normal and oligospermic men. Fertil Steril 29:320–327
Vigersky RA, Glass AR (1981) Effects of delta 1-testolactone on the pituitary-testicular axis in oligospermic men. J Clin Endocrinol Metab 52:897–902
Von Mauss J (1974) Ergebnisse der Behandlung von Fertilitätsstörungen des Mannes mit Mesterolon oder einem Placebo. Arzneimittelforschung 24:1338–1442
WHO (1989) Mesterolone and idiopathic male infertility: a double-blind study. World Health Organization Task Force on the Diagnosis and Treatment of Infertility. Int J Androl 12:254–264
WHO (1992) A double-blind trial of clomiphene citrate for the treatment of idiopathic male infertility. Int J Androl 15: 299–307
Winters SJ, Troen P (1982) Gonadotropin therapy in male infertility. In: Bain J, Schill WB, Schwartzstein L (eds) Treatment of male infertility. Springer, Berlin Heidelberg New York, pp 85–101

II.4.7 Hormonal Male Contraception

D.J. Handelsman, G.M.H. Waites

Summary

Reliable and reversible hormonal contraceptive methods for men, comparable to modern female methods, have been identified, and selected regimens are under active development through the collaboration of andrologists, public sector agencies and pharmaceutical industries.

- Clinical studies employing prototype drugs have demonstrated that the hormonal approach to switching off spermatogenesis provides contraceptive efficacy and is reversible with short-term safety.
- No regimen yet achieves consistent azoospermia in all men, although testosterone administration to men in China and Indonesia gets close.
- Combination regimens involving a second gonadotrophin-suppressing agent, usually a progestin, combined with testosterone achieve close to the ideal of universal suppression of spermatogenesis and contraceptive efficacy.

II.4.7.1 Introduction

Pituitary gonadotrophin [luteinizing hormone (LH), follicle-stimulating hormone (FSH)] secretion leading to high levels of intratesticular testosterone is essential for inducing spermatogenesis. Yet, because the hypothalamo–pituitary testicular axis is a tightly regulated negative feedback system, exogenous testosterone has the seemingly paradoxical effect of switching off spermatogenesis by suppressing pituitary gonadotrophin secretion and thereby depleting intratesticular testosterone (Handelsman 2005). Androgen-induced reversible suppression of human spermatogenesis has long been known (Heckel 1939). Extensive dose-finding and feasibility studies have established that injections of testosterone (T) esters, mostly involving weekly intramuscular injections of testosterone enanthate in an oily vehicle, induced azoospermia in most but not all men (Patanelli 1977; Schearer et al. 1978).

While these studies demonstrated that the hormonal approach was reversible and had reassuring short-term safety, the degree of sperm suppression required to provide acceptable contraceptive efficacy remained uncertain (Patanelli 1977). This issue was resolved by two large World Health Organization (WHO) clinical trials, the first male contraceptive efficacy studies, which established that azoospermia induced by weekly injections of testosterone enanthate provided highly reliable and reversible contraception (WHO 1990, 1996;

Waites 2003). More recently, a second contraceptive efficacy study using a depot androgen/progestin combination found high levels of spermatogenic suppression with all men achieving azoospermia and no pregnancies occurring among 55 couples during 35.5 person years of exposure (Turner et al. 2003).

II.4.7.2 Androgens Alone as Hormonal Contraceptives

Testosterone is potentially the ideal single contraceptive agent as it provides both gonadotrophin suppression and androgen replacement (Nieschlag et al. 2004). The WHO clinical trials involving 671 men in 10 countries established that 98% of all men had sperm suppression to <3 million/ml by 3–4 months (a similar rate to that after vasectomy) and that no pregnancies occurred when the men were azoospermic (WHO 1990, 1996). In the subgroup with residual sperm (0.1–3 million/ml) in the ejaculate, there were only four pregnancies in 49.5 person years; the contraceptive failure rate in the non-azoospermic subgroup (~8% per annum) was proportional to residual sperm concentration. Based on these results, the ideal goal is to achieve universal azoospermia, although the realistic minimal objective is to have <1 million residual sperm per millilitre to give an acceptable failure rate (Nieschlag 2002).

These WHO trials also revealed that >90% Asian men suppressed to azoospermia compared to only ~60% of Caucasian men, an unexplained population variation in testosterone-induced azoospermia (Handelsman et al. 1995). After cessation of testosterone, sperm reappeared within 3 months and returned to normal sperm output by 6 months. Discontinuations for acne, weight gain, polycythaemia or behavioural effects were few and readily reversible, as were changes in haemoglobin, testis size and plasma urea. There was no short-term evidence of liver, prostate or cardiovascular disorders (WHO 1990, 1996; Wu et al. 1996).

II.4.7.3 Pharmacokinetic Considerations

Weekly injections are clearly impractical and testosterone enanthate caused supraphysiological levels of testosterone which may have contributed to the incomplete spermatogenic suppression. Longer-acting depot preparations with more stable steady-state pharmacokinetics have therefore been developed: subdermal T pellets (Handelsman et al. 1990), T-loaded biodegradable microspheres (Amory et al. 2002), and the newer injectable preparations, T undecanoate (Gu et al. 2002) and T buciclate (Behre et al. 1995). All sustain physiological T levels for 2–6 months. Monthly injections of T undecanoate have demonstrated high contraceptive efficacy in Chinese men (Gu et al. 2002). Although synthetic androgens, including esters and a 7-methyl derivative of nandrolone, have been trialled by parenteral and oral routes, none yet offers greater efficacy or safety than testosterone itself (Kamischke and Nieschlag 2004; Handelsman 2005).

II.4.7.4 Safety

The safety of exogenous androgen administration concerns potential effects on cardiovascular and prostatic disease and idiosyncratic effects such as polycythaemia and sleep apnoea. The available short-term studies have generally revealed no safety concerns but long-term surveillance of actual disease endpoints rather than surrogate markers would be required, as it was for female hormonal contraception. The relationship between androgens and prostatic disease and any influence of exogenous androgens remains poorly understood. Prospective studies show little direct relationship between endogenous T levels and prostatic disease (Shaneyfelt et al. 2000). In situ prostate cancer is common in older men whereas rates of invasive prostate cancer vary considerably between populations despite similar blood T concentrations. Similarly, the relationship between androgens and cardiovascular disease are complex and poorly understood (Liu et al. 2003; Wu and von Eckardstein 2003) so that the risks, if any, from exogenous androgens in normal men cannot be predicted with any certainty. Idiosyncratic androgen effects such as polycythaemia and sleep apnoea are rare (<1%) and age-dependent so that the use of physiological doses of, and delivery systems for, T in a relatively young population minimize these risks. Clearly, for contraceptive purposes, it is prudent not to exceed physiological levels of androgen and to monitor long-term for cardiovascular and prostatic disease risk (Nieschlag et al. 2004; Handelsman 2005).

II.4.7.5 Combination Regimens as Hormonal Contraceptives

Second, non-androgenic, agents that suppress gonadotrophins include progestins, oestrogens and gonadotrophin-releasing hormone (GnRH) antagonists. Progestins are more affordable and numerous synthetic progestins are used in female contraception with oestrogen replacement therapy. They are potent inhibitors of gonadotrophin secretion and of endogenous T, and suppress spermatogenesis but require androgen supplementation to avoid androgen deficiency (Heller et al. 1959; Frick et al. 1981). In practice, androgen-progestin combinations achieve equally high rates of azoospermia as with androgens alone, approaching uniform suppression in all populations. This reduces the practical importance of the population differences for contraception found with androgens alone, although it has implications for understanding population differences in hormone-dependent diseases.

II.4.7.6 Efficacy of Combination Regimens

Such combinations have shown important improvements in the efficacy of spermatogenic suppression (Bebb et al. 1996; Handelsman et al. 1996; Meriggiola et al. 1996) possibly by reducing the impact of residual T in supporting persistent spermatogenesis (Bouchard and Garcia 1987; Behre et al. 1992). Many studies with medroxyprogesterone acetate (MPA) given orally or by injection, combined with T by injection or by dermal gels, produce azoospermia (Patanelli 1977; Schearer et al. 1978). The azoospermia is nearly uniform in Indonesian men (Pangkahila 1991; WHO 1993), as it is in Caucasian men when the T is given as a depot implant (Handelsman et al. 1996).

Oral progestins, e.g. levonorgestrel (Foegh 1983; Bebb et al. 1996; Anawalt et al. 1999) and norethisterone (Guerin and Rollet 1988; Lobel et al. 1989) and cyproterone acetate (Meriggiola et al. 1996, 1998) have high efficacy when combined with T. Highly effective suppression of spermatogenesis also occurs with depot progestins, e.g. norgestrel (Gonzalo et al. 2002), etonogestrel (Anderson et al. 2002), depot injectable MPA (Handelsman et al. 1996; Turner et al. 2003) or norethisterone (Kamischke et al. 2002) when combined with T. A contraceptive efficacy study using a depot androgen/progestin combination found high levels of spermatogenic suppression, with all men achieving azoospermia and no pregnancies occurring among 55 couples during 35.5 person years of exposure (Turner et al. 2003).

Spermatogenesis recovers to normal post treatment but at a slower rate than with androgen alone, possibly due to prolonged residual depot effects (Handelsman 2005).

II.4.7.7 Gonadotrophin Blockade: GnRH Analogues

GnRH agonists or GnRH antagonists when combined with T replacement suppress gonadotrophins and spermatogenesis. GnRH superactive agonists achieve this by gradual desensitization of the GnRH receptors, a paradoxical response that takes days to weeks until the initial stimulation of gonadotrophin and T secretion abate, after which prolonged use achieves functional antagonism with lowered gonadotrophin and testosterone secretion. However, GnRH agonists remain partial agonists and these more affordable analogues rarely achieve azoospermia (Bouchard and Garcia 1987; Lunn et al. 1990; Behre et al. 1992). Pure GnRH antagonists, on the other hand, sustain immediate competitive blockade of GnRH receptors (Marshall et al. 1986) and in combination with T produce rapid, sustained and reversible spermatogenesis in men (Pavlou et al. 1991; Tom et al. 1992). Although modern GnRH antagonists retain some local irritation at the injection site, they otherwise have few side-effects and prolonged depot release formulations are under development, as are non-peptide GnRH antagonists.

II.4.7.8 Immunoneutralization as a Contraceptive Approach

Immunoneutralization of GnRH is not likely to be a safe and effective option for contraception (Handelsman 2005). However, immunological blockade of FSH action by vaccination theoretically offered the attractive possibility of inhibiting spermatogenesis by disrupting Sertoli cell function but without inhibiting endogenous T production. Although FSH was considered essential for human spermatogenesis, spermatogenesis and fertility persist in rodents (Singh et al. 1995; Kumar et al. 1997; Dierich et al. 1998) and humans (Tapanainen et al. 1997) lacking FSH bioactivity. Hence even complete FSH blockade might produce insufficient reduction in sperm output and function required for adequate contraceptive efficacy (Nieschlag 1986). In addition to the usual safety concerns of contraceptive vaccines, including autoimmune hypophysitis, orchitis or immune-complex disease, an FSH vaccine might be overcome by reflex increases in pituitary FSH secretion.

References

Amory JK, Anawalt BD, Blaskovich PD, Gilchriest J, Nuwayser ES, Matsumoto AM (2002) Testosterone release from a subcutaneous, biodegradable microcapsule formulation (Viatrel) in hypogonadal men. J Androl 23:84–91

Anawalt BD, Bebb RA, Bremner WJ, Matsumoto AM (1999) A lower dosage levonorgestrel and testosterone combination effectively suppresses spermatogenesis and circulating gonadotropin levels with fewer metabolic effects than higher dosage combinations. J Androl 20:407–414

Anderson RA, Kinniburgh D, Baird DT (2002) Suppression of spermatogenesis by etonogestrel implants with depot testosterone: potential for long-acting male contraception. J Clin Endocrinol Metab 87:3640–3649

Bebb RA, Anawalt BD, Christensen RB, Paulsen CA, Bremner WJ, Matsumoto AM (1996) Combined administration of levonorgestrel and testosterone induces more rapid and effective suppression of spermatogenesis than testosterone alone: a promising male contraceptive approach. J Clin Endocrinol Metab 81:757–762

Behre HM, Nashan D, Hubert W, Nieschlag E (1992) Depot gonadotropin-releasing hormone agonist blunts the androgen-induced suppression of spermatogenesis in a clinical trial of male contraception. J Clin Endocrinol Metab 74:84–90

Behre HM, Baus S, Kliesch S, Keck C, Simoni M, Nieschlag E (1995) Potential of testosterone buciclate for male contraception: endocrine differences between responders and nonresponders. J Clin Endocrinol Metab 80:2394–2403

Bouchard P, Garcia E (1987) Influence of testosterone substitution on sperm suppression by LHRH agonists. Hormone Res 28:175–180

Dierich A, Sairam MR, Monaco L, Fimia GM, Gansmuller A, LeMeur M, Sassone-Corsi P (1998) Impairing follicle-stimulating hormone (FSH) signalling in-vivo: targeted disruption of the FSH receptor leads to aberrant gametogenesis and hormonal imbalance. Proc Natl Acad Sci USA 95: 13612–13617

Foegh M (1983) Evaluation of steroids as contraceptives in men. Acta Endocr Suppl 260:1–48

Frick J, Danner C, Joos H, Kunit G, Luukkainen T (1981) Spermatogenesis in men treated with subcutaneous application of levonorgestrel and estrone rods. J Androl 2:331–338

Gonzalo IT, Swerdloff RS, Nelson AL, Clevenger B, Garcia R, Berman N, Wang C (2002) Levonorgestrel implants (Norplant II) for male contraception clinical trials: combination with transdermal and injectable testosterone. J Clin Endocrinol Metab 87:3562–3572

Gu YQ, Wang XH, Xu D, Peng L, Cheng LF, Huang MK, Huang ZJ, Zhang GY (2002) A multicenter contraceptive efficacy study of injectable testosterone undecanoate in healthy Chinese men. J Clin Endocrinol Metab 88:562–568

Guerin JF, Rollet J (1988) Inhibition of spermatogenesis in men using various combinations of oral progestagens and percutaneous or oral androgens. Int J Androl 11:187–199

Handelsman DJ (2006) Male contraception. In: DeGroot LJ (ed) Endocrinology, 5th edn. Saunders, Philadelphia

Handelsman DJ, Conway AJ, Boylan LM (1990) Pharmacokinetics and pharmacodynamics of testosterone pellets in man. J Clin Endocrinol Metab 71:216–222

Handelsman DJ, Farley TMM, Peregoudov A, Waites GMH, WHO Task Force On Methods For The Regulation Of Male Fertility (1995) Factors in nonuniform induction of azoospermia by testosterone enanthate in normal men. Fertil Steril 63:125–133

Handelsman DJ, Conway AJ, Howe CJ, Turner L, Mackey MA (1996) Establishing the minimum effective dose and additive effects of depot progestin in suppression of human spermatogenesis by a testosterone depot. J Clin Endocrinol Metab 81:4113–4121

Heckel NJ (1939) Production of oligospermia in a man by the use of testosterone propionate. Proc Soc Exp Biol Med 40:658–659

Heller CG, Moore DJ, Paulsen CA, Nelson WO, Laidlaw WM (1959) Effects of progesterone and synthetic progestins on the reproductive physiology of normal men. Fed Proc 18:1057–1064

Kamischke A, Nieschlag E (2004) Progress towards hormonal male contraception. Trends Pharmacol Sci 25:49–57

Kamischke A, Heuermann T, Kruger K, von Eckardstein S, Schellschmidt I, Rubig A, Nieschlag E (2002) An effective hormonal male contraceptive using testosterone undecanoate with oral or injectable norethisterone preparations. J Clin Endocrinol Metab 87:530–539

Kumar TR, Wang Y, Lu N, Matzuk MM (1997) FSH is required for ovarian follicle maturation but not for male fertility. Nat Genet 15:201–204

Liu PY, Death AK, Handelsman DJ (2003) Androgens and cardiovascular disease. Endocr Rev 24:313–340

Lobel B, Olivo JF, Guille F, D Le Lanou (1989) Contraception in men: efficacy and immediate toxicity, a study of 18 cases. Acta Urol Belg 57:117–124

Lunn SF, Dixson AF, Sandow J, Fraser HM (1990) Pituitary-testicular function is suppressed by an LHRH antagonist but not by an LHRH agonist in the marmoset monkey. J Endocrinol 125:233–239

Marshall GF, Akhtar FB, Weinbauer GF, Nieschlag E (1986) Gonadotrophin-releasing hormone (GnRH) overcomes GnRH antagonist-induced suppression of LH secretion in primates. J Endocrinol 110:145–150

Meriggiola MC, Bremner WJ, Paulsen CA, Valdiserri A, Incorvaia L, Motta R, Pavani A, Capelli M, Flamigni C (1996) A combined regimen of cyproterone acetate and testosterone enanthate as a potentially highly effective male contraceptive. J Clin Endocrinol Metab 81:3018–3023

Meriggiola MC, Bremner WJ, Constantino A, Di Cintio G, Flamigni C (1998) Low dose of cyproterone acetate and testosterone enanthate for contraception. Hum Reprod 13:1225–1229

Nieschlag E (1986) Reasons for abandoning immunization against FSH as an approach to male fertility regulation. In: Zatuchni GI, Goldsmith A, Spieler JM, Sciarra JJ (eds) Male contraception: advances and future prospects. Harper and Row, Philadelphia, pp 395–400

Nieschlag E (2002) Sixth Summit Meeting Consensus: Recommendations for Regulatory Approval for Hormonal Male Contraception. Int J Androl 25:375

Nieschlag E, Kamische A, Behre HM (2004) Hormonal male contraception: the essential role of testosterone. In: Nieschlag E, Behre HM (eds) Testosterone – action, deficiency, substitution, 3rd edn. Cambridge University Press, Cambridge, pp 685–714

Pangkahila W (1991) Reversible azoospermia induced by an androgen-progestagen combination regimen in Indonesian men. Int J Androl 44:248–256

Patanelli DJ (ed) (1977) Hormonal control of fertility. US Department of Health Education and Welfare, Washington

Pavlou SN, Brewer K, Farley MG, Lindner J, Bastias MC, Rogers BJ, Swift LL, Rivier JE, Vale WW, Conn PM, Herbert CM (1991) Combined administration of a gonadotropin-releasing hormone antagonist and testosterone in men induces reversible azoospermia without loss of libido. J Clin Endocrinol Metab 73:1360–1369

Schearer SB, Alvarez-Sanchez F, Anselmo J, Brenner P, Coutinho E, Latham-Faundes A, Frick J, Heinild B, Johansson EDB (1978) Hormonal contraception for men. Int J Androl (Suppl 2):680–712

Shaneyfelt T, Husein R, Bubley G, Mantzoros CS (2000) Hormonal predictors of prostate cancer: a meta-analysis. J Clin Oncol 18:847–853

Singh J, O'Neill C, Handelsman DJ (1995) Induction of spermatogenesis by androgens in gonadotropin-deficient (*hpg*) mice. Endocrinology 136:5311–5321

Tapanainen JS, Aittomaki K, Min J, Vasivou T, Huhtaniemi IT (1997) Men homozygous for an inactivating mutation of the follicle-stimulating hormone (FSH) receptor present variable suppression of spermatogenesis and fertility. Nat Genet 15:205–206

Tom L, Bhasin S, Salameh W, Steiner B, Peterson M, Sokol R, Rivier J, Vale WW, Swerdloff RS (1992) Induction of azoospermia in normal men with combined Nal-Glu GnRH antagonist and testosterone enanthate. J Clin Endocrinol Metab 75:476–483

Turner L, Conway AJ, Jimenez M, Liu PY, Forbes E, McLachlan RI, Handelsman DJ (2003) Contraceptive efficacy of a depot progestin and androgen combination in men. J Clin Endocrinol Metab 88:4659–4667

Waites GMH (2003) Development of methods of male contraception: impact of the World Health Organization Task Force. Fertil Steril 80:1–15

WHO Task Force on Methods for the Regulation of Male Fertility (1990) Contraceptive efficacy of testosterone-induced azoospermia in normal men. Lancet 336:955–999
WHO Task Force on Methods for the Regulation of Male Fertility (1993) Comparison of two androgens plus depot-medroxyprogesterone acetate for suppression to azoospermia in Indonesian men. Fertil Steril 60:1062–1068
WHO Task Force on Methods for the Regulation of Male Fertility (1996) Contraceptive efficacy of testosterone-induced azoospermia and oligozoospermia in normal men. Fertil Steril 65:821–829
Wu FCW, von Eckardstein A (2003) Androgens and coronary artery disease. Endocr Rev 24:183–217
Wu FCW, Farley TMM, Peregoudov A, Waites GMH, WHO Task Force on Methods for the Regulation of Male Fertility (1996) Effects of testosterone enanthate in normal men: experience from a multicenter contraceptive efficacy study. Fertil Steril 65:626–636

II.4.8 Treatment of Gender Dysphoria

L.J.G. Gooren

Summary

Hormonal sex reassignment of transsexuals aims to reduce the hormonally induced secondary sex characteristics of the original sex and to induce the secondary sex characteristics of the new sex.

- In male-to-female transsexuals a complete reduction of androgen action favours feminizing effects of oestrogens. The risk of venous thrombosis is high with ethinyloestradiol but much lower with transdermal or oral 17β-oestradiol. Development of prolactinomas has been observed, usually with an overdose of oestrogens. Breast cancer, though infrequent, remains a risk.
- Female-to-male transsexuals receive high-dose testosterone treatment. If menstrual periods are not suppressed a progestin may be added. Side-effects are acceptable but extirpation of ovaries and internal genitalia in due course is recommended as a safeguard against malignant development.
- Transsexualism is increasingly diagnosed in juveniles. Hormonal treatment to delay pubertal development of their original sex may be an option.

Transsexualism is the condition in which a person with apparently normal somatic sexual differentiation of one gender is convinced that he or she is actually a member of the opposite gender. It is associated with an irresistible urge to be that gender hormonally, anatomically and psychosocially.

In 2004, the international organization involved with professional help to transsexuals, the Harry Benjamin International Gender Dysphoria Association, drafted Standards of Care (SOC) available at http://www.hbigda.org. The major purpose of the SOC is to articulate this organization's professional consensus about the psychological, medical and surgical management of gender identity disorders. These standards provide guidance to professionals practising in this area, who often work in isolation from mainstream medicine. It may also be of help in legal medicine to identify professional standards. Persons with gender identity disorders, their families and social institutions may use the SOC as a means to understand the current thinking of professionals.

Before initiating hormonal or surgical treatment that will change a person's gender, the physician should counsel the patient about realistic expectations from treatment. The only benefit sex reassignment can bring is relief of gender dysphoria; all human problems outside the area of gender dysphoria will remain. Unrealistic expectations that subjects may have of the success of hormonal and surgical treatment for their transition to the desired sex must be addressed. Contacts with other transsexuals who are already in the process of changing over to the new sex or who have completed this process may be helpful in shaping a subject's expectations of what can be achieved and what problems, personally and socially, may arise in the transition to the new sex.

II.4.8.1 Real Life Test

When hormone treatment starts, or maybe even earlier, the "real life test" should begin. It is an extended period of full-time living as a member of the desired sex. The "real life test" allows the subject and the attending professional to monitor the experience in the new sex status as he/she habituates his/her responses to other people. Without this test of how others react and how he/she reacts to others, the subject knows only his/her private convictions and fantasies of being a member of the opposite sex. Convictions and fantasies may be unrealistic and may lead to magical expectations of life in the new sex.

Embarking on the "real life test" may be done in a stepwise fashion; for instance, first in a trusted environment and later in public. The subject should have lived at least one full year full-time in the new sex before irreversible surgical reassignment is considered.

The "real life test" may be prolonged if too many hurdles present themselves during the test period. During the "real life test" the subject should stay in contact with a mental health professional to allow assessment of the success of the test and to discuss how to overcome problems that almost inevitably arise during this period.

II.4.8.2 Hormonal Sex Reassignment

Hormonal reassignment has two aims (Levy et al. 2003):

- To reduce the hormonally induced secondary sex characteristics of the original sex as much as possible, though complete elimination is rare. As an example, in male-to-female transsexuals, the previous effects of androgens on the skeleton, such as the greater height of men than women, the size and shape of hands, feet, jaws and pelvis, cannot be reversed. Conversely, the relatively lower height and the broader hip configuration of female-to-male transsexuals compared to men will not change with androgen treatment.
- To induce the secondary sex characteristics of the new sex.

II.4.8.2.1 Male-to-Female

To male-to-female transsexuals, elimination of sexual hair growth, induction of breast formation and a more female fat distribution are essential. To accomplish this, a near-complete reduction of the biological effects of androgens is required. Administration of oestrogens alone will suppress gonadotrophin output and therefore androgen production, but dual therapy with one compound that suppresses androgen secretion or action and a second compound that supplies oestrogen is more effective.

Suppression of Androgen Secretion or Action

Several agents are available to inhibit androgen secretion or action. In Europe, the most widely used drug is cyproterone acetate (usually 50 mg twice daily), a progestational compound with antiandrogenic properties. If it is not available, medroxyprogesterone acetate, 5–10 mg/day, is an alternative, although less effective. Nonsteroidal antiandrogens, such as flutamide and nilutamide, are also used, but they increase gonadotrophin secretion, causing increased secretion of testosterone and oestradiol; the latter is a desirable effect in this context. Spironolactone (100 mg twice daily), a diuretic with antiandrogenic properties, has similar effects. Long-acting gonadotrophin-releasing hormone (GnRH) agonists, used as monthly injections, also inhibit gonadotrophin secretion. Finasteride (5 mg/day), a 5-α-reductase inhibitor, might also be considered.

Oestrogen

There is a wide range of oestrogens from which to choose. Oral ethinyloestradiol (50–100 μg/day) is a potent and inexpensive oestrogen, but it may cause venous thrombosis, particularly in subjects over 40 years (van Kesteren et al. 1997; Moore et al. 2003; Toorians et al. 2003) and should no longer be used. Oral 17β-oestradiol valerate 2–4 mg per day or transdermal 17β-oestradiol, 100 μg twice a week, is the treatment of choice (Toorians et al. 2003).

Consequences

There are a variety of consequences of hormonal therapy in male-to-female transsexuals:

- Sexual hair – adult male beard growth is very resistant to inhibition by combined hormonal intervention, and in Caucasian subjects additional measures to eliminate facial hair are necessary. Sexual hair growth on other parts of the body respond more favourably (Giltay and Gooren 2000).
- Breast development – breast formation starts almost immediately after initiation of oestrogen administration and goes through periods of growth and standstill. Androgens have an inhibitory effect on breast formation and, therefore, oestrogens will be most effective in a milieu devoid of androgen action. After 2 years of oestrogen administration, no further development can be expected. It is quantitatively satisfactory in 40–50 % of the subjects. The attained size is often disproportional to the male dimension of the chest and height of the subject, so the subject may desire surgical breast augmentation. Older age also impedes full breast formation.
- Skin – androgen deprivation leads to a decreased activity of the sebaceous glands, which may result in a dry skin or brittle nails (Giltay and Gooren 2000).
- Body composition – following androgen deprivation there is an increase in subcutaneous fat and a decrease in lean body mass. Body weight usually increases.
- Testes – lacking gonadotrophic stimulation, the testes become atrophic and may enter the inguinal canal, which may cause discomfort.
- Prostate – atrophy of the prostate may produce transient dribbling following micturition. This is usually temporary.

- Voice – antiandrogens and oestrogens have no effect on the properties of the voice, so male-to-female transsexuals may wish to consult a specialized phoniatric centre for speech therapy. Maleness of the voice is not so much determined by the pitch of the voice as by chest resonance and volume. Speech therapy may lead to more feminine speech (de Bruin et al. 2000). Laryngeal surgery may change the pitch of the voice but reduces its range.

Long-term Therapy

After reassignment surgery, including orchiectomy, hormone therapy must be continued. Some subjects still experience growth of sexual hair in a male pattern, and antiandrogens appear to be effective in reducing it, although the dose may be reduced. Continuous oestrogen therapy is required to avoid symptoms of hormone deprivation and, most importantly, to prevent osteoporosis (van Kesteren et al. 1998). We have found that oestrogens alone are capable of maintaining bone mass in male-to-female transsexuals. There was an inverse relationship between serum luteinizing hormone (LH) concentrations and bone mineral density, so serum LH may serve as an indicator of the adequacy of sex steroid administration.

II.4.8.2.2 Female-to-Male

The goal of treatment in female-to-male transsexuals is to induce virilization, including a male pattern of sexual hair and male physical contours, and to stop menses. The principal hormonal treatment is a testosterone preparation. The most commonly used preparations are testosterone esters in doses of 200 – 250 mg intramuscularly every 2 weeks. Recently, transdermal testosterone gels have become available. Occasionally menstrual bleeding does not cease with this regimen, and addition of a progestational agent is necessary. If a transdermal testosterone preparation is used, addition of a progestational agent is nearly always necessary.

Consequences

There are a variety of consequences of hormonal therapy in female-to-male transsexuals:

- Hair – the development of sexual hair follows essentially the pattern observed in pubertal boys: first the upper lip, then chin, then cheeks, etc. (Giltay and Gooren 2000). The degree of hirsutism can usually be predicted from the degree and pattern in male members of the same family. The same applies to the occurrence of alopecia androgenica.
- Voice – deepening of the voice occurs after 6 – 10 weeks of androgen administration and is irreversible. Androgen administration leads to a reduction of subcutaneous fat but increases abdominal fat. The increase in lean body mass is on average 4 kg, and the increase in body weight is usually greater.
- Acne – acne occurs in approximately 40 %, usually very pronounced on the back, similar to that observed in hypogonadal men starting androgen treatment past the age of normal puberty (Giltay and Gooren 2000).
- Clitoral enlargement – clitoral enlargement occurs in all, but the degree varies. In approximately 5 – 8 %, the size becomes sufficient for vaginal intercourse.
- Libido – most subjects will note an increase.
- Other – ovaries show polycystic changes, and androgen administration may decrease glandular activity of the breasts but does not reduce their size.

After bilateral oophorectomy, androgen therapy must be continued to maintain virilization and prevent osteoporosis (van Kesteren et al. 1998). Suppression of the serum LH concentration to within the normal range can be used to indicate the adequacy of androgen administration.

II.4.8.3 Side-Effects of Hormonal Sex Reassignment

In a review of 816 male-to-female transsexuals and 293 female-to-male transsexuals (total exposure 10,152 patient years), mortality was no higher than in a comparison group (van Kesteren et al. 1997). However, cross-sex hormone administration may be associated with side-effects (Futterweit 1998):

- Venous thromboembolism – the incidence of these side-effects was 2 – 6 % in male-to-female transsexuals treated with oral ethinyloestradiol. In vitro studies show that this thrombogenic effect is typical of oral ethinyloestradiol but not of oral 17β-oestradiol (Toorians et al. 2003). Because immobilization is also a risk factor for venous thromboembolic events, oestrogen administration should be discontinued 3 – 4 weeks before elective surgical interventions. Once subjects are fully mobilized again, oestrogen therapy may be resumed.
- Atherosclerosis – although the considerable sex difference in the prevalence of cardiovascular disease between men and women would lead one to expect an effect of hormonal treatment, the actual risk remains to be established. The effects of

oestrogen administration to male-to-female and of androgens to female-to-male transsexuals on biochemical risk markers have been studied. It appeared that oestrogen administration had more negative effects on these risk markers than androgens (Elbers et al. 2003).

- Lactotroph adenoma – four cases of lactotroph adenoma (prolactinoma) following high-dose oestrogen administration have been reported in subjects who had normal serum prolactin concentrations before therapy (van Kesteren et al. 1997). Though causality has not been established, we recommend that serum prolactin levels continue to be monitored in oestrogen-treated male-to-female transsexuals, also in the long-term.
- Breast cancer – there are two reports of male-to-female transsexuals who were found to have breast carcinomas while they were receiving oestrogen treatment (van Kesteren et al. 1997). In recent years no cases have been observed, but self examination of the breast must be part of the monitoring of oestrogen administration, following the same guidelines that exist for other women.
- Prostate cancer – three cases of prostate cancer in male-to-female transsexuals taking oestrogen have been reported (Van Haarst et al. 1998). It is not clear whether these cancers were oestrogen-sensitive or whether they were present before oestrogen administration started and progressed to become hormone-independent.
- Ovarian cancer – we recently observed two cases of ovarian carcinoma in a long-term, testosterone-treated, female-to-male transsexual. Ovaries of female-to-male transsexuals taking androgens show similarities with polycystic ovaries, which are also more likely to develop malignancies. Therefore, it seems reasonable to remove the ovaries of androgen-treated female-to-male transsexuals after a successful transition to the male role.
- Contraindications – because of the potential side-effects described above, hormonal treatment is contraindicated in certain situations. Contraindications to oestrogen use are a strong family history of breast cancer or a lactotroph adenoma, and to androgen-use lipid disorders with cardiovascular complications. Contraindications against the use of high doses of either sex steroid are cardiovascular disease, cerebrovascular disease, thromboembolic disease, marked obesity, poorly controlled diabetes mellitus, and active liver disease (Futterweit 1998; Levy et al. 2003; Moore et al. 2003).

II.4.8.4 Juvenile Gender Dysphoria

Adult transsexuals often recall that their gender dysphoria started early in life, well before puberty. Children with gender identity problems increasingly come to the attention of the psychomedical care system. A reliable estimation indicates that only about 20% will become transsexuals in adolescence (Cohen-Kettenis and van Goozen 1998). Homosexuality will be more often the outcome.

If, in expert opinion, a child's cross-sex gender identity will not change during long-term follow-up the individual may be spared the torment of (full) pubescent development of the "wrong" secondary sex characteristics (Cohen-Kettenis and van Goozen 1998). Depot forms of luteinizing hormone releasing hormone (LHRH) antagonists/agonists, following the regimen in children with precocious puberty, can be used when clear signs of sexual maturation are evident in order to delay pubertal development until an age that a balanced and responsible decision can be made to transition to the other sex (Gooren and Dellemarre van de Waal 1996).

References

Cohen-Kettenis PT (2001) Gender identity disorder in DSM? J Am Acad Child Adolesc Psychiatry 40:391

Cohen-Kettenis PT, van Goozen SH (1998) Pubertal delay as an aid in diagnosis and treatment of a transsexual adolescent. Eur Child Adolesc Psychiatry 7:246–248

de Bruin MD, Coerts MJ, Greven AJ (2000) Speech therapy in the management of male-to-female transsexuals. Folia Phoniatr Logop 52:220–227

Elbers JM, Giltay EJ, Teerlink T, Scheffer PG, Asscheman H, Seidell JC et al (2003) Effects of sex steroids on components of the insulin resistance syndrome in transsexual subjects. Clin Endocrinol (Oxf) 58:562–571

Futterweit W (1998) Endocrine therapy of transsexualism and potential complications of long-term treatment. Arch Sex Behav 27:209–226

Giltay EJ, Gooren LJ (2000) Effects of sex steroid deprivation/administration on hair growth and skin sebum production in transsexual males and females. J Clin Endocrinol Metab 85:2913–2921

Gooren L, Delemarre- van de Waal H (1996) Memo on the feasibility of endocrine interventions in juvenile transsexuals. J Psychol Hum Sex 8:69–74

Levy A, Crown A, Reid R (2003) Endocrine intervention for transsexuals. Clin Endocrinol (Oxf) 59:409–418

Moore E, Wisniewski A, Dobs A (2003) Endocrine treatment of transsexual people: a review of treatment regimens, outcomes, and adverse effects. J Clin Endocrinol Metab 88: 3467–3473

Toorians AW, Thomassen MC, Zweegman S, Magdeleyns EJ, Tans G, Gooren LJ et al (2003) Venous thrombosis and changes of hemostatic variables during cross-sex hormone treatment in transsexual people. J Clin Endocrinol Metab 88:5723–5729

Van Haarst EP, Newling DW, Gooren LJ, Asscheman H, Prenger

DM (1998) Metastatic prostatic carcinoma in a male-to-female transsexual. Br J Urol 81:776
van Kesteren PJ, Asscheman H, Megens JA, Gooren LJ (1997) Mortality and morbidity in transsexual subjects treated with cross-sex hormones. Clin Endocrinol (Oxf) 47:337–342
van Kesteren P, Lips P, Gooren LJ, Asscheman H, Megens J (1998) Long-term follow-up of bone mineral density and bone metabolism in transsexuals treated with cross-sex hormones. Clin Endocrinol (Oxf) 48:347–354

II.4.9 Treatment of Sexual Dysfunction

L.J.G. Gooren

Summary

The introduction of the phosphodiesterase type 5 inhibitors (PDE inhibitors) has been a major step forward in the treatment of erectile dysfunction (ED). Though efficacious and safe, 50% of men discontinue treatment, largely because other sexological issues have not been properly addressed. To predict onset and duration of action, insight into the pharmacokinetics of the PDE inhibitors is required.

- In men whose testosterone levels are low, testosterone substitution may booster the efficacy of PDE inhibitors.
- Before receiving PDE inhibitor the cardiovascular status of a patient must be assessed.

The main action of testosterone is on the central nervous system. It improves libido and mood. Levels in the low-normal range suffice.

Hyperprolactinaemia impairs sexual interest and leads to secondary ED. Dopamine agonists are the treatment of choice.

Men with paraphilias may be treated with drugs that lower androgen action if the desire to act out their paraphilia is high.

II.4.9.1 Erectile Dysfunction

The availability of a highly efficacious and relatively safe compound such as the phosphodiesterase type 5 inhibitor sildenafil has had a profound impact on diagnosis and treatment of erectile dysfunction (ED). Once the domain of the urologist attempting to define the precise aetiology, ED is now largely treated by first-line physicians, without much of a diagnostic work-up. Despite the simplicity and safety of the present therapy of ED, approximately 50% of patients discontinue treatment. The reasons for discontinuations lie mostly in an incomplete evaluation of the sexual problem. Hypogonadism, ejaculatory dysfunction, lower urinary tract symptoms, depression, and last but not least partner issues may all be components of the sexual dysfunction of the patient, and apparently restoration of erectile function does not necessarily imply restoration of a happy sex life (Montorsi and Althof 2004). Nevertheless, the introduction of the phosphodiesterase type 5 inhibitors has substantially improved the therapeutic options for ED.

II.4.9.1.1 Phosphodiesterase Type 5 Inhibitors

The identification of pathways in the physiology of erection and the discovery of the importance of nitric oxide (NO) and its downstream effects lie at the basis of the development of the phosphodiesterase type 5 inhibitors (PDE inhibitors). Subsequent to sexual stimulation, NO arising from the nerve endings of non-adrenergic non-cholinergic innervation of the corpus cavernosum activates guanylyl cyclase, an enzyme that catalyses the conversion of GTP to cGMP. At the cellular level cGMP is broken down to 5-GMP by phosphodiesterase type 5. Via a molecular cascade cGMP lowers intracellular calcium and vascular smooth muscle of the corpus cavernosum relaxes, resulting in an increased penile blood flow thus facilitating the initiation and maintenance of an erection.

The pharmacological action of PDE inhibitors manifests itself only when a person is sexually aroused, which distinguishes this class of drugs from intracavernosal injections. This is also important information for the user (Seftel 2004).

The efficacy and relative safety of PDE inhibitors is well documented now. They have a common mode of action, the inhibition of PDE 5. Selectivity and tissue localization of the PDE inhibitors determine the side-effect profiles and safety.

There are presently three PDE inhibitors available for prescription: sildenafil, vardenafil and tadalafil. All are efficacious, but there are differences in pharmacokinetic profile, interactions with food and drugs, and possible side-effects. Taking nitrate medications is an absolute contraindication to the use of PDE inhibitors since PDE inhibitors increase the potential for excessively low blood pressure. Low blood pressure, though to a lesser degree, has also been observed with PDE inhibitors in men taking alpha adrenoreceptor antagonists, such as doxazosin, prazosin, terazosin, alfuzosin or tamsulosin, which are used as antihypertensive agents or for symptomatic relief of lower urinary tract symptoms (LUTS). The latter is relevant since sexual dysfunction is not rare in men with LUTS, both significantly increasing with age, and possibly sharing aetiological factors (Rosen et al. 2003). Drugs such as erythromycin, ketoconazole and itraconazole, and protease inhibitors used in HIV treatment such as saquinavir, indinavir and ritovir may slow liver metabolism of PDE inhibitors and may increase plasma levels and the effect of PDE inhibitors. Grapefruit juice may have a similar effect on liver metabolism. Lower doses must be used in patients with liver and/or kidney disease.

Sildenafil and vardenafil work best if no (fatty) food has been taken within the previous 2 h, while tadalafil can be used without regard to food.

Common adverse effects attributable to vasodilatory effects include headache, flushing, stuffy nose, stomach pain, back pain (tadalafil) and indigestion. Visual problems (for example, blurred vision, increased sensitivity to light, bluish haze, or temporary difficulty distinguishing between blue and green) may occur, more often with sildenafil since the latter is less selective in inhibiting phosphodiesterase 6 in the retina.

The prescribed tablet strength is swallowed 30 – 60 min before sexual activity. Tadalafil has a longer duration of increased sensitivity for developing an erection (up to 24 – 36 h) compared with sildenafil and vardenafil (up to 4 – 12 h).

There is no convincing evidence that the three available PDE inhibitors differ significantly in their clinical efficacy. For sildenafil (50 and 100 mg) and tadalafil (10 and 20 mg) there is a dose–response relationship, which is not so much the case for vardenafil (10 and 20 mg) (Carson et al. 2004). In general starting with the lowest dose of PDE inhibitors is recommended.

The feature that distinguishes the three PDE inhibitors is their pharmacokinetic profile, which impacts on their clinical use, in terms of the initiation of optimal pharmacological effect and duration of pharmacological action [for review see Porst (2004)]. The time to maximal plasma concentration (in minutes) is on average 60 (variation 30 – 120) for sildenafil, 120 (variation 30 – 720!) for tadalafil and 60 (variation 30 – 120) for vardenafil. These are statistical data and individual patients may experience a faster onset of action. This information lets patients plan prospective sexual action. Another significant pharmacokinetic variable is the half-life of the drug, which provides an indication of how long the drug can be expected to be pharmacologically active after ingestion. The half-life of sildenafil 100 mg is 3 – 4 h; for tadalafil, 20 mg 17 hours; and for vardenafil, 3 – 6 h. This information lets the patient make reasonable assumptions about how long they can expect the ingested compound to be pharmacologically active.

It is not rare for patients to wish to "experiment" with the available PDE inhibitors to find the drug that suits them best. Patients do have distinctly different sexual habits with regard to timing of sexual activity. Another consideration is the "readiness" of the patients when sexual activity is initiated by the partner.

The above information on dose–response effects (sildenafil and tadalafil), the interaction with (particularly fat-rich) food in slowing absorption, and the pharmacokinetic profiles may provide guidance. Patients who, in a series of at least four attempts to have intercourse, do not respond to the maximum dose of one of the PDE inhibitors are unlikely to respond to the others.

Naturally, patients starting treatment with a PDE inhibitor will experience some anxiety about whether the new drug will indeed induce an erection. Anxiety may reduce sexual arousal, which is a necessary condition for the desired pharmacological action of PDE inhibitors. Therefore, in case the patient recognizes this as a potential problem, testing the efficacy of the drug first with masturbation may be recommended.

At least 50 % of patients suffering from ED have endothelial dysfunction, and there are early indications that chronic treatment with PDE inhibitors might improve their vascular function (Jackson 2003; Reffelmann and Kloner 2003). At the same time chronic use would obviate the need to take a PDE inhibitor before engaging in sexual activity.

II.4.9.1.2 PDE Inhibitors and the Cardiovascular System

When the first PDE inhibitor sildenafil was introduced there was great concern about the cardiovascular safety of this class of drugs. In many a patient the aetiology of ED is (also) based on vascular disease. The availability of the drug prompted patients to resume sexual activity after prolonged periods of inactivity. The pharmacological action of PDE inhibitors is vasodilatory. Fears arose that these elements would lead to myocardial ischaemia or infarction when intercourse was attempted. Fortunately, these concerns have remained unsubstantiated. Placebo-controlled studies fail to show a higher cardiovascular morbidity/mortality in patients using PDE inhibitors (Hutter 2004; Kloner 2004). Naturally, before starting PDE inhibitors, the cardiovascular risks of the patient must be assessed. Factors such as hypertension, biochemical risk markers, angina pectoris, arrhythmias, cardiomyopathy, congestive heart failure and a history of myocardial infarction and the time elapsed since and whether these conditions are adequately treated must be weighed. The Princeton Consensus Panel has drafted an algorithm for stratification of cardiac patients as being at low, intermediate or high risk of using PDE inhibitors for ED (DeBusk et al. 2000;

Seftel 2004; Seftel et al. 2004). Patients with intermediate and high risks may benefit from a cardiological evaluation to optimize their cardiac condition. A rule of thumb indicator is whether a patient can walk 1 km in 10 min without cardiac symptoms, an equivalent of the physical exertion of sexual intercourse.

Patients should be instructed to report use of a PDE inhibitor in the foregoing 24 h (sildenafil / vardenafil) or 48 h (tadalafil) when a cardiovascular emergency occurs that might need treatment with nitrates.

II.4.9.1.3 Centrally Acting Oral Agents

Increasing understanding of the physiology of erections and particularly the role of the central nervous system has led to the development of apomorphine hydrochloride. This compound targets structures in the central nervous system associated with erectile function. Apomorphine is a non-specific dopaminergic receptor agonist that acts at the paraventricular nucleus of the hypothalamus (Altwein and Keuler 2001; Martinez et al. 2003). Apomorphine is available in a sublingual formulation at doses of 2 and 3 mg. Apomorphine is a fast acting agent (maximum plasma concentrations at 15–20 min) that has been shown in various clinical trials to be more effective at achieving erections firm enough for intercourse compared to placebo. But its efficacy is less than that of the PDE inhibitors (Heaton and Altwein 2001). Side-effects have been reported in clinical trials. At 6 mg dosages of apomorphine nausea has been reported in up to 34% of patients (Bukofzer and Livesey 2001). At the approved dosage of 2 and 3 mg the incidence of nausea decreases to only 7%. Other significant known side-effects include headache, dizziness and yawning.

II.4.9.1.4 Intracavernosal Agents

Nowadays before patients resort to intracavernosal therapy, they have usually tried oral therapy unsuccessfully. For intracavernosal injections a patient or his partner must possess adequate manual dexterity to carry out the penile injections. Patients must receive information on the potential adverse effects of the injections. Side-effects include penile scarring, pain, ecchymosis and prolonged erection. The incidence of these side-effects depends on the agent injected. The most common agents used in practice include prostaglandin E_1, papaverine and phentolamine, and the α-blocker moxisylyte.

Phentolamine, which is an alpha adrenergic antagonist, has a very poor erectile response in humans when used on its own. It is therefore usually combined with either papaverine alone (Bimix) or with papaverine and prostaglandin E_1 (Trimix). Papaverine is a nonspecific phosphodiesterase inhibitor that causes an increase in both intracellular cAMP and cGMP. Increases in these molecules cause a relaxation in penile smooth muscle and eventual erection.

Prostaglandin E_1 modulates adenyl cyclase to increase cAMP concentrations. This in turn leads to a decrease in intracellular free calcium and smooth muscle relaxation in the penis (Porst 1996). Although prostaglandin E_1 leads to significantly fewer occurrences of penile fibrosis and priapism, some studies quote a 13% incidence of penile pain with injection of this medication. In an effort to reduce the adverse effects of these medications used alone, combination therapy with a mixture of phentolamine, papaverine and prostaglandin E_1 (Trimix) at lower doses often will provide a higher efficacy, lower incidence of pain and lower cost per dose (Bennett et al. 1991).

II.4.9.1.5 Intraurethral Agents

Prostaglandin E_1 (PGE_1) (trade name MUSE) is the most common agent used for this purpose, and by delivering the active compound into the urethra there is transportation of the compound into the corpus spongiosum and later into the corpora cavernosum where smooth muscle relaxation occurs.

Efficacy rates are variable: from a 13.6% response to a 64% response (when a constriction band is used) (Hellstrom et al. 1996). The most common side-effect of intraurethral agents is local penile pain which occurs in more than one-third of patients. Urinary tract infection, dizziness, penile pain and urethral bleeding are other known side-effects.

II.4.9.1.6 Non-pharmacologic Treatment

Non-pharmacologic options may be offered as second-line treatment in lieu of intraurethral or intracavernosal injection for patients who do not respond to or cannot tolerate oral therapy. Vacuum erection devices increase corporal blood flow, and a constrictor ring is then used to retain this blood within the penis. Satisfaction is variable (27–74%), and this technique can cause discomfort and bruising of the penis (Hatzichristou and Pescatori 2001).

Surgical options exist for patients with ED. Penile arterial bypass surgery is appropriate in only a select group of patients (men under 35 years of age who have no generalized vascular disease and in whom an isolated injury has obstructed blood flow). Penile implants are available for patients who have not responded to more conservative treatment. This procedure is invasive, irreversible and subject to complications such as infection, erosion and mechanical failure. There is, however, a high rate of patient and partner satisfaction (Hatzichristou and Pescatori 2001).

II.4.9.2 Retarded Ejaculation

Retarded ejaculation is not infrequent in the ageing male. It may be related to a decrease in sexual arousability, often associated with ageing. In general, measures to improve erectile function will also benefit retarded ejaculation. It is also often found in men with lower urinary tract symptoms and there is some preliminary evidence that an alpha adrenoreceptor blocker such as alfuzosin might alleviate the complaint. It may be associated with the use of psychotropic drugs such as serotonin reuptake inhibitors and monoamine oxidase inhibitors.

II.4.9.3 Rapid Ejaculation

Rapid or premature ejaculation is difficult to treat (Waldinger 2004). The complaint may be presented as ED by patients who are unable to attain sufficient penile rigidity after rapid ejaculation. Several oral agents, such as selective serotonin reuptake inhibitors, monoamine oxidase inhibitors and tricyclic antidepressants (e.g. imipramine and clomipramine) or topical anaesthetic agents (e.g. lidocaine) have been recommended (Montague et al. 2004). Of late sildenafil has also been helpful. Sexual counselling may help the patient to have better control of the ejaculatory response.

II.4.9.4 Testosterone Treatment

The evidence for testosterone-induced masculinization of certain aspects of sexual behaviour in men is persuasive. Although clinicians have long been impressed with the influence of androgen replacement on sexual functioning of androgen-deficient men, scientific proof that androgen plays a role in human sexuality is a product of the 1970s and 1980s (Bancroft 2002).

Most of the information has been collected from androgen withdrawal/replacement studies of hypogonadal men. It is now clear that androgens are fundamental to normal sexual behaviour in men, although they do not have a simple on/off effect on sexual functions, and are not the only factor involved in male sexual behaviour (Gooren and Kruijver 2002).When androgen production is deficient from the foetal/prepubertal stage, as in hypogonadotrophic hypogonadism and Klinefelter syndrome, the response to androgen replacement during puberty or later may be manifestly impaired, expressing itself as relative sexual inertia. The reason probably is that emotional, cognitive and social learning are also elements of the manifestations of testosterone on adolescent and adult sexuality (Gooren and Kruijver 2002).

The distinction between sexual interest and erectile function and its subdivision has helped considerably in clarifying the role of androgens in male function (Bancroft and Wu 1983; Bancroft 2002).

Spontaneous erections, particularly those that occur during sleep (nocturnal penile tumescence, NPT), and probably fantasy-induced erections are androgen-dependent, whereas erections in response to erotic (e.g. visual or tactile) stimuli are relatively androgen-independent (Bancroft and Wu 1983). These early studies addressed, however, maximum increase in penile circumference as the only parameter, but more recent work suggests that androgens affect penile responses to erotic stimuli with regard to duration of response, degree of rigidity and speed of detumescence (Carani et al. 1996). In men the principal target of androgens appears to be sexual interest or appetite (Bancroft and Wu 1983; Bancroft 2002). Androgens may enhance the persistence of attention to eroticism, which, in turn, may affect sexual behaviour. It has been argued that androgen influences pleasurable awareness during sexual activity, possibly by enhancing sensory (genital) function.

It is not known how the effects of androgens on the central nervous system are mediated. Preliminary evidence suggests that there may be a noradrenergic mediation of sexual arousal, involving both central arousal and peripheral inhibition of erectile responses (Bancroft 1995).

Although it has been convincingly established that the main effect of androgens on male sexual functioning is on the central nervous system, additional evidence now suggests that they also affect nitric oxide synthase in the corpus cavernosum [nitric oxide induces smooth muscle relaxation of the penile vasculature, essential for penile erection (Morelli et al. 2004)] and that androgen administration may be helpful in men who respond poorly to treatment of ED with phosphodiesterase inhibitors (Foresta et al. 2004). So there seems to be a point in treating men with low or low-normal plasma testosterone, who do not respond well to phosphodiesterase inhibitors, with testosterone.

In most studies, 60–70% of the reference values of testosterone were sufficient to maintain sexual functions in adult men (Gooren 1987; Buena et al. 1993). One study suggested that thresholds for NPT are even lower than those for normal sexual functioning (Carani et al. 1996). From this it follows that in men with sexual dysfunction and normal androgen levels, additional testosterone is likely to be of no help, although a short-lived beneficial effect from additional testosterone in eugonadal men who complained of lack of sexual interest has been found (Anderson et al. 1992) and confirmed in men receiving testosterone in a male contraceptive study (Alexander et al. 1997), but the follow-up was limited to 6 weeks. There is no evidence that long-term high testosterone levels enhance male sexual function. In general it has been difficult to establish a relationship in men between circulating testosterone levels (above a certain therapeutic threshold) and levels of sexual responses (Gooren 1987; Buena et al. 1993).

Information on the timing of onset of behavioural effects after withdrawal of androgens is limited. With both naturally occurring and pharmacologically induced hypotestosteronaemia, behavioural effects and a reduction in seminal emission become clear after 2 weeks and reach a maximum after 4 weeks or later. A sexually active partner may be a factor in prolongation of sexual activity (Bancroft 2002). In the majority of men the ejaculatory capacity is profoundly decreased after androgen withdrawal, affecting sexual behaviour in its own right (Bancroft 2002).

Restoration of testosterone effects is probably somewhat quicker, approximately over 1 – 2 weeks, and there may be a relationship with the duration of foregoing androgen deficiency (Bancroft 2002).

Testosterone is currently available in oral, intramuscular, subcutaneous and transdermal preparations. Recent advances in testosterone replacement therapy include testosterone gels, which provide flexibility in dosing and minimal skin irritation resulting in good compliance, and the development of longer acting intramuscular preparations (testosterone undecanoate), which result in more stable testosterone levels with longer injection intervals up to 12 weeks (Gooren and Bunck 2004).

In summary, it is certain that androgens are powerful modulators of the biochemistry of peripheral structures related to sexual functioning and the brain, thus modulating behaviour. Their effects are strongly intertwined with idiosyncratic aspects of the person concerned: they enhance sexual motivation in men, be it a heterosexual, homosexual or paraphilic man. The blood level of testosterone critical for normal male sexual function varies between individuals. In most males, 60 – 70 % of the reference values was sufficient (Gooren 1987; Buena et al. 1993). In men with sexual dysfunction and normal androgen levels, additional testosterone is likely to be of no help, although a short-lived beneficial effect from additional testosterone in eugonadal men who complained of lack of sexual interest has been found.

II.4.9.5 Pubertal Development

Pubertal development is associated with a gradual though variable increase in sexual interest and activity, but it has been difficult to relate levels of androgens to the development of adolescent sexuality, probably because there is a fair but individually different amount of socially influenced learning which impacts on this hormone–behaviour relation. Physical pubertal development may be a better predictor of sexual interest and behaviour than free testosterone (Finkelstein et al. 1998; Halpern et al. 1998) but one study was able to demonstrate a more direct relationship between salivary/plasma testosterone and sexual activity (Udry et al. 1985).

II.4.9.6 Sexual Function and Ageing

Sexual functions decline with ageing. Ageing as such is the best predictor of ED, with diabetes mellitus and atherosclerotic cardiovascular diseases further increasing the risk (Johannes et al. 2000).

Ageing is also associated with a variable decline in bioavailable testosterone levels, but levels remain well above minimum testosterone levels for normal sexual functioning established in younger men. The hypothesis has been advanced that ageing men are less sensitive to the actions of testosterone (Schiavi and Rehman 1995), but as indicated above testosterone is not the first-line treatment in elderly men with ED, but it may be adjuvant treatment when phosphodiesterase inhibitors are not helpful and plasma testosterone is low.

II.4.9.7 Hyperprolactinaemia

The role of prolactin in males is not well understood. No convincing evidence has emerged that a lower than normal prolactin level impairs sexual functioning in humans (Carani et al. 1996). In women the initial symptom of hyperprolactinaemia is mostly a disturbance in reproductive physiology (amenorrhoea, infertility), leading to a relatively early discovery of the condition. Interference with female sexual functioning has been reported but is less clear-cut than in men. It may be manifested as a depressive disorder affecting orgasmic capacity, which improves upon treatment with dopamine agonists.

In men, sexual dysfunction, but more often symptoms of a pituitary tumour may lead to the discovery of hyperprolactinaemia. This condition accounts for less than 2 % of cases of sexual dysfunction in men (Carani et al. 1996). About 80 – 90 % of men with chronic hyperprolactinaemia have complaints such as loss of libido, erectile weakness (De Rosa et al. 2004) and, frequently, difficulty ejaculating (Meston and Frohlich 2000). The mechanism by which hyperprolactinaemia impairs sexual function is not completely understood. In cases of associated testosterone deficiency, testosterone substitution did not reverse the symptoms (Carani et al.

1996). Dopaminergic drugs restored sexual function even before testosterone levels had risen to normal (De Rosa et al. 2004).

Most experts now believe that hyperprolactinaemia impairs sexual function through a CNS mechanism by interference with neurotransmitter activity, in particular dopamine and endogenous opioids (Meston and Frohlich 2000). In some men with sexual complaints, serum prolactin levels may be found to be elevated in the presence of normal gonadotrophin and testosterone levels. They may have macroprolactinaemia, and their sexual problems cannot be ascribed to their spurious hyperprolactinaemia (Schlechte 2002).

Administration of antipsychotic drugs is not rarely associated with marked hyperprolactinaemia. And it is increasingly clear that this drug-induced hyperprolactinaemia may produce galactorrhoea, gynaecomastia, sexual dysfunction and mood disturbances (Halbreich et al. 2003). The condition is often not diagnosed since the psychological effects are viewed as part of the disease requiring antipsychotic medication. In cases of clinically relevant hyperprolactinaemia, the dose of the antipsychotic drug may be lowered or an alternative drug must be chosen.

II.4.9.8 Paraphilias and their Pharmacologic Treatment

Persons with a paraphilia are compulsively responsive to and dependent on an unusual and often personally or socially unacceptable sexual stimulus for sexual arousal and orgasm. No known correlation between paraphilic behaviour and an endocrine condition, past or present, has been detected (Gijs and Gooren 1996). Paraphilias occur predominantly in men but also may occur in women. There is no convincing evidence that circulating testosterone levels are higher in (violent) sex offenders than controls (Gijs 1996). The socially intolerable paraphilias (such as rape, exhibitionism and paedophilia) may bring persons into conflict with the law, and (forensic) medicine may play a part in pharmacological interventions aimed at helping paraphiliacs. When dealing with this category it is mandatory to observe professional neutrality. As in normal persons, testosterone lowers the threshold of occurrence of erotosexual imagery and sexual activity in paraphiliacs. However, it has no effect on the contents of the imagery (Gijs and Gooren 1996). Anti-androgens may be of benefit, particularly for those paraphilias characterized by intense and frequent sexual desire and arousal. To be effective, hormonal treatment must be accompanied by sexologic counselling. The most widely used drug in the United States is medroxyprogesterone acetate, and in Canada and Europe cyproterone acetate. Luteinizing hormone-releasing hormone (LHRH) agonists have also been successfully used (Reilly et al. 2000). Both are available in injectable form, thus facilitating greater compliance with the treatment programme. Long-term androgen deprivation may lead to osteopenia (Grasswick and Bradford 2003). Some forms of paraphilia are not so much characterized by sexual desire but are obsessive-compulsive or impulse control disorders or are acted out in depressive mood states, and do not respond well to anti-androgenic intervention. These can be successfully treated with psychotropic drugs such as modern antidepressants in view of the role of the dopaminergic system in motivational processes.

References

Alexander GM, Swerdloff RS, Wang C et al (1997) Androgen-behavior correlations in hypogonadal men and eugonadal men. I. Mood and response to auditory sexual stimuli. Horm Behav 31:110–119

Altwein JE, Keuler FU (2001) Oral treatment of erectile dysfunction with apomorphine SL. Urol Int 67:257–263

Anderson RA, Bancroft J, Wu FC (1992) The effects of exogenous testosterone on sexuality and mood of normal men. J Clin Endocrinol Metab 75:1503–1507

Bancroft J (1995) Are the effects of androgens on male sexuality noradrenergically mediated? Some consideration of the human. Neurosci Biobehav Rev 19:325–330

Bancroft J (2002) Biological factors in human sexuality. J Sex Res 39:15–21

Bancroft J, Wu FC (1983) Changes in erectile responsiveness during androgen replacement therapy. Arch Sex Behav 12: 59–66

Bennett AH, Carpenter AJ, Barada JH (1991) An improved vasoactive drug combination for a pharmacological erection program. J Urol 146:1564–1565

Buena F, Swerdloff RS, Steiner BS et al (1993) Sexual function does not change when serum testosterone levels are pharmacologically varied within the normal male range. Fertil Steril 59:1118–1123

Bukofzer S, Livesey N (2001) Safety and tolerability of apomorphine SL (Uprima). Int J Impot Res 13 (Suppl 3):S40–S44

Carani C, Granata AR, Fustini MF, Marrama P (1996) Prolactin and testosterone: their role in male sexual function. Int J Androl 19:48–54

Carson C, Giuliano F, Goldstein I et al (2004) The "effectiveness" scale – therapeutic outcome of pharmacologic therapies for ED: an international consensus panel report. Int J Impot Res 16:207–213

DeBusk R, Drory Y, Goldstein I et al (2000) Management of sexual dysfunction in patients with cardiovascular disease: recommendations of The Princeton Consensus Panel. Am J Cardiol 86:175–181

De Rosa M, Zarrilli S, Vitale G et al (2004) Six months of treatment with cabergoline restores sexual potency in hyperprolactinemic males: an open longitudinal study monitoring nocturnal penile tumescence. J Clin Endocrinol Metab 89:621–625

Finkelstein JW, Susman EJ, Chinchilli VM et al (1998) Effects of estrogen or testosterone on self-reported sexual responses and behaviors in hypogonadal adolescents. J Clin Endocrinol Metab 83:2281–2285

Foresta C, Caretta N, Rossato M, Garolla A, Ferlin A (2004) Role of androgens in erectile function. J Urol 171 (6 Pt 1): 2358–2362

Gijs L, Gooren LJ (1996) Hormonal and psychopharmacological interventions in the treatment of paraphilias: an update. J Sex Res 33:273–290

Gooren LJ (1987) Androgen levels and sex functions in testosterone-treated hypogonadal men. Arch Sex Behav 16: 463–473
Gooren LJ, Bunck MC (2004) Androgen replacement therapy: present and future. Drugs 64:1861–1891
Gooren LJ, Kruijver FP (2002) Androgens and male behavior. Mol Cell Endocrinol 198:31–40
Grasswick LJ, Bradford JM (2003) Osteoporosis associated with the treatment of paraphilias: a clinical review of seven case reports. J Forensic Sci 48:849–855
Halbreich U, Kinon BJ, Gilmore JA, Kahn LS (2003) Elevated prolactin levels in patients with schizophrenia: mechanisms and related adverse effects. Psychoneuroendocrinology 28 (Suppl 1):53–67
Halpern CT, Udry JR, Suchindran C (1998) Monthly measures of salivary testosterone predict sexual activity in adolescent males. Arch Sex Behav 27:445–465
Hatzichristou DG, Pescatori ES (2001) Current treatments and emerging therapeutic approaches in male erectile dysfunction. BJU Int 88 (Suppl 3):11–17
Heaton JP, Altwein JE (2001) The role of apomorphine SL in the treatment of male erectile dysfunction. BJU Int 88 (Suppl 3):36–38
Hellstrom WJ, Bennett AH, Gesundheit N et al (1996) A double-blind, placebo-controlled evaluation of the erectile response to transurethral alprostadil. Urology 48:851–856
Hutter AM Jr. (2004) Role of the cardiologist: clinical aspects of managing erectile dysfunction. Clin Cardiol 27 (4 Suppl 1): I3–I7
Jackson G (2003) Erectile dysfunction: a window of opportunity for preventing vascular disease? Int J Clin Pract 57:747
Johannes CB, Araujo AB, Feldman HA, Derby CA, Kleinman KP, McKinlay JB (2000) Incidence of erectile dysfunction in men 40 to 69 years old: longitudinal results from the Massachusetts male aging study. J Urol 163:460–463
Kloner RA (2004) Novel phosphodiesterase type 5 inhibitors: assessing hemodynamic effects and safety parameters. Clin Cardiol 27 (4 Suppl 1):I20–I25
Martinez R, Puigvert A, Pomerol JM, Rodriguez-Villalba R (2003) Clinical experience with apomorphine hydrochloride: the first 107 patients. J Urol 170(6 Pt 1):2352–2355
Meston CM, Frohlich PF (2000) The neurobiology of sexual function. Arch Gen Psychiatry 57:1012–1030
Montague DK, Jarow J, Broderick GA et al (2004) AUA guideline on the pharmacologic management of premature ejaculation. J Urol 172:290–294
Montorsi F, Althof SE (2004) Partner responses to sildenafil citrate (Viagra) treatment of erectile dysfunction. Urology 63: 762–767
Morelli A, Filippi S, Mancina R et al (2004) Androgens regulate phosphodiesterase type 5 expression and functional activity in corpora cavernosa. Endocrinology 145:2253–2263
Porst H (1996) The rationale for prostaglandin E1 in erectile failure: a survey of worldwide experience. J Urol 155: 802–815
Porst H (2004) [Erectile dysfunctionNew drugs with special consideration of the PDE 5 inhibitors]. Urologe A43: 820–828
Reffelmann T, Kloner RA (2003) Therapeutic potential of phosphodiesterase 5 inhibition for cardiovascular disease. Circulation 108:239–244
Reilly DR, Delva NJ, Hudson RW (2000) Protocols for the use of cyproterone, medroxyprogesterone, and leuprolide in the treatment of paraphilia. Can J Psychiatry 45:559–563
Rosen R, Altwein J, Boyle P et al (2003) Lower urinary tract symptoms and male sexual dysfunction: the multinational survey of the aging male (MSAM-7). Eur Urol 44:637–649
Schiavi RC, Rehman J (1995) Sexuality and aging. Urol Clin North Am 22:711–726
Schlechte JA (2002) The macroprolactin problem. J Clin Endocrinol Metab 87:5408–5409
Seftel AD (2004) Phosphodiesterase type 5 inhibitor differentiation based on selectivity, pharmacokinetic, and efficacy profiles. Clin Cardiol 27 (4 Suppl 1):I14–I19
Seftel AD, Mohammed MA, Althof SE (2004) Erectile dysfunction: etiology, evaluation, and treatment options. Med Clin North Am 88:387–416
Udry JR, Billy JO, Morris NM, Groff TR, Raj MH (1985) Serum androgenic hormones motivate sexual behavior in adolescent boys. Fertil Steril 43:90–94
Waldinger MD (2004) Lifelong premature ejaculation: from authority-based to evidence-based medicine. BJU Int 93: 201–207

II.4.10 Therapeutic Options for Benign Prostate Hyperplasia (BPH) and Prostatic Cancer

S.K.W. Leung, S.A. McNeill

Summary

The management of symptomatic benign prostate hyperplasia (BPH) includes:

- Watchful waiting – suitable management of patients with mild symptoms of BPH (International Prostate Symptom Score, IPSS ≤ 7) or patients with moderate or severe symptoms (IPSS ≥ 8) but with minimal bother.
- Medical therapy – suitable management of patients with moderate or severe symptoms with bother.
- Alpha-blockers – alfuzosin, tamsulosin, terazosin and doxazosin are similarly effective and have quicker onset of action.
- 5α-Reductase inhibitors – finasteride and dutasteride are suitable for patients with lower urinary tract symptoms (LUTS) associated with demonstrable prostatic enlargement but the onset of action is slower.
- Combination therapy – combination of alpha-blocker and a 5α-reductase inhibitor suitable in patients with LUTS associated with demonstrable prostatic enlargement.
- Minimally invasive therapy – thermal, radiofrequency or laser are the energy sources used. The efficacies of these modalities are not conclusively proven yet.
- Surgical therapy – suitable for patients who have bothersome symptoms and for those who have developed complications of BPH. This may be open or endoscopic surgery.

The management of locally advanced prostate cancer includes:

- Active monitoring – suitable for patients with low volume and well differentiated prostate cancer with less than 10 years of life expectancy.
- Radical prostatectomy – suitable for patients with localized prostate cancer with more than 10 years of life expectancy.
- Radical radiotherapy – suitable for patients with localized prostate cancer and the results are comparable to those for radical prostatectomy.
- Brachytherapy – suitable for patients with localized low-grade small volume prostate cancer.

The management of locally advanced prostate cancer and metastatic disease includes:

- Surgical castration – the procedure is well tolerated and is effective at lowering testosterone.
- Oestrogen – decrease dosing decreases the risk of cardiovascular toxicity but testosterone levels do not fall to castration levels.
- Luteinizing hormone releasing hormone agonist (LHRHa) – as effective as surgical castration in lowering testosterone levels but can cause an initial flare in tumour growth and therefore initiation of therapy should be covered with 4 weeks of anti-androgen therapy.
- Non-steroidal anti-androgens – bicalutamide is currently being evaluated for monotherapy use in the management of advanced prostate cancer.
- Steroidal anti-androgens – cyproterone acetate causes a decrease in serum androgens and therefore may reduce libido and sexual potency.
- Maximal androgen blockade – patients with severe symptoms due to local cancer spread or metastatic disease or very high prostate specific antigen (PSA) and alkaline phosphatase may achieve quicker symptom control.

The management of hormone relapsed prostate cancer includes:

- Anti-androgen withdrawal – withdrawal of anti-androgen may improve clinical symptoms.
- Second-line hormonal therapy – agents such as oestrogens and steroids may provide a useful symptomatic response.
- Cytotoxic chemotherapy – there are a number of agents evaluated with initial promising results.
- Palliative management – bone pain can be alleviated with local radiotherapy or intravenous strontium. Zoledronic acid, a bisphosphonate, reduces bone pain and delays the onset of skeletal complications. Spinal cord compression is an emergency and is treated with high-dose steroids, local radiotherapy, surgical decompression or percutaneous vertebroplasty.

II.4.10.1 Diagnosis

II.4.10.1.1 Symptoms

- Obstructed symptoms – hesitancy, weak stream, straining, feeling of incomplete emptying and overflow incontinence.
- Irritative symptoms – urgency, frequency, nocturia and urge incontinence.
- International Prostate Symptom Score (IPSS) – structured questionnaire for the assessment of lower urinary tract symptoms (LUTS): mild (0–7), moderate (8–19) and severe (20–35).

The challenge is to establish whether the symptoms are due to benign prostate hyperplasia (BPH) as there are many non-prostatic causes of LUTS. Initial evaluation should start with a general medical history regarding general health, medical conditions that lead to bladder dysfunction or excessive urine production, and family history of prostate disease (BPH and prostate cancer). A specific urinary tract history should also be taken and this would focus on BPH symptoms such as hesitancy, frequency, nocturia, post-micturition dribbling, haematuria, urinary tract infection and urinary retention. The patient's medication needs to be reviewed for drugs that may affect bladder function such as anticholinergics (e.g. chlorpheniramine), which may impair bladder contractility, and α-sympathomimetics (e.g. pseudoephedrine), which may increase outflow resistance.

Several structured symptom questionnaires have been developed, points being assigned for each answer and the sum of which comprises the symptom score. The IPSS (Barry et al. 1992) is the most widely used and recommended questionnaire for the assessment of

Table II.4.3. International Prostate Symptom Score (IPSS) questionnaire with quality of life question

	Not at all	Less than 1 time in 5	Less than half the time	About half the time	More than half the time	Almost always	Your score
1. Incomplete emptying Over the past month, how often have you had a sensation of not emptying your bladder completely after you finish urinating?	0	1	2	3	4	5	
2. Frequency Over the past month, how often have you had to urinate again less than 2 h after you finish urinating?	0	1	2	3	4	5	
3. Intermittency Over the past month, how often have you found you stopped and started again several times when you urinated?	0	1	2	3	4	5	
4. Urgency Over the past month, how often have you found it difficult to postpone urination?	0	1	2	3	4	5	
5. Weak stream Over the past month, how often have you had a weak urinary stream?	0	1	2	3	4	5	
6. Straining Over the past month, how often have you had to push or strain to begin urination?	0 None	1 1 time	2 2 times	3 3 times	4 4 times	5 5 or more times	
7. Nocturia Over the past month, how many times did you most typically get up to urinate from the time you went to bed at night until the time you got up in the morning?	0	1	2	3	4	5	
Total symptom score							

Quality of life due to urinary symptoms	Delighted	Pleased	Mostly satisfied	Mixed – equally satisfied	Mostly dissatisfied	Unhappy	Terrible
If you were to spend the rest of your life with your urinary condition just the way it is now, how would you feel about it? (Circle number)	0	1	2	3	4	5	6

LUTS associated with BPH (Denis et al. 1998). It consists of seven questions relating to the symptoms of BPH and one further quality of life question (Table II.4.3). By using this system, the symptoms can be classified as mild (0–7), moderate (8–19) or severe (20–35). However, the IPSS does not correlate well with other indices of lower urinary tract dysfunction (e.g. flow rates) but is a useful tool for obtaining baseline symptom severity, assessing the response to treatment and detecting the progression of symptoms in patients managed by watchful waiting.

II.4.10.1.2 Physical Examination

- Digital rectal examination (DRE) – simple and cost-effective method for assessing the prostate (size, consistency and surface texture are noted).
- PSA – performed for patients in whom the diagnosis of prostate cancer would alter management. A level of ≥4 ng/ml is abnormal but there are age-specific reference ranges.
- Uroflowmetry – this is an electronic measurement of urinary flow and the lower the maximum flow rate, the higher the probability of bladder outlet obstruction.
- Pressure-flow studies – this invasive test differentiates between patients with detrusor failure (e.g. due to neuropathic disease) and bladder outlet obstruction.
- Urethrocystoscopy – invasive test to allow visualization of the lower urinary tract.
- Transrectal ultrasound of prostate – allows assessment of size and shape of prostate to plan invasive treatment and is used to guide needle biopsies of the prostate.
- Upper tract imaging – useful to rule out upper tract pathology if the patient has reported haematuria or urea and creatinine are deranged.

The abdomen should be carefully examined to assess whether a full bladder is palpable and whether there is evidence of phimosis, which may obstruct urinary flow. DRE is a simple method for assessing prostate health. The normal prostate is about the size of a walnut and has the same rubbery consistency as the tip of the nose. Symmetrical enlargement with a smooth and elastic consistency and preservation of the midline sulcus is consistent with BPH. However, prostate cancer may result in a nodular prostate that can be stony and asymmetrical. A tender prostate suggests prostatitis. DRE tends to underestimate the volume of the prostate especially in those greater than 30 ml (Roehrborn et al. 1997).

II.4.10.1.3 Investigations

Urinalysis should be performed by dipstick testing or by microscopic examination to screen for haematuria or urinary tract infection (UTI). Bladder cancer, carcinoma in situ of the bladder, UTIs, urethral strictures and bladder stones can produce LUTS in men. Although pyuria or haematuria is not always present in these conditions, a normal urinalysis makes these diagnoses less likely (Messing et al. 1992).

The measurement of serum creatinine has been recommended in patients with LUTS. This is to rule out renal insufficiency caused by obstructive uropathy (Denis et al. 1998). It may also be necessary to check the creatinine values prior to imaging studies that require intravenous contrast. Also it is well established that patients with a degree of renal insufficiency have a higher risk of post-operative complications (Mebust et al. 1989).

Prostate cancer can also occur in patients with BPH. Measurement of PSA should be performed for patients for whom the detection of prostate cancer would alter management. This measurement should not be performed soon after DRE as PSA may be falsely elevated (Lechevallier et al. 1999). Some physicians consider a PSA level of greater than 4 ng/ml abnormal whereas others use age-specific reference ranges which reflect the fact that prostate size and PSA increase with age. Age 50–59, 3.5 ng/ml; age 60–69, 4.5 ng/ml; age 70–79, 6.5 ng/ml (Oesterling et al. 1993). However it is the rapid increase in PSA with time that is a particularly alarming and reliable sign of cancer development. Undertaking both PSA and DRE is a relatively sensitive way to exclude prostate cancer as a diagnosis. Unfortunately, PSA is not a specific test for prostate cancer as approximately 25 % of men with BPH have a serum PSA greater than 4 ng/ml. Due to this overlap in serum PSA in men with BPH and clinically localized prostate cancer, PSA velocity, free/total PSA ratio, complexed PSA (cPSA), and PSA density measurements have been developed in attempts to improve diagnostic specificity (Mikolajczyk et al. 2002). It is also known that patients with higher serum PSA have a higher risk of future growth of the prostate, worsening symptoms, decrease in flow rate, acute urinary retention and BPH-related surgery (Roehrborn et al. 1999, 2000, 2001).

II.4.10.1.4 Additional Diagnostic Tests

Patients with a normal initial evaluation and mild symptoms that are not bothersome do not usually require further investigation or treatment. They may be offered advice on lifestyle and fluid intake and discharged. Those with more bothersome symptoms should be assessed further using the additional tests outlined here.

II.4.10.1.5 Urinary Flow Rate

This is measured with a flowmeter and is an electronic measurement of urinary flow throughout the course of micturition. Modern flowmeters produce not only a flow trace but also a printout of the important parameters (Fig. II.4.31). Flow rate measurements on a voided volume of less than 150 ml may not provide a true indication of the patient's flow, as the maximum flow rate increases with volume up to this point (Drach et al. 1979). The peak flow (Q_{max}), measured in millilitres per second, identifies patients with BPH more specifically than average flow rate (Q_{ave}) (Gleason et al. 1982). Maximum urinary flow rates have been shown to decrease gradually with age and a Q_{max} of between 10 and 15 ml/s may be considered normal in men aged 70–80 years (Girman et al. 1993). Symptoms and symptom score analysis do not correlate strongly with uroflowmetry measurements and, due to test and re-test variability, there is not a flow rate "cut off point" for decision making.

II.4.10.1.6 Post Void Residual

Post void residual (PVR) is defined as the amount of urine left behind in the bladder after micturition. The PVR is usually measured with transabdominal ultrasound but can be measured invasively with catheterization. Large variations in measurements of PVR in the same patient have been documented (Bruskewitz et al. 1982). Most clinical studies have demonstrated that PVR correlates poorly with other signs and symptoms of BPH (Abrams and Griffiths 1979) although a PVR >50 ml has been shown to be associated with a threefold increase in the risk of acute urinary retention (Jacobsen et al. 1997).

II.4.10.1.7 Pressure-Flow Studies

The recording of detrusor pressure during bladder filling and voiding requires either urethral or suprapubic catheterization. Pressure-flow studies or urodynamic studies differentiate between the patients who have detrusor failure and those who have bladder outlet obstruction (BOO). They should be considered in patients in whom the initial evaluation, uroflowmetry and PVR cannot confirm BOO, particularly when invasive therapy is being considered (Denis et al. 1998). Pressure-flow studies are also useful in patients with neurological disease whose LUTS may have detrusor failure or in patients who have not responded to previous treatment. The key measure-

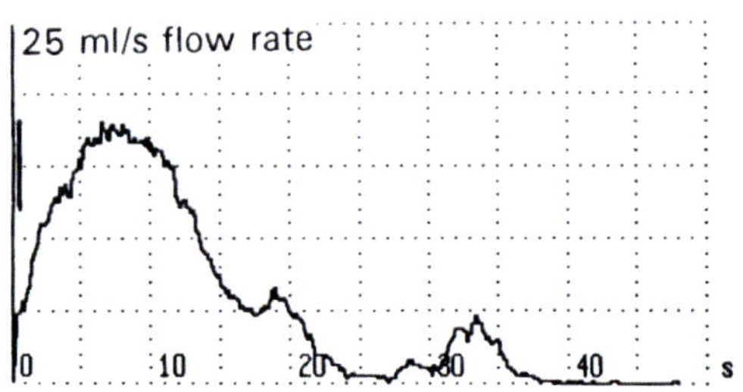

Results of UROFLOWMETRY

T_{100}	37	s
T_Q	36	s
T_{Qmax}	6	s
Q_{max}	18.1	ml/s
Q_{ave}	7.0	ml/s
V_{comp}	257	ml

Fig. II.4.31. Uroflowmetry tracing

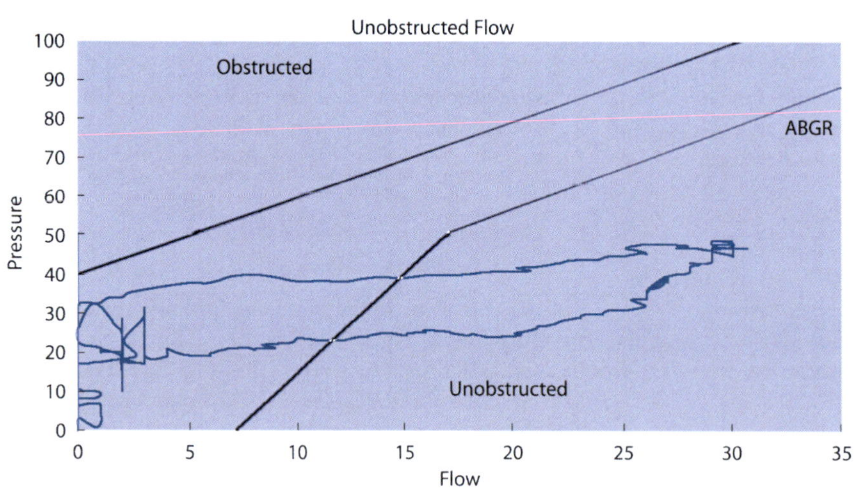

Fig. II.4.32. ICS nomogram

ment is the pressure generated by the contracting bladder muscle at maximum flow corrected for rectal pressure to remove artefact from intra-abdominal pressure. These measurements are then plotted on the ICS nomogram (see Fig. II.4.32), which can then be used to classify the patient as obstructed, unobstructed or equivocal.

II.4.10.1.8 Urethrocystoscopy

Urethrocystoscopy is recommended for men who either have bothersome symptoms and a history of haematuria, bladder cancer, or previous urethral stricture or prior to transurethral resection of the prostate (TURP). It permits direct examination of the lower urinary tract and, when performed under local anaesthesia, can be useful in planning the best invasive (surgical) therapy. Urethral strictures, bladder stones, high bladder neck, diverticulae and other bladder pathologies may be identified and subsequent surgical interventions planned as required. The main side-effects of this procedure are patient discomfort and, infrequently, urinary tract infection, bleeding and urinary retention.

II.4.10.1.9 Transrectal Ultrasound of the Prostate

Transrectal ultrasound examination of the prostate may be used to assess the size and shape of the prostate, which can be important in selecting patients for minimally invasive therapies such as transurethral microwave heat treatments or identifying patients with very large prostates who would be better served by open prostatectomy. Anatomical considerations such as intravesical lobes may impact on the choice of a TURP or incision of prostate. However, the most common indication for transrectal ultrasound of the prostate is as a means of guiding systematic prostate biopsies. These are performed if there are abnormalities on DRE and/or the PSA is elevated. To minimize the risk of sepsis the procedure is covered with oral antibiotics, usually of the quinolone family, to be taken at least an hour prior to biopsy and later that evening. Patients may also experience haemospermia or haematuria for some days or weeks after the biopsy (Desmond et al. 1993).

II.4.10.1.10 Upper Urinary Tract Imaging

Imaging of the upper urinary tract is recommended in the patient with a history of urolithiasis, haematuria, urinary tract infection and renal insufficiency but, because the diagnostic yield is low, it is not used routinely in the assessment of BPH. If imaging is indicated, it has been suggested that ultrasonography and a kidney-ureter-bladder (KUB) plain radiographic film be performed (Hendrikx et al. 1988).

II.4.10.2 Management of BPH

Open prostatectomy and TURP was the widely accepted treatment for BPH before the advent of medical treatments in the 1970s (Caine et al. 1976). Currently TURP is still considered the "gold standard" for the treatment of symptomatic BPH. However, there are now many acceptable alternatives to surgical intervention that are less costly per treatment and have less associated morbidity. As the aim of intervention in the patient with bothersome symptoms from BPH is to improve the quality of life, the lower morbidity of these alternative therapies is a very important factor in patient-driven decisions.

II.4.10.3 Watchful Waiting

Watchful waiting is a policy of careful monitoring for the progression of symptoms and possible complications of BPH but there is no active intervention. Patients should be advised to void completely and to decrease their intake of alcohol- and caffeine-containing beverages late in the day. They should also avoid over-the-counter cold and allergy medication for the reasons stated in the introduction. They are advised to report any changes in symptoms promptly. Patients are usually re-examined annually and the initial evaluation repeated at that time.

II.4.10.4 Pharmacologic Therapy

There are two main classes of medication currently in use for the treatment of symptomatic BPH: these are alpha-adrenergic blockers and 5α-reductase inhibitors. Phytotherapy describes the use of plant extracts and is used widely in some parts of the world. The extract of the American dwarf palm *Serenoa repens* is the most commonly used phytotherapy agent for BPH and the *n*-hexane liposterolic extract of *Serenoa repens*, Permixon (which is manufactured in France), is the product that has been most rigorously investigated to date. A meta-analysis of several open, blind, placebo-controlled and comparative clinical trials of Permixon showed statistically significant improvement in symptoms in men with LUTS compared with placebo and equivalence with finasteride and the alpha-blocker tamsulosin with a lower risk of androgen-dependent unwanted side-effects (Boyle et al. 2004). However, we will focus our discussion on the commonly prescribed medications for symptomatic BPH.

II.4.10.4.1 Alpha-Adrenergic Blockers

The rationale for alpha-adrenergic blocker use in the treatment of BPH is based on the findings that bladder outlet obstruction (BOO) from BPH is caused by the bulk of the prostate adenoma, the static component, and by the increased prostatic tone mediated by the alpha$_1$-adrenoceptors (α_1AR) in prostatic smooth muscle tissue and bladder neck, termed the dynamic component (Caine 1986). By blocking the alpha-adrenergic receptors at the bladder neck and prostate these medications decrease the prostate tone and decrease the pressure developed in the urethra, which results in diminished BOO (Shapiro et al. 1992).

Phenoxybenzamine is a non-selective alpha-adrenergic blocker which blocks both alpha$_1$ and alpha$_2$-adrenoceptors and was used in initial clinical studies. It was demonstrated that symptoms and urinary flow rate improved but this was associated with significant cardiovascular side-effects in 30% of patients (Caine et al. 1978). Selective alpha$_1$-adrenoceptor blockers such as prazosin, terazosin, doxazosin and the current uroselective medications alfuzosin and tamsulosin have minimal cardiovascular side-effects.

The American Urological Association has conducted a meta-analysis of alpha-blocker studies which demonstrates that the therapeutic efficacy of all contemporary alpha-blockers appears similar in terms of symptom improvement, quality of life and urinary flow rate (Table II.4.4) (American Urological Association 2003). Alfuzosin and tamsulosin are uroselective and therefore do not require titration of dose and, hence, they are the most widely prescribed in the UK. The alpha-blockers have a quick onset of action with rapid symptom improvement and are associated with a reduction in rates of surgery in developed countries. The most common adverse events associated with alpha-blockers are a 4.4% incidence of dizziness and postural hypotension (McConnell et al. 2003). However, tamsulosin has found to have a 5–10% incidence of retrograde or delayed ejaculation (Schulman et al. 1999).

II.4.10.4.2 5α-Reductase Inhibition

The rationale for the use of 5α-reductase inhibition (5ARI) is based on the observation that the embryonic development of the prostate depends upon the androgen dihydrotestosterone (DHT) (Peterson et al. 1977). Testosterone is converted to the more potent DHT by the enzyme 5α-reductase. DHT is a powerful ligand for the androgen receptor in the epithelial cells of the prostate and removal or suppression of DHT removes stimulus for cell growth and replication. This has been shown to decrease prostate volume, improve symptom scoring and urinary flow rate and decrease the risk of developing acute urinary retention and BPH-related surgery for both the currently available 5ARIs (Table II.4.5) (Roehrborn et al. 1999; Debruyne et al. 2004). Two 5ARIs are available, finasteride and dutasteride, and they differ in their inhibition of type 1 and type 2 isoenzymes of 5α-reductase. Finasteride is a mono-

Table II.4.4. Outcome parameters with alpha-blockers: changes in symptom score and peak urinary flow rate

Alpha-blockers	AUA/IPSS 3–9 months	10–16 months	>16 months	Peak flow rate (Q_{max}) 3–9 months	10–16 months	>16 months
Alfuzosin	-4.44			2.05		
Doxazosin	-5.10	-5.63		3.11	2.98	1.90[a]
Tamsulosin	-4.63	-7.53[a]		1.85	1.86[a]	
Terazosin	-6.22	-5.99		2.51	1.94	2.61[a]

[a] These numbers are based on single-arm analysis – no RCT data available

Table II.4.5. Outcome parameters with 5α-reductase inhibitors (*5ARIs*): changes in symptom score, urinary flow rate, prostate volume and risk of AUR and BPH-related surgery (Marberger et al. 2004)

Study	Patients	Agent	Change in AUA-SI score	Change in peak flow (ml/s)	Change in prostate volume (%)	Reduction in risk of AUR (%)	Reduction in risk of BPH-related surgical intervention (%)
PLESS (McConnell et al. 1998)	3040	Finasteride	3.3	+1.9	−18	57	55
		Placebo	1.3	+0.2	+14		
Dutasteride study (Roehrborn et al. 2002)	4325	Dutasteride	4.5	+2.2	−25.7	57	48
		Placebo	2.3	+0.6	+1.7		

inhibitor of 5AR type 2 whereas dutasteride is a dual inhibitor of both isoenzyme types. The side-effects of the 5ARIs are decreased libido, ejaculatory disorder and impotence affecting 3–5% of patients (Gormley et al. 1992). The results of the Prostate Cancer Prevention Trial demonstrated that long-term use of finasteride is associated with a 25% reduction in the prevalence of prostate cancer but this is balanced by the finding of an increase by a factor of 1.7 in the risk of high-grade tumour among those in whom cancer develops (Thompson et al. 2003a, 2003b).

II.4.10.4.3 Role of Combination Therapy with Alpha$_1$-Blockers and 5α-Reductase Inhibitors

The publication of the 4-year Medical Therapy of Prostatic Symptoms (MTOPS) study, which randomized 3047 men with BPH to treatment with finasteride, doxazosin, a combination of both, or placebo has provided insight into the relative long-term benefits of the two different types of medical therapy alone or in combination. This study confirms that all active treatment arms were associated with significant improvement in symptoms and overall progression. Of the monotherapies, only treatment with 5α-reductase inhibitors demonstrated significant reductions in the risk of acute urinary retention and the progression to invasive therapy. Doxazosin monotherapy resulted in an improvement in symptoms that was significantly greater than with finasteride monotherapy, but inferior to combination therapy. Doxazosin was noted to delay the time to progression of acute urinary retention and the need for invasive therapy but did not significantly reduce the long-term risk of either event. As combination therapy and monotherapy with finasteride were associated with significant reductions in prostate size, whilst there was no observed change in the prostate size in the doxazosin arm, it would appear that 5α-reductase inhibitors alter the natural history of BPH by reducing the size of the prostate (McConnell et al. 2003).

II.4.10.4.4 Summary

BPH is a progressive disease in ageing men and those who are most likely to progress to acute urinary retention or surgery have larger prostates. The aims of treatment of BPH are to alleviate symptoms and prevent progression of the disease. Alpha-blockers have a relatively quick onset of action and should be considered in patients who are symptomatic, whilst only the 5α-reductase inhibitors have been shown to reduce the progression of BPH. Consequently, 5α-reductase inhibitors should be used in combination with alpha-blockers in patients with larger prostate volumes of >30 ml. The 5α-reductase inhibitors have a relatively slow onset of action and the maximum effect is reached at about 6 months. Short-term combination therapy can be useful for patients with enlarged prostates requiring rapid symptom control whereas longer-term combination therapy may benefit patients with severe symptoms with enlarged prostates. The optimum duration of combination therapy may be as short as 6 months.

II.4.10.5 Minimally Invasive Therapies

II.4.10.5.1 Thermal-Based Treatments

Thermal-based treatments use high temperatures to produce coagulation necrosis of prostate tissue. Microwave technology has been used to produce heat but other methods, such as using radiofrequency waves, hot water, high intensity ultrasound and interstitial laser, have been used to similar effect. Thermotherapy refers to a temperature above 45 °C and causes tissue necrosis, whereas treatment temperatures of less than 45 °C are termed hyperthermia and do not. A multicentre sham-controlled study of technologies using hyperthermia found neither the transurethral nor transrectal treatment to be superior to sham treatments in subjective or objective criteria (Abbou et al. 1995).

Thermotherapy, or transurethral microwave therapy (TUMT), is delivered by the Prostatron. This uses a combination of heat delivered transurethrally and a water balloon to lower prostatic temperature, thereby preventing urethral damage and pain. The efficacy of TUMT has been assessed in several trials though long-term, multicentre studies are lacking (Ahmed et al. 1997; D'Ancona et al. 1997). Whilst it is clear that TUMT is not as effective as TURP in improving the symptom scores and peak flow rate, the improvement in symptoms seems to be related to the energy used. The complications are less than those seen with TURP, with prolonged catheterization and urinary tract infection being the most common. It seems that higher energy devices will be used in the future but continued long-term studies are required to assess this modality of treatment fully.

II.4.10.5.2 Transurethral Needle Ablation

Transurethral needle ablation (TUNA) uses radiofrequency (RF) waves to heat prostatic tissue. The RF energy is delivered into the prostatic tissue via two needles at the tip of the TUNA catheter. A randomized trial comparing TUNA with TURP demonstrated that the symptom improvement was similar to that achieved with TURP but that the improvement in peak urinary flow rate was not as great. The most commonly reported side-effects were bleeding (32.3%) and urinary tract infection (7.7%). Sexual dysfunction is noted to be rare and there have not been any reported cases of incontinence in any series (Bruskewitz et al. 1998). Again the long-term efficacy of this treatment has not been clearly evaluated as there are no large series with long-term follow-up.

II.4.10.5.3 Laser Treatment

Laser energy can be used to produce coagulation necrosis, vaporization of tissue or resection of tissue. Urologists at present do not agree on the most effective means to deliver laser energy. Some techniques produce tissue coagulation, which causes a delayed sloughing of tissue, whereas other techniques cause immediate vaporization of tissue. Comparisons with TURP have demonstrated that, in the short-term, symptom scores and peak flow rate are equivalent to TURP but the rates of post-operative urinary retention and the need for unplanned catheterization are greater than for TURP. Transurethral holmium laser resection/enucleation is a relatively new technique and it has been demonstrated that, in the hands of an experienced surgeon, the results are comparable to those achieved with open prostatectomy (Kuntz and Lehrich 2002). Long-term data are lacking for these techniques and cost constraints may limit the widespread usage of this technology.

II.4.10.6 Surgical Treatment

II.4.10.6.1 Open Prostatectomy

An open prostatectomy is performed through a lower abdominal incision which is placed either in the midline or transverse suprapubic, and the prostate adenoma is enucleated either through the bladder (transvesical prostatectomy) or through the prostate capsule (Millin's prostatectomy). This procedure is usually performed in patients with very large prostates (> 100 g) and data have shown that symptoms improve markedly. The procedure is more invasive and requires a longer hospital stay than TURP.

II.4.10.6.2 Transurethral Resection of the Prostate

TURP is carried out via a resectoscope with a diathermy loop that removes slivers of prostate tissue. The procedure involves a hospital stay of 2–3 days and is performed under general or spinal anaesthesia. The efficacy of this procedure was evaluated definitively in the Veterans Cooperative Study, which demonstrated that 91% of patients had no complications during the first 30 days after surgery, and that the outcomes of surgery were best for patients who were most bothered by their symptoms. Importantly, the study demonstrated there was no difference between the watchful waiting and surgical treatment groups with respect to incontinence and impotence (Wasson et al. 1995). At present, TURP is still considered the "gold standard" against which all invasive procedures are judged.

II.4.10.6.3 Transurethral Incision of the Prostate

Transurethral incision of the prostate is suitable for small prostates with a high bladder neck and no middle lobe enlargement. An incision is made from below the ureteric orifice on both sides and taken through the bladder neck to just proximal to the verumontanum. The results of this procedure are excellent with the incidence of complications being low (Bruskewitz et al. 1998).

II.4.10.7 Complications of Surgical Treatments

II.4.10.7.1 Primary Haemorrhage

This occurs within 24 h of surgery and is related to the surgery itself. There is a need for routine cross-matching, because 5–15% require a blood transfusion after the procedure. Patients who are taking anticoagulants must be identified and steps taken to stop the medication prior to surgery. Warfarin, for example, is usually stopped 5 days preoperatively and anticoagulation covered with heparin. Aspirin should also be stopped 2 weeks prior to surgery.

II.4.10.7.2 Secondary Haemorrhage

This generally happens 10–14 days postoperatively and is a common occurrence. The patient is advised to increase his oral intake of fluid and take appropriate antibiotics as required. Occasionally, the patient may experience a clot retention, in which case urgent catheterization is required.

II.4.10.7.3 Urethral Stricture

This can occur in 3–6% of patients and the most affected sites are the external meatus, the bladder neck and the bulbar urethra. Urethral strictures usually present 4–5 months after surgery when the patient experiences symptoms of outflow obstruction. Depending on the length and anatomy of the stricture, the treatment may be bouginage or urethotomy to reconstructive surgery of the urethra.

II.4.10.7.4
Retrograde Ejaculation

This is the most common sexual dysfunction after TURP. The incidence is about 70% but only 10% in transurethral incision of the prostate (TUIP). Therefore, patients should be counselled regarding this fact prior to surgery.

II.4.10.8
Therapeutic Options for Prostate Cancer

II.4.10.8.1
Staging of Prostate Cancer

- TRUS and prostate biopsy – allows visual assessment and histological confirmation of prostate cancer
- MRI/CT – assessment of local and metastatic spread
- Isotope bone scan – confirms or excludes skeletal deposits from metastatic prostate cancer
- Pelvic lymph node dissection – most accurate method of assessing metastatic spread to lymph nodes but most clinicians rely on cross-sectional radiological imaging.

II.4.10.8.2
Transrectal Ultrasound and Prostate Biopsy

The early diagnosis of prostate cancer is suspected if there are abnormalities in DRE and/or PSA measurement. Histological confirmation is then sought of the diagnosis by transrectal ultrasound (TRUS) directed biopsies. The procedure should be covered with two doses of oral antibiotics, usually of the quinolone family, to be taken at least an hour prior to biopsy and later that evening. This is to prevent septic complications, which may occur in up to 3% of patients. Patients should also be warned that they may experience haemospermia or haematuria for some days or weeks after the biopsy (Desmond et al. 1993).

II.4.10.8.3
Histological Grading System

The most widely used and recognized grading system for prostate cancer is the Gleason scoring system (Fig. II.4.33). It is based on the low-powered microscopy description of the cancer architecture and this has been correlated with the pathological extent of the disease. Higher Gleason grades (4 or 5), or a Gleason sum grade of greater than 7 has been shown to be predictive of a poor prognosis (Stamey et al. 1999).

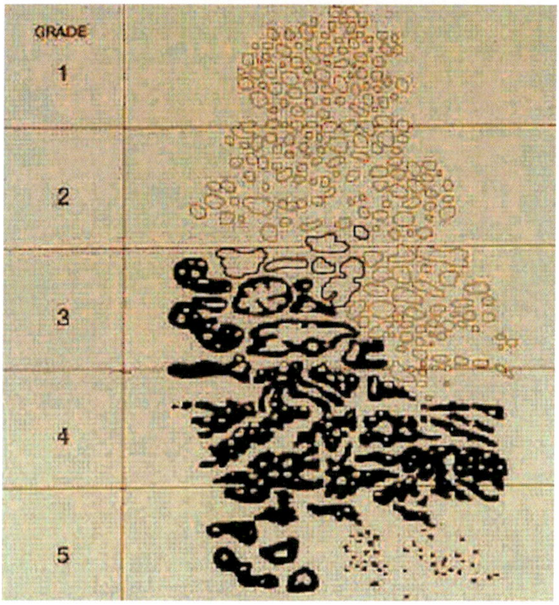

Fig. II.4.33. Gleason Pathological Grading System

II.4.10.8.4
Clinical Staging System

TNM classification for clinical staging of prostate cancer is the most widely used system (see Table II.4.6). It was updated in 2002. The distinction between intracapsular (T1–T2) and extracapsular (T3–T4) disease has a significant impact on treatment decision (Table II.4.6).

II.4.10.8.5
Magnetic Resonance Imaging

Magnetic resonance imaging is now of such a high standard that, with endorectal surface coils, it appears to be the most accurate non-invasive method in detecting locally advanced disease (Fig. II.4.34). It would be appropriate in a selected group of patients when curative treatment is an option and more precise staging will affect the treatment offered.

II.4.10.8.6
Computed Tomography Scanning

Computed tomography (CT) is also useful for assessing local tumour invasion but has the added benefit of

Table II.4.6. Tumour node metastasis (TNM) classification of prostate cancer

Classification	Primary tumour
T	
TX	Primary tumour cannot be assessed
T0	No evidence of primary tumour
T1	Clinically unapparent tumour not palpable or visible with imaging
T1a	Tumour an incidental finding at TURP involving 5% or less of resected tissue
T1b	Tumour an incidental finding at TURP in more than 5% of resected tissue
T1c	Tumour identified by needle biopsy
T2	Tumour confined to the prostate
T2a	Tumour involves less than one-half of one lobe
T2b	Tumour involves more than one-half of one lobe
T2c	Tumour involves both lobes
T3	Tumour extends through prostate capsule
T3a	Extracapsular extension (unilateral or bilateral)
T3b	Tumour invades seminal vesicle(s)
T4	Tumour is fixed or invades adjacent structures other than seminal vesicles: bladder neck, external sphincter, rectum, levator ani and/or pelvic wall
N	Regional lymph nodes
Nx	Regional lymph nodes cannot be assessed
N0	No regional lymph node metastasis
N1	Regional lymph node metastasis
M	Distant metastasis
Mx	Distant metastasis cannot be assessed
M0	No distant metastasis
M1	Distant metastasis
M1a	Non regional lymph node(s)
M1b	Bone(s)
M1c	Other site(s)

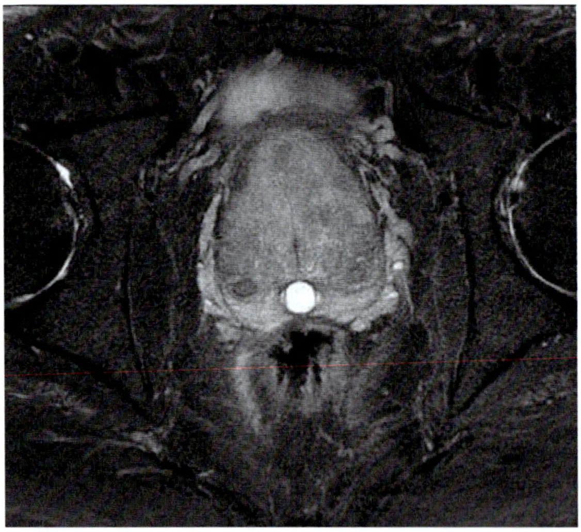

Fig. II.4.34. MRI of prostate

permitting fine needle aspiration of suspected nodal involvement. It is also useful in planning for radiotherapy.

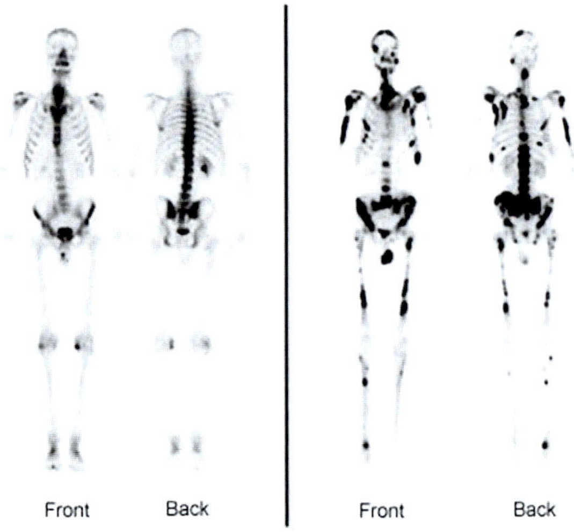

Fig. II.4.35. Normal bone scan on *left*, metastasis demonstrated on *right*

II.4.10.8.7 Bone Isotope Scanning

Bone isotope scanning is the most sensitive method for detecting the presence of bone metastases (Fig. II.4.35). They are seldom positive if the PSA measurement is below 20 ng/ml and almost never when the value is less than 10 ng/ml.

II.4.10.8.8 Pelvic Lymph Node Dissection

Accurate nodal staging is important as the presence of lymph node metastasis precludes curative therapy. Pelvic lymph node dissection remains the most accurate method of assessing nodal metastasis and may be indicated if there is sufficient suspicion of nodal metastasis on imaging, serum PSA >20 ng/ml and Gleason grade 8–10 (Sgrignoli et al. 1994); however, it is more common for surgeons and oncologists to rely on cross-sectional imaging to assess lymph node involvement.

II.4.10.9 Management of Localized Prostate Cancer

II.4.10.9.1 Active Monitoring

Active monitoring describes a treatment strategy of careful monitoring for progression of the disease with postponement of treatment until it is required. This strategy may be appropriate in patients with prostate cancer that is low volume and well differentiated (i.e. Gleason score ≤4), especially in patients who have less than 10 years life expectancy and have significant co-morbid factors (Kirby 1998). The precise strategy of follow-up for active monitoring varies from centre to centre. Most would undertake PSA measurement at 3-monthly intervals initially, extending this to 6-monthly assay and then annually in patients with stable PSA. However, active treatment should be considered if serum PSA is rising. Others follow a more aggressive strategy with repeat TRUS-guided prostate biopsies annually (Carter et al. 2002).

II.4.10.9.2 Radical Prostatectomy

Radical prostatectomy is the surgical treatment of prostate cancer and involves the removal of the entire prostate gland and both seminal vesicles. The indications for this treatment are in patients with localized prostate cancer with a life expectancy of more than 10 years. Radical prostatectomy was unpopular as there were concerns of the morbidity associated with the procedure but continence and potency-preserving modifications of the original technique have resulted in decreased complication rates. The retropubic approach is most commonly used as it allows for simultaneous pelvic lymph node assessment to be carried out.

The postoperative complications that patients need to be made aware of are a 7.7% risk of incontinence that persists for more than 1 year, a 9.0% risk of urethral stricture and a 50% risk of erectile dysfunction (Walsh et al. 1994). Patients require to be carefully selected for nerve sparing radical prostatectomy as a higher risk of local recurrence is present if the disease is not truly organ-confined and the surgical margins are positive. If the surgical margins are clear, the postoperative PSA reduces to <0.1 ng/ml. Therefore, any detectable PSA after radical prostatectomy indicates residual or recurrence of cancer and further treatment should be considered, such as radiotherapy or androgen blockade (Huland et al. 1994). Long-term studies have demonstrated the 15-year cancer-specific survival rate of 90% (Han et al. 2001).

II.4.10.9.3 External Beam Radiation Therapy

External beam radiation therapy, for patients with localized prostate cancer, has been shown to produce treatment results that are comparable to results achieved with radical prostatectomy. The long-term disease-free survival rate is 70–90% (Zietman et al. 1995; Hahn et al. 1996). The adverse side-effects associated with this treatment are urinary frequency due to radiation cystitis, bowel upset due to radiation proctitis and the risk of erectile dysfunction.

II.4.10.9.4 External Beam Radiation Therapy and Adjuvant Hormonal Therapy

Adjuvant hormonal ablation therapy with LHRHa prior to and during external beam radiation has been shown to offer better outcomes than radiotherapy alone (Bolla 1999). The clinical disease-free survival rate was improved from 40% to 75%. The study noted that hot flushes occurred in 33% of the combined therapy group compared to the radiotherapy group. Consequently, most patients undergoing external radiotherapy for prostate cancer now receive adjuvant hormone ablation.

II.4.10.9.5 Three-Dimensional Conformal Radiation Therapy

Three-dimensional conformal radiation therapy (3D-CRT) allows more accurate targeting of radiation at cancer tissues, thereby increasing the radiation dose to these sites and sparing normal tissue. This then lowers the toxicity and morbidity of the treatment. Studies have demonstrated up to 90% biochemical freedom from failure (i.e. PSA <0.1 ng/ml) for 5 years (Anderson et al. 1998).

II.4.10.9.6 Interstitial Radiotherapy or Brachytherapy

Interstitial radiotherapy describes the technique of placing a radioactive source within the prostate, allowing the delivery of a high dose of radiation to the prostate and sparing surrounding tissues.

High dose rate (HDR) interstitial radiotherapy involves an operation for the placement of needles within the prostate and short-term results have demonstrated comparable results to those of surgery and external beam radiotherapy (Khan et al. 1992). The incidence of side-effects such as proctitis seems to be higher and this may be suitable for patients with advanced rather than localized disease.

Low dose rate (LDR) interstitial therapy can be administered in an outpatient setting and involves placement of radioactive sources within the prostate under ultrasound guidance. The long-term side-effect profile is better than that of HDR therapy with <1–2% reporting incontinence and 1–2% of patients reporting proctitis (Blasko et al. 1996). Results have indicated that at 9 years the biochemical control rate was 83.5% in localized prostate cancer (Blasko et al. 2000).

II.4.10.9.7 Neoadjuvant Therapy Prior to Curative Treatment

This describes therapy given prior to definitive treatment with the modalities outlined above. As prostate cancer is an androgen-dependent tumour, neoadjuvant hormone treatment is an attractive prospect. It has been shown in vitro that prostate cancer cells undergo apoptosis, or cell death, when androgens are withdrawn (Kyprianou et al. 1990).

II.4.10.9.8
Neoadjuvant Therapy Prior to Surgery

In a number of studies, it was demonstrated that there was a significantly lower number of positive surgical margins in patients treated with neoadjuvant therapy (NAT). Unfortunately, follow-up results did not demonstrate a reduced PSA failure rate. When considering surgical technique, it was noted that surgery was slightly more difficult in patients who had received LHRHa prior to surgery (Soloway et al. 1995).

II.4.10.9.9
Neoadjuvant Therapy Prior to Radiotherapy

The current studies regarding NAT prior to radiotherapy have demonstrated that, in the initial 5 years of follow-up, the NHT group had improved local control and disease progression rates but, unfortunately, an update could not demonstrate improved overall survival (Pilepich et al. 1995).

II.4.10.10
Management of Locally Advanced Prostate Cancer and Metastatic Disease

Hormonal therapy is indicated in patients with locally advanced prostate cancer. Hormonal therapy describes any treatment that reduces the level of testosterone. Huggins and Hodges (1941) demonstrated the androgen dependence of prostate cancer. Whilst hormone-based therapy does not cure prostate cancer, it can diminish the size of the cancer and slow the growth and spread of metastasis. It is now generally agreed that prompt intervention with hormone therapy as soon as locally advanced or metastatic disease is diagnosed will be beneficial in terms of overall survival, but this must be balanced against the side-effects of these therapies (The Medical Research Council Prostate Cancer Working Party Investigators Group 1997). As with all forms of treatment for prostate cancer the response to treatment with hormone manipulation may be assessed and monitored by assay of serial serum PSA levels.

II.4.10.10.1
Surgical Castration

Bilateral orchiectomy is the gold standard against which all other hormone treatments must be compared. The surgical procedure is well tolerated by patients and can be performed under a short general anaesthetic or local anaesthesia. About 80% of patients have an excellent response to this mode of treatment with a mean duration of effectiveness of 2.5 years. The disadvantages of this treatment are the psychological effect of losing the testes and surgical morbidity. The main side-effects of testosterone suppression, whether surgical or chemically induced, are erectile dysfunction, hot flushes and occasionally breast tenderness.

II.4.10.10.2
Oestrogens

Oestrogens reduce the level of testosterone by acting on the negative feedback mechanism in the pituitary-gonadal axis. It blocks the secretion of luteinizing hormone (LH) and follicle-stimulating hormone (FSH). The most commonly used oestrogen is diethylstilboestrol (DES), but used at a dose of 5 mg/day, this produces significant cardiovascular toxicity. This risk is reduced with doses of 1 mg/day, particularly when low-dose aspirin is prescribed in conjunction, but serum testosterone levels do not fall to the levels seen in castrated patients (Shearer et al. 1973; Garnick 1986). As yet, further studies are required to elucidate the role of oestrogens in the treatment of prostate cancer (Iversen 1998).

II.4.10.10.3
LHRH Analogues

Luteinizing hormone releasing hormone analogues (LHRHa) such as leuprolide, buserelin and goserelin have been shown to be as effective as surgical castration in suppressing serum testosterone and do not increase the risk of cardiovascular toxicity. LHRHa are chemically similar to oestrogens and interfere with the negative feedback mechanism of the pituitary–gonadal axis. However, they also cause an initial rise in LH and FSH release from the pituitary and thereby testosterone production increases. This is described as the "flare phenomenon" as this can cause an increase in prostate tumour growth. Therefore, 4 weeks of adjuvant treatment with an anti-androgen such as bicalutamide (50 mg once daily), starting 1 week prior to the first injection of LHRHa, is recommended to prevent deleterious consequences of tumour flare associated with the brief rise in testosterone levels. LHRHa are given as a monthly or 3-monthly subcutaneous depot injection. The major side-effects of hormone treatment are loss of libido and impotence. Hot flushes and gynaecomastia occur to varying degrees.

II.4.10.10.4 Anti-Androgens

Anti-androgens are a group of compounds that inhibit the action of androgens at the cellular level. They may be used in conjunction with LHRHa to achieve what is known as "maximal androgen blockade", which is discussed later. Anti-androgens are classified according to their chemical structure with cyproterone acetate as a steroidal anti-androgen and nilutamide, flutamide and bicalutamide as non-steroidal anti-androgens. All of these compounds compete for androgen receptors but steroidal anti-androgens also lower LH and testosterone levels, which may lead to impotence and loss of libido. The non-steroidal anti-androgens, on the other hand, tend to increase serum testosterone due to increased gonadotrophin secretion (Soloway and Matzkin 1993).

II.4.10.10.5 Non-Steroidal Anti-Androgens

Nilutamide is not recommended for monotherapy and currently there is no evidence to support its use in this context. Flutamide has been used as monotherapy for metastatic prostate cancer but currently its use is recommended only in combination with either surgical or medical castration (Decensi et al. 1991). Bicalutamide has been compared with surgical and medical castration in several studies and has been found to be less effective in terms of time to progression and median survival (Bales and Chodak 1996). The role of bicalutamide as monotherapy is currently being investigated in the largest clinical trial in prostate cancer to date. The Bicalutamide Early Prostate Cancer Programme has not matured yet but will provide invaluable insight into the effect of early hormonal treatment on survival (See et al. 2001, 2002). A common side-effect of bicalutamide therapy is the occurrence of bothersome gynaecomastia, requiring complementary treatment with local radiotherapy, medical treatment (anti-oestrogens, e.g. tamoxifen) or surgery (Iversen et al. 2000).

II.4.10.10.6 Steroidal Anti-Androgens

Cyproterone acetate is a potent steroidal anti-androgen and causes suppression of testosterone and LH secretion. This has been evaluated in a number of earlier studies showing that, compared to treatment with DES, there was no difference with respect to cancer progression or overall survival (Pavone-Macaluso et al. 1986). The side-effect profiles of this treatment are loss of libido and potency. Abnormal liver function tests have been observed with long-term use (Schroder et al. 2000).

II.4.10.10.7 Maximal Androgen Blockade

Maximal androgen blockade (MAB) or total androgen suppression is the simultaneous suppression/blockade of both testicular and adrenal androgens as first-line treatment. This modality of treatment has been studied extensively and results from the majority of studies demonstrate that the 5-year survival with MAB amounted to 25.4% versus 23.4% with castration or LHRHa therapy; this difference did not reach statistical significance (Prostate Cancer Trialist' Collaborative Group 2000). The studies, however, demonstrate that patients receiving MAB achieved a quicker response to clinical symptoms and markers. Therefore, there may be an indication for MAB in patients who have severe symptoms due to local cancer spread or metastasis and very high PSA and alkaline phosphatase.

II.4.10.11 Treatment of Hormone Relapsed Prostate Cancer

Hormone relapsed prostate cancer is defined as cancer that returns after initial hormone therapy. There are many different terms for this, such as hormone-resistant or refractory prostate cancer, androgen- or hormone-independent prostate cancer. Analysis of the many studies examining the outcomes of treatment for hormone relapsed prostate cancer demonstrate that the mean time to progression ranges from 12 to 18 months and the mean time for survival ranges from 2 to 3 years (Eisenberger et al. 1986, 1998; Denis et al. 1993).

II.4.10.11.1 Anti-Androgen Withdrawal

It has been noted that withdrawal of anti-androgen can result in improved clinical symptoms and a decrease in PSA (Scher and Kelly 1993). This was initially seen with flutamide therapy and has been reported with bicalutamide therapy (Small and Carroll 1994). Therefore, in patients treated with anti-androgens who are diagnosed with hormone relapsed prostate cancer by serial rises in their serum PSA, the initial step should be to consider discontinuing therapy and to monitor PSA levels closely before considering the next treatment option.

II.4.10.11.2
Second-Line Hormonal Therapy

Several studies have examined this treatment modality and have concluded that the median duration of response ranged between 2 and 4 months. The compounds used have been diethylstilbestrol (DES), ketoconazole and corticosteroids (Storlie et al. 1995).

II.4.10.11.3
Cytotoxic Chemotherapy

Chemotherapy can be given more safely and is better tolerated now that supportive care has been improved with the use of haematological growth factors and anti-emetics. Several combinations of chemotherapy agents have been assessed and there has been an encouraging initial result. A study in 1995 demonstrated that treatment with mitoxantrone (related to anthracycline) combined with prednisolone resulted in a significant improvement in quality of life issues (Tannock et al. 1996). Treatment with estramustine in combination with different compounds has also been studied and results have been promising. Cyclophosphamide is an alkylating agent and it has been found that an oral preparation of this agent is less toxic than intravenous treatment and seems to have greater efficacy (Maulard-Durdux et al. 1996). Recent data regarding treatment with docetaxel and prednisolone have shown an improvement in survival compared to mitoxantrone and prednisolone therapy (Tannock et al. 2004).

II.4.10.11.4
Palliative Management of Bone Pain and Spinal Cord Compression

Metastatic prostate cancer frequently involves bone and one of the most common clinical problems is bone pain. The focal area should be assessed with plain radiographs and possibly a bone scan to rule out pathological fractures, especially in weight-bearing bones. Localized radiotherapy has been shown to control focal bone pain. If the deposits are diffuse, then intravenous strontium-89 can improve symptoms (Laing et al. 1991). A study demonstrated that zoledronic acid, a bisphosphonate, has clinical benefit in patients with advanced disease. It was shown that there was a reduction in bone pain and a delay of onset of skeletal complications (Saad et al. 2002). Growth of metastatic bone deposits may also cause spinal cord compression or interfere with haematological function if the bone marrow is replaced with cancerous tissue. The incidence of spinal cord compression is quite high and early recognition and treatment is required to avoid the serious sequelae of loss of sphincter control of the bladder and bowel or complete paraplegia. Emergency treatment involves high-dose corticosteroids, external beam radiotherapy and possible surgical decompression (Sorensen et al. 1990). Percutaneous vertebroplasty is a minimally invasive technique whereby acrylate cement is injected into the compressed vertebra to relieve pain and to provide strength (Weill et al. 1996). There is considerable experience in continental Europe but limited experience in the United Kingdom in this technique (Hide and Gangi 2004).

II.4.10.11.5
The Future

The management of hormone relapsed prostate cancer remains a challenge for clinicians due to the fact that no second-line therapy has been found to be as efficacious as androgen ablation has been for first-line treatment. Currently, important advances are being made in the fields of molecular and cell biology of prostate cancer and new drugs are being developed, which will increase our understanding of hormone relapsed prostate cancer and help improve care for these patients.

References

Abbou CC, Payan C et al (1995) Transrectal and transurethral hyperthermia versus sham treatment in benign prostatic hyperplasia: a double-blind randomized multicentre clinical trial. The French BPH Hyperthermia. Br J Urol 76:619–624

Abrams PH, Griffiths DJ (1979) The assessment of prostatic obstruction from urodynamic measurements and from residual urine. Br J Urol 51:129–134

Ahmed M, Bell T et al (1997) Transurethral microwave thermotherapy (Prostatron version 2.5) compared with transurethral resection of the prostate for the treatment of benign prostatic hyperplasia: a randomized, controlled, parallel study. Br J Urol 79:181–185

American Urological Association (2003) AUA guideline on the management of benign prostatic hyperplasia. American Urological Association, New York

Anderson PR, Hanlon AL et al (1998) Perineural invasion and Gleason 7–10 tumors predict increased failure in prostate cancer patients with pretreatment PSA < 10 ng/ml treated with conformal external beam radiation therapy. Int J Radiat Oncol Biol Phys 41:1087–1092

Bales GT,Chodak GW (1996) A controlled trial of bicalutamide versus castration in patients with advanced prostate cancer. Urology 47(1A Suppl):38–43; discussion 48–53

Barry MJ, Fowler FJ Jr et al (1992) The American Urological Association symptom index for benign prostatic hyperplasia. The Measurement Committee of the American Urological Association. J Urol 148:1549–1557; discussion 1564

Blasko JC,Ragde H et al (1996) Should brachytherapy be considered a therapeutic option in localized prostate cancer? Urol Clin North Am 23:633–650

Blasko JC, Grimm PD et al (2000) Palladium-103 brachytherapy for prostate carcinoma. Int J Radiat Oncol Biol Phys 46: 839–850

Bolla M (1999) Adjuvant hormonal treatment with radiotherapy for locally advanced prostate cancer. Eur Urol 35 (Suppl 1): 23–25; discussion 26

Boyle P, Robertson C et al (2004) Updated meta-analysis of clinical trials of Serenoa repens extract in the treatment of symptomatic benign prostatic hyperplasia. BJU Int 93: 751–756

Bruskewitz RC, Iversen P et al (1982) Value of postvoid residual urine determination in evaluation of prostatism. Urology 20:602–604

Bruskewitz R, Issa MM et al (1998) A prospective, randomized 1-year clinical trial comparing transurethral needle ablation to transurethral resection of the prostate for the treatment of symptomatic benign prostatic hyperplasia. J Urol 159:1588–1593; discussion 1593–1594

Caine M (1986) The present role of alpha-adrenergic blockers in the treatment of benign prostatic hypertrophy. J Urol 136:1–4

Caine M,Pfau A et al (1976) The use of alpha-adrenergic blockers in benign prostatic obstruction. Br J Urol 48:255–263

Caine M,Perlberg S et al (1978) A placebo-controlled double-blind study of the effect of phenoxybenzamine in benign prostatic obstruction. Br J Urol 50:551–554

Carter HB, Walsh PC et al (2002) Expectant management of nonpalpable prostate cancer with curative intent: preliminary results. J Urol 167:1231–1234

D'Ancona FC, Francisca EA et al (1997) High energy thermotherapy versus transurethral resection in the treatment of benign prostatic hyperplasia: results of a prospective randomized study with 1 year of followup. J Urol 158: 120–125

Debruyne F,Barkin J et al (2004) Efficacy and safety of long-term treatment with the dual 5alpha-reductase inhibitor dutasteride in men with symptomatic benign prostatic hyperplasia. Eur Urol 46:488–495

Decensi A,Guarneri D et al (1991) Phase II study of the pure non-steroidal antiandrogen nilutamide in prostatic cancer. Italian Prostatic Cancer Project (PONCAP). Eur J Cancer 27:1100–1104

Denis LJ, Carnelro de Moura JL et al (1993) Goserelin acetate and flutamide versus bilateral orchiectomy: a phase III EORTC trial (30853). EORTC GU Group and EORTC Data Center. Urology 42:119–129; discussion 129–130

Denis L,Griffiths K et al (1998) Proceedings of the 4th International Consultation on benign prostatic hyperplasia (BPH). 2–5 July 1997, Plymouth, UK

Desmond PM,Clark J et al (1993) Morbidity with contemporary prostate biopsy. J Urol 150(5 Pt 1):1425–1426

Drach GW, Layton TN et al (1979) Male peak urinary flow rate: relationships to volume voided and age. J Urol 122: 210–214

Eisenberger MA, O'Dwyer PJ et al (1986) Gonadotropin hormone-releasing hormone analogues: a new therapeutic approach for prostatic carcinoma. J Clin Oncol 4:414–424

Eisenberger MA, Blumenstein BA et al (1998) Bilateral orchiectomy with or without flutamide for metastatic prostate cancer. N Engl J Med 339:1036–1042

Garnick MB (1986) Leuprolide versus diethylstilbestrol for previously untreated stage D2 prostate cancer. Results of a prospectively randomized trial. Urology 27(1 Suppl):21–28

Girman CJ, Panser LA et al (1993) Natural history of prostatism: urinary flow rates in a community-based study. J Urol 150:887–892

Gleason DM, Bottaccini MR et al (1982) Urinary flow velocity as an index of male voiding function. J Urol 128:1363–1367

Gormley GJ, Stoner E et al (1992) The effect of finasteride in men with benign prostatic hyperplasia. The Finasteride Study Group. N Engl J Med 327:1185–1191

Hahn P, Baral E et al (1996) Long-term outcome of radical radiation therapy for prostatic carcinoma: 1967–1987. Int J Radiat Oncol Biol Phys 34:41–47

Han M, Partin AW et al (2001) Long-term biochemical disease-free and cancer-specific survival following anatomic radical retropubic prostatectomy. The 15-year Johns Hopkins experience. Urol Clin North Am 28:555–565

Hendrikx AJ,Doesburg WH et al (1988) Effectiveness of ultrasound in the preoperative evaluation of patients with prostatism. Prostate 13:199–208

Hide IG, Gangi A (2004) Percutaneous vertebroplasty: history, technique and current perspectives. Clin Radiol 59: 461–467

Huggins C, Hodges CV (1941) Studies on prostate cancer. I. The effect of castration, of estrogen and of androgen injection on serum phosphatase in metastatic cancer of the prostate. Cancer Res 1:293–297

Huland H, Hubner D et al (1994) Systematic biopsies and digital rectal examination to identify the nerve-sparing side for radical prostatectomy without risk of positive margin in patients with clinical stage T2, N0 prostatic carcinoma. Urology 44:211–214

Iversen P (1998) Orchidectomy and oestrogen therapy revisited. Eur Urol 34 (Suppl 3):7–11

Iversen P, Tyrrell CJ et al (2000) Bicalutamide monotherapy compared with castration in patients with nonmetastatic locally advanced prostate cancer: 6.3 years of followup. J Urol 164:1579–1582

Jacobsen SJ, Jacobson DJ et al (1997) Natural history of prostatism: risk factors for acute urinary retention. J Urol 158: 481–487

Khan K, Thompson W et al (1992) Transperineal percutaneous iridium-192 interstitial template implant of the prostate: results and complications in 321 patients. Int J Radiat Oncol Biol Phys 22:935–939

Kirby R (1998) Treatment options for early prostate cancer. Urology 52:948–962

Kuntz RM, Lehrich K (2002) Transurethral holmium laser enucleation versus transvesical open enucleation for prostate adenoma greater than 100 gm.: a randomized prospective trial of 120 patients. J Urol 168(4 Pt 1):1465–1469

Kyprianou N, English HF et al (1990) Programmed cell death during regression of PC-82 human prostate cancer following androgen ablation. Cancer Res 50:3748–3753

Laing AH, Ackery DM et al (1991) Strontium-89 chloride for pain palliation in prostatic skeletal malignancy. Br J Radiol 64:816–822

Lechevallier E, Eghazarian C et al (1999) Effect of digital rectal examination on serum complexed and free prostate-specific antigen and percentage of free prostate-specific antigen. Urology 54:857–861

Marberger M, Harkaway R et al (2004) Optimising the medical management of benign prostatic hyperplasia. Eur Urol 45:411–419

Maulard-Durdux C, Dufour B et al (1996) Phase II study of the oral cyclophosphamide and oral etoposide combination in hormone-refractory prostate carcinoma patients. Cancer 77:1144–1148

McConnell JD,Bruskewitz R et al (1998) The effect of finasteride on the risk of acute urinary retention and the need for surgical treatment among men with benign prostatic hyperplasia. Finasteride Long-Term Efficacy and Safety Study Group. N Engl J Med 338:557–563

McConnell JD, Roehrborn CG et al (2003) The long-term effect of doxazosin, finasteride, and combination therapy on the clinical progression of benign prostatic hyperplasia. N Engl J Med 349:2387–2398

Mebust WK, Holtgrewe HL et al (1989) Transurethral prostatectomy: immediate and postoperative complications. A cooperative study of 13 participating institutions evaluating 3,885 patients. J Urol 141:243–247

Messing EM, Young TB et al (1992) Home screening for hematuria: results of a multiclinic study. J Urol 148(2 Pt 1):289–292

Mikolajczyk SD, Marks LS et al (2002) Free prostate-specific antigen in serum is becoming more complex. Urology 59:797–802
Oesterling JE, Jacobsen SJ et al (1993) Serum prostate-specific antigen in a community-based population of healthy men. Establishment of age-specific reference ranges. J Am Med Assoc 270:860–864
Pavone-Macaluso M, de Voogt HJ et al (1986) Comparison of diethylstilbestrol, cyproterone acetate and medroxyprogesterone acetate in the treatment of advanced prostatic cancer: final analysis of a randomized phase III trial of the European Organization for Research on Treatment of Cancer Urological Group. J Urol 136:624–631
Peterson RE, Imperato-McGinley J et al (1977) Male pseudohermaphroditism due to steroid 5-alpha-reductase deficiency. Am J Med 62:170–191
Pilepich MV, Krall JM et al (1995) Androgen deprivation with radiation therapy compared with radiation therapy alone for locally advanced prostatic carcinoma: a randomized comparative trial of the Radiation Therapy Oncology Group. Urology 45:616–623
Prostate Cancer Trialist' Collaborative Group (2000) Maximum androgen blockade in advanced prostate cancer: an overview of the randomised trials. Lancet 355:1491–1498
Roehrborn CG, Girman CJ et al (1997) Correlation between prostate size estimated by digital rectal examination and measured by transrectal ultrasound. Urology 49:548–557
Roehrborn CG, Boyle P et al (1999) Serum prostate-specific antigen and prostate volume predict long-term changes in symptoms and flow rate: results of a four-year, randomized trial comparing finasteride versus placebo. PLESS Study Group. Urology 54:662–669
Roehrborn CG, McConnell J et al (2000) Serum prostate specific antigen is a strong predictor of future prostate growth in men with benign prostatic hyperplasia. PROSCAR long-term efficacy and safety study. J Urol 163:13–20
Roehrborn CG,Malice M et al (2001) Clinical predictors of spontaneous acute urinary retention in men with LUTS and clinical BPH: a comprehensive analysis of the pooled placebo groups of several large clinical trials. Urology 58: 210–216
Roehrborn CG, Boyle P et al (2002) Efficacy and safety of a dual inhibitor of 5-alpha-reductase types 1 and 2 (dutasteride) in men with benign prostatic hyperplasia. Urology 60:434–441
Saad F, Gleason DM et al (2002) A randomized, placebo-controlled trial of zoledronic acid in patients with hormone-refractory metastatic prostate carcinoma. J Natl Cancer Inst 94:1458–1468
Scher HI, Kelly WK (1993) Flutamide withdrawal syndrome: its impact on clinical trials in hormone-refractory prostate cancer. J Clin Oncol 11:1566–1572
Schroder FH, Collette L et al (2000) Prostate cancer treated by anti-androgens: is sexual function preserved? EORTC Genitourinary Group. European Organization for Research and Treatment of Cancer. Br J Cancer 82:283–290
Schulman CC, Cortvriend J et al (1999) Tamsulosin: 3-year long-term efficacy and safety in patients with lower urinary tract symptoms suggestive of benign prostatic obstruction: analysis of a European, multinational, multicenter, open-label study. European Tamsulosin Study Group. Eur Urol 36:609–620
See WA, McLeod D et al (2001) The bicalutamide Early Prostate Cancer Program. Demography 6:43–47
See WA,Wirth MP et al (2002) Bicalutamide as immediate therapy either alone or as adjuvant to standard care of patients with localized or locally advanced prostate cancer: first analysis of the early prostate cancer program. J Urol 168: 429–435
Sgrignoli AR, Walsh PC et al (1994) Prognostic factors in men with stage D1 prostate cancer: identification of patients less likely to have prolonged survival after radical prostatectomy. J Urol 152:1077–1081
Shapiro E, Hartanto V et al (1992) The response to alpha blockade in benign prostatic hyperplasia is related to the percent area density of prostate smooth muscle. Prostate 21:297–307
Shearer RJ, Hendry WF et al (1973) Plasma testosterone: an accurate monitor of hormone treatment in prostatic cancer. Br J Urol 45:668–677
Small EJ, Carroll PR (1994) Prostate-specific antigen decline after casodex withdrawal: evidence for an antiandrogen withdrawal syndrome. Urology 43:408–410
Soloway MS, Matzkin H (1993) Antiandrogenic agents as monotherapy in advanced prostatic carcinoma. Cancer 71 (Suppl 3):1083–1088
Soloway MS, Sharifi R et al (1995) Randomized prospective study comparing radical prostatectomy alone versus radical prostatectomy preceded by androgen blockade in clinical stage B2 (T2bNxM0) prostate cancer. The Lupron Depot Neoadjuvant Prostate Cancer Study Group. J Urol 154(2 Pt 1): 424–428
Sorensen PS, Borgensen SE et al (1990) Metastatic epidural spinal cord compression: results of treatment and survival. Cancer 65:1502–1510
Stamey TA, McNeal JE et al (1999) Biological determinants of cancer progression in men with prostate cancer. J Am Med Assoc 281:1395–1400
Storlie JA, Buckner JC et al (1995) Prostate specific antigen levels and clinical response to low dose dexamethasone for hormone-refractory metastatic prostate carcinoma. Cancer 76:96–100
Tannock IF, Osoba D et al (1996) Chemotherapy with mitoxantrone plus prednisone or prednisone alone for symptomatic hormone-resistant prostate cancer: a Canadian randomized trial with palliative end points. J Clin Oncol 14:1756–1764
Tannock IF, de Wit R et al (2004) Docetaxel plus prednisone or mitoxantrone plus prednisone for advanced prostate cancer. N Engl J Med 351:1502–1512
The Medical Research Council Prostate Cancer Working Party Investigators Group (1997) Immediate versus deferred treatment for advanced prostatic cancer: initial results of the Medical Research Council Trial. Br J Urol 79:235–246
Thompson IM, Goodman PJ et al (2003a) The influence of finasteride on the development of prostate cancer. N Engl J Med 349:215–224
Thompson IM, Klein EA et al (2003b) Prevention of prostate cancer with finasteride: US/European perspective. Eur Urol 44:650–655
Walsh PC, Partin AW et al (1994) Cancer control and quality of life following anatomical radical retropubic prostatectomy: results at 10 years. J Urol 152(5 Pt 2):1831–1836
Wasson JH, Reda DJ et al (1995) A comparison of transurethral surgery with watchful waiting for moderate symptoms of benign prostatic hyperplasia. The Veterans Affairs Cooperative Study Group on Transurethral Resection of the Prostate. N Engl J Med 332:75–79
Weill A, Chiras J et al (1996) Spinal metastases: indications for and results of percutaneous injection of acrylic surgical cement. Radiology 199:241–247
Zietman AL, Coen JJ et al (1995) The treatment of prostate cancer by conventional radiation therapy: an analysis of long-term outcome. Int J Radiat Oncol Biol Phys 32:287–292

II.4.11 Partial Androgen Deficiency of the Ageing Male (PADAM) and Testosterone Supplementation: Use, Misuse or Abuse?

D. Vanderschueren

Summary

- Testosterone (T) supplementation is only indicated in elderly men with well-defined underlying testicular, pituitary or hypothalamic disease.
- T supplementation in elderly men without well-defined underlying testicular, pituitary or hypothalamic disease and with T concentrations below or just below the young reference range is still in an experimental stage.
- The threshold for T for different symptoms and complaints and/or tissue dysfunctions is still poorly defined. This threshold may show interindividual variation.
- Supraphysiological T supplementation should be avoided in the elderly. If T treatment is to be considered, replacement should be physiological.
- Monitoring of prostatic disease and haematocrit during T therapy is of utmost importance.
- New treatment modalities should avoid stimulating the prostate but should maintain the benefits of androgen receptor stimulation in other organs (mood, sexual function, bone).

II.4.11.1 Introduction

The benefits of testosterone (T) replacement are well defined in hypogonadal men. Hypogonadal men indeed gain bone and muscle and lose fat following T substitution. Moreover, they also report increased energy and improved sexual function during T treatment. For this reason, T substitution is essential for the quality of life of hypogonadal men (Morley and Perry 2003).

However, many of the symptoms of hypogonadism, such as diminished libido, depression, less energy, muscle wasting, visceral fat accumulation and osteoporosis, are also reminiscent of ageing. Ageing is associated with hormonal changes, therefore it is tempting to speculate that some of these age-related symptoms are explained by hormonal changes such as a decrease of total and bioavailable T (Table II.4.7). Thus, it is no surprise that T supplementation is also promoted in elderly men with age-related partial androgen deficiency (PADAM). In accordance, the use of T has increased beyond the well established indication of male hypogonadism (Hayes 2000). Still, potential indiscriminate use of T in elderly men may carry risks. Consequently, it is of utmost importance to clearly define the benefits versus the risks of T treatment in elderly men. The aim of this chapter is to evaluate to what extent the available scientific literature is already able to answer the following critical questions:

- Who in the elderly population is to benefit from T replacement?
- What is the expected benefit of T replacement in elderly men?
- What are the risks/side-effects of T replacement?
- What type of T replacement should be used in elderly men?
- How long should we administer T in the elderly?

During ageing, T levels decrease 1 – 2 %/year but the decrease is greater for bioavailable T because of an age-related increase in the levels of sex hormone binding globulin. Although serum oestradiol concentrations remain constant, the levels of bioavailable oestradiol also tend to decrease. About 20 % of men older than 60 may experience T levels lower than the young normal range. Most of these elderly men with partial androgen deficiency have, however, only mildly decreased T concentrations.

Table II.4.7. Most relevant age-related changes in sex steroid concentrations in men

Testosterone	↓
Sex hormone binding globulin	↑
Bioavailable testosterone	↓↓
5α-Dihydrotestosterone	↔
17β-Oestradiol	↔
Bioavailable 17β-oestradiol	↓
Dehydroepiandrosterone sulphate	↓↓

↓ = decreased; ↑ = increased; ↔ = no change

II.4.11.2 Who is to Benefit from T Replacement? What is the Target Population?

According to a meta analysis, there are no data available to support the unlimited use of T in every man older than 60 regardless of symptoms and/or complaints or T levels (Gruenewald and Matsumoto 2003).

The only randomized controlled trial in asymptomatic eugonadal elderly men evaluated the effects of a modest oral dose of T undecanoate (80 mg) during 8 months. Unfortunately, this trial was designed only to evaluate the safety of T [effect on prostate volume (increase), urinary symptoms (no change) and prostate specific antigen (PSA) levels (no change)] and not to show benefit (Holmang et al. 1993). Therefore, all major reviews published on this issue show general agreement with respect to their conclusion that the practice of T supplementation in elderly men is still in an experimental stage (Tenover 1999; Vermeulen 2001; Gooren 2003; Gruenewald and Matsumoto 2003; Swerdloff and Wang 2004).

The first and most relevant challenge concerning T supplementation is to define the target population in the ageing male population. A first approach is to target those elderly men with hypogonadal symptoms or complaints. Unfortunately, these symptoms are not specific for the elderly population. Indeed, questionnaires such as the ADAM score (**a**ndrogen **d**eficiency in the **a**geing **m**ale) have been designed to detect undiagnosed hypogonadal men in the population (Morley et al. 2000). Many men with a positive ADAM score are, however, not hypogonadal but often depressed (Delhez et al. 2003). Therefore, at present, no reliable clinical method allows the clinician to make an accurate distinction between hypogonadal symptoms and complaints related to depression, other chronic illness or simply age-related dysfunction. Some authors have used low bone density as a surrogate marker of fracture risk in order to select elderly men who may benefit from androgen replacement. Bone density is indeed a useful marker for follow-up of androgenicity in hypogonadal men (Vanderschueren et al. 2004). Still, in elderly men bone density may be determined more by genetic background, calcium intake, physical activity, concomitant diseases and vitamin D status than by androgen levels. Hence, another approach is to screen elderly men for hypogonadism regardless of symptoms or complaints in order to detect those men who have serum T levels below a certain threshold. Again, such an approach creates the problem of defining a threshold, if it exists. A threshold is an absolute serum level of T below which certain symptoms/complaints occur or the function of androgen target tissues becomes problematic. Such a threshold for T may differ according to selected symptoms and/or tissues. For instance, bone may have a lower threshold for T than more androgen-sensitive tissues such as the prostate. Indeed, in aged orchiectomized male rats, low doses of T that only minimally stimulate the prostate or seminal vesicles are able to maintain both bone density and lean body mass (Vanderschueren et al. 2000). Whether such a tissue-specific threshold also exists in older men is still unknown. Probably 20% of all men older than 60 will have a serum T level below 2 SD of the mean concentrations of young healthy men. Most of these men have T concentrations only mildly below this young normal range, but still far above the castrate range. The question therefore remains as to whether this relatively limited lowering of T levels below the young normal limit may induce symptoms and/or tissue dysfunction. For instance, many elderly men with a T level below 2 SD for young men still report normal sexual function. Sexual dysfunction becomes a typical and constant complaint only when T decreases into the low castrate range, most often in the context of testicular or pituitary disease. These clinical observations suggest that T levels below the normal range in young men may be sufficient to maintain at least some, if not most, androgen-related functions in the elderly. An alternative and opposite point of view is that some elderly men with T levels within the normal range of young men may still have significantly less T than they had say 20 years previously. At present we cannot rule out that such men, even when their T concentrations are within normal limits, may also benefit from T substitution. The threshold for T may therefore not only be tissue or symptom specific but also different from one individual to another (Kelleher et al. 2004). Men with a specific genetic constitution may also be more vulnerable than others to the effects of androgen deficiency. Population studies looking at relevant genetic polymorphisms for androgen metabolism with respect to symptoms of androgen deficiency and/or the response to androgen replacement are still lacking and therefore needed in this context.

In conclusion, the target population of elderly men who may benefit from T replacement is yet to be defined. There is no agreement on whether we should use symptoms, surrogate markers of risk, questionnaires or simply T levels (with or without genetic markers in the future) in order to decide whether to start T supplementation in older men. Therefore, it is no surprise that every randomized trial published thus far has used different inclusion criteria. As a result, no two studies are comparable, making it impossible to define any target population for T supplementation at present. Therefore, the elderly men who should receive T replacement are those with a well-defined testicular, pituitary or hypothalamic disease that induces clear-cut hypogonadism and related symptoms.

II.4.11.3 What is the Expected Benefit of T Replacement in Elderly Men?

Patients and clinicians both expect an improvement of relevant clinical endpoints. Ideally, in the context of T supplementation, older men should therefore have im-

Table II.4.8. Effects of testosterone (T) supplementation on clinical and subclinical endpoints in the elderly. In many circumstances both an increase and no change or a decrease and no change have been reported. For more detailed information, please read the excellent review of Gruenewald and Matsumoto (2003)

Endpoint: Insufficient data	↔	↔/↓	↓	↑/↔	↑
Prostate cancer	Urinary symptoms	–	–	PSA level	Prostate size? (beware subclinical prostate cancer)
Fractures	–	–	–	Bone density	–
Cardiovascular events	HDL cholesterol	LDL cholesterol/ angina pectoris frequency	–	–	Short-term vasodilatation/ improvement in ECG in angina pectoris
–	–	–	–	Cognitive tests, mood	Subjective perception of energy
–	Sleep apnoea	–	–	Sexual function	–
–	–	–	Fat mass	Muscle strength	Lean mass
–	–	–	–	–	Haemoglobin (beware polycythaemia)

↓ = decreased; ↑ = increased; ↔ = no change

proved mood, energy, sexual and cognitive function, no more prostate cancer and fewer cardiovascular events and fractures. Again, however, there are no firm data with respect to T supplementation in elderly men and cardiovascular events, prostate cancer, fractures or cognitive function (Table II.4.8). Except for reports of a subjective improvement of strength and energy, insufficient information about other clinical benefits of T supplementation in the elderly is available.

In the absence of firm data on clinical benefit, subclinical endpoints may to the same extent serve as surrogate markers of relevant clinical improvement (Table II.4.8). In accordance with its action on body composition in hypogonadal men, T substitution increases muscle mass and decreases fat in older men. Whether insulin resistance and the cardiovascular risk profile improve in line with these potential beneficial changes in body composition remains uncertain. It is also not clear if muscle strength improves and whether such improvement is clinically relevant.

T replacement may improve bone density, however probably only in those elderly men with very low T levels. In one study even, the effect of T was not significantly better than calcium supplementation. Whether an improvement of bone density also translates into a clinically relevant decrease of fracture risk is not yet known (for extended reading see Vanderschueren et al. 2004). Unfortunately, areal bone mineral density also remains a poorly validated marker of osteoporosis risk in elderly men.

Short-term administration of T may increase coronary blood flow, reduce ECG changes during exercise testing in angina patients and even mildly decrease low-density lipoprotein (LDL). It remains unsolved whether T (especially long-term supplementation) in terms of cardiovascular risk assessment is safe and beneficial (Wu and von Eckardstein 2003).

T may increase prostate volume and PSA, however within normal limits and without a significant increase of clinical urinary symptoms. To date, there are no alarming data with respect to T supplementation on the progression or development of prostate disease and/or symptoms. Two major concerns remain. The first concern is that the duration of T supplementation and the number of subjects included are still limited. Therefore, the statistical power is not sufficient to exclude the possibility that T supplementation in elderly men will increase the incidence of prostate disease. A second major concern in this context is the high frequency of silent subclinical prostate cancer, especially in the very elderly. Subclinical prostate cancer is by definition not detectable at the start of T supplementation and may grow at a faster rate than expected.

II.4.11.4 What are the Risks/Side-Effects of T Replacement?

The most well documented and easily detectable side-effect of T replacement is polycythaemia. Other potential risks such as gynaecomastia and sleep apnoea do not represent a clinical problem. In addition, no negative effects of T on lipoproteins are reported in the elderly population (Table II.4.8). The major concern therefore remains the prostate. Although data on prostate size, urinary symptoms, PSA level and prostate cancer have been not alarming thus far, information is still limited in the background of the high prevalence of subclinical prostate cancer in the elderly.

II.4.11.5
What Type of T Replacement Should be Used in Elderly Men?

Multiple T preparations (injectable, oral or transdermal) are available for the treatment of elderly men (Table II.4.9). These forms of treatment can differ in their risk profile. The available data suggest that administration of supraphysiological doses of T should be avoided in order to limit side-effects that may be more apparent in the elderly. The most well documented side-effect in this context is polycythaemia, which may occur in 6–12% of the elderly population following T treatment. Restoration of the often modest anaemia observed during hypogonadism by T replacement is of course beneficial but polycythaemia should be avoided especially in the elderly (Table II.4.8). Supraphysiological concentrations often result from intramuscular administration (Table II.4.9), which is still the most common mode of T treatment.

Table II.4.9. Most common types of T replacement in elderly men

Preparation	Mode of administration	Dose/frequency
Testosterone enanthate	Intramuscular	100–200 mg every 2 weeks
Testosterone undecanoate	Oral	120–160 mg daily
Testosterone gel or patch	Transdermal	5–10 mg daily

II.4.11.6
How Long Should we Administer T in the Elderly?

Clearly, the goal of T supplementation, if it works, should be to treat men older than 60 for the rest of their life in order to increase their quality of life. However, there are no studies on T supplementation of longer than 3 years. Many side-effect and/or benefits may occur after a longer duration of T treatment. Results from the Women's Health Initiative Study have shown that some risks of hormone replacement in postmenopausal women, such as breast cancer, may become evident only after 5 years. Therefore, long-term T supplementation studies are needed to assess the benefits and risks.

II.4.11.7
Conclusions and Research Agenda

Many questions remain unresolved with respect to T supplementation in the elderly. It is unlikely, in the absence of clinically relevant testicular, pituitary or hypothalamic disease, that a list of symptoms or complaints and/or a T level below a certain threshold will inform us as to who should receive T supplementation. Moreover, the benefits of T treatment will probably be less evident than in the frankly hypogonadal and mainly subclinical men. In such a context, side-effects should be clearly limited. It is evident that some of the risks are related to supraphysiological T treatment which therefore should be avoided in the elderly. The main issue of concern during T supplementation will remain the prostate as long as we use T that is converted into dihydrotestosterone and therefore will stimulate prostate growth. Although not alarming, available data are insufficiently reassuring with respect to the risks of therapy, especially for prostate cancer. Large-scale studies of long(er) duration will be needed if T replacement is to be used in the elderly. An alternative challenge for the pharmaceutical industry is to develop selective androgen receptor modulators, analogous to selective oestrogen receptor modulators, which do not stimulate prostate tissue.

References

Delhez M, Hansenne M, Legros JJ (2003) Andropause and psychopathology: minor symptoms rather than pathological ones. Psychoneuroendocrinology 28:863–874

Gooren L (2003) Androgen deficiency in the aging male: benefits and risks of androgen supplementation. J Steroid Biochem Mol Biol 85:349–355

Gruenewald DA, Matsumoto AM (2003) Testosterone supplementation therapy for older men: potential benefits and risks. J Am Geriatr Soc 51:101–115

Hayes FJ (2000) Testosterone-fountain of youth or drug of abuse. J Clin Endocrinol Metab 85:3020–3023

Holmang S, Marin P, Lindstedt G, Hedelin H (1993) Effect of long-term oral testosterone undecanoate treatment on prostate volume and serum prostate-specific antigen concentration in eugonadal middle-aged men. Prostate 23:99–106

Kelleher S, Conway AJ, Handelsman DJ (2004) Blood testosterone threshold for androgen deficiency symptoms. J Clin Endocrinol Metab 89:3813–3817

Morley JE, Perry HM (2003) Androgen treatment of male hypogonadism in older males. J Steroid Biochem Mol Biol 85:367–373

Morley JE, Charlton E, Patrick P, Kaiser FE, Cadeau P, McCready D, Perry HM 3rd (2000) Validation of a screening questionnaire for androgen deficiency in aging males. Metabolism 49:1239–1242

Swerdloff RS, Wang C (2004) Androgens and the ageing male. Best Pract Res Clin Endocrinol Metab 18:349–362

Tenover JL (1999) Testosterone replacement therapy in older adult men. Int J Androl 22:300–306

Vanderschueren D, Vandenput L, Boonen S, Van Herck E, Swinnen JV, Bouillon R (2000) An aged rat model of partial androgen deficiency: prevention of both loss of bone and lean body mass by low-dose androgen replacement. Endocrinology 141:1642–1647

Vanderschueren D, Vandenput L, Boonen S, Lindberg MK, Bouillon R, Ohlsson C (2004) Androgens and bone. Endocr Rev 25:389–425

Vermeulen A (2001) Androgen replacement therapy in the aging male–a critical evaluation. J Clin Endocrinol Metab 86:2380–2390

Wu FC, von Eckardstein A (2003) Androgens and coronary artery disease. Endocr Rev 24:183–217

II.4.12 Abuse of Androgens

H.-C. Schuppe, A. Jung, W.-B. Schill

Summary

The attraction of anabolic-androgenic steroids for both professional and recreational athletes is to improve muscle mass, strength and endurance. Moreover, an increasing number of men take anabolic-androgenic steroids primarily as lifestyle drugs in an effort to enhance their appearance and sense of well-being. Most frequently misused compounds are 17β-hydroxyl esters of testosterone, 19-nortestosterone, methenolone, and the hepatotoxic 17α-alkylated derivatives stanozolol and methandienone. A typical administration regimen includes combinations of various anabolic-androgenic steroids taken intermittently at doses that exceed those required for androgen replacement therapy in male hypogonadism up to 100-fold. Among the well-known side-effects, suppression of the hypothalamic-pituitary-gonadal axis resulting in inhibition of spermatogenesis, testicular atrophy and disturbed sexual function as well as gynaecomastia are most important in clinical andrology. Hormonal dysregulation and changes in semen parameters are considered to be reversible after drug withdrawal; however, recovery of spermatogenesis can require more than 12 months or may even be absent after long-term abuse. Considering that anabolic-androgenic steroids represent a major health risk in the general population, including adolescents, increasing efforts for prevention of abuse are needed. Prescription of anabolic-androgenic steroids to healthy men by physicians is ethically and medico-legally unacceptable.

II.4.12.1 Introduction

Androgens are required for prenatal sexual differentiation and pubertal development of the male phenotype. In the adult male, testosterone plays a key role in maintaining specific reproductive tissues including spermatogenesis at the testicular level. Moreover, androgens significantly stimulate sexual function and behaviour. It is well known that testosterone replacement therapy in hypogonadal men increases nitrogen retention, lean body mass and body weight (Bagatell and Bremner 1996). Reversal of androgen deficiency is associated with beneficial effects on muscle strength, bone mineral density, erythropoiesis and mood. In contrast, it has been a matter of debate whether androgens can improve muscle strength and performance in healthy, eugonadal men (Wilson 1988; Elashoff et al. 1991; Bagatell and Bremner 1996). More recent studies, however, indicate that testosterone has direct anabolic effects on skeletal muscles reflected by an increase in muscle mass due to muscle fibre hypertrophy (Bhasin et al. 2001, 2004). Notably, administration of supraphysiological doses of testosterone in healthy men, especially when combined with strength training, increases fat-free mass as well as muscle size and maximal voluntary strength (Bhasin et al. 1996).

The observation that testosterone and other androgens exert anabolic effects has led to their use as performance-enhancing drugs among athletes since the 1950s. Today, abuse of anabolic-androgenic steroids (AAS) is no longer restricted to competitive sports but represents a major health risk in the general population including adolescents.

II.4.12.2 Anabolic-Androgenic Steroids

Since it is rapidly metabolized in the liver, testosterone is virtually inactive when taken orally. The search for clinically useful testosterone preparations in the past 60 years has yielded a wide range of synthetic derivatives (Kochakian 1976; Bagatell and Bremner 1996; Mottram and George 2000; Fig. II.4.36). Common modifications of testosterone suitable for intramuscular injection in oily vehicles are 17β-hydroxyl esters, whereas alkylation at position 17α renders the molecule orally active. Further modifications comprise 19-nortestosterone (nandrolone) and its derivatives as well as 1α-alkylated compounds. With regard to possible clinical indications beyond androgen-replacement therapy in males, many attempts have been made to develop steroids with predominant nitrogen-retaining, anabolic and less androgenic properties. As yet, however, there are no pure anabolic steroids available. Nevertheless, AAS represent the most prevalent performance-enhancing drugs illicitly used in competitive and non-competitive sports (Mottram and George 2000; Verroken 2000; Dawson 2001). Apart from the testosterone esters, the most frequently administered compounds are nandrolone, methenolone, and the 17α-alkylated derivatives methandienone, stanozolol, and methyltestosterone (see Fig. II.4.36). Moreover, new "designer steroids" have to be considered as illustrated by the recent identification of tetrahydrogestrinone (THG; Catlin et al. 2004; Noakes 2004). This compound, which proved to be a highly potent androgen in a yeast-based in vitro bioassay system, had been distributed without any prior biological or toxicological evaluation (Death et al. 2004).

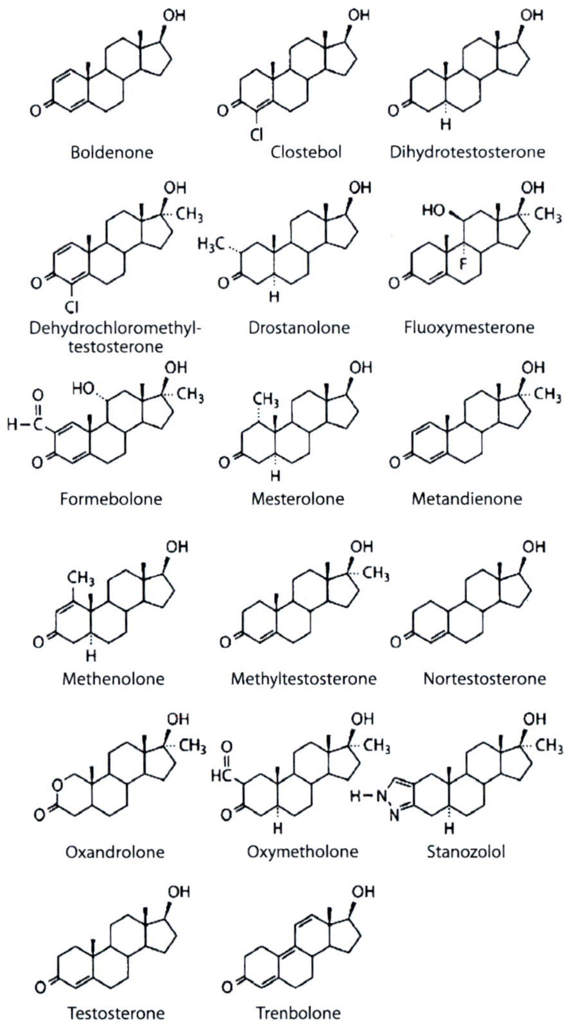

Fig. II.4.36. Structure of anabolic-androgenic steroids frequently detected in international doping tests. Figure taken from Schänzer W (1998) Abuse of androgens and detection of illegal use. In: Nieschlag E, Behre HM (eds) Testosterone – action, deficiency, substitution, 2nd edn. Springer, Berlin Heidelberg New York, pp 545–565

II.4.12.2.1 Are There Clinical Indications for Anabolic-Androgenic Steroids?

The efficacy and safety of testosterone preparations for treatment of male hypogonadism are well established (Nieschlag et al. 2004; see Chap. II.4.13). Androgenic steroids, however, were initially recognized for their anabolic effects and have been widely used in clinical medicine. Before bone marrow transplantation and recombinant erythropoietin became available, AAS played an important role in the treatment of haematologic disorders such as various types of anaemias (Bagatell and Bremner 1996; Basaria et al. 2001). Furthermore, the beneficial effects of these compounds have been observed in patients suffering from cachexia associated with severe burns as well as chronic diseases such as renal and hepatic failure, cancer, or pulmonary disease (Basaria et al. 2001; Liu and Handelsman 2004). Recent studies suggest that AAS can be used for the treatment of wasting associated with human immunodeficiency virus/acquired immunodeficiency syndrome. Compounds such as danazol are important therapeutic options in the management of hereditary angioedema.

II.4.12.2.2 Historical and Epidemiological Aspects of Abuse

The use of performance-enhancing medicinal products by athletes can be traced back to the ancient Olympic Games (Verroken 2000). In the 1950s, weightlifters were probably the first to take testosterone derivatives without any medical indication in order to increase muscle mass and strength. Since then, the abuse of AAS rapidly spread to other disciplines of competitive sports in spite of early warnings concerning serious adverse effects (Wade 1972; Wilson 1988; Verroken 2000; Dawson 2001). In some countries, such as the former German Democratic Republic, athletes were even systematically subjected to unethical and secret programmes of hormonal doping by the government (Franke and Berendonk 1997).

In 1968, the International Olympic Committee (IOC) released the first anti-doping rules. The list of illicit compounds, however, included only stimulants and narcotics. Synthetic AAS were prohibited in 1974 when the first methods to detect abuse of these compounds became available (Verroken 2000; Schänzer 2004). Notably, testosterone itself was not banned until 1984. Later definitions of doping are more general and comprise a wide range of different performance-enhancing drugs and methods (IOC 1999; Verroken 2000): "Doping is (1) the use of an expedient (substance or method) that is potentially harmful to athletes' health and/or capable of enhancing their performance, or (2) the presence in the athletes' body of a prohibited substance or evidence of the use thereof or evidence of the use of a prohibited method".

With regard to different disciplines, the highest prevalence of abuse is found among bodybuilders and weightlifters, followed by track-and-field athletes, cyclists and swimmers (Wilson 1988; Schänzer 1998). The overall statistics of doping tests performed by laboratories accredited by the IOC and World Anti-Doping Agency during competition and training revealed approximately 1% of samples positive for AAS over the last decade (Verroken 2000; Schänzer 2004). On the other hand, enquiries after the Seoul Olympics of 1988 provided suggestive evidence that more than 50% of the athletes had been illicitly using performance-enhancing drugs (Dawson 2001).

The inappropriate use of AAS, however, is not restricted to high level competitive sports. It has been assumed that more than 25% of men attending gyms take AAS and other performance-enhancing drugs, and a prevalence of up to 80% was reported for male amateur bodybuilders (Johnson 1990; Boos et al. 1998). Moreover, occupational users such as doormen, police and prison warders have to be considered (Dawson 2001). Several surveys concerning adolescents between the ages of 11 and 18 showed that 3–12% of boys and 1–2% of girls had used or were using AAS (Buckley et al. 1988; Handelsman and Gupta 1997; Bahrke et al. 2000). According to data from the UK, AAS are the third most common drugs behind cannabis and amphetamines offered to schoolchildren (Dawson 2001). Although concise epidemiological data are lacking, the available pieces of information indicate that abuse of AAS is dramatically increasing among the general population. AAS have become lifestyle drugs and abuse is often associated with that of other compounds such as narcotics as well as alcohol consumption and smoking (Durant et al. 1993; Boos et al. 1998; Bahrke et al. 2000).

II.4.12.2.3 Aims and Psychopathology of Abuse

The attraction of AAS for both professional and recreational athletes is to increase muscle mass – and thus strength, sprinting speed and endurance – beyond the level achievable by any training regimen or complex non-pharmaceutical interventions including special diets (Dawson 2001; Noakes 2004). Occupational users such as security personnel have the objective that they must increase their strength both to threaten and protect others. An increasing number of men, however, take AAS primarily in an effort to enhance their appearance and sense of well-being (Pope et al. 2000; Dawson 2001). Notably, men have reported a great desire for larger, more muscular bodies. Although highly muscular, these men are often dissatisfied with their body image and perceive themselves as underweight (Drenowski and Yee 1987; Pope et al. 2000). Several studies revealed that bodybuilders, as compared to other athletes, display an increased preoccupation with their body appearance, similar to that observed among patients with eating disorders such as anorexia nervosa, but with a "reversed" focus of gaining muscle (Blouin and Goldfield 1995; Mangweth et al. 2001). Thus, abuse of AAS and obsessive exercising associated with body image dissatisfaction may reflect a body dysmorphic disorder according to DSM-IV (American Psychiatric Association 1994, Diagnostic and statistical manual of mental disorders). The pathological belief of not having enough musculature found among weightlifters and bodybuilders has been coined "biggerexia" or "muscle dysmorphia" (Pope et al. 2000; Choi et al. 2002).

II.4.12.3 Patterns of Abuse

Athletes and recreational bodybuilders who abuse AAS believe that higher doses of these compounds produce greater effects on the muscle than lower doses (Wilson 1988; Knuth et al. 1989; Bagatell and Bremner 1996; Boos et al. 1998; Mottram and George 2000; Dawson 2001). Therefore, typical administration regimens differ markedly from those applied clinically, as illustrated by respective "recommendations" available from publications such as the "Underground steroid handbook" (Duchaine 1989), magazines for bodybuilders, or via the internet. Various combinations of both intramuscular and oral AAS including 17α-alkylated compounds are taken intermittently and in progressively increasing doses ("stacking"; compounds frequently used are shown in Fig. II.4.36). Treatment cycles of 4–18 weeks are followed by variable drug-free intervals lasting as long as a year. The doses of AAS administered exceed those required for androgen replacement therapy in male hypogonadism up to 100-fold. For maximal effect, AAS are used in combination with other hormones such as insulin, growth hormone, insulin-like growth factor, or thyroid hormones (Mottram and George 2000; Dawson 2001; Noakes 2004). In order to "prevent" untoward effects of AAS, human chorionic gonadotrophin (hCG), anti-oestrogens such as tamoxifen, or diuretics are administered.

The exact magnitude of benefit from the above-mentioned regimens combining various AAS or concomitant use of other compounds is unknown (Noakes 2004). Due to the secrecy that surrounds the use of performance-enhancing drugs, objective data are scarce. Whether or not steroids with strong anabolic properties are more effective than testosterone preparations in increasing muscle mass, strength and endurance remains to be elucidated. Controlled prospective investigations under appropriate conditions, however, remain prohibited for ethical reasons.

Although several AAS such as 17α-alkylated compounds are no longer used in clinical medicine and have been officially withdrawn because of severe adverse effects, they are still available on the black market or may be ordered via the internet. Moreover, preparations approved only for veterinary use are administered. In particular, the unknown quality of illegally produced AAS is a matter of concern. On the other hand, it has been estimated that in 15% of cases AAS are prescribed by physicians or released by pharmacists (Boos et al. 1998).

Pro-hormones of testosterone as well as derivatives of dihydrotestosterone and nortestosterone have been marketed as nutritional supplements and are advertised to be as effective as testosterone (Schänzer 2004). However, only high doses of such compounds given orally may result in significant increases in serum testosterone. Other nutritional supplements, which are offered as drug-free alternatives for performance improvement, have been shown to contain substantial concentrations of non-labelled AAS (Geyer et al. 2004). Unintentional use of such preparations by athletes may result in positive doping tests.

II.4.12.3.1 Adverse Effects of Anabolic-Androgenic Steroids

The untoward effects of AAS depend on both the type and dose administered (Bagatell and Bremner 1996). In general, replacement doses and the administration of testosterone esters are associated with fewer complications than is the use of 17α-alkylated derivatives, particularly at excessive doses. Both androgenic and oestrogenic as well as non-hormonal toxic effects of the original compounds and their metabolites have to be considered. Available studies in this field, however, may not sufficiently reflect the sequelae of long-term abuse, especially considering the non-standardized doses and combinations of AAS administered. Moreover, there is no reporting of side-effects to a central body (Dawson 2001).

The most common adverse effects of AAS encountered among athletes, bodybuilders and other male abusers are compiled in Table II.4.10. The top ten complaints self-reported by men calling an anti-doping hot-line in Sweden were aggressiveness, depression, acne, gynaecomastia, anxiousness, potency problems, testicular atrophy, sleep disorders, fluid retention and mood disturbances (Eklof et al. 2003).

For the clinical andrologist, suppression of the hypothalamic–pituitary–gonadal axis and subsequent infertility are of major importance: based on the negative feedback mechanism, secretion of gonadotrophins and endogenous testosterone is impaired, resulting in inhibition of spermatogenesis with oligo- or azoospermia (Schürmeyer et al. 1984). Moreover, percentages of motile and morphologically normal spermatozoa may be significantly reduced (Knuth et al. 1989; Torres-Calleja et al. 2001). Recent observations suggest that concomitant abuse of hCG may further impair spermatogenesis and thus sperm morphology (Karila et al. 2004). Testicular atrophy and disturbed sexual function with loss of libido and erectile dysfunction are also frequent signs and symptoms of AAS-induced hypogonadism (Wilson 1988).

AAS-induced hormonal dysregulation and changes in semen parameters are considered to be reversible after drug withdrawal (Schürmeyer et al. 1984; Knuth et al. 1989). The recovery of spermatogenesis, however, can require more than 12 months (Gazvani et al. 1997). Other case reports indicate that hypogonadotrophic hypogonadism may even be irreversible (Van Breda et al. 2003; Jung et al. 2003). In this context, the multifactorial aetiology of male infertility and the impact of pre-existing or concomitant disorders of reproductive functions should be noted (see Chaps. I.3).

With regard to therapy, clomiphene citrate has been used to reverse hypogonadism (Tan and Vasudevan 2003). Men with primary infertility due to persistent azoospermia after abuse of AAS were successfully treated with hCG either alone or in combination with human menopausal gonadotrophin (hMG), in one case

Table II.4.10. Adverse effects of anabolic-androgenic steroids in males[a]

Hypothalamic-pituitary-gonadal axis	Suppression of gonadotrophin secretion Testicular atrophy Oligo- or azoospermia, infertility Testosterone deficiency Decreased libido
Breast	Gynaecomastia
Haematopoiesis	Polycythaemia Thrombo-embolic complications
Cardiovascular system	Cardiomyopathy, sudden cardiac death
Liver[b]	Hepatocellular and intrahepatic cholestasis Peliosis hepatis (haemorrhagic liver cysts) Hepatocellular adenoma/carcinoma
Metabolism	Reduction in plasma HDL cholesterol levels, increase in LDL cholesterol level Hyperinsulinaemia
Bone	Premature closure of epiphyses (in adolescents)
Skin	Acne Androgenetic alopecia
Psychological disorders	Mood disturbances, depression, psychotic symptoms (withdrawal syndromes), increased aggression (?)

[a] Adapted from Jockenhövel (2002) [b] Especially after administration of 17α-alkylated derivatives

assisted reproductive techniques were required to achieve a pregnancy (Turek et al. 1995; Jung et al. 2003; Menon 2003).

Gynaecomastia is one of the most common adverse effects of AAS, especially when compounds undergoing aromatization to oestrogens are administered (Eklof et al. 2003). Breast changes often persist after withdrawal of AAS and may require mastectomy. The hallmark of skin-related adverse reactions of AAS is acne vulgaris including severe forms such as acne fulminans with its deleterious sequelae (Assmann et al. 1999). Hepatotoxicity is related mainly to high doses of 17α-alkylated compounds (Bagatell and Bremner 1996). Hepatocellular and intrahepatic cholestasis may result in severe jaundice and hepatic failure; moreover, peliosis hepatis as well as the development of hepatocellular adenoma or carcinoma have been reported (Soe et al. 1992). Furthermore, administration of high doses of AAS causes unfavourable changes in lipid metabolism leading to an increased atherogenic lipid profile (Hartgens et al. 2004). It is a matter of debate, however, whether long-term abuse of AAS is associated with a significantly increased risk of cardiovascular disease, thrombogenicity and embolic complications. On the other hand, stroke, myocardial infarction and sudden deaths due to cardiomyopathy have been reported in young men abusing AAS (Bagatell and Bremner 1996). Studies in power athletes indicate that the abuse of AAS is associated with myocardial hypertrophy in a dose-dependent manner (Karila et al. 2003). The changes in left ventricular mass were potentiated by concomitant use of growth hormone. It should be noted that AAS also affect psyche and behaviour (Pope and Katz 1994; Brower 2002). Apart from mood disturbances, increments of aggressive behaviour, dependence as well as withdrawal syndromes with depression, hypomania or psychotic features have been observed. Whether these symptoms result from AAS abuse or reflect an underlying psychopathology of the patient is unclear (see above).

II.4.12.3.2 Detection of Abuse

Doping control in competition sports is organized by national and international sport federations, the IOC and the World Anti-Doping Agency including "out-of-competition testing programmes" (Schänzer 2004). Test samples have to be processed in accredited laboratories according to standardized protocols. Concerning the identification of AAS, analysis of urine samples by gas chromatography and high resolution mass spectrometry after appropriate sample preparation represent the main analytical tools (Saugy et al. 2000; Schänzer 2004). In order to increase the accuracy of analytical results, derivatization methods and selected ion monitoring profiles are employed. Moreover, the highly complex metabolism of AAS as well as the pharmacokinetics of parent compounds and their excreted metabolites have to be considered. Detection of more than 20 metabolites after administration of one single AAS is not unusual (Schänzer 2004). With regard to the abuse of endogenously produced AAS, e.g. testosterone, the ratio of testosterone to epitestosterone excreted in urine is determined and appears significantly increased after administration of exogenous testosterone. Respective results, however, require further confirmation by additional methods such as gas chromatography-combustion-isotype ratio mass spectrometry. In the future, bioassays may become important tools, especially to detect novel designer steroids (Handelsman 2004).

References

American Psychiatric Association (1994) Diagnostic and statistical manual of mental disorders, 4th edn. American Psychiatric Association, Washington

Assmann T, Arens A, Becker-Wegerich P, Schuppe HC, Lehmann P (1999) Acne fulminans, sternoclavicular bone lesions and azoospermia following abuse of anabolic steroids [in German]. Z Hautkr 74:570–572

Bagatell CJ, Bremner WJ (1996) Androgens in men – uses and abuses. N Engl J Med 334:707–714

Bahrke M, Yesalis CE, Kopstein AN, Stephens JA (2000) Risk factors for anabolic-androgenic steroid use among adolescents. Sports Med 29:1–9

Basaria S, Wahlstrom JT, Dobs AS (2001) Clinical review 138: anabolic-androgenic steroid therapy in the treatment of chronic diseases. J Clin Endocrinol Metab 86:5108–5117

Bhasin S, Storer TW, Berman N, Callegari C, Clevenger B, Phillips J, Bunnel TJ, Tricker R, Shirazi A, Casaburi R (1996) The effects of supraphysiologic doses of testosterone on muscle size and strength in normal men. N Engl J Med 335:1–7

Bhasin S, Woodhouse L, Storer TW (2001) Proof of the effect of testosterone on skeletal muscle. J Endocrinol 170:27–38

Bhasin S, Storer TW, Singh AB, Woodhouse L, Singh R, Artaza J, Taylor WE, Sinha-Hikim I, Jasuja R, Gonzalez-Cadavid N (2004) Testosterone effects on the skeletal muscle. In: Nieschlag E, Behre HM (eds) Testosterone – action, deficiency, substitution, 3rd edn. Cambridge University Press, Cambridge, pp 715–735

Blouin AG, Goldfield GS (1995) Body image and steroid use in male bodybuilders. Int J Eat Disord 18:159–165

Boos C, Wulff P, Kujath P, Bruch H-P (1998) Drug abuse among recreational athletes in leisure sports [in German]. Dt Ärztebl 95:A953–A957

Brower KJ (2002) Anabolic steroid abuse and dependence. Curr Psychiatry Rep 4:377–387

Buckley WE, Yesalis CE, Friedl KE, Anderson WA, Streit AL, Wright JE (1988) Estimated prevalence of anabolic steroid use among male high school seniors. J Am Med Assoc 260:3441–3445

Catlin DH, Sekera MH, Ahrens BD, Starcevic B, Chang YC, Hatton CK (2004) Tetrahydrogestrinone: discovery, synthesis, and detection in urine. Rapid Commun Spectrom 18: 1245–1249

Choi PY, Pope HG Jr, Olivardia R (2002) Muscle dysmorphia: a new syndrome in weightlifters. Br J Sports Med 36:375–376

Dawson RT (2001) Drugs in sport – the role of the physician. J Endocrinol 170:55–61

Death AK, McGrath KC, Kazlauskas R, Handelsman DJ (2004) Tetrahydrogestrinone is a potent androgen and progestin. J Clin Endocrinol Metab 89:2498 - 2500
Drenowski A, Yee DK (1987) Men and body image: are males satisfied with their body weight? Psychosom Med 49:626 - 634
Duchaine D (1989) Underground steroid handbook II. HLR Technical Books, Venice
Durant RH, Rickert VI, Ashworth CS, Newman C, Slavens G (1993) Use of multiple drugs among adolescents who use anabolic steroids. N Engl J Med 328:922 - 926
Eklof AC, Thurelius AM, Garle M, Rane A, Sjoqvist F (2003) The anti-doping hot-line, a means to capture the abuse of doping agents in the Swedish society and a new service function in clinical pharmacology. Eur J Clin Pharmacol 59: 571 - 577
Elashoff JD, Jacknow AD, Shain SG, Braunstein GD (1991) Effects of anabolic-androgenic steroids on muscular strength. Ann Intern Med 115:387 - 393
Franke WW, Berendonk B (1997) Hormonal doping and androgenization of athletes: a secret program of the German Democratic Republic government. Clin Chem 43:1262 - 1279
Gazvani MR, Buckett W, Luckas MJM, Aird IA, Hipkin LJ, Lewis-Jones DI (1997) Conservative management of azoospermia following steroid abuse. Hum Reprod 12:1706 - 1708
Geyer H, Parr MK, Mareck U, Reinhart U, Schrader Y, Schänzer W (2004) Analysis of non-hormonal nutritional supplements for anabolic-androgenic steroids - results of an international study. Int J Sports Med 25:124 - 129
Handelsman DJ (2004) Designer androgens in sport: when too much is never enough. Sci STKE 244:41
Handelsman DJ, Gupta (1997) Prevalence and risk factors for anabolic-androgenic steroid abuse in Australian high school students. Int J Androl 20:159 - 164
Hartgens F, Rietjens G; Keizer HA, Kuipers H, Wolffenbuttel BH (2004) Effects of androgenic-anabolic steroids on apolipoproteins and lipoprotein (a). Br J Sports Med 38:253 - 259
International Olympic Committee (1999) Lausanne declaration on doping in sport. IOC, Lausanne
Jockenhövel F (2002) Männlicher Hypogonadismus - aktuelle Aspekte der Androgensubstitution, 2nd edn. Uni-Med, Bremen
Johnsen MD (1990) Anabolic steroid use in adolescent athletes. Pediatr Clin North Am 37:1111 - 1123
Jung A, Schill WB, Schuppe HC (2003) Persistent hypogonadotrophic hypogonadism after abuse of anabolic steroids [in German]. JDDG 1 (Suppl 1):S43
Karila T, Karjalainen JE, Mantysaari MJ, Viitasalo MT, Seppälä T (2003) Dose-dependent increase in left ventricular mass in power athletes and this effect is potentiated by concomitant use of growth hormone. Int J Sports Med 24:337 - 343
Karila T, Hovatta O, Seppälä T (2004) Concomitant abuse of anabolic androgenic steroids and human chorionic gonadotrophin impairs spermatogenesis in power athletes. Int J Sports Med 25:257 - 263
Knuth UA, Maniera H, Nieschlag E (1989) Anabolic steroids and semen parameters in bodybuilders. Fertil Steril 52:1041 - 1047
Kochakian CD (1976) Anabolic-androgenic steroids. In: Handbook of experimental pharmacology, Vol 43. Springer, Berlin Heidelberg New York
Liu PY, Handelsman DJ (2004) Androgen therapy in non-gonadal disease. In: Nieschlag E, Behre HM (eds) Testosterone - action, deficiency, substitution, 3rd edn. Cambridge University Press, Cambridge, pp 445 - 495
Mangweth B, Pope HG, Kemmler G, Ebenbichler C, Hausmann A, De Col C, Kreutner B, Kinzl J, Biebl W (2001) Body image and psychopathology in male bodybuilders. Psychother Psychosom 70:38 - 43
Menon DK (2003) Successful treratment of anabolic steroid-induced azoospermia with human chorionic gonadotropin and human menopausal gonadotropin. Fertil Steril 79 (Suppl 3):1659 - 1661
Mottram DR, George AJ (2000) Anabolic steroids. Baillieres Best Pract Res Clin Endocrinol Metab 14:55 - 69
Nieschlag E, Behre HM, Bouchard P, Corrales JJ, Jones TH, Stalla GK, Webb SM, Wu FCW (2004) Testosterone replacement therapy: current trends and future directions. Hum Reprod Update 10:409 - 419
Noakes TD (2004) Tainted glory - doping and athletic performance. N Engl J Med 351:847 - 849
Pope HG, Katz DL (1994) Psychiatric and medical effects of anabolic-androgenic steroid abuse. Arch Gen Psychiatry 51: 375 - 382
Pope HG, Phillips KA, Olivardia R (2000) The Adonis complex: the secret crisis of male body obsession. Free Press, New York
Saugy M, Cardis C, Robinson N, Schweizer C (2000) Test methods: anabolics. Baillieres Best Pract Res Clin Endocrinol Metab 14:111 - 133
Schänzer W (1998) Abuse of androgens and detection of illegal use. In: Nieschlag E, Behre HM (eds) Testosterone - action, deficiency, substitution, 2nd edn. Springer, Berlin Heidelberg New York, pp 545 - 565
Schänzer W (2004) Abuse of androgens and detection of illegal use. In: Nieschlag E, Behre HM (eds) Testosterone - action, deficiency, substitution, 3rd edn. Cambridge University Press, Cambridge, pp 715 - 735
Schürmeyer TH, Knuth UA, Belkien L, Nieschlag E (1984) Reversible azoospermia induced by anabolic steroid 19-nortestosterone. Lancet 1:417 - 420
Soe KL, Soe M, Gluud C (1992) Liver pathology associated with the use of anabolic-androgenic steroids. Liver 12:73 - 79
Tan RS, Vasudevan D (2003) Use of clomiphene citrate to reverse premature andropause secondary to steroid abuse. Fertil Steril 79:203 - 205
Torres-Calleja J, Gonzales-Unzaga M, DeCelis-Carrillo R, Calzada-Sanchez L, Pedron N (2001) Effect of androgenic anabolic steroids on sperm quality and serum hormone levels in adult male bodybuilders. Life Sci 68:1769 - 1774
Turek PJ, Williams RH, Gilbaugh JH, Lipshultz LI (1995) The reversibility of anabolic steroid-induced azoospermia. J Urol 153:1628 - 1630
Van Breda E, Keizer HA, Kuipers H, Wolffenbuttel BH (2003) Androgenic anabolic steroid use and severe hypothalamic-pituitary dysfunction: a case study. Int J Sports Med 24:195 - 196
Verroken M (2000) Drug use and abuse in sport. Baillieres Best Pract Res Clin Endocrinol Metab 14:1 - 23
Wade N (1972) Anabolic steroids: doctors denounce them but athletes aren't listening. Science 176:1399 - 1403
Wilson JD (1988) Androgen abuse by athletes. Endocr Rev 9:181 - 199

II.4.13 Exotic Hormones

F. Comhaire, A. Mahmoud

Summary

During male ageing important changes occur in the neuroendocrine environment. The most remarkable are the decreased secretion of melatonin, growth hormone, dehydroepiandrosterone (DHEA) and testosterone. Hormone replacement therapy (HRT) with each of these substances has been proposed, but few data are available on the long-term effects.

Today, HRT with testosterone seems to offer the most promising prospect. New delivery systems are under development that can restore physiological testosterone levels in blood, including day-night variability. However, melatonin and DHEA may be of benefit in particular circumstances.

- Regular exercise and reduced nutritional calorie intake are **important elements** of the "healthy lifestyle" of ageing persons.
- Hormone replacement therapy with growth hormone needs further studies, and should not be recommended as yet.
- Androgen replacement therapy may be beneficial for ageing men with clear-cut hypoandrogenism.
- There are hardly any arguments to recommend delivery of DHEA to ageing or elderly men.

II.4.13.1 Introduction

Thanks to better hygiene and up-to-date medicine fewer people die at an early age. However, those who survive do not live longer than in the past. The increased "average life expectancy" observed over recent decades does not imply that mankind really lives longer (Callahan 2000). In the USA, and probably in Europe as well, the median number of remaining years of life for all 80 year olds is approximately 7.0 years; for 85 year olds, it is 5.0 years. So, clearly, in order to live until a very old age, one must reach an old age first. This truism highlights the need for systems and strategies to maintain a reasonable health condition until old age.

There are several theories attempting to explain the ageing phenomenon.

Programmed deterioration of the neuroendocrine and/or the immune systems may be related to the finite capacity of cells to divide and thus "renew" the systems. The reasons for the finiteness of cell replication are not well known, but there are arguments that progressive shortening of the telomeres, which are situated at the extremity of the chromosomes, is involved (review see Klapper et al. 2001).

Wear and tear of tissues and cells are, among other factors, related to damage caused by reactive oxygen species to both the cell membrane and its contents, particularly the mitochondria (Calabrese et al. 2001), which generate energy, and DNA.

A reasonable strategy that aims to delay the epiphenomena of ageing should maintain or restore a "normal" hormonal equilibrium, and counteract the mechanisms causing wear and tear (Chap. II.4.14).

II.4.13.2 Hormonal Changes in Ageing Men

In men, age-related changes occur in serum hormone levels, as shown in Table II.4.11.

II.4.13.2.1 Melatonin

The pineal gland secretes melatonin, which regulates the biological clock in seasonal breeders, and in humans. Melatonin is present in children and may exert a suppressive effect on pituitary gonadotrophin secretion during pre-puberty. In adults, the nocturnal secretion of melatonin also seems to depend on the pineal gland, while the "background" secretion of this hormone during the day originates instead from the gastrointestinal tract (Messner et al. 2001; Bubenik 2002).

Melatonin plays a role in the night-time regulation of metabolism that is slowed down during sleep. The increase in body temperature that occurs during vigorous exercise is counteracted by the anti-pyretic action of melatonin.

Table II.4.11. Age-related changes in serum hormones in men. (*ACTH* Adrenocorticotrophin, *DHEA* dehydroepiandrosterone, *FSH* follicle-stimulating hormone, *LH* luteinizing hormone, T_3 *triiodothyronine*, T_4 *thyroxine*, *TSH* thyroid-stimulating hormone)

Hormone	Change
Melatonin	↓
Growth hormone	= N
Insulin-like growth factor I (somatomedin C)	↓
ACTH and cortisol	= N
DHEA	↓
TSH and T_4	= N
T_3	↓
LH	= N
FSH	↑
Total and free testosterone	↓
Inhibin B	↓

II.4.13.2.2 Growth Hormone

Growth hormone (GH) is secreted by the pituitary gland, under stimulation of growth hormone releasing hormone (GHRH) produced by the hypothalamus. Growth hormone circulates in blood and is converted in the liver and in other tissues to what was previously called somatomedin C, but is now referred to as insulin-like growth factor 1 (IGF 1). It is IGF 1 that stimulates cell proliferation and protein synthesis. In synergism with thyroid hormones, GH stimulates skeletal growth and tissue growth through IGF 1. Growth hormone in synergism with cortisol increases lipolysis of fat tissue, and has a "diabetogenic" effect by increasing blood sugar levels (Lo et al. 2001).

In ageing men the levels of GH decrease, because of a decreased responsiveness of the pituitary to stimulation by GHRH. In physiological circumstances the release of GH is stronger during sleep. Since sleep is often fragmented in the elderly, nocturnal GH secretion is reduced. Both testosterone and oestradiol stimulate GH secretion. In ageing men and women, the secretion of sex hormones decreases, reducing the GH secretion. A strong natural stimulus of GH secretion is exercise. Since many ageing persons reduce their exercising, this equally decreases GH secretion.

In fact, the GH level in blood decreases by an average of 14% per decade of life. This results in lower lipolytic action and increased body fat, as well as decreased protein synthesis with decreasing lean body mass.

II.4.13.2.3 Adrenal Hormones

The secretion of **adrenocorticotrophin** (**ACTH**) and **cortisol** changes little with age. It has been reported that stress and depression cause a longer-lasting increase of cortisolemia in ageing persons than in the young. This is attributed to mitigated counterregulation mechanisms reducing ACTH at the hypothalamic level. The longer-lasting cortisol response to stress and depression may accelerate ageing and may precipitate degeneration of neurons of the central nervous system (Newcomer et al. 1994). In view of their exaggerated susceptibility to stress, efforts should be made to avoid submitting ageing persons to stressful circumstances. Also, depressive mood changes (weariness of life) must be diagnosed and treated appropriately.

Another important adrenal hormone is **dehydroepiandrosterone** (**DHEA**). Aside from being a direct precursor hormone of oestradiol and of testosterone in target tissues (Labrie et al. 2001), DHEA has central nervous effects and is metabolized in the limbic system and hippocampal-hypothalamic region (Hunt et al. 2000). It has been suggested that persons who attain a very high age in a relatively healthy condition tend to have a higher DHEA (sulphate) level in blood. Indeed, during ageing the concentration of DHEA(S) decreases (Montanini et al. 1988), but the rate of decline is different from one person to another. It is impossible to assess whether the higher DHEA level in the "fit" elderly is the cause or rather the result of their good physical condition (Hinson et al. 2003).

II.4.13.2.4 Testicular Function

Testicular function dramatically decreases during ageing. This item is covered in extenso by Kaufman (Chap. I.11.1) and by Vanderschueren (Chap. II.4.11).

II.4.13.3 Treatment Options

The diagnosis of hormone deficiency must always be based on the measurement of the hormone levels in blood before hormone replacement therapy is introduced. Measurement of melatonin is not part of routine evaluation, because it requires multiple sampling during the night. In addition, there are few consequences of decreased melatonin levels that need treatment.

The assessment of GH and IGF 1, of DHEA-sulphate and of total and free testosterone should be performed on blood taken in the morning, in view of the significant day–night variability. Interpretation of the results requires good insight into the endocrine mechanisms involved in ageing, and must be related to the signs and symptoms.

Melatonin was proven to "reset" the sleep pattern of blind persons (who cannot perceive light) (Sack et al. 2000) and has been advocated for the readjustment of the sleep pattern caused by "jet-lag". Melatonin has been marketed as a natural sleeping pill at a dose of 3–10 mg, and it seems to be safe for this indication. However, the evening administration of melatonin to hypertensive patients treated with calcium channel blockers may increase blood pressure and heart rate throughout a 24-h period (Lusardi et al. 2000).

Much higher doses, up to 100 mg per day, seem to exert antioxidant effects. Also, these pharmacological doses have been reported to sometimes act beneficially as adjuvant therapy in patients with untreatable cancers. However, the latter is based on uncontrolled observations (Lissoni et al. 1994; Lissoni 1998).

The best method to "rejuvenate" the **growth hormone–IGF 1 axis** is to encourage exercise and to control body weight. Particular amino acids (such as arginine) have been advocated to stimulate GH secretion, but this effect has not yet been objectively proven. Substitution of sex hormones and of DHEA will also increase GH secretion (Genazzani et al. 2001).

Treatment by injections of GH has been shown to increase lean body mass and muscle force in hypopituitary adults (Weaver et al. 1995) and in obese men (Johannsson et al. 1997). The results of studies supporting this claim need confirmation. However, GH may be diabetogenic, particularly in the elderly, who have a decreased secretory reserve capacity of Langerhans' island beta cells. Hence, physiological doses of GH, which would not promote diabetes in young persons, may do so in ageing men. In addition it is documented that patients suffering from acromegaly, caused by excessive GH secretion, run a higher risk of cancer in general (Higuchi et al. 2000; Baris et al. 2002), and of colon cancer in particular (Orme et al. 1998). Whether long-term hormone replacement therapy with GH increases the cancer risk is not known. Growth hormone substitution in ageing men remains controversial.

Hormone replacement therapy using DHEA has been reported to improve mood and to reduce fatigue when it is given to patients with Addison's disease, who – by virtue of their adrenal insufficiency – have an extremely low DHEA(S) concentration in blood (Hunt et al. 2000). A similar effect was observed in healthy elderly women, but not in elderly men (Wolf et al. 1997). HRT with DHEA was shown to exert a positive influence on bone metabolism and to maintain, or to some extent restore, mineral bone density (Villareal et al. 2000). The latter is probably related to the DHEA being converted to oestrogen (Legrain et al. 2000; Labrie et al. 1997, 2001; Weill-Engerer et al. 2003). As far as DHEA supplementation to ageing men is concerned, it should be remembered that metabolism of this steroid generates both oestrogen and androgen (Genazzani et al. 2001). Ageing men have a relatively excessive oestrogen/testosterone ratio in blood, and it remains to be assessed whether DHEA substitution is beneficial or constitutes a risk for coronary heart disease (Hautanen et al. 1994; Khaw 1996; Arlt et al. 1999; Porsova-Dutoit et al. 2000; Thijs et al. 2003; Tchernof and Labrie 2004).

Before DHEA is administered, a thorough clinical investigation is mandatory. Women with oestrogen-sensitive cancers should not receive this substance. Activation of their tumour may occur in men suffering from overt or hidden prostate cancer when DHEA is given (Schiller et al. 1991; Koh et al. 2001). Careful follow-up during DHEA supplementation is mandatory, and it can be questioned whether DHEA is useful in ageing persons with a normal DHEA(S) level in serum (Nippoldt and Nair 1998).

II.4.13.4 Conclusion

From the (neuro)-endocrine viewpoint, several strategies can be adopted to counteract ageing. Lifestyle factors include encouragement of exercise and adaptation of nutrition, among other things, in order to avoid obesity. Possible hormone replacement therapy may be part of a more general approach to ageing which should probably include some form of nutritional supplementation as well.

Hormone replacement therapy with GH, GHRH or IGF 1 needs further study. The possible side-effects of GH call for prudence.

Optimal hormone replacement therapy using testosterone may have the potential of offering long-term benefit to the ageing male. Among other things, it may prevent osteoporosis, vascular disease, mental degeneration and muscle wastage. Hormone replacement therapy is unlikely to induce prostate hyperplasia or invasive prostate cancer (Comhaire and Mahmoud 2004). It may improve the quality of life, though long-term studies are needed to sustain these expectations.

There may be arguments in favour of using DHEA, though it seems preferable to apply this hormone in the ageing female rather than the ageing male.

In no way can any hormone treatment be considered a panacea that would be suitable for everybody. Hormone replacement therapy needs careful medical indication and follow-up, and should not be made available as an over-the-counter product.

Finally, it must be clear that hormone replacement therapy will probably not increase the life span of men. It is justified to presume that it may improve their quality of life and, perhaps, reduce the risk of particular life-threatening diseases.

References

Arlt W, Haas J, Callies F, Reincke M, Hubler D, Oettel M, Ernst M, Schulte HM, Allolio B (1999) Biotransformation of oral dehydroepiandrosterone in elderly men: significant increase in circulating estrogens. J Clin Endocrinol Metab 84:2170–2176

Baris D, Gridley G, Ron E, Weiderpass E, Mellemkjaer L, Ekbom A, Olsen JH, Baron JA, Fraumeni JF Jr. (2002) Acromegaly and cancer risk: a cohort study in Sweden and Denmark. Cancer Causes Control 13:395–400

Bubenik GA (2002) Gastrointestinal melatonin: localization, function, and clinical relevance. Dig Dis Sci 47:2336–2348

Calabrese V, Scapagnini G, Giuffrida SA, Bates TE, Clark JB (2001) Mitochondrial involvement in brain function and dysfunction: relevance to aging, neurodegenerative disorders and longevity. Neurochem Res 26:739–764

Callahan D (2000) Death and the research imperative. N Engl J Med 342:654–656

Comhaire F, Mahmoud A (2004) Preventing diseases of the prostate in the elderly using hormones and nutriceuticals. Aging Male 7:155–169

Genazzani AD, Stomati M, Strucchi C, Puccetti S, Luisi S, Genazzani AR (2001) Oral dehydroepiandrosterone supplementation modulates spontaneous and growth hormone-releasing hormone-induced growth hormone and insulin-like growth factor-1 secretion in early and late postmenopausal women. Fertil Steril 76:241–248

Hautanen A, Manttari M, Manninen V, Tenkanen L, Huttunen JK, Frick MH, Adlercreutz H (1994) Adrenal androgens and

testosterone as coronary risk factors in the Helsinki Heart Study. Atherosclerosis 105:191–200
Higuchi Y, Saeki N, Iuchi T, Uchino Y, Tatsuno I, Uchida D, Tanaka T, Noguchi Y, Nakamura S, Yasuda T, Yamaura A, Sunami K, Oka Y, Uozumi A (2000) Incidence of malignant tumors in patients with acromegaly. Endocr J 47 [Suppl]:S57–S60
Hinson JP, Brooke A, Raven PW (2003) Therapeutic uses of dehydroepiandrosterone. Curr Opin Investig Drugs 4:1205–1208
Hunt PJ, Gurnell EM, Huppert FA, Richards C, Prevost AT, Wass JA, Herbert J, Chatterjee VK (2000) Improvement in mood and fatigue after dehydroepiandrosterone replacement in Addison's disease in a randomized, double blind trial. J Clin Endocrinol Metab 85:4650–4656
Johannsson G, Marin P, Lonn L, Ottosson M, Stenlof K, Bjorntorp P, Sjostrom L, Bengtsson BA (1997) Growth hormone treatment of abdominally obese men reduces abdominal fat mass, improves glucose and lipoprotein metabolism, and reduces diastolic blood pressure. J Clin Endocrinol Metab 82:727–734
Khaw KT (1996) Dehydroepiandrosterone, dehydroepiandrosterone sulphate and cardiovascular disease. J Endocrinol 150 [Suppl]:S149–S153
Klapper W, Parwaresch R, Krupp G (2001) Telomere biology in human aging and aging syndromes. Mech Ageing Dev 122:695–712
Koh E, Kanaya J, Namiki M (2001) Adrenal steroids in human prostatic cancer cell lines. Arch Androl 46:117–125
Labrie F, Belanger A, Cusan L, Candas B (1997) Physiological changes in dehydroepiandrosterone are not reflected by serum levels of active androgens and estrogens but of their metabolites: intracrinology. J Clin Endocrinol Metab 82:2403–2409
Labrie F, Luu-The V, Labrie C, Simard J (2001) DHEA and its transformation into androgens and estrogens in peripheral target tissues: intracrinology. Front Neuroendocrinol 22:185–212
Legrain S, Massien C, Lahlou N, Roger M, Debuire B, Diquet B, Chatellier G, Azizi M, Faucounau V, Porchet H, Forette F, Baulieu EE (2000) Dehydroepiandrosterone replacement administration: pharmacokinetic and pharmacodynamic studies in healthy elderly subjects. J Clin Endocrinol Metab 85:3208–3217
Lissoni P (1998) Melatonin and cancer treatment. In: Watson RR (eds) Melatonin in the promotion of health. CRC, London, pp 175–190
Lissoni P, Meregalli S, Fossati V, Paolorossi F, Barni S, Tancini G, Frigerio F (1994) A randomized study of immunotherapy with low-dose subcutaneous interleukin-2 plus melatonin vs chemotherapy with cisplatin and etoposide as first-line therapy for advanced non-small cell lung cancer. Tumori 80:464–467
Lo JC, Mulligan K, Noor MA, Schwarz JM, Halvorsen RA, Grunfeld C, Schambelan M (2001) The effects of recombinant human growth hormone on body composition and glucose metabolism in HIV-infected patients with fat accumulation. J Clin Endocrinol Metab 86:3480–3487
Lusardi P, Piazza E, Fogari R (2000) Cardiovascular effects of melatonin in hypertensive patients well controlled by nifedipine: a 24-hour study. Br J Clin Pharmacol 49:423–427
Messner M, Huether G, Lorf T, Ramadori G, Schworer H (2001) Presence of melatonin in the human hepatobiliary-gastrointestinal tract. Life Sci 69:543–551
Montanini V, Simoni M, Chiossi G, Baraghini GF, Velardo A, Baraldi E, Marrama P (1988) Age-related changes in plasma dehydroepiandrosterone sulphate, cortisol, testosterone and free testosterone circadian rhythms in adult men. Horm Res 29:1–6
Newcomer JW, Craft S, Hershey T, Askins K, Bardgett ME (1994) Glucocorticoid-induced impairment in declarative memory performance in adult humans. J Neurosci 14:2047–2053
Nippoldt TB, Nair KS (1998) Is there a case for DHEA replacement? Baillieres Clin Endocrinol Metab 12:507–520
Orme SM, McNally RJ, Cartwright RA, Belchetz PE (1998) Mortality and cancer incidence in acromegaly: a retrospective cohort study. United Kingdom Acromegaly Study Group. J Clin Endocrinol Metab 83:2730–2734
Porsova-Dutoit I, Sulcova J, Starka L (2000) Do DHEA/DHEAS play a protective role in coronary heart disease? Physiol Res 49 [Suppl 1]:S43–S56
Sack RL, Brandes RW, Kendall AR, Lewy AJ (2000) Entrainment of free-running circadian rhythms by melatonin in blind people. N Engl J Med 343:1070–1077
Schiller CD, Schneider MR, Hartmann H, Graf AH, Klocker H, Bartsch G (1991) Growth-stimulating effect of adrenal androgens on the R3327 Dunning prostatic carcinoma. Urol Res 19:7–13
Tchernof A, Labrie F (2004) Dehydroepiandrosterone, obesity and cardiovascular disease risk: a review of human studies. Eur J Endocrinol 151:1–14
Thijs L, Fagard R, Forette F, Nawrot T, Staessen JA (2003) Are low dehydroepiandrosterone sulphate levels predictive for cardiovascular diseases? A review of prospective and retrospective studies. Acta Cardiol 58:403–410
Villareal DT, Holloszy JO, Kohrt WM (2000) Effects of DHEA replacement on bone mineral density and body composition in elderly women and men. Clin Endocrinol (Oxf) 53:561–568
Weaver JU, Monson JP, Noonan K, John WG, Edwards A, Evans KA, Cunningham J (1995) The effect of low dose recombinant human growth hormone replacement on regional fat distribution, insulin sensitivity, and cardiovascular risk factors in hypopituitary adults. J Clin Endocrinol Metab 80:153–159
Weill-Engerer S, David JP, Sazdovitch V, Liere P, Schumacher M, Delacourte A, Baulieu EE, Akwa Y (2003) In vitro metabolism of dehydroepiandrosterone (DHEA) to 7alpha-hydroxy-DHEA and Delta5-androstene-3beta,17beta-diol in specific regions of the aging brain from Alzheimer's and non-demented patients. Brain Res 969:117–125
Wolf OT, Neumann O, Hellhammer DH, Geiben AC, Strasburger CJ, Dressendorfer RA, Pirke KM, Kirschbaum C (1997) Effects of a two-week physiological dehydroepiandrosterone substitution on cognitive performance and well-being in healthy elderly women and men. J Clin Endocrinol Metab 82:2363–2367

II.4.14 Anti-Ageing Nutrition and Food Supplements

F. Comhaire, A. Mahmoud

Summary

In addition to adopting a healthy lifestyle, ageing men can promote their good physical and mental condition by using particular food supplements. The maximum lifespan seems to be genetically determined for each individual person, whereas the quality of life of elderly people can probably be influenced by external factors. The prevention and correction of obesity, regular engagement in moderate physical activities and the early identification and treatment of "diseases of the elderly", such as hypertension, diabetes and certain forms of cancer, are of essential importance. Correction of specific hormone deficiencies may be indicated.

In addition, certain nutritional supplements may be used to counter "wear and tear" phenomena by reversing the cellular damage resulting from environmental toxins and oxidative overload. To do this, "nutriceuticals" are used. These formulations consist of vitamins, minerals and judiciously selected and prepared non-toxic plant extracts. They are taken in quantities that do not exceed the recommended daily dosage, to avoid toxicity. The simultaneous implementation of well-selected agents results in synergistic effects.

In addition to a healthy lifestyle, ageing men can promote their good physical and mental condition by using particular food supplements.

Nutriceuticals aim to prevent or delay the occurrence of common diseases, maintain optimal organ function and counteract the "wear and tear" caused by reactive oxygen species.

The judicious combination of vitamins, minerals and plant extracts helps maintain adequate brain function and bone strength, and may protect against common vascular and prostate diseases.

Since a large proportion of the ageing population lives in an environment that is highly polluted by agents that accelerate the ageing processes, it may be useful to start nutriceutical intake rather early in life (between 40 and 50 years of age).

II.4.14.1 Introduction

There are several phenomena that are held responsible for the signs and symptoms of ageing, such as changed neuroendocrine status, immunological processes and "wear and tear", a kind of cellular wearing out as a result of oxidative damage, among other things. The last is related to the continuous production of oxygen radicals, which are derivatives of oxygen that can harm the cell membrane, the mitochondria and the DNA. This changes the composition of the phospholipids of the cell membrane, which becomes less fluid. Both the enzyme functions and the receptor activity, which are linked to the cell membrane, decrease. The production of ATP in the mitochondria becomes less efficient, whereby the energy available for cells reduces. Redox imbalance is also involved in the impairment of the immune system seen in the elderly (Daynes et al. 2003). Oxidative damage to DNA causes genetic changes that can be mutagenic and, in some circumstances, promote the occurrence of cancer (Jakobisiak et al. 2003; Martinez et al. 2003; Ohshima et al. 2003).

On the one hand, the average life expectancy of the elderly has increased over the last few decades; on the other hand, all sorts of "diseases of old age" are occurring ever more often – even at relatively young ages – as a result of changed lifestyles and of environmental factors. Typical examples are the diseases related to obesity and sedentary lifestyle such as diabetes, arteriosclerosis, and all sorts of forms of cancer. The phenomenal increase of cancer is attributed to continual exposure to ever-larger amounts of numerous chemical agents in the environment and in our food.

Adaptation of lifestyle, the encouragement of physical movement (Westerlind 2003) and appropriate nutrition, and the early detection and treatment of "diseases of old age" benefit the quality of life and extend an individual's life expectancy. Unfortunately, it will be several decades before exposure to harmful environmental factors is substantially reduced. In the meantime, we must strive to limit or counter their influence and that of the already mentioned oxidative cellular damage.

II.4.14.2 Components of Nutriceuticals

By way of example, here is the composition of some nutriceuticals that are presently available on the market as OTC or "over-the-counter" products (AndroCell®, Biodynamics, Oostende, Belgium; Androxir®, Nutriphyt, Oostkamp, Belgium).

II.4.14.2.1 Plant Extracts

Vinca minor (Common Periwinkle)

Extract of *Vinca minor*, from which the toxic alkaloids have been removed, has long been used because of its

II.4

favourable effect on the brain's blood circulation (Hadjiev and Yancheva 1976; Karpati and Szporny 1976; Solti et al. 1976). The vinca extract also stimulates glucose metabolism in the brain cells (Tesseris et al. 1975; Vamosi et al. 1976; Matkovics et al. 1991). Animal experiments have demonstrated these effects, and a favourable effect on memory in humans has also been documented.

For Men: *Serenoa repens* (Saw Palmetto)

The lipido-sterolic extract from *Serenoa repens* is used because of its favourable effect on the prostate gland. The extract changes the phospholipid composition of the nuclear membrane whereby the reductase activity is inhibited and the conversion of testosterone into 5α-dihydrotestosterone (which is 10 times more androgen active than testosterone itself) is decreased (Weisser et al. 1996, 1997). This effect is lower than that of the pharmaceutical 5α-reductase inhibitors finasteride and dutasteride. Still, the therapeutic result of treatment with serenoa extract on lower urinary tract symptoms (LUTS) or "prostatic complaints" is comparable with that of both finasteride (Wilt et al. 2000) and the α_1-blocker tamsulosin (for references and review article see Comhaire and Mahmoud 2004).

Serenoa extract reduces the prostate volume (Romics et al. 1993; Kondas et al. 1996; Stepanov et al. 1999; Bayne et al. 2000; Boyle et al. 2000; Vacherot et al. 2000) albeit to a lesser degree than the reductase inhibitors, and it induces apoptosis, reduces the proliferation of stroma cells and neutralizes the inflammatory leukotriene B_4. Serenoa extract is used in the treatment of benign prostate hyperplasia (BPH) and, in contrast to the pharmaceutical 5α-reductase inhibitors, does not reduce the libido. The serum concentration of prostate specific antigen (PSA) is not decreased by serenoa extract, while the pharmaceutical reductase inhibitors approximately halve the PSA value in blood. This complicates the monitoring of the PSA value in the context of preventing prostate carcinoma.

It thus seems logical to use serenoa extract to prevent prostate hyperplasia (Cristoni et al. 2000), but there have been no controlled studies in this regard.

An extract of the pumpkin pit (*Cucurbita pepo*) is sometimes added to the serenoa extract with the intention of enhancing the effect on prostatic complaints by additional inhibition of 5α-reductase and aromatase.

Linum

Linum is obtained from linseed oil. It contains lignans, which are converted by the intestinal flora into enterodiol and enterolactone (Denis et al. 1999). Both substances have discrete phytoestrogenic effects. The enterolactone, however, is primarily an inhibitor of aromatase. Administration of linum results in a reduced total oestrogenic effect because the production of the very active oestrogens (primarily oestrone and oestradiol) is inhibited. In women, the supplementary administration of lignans increases the urinary 2:16 alpha-hydroxyoestrone ratio (see below) (Haggans et al. 1999, 2000; Brooks et al. 2004), which is associated with a decreased risk of invasive breast cancer (Muti et al. 2000). Indeed, epidemiological studies show a link between a high level of enterolactone in the blood and a reduced chance of breast cancer (Adlercreutz 1988).

In the ageing man, the testosterone concentration declines more than the oestradiol concentration. Moreover, aromatase activity increases as a result of increased tissue fat, which leads to increased disturbance of the equilibrium between oestrogens and androgens. The relative hyperoestrogenism of the older man is associated with a higher risk of coronary problems and prostate pathology. Inhibition of aromatase activity with the aid of linum can restore the oestrogen–androgen balance. In epidemiological studies, it has been established that men with a high enterolactone level in the blood do, indeed, run less risk of a heart attack than those with a low level.

Soya Isoflavones

The primary soya isoflavones, daidzein and genistein, are often used in nutritional supplements for both men and women for the prevention of, respectively, prostate cancer and breast cancer. These isoflavones are weak oestrogens. They bond more strongly on the beta than on the alpha oestrogen receptor. They generate interesting effects and work as a relative anti-oestrogen in women during the reproductive phase of their lives. They also cause a shift in oestrogen metabolism from the 16-hydroxy oestrogens, which are rather oncogenic, to the 2-hydroxy oestrogens, which are said to have a protective effect against breast cancer. The isoflavones inhibit tyrosine kinase, which plays an important role during invasive cell migration upon metastasis.

Less prostate and breast cancer is observed in people who, during their entire lives, have taken in many soya isoflavones in their diet. However, administering soya isoflavones to older men does not appear to be appropriate in view of the relative hyperoestrogenism that is present in many of them. Indeed, the amount of circulating oestrogen will even increase, which, among other things, results in an increase of the concentration of sex hormone binding globulin (SHBG). This leads to a relatively large reduction of the content of free testosterone in the blood. The oestrogen–androgen equilibrium would be even more disturbed, which could increase the risk of cardiovascular disease.

A similar argument applies to Ginseng extracts, which also have significant oestrogenic activity.

Finally, a higher concentration of daidzein and genistein was measured in the blood of patients with prostate cancer than in a control group of men without this disease (Akaza et al. 2002).

II.4.14.2.2 Minerals

Zinc (Chelate)

Zinc, together with vitamin B_6, plays an important role in the conversion of the essential omega-3 short-chain fatty acids – such as the 18:3 ω3 (alpha linolenic acid) in long-chain polyunsaturated fatty acids, in particular eicosapentaenoic acid (EPA) and the docosahexaenoic acid or cervonic acid (DHA; 22:3 ω3). The anti-inflammatory properties of the latter have been repeatedly demonstrated in patients with rheumatoid arthritis and other conditions (Adam 2003). Zinc and vitamin B_6 are necessary for the elongase and desaturase processes that are active in this conversion. For postmenopausal women, the administration of zinc can be combined with supplementary intake of linseed oil, which is an important source of alpha linolenic acid. The supplementary administration of linseed oil is not recommended for the older man.

Selenium (Methionine)

Selenium has a strong antioxidant effect that protects against oxidative DNA damage. Several studies point to the connection between a low selenium content in the blood and an increased risk of dying as a result of cancer (Kornitzer et al. 2004). Prospective research has also demonstrated a protective effect of selenium against prostate cancer (Combs 2004; Dagnelie et al. 2004; Li et al. 2004).

II.4.14.2.3 Vitamins and Lipoic Acid

Antioxidant Vitamins

Vitamin C, vitamin E and lipoic acid repair the equilibrium between oxidative overload and the anti-oxidative capacity of the body. The oxidative overload can result from tobacco use, from intercurrent inflammatory or infectious conditions, from exposure to toxic environmental factors (including pesticides) and heavy metals, and from hypertension or diabetes. The oxidative overload causes an accelerated conversion of LDL cholesterol to oxidated LDL cholesterol, which, in the vascular wall, is phagocytosed by macrophages, which are themselves converted to foam cells. This promotes the development of arteriosclerosis. A correctly dosed composition of antioxidants retards the conversion of the LDL cholesterol to its oxidated form (Bernard et al. 2003), which could inhibit the occurrence of arteriosclerosis. Vitamin C also reduces the stress-induced constriction of the coronary arteries, and improves endothelial function.

The results of various prospective studies concerning an anti-arteriosclerosis effect of vitamin C and vitamin E are contradictory, so meta-analysis could not show a positive effect. However, this conclusion must be qualified since, in the various studies, highly divergent doses of vitamins E and C were used. In addition, use was often made of synthetic vitamin E, which differs significantly from the natural tocopherols in biological activity.

Natural "vegetable" vitamin E consists of various isomers whereby the ratio between the alpha and gamma forms is apparently important for an optimal antioxidative effect. The natural tocopherols are up to 8 times more active than the synthetic alpha-d-tocopherol. In addition, a high concentration of the latter reduces the concentration of gamma tocopherol (Cooney et al. 1993; Freeman et al. 2000; Giovannucci 2000; Helzlsouer et al. 2000). Administration of nutritional supplements with a high dose of synthetic alpha-d-tocopherol can result in a paradoxically unfavourable effect, for example, as far as preventing certain forms of cancer is concerned (Behrens and Madere 1987; Handelman et al. 1994). In contrast, administration of natural vitamin E, with the correct proportion of gamma tocopherol, manifested a protective effect, particularly in the prevention of prostate cancer. It has also been demonstrated that administration of vitamin E reduces the concentration of mutagenic oxidated DNA (8-OH-2-deoxyguanosine) in cells (Comhaire et al. 2000).

Particularly important is the dosage of vitamin C that is administered: more is not always better! Indeed, high doses of vitamin C can cause a pro-oxidative effect by increasing the content of free Fe^{2+}, which, via the Haber-Weiss and Fenton reactions, generates free oxygen radicals. It has been shown that cyclooxygenase-2 (COX2) is involved in the induction of DNA damage and that vitamin C promotes it (Blair 2004). On the other hand, the administration of a balanced combination of antioxidants increases the serum concentration of ferritin whereby the free Fe^{2+} is more strongly bonded and so can have less of a pro-oxidative effect (Fig. II.4.37).

Vitamin E is fat-soluble and is regenerated by the water-soluble vitamin C. Lipoic acid is both fat- and water-soluble and has a high "buffering" capacity, i.e. it can take up many oxygen radicals.

Prospective cohort and intervention studies have shown that the combined administration of vitamins E and C significantly reduces the risk of Alzheimer's disease (Zandi et al. 2004). Vitamin E also increases the immunological resistance of the elderly (Lesourd

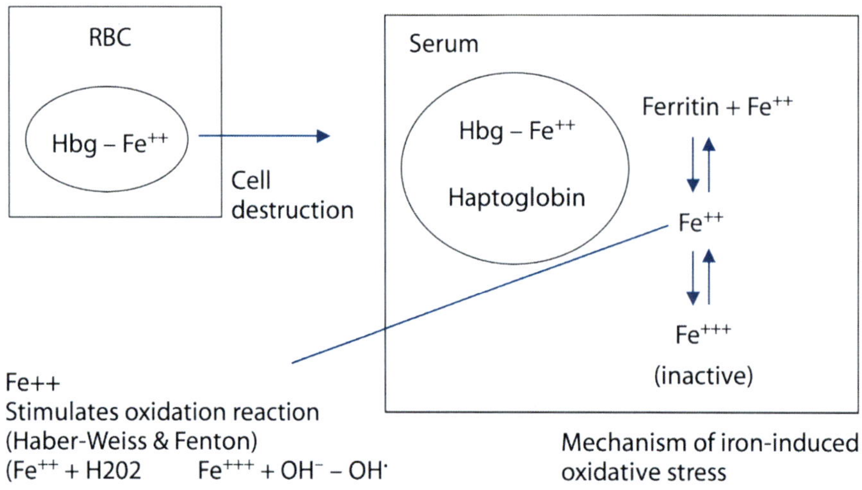

Fig. II.4.37. Mechanism of iron-induced oxidative stress. When red blood cells (RBC) are disintegrated, the complex haemoglobin-iron (Hbg-Fe^{++}) ist released into the circulation. In serum, this complex is bound to haptoglobin. Iron can escape from the haemoglobin-haptoglobin-iron complex and circulates as free iron++ (Fe^{++}) and as iron bound to ferritin (ferritin-iron complex). The free iron++ stimulates the Haber-Weiss and Fenton reactions that generate highly active oxygen radicals. The free iron++ in serum is in equilibrium with the inactive iron+++ (Fe^{++}). The latter equilibrium is shifted towards more iron++ under the influence of high dose vitamin C administration. Hence, the Haber-Weiss and Fenton reactions are stimulated, generating excess free oxygen radicals. On the other hand, adequate anti-oxidant treatment increases the ferritin concentration in serum, enhancing the proportion of bound iron++ and decreasing the level of free iron++. This results in lower production of free radicals. The latter is probably one of the mechanisms by which anti-oxidants can exert their tissue-protective effects

2004) and of patients with HIV infection (Fawzi et al. 2004).

Vitamin A and retinol are not contained in the formulations presented here. Indeed, these substances are used in large quantities in cattle raising and for food preservation. Through these routes, they are sufficiently present in our diet (Kornitzer and Bara 1989). Large quantities of them have a hepatotoxic effect. Moreover, the addition of vitamin A turned out to nullify the protection provided by vitamins E and C in AIDS patients (Fawzi et al. 2004).

Vitamins B_6, B_9 (Folic Acid) and B_{12}

Vitamin B_6 plays an important role in the elongation and desaturation of the unsaturated short-chain fatty acids (see above). The combination of the three B vitamins reduces the concentration of homocysteine in the blood (Clarke and Armitage 2000). A high homocysteine level is an independent risk factor not only for arteriosclerosis and cardiovascular disease (Nygard et al. 1997; Klerk et al. 2002) but also for osteoporotic bone fractures. The prevalence of bone fractures is 4 times higher in men in the highest homocysteine quartile than in those in the lowest quartile (McLean et al. 2004; van Meurs et al. 2004).

Interventions that reduce the homocysteine level in persons with a high basal blood value, particularly administering a combination of vitamins B_6, B_9 and B_{12}, could reduce the risk of fractures in the elderly and also have a protective effect against coronary illness (Vermeulen et al. 2000; Thambyrajah et al. 2001; Schnyder et al. 2002; Dinckal et al. 2003).

Ubiquinone Q10 Oxidoreductase

The oxido-reductase ubiquinone Q10 plays an important role in the production of adenosine triphosphate (ATP). Q10 promotes muscle function and is necessary for the proper operation of the heart muscle. A deficiency of Q10 or inhibition of its enzymatic functioning can cause heart failure. The apolar polychlorinated biphenyls (PCBs) inhibit the oxido-reductive operation of Q10. PCBs have been present in our diet for decades and accumulate in the body, and they are possibly involved in the increased prevalence of heart failure in the population. The supplementary administration of Q10 can compensate for the deficient muscle contractility and thus combat the occurrence of heart failure due to environmental contamination thanks to its positive inotropic effect.

The statins develop their cholesterol-reducing effect by the inhibition of hydroxy-3-methyl-3-glutaryl-coenzymA-reductase (HMG-Co-A-reductase). However, this enzyme is necessary for the synthesis of Q10, and the administration of primarily fat-soluble statins (atorvastatin, fluvastatin and simvastatin) significantly reduces the amount of Q10 in the cells (Lankin et al. 2003; Passi et al. 2003). This decreases the production of ATP, which explains the muscle complaints (Bolego et al. 2002; Farmer 2003; Schaefer et al. 2004) and the feeling of fatigue which are quite often mentioned by patients during treatment with statins. In addition, a higher degree of myocardial stunning has been observed after short coronary ischaemia was induced in dogs that had been pre-treated with fat-soluble statins (Ichihara et al. 1999; Satoh and Ichihara 2000). It is not clear whether such a phenomenon also occurs in humans. The administration of a nutritional supplement with Q10 can prevent ATP deficiency in the heart muscle cells (Oranje et al. 2001) and thus protect or improve the pumping function of the heart during treatment with statins.

Vitamin D

In elderly people admitted to a care institution, the risk of fall incidents could be reduced significantly by the administration of a vitamin D supplement (Bischoff-Ferrari et al. 2004). This is ascribed to improved muscle strength rather than to any effect on the bones.

II.4.14.2.4 Other Substances

The substances enumerated below are not included in the "basic formulation", but can be applied to prevent functional deficiency among the elderly.

Chondroitin Sulphate and Glucosamine Sulphate

These compounds are administered to inhibit the evolution of arthrosis (Richy et al. 2003). Their beneficial effect is indeed statistically demonstrated in prospective clinical studies, but their influence on arthrosis complaints varies (McAlindon et al. 2000). Whether the early administration of these compounds in the form of a nutritional supplement can prevent, retard, or inhibit the generation of arthrosis has not been unequivocally demonstrated.

Carnitines support the transport of long-chain fatty acids from the cytoplasm to the mitochondria, which can enhance energy production in the cells and will combat fatigue.

With the extracts of **Crataegus** (hawthorn) (De Smet 2002) and **Scilla maritima** (sea onion) (Rötter 1958; Dias et al. 2000) a positive inotropic effect has been demonstrated.

Extracts from the bark of the **Salix** (willow) and of the **Pinus maritima** (French maritime pine) develop an anti-inflammatory effect.

Extract from **Peumus boldus** (boldo) protects liver cells against toxic damage (Speisky and Cassels 1994; Kringstein and Cederbaum 1995; Zhao et al. 2002; Schmeda-Hirschmann et al. 2003).

Extract from **Lespedeza bicolor** supports kidney function and was actually used in the past in the treatment of patients with kidney insufficiency.

A favourable effect of **Cordyceps sinensis** extract on the efficiency of insulin has been demonstrated (Balon et al. 2002; Zhao et al. 2002), as have an increase of physical performance capacity (Koh et al. 2003) and a slight stimulation of testosterone production in male laboratory animals (Huang et al. 2001a, b, 2004; Hsu 2003).

It is important to point out that the substances cited above have no demonstrable toxic side-effects, at least not when correctly extracted products are used that are not contaminated with pesticides or other environmental contaminants and when undesirable alkaloids have been removed during their preparation.

II.4.14.2.5 Discussion

A "healthy lifestyle" with sufficient physical movement, a balanced diet, a controlled caloric intake to combat obesity and the early detection and treatment of "diseases of the elderly" are the cornerstones of a strategy that can improve the well-being and the quality of life of elderly people.

Living in a strongly polluted environment, people are protractedly exposed to numerous agents, many of which are carcinogenic and/or disturb the hormones and which, in any case, can upset the proper operation of cells and organs. This takes its toll on health at an advanced age.

There is strong, albeit indirect, evidence that the use of certain nutritional supplements can counter the unfavourable influence of this exposure, at least to some degree. In addition, serious scientific research has shown that complementing the diet with a balanced supplement cannot prevent the occurrence of certain phenomena and diseases of ageing, but can delay or slow them down.

References

Adam O (2003) Dietary fatty acids and immune reactions in synovial tissue. Eur J Med Res 8:381–387

Adlercreutz H (1988) Lignans and phytoestrogens. Possible preventive role in cancer. Front Gastrointest Res 14:165–176

Akaza H, Miyanaga N, Takashima N, Naito S, Hirao Y, Tsukamoto T, Mori M (2002) Is daidzein non-metabolizer a high risk for prostate cancer? A case-controlled study of serum soybean isoflavone concentration. Jpn J Clin Oncol 32: 296–300

Balon TW, Jasman AP, Zhu JS (2002) A fermentation product of *Cordyceps sinensis* increases whole-body insulin sensitivity in rats. J Altern Complement Med 8:315–323

Bayne CW, Ross M, Donnelly F, Habib FK (2000) The selectivity and specificity of the actions of the lipido-sterolic extract of *Serenoa repens* (Permixon) on the prostate. J Urol 164: 876–881

Behrens WA, Madere R (1987) Mechanisms of absorption, transport and tissue uptake of RRR-alpha-tocopherol and d-gamma-tocopherol in the white rat. J Nutr 117:1562–1569

Bernard D, Christophe A, Delanghe J, Langlois M, de Buyzere M, Comhaire F (2003) The effect of supplementation with an antioxidant preparation on LDL-oxidation is determined by haptoglobin polymorphism. Redox Rep 8:41–46

Bischoff-Ferrari HA, Dawson-Hughes B, Willett WC, Staehelin HB, Bazemore MG, Zee RY, Wong JB (2004) Effect of Vitamin D on falls: a meta-analysis. J Am Med Assoc 291:1999–2006

Blair I (2004) First evidence COX-2 enzymes can regulate DNA

damage. ASBMB Annual Meeting and 8th IUBMB Conference, 12–16 June 2004, Boston, Mass., http://www.bio.com
Bolego C, Baetta R, Bellosta S, Corsini A, Paoletti R (2002) Safety considerations for statins. Curr Opin Lipidol 13: 637–644
Boyle P, Robertson C, Lowe F, Roehrborn C (2000) Meta-analysis of clinical trials of permixon in the treatment of symptomatic benign prostatic hyperplasia. Urology 55:533–539
Brooks JD, Ward WE, Lewis JE, Hilditch J, Nickell L, Wong E, Thompson LU (2004) Supplementation with flaxseed alters estrogen metabolism in postmenopausal women to a greater extent than does supplementation with an equal amount of soy. Am J Clin Nutr 79:318–325
Clarke R, Armitage J (2000) Vitamin supplements and cardiovascular risk: review of the randomized trials of homocysteine-lowering vitamin supplements. Semin Thromb Hemost 26:341–348
Combs GF (2004) Status of selenium in prostate cancer prevention. Br J Cancer 91:195–199
Comhaire F, Mahmoud A (2004) Preventing diseases of the prostate in the elderly using hormones and nutriceuticals. Ageing Male 7:155–169
Comhaire FH, Christophe AB, Zalata AA, Dhooge WS, Mahmoud AM, Depuydt CE (2000) The effects of combined conventional treatment, oral antioxidants and essential fatty acids on sperm biology in subfertile men. Prostaglandins Leukot Essent Fatty Acids 63:159–165
Cooney RV, Franke AA, Harwood PJ, Hatch-Pigott V, Custer LJ, Mordan LJ (1993) Gamma-tocopherol detoxification of nitrogen dioxide: superiority to alpha-tocopherol. Proc Natl Acad Sci USA 90:1771–1775
Cristoni A, Di Pierro F, Bombardelli E (2000) Botanical derivatives for the prostate. Fitoterapia 71 [Suppl 1]:S21–S28
Dagnelie PC, Schuurman AG, Goldbohm RA, Van den Brandt PA (2004) Diet, anthropometric measures and prostate cancer risk: a review of prospective cohort and intervention studies. BJU Int 93:1139–1150
Daynes RA, Enioutina EY, Jones DC (2003) Role of redox imbalance in the molecular mechanisms responsible for immunosenescence. Antioxid Redox Signal 5:537–548
De Smet PA (2002) Herbal remedies. N Engl J Med 347:2046–2056
Denis L, Morton MS, Griffiths K (1999) Diet and its preventive role in prostatic disease. Eur Urol 35:377–387
Dias C, Borralho Graca JA, Lurdes GM (2000) *Scilla maderensis*, TLC screening and positive inotropic effect of bulb extracts. J Ethnopharmacol 71:487–492
Dinckal MH, Aksoy N, Aksoy M, Davutoglu V, Soydinc S, Kirilmaz A, Dinckal N, Akdemir I (2003) Effect of homocysteine-lowering therapy on vascular endothelial function and exercise performance in coronary patients with hyperhomocysteinaemia. Acta Cardiol 58:389–396
Farmer JA (2003) Statins and myotoxicity. Curr Atheroscler Rep 5:96–100
Fawzi WW, Msamanga GI, Spiegelman D, Wei R, Kapiga S, Villamor E, Mwakagile D, Mugusi F, Hertzmark E, Essex M, Hunter DJ (2004) A randomized trial of multivitamin supplements and HIV disease progression and mortality. N Engl J Med 351:23–32
Freeman VL, Meydani M, Yong S, Pyle J, Wan Y, Arvizu-Durazo R, Liao Y (2000) Prostatic levels of tocopherols, carotenoids, and retinol in relation to plasma levels and self-reported usual dietary intake. Am J Epidemiol 151:109–118
Giovannucci E (2000) Gamma-tocopherol: a new player in prostate cancer prevention? J Natl Cancer Inst 92:1966–1967
Hadjiev D, Yancheva S (1976) Rheoencephalographic and psychological studies with ethyl apovincaminate in cerebral vascular insufficiency. Arzneimittelforschung 26:1947–1950
Haggans CJ, Hutchins AM, Olson BA, Thomas W, Martini MC, Slavin JL (1999) Effect of flaxseed consumption on urinary estrogen metabolites in postmenopausal women. Nutr Cancer 33:188–195
Haggans CJ, Travelli EJ, Thomas W, Martini MC, Slavin JL (2000) The effect of flaxseed and wheat bran consumption on urinary estrogen metabolites in premenopausal women. Cancer Epidemiol Biomarkers Prev 9:719–725
Handelman GJ, Epstein WL, Peerson J, Spiegelman D, Machlin LJ, Dratz EA (1994) Human adipose alpha-tocopherol and gamma-tocopherol kinetics during and after 1 y of alpha-tocopherol supplementation. Am J Clin Nutr 59:1025–1032
Helzlsouer KJ, Huang HY, Alberg AJ, Hoffman S, Burke A, Norkus EP, Morris JS, Comstock GW (2000) Association between alpha-tocopherol, gamma-tocopherol, selenium, and subsequent prostate cancer. J Natl Cancer Inst 92:2018–2023
Hsu CC, Huang YL, Tsai SJ, Sheu CC, Huang BM (2003) In vivo and in vitro stimulatory effects of *Cordyceps sinensis* on testosterone production in mouse Leydig cells. Life Sci 73:2127–2136
Huang BM, Hsu CC, Tsai SJ, Sheu CC, Leu SF (2001a) Effects of *Cordyceps sinensis* on testosterone production in normal mouse Leydig cells. Life Sci 69:2593–2602
Huang BM, Ju SY, Wu CS, Chuang WJ, Sheu CC, Leu SF (2001b) *Cordyceps sinensis* and its fractions stimulate MA-10 mouse Leydig tumor cell steroidogenesis. J Androl 22:831–837
Huang BM, Hsiao KY, Chuang PC, Wu MH, Pan HA, Tsai SJ (2004) Upregulation of steroidogenic enzymes and ovarian 17beta-estradiol in human granulosa-lutein cells by *Cordyceps sinensis* mycelium. Biol Reprod 70:1358–1364
Ichihara K, Satoh K, Yamamoto A, Hoshi K (1999) [Are all HMG-CoA reductase inhibitors protective against ischemic heart disease?]. [Japanese] Nippon Yakurigaku Zasshi Folia Pharmacol Jpn 114 [Suppl 1]:142P–149P
Jakobisiak M, Lasek W, Golab J (2003) Natural mechanisms protecting against cancer. Immunol Lett 90:103–122
Karpati E, Szporny L (1976) General and cerebral haemodynamic activity of ethyl apovincaminate. Arzneimittelforschung 26:1908–1912
Klerk M, Verhoef P, Clarke R, Blom HJ, Kok FJ, Schouten EG (2002) MTHFR 677C->T polymorphism and risk of coronary heart disease: a meta-analysis. J Am Med Assoc 288: 2023–2031
Koh JH, Kim KM, Kim JM, Song JC, Suh HJ (2003) Antifatigue and antistress effect of the hot-water fraction from mycelia of *Cordyceps sinensis*. Biol Pharm Bull 26:691–694
Kondas J, Philipp V, Dioszeghy G (1996) Sabal serrulata extract (Strogen forte) in the treatment of symptomatic benign prostatic hyperplasia. Int Urol Nephrol 28:767–772
Kornitzer M, Bara L (1989) Clinical and anthropometric data, blood chemistry and nutritional patterns in the Belgian population according to age and sex. For the B.I.R.N.H. Study Group. Acta Cardiol 44:101–144
Kornitzer M, Valente F, De Bacquer D, Neve J, De Backer G (2004) Serum selenium and cancer mortality: a nested case-control study within an age- and sex-stratified sample of the Belgian adult population. Eur J Clin Nutr 58:98–104
Kringstein P, Cederbaum AI (1995) Boldine prevents human liver microsomal lipid peroxidation and inactivation of cytochrome P4502E1. Free Radic Biol Med 18:559–563
Lankin VZ, Tikhaze AK, Kukharchuk VV, Konovalova GG, Pisarenko OI, Kaminnyi AI, Shumaev KB, Belenkov YN (2003) Antioxidants decreases the intensification of low density lipoprotein in vivo peroxidation during therapy with statins. Mol Cell Biochem 249:129–140
Lesourd B (2004) Nutrition: a major factor influencing immunity in the elderly. J Nutr Health Aging 8:28–37

Li H, Stampfer MJ, Giovannucci EL, Morris JS, Willett WC, Gaziano JM, Ma J (2004) A prospective study of plasma selenium levels and prostate cancer risk. J Natl Cancer Inst 96:696–703

Martinez GR, Loureiro AP, Marques SA, Miyamoto S, Yamaguchi LF, Onuki J, Almeida EA, Garcia CC, Barbosa LF, Medeiros MH, Di Mascio P (2003) Oxidative and alkylating damage in DNA. Mutat Res 544:115–127

Matkovics B, Szabo L, Kiss B, Szpornyi L (1991) Effect of ethyl apovincaminate on the utilization of ^{14}C-glucoses by rat brain in vitro. Arzneimittelforschung 41:107–108

McAlindon TE, LaValley MP, Gulin JP, Felson DT (2000) Glucosamine and chondroitin for treatment of osteoarthritis: a systematic quality assessment and meta-analysis. J Am Med Assoc 283:1469–1475

McLean RR, Jacques PF, Selhub J, Tucker KL, Samelson EJ, Broe KE, Hannan MT, Cupples LA, Kiel DP (2004) Homocysteine as a predictive factor for hip fracture in older persons. N Engl J Med 350:2042–2049

Muti P, Bradlow HL, Micheli A, Krogh V, Freudenheim JL, Schunemann HJ, Stanulla M, Yang J, Sepkovic DW, Trevisan M, Berrino F (2000) Estrogen metabolism and risk of breast cancer: a prospective study of the 2:16alpha-hydroxyestrone ratio in premenopausal and postmenopausal women. Epidemiology 11:635–640

Nygard O, Nordrehaug JE, Refsum H, Ueland PM, Farstad M, Vollset SE (1997) Plasma homocysteine levels and mortality in patients with coronary artery disease. N Engl J Med 337:230–236

Ohshima H, Tatemichi M, Sawa T (2003) Chemical basis of inflammation-induced carcinogenesis. Arch Biochem Biophys 417:3–11

Oranje WA, Sels JP, Rondas-Colbers GJ, Lemmens PJ, Wolffenbuttel BH (2001) Effect of atorvastatin on LDL oxidation and antioxidants in normocholesterolemic type 2 diabetic patients. Clin Chim Acta 311:91–94

Passi S, Stancato A, Aleo E, Dmitrieva A, Littarru GP (2003) Statins lower plasma and lymphocyte ubiquinol/ubiquinone without affecting other antioxidants and PUFA. Biofactors 18:113–124

Richy F, Bruyere O, Ethgen O, Cucherat M, Henrotin Y, Reginster JY (2003) Structural and symptomatic efficacy of glucosamine and chondroitin in knee osteoarthritis: a comprehensive meta-analysis. Arch Intern Med 163:1514–1522

Romics I, Schmitz H, Frang D (1993) Experience in treating benign prostatic hypertrophy with Sabal serrulata for one year. Int Urol Nephrol 25:565–569

Rötter W (1958) [Indications for therapy with digitaloids (*Scilla maritima*).]. Münch Med Wochenschr 100:812–815

Satoh K, Ichihara K (2000) Lipophilic HMG-CoA reductase inhibitors increase myocardial stunning in dogs. J Cardiovasc Pharmacol 35(2):256–262

Schaefer WH, Lawrence JW, Loughlin AF, Stoffregen DA, Mixson LA, Dean DC, Raab CE, Yu NX, Lankas GR, Frederick CB (2004) Evaluation of ubiquinone concentration and mitochondrial function relative to cerivastatin-induced skeletal myopathy in rats. Toxicol Appl Pharmacol 194:10–23

Schmeda-Hirschmann G, Rodriguez JA, Theoduloz C, Astudillo SL, Feresin GE, Tapia A (2003) Free-radical scavengers and antioxidants from Peumus boldus Mol. ("Boldo"). Free Radic Res 37:447–452

Schnyder G, Roffi M, Flammer Y, Pin R, Hess OM (2002) Effect of homocysteine-lowering therapy with folic acid, vitamin B12, and vitamin B6 on clinical outcome after percutaneous coronary intervention: the Swiss Heart study: a randomized controlled trial. J Am Med Assoc 288:973–979

Solti F, Iskum M, Czako E (1976) Effect of ethyl apovincaminate on the cerebral circulation. Studies in patients with obliterative cerebral arterial disease. Arzneimittelforschung 26: 1945–1947

Speisky H, Cassels BK (1994) Boldo and boldine: an emerging case of natural drug development. Pharmacol Res 29:1–12

Stepanov VN, Siniakova LA, Sarrazin B, Raynaud JP (1999) Efficacy and tolerability of the lipidosterolic extract of *Serenoa repens* (Permixon) in benign prostatic hyperplasia: a double-blind comparison of two dosage regimens. Adv Ther 16:231–241

Tesseris J, Roggen G, Caracalos A, Triandafillou D (1975) Effects of vincamin on cerebral metabolism. Eur Neurol 13: 195–202

Thambyrajah J, Landray MJ, Jones HJ, McGlynn FJ, Wheeler DC, Townend JN (2001) A randomized double-blind placebo-controlled trial of the effect of homocysteine-lowering therapy with folic acid on endothelial function in patients with coronary artery disease. J Am Coll Cardiol 37:1858–1863

Vacherot F, Azzouz M, Gil-Diez-De-Medina S, Colombel M, De La TA, Lefrere Belda MA, Abbou CC, Raynaud JP, Chopin DK (2000) Induction of apoptosis and inhibition of cell proliferation by the lipido-sterolic extract of Serenoa repens (LSESr, Permixon) in benign prostatic hyperplasia. Prostate 45:259–266

Vamosi B, Molnar L, Demeter J, Tury F (1976) Comparative study of the effect of ethyl apovincaminate and xantinol nicotinate in cerebrovascular diseases. Immediate drug effects on the concentrations of carbohydrate metabolites and electrolytes in blood and CSF. Arzneimittelforschung 26:1980–1984

van Meurs JB, Dhonukshe-Rutten RA, Pluijm SM, van der KM, de Jonge R, Lindemans J, de Groot LC, Hofman A, Witteman JC, van Leeuwen JP, Breteler MM, Lips P, Pols HA, Uitterlinden AG (2004) Homocysteine levels and the risk of osteoporotic fracture. N Engl J Med 350:2033–2041

Vermeulen EG, Stehouwer CD, Twisk JW, van den BM, de Jong SC, Mackaay AJ, van Campen CM, Visser FC, Jakobs CA, Bulterjis EJ, Rauwerda JA (2000) Effect of homocysteine-lowering treatment with folic acid plus vitamin B6 on progression of subclinical atherosclerosis: a randomised, placebo-controlled trial. Lancet 355:517–522

Weisser H, Tunn S, Behnke B, Krieg M (1996) Effects of the Sabal serrulata extract IDS 89 and its subfractions on 5 alpha-reductase activity in human benign prostatic hyperplasia. Prostate 28:300–306

Weisser H, Behnke B, Helpap B, Bach D, Krieg M (1997) Enzyme activities in tissue of human benign prostatic hyperplasia after three months' treatment with the Sabal serrulata extract IDS 89 (Strogen) or placebo. Eur Urol 31:97–101

Westerlind KC (2003) Physical activity and cancer prevention–mechanisms. Med Sci Sports Exerc 35:1834–1840

Wilt TJ, Ishani A, Rutks I, MacDonald R (2000) Phytotherapy for benign prostatic hyperplasia. Public Health Nutr 3:459–472

Zandi PP, Anthony JC, Khachaturian AS, Stone SV, Gustafson D, Tschanz JT, Norton MC, Welsh-Bohmer KA, Breitner JC (2004) Reduced risk of Alzheimer disease in users of antioxidant vitamin supplements: the Cache County Study. Arch Neurol 61:82–88

Zhao CS, Yin WT, Wang JY, Zhang Y, Yu H, Cooper R, Smidt C, Zhu JS (2002) CordyMax Cs-4 improves glucose metabolism and increases insulin sensitivity in normal rats. J Altern Complement Med 8:309–314

II.4.15 Nutriceuticals and Food Supplements in the Treatment of the Infertile Man

F. Comhaire, A. Mahmoud

Summary

- Male infertility commonly results from synergistic negative influences of several groups of factors.
- External factors related to lifestyle and environmental exposure reinforce the effects of congenital or acquired testicular damage through direct toxicity, hormone disruption and overload of reactive oxygen species.
- Combating obesity, correcting inappropriate diet and cutting out tobacco and alcohol use are part of the holistic approach to the infertile male.
- Nutriceuticals are judiciously formulated food supplements containing particular vitamins, antioxidants, minerals and plant extracts.
- There is strong evidence that complementary treatment with an appropriate nutriceutical improves the fertilizing potential of subfertile patients.

II.4.15.1 Introduction

The introduction of **assisted reproductive technology (ART)**, namely in vitro fertilization (IVF; Steptoe and Edwards 1978) and intracytoplasmic sperm injection (ICSI; Palermo et al. 1992) caused a true revolution in reproductive medicine, while also revealing the magnitude of the "male factor" contributing to couple infertility. Conventional treatment of the infertile male was considered outdated by some, but others have continued unravelling the mechanisms involved in men's defective reproductive capacity. Concerns have repeatedly been raised about economical and ethical aspects (Comhaire 2000; Katz et al. 2002) as well as the side-effects of ART (Lambert 2002; Schieve et al. 2004). IVF and ICSI were found to be associated with an increased prevalence of genetic defects (Edwards and Ludwig 2003), major congenital malformations (Kent-First et al. 1996; van der Ven et al. 1998; Sutcliffe et al. 1999; Koudstaal et al. 2000; Wennerholm et al. 2000; Hansen et al. 2002; Green 2004), impaired development (Stromberg et al. 2002; Pinborg et al. 2004) and increased risk of retinoblastoma (Moll et al. 2003) as well as other malignant tumours (DeBaun et al. 2003; Maher et al. 2003) in the offspring. Today, it seems that the wheel has turned a full circle, and that clinical andrology has recaptured its well-deserved place in the armamentarium for the treatment of couple infertility.

II.4.15.2 Role of Lifestyle and Nutritional Factors

Similar to other diseases, male infertility is a disease that develops as a result of multiple pathogenic factors (Chap. I.3). Thereby, four major groups of factors seem to act in synergy: genetic defects or constitution, lifestyle factors, professional and/or environmental exposure and diseases of the urethro-genital region or endocrine system.

The field of genetics is rapidly expanding and includes numerical and structural abnormalities of the chromosomal make-up, as well as microdeletions of the Y chromosome (Tiepolo and Zuffardi 1976; Ma et al. 1992). Certain genetic microdeletions may cause infertility, depending on the coincidental presence of unfavourable lifestyle factors or exposure to toxic substances or hormone disrupters (Chap. II.2.2). These, and the genital diseases, have been shown to increase the load of reactive oxygen species (ROS) to the ejaculate and the spermatozoa, resulting in increased chromosome fractionation (Hughes et al. 1998; Irvine et al. 2000) and excessive production of oxidized DNA (8-hydroxy 2-deoxyguanosine) (Fraga et al. 1991). The latter induces transition mutagenesis.

The membrane of spermatozoa of fertile men contains a high concentration of docosahexaenoic acid (DHA, also called: cervonic acid, 22:6ω3) that renders fluidity to the membrane. Fluidity is necessary for the acrosome reaction to occur and for membrane fusion of the sperm head and the oocyte. The sperm membrane of infertile men contains less DHA, reducing the fluidity and fusogenic capacity. On the other hand, DHA has a strong oxidative potential because of its large number of double bonds. The serum of infertile men presents an imbalance between oxidative overload and decreased antioxidative capacity, as demonstrated by the higher oxidative sensitivity of LDL cholesterol in infertile compared to fertile men. Oxidative overload changes the phospholipid composition of the sperm membrane (Zalata et al. 1998), reducing its DHA content and fluidity, and resulting in reduced fusogenic capacity as well as acrosome reactivity.

Inappropriate nutrition, abuse of alcohol, tobacco or recreational drugs, tight clothing and hot baths have been incriminated among lifestyle factors. Also, a higher proportion of men with infertile as opposed to fertile semen were found to have a body mass index in excess of the optimal value of 25 kg/m^2, and are overweight or obese. They consume fewer ω-3 fatty acids than fertile men, and the ratio of ω-3 over ω-6 fatty acids commonly is suboptimal. A significant positive correlation was established between the consumption of α-linolenic acid (18:3 ω3) on the one hand, and sperm concentration and type (a) motility on the other hand (Christophe et al. 1998). In contrast, there was a negative correlation between these sperm characteristics and the consumption of highly polyunsaturated fatty acids (including DHA). This suggests that the oxidative stress existing in infertile men can induce the oxidative cascade when there is a high intake of the latter fatty acids, which are more vulnerable than the shorter chain and less unsaturated fatty acids, such as α-linolenic acid. Finally, it was demonstrated that testicular tissue, Sertoli cells in particular, contain more desaturase (Saether et al. 2003) and elongase (Cinti et al. 1992) than other body tissues – enzymes that convert α-linolenic acid into the long-chain polyunsaturated fatty acids (Hurtado de Catalfo and de Gomez Dumm 2002; Tran et al. 2003). This process generates higher concentrations of DHA locally.

Exposure to professional toxicants was proven to impair sperm quality, including heavy metals such as lead (Bonde et al. 2002), and carbon disulphide (Vanhoorne et al. 1994). However, it is exposure to environmental agents with hormone-disrupting effects, mainly pseudo- or xeno-oestrogens and anti-androgens, that has caused most concern recently (Chap. II.2.2). The obvious, though regional, deterioration both of sperm variables and fertility, and the parallel increase in the prevalence of testicular cancer have been linked to an increased internal exposure to synthetic chemical substances that mimic or enhance the effects of oestrogens by binding to the human oestrogen receptor or by influencing oestrogen metabolism (for review see: Sharpe 2003; Skakkebaek 2004).

II.4.15.3 Pivotal Role of Inhibin B

Inhibin B is a secretion product of Sertoli cells which plays an important role in both endocrine feedback, inhibiting the pituitary secretion of follicle-stimulating hormone (FSH), and the local regulation of spermatogenesis (Chap. II.1.3). Whereas the serum inhibin B concentration is significantly related to sperm concentration (for review see Meachem et al. 2001), there is evidence for a direct suppressive effect of inhibin B on spermatogenesis (van Dissel-Emiliani et al. 1989). Both in vitro tests (Depuydt et al. 1999) and in vivo data (Mahmoud et al. 1998, 2000) indicate that oestrogens and certain heavy metals, such as lead, may inappropriately stimulate the secretion of inhibin B by Sertoli cells. This results in decreased sperm production, in the presence of normal serum concentrations of inhibin B and FSH.

During treatment with the strong antioxidant astaxanthin, which reduces the concentration of reactive oxygen species, the serum concentration of inhibin B was reduced although the sperm concentration did not change (Comhaire and Mahmoud 2004). This suggests that ROS stimulates inhibin B secretion by Sertoli cells, similar to the effect of oestrogens.

Decreasing the secretion of inhibin B by reducing the oestrogen load and the exposure to ROS may be a target of medical treatment.

II.4.15.4 Food Supplementation

II.4.15.4.1 Fatty Acids

Since there is a positive correlation between the intake of α-linolenic acid (ALA) and sperm concentration and motility, and since the food intake of essential fatty acids of the ω-3 group was found to be suboptimal among subfertile men, it seems logical to supplement these patients with ALA, namely by giving them linseed oil, also called flaxseed oil. In association with the co-factors zinc and vitamin B_6, which enhance the activity of enzymes elongase and desaturase, ALA will be converted in situ into the long-chain, highly unsaturated ω-fatty acids, namely eicosapentaenoic acid (EPA) and docosahexaenoic acid (DHA). The fluidity of the sperm membrane will improve and the acrosome reaction and fusogenic capacity of the spermatozoa will increase (Comhaire et al. 2000).

Alternatively, supplementation with fish oil can be considered a source of the highly unsaturated long-chain fatty acids EPA and DHA. These fatty acids are, however, highly susceptible to oxidative damage initiating an undesirable chain reaction of lipo-oxidation. If fish oil is given as food supplementation, it is mandatory to ascertain a favourable internal antioxidant environment.

II.4.15.4.2 Antioxidants

Subfertile patients were found to present an imbalance between excessive oxidative stress as compared to a reduced antioxidant capacity (Christophe et al. 1998). Food supplementation with antioxidants significantly and persistently improves the balance between oxidative overload and antioxidant defense (Bernard et al. 2003). Also, treatment with either acetylcysteine (600 mg per day orally) or an antioxidant mixture significantly reduces the level of reactive oxygen species (ROS) in semen (Comhaire et al. 2000). In combination with fish oil, antioxidant treatment increases sperm concentration and significantly reduces the concentration of oxidized DNA (8-hydroxy 2-deoxyguanosine) in spermatozoa of subfertile men. The fatty acid composition of the phospholipids of the sperm membrane is shifted toward EPA and DHA, enhancing membrane fluidity, which results in increased induced, but not spontaneous, acrosome reactivity. This treatment increases the spontaneous conception rate, particularly in couples where the subfertile men are smokers. Also, vitamin E supplementation improves the in vitro function of spermatozoa as assessed in the zona-free hamster oocyte test (Kessopoulou et al. 1995).

Supplementation with vitamin C to smokers with abnormal sperm quality was reported to improve semen quality (Dawson et al. 1992), whereas no such effect was seen in another trial using high-dose vitamin C (Rolf et al. 1999). The latter may be related to the known pro-oxidative effect of high-dose vitamin C (Fraga et al. 1991), particularly in men with haptoglobin type 1–2 or 2–2 (Bernard et al. 2003).

When added in vitro, or given orally (Lewin and Lavon 1997), the oxido-reductase ubiquinone Q10 increased sperm motility in cases with asthenozoospermia. Also other antioxidants such as selenium (Scott et al. 1998) and glutathione (Lenzi et al. 1993) were found to improve sperm motility in subgroups of patients.

Astaxanthin is a lipophilic carotenoid produced by the algae *Haematococcus pluvialis*, and has a strong antioxidant capacity (Iwamoto et al. 2000; Goto et al. 2001). In a pilot double-blind randomized trial, natural astaxanthin (AstaReal®, Gustavsberg, Sweden) was given to the male partners of infertile couples, whose semen characteristics were below the WHO recommended reference values. The food supplement resulted in a significant reduction of seminal ROS and serum inhibin B concentration among treated cases, while no changes occurred in the placebo controls. Rapid linear progressive motility significantly increased and sperm morphology showed a non-significant improvement in the astaxanthin group. In the treated group the total and monthly pregnancy rates were 54.5% and 23.1% respectively, as compared to 11.1% and 3.6% in the placebo group (Comhaire et al. 2005).

II.4.15.4.3
Carnitine

L-Carnitine plays a pivotal role in the transport mechanisms that are necessary for the passage of long-chain fatty acids from the cellular cytosol into the mitochondrial matrix, where they are oxidized, generating energy (Wildman and Medeiros 2000) and stimulating the respiratory chain complexes (Ruiz-Pesini et al. 2001). Free carnitine and acetyl-L-carnitine play an important role in the post-gonadal maturation of mammalian spermatozoa (Jeulin and Lewin 1996), and the ratio of acetyl-carnitine/carnitine was different in extract of sperm with good or poor motility (Golan et al. 1984; Bartellini et al. 1987). Acetyl-L-carnitine is the prominent carnitine in spermatozoa and its concentration was lower in semen of infertile men (Kohengkul et al. 1977; Soufir et al. 1984). The free carnitine concentration in seminal plasma was significantly correlated with sperm concentration and motility (Menchini-Fabris et al. 1984), and sperm motility could be stimulated by the addition of acetyl-carnitine in vitro (Tanphaichitr 1977).

Treatment with a food supplement containing a combination of L-carnitine (2 g per day) and acetyl-L-carnitine (1 g per day) together with fructose and citric acid (Proxeed®, Sigma-tau Health Science, Rome, Italy) was reported to increase sperm concentration and forward progressive motility in both open-label trials (Moncada et al. 1992; Costa et al. 1994; Vitali et al. 1995) and a double-blind cross-over trial (Lenzi et al. 2003). In one open-label trial a total spontaneous pregnancy rate of 6.7% in 3 months was registered (Voliani et al. 2001). The monthly conception rate calculated in a meta-analysis of published trials was 2.3% (Comhaire and Mahmoud 2004). In a double-blind trial, the complementary intake of Proxeed® did not influence the outcome of conventional treatment, neither in terms of improving sperm characteristics, nor regarding the pregnancy rate (Comhaire et al. unpublished).

II.4.15.4.4
Folic Acid and Zinc

Folic acid and zinc have been given orally, both to men with normal sperm quality and to patients with moderate oligozoospermia during a placebo-controlled trial (Wong et al. 2002). This combination was found to significantly increase sperm concentration (by an average of 60%) and morphology in the subfertile men. Changes occurred though the blood levels of the substances were not deficient before treatment. It remains, however, to be established whether the administration of the combination of folic acid and zinc will improve fertility.

II.4.15.4.5
Seed Oil and Lignans

Aside from α-linolenic acid (see above), linseed (or flaxseed) oil contains several lignans that are converted in the intestine into enterodiol and enterolactone. These are phytoestrogens with a very weak oestrogenic effect, but enterolactone has moderate aromatase inhibitory activity, reducing the conversion of androgens (androstenedione and testosterone) into the potent oestrogens oestrone and oestradiol (Adlercreutz et al. 1993; Wang et al. 1994). As a result, food supplementation with linseed oil or lignans decreases the body burden of oestrogens. Men combining oligozoospermia with normal serum concentrations of FSH and inhibin B were found to commonly present relative hyper-oestrogenism, possibly connected to being overweight (Mahmoud et al. 1998), which can be corrected by lignans.

II.4.15.4.6 Plant Extracts

Using immunohistochemical techniques, Mayerhofer et al. (2002) demonstrated that the cyclooxygenase isoenzyme 2 (COX2), which converts arachidonic acid (20:4ω6) into the inflammatory prostaglandin E_2, is present in the testicular interstitial tissue of patients with idiopathic oligozoospermia, but not in men with normal spermatogenesis. Extract of the bark of *Pinus maritima* (Pycnogenol®) contains substances that inhibit the COX enzyme (Baumann et al. 1980; Rohdewald 2002), reduce mRNA levels for the inflammatory cytokine interleukin 1β (Cho et al. 2001) and protect the effects of vitamin E on endothelial cells (Virgili et al. 1998). In an open-label trial, oral administration of 200 mg per day of this extract improved sperm morphology by an average of 99 % (Roseff and Gulati 1999).

The extract of *Lepidium meyenii* (also called Maca), a plant growing in the central Andean region of Peru, increases sexual function of male mice and rats (Zheng et al. 2000), and invigorates spermatogenesis at the mitotic stages (Gonzales et al. 2001a). When given to men with normal spermatogenesis, the extract significantly increased sperm production (+ 85%) and motility (+ 15%) without interfering with endocrine regulation (Gonzales et al. 2001b).

Evidently, extracts of particular plants display interesting effects that may show promise for the future.

II.4.15.4.7 Arginine and Kallikrein

For several years arginine (De Aloysio et al. 1982; Aydin et al. 1995) and kallikrein (Schill 1979; Schill et al. 1979) have been promoted for the treatment of men with oligozoospermia. The alleged favourable effects of these supplements for the routine treatment of patients with idiopathic oligozoospermia have been questioned in other trials (Pryor et al. 1978; Comhaire and Vermeulen 1983; Glezerman et al.1993; Keck et al. 1994).

II.4.15.5 Conclusions

Several controlled and well-validated trials provide evidence that food supplementation with particular substances can improve the semen quality and function of subfertile men. These include the antioxidants astaxanthin, tocopherol and ubiquinone Q10, essential fatty acids of the ω-3 group, zinc and folic acid. There is suggestive evidence that certain plant extracts and lignans may equally exert beneficial effects. Supplementation with a nutriceutical (Qualisperm®, Nutriphyt, Oostkamp, Belgium) containing these substances increases the probability of spontaneous conception and successful pregnancy. Although the exact mechanisms of action of these supplements on spermatogenesis and sperm function remain to be unravelled, a direct effect on Sertoli cells (Fig. II.4.38) and an effect via epididymal function seem conceivable. Nutriceutical food supplementation should also be considered before IVF and ICSI, in order to reduce the oxidative damage to sperm DNA.

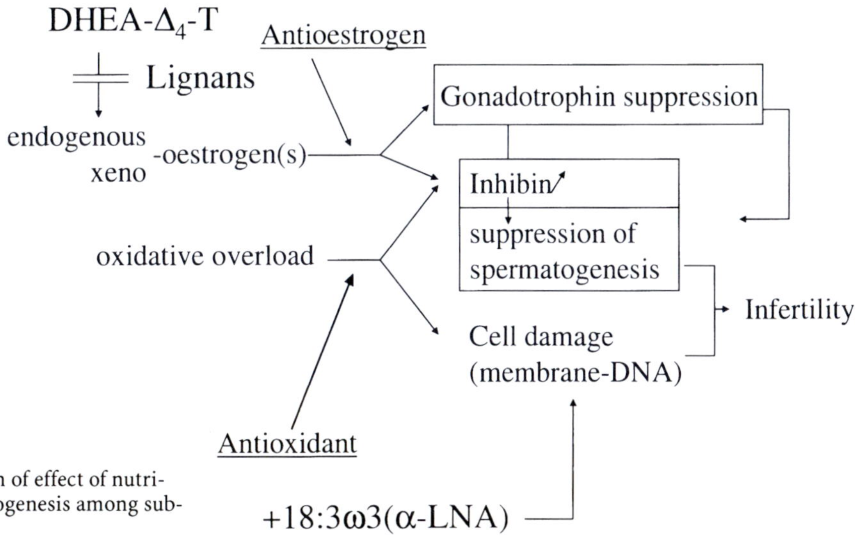

Fig. II.4.38. Proposed mechanism of effect of nutriceuticals in improving spermatogenesis among subfertile men

References

Adlercreutz H, Bannwart C, Wahala K, Makela T, Brunow G, Hase T, Arosemena PJ, Kellis JT Jr., Vickery LE (1993) Inhibition of human aromatase by mammalian lignans and isoflavonoid phytoestrogens. J Steroid Biochem Mol Biol 44: 147–153

Aydin S, Inci O, Alagol B (1995) The role of arginine, indomethacin and kallikrein in the treatment of oligoasthenospermia. Int Urol Nephrol 27:199–202

Bartellini M, Canale D, Izzo PL, Giorgi PM, Meschini P, Menchini-Fabris GF (1987) L-Carnitine and acetylcarnitine in human sperm with normal and reduced motility. Acta Eur Fertil 18:29–31

Baumann J, von Bruchhausen F, Wurm G (1980) Flavonoids and related compounds as inhibition of arachidonic acid peroxidation. Prostaglandins 20:627–639

Bernard D, Christophe A, Delanghe J, Langlois M, de Buyzere M, Comhaire F (2003) The effect of supplementation with an antioxidant preparation on LDL-oxidation is determined by haptoglobin polymorphism. Redox Rep 8:41–46

Bonde JP, Joffe M, Apostoli P, Dale A, Kiss P, Spano M, Caruso F, Giwercman A, Bisanti L, Porru S, Vanhoorne M, Comhaire F, Zschiesche W (2002) Sperm count and chromatin structure in men exposed to inorganic lead: lowest adverse effect levels. Occup Environ Med 59:234–242

Cho KJ, Yun CH, Packer L, Chung AS (2001) Inhibition mechanisms of bioflavonoids extracted from the bark of *Pinus maritima* on the expression of proinflammatory cytokines. Ann NY Acad Sci 928:141–156

Christophe A, Zalata A, Mahmoud A, Comhaire F (1998) Fatty acid composition of sperm phospholipids and its nutritional implications. Middle East Fertil Soc J 3:46–53

Cinti DL, Cook L, Nagi MN, Suneja SK (1992) The fatty acid chain elongation system of mammalian endoplasmic reticulum. Prog Lipid Res 31:1–51

Comhaire F (2000) Clinical andrology: from evidence-base to ethics. The "E" quintet in clinical andrology. Hum Reprod 15:2067–2071

Comhaire FH, Mahmoud AM (2004) Editorial commentary. J Androl 25:771–772

Comhaire F, Vermeulen L (1983) Effect of high dose oral kallikrein treatment in men with idiopathic subfertility: evaluation by means of in vitro penetration test of zona free hamster ova. Int J Androl 6:168–172

Comhaire FH, Christophe AB, Zalata AA, Dhooge WS, Mahmoud AM, Depuydt CE (2000) The effects of combined conventional treatment, oral antioxidants and essential fatty acids on sperm biology in subfertile men. Prostaglandins Leukot Essent Fatty Acids 63:159–165

Comhaire FH, Garem YFE, Mahmoud A, Eertmans F, Schoonjans F (2005) Combined conventional/antioxidant "Astaxanthin" treatment for male infertility: a double blind randomized trial. Asian J Androl 7:257–262

Costa M, Canale D, Filicori M, D'lddio S, Lenzi A (1994) L-Carnitine in idiopathic asthenozoospermia: a multicenter study. Italian Study Group on Carnitine and Male Infertility. Andrologia 26:155–159

Dawson EB, Harris WA, Teter MC, Powell LC (1992) Effect of ascorbic acid supplementation on the sperm quality of smokers. Fertil Steril 58:1034–1039

De Aloysio D, Mantuano R, Mauloni M, Nicoletti G (1982) The clinical use of arginine aspartate in male infertility. Acta Eur Fertil 13:133–167

DeBaun MR, Niemitz EL, Feinberg AP (2003) Association of in vitro fertilization with Beckwith-Wiedemann syndrome and epigenetic alterations of LIT1 and H19. Am J Hum Genet 72:156–160

Depuydt CE, Mahmoud AM, Dhooge WS, Schoonjans FA, Comhaire FH (1999) Hormonal regulation of inhibin B secretion by immature rat Sertoli cells in vitro: possible use as a bioassay for estrogen detection. J Androl 20:54–62

Edwards RG, Ludwig M (2003) Are major defects in children conceived in vitro due to innate problems in patients or to induced genetic damage? Reprod Biomed Online 7:131–138

Fraga CG, Motchnik PA, Shigenaga MK, Helbock HJ, Jacob RA, Ames BN (1991) Ascorbic acid protects against endogenous oxidative DNA damage in human sperm. Proc Natl Acad Sci USA 88:11003–11006

Glezerman M, Lunenfeld E, Potashnik G, Huleihel M, Soffer Y, Segal S (1993) Efficacy of kallikrein in the treatment of oligozoospermia and asthenozoospermia: a double-blind trial. Fertil Steril 60:1052–1056

Golan R, Weissenberg R, Lewin LM (1984) Carnitine and acetylcarnitine in motile and immotile human spermatozoa. Int J Androl 7:484–494

Gonzales GF, Ruiz A, Gonzales C, Villegas L, Cordova A (2001a) Effect of *Lepidium meyenii* (Maca) roots on spermatogenesis of male rats. Asian J Androl 3:231–233

Gonzales GF, Cordova A, Gonzales C, Chung A, Vega K, Villena A (2001b) *Lepidium meyenii* (Maca) improved semen parameters in adult men. Asian J Androl 3:301–303

Goto S, Kogure K, Abe K, Kimata Y, Kitahama K, Yamashita E, Terada H (2001) Efficient radical trapping at the surface and inside the phospholipid membrane is responsible for highly potent antiperoxidative activity of the carotenoid astaxanthin. Biochim Biophys Acta 1512:251–258

Green NS (2004) Risks of birth defects and other adverse outcomes associated with assisted reproductive technology. Pediatrics 114:256–259

Hansen M, Kurinczuk JJ, Bower C, Webb S (2002) The risk of major birth defects after intracytoplasmic sperm injection and in vitro fertilization. N Engl J Med 346:725–730

Hughes CM, Lewis SE, McKelvey-Martin VJ, Thompson W (1998) The effects of antioxidant supplementation during Percoll preparation on human sperm DNA integrity. Hum Reprod 13:1240–1247

Hurtado de Catalfo GE, de Gomez Dumm IN (2002) Polyunsaturated fatty acid biosynthesis from [1–14 C]20:3 n-6 acid in rat cultured Sertoli cells. Linoleic acid effect. Int J Biochem Cell Biol 34:525–532

Irvine DS, Twigg JP, Gordon EL, Fulton N, Milne PA, Aitken RJ (2000) DNA integrity in human spermatozoa: relationships with semen quality. J Androl 21:33–44

Iwamoto T, Hosoda K, Hirano R, Kurata H, Matsumoto A, Miki W, Kamiyama M, Itakura H, Yamamoto S, Kondo K (2000) Inhibition of low-density lipoprotein oxidation by astaxanthin. J Atheroscler Thromb 7:216–222

Jeulin C, Lewin LM (1996) Role of free L-carnitine and acetyl-L-carnitine in post-gonadal maturation of mammalian spermatozoa. Hum Reprod Update 2:87–102

Katz P, Nachtigall R, Showstack J (2002) The economic impact of the assisted reproductive technologies. Nat Cell Biol 4 [Suppl]:s29–s32

Keck C, Behre HM, Jockenhövel F, Nieschlag E (1994) Ineffectiveness of kallikrein in treatment of idiopathic male infertility: a double-blind, randomized, placebo-controlled trial. Hum Reprod 9:325–329

Kent-First MG, Kol S, Muallem A, Ofir R, Manor D, Blazer S, First N, Itskovitz-Eldor J (1996) The incidence and possible relevance of Y-linked microdeletions in babies born after intracytoplasmic sperm injection and their infertile fathers. Mol Hum Reprod 2:943–950

Kessopoulou E, Powers HJ, Sharma KK, Pearson MJ, Russell JM, Cooke ID, Barratt CL (1995) A double-blind randomized placebo cross-over controlled trial using the antioxidant vi-

tamin E to treat reactive oxygen species associated male infertility. Fertil Steril 64:825–831
Kohengkul S, Tanphaichitr V, Muangmun V, Tanphaichitr N (1977) Levels of L-carnitine and L-*O*-acetylcarnitine in normal and infertile human semen: a lower level of L-*O*-acetycarnitine in infertile semen. Fertil Steril 28:1333–1336
Koudstaal J, Bruinse HW, Helmerhorst FM, Vermeiden JP, Willemsen WN, Visser GH (2000) Obstetric outcome of twin pregnancies after in-vitro fertilization: a matched control study in four Dutch University hospitals. Hum Reprod 15:935–940
Lambert RD (2002) Safety issues in assisted reproduction technology: the children of assisted reproduction confront the responsible conduct of assisted reproductive technologies. Hum Reprod 17:3011–3015
Lenzi A, Culasso F, Gandini L, Lombardo F, Dondero F (1993) Placebo-controlled, double-blind, cross-over trial of glutathione therapy in male infertility. Hum Reprod 8:1657–1662
Lenzi A, Lombardo F, Sgro P, Salacone P, Caponecchia L, Dondero F, Gandini L (2003) Use of carnitine therapy in selected cases of male factor infertility: a double-blind crossover trial. Fertil Steril 79:292–300
Lewin A, Lavon H (1997) The effect of coenzyme Q10 on sperm motility and function. Mol Aspects Med 18 [Suppl]:S213–S219
Ma K, Sharkey A, Kirsch S, Vogt P, Keil R, Hargreave TB, McBeath S, Chandley AC (1992) Towards the molecular localisation of the AZF locus: mapping of microdeletions in azoospermic men within 14 subintervals of interval 6 of the human Y chromosome. Hum Mol Genet 1:29–33
Maher ER, Afnan M, Barratt CL (2003) Epigenetic risks related to assisted reproductive technologies: epigenetics, imprinting, ART and icebergs? Hum Reprod 18:2508–2511
Mahmoud AM, Comhaire FH, Depuydt CE (1998) The clinical and biologic significance of serum inhibins in subfertile men. Reprod Toxicol 12:591–599
Mahmoud A, Kiss P, Kaufman JM, Comhaire F, Asclepios (2000) The influence of age and lead exposure on inhibin B serum levels in men. Int J Androl 23 [Suppl 1]:PO94
Mayerhofer A, Meineke V, Köhn FM, Frungieri M (2002) O-03 Cyclooxygenase (COX-2) in male infertility: a new link between prostaglandins and testicular fibrosis? Andrologia 34:272–273
Meachem SJ, Nieschlag E, Simoni M (2001) Inhibin B in male reproduction: pathophysiology and clinical relevance. Eur J Endocrinol 145:561–571
Menchini-Fabris GF, Canale D, Izzo PL, Olivieri L, Bartelloni M (1984) Free L-carnitine in human semen: its variability in different andrologic pathologies. Fertil Steril 42:263–267
Moll AC, Imhof SM, Cruysberg JR, Schouten-van Meeteren AY, Boers M, van Leeuwen FE (2003) Incidence of retinoblastoma in children born after in-vitro fertilisation. Lancet 361:309–310
Moncada ML, Vicari E, Cimino C, Calogero AE, Mongioi A, D'Agata R (1992) Effect of acetylcarnitine treatment in oligoasthenospermic patients. Acta Eur Fertil 23:221–224
Palermo G, Joris H, Devroey P, Van Steirteghem AC (1992) Pregnancies after intracytoplasmic injection of single spermatozoon into an oocyte. Lancet 340:17–18
Pinborg A, Loft A, Schmidt L, Greisen G, Rasmussen S, Andersen AN (2004) Neurological sequelae in twins born after assisted conception: controlled national cohort study. BMJ 329:311
Pryor JP, Blandy JP, Evans P, Chaput DSD, Usherwood M (1978) Controlled clinical trial of arginine for infertile men with oligozoospermia. Br J Urol 50:47–50
Rohdewald P (2002) A review of the French maritime pine bark extract (Pycnogenol), a herbal medication with a diverse clinical pharmacology. Int J Clin Pharmacol Ther 40:158–168
Rolf C, Cooper TG, Yeung CH, Nieschlag E (1999) Antioxidant treatment of patients with asthenozoospermia or moderate oligoasthenozoospermia with high-dose vitamin C and vitamin E: a randomized, placebo-controlled, double-blind study. Hum Reprod 14:1028–1033
Roseff SJ, Gulati R (1999) Improvement of sperm quality by Pycnogenol. Eur Bull Drug Res 7:33–36
Ruiz-Pesini E, Alvarez E, Enriquez JA, Lopez-Perez MJ (2001) Association between seminal plasma carnitine and sperm mitochondrial enzymatic activities. Int J Androl 24:335–340
Saether T, Tran TN, Rootwelt H, Christophersen BO, Haugen TB (2003) Expression and regulation of delta5-desaturase, delta6-desaturase, stearoyl-coenzyme A (CoA) desaturase 1, and stearoyl-CoA desaturase 2 in rat testis. Biol Reprod 69:117–124
Schieve LA, Rasmussen SA, Buck GM, Schendel DE, Reynolds MA, Wright VC (2004) Are children born after assisted reproductive technology at increased risk for adverse health outcomes? Obstet Gynecol 103:1154–1163
Schill WB (1979) Treatment of idiopathic oligozoospermia by kallikrein: results of a double-blind study. Arch Androl 2:163–170
Schill WB, Krizic A, Rjosk H (1979) Determination of various semen parameters and sex hormone levels in subfertile men during kallikrein therapy. Adv Exp Med Biol 120A:537–546
Scott R, MacPherson A, Yates RW, Hussain B, Dixon J (1998) The effect of oral selenium supplementation on human sperm motility. Br J Urol 82:76–80
Sharpe RM (2003) The "oestrogen hypothesis" – where do we stand now? Int J Androl 26:2–15
Skakkebaek NE (2004) Testicular dysgenesis syndrome: new epidemiological evidence. Int J Androl 27:189–191
Soufir JC, Ducot B, Marson J, Jouannet P, Feneux D, Soumah A, Spira A (1984) Levels of seminal free L(–) carnitine in fertile and infertile men. Int J Androl 7:188–197
Steptoe PC, Edwards RG (1978) Birth after the reimplantation of a human embryo. Lancet 2:366
Stromberg B, Dahlquist G, Ericson A, Finnstrom O, Koster M, Stjernqvist K (2002) Neurological sequelae in children born after in-vitro fertilisation: a population-based study. Lancet 359:461–465
Sutcliffe AG, Taylor B, Li J, Thornton S, Grudzinskas JG, Lieberman BA (1999) Children born after intracytoplasmic sperm injection: population control study. Br Med J 318:704–705
Tanphaichitr N (1977) In vitro stimulation of human sperm motility by acetylcarnitine. Int J Fertil 22:85–91
Tiepolo L, Zuffardi O (1976) Localization of factors controlling spermatogenesis in the nonfluorescent portion of the human Y chromosome long arm. Hum Genet 34:119–124
Tran TN, Retterstol K, Christophersen BO (2003) Metabolism of long-chain polyunsaturated fatty acids in testicular cells. In: De Vriese SR, Christophe AB (eds) Male fertility and lipid metabolism. AOCS, Illinois, pp 11–22
van der Ven K, Peschka B, Montag M, Lange R, Schwanitz G, van der Ven HH, van der Ven K (1998) Increased frequency of congenital chromosomal aberrations in female partners of couples undergoing intracytoplasmic sperm injection. Hum Reprod 13:48–54
van Dissel-Emiliani FM, Grootenhuis AJ, De Jong FH, de Rooij DG (1989) Inhibin reduces spermatogonial numbers in testes of adult mice and Chinese hamsters. Endocrinology 125:1899–1903
Vanhoorne M, Comhaire F, De Bacquer D (1994) Epidemiological study of the effects of carbon disulfide on male sexuality and reproduction. Arch Environ Health 49:273–278

Virgili F, Kim D, Packer L (1998) Procyanidins extracted from pine bark protect alpha-tocopherol in ECV 304 endothelial cells challenged by activated RAW 264.7 macrophages: role of nitric oxide and peroxynitrite. FEBS Lett 431:315–318
Vitali G, Parente R, Melotti C (1995) Carnitine supplementation in human idiopathic asthenospermia: clinical results. Drugs Exp Clin Res 21:157–159
Voliani S, Bertozzi MA, Rossi P, Menchini-Fabris GF (2001) The treatment of male infertility with L-carnitine/L-acetyl carnitine. XVII National Congress, Societa Italiana Andrologia SIA, Venezia 2001, 8:122
Wang C, Makela T, Hase T, Adlercreutz H, Kurzer MS (1994) Lignans and flavonoids inhibit aromatase enzyme in human preadipocytes. J Steroid Biochem Mol Biol 50:205–212
Wennerholm U, Bergh C, Hamberger L, Lundin K, Nilsson L, Wikland M, Kallen B (2000) Incidence of congenital malformations in children born after ICSI. Hum Reprod 15:944–948
Wildman REC, Medeiros DM (2000) Advanced human nutrition. CRC, London, pp 370–371
Wong WY, Merkus HM, Thomas CM, Menkveld R, Zielhuis GA, Steegers-Theunissen RP (2002) Effects of folic acid and zinc sulfate on male factor subfertility: a double-blind, randomized, placebo-controlled trial. Fertil Steril 77:491–498
Zalata AA, Christophe AB, Depuydt CE, Schoonjans F, Comhaire FH (1998) The fatty acid composition of phospholipids of spermatozoa from infertile patients. Mol Hum Reprod 4:111–118
Zheng BL, He K, Kim CH, Rogers L, Shao Y, Huang ZY, Lu Y, Yan SJ, Qien LC, Zheng QY (2000) Effect of a lipidic extract from *Lepidium meyenii* on sexual behavior in mice and rats. Urology 55:598–602

II.4.16 Assisted Reproductive Techniques

W. Ombelet

Summary

There is good evidence in the literature in favour of intrauterine insemination (IUI) as the best first-line treatment and most cost-effective procedure in cases of mild and moderate male factor subfertility before starting more invasive and expensive techniques such as in vitro fertilization (IVF) and intracytoplasmic sperm injection (ICSI). On the other hand, it seems very difficult to isolate individual semen parameters predicting the likelihood of pregnancy after IUI. A review of the literature confirmed that sperm morphology using strict criteria and the inseminating motile sperm count (IMC) are the most important sperm parameters for assessing the real impact of semen quality on IUI outcome. A universal threshold level above which IUI can be performed with acceptable pregnancy rates has not been determined yet, although IUI success seems to be impaired with fewer than 5% normal spermatozoa using strict criteria and with an IMC of less than one million.

In cases of severe male subfertility, it is not only the number of motile spermatozoa recovered after washing but also the number of oocytes retrieved that will guide the laboratory as to which procedure (IVF or ICSI) will be chosen. Only absolute immotility of spermatozoa seems to reduce the fertilization rate after ICSI.

Epididymal aspiration of sperm and/or testicular sperm extraction can successfully be applied in most cases of azoospermia. These techniques revolutionized the treatment of azoospermic patients. For obstructive azoospermia, fertilization and pregnancy rates are comparable with those achieved with ejaculated sperm. The results with frozen testicular sperm are comparable to those obtained with fresh testicular sperm. In men with non-obstructive azoospermia, ICSI seems to be less successful.

Approximately 10–15% of women will receive infertility treatment during their lifetime and in more than one-third of cases male infertility is involved. Of all subfertile couples, only 1–2% will undergo treatment with assisted reproductive technologies (ART). The increasing availability of ART during the past 20 years has received a lot of public attention, not least because of the ethical implications, the high costs associated with these treatments, the impact of age and multiple births on costs, the inequities in access to infertility services in many countries and the issue of safety. On the other hand, the true value of treatment modalities of infertility is poorly understood because there are many different measures of quality and effectiveness. Success of infertility treatment is generally described as "cumulative pregnancy rate" (andrological surgery, varicocele treatment, etc.) or pregnancy rate per treatment cycle (IVF, ICSI, IUI). For ART it is important to be aware of the complex weave of secondary issues to consider such as neonatal outcome, short- and long-term infant morbidity and maternal complications, all of which are closely linked to the higher incidence of multiple pregnancies. Consequently, ART (especially IVF and ICSI) account for 0.4–0.8% of the total health care costs in the USA.

II.4.16.1 IUI and Male Infertility

When male infertility is found in couples with long-standing infertility, expectant treatment seems to be disappointing, with a spontaneous conception rate of less than 2% per cycle (Collins et al. 1995). From a theoretical point of view, increasing the number of motile spermatozoa at the site of fertilization, especially when sperm quality is suboptimal, should increase the probability of conception. Cohlen et al. (2000) showed that in cases of male subfertility IUI is an effective treatment option as compared to controls. A meta-analysis of six studies showed a statistically significant improvement of conception rates favouring IUI, although the pregnancy rate per completed IUI cycle varied from 0% to 8.7%. In another meta-analysis, the results were also significantly better for IUI when mild ovarian stimulation had been used (Cohlen et al. 2000). According to Cohlen (2005), IUI should only be applied in couples who have a reasonable probability of achieving an ongoing pregnancy after IUI, and couples should make the decision themselves in dialogue with their physicians.

II.4.16.2 Male Infertility: IUI Versus IVF/ICSI

Whereas ICSI is the most successful treatment option per cycle in most cases of moderate and severe male infertility, simpler methods of assisted reproduction such as IUI have to be weighed against ICSI, taking into account not only the immediate success rate but also the cost-effectiveness of the different strategies. IUI is less invasive, less stressful, less expensive and more cost-effective compared to IVF/ICSI. A number of studies have been performed focusing on the cost-effectiveness of IUI when compared to IVF (Peterson et al. 1994; Zayed et al. 1997; Van Voorhis et al. 1997, 2001; Goverde et al. 2000; Philips et al. 2000). In all studies, three cycles of IUI were as successful as, but much cheaper than one IVF/ICSI cycle.

In a prospective randomized controlled trial, Goverde et al. (2000) observed that three cycles of IUI offered the same likelihood of a successful pregnancy as IVF. According to their results, IUI is a more cost-effective approach for moderate male factor infertility when compared to IVF. This important message was confirmed by another study performed in the UK (Philips et al. 2000). In the latter study the authors complemented existing clinical guidelines by including cost-effectiveness of different treatment options for infertility in the UK. A series of decision-analytical models was developed to reflect current diagnostic and treatment pathways for the different causes of infertility. They also concluded that IUI during stimulated cycles is a cost-effective approach for the treatment of couples with unexplained and/or moderate male factor infertility.

The effectiveness of IUI was also reported in a large retrospective analysis of almost 10,000 IUI cycles in which male factor infertility was associated with a high pregnancy rate of 8.2% per cycle in a population with an average female age of 39 years (Stone et al. 2002).

Most studies reported a significant decline in success rate per cycle after the third or fourth IUI cycle (Comhaire et al.1994; Plosker et al. 1994; Ombelet et al. 1996; Khalil et al. 2001). The unsuccessful couples seem not to benefit from this method of treatment and should be advised to start with other treatment options such as IVF and/or ICSI. A Cochrane review also showed that performing two intrauterine inseminations on subsequent days yielded no benefit over single intrauterine insemination (Cantineau et al. 2003).

In selecting couples with male factor infertility to be treated with IUI or IVF/ICSI, it would be of interest to establish cut-off values of semen parameters above which IUI is an effective alternative to IVF/ICSI.

We previously demonstrated that in a selected group of patients with normal ovarian response to clomiphene (CC) stimulation, individual sperm parameters, including inseminating motile count (IMC or number of motile spermatozoa after the washing procedure) and sperm morphology, turned out to be of little prognostic value in predicting success for the group as a whole (Ombelet et al. 1997). However, sperm morphology becomes a very useful predictive tool in a subgroup of patients with an IMC of less than one million. In terms of therapeutic strategy, this implies that above the cut-off value of one million motile spermatozoa recovered after washing, CC-IUI can be promoted as a first-line therapy with a cumulative ongoing pregnancy rate (OPR) of 24% after three cycles. On the other hand, in cases with fewer than one million motile spermatozoa, CC-IUI remains important as a first-line option provided the sperm morphology score is 4% or more (cumulative OPR of 21.9% after three IUI cycles). A proposed algorithm for couples with male infertility and without tubal factor is shown in Fig. II.4.39.

In order to investigate the threshold levels of sperm parameters above which the pregnancy rate after IUI is significantly better, we performed a Medline literature search for the period from 1983 until 2002 (Ombelet et al. 2003).

According to this review, IMC and sperm morphology are the most valuable sperm parameters for predicting IUI outcome. A trend towards increasing conception rates with increasing IMC was found. However, the cut-off value above which IUI seems to be successful ranges from 0.3 to 20 million. This finding highlights the importance of confounding factors influencing the success rate such as female age, duration of subfertility, etc.

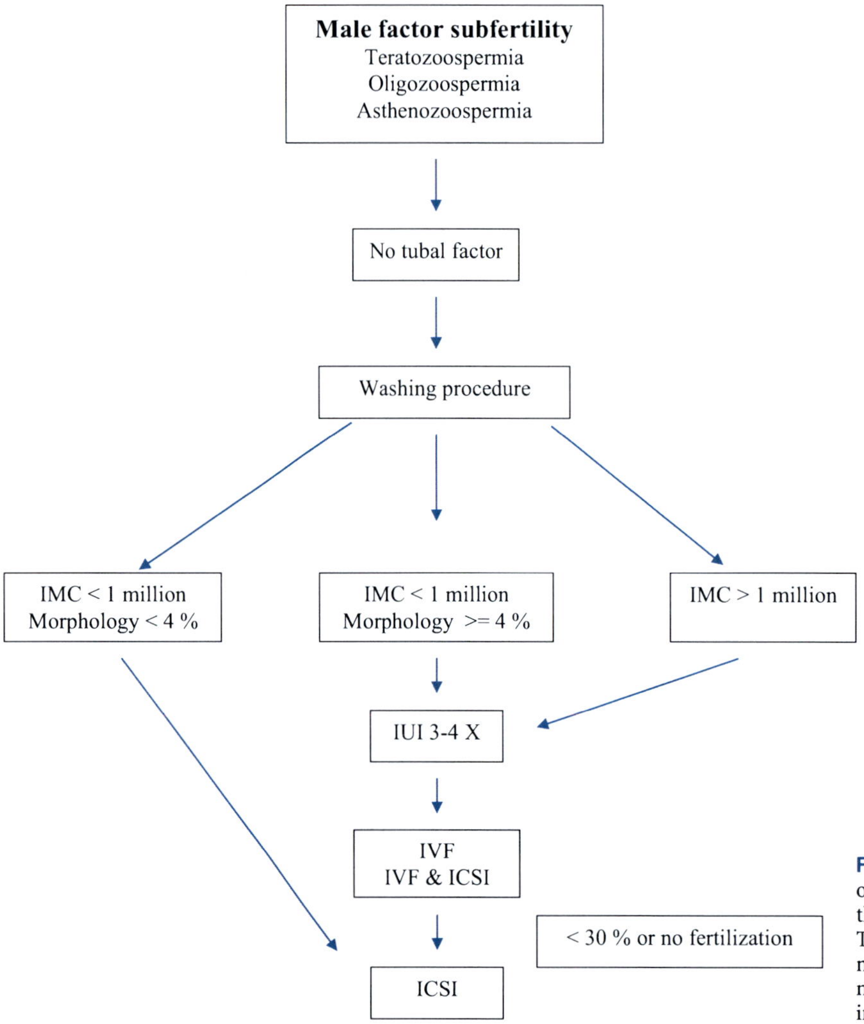

Fig. II.4.39. Proposed algorithm of male subfertility treatment at the Genk Institute for Fertility Technology. (*IMC* Inseminating motile count or the number of motile spermatozoa after washing procedure)

Our analysis also confirmed the results of a previously reported meta-analysis showing a significant improvement in pregnancy rates above the 4% normal morphology threshold using strict criteria (Van Waart et al. 2001). According to our Medline search, the cut-off level for total progressive sperm motility before sperm preparation ranged between 30% and 50%. Two other parameters influencing the pregnancy rate after IUI were the hypo-osmotic swelling (HOS) test (threshold: > 50%) and sperm DNA fragmentation (threshold: < 12%). The sperm chromatin structure assay (SCSA) also seems to provide an objective assessment of sperm chromatin integrity and may become an important marker in IUI in the near future.

There is a widespread belief among fertility specialists that an increased use of artificial insemination with controlled ovarian hyperstimulation (COH) will lead to an uncontrolled increase in multiple pregnancies. To investigate the impact of controlled ovarian stimulation with IUI on the number of multiple pregnancies in Flanders, we used the data from the "Studiecentrum voor perinatale Epidemiologie" (SPE). The SPE collects data on the medical and obstetric history, and on perinatal events of each hospital delivery in Flanders of more than 21 weeks of gestational age or ≥500 g at birth.

A retrospective analysis of 363,187 deliveries between 1997 and 2002 showed that infertility treatment with ovarian stimulation, including IVF and non-IVF procedures, was responsible for 3.9% of all registered deliveries. Of all multiple pregnancies following ovarian stimulation, IVF/ICSI was performed in 66.7%, COH with timed coitus (COH-TC) in 23.7% and COH-IUI in 9.6% of cases (Fig. II.4.40a). The low figure for COH-IUI can be explained by the fact that most centres in Flanders use clomiphene citrate rather than gonadotrophins in IUI cycles (Ombelet et al. 2003; unpublished data, questionnaire for the Flemish Society of Obstetrics and Gynaecology). Concerning the different treatment procedures, the multiple birth rate was

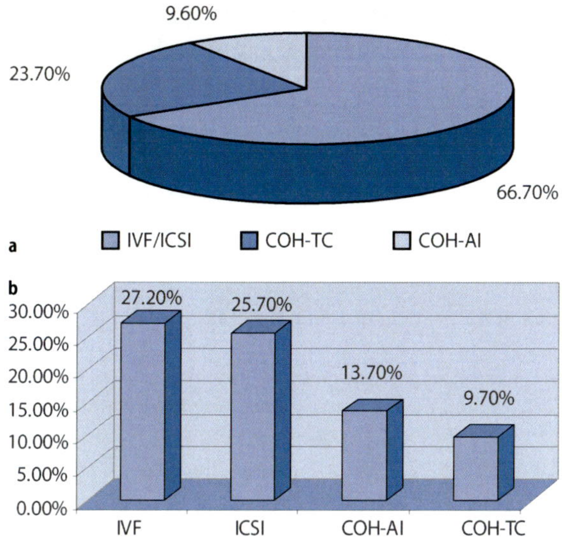

Fig. II.4.40a, b. a SPE data on 363,187 deliveries in Flanders between 1997 and 2002: incidence of multiple pregnancy rate after IVF/ICSI, COH + TC, COH + AI. (*AI* Artificial insemination, *COH* controlled ovarian hyperstimulation, *ICSI* intracytoplasmic sperm injection, *IVF* in vitro fertilization, *SPE* Study Center for Perinatal Epidemiology, *TC* timed coitus). **b** SPE data on 13,120 deliveries following hormonal treatment in Flanders between 1997 and 2002: relative contribution of different methods of infertility treatment in the "multiple pregnancy population"

27.2% for IVF, 25.7% for ICSI, 13.7% for COH-IUI and 9.7% for COH-TC respectively (Fig. II.4.40b). These data show that the criticism mentioned in some reports about the high risk of multiple pregnancies following non-IVF assisted reproduction can easily be overcome by using low-dose hormonal stimulation. According to our data, IVF and ICSI remain the most important contributors to the high incidence of multiple gestation following ART.

II.4.16.3 IVF and ICSI

The first observation showing that IVF could successfully be applied to treat male factor infertility was reported by Fishel and Edwards (1982). This was confirmed by a series of reports indicating the value of IVF in such cases. Conventional IVF refers to incubation of the oocyte–cumulus complex in a washed sperm suspension of approximately 200,000 motile spermatozoa. The number of motile spermatozoa recovered after washing as well as the number of oocytes retrieved will indicate to the laboratory which procedure (IVF or ICSI) should be chosen for each specific couple. In order to achieve increased rates of conception, conventional IVF has been modified and refined. For cases with severe teratozoospermia (fewer than 5% normal forms using strict criteria), a higher insemination concentration of more than 400,000 spermatozoa per oocyte might improve the fertilization rate significantly (Oehninger et al.1988), although the pregnancy rate was not improved in that particular study. Another option, in cases of severe oligozoospermia, is the use of microdrop IVF. This technique is usually applied when the volume of sperm available for insemination is very low, but the sperm quality is acceptable. A possible adverse effect of both techniques might be the exposure of the oocytes and developing embryos to relatively high concentrations of reactive oxygen species (ROS) generated by increased numbers of immotile and morphologically abnormal spermatozoa.

Even with the skilled use of IVF, severe male infertility was considered to be untreatable in most cases before the introduction of ICSI, i.e. the injection of one spermatozoon into each single oocyte (Palermo et al. 1992). The first results indicated the same success rate for moderate versus severe male infertility when ICSI was used. Comparable results were reported for ICSI in severe cases of oligo-astheno-teratozoospemia (OAT) when compared to conventional IVF in couples without male factor infertility. Thanks to ICSI, treating couples with severe male infertility has become possible not only using ejaculated spermatozoa, but also using sperm recovered from the epididymis, the testis or even from the seminiferous tubules. In the view of some clinicians, the detection of the underlying pathology responsible for deficient spermatogenesis has become irrelevant since they consider that this does not affect the choice of treatment at least in the majority of cases. Nowadays it seems that only absolute immotility of spermatozoa reduces the fertilization rate after ICSI, and this is probably not caused by the immotility itself, but rather the non-viability of spermatozoa.

Another important advantage of ICSI is the possibility of freezing semen samples before a patient undergoes chemotherapy and/or radiation for cancer. If sperm quality is poor at that moment, ICSI will be the method of choice later on. Subsequently, there is no delay in cancer treatment and future fertility is preserved.

II.4.16.4 Azoospermia: MESA, PESA, TESE and TESA

The first successful attempt at ICSI using epididymal sperm (MESA or microsurgical epididymal sperm aspiration) was reported by Silber et al. (1994) and Tournaye et al. (1994). It seems that the results in terms of probability of conception are significantly better with MESA than after vaso-epididymostomy in the case of obstructive azoospermia. Furthermore, many reports have shown that the cause of obstruction is not impor-

Table II.4.12. Sperm retrieval in obstructive azoospermia: Pros and cons of microsurgical epididymal sperm aspiration (*MESA*) and percutaneous epididymal sperm aspiration (*PESA*)

MESA	PESA
More sperm	Fewer sperm
Easier to freeze	More difficult to process
Easier to schedule	Difficult to schedule
Single procedure	Repeated procedures possible
More invasive	Less invasive
More costly	Less costly
Operating room (microscope)	Office procedure
Microsurgical skills needed	No microsurgical skills needed

tant when considering the success rate with MESA. An alternative method for epididymal aspiration of sperm is PESA (percutaneous epididymal sperm aspiration), being less invasive and less costly than MESA. The pros and cons of MESA and PESA are summarized in Table II.4.12.

Despite the good results with MESA and PESA, many studies have shown that ICSI with testicular spermatozoa retrieved by TESE (testicular sperm extraction) could also be successfully applied in almost all cases of azoospermia. This technique really revolutionized the treatment of azoospermic patients. The most popular methods of sperm retrieval are conventional "open biospy" retrieval (TESE), FNA (fine needle aspiration) or TESA (testicular sperm aspiration). In patients with normal spermatogenesis it seems that FNA and TESE give comparable results (Tournaye 1997).

Another breakthrough was the finding that epididymal and testicular sperm could be frozen, stored and subsequently used in future ICSI cycles.

For obstructive azoospermia, fertilization and pregnancy rates are comparable with those using ejaculated spermatozoa, and results with frozen sperm are comparable to those obtained with fresh testicular sperm. However, ICSI seems to be less successful in men with non-obstructive azoospermia. In the majority of cases of patients with testicular failure, such as Sertoli cell only syndrome, cryptorchidism, maturation arrest and azoospermia post-chemotherapy, only a small but still sufficient number of spermatozoa can be extracted and utilized for ICSI, with satisfactory albeit lower results compared to obstructive azoospermia cases. Reports comparing ICSI with fresh and with frozen testicular sperm from non-obstructive azoospermia are very scarce. Success may depend on the strategy of the centre to allocate patients to ICSI with frozen sperm (very restrictive versus poorly restrictive). Compared to the use of fresh TESE spermatozoa, there seems to be an increased risk of post-thaw loss of sperm motility causing fertilization failure.

The use of testicular sperm for ICSI is also a treatment option that can be offered to azoospermic males with hypogonadotrophic hypogonadism who do not respond or are reluctant to continue long-term hormonal treatment. A recently reported systematic review showed that even in non-mosaic and mosaic Klinefelter patients, chromosomally normal sperm cells can be extracted from testicular tissue and used for ICSI. Therefore, the application of ART to Klinefelter patients may be offered as a possible method of achieving reproduction with a limited risk of transmitting a chromosomal abnormality to the offspring (Denschlag et al. 2004). Nonetheless, the success rate of ICSI in cases with Klinefelter syndrome is low, and patients must be informed about this. Also, amniocentesis should be recommended in case a pregnancy is attained.

It is generally accepted that genetic testing is mandatory in all cases of azoospermia and severe oligozoospermia (<5 million per ml). Deletions in the azoospermia factor (AZF) locus on the long arm of the Y chromosome (region q11.23) are observed in about 15% of men with azoospermia and in 10% of men with severe oligozoospermia (Reijo et al. 1996). Microdeletion of the entire AZFa or AZFb regions of the Y chromosome portends an exceptionally poor prognosis for sperm retrieval, whereas the majority of men with AZFc deletion have spermatozoa within their semen or in the testes available for use in IVF/ICSI. Patients with AZFc microdeletions seem to have IVF/ICSI outcomes

Table II.4.13. Most important genetic abnormalities associated with male sub(in)fertility

Gene abnormalities		
Syndrome/ condition	**Genotype/inheritance**	**Frequency**
Cystic fibrosis	Autosomal recessive CFTR gene Chromosome 7q31.2	1/2500
Immotile cilia (Kartagener)	Autosomal recessive Chromosome 1q35.1	1/30,000
Kallmann	X-linked recessive KAL-locus Chromosome Xp22.3	1/30,000
Myotonic dystrophy	Autosomal dominant/variable penetrance Chromosome 19q13.3	1/8000
Numerical and structural abnormalities		
Syndrome/ condition	**Genotype**	**Frequency**
Klinefelter	47,XXY or mosaic 47,XXY/46,XY	1/1000
Noonan	Autosomal dominant Mosaicism 46,XY/XO and chromosome 12q22ter	1/2000
Y deletions	Deletion AZF locus Yq11.21	1/8000

comparable to those of controls with normal Y chromosomes (Hopps et al. 2003). A list of the most frequent genetic abnormalities associated with male sub- or infertility is shown in Table II.4.13. However, counselling of the couple is mandatory since a possible male offspring will carry the genetic abnormality, and therefore be infertile as well when Y deletions are involved.

II.4.16.5 Art: Prevention of Multiple Pregnancies

The aim of infertility treatment is not just to achieve a successful conception, but to offer the parents a healthy and normal child. The major complication of ART is the high incidence of multiple pregnancies. For IVF and ICSI, transferring multiple embryos into the uterus maximizes pregnancy rates, at the expense however of an unacceptably high multiple pregnancy rate. The most important causal factor is undoubtedly the number of embryos transferred. After the transfer of three, four and five embryos the incidence of triplet pregnancies is respectively 8%, 11% and 15% (Cohen 2003). Nowadays, the policy of elective single embryo transfer (eSET) in stimulated cycles is becoming more popular and is the most efficacious measure to reduce the incidence of twin pregnancies (Wolner-Hanssen and Rydhstroem 1998; Gerris et al. 1999; Van Royen et al. 1999; Tiitinen et al. 2001; De Sutter et al. 2003). In a large retrospective study it was shown that with the implementation of eSET multiple pregnancy delivery rates could drop from 25% to 5% (Tiitinen et al. 2003).

Accessibility to IVF/ICSI services remains another important problem and, to a large extent, this can be explained by the high cost of a single IVF cycle in most countries (Fauser et al. 2002). The use of ART is more common in countries that subsidize expenses, and in many countries basic fertility services are provided through public funding, but IVF provision is limited or absent (Hughes and Giacomini 2001). Furthermore, insurance coverage for IVF services seems to be associated with increased utilization of IVF and with a decreasing number of embryos transferred (Reynolds et al. 2003). On 1 July, 2003, the Belgian government started reimbursing the laboratory expenses for IVF-ICSI in couples with a female age of less than 43 years and for a maximum of six treatment cycles in a lifetime. This strategy was only acceptable and affordable by the government if the number of embryos transferred was limited, subsequently leading to a decrease in perinatal costs associated with multiple pregnancies. This project tried to meet the needs of most infertile couples without additional costs and it is a good example of cost-efficient health care through responsibilization (Ombelet et al. 2005).

Unfortunately, a high multiple pregnancy rate is associated not only with IVF and ICSI, but also with non-IVF procedures, such as ovarian hyperstimulation with or without artificial insemination. Because IUI is a successful, simpler, less invasive and cheaper first-line treatment compared to IVF, it is nowadays the most frequently used treatment option worldwide. However, because of the widespread use of gonadotrophins, induction of ovulation, with or without IUI, has become the main cause of multiple pregnancies related to infertility treatment in the USA (Gleicher et al. 2000; Evans et al. 2001; Tur et al. 2001).

Ovulation induction can be achieved with clomiphene citrate (CC), a good first-line option since ovulation can be induced in about 50–70% of cases, with a multiple pregnancy rate of 6–8% (Ombelet et al. 1996, 1997; Sovino et al. 2002). Gonadotrophins are necessary in clomiphene-resistant cases and yield better pregnancy rates compared to CC, but at the expense of a higher multiple pregnancy rate of more than 15% in most studies. Low dosage gonadotrophin protocols are being tested and seem to result in a lower multiple birth rate without influencing the ongoing pregnancy rate too much (Dhaliwal et al. 2002; Alsina et al. 2003).

Another elegant option is to start ovarian stimulation on cycle day 6 or even later. In a prospective randomized study, Hohmann et al. (2001) showed that when follicle-stimulating hormone (FSH) injections were started on cycle day 7, monofollicular growth was observed more often compared to patients with FSH given from day 3 or day 5 on. It seems that the proper timing of initiation of exogenous FSH may be an important tool for optimizing ovarian stimulation and for selecting the best moment for insemination in IUI.

II.4.16.6 Conclusion

IUI should be promoted as the best first-line treatment in almost all cases of mild and moderate male infertility provided at least one tube is patent and a motile sperm count of more than 0.3 to 1 million can be obtained after sperm preparation. After three or four unsuccessful attempts, IVF or ICSI should be advised. The decision of whether to perform regular IVF or ICSI depends on the number of oocytes retrieved, the number of motile spermatozoa after washing and sperm morphology.

Most cases of azoospermia can be treated with ICSI using spermatozoa obtained after MESA or TESE. Otherwise, insemination with donor semen remains an alternative treatment option. Genetic testing is advisable in all cases of severe OAT and/or azoospermia.

References

Alsina JC, Balda JAR, Sarrio AR, Fernandez AR, Trigo IC, Parga JLG, Batres CG, Escudero JR (2003) Ovulation induction with a starting dose of 50 IU of recombinant follicle stimulating hormone in WHO group II anovulatory women: the IO-50 study, a prospective, observational, multicentre, open trial. Br J Obstet Gynaecol 110:1072–1077

Cantineau AE, Heineman MJ, Cohlen BJ (2003) Single versus double intrauterine insemination (IUI) in stimulated cycles for subfertile couples. Cochrane Database Syst Rev 1:CD003854

Cohen J (2003) Associated multiple gestation – ART. Clin Obstet Gynecol 46:363–374

Cohlen BJ (2005) Should we continue performing intrauterine inseminations in the year 2004? Gynecol Obstet Invest 59:3–13

Cohlen BJ, Vandekerckhove P, te Velde ER, Habbema JD (2000) Timed intercourse versus intra-uterine insemination with or without ovarian hyperstimulation for subfertility in men. Cochrane Database Syst Rev CD000360

Collins JA, Bustillo M, Visscher RD, Lawrence LD (1995) An estimate of the cost of in vitro fertilization services in the United States in 1995. Fertil Steril 64:538–545

Comhaire F, Milingos S, Liapi A, Gordts S, Campo R, Depypere H, Dhont M Schoonjans F (1994) The effective cumulative pregnancy rate of different modes of treatment of male infertility. Andrologia 27:217–221

Denschlag D, Tempfer C, Kunze M, Wolff G, Keck C (2004) Assisted reproductive techniques in patients with Klinefelter syndrome: a critical review. Fertil Steril 82:775–779

De Sutter P, Van der Elst J, Coetsier T, Dhont M (2003) Single embryo transfer and multiple pregnancy rate reduction in IVF/ICSI: a 5-year appraisal. Reprod Biomed Online 6: 464–469

Dhaliwal LK, Sialy RK, Gopalan S, Majumdar S (2002) Minimal stimulation protocol for use with intrauterine insemination in the treatment of infertility. J Obstet Gynaecol Res 28: 295–299

Evans MI, Berkowitz RL, Wapner RJ, Carpenter RJ, Goldberg JD, Ayoub MA, Horenstein J, Dommergues M, Brambati B, Nicolaides KH, Holzgreve W, Timor-Tritsch IE (2001) Improvement in outcomes of multifetal pregnancy reduction with increased experience. Am J Obstet Gynecol 184:97–103

Fauser BC, Bouchard P, Coelingh Bennink HJ, Collins JA, Devroey P, Evers JL, van Steirteghem A (2002) Alternative approaches in IVF. Hum Reprod Update 8:1–9

Fishel SB, Edwards RG (1982) Essentials of fertilisation. In: Edwards RG, Purdy JM (eds) Human conception in vitro. Academic Press, London, pp 157–179

Gerris J, De Neubourg D, Mangelschots K, Van Royen E, Van de Meerssche M, Valkenburg M (1999) Prevention of twin pregnancy after in-vitro fertilization or intracytoplasmic sperm injection based on strict embryo criteria: a prospective randomized clinical trial. Hum Reprod 14:2581–2587

Gleicher N, Oleske DM, Tur-Kaspa I, Vidali A, Karande V (2000) Reducing the risk of high-order multiple pregnancy after ovarian stimulation with gonadotropins. N Engl J Med 343:2–7

Goverde AJ, McDonnell J, Vermeiden JP, Schats R, Rutten FF, Schoemaker J (2000) Intrauterine insemination or in-vitro fertilisation in idiopathic subfertility and male subfertility: a randomized trial and cost-effectiveness analysis. Lancet 355:13–18

Griffin M, Panak WF (1998) The economic cost of infertility-related services: an examination of the Massachusetts infertility insurance mandate. Fertil Steril 70:22–29

Hohmann FP, Laven JS, de Jong FH, Eijkemans MJ, Fauser BC (2001) Low-dose exogenous FSH initiated during the early, mid or late follicular phase can induce multiple dominant follicle development. Hum Reprod 16:846–854

Hopps CV, Mielnik A, Goldstein M, Palermo GD, Rosenwaks Z, Schlegel PN (2003) Detection of sperm in men with Y chromosome microdeletions of the AZFa, AZFb and AZFc regions. Hum Reprod 18:1660–1665

Hughes EG, Giacomini M (2001) Funding in vitro fertilization treatment for persistent subfertility: the pain and the politics. Fertil Steril 76:431–442

Khalil MR, Rasmussen PE, Erb K, Laursen SB, Rex S, Westergaard LG (2001) Homologous intrauterine insemination. An evaluation of prognostic factors based on a review of 2473 cycles. Acta Obstet Gynecol Scand 80:74–81

Oehninger S, Acosta AA, Morshedi M, Veeck L, Swanson RJ, Simmons K, Rosenwaks Z (1988) Corrective measures and pregnancy outcome in in vitro fertilization in patients with severe sperm morphology abnormalities. Fertil Steril 50: 283–287

Ombelet W, Cox A, Janssen,M, Vandeput H, Bosmans E (1996) Artificial insemination (AIH) artificial insemination 2: using the husband's sperm. In: Acosta AA, Kruger TF (eds) Diagnosis and therapy of male factor in assisted reproduction. Parthenon, London, pp 397–410

Ombelet W, Vandeput H, Van de Putte G, Cox A, Janssen M, Jacobs P, Bosmans E, Steeno O, Kruger T (1997) Intrauterine insemination after ovarian stimulation with clomiphene citrate: predictive potential of inseminating motile count and sperm morphology. Hum Reprod 12:1458–1463

Ombelet W, Deblaere K, Bosmans E, Cox A, Jacobs P, Janssen M, Nijs M (2003) Semen quality and intrauterine insemination. Reprod Biomed Online 7:485–492

Ombelet W, De Sutter P, Van der Elst J, Martens G (2005) Multiple gestation and infertility treatment: registration, reflection and reaction–the Belgian project. Hum Reprod Update 11:3–14

Palermo G, Joris H, Devroey P, Van Steirteghem AC (1992) Pregnancies after intracytoplasmic injection of single spermatozoon into an oocyte. Lancet 340:17–18

Peterson CM, Hatasaka HH, Jones KP, Poulson AM Jr, Carrell DT, Urry RL (1994) Ovulation induction with gonadotropins and intrauterine insemination compared with in vitro fertilization and no therapy: a prospective, nonrandomized, cohort study and meta-analysis. Fertil Steril 62:535–544

Philips Z, Barraza-Llorens M, Posnett J (2000) Evaluation of the relative cost-effectiveness of treatments for infertility in the UK. Hum Reprod 15:95–106

Plosker SM, Jacobson W, Amato P (1994) Prediction and optimizing success in an intra-uterine insemination programme. Hum Reprod 9:2014–2021

Reijo R, Alagappan RK, Patrizio P, Page DC (1996) Severe oligozoospermia resulting from deletions of azoospermia factor gene on Y chromosome. Lancet 347:1290–1293

Reynolds MA, Schieve LA, Jeng G, Peterson HB (2003) Does insurance coverage decrease the risk for multiple births associated with assisted reproductive technology? Fertil Steril 80:16–23

Silber SJ, Nagy ZP, Liu J, Godoy H, Devroey P, Van Steirteghem AC (1994) Conventional in vitro fertilization versus intracytoplasmic sperm injection for patients requiring microsurgical sperm aspiration. Hum Reprod 9:1705–1709

Sovino H, Sir-Petermann T, Devoto L (2002) Clomiphene citrate and oulation induction. Reprod Biomed Online 4:303–310

Stone J, Eddleman K, Lynch L, Berkowitz RL (2002) A single center experience with 1000 consecutive cases of multifetal pregnancy reduction. Am J Obstet Gynecol 187:1163–1167

Stovall DW, Allen BD, Sparks AET, Syrop CH, Saunders RG, Van Voorhis BJ (1999) The cost of infertility evaluation and therapy: findings of a self-insured university healthcare plan. Fertil Steril 72:778–784

Tiitinen A, Halttunen M., Härkki P, Vuoristo P, Hyden-Granskog C (2001) Elective single embryo transfer: the value of cryopreservation. Hum Reprod 16:1140–1144

Tiitinen A, Unkila-Kallio L, Halttunen M, Hyden-Granskog C (2003) Impact of elective single embryo transfer on the twin pregnancy rate. Hum Reprod 18:1449–1453

Tournaye H (1997) Use of testicular sperm for the treatment of male infertility. Baillieres Clin Obstet Gynaecol 11:753–762

Tournaye H, Devroey P, Liu J, Nagy Z, Lissens W, Van Steirteghem A (1994) Microsurgical epididymal sperm aspiration and intracytoplasmic sperm injection: a new effective approach to infertility as a result of congenital bilateral absence of the vas deferens. Fertil Steril 61:1045–1051

Tur R, Barri PN, Coroleu B, Buxaderas R, Martinez F, Balasch J (2001) Risk factors for high-order multiple implantation after ovarian stimulation with gonadotrophins: evidence from a large series of 1878 consecutive pregnancies in a single centre. Hum Reprod 16:2124–2129

Van Royen E, Mangelschots K, De Neubourg D, Valkenburg M, Van de Meerssche M, Ryckaert G, Eestermans W, Gerris J (1999) Characterization of a top quality embryo, a step towards single-embryo transfer. Hum Reprod 14:2345–2349

Van Voorhis BJ, Sparks AET, Allen BD, Stovall DW, Syrop CH, Chapler FK (1997) Cost-effectiveness of infertility treatments: a cohort study. Fertil Steril 67:830–836

Van Voorhis BJ, Barnett M, Sparks AET, Syrop CH, Rosenthal G, Dawson J (2001) Effect of the totile motile sperm count on the efficacy and cost-effectiveness of intrauterine insemination and in vitro fertilization. Fertil Steril 75:661–668

Van Waart J, Kruger TF, Lombard CJ, Ombelet W (2001) Predictive value of normal sperm morphology in intrauterine insemination (IUI): a structured literature review. Hum Reprod 7:495–500

Wolner-Hanssen P, Rydhstroem H (1998) Cost-effectiveness analysis of in-vitro fertilization: estimated costs per successful pregnancy after transfer of one or two embryos. Hum Reprod 13:88–94

Zayed F, Lenton EA, Cooke ID (1997) Comparison between stimulated in-vitro fertilization and stimulated intrauterine insemination for the treatment of unexplained and mild male factor infertility. Hum Reprod 12:2408–2413

II.4.17 Cryopreservation of Spermatozoa and Testicular Tissue Including Autotransplantation of Germinal Epithelium

F.-M. Köhn

Summary

Assisted reproduction techniques have widened the indications for human sperm cryopreservation, because semen quality is no longer a limiting factor. Therefore, cryopreservation can now be used more often than in the past by cancer patients for the purpose of fertility protection.

Since the fertilizing capacity of cryopreserved testicular and epididymal spermatozoa is comparable to that of ejaculated spermatozoa, the most evident advantage of cryopreservation techniques is that active spermatogenesis can be identified before the female partner undergoes any stimulation protocol.

- Cryopreservation of human ejaculates is a well-established medical procedure to maintain the fertilizing potential of spermatozoa during storage in liquid nitrogen.
- Pregnancies have been achieved with semen samples cryopreserved for more than 15 years.
- There is no doubt that pre-therapy storage of semen from cancer patients is an important medical task, all the more since the prognosis and life expectancy of those with Hodgkin's disease and testicular tumours is very good today.
- Since intracytoplasmic sperm injection (ICSI) requires only one living spermatozoon per oocyte, cut-off values of standard semen parameters prior to cryopreservation of samples are no longer necessary.
- There is no marker available to predict the freezability of individual semen samples; in general, however, the survival rate 1 h after thawing of frozen semen is between 50 and 60 %.
- Cryopreservation of ejaculated, epididymal and testicular spermatozoa does not affect ICSI results in terms of fertilization and pregnancy rates; however, the data about testicular spermatozoa are contradictory because single studies have reported reduced fertilizing capacity of testicular spermatozoa with no decrease in pregnancy rates.
- A major problem of cancer patients is that 50 % of them may have a disease-intrinsic suppression of spermatogenesis.
- Sperm cryopreservation should also be recommended to oncological patients younger than 15 years, if they are able to produce a semen sample.
- Protection of fertility in childhood cancer patients by later autotransplantation of cryopreserved testicular stem cells will probably be a future option for this patient group.

II.4.17.1 Introduction

Cryopreservation of human ejaculates is a well-established medical procedure to maintain the fertilizing potential of spermatozoa during storage in liquid nitrogen (–196 °C). Pregnancies have been achieved with semen samples cryopreserved for more than 15 years. Modern trends in assisted reproduction technologies (ART) have influenced the indications for human sperm cryobanking. In addition to cryopreservation of donor spermatozoa for artificial insemination or cryobanking of ejaculates from cancer patients, new indications include the storage of epididymal or testicular spermatozoa prior to intracytoplasmic sperm injection (ICSI). The most important benefits of cryopreservation in combination with ART are:

- Biological material can be stored and is available for more than one microinjection without repeated surgery.
- Surgery to achieve testicular or epididymal spermatozoa and oocyte retrieval do not have to be performed at the same time.

The different aspects of cryobanking of human semen have been described in detail by Sherman (1986), Schill and Bollmann (1986), Brotherton (1990), Quinn (1993), Van der Elst et al. (1997), Agca and Critser (2002), Hovatta (2003) and Anger et al. (2003). Cryobanking of semen has received greatest promotion through the emergence of acquired immunodeficiency syndrome (AIDS), for which the use of fresh semen for donor insemination is no longer acceptable. It has been shown that transmission of HIV to recipients of donor semen in artificial insemination is possible (Stewart et al. 1985). To avoid any transmission of HIV, donor semen should be held in quarantine for at least 3 months before testing of donor's blood shows that it is negative for HIV antibodies. Thus, frozen semen in artificial insemination by donor has to be used in order to meet the standards of cryobanking as established by the American Association of Tissue Banks (Linden and Centola 1997) and the British Andrology Society (1999), although Payne and Lamb (2004) recommended a revision of these guidelines to allow the use of fresh semen by informed recipients based on their cost-effectiveness analysis comparing the use of frozen semen with the use of fresh semen from the same donors without a second antibody test.

Many other organisms have been reported to survive the freezing/thawing procedure such as *Neisseria gonorrhoeae*, *Treponema pallidum*, *Chlamydia trachomatis*, *Ureaplasma urealyticum*, *Mycoplasma hominis*, streptococci, cytomegalovirus, hepatitis viruses, herpesvirus, adenovirus, papillomavirus, *Trichomonas vaginalis*, *Aspergillus* species and *Candida albicans*. Therefore, contamination of the liquid nitrogen and cross-contamination of other samples during semen cryopreservation are possible hazards, especially because some cryovials absorb liquid nitrogen (Clarke 1999). It is recommended that straws and ampoules should be sealed and free from external contamination (British Andrology Society 1999).

There is no doubt that pre-therapy storage of semen from cancer patients is an important medical task, all the more since the prognosis and life expectancy of those with Hodgkin's disease and testicular tumours is very good today (Köhn and Schill 1988). As ICSI requires only one living spermatozoon per oocyte, cut-off values of standard semen parameters prior to cryopreservation of semen samples are no longer necessary. Even ejaculates of poorest quality can now be stored in liquid nitrogen (Schill and Köhn 1997).

II.4.17.2 Basic Principles of Cryobiology

During the freezing of cells, ice formation of the medium does not occur uniformly. Even at –30 to –40 °C there are liquid compartments in which the electrolytes concentrate. As a consequence of this osmotic gradient, water escapes from the cell, which results in shrinkage. Because of their low amount of cytoplasm and small volume, spermatozoa have an advantage over larger cells. The speed of freezing is decisive. Too high or too low a cooling rate results in intracellular ice crystal formation. Ice crystal formation has also been observed during long-term storage of semen samples below –70 °C. Thus, cell damage during freezing and thawing is caused both by osmotic factors and mechanical stimuli during ice crystallization.

II.4.17.3 Indications for Human Sperm Cryopreservation

Clinical applications for cryopreservation can be summarized as follows:

1. Possibility of timed multiple inseminations of donor semen or husband's semen, including microbiological testing of semen or blood prior to insemination to exclude sexually transmitted diseases.
2. Preservation of semen before surgical, chemical or radiological cancer therapy leading to subsequent sterility.
3. Storage of semen in the temporary or permanent absence of the donor or husband.
4. Storage of semen before vasectomy.
5. Use of cryobanking in reproductive medicine (microsurgical epididymal sperm aspiration, MESA; testicular sperm extraction, TESE).

New indications may also include testicular cryopreservation in boys prior to chemotherapy or radiation therapy. However, this technique still presents practical and ethical dilemmas (Bahadur et al. 2000).

II.4.17.4 Sperm Preparation Techniques Before Cryopreservation

To minimize cryoinjury in human spermatozoa, sufficient concentrations of cryoprotectants to control the rise in salt concentration and to increase the unfrozen volume during cooling are necessary (Hammerstedt et al. 1990; Gilmore et al. 1997). After initial studies with dimethyl sulphoxide (DMSO) as the cryoprotectant medium, glycerol at 5–7% per volume is now used almost universally (Critser et al. 1988; Brotherton 1990). To store semen, containers for deep freezing are screw-cap plastic ampoules and plastic straws (French: paillettes) containing 0.25 or 0.5 ml semen mixture.

In contrast to caffeine and kallikrein, which were used in the past to stimulate sperm motility and the fertilizing capacity of cryostored human spermatozoa (Schill et al. 1979), the phosphodiesterase inhibitor pentoxifylline has received considerable attention (Bell et al. 1993; Mbizvo et al. 1993; Brennan and Holden 1995; Sharma et al. 1996). The drug is used for systemic treatment of patients with cardiovascular diseases (Trental® or Torental®) and has a higher water solubility than caffeine, which increases its usability (Tournaye et al. 1995). Treatment of spermatozoa with pentoxifylline after thawing has significantly better effects on sperm motility than incubation with pentoxifylline before freezing, but there are no convincing data on its possible influence on pregnancy rates after insemination (Stanic et al. 2002). Apart from the effects on sperm motility, pentoxifylline is also reported to augment the acrosome reaction (Tesarik et al. 1992). Nassar et al. (1998) demonstrated that this induction is not due to a Ca^{2+} influx into the sperm cell, which is thought to stimulate the acrosome reaction (Blackmore et al. 1991). The intracellular concentration ($[Ca^{2+}]_i$) even decreased following the pentoxifylline treatment. Since cyclic adenosine monophosphate (cAMP) is intimately involved as a second messenger in the induction of the acrosome reaction (De Jonge et al. 1991), non-specific inhibition of phosphodiesterases by this methylxanthine will increase the intracellular cAMP levels and therefore induce the acrosome reaction. Pentoxifylline also enhances the capacity of spermatozoa to bind to the zona pellucida (Yogev et al. 1995; Paul et al. 1996), although this improvement may be more likely the result of increased progressive sperm motility, as indicated by straight line velocity (VSL) and average path velocity (VAP). These spermatozoa are from a sperm population that did not initiate the acrosome reaction with its characteristic change in movement before treatment with pentoxifylline (Yogev et al. 2000).

The conflicting results on the effectiveness of pentoxifylline treatment raised questions about the embryotoxicity of this substance, especially since possible pentoxifylline-induced adverse effects on spermatozoa (Centola et al. 1995) and mouse embryo development (Tournaye et al. 1993a, b) have been reported. In contrast, Lacham-Kaplan and Trounson (1993) did not observe any such negative effects on embryonic development after insemination of the oocytes with spermatozoa incubated in 3 mM pentoxifylline. Finally, short-term incubation of spermatozoa with subsequent washing of the male germ cells did not produce such adverse effects in intrauterine insemination (IUI) or ICSI (Terriou et al. 2000). An alternative approach to increase sperm motility or the number of motile spermatozoa was to administer the drug orally over a period of 3–6 months (Schill 1986). In a placebo-controlled study including 47 normogonadotrophic men with idiopathic asthenozoospermia, Merino et al. (1997) showed a significant increase in progressive motility in men who received 1200 mg of pentoxifylline per day over 6 months. Clinical data about fertilization and pregnancy, however, are not yet available.

Another important point that must not be underestimated in explaining the controversial effects of pentoxifylline is the fact that this drug is a non-specific phosphodiesterase (PDE) inhibitor. Considering that 11 different families of this enzyme have been described (O'Donnell 2000) – of which PDE-1 and PDE-4 are present in human spermatozoa and stimulate different sperm functions, i.e. acrosome reaction and motility, (Fisch et al. 1998) – non-specific inhibition of the PDEs will obviously result in both stimulation of motility and the acrosome reaction. Depending on the conditions and most importantly on the time of stimulation and the concentration of pentoxifylline in the medium, overstimulation will definitely result in premature acrosome reaction. Hence, overstimulated spermatozoa for an IUI or IVF treatment will not fertilize oocytes because they are no longer able to bind to the zona pellucida. This problem might be overcome by the use of a non-embryotoxic PDE-4 inhibitor to stimulate sperm motility only. Unfortunately, to our knowledge, no further progress has been made in this regard.

Another possibility to increase the percentage of living spermatozoa after cryopreservation was thought to be separation of motile spermatozoa before freezing (Kaneko et al. 1990; Bongso et al. 1993; Pérez-Sánchez et al. 1994).

Pre-freezing selection of motile spermatozoa by preparation techniques such as glass wool filtration, sedimentation migration or underlay does not improve the recovery rate after thawing. Concentration of spermatozoa by centrifugation results in slightly higher numbers of motile spermatozoa per microlitre after thawing. However, more samples do not show any motility (Köhn et al. 1997). Selection of motile spermatozoa by swim-up prior to the freezing procedure resulted in higher post-thaw progression, velocity and percentages of spermatozoa with intact acrosomes (Esteves et al. 2000). These effects seem to be due to lower nitric oxide production in semen samples that have been prepared by swim-up (Chan et al. 2004).

In cases of severe oligozoospermia or non-obstructive azoospermia only few ejaculated or testicular spermatozoa are available. Since it may be difficult to recover these spermatozoa after freezing and thawing, zonae pellucidae or cryoloops can be used as vehicles for their cryopreservation (Hsieh et al. 2000; Schuster et al. 2003).

II.4.17.5 Effects of Freezing on Sperm Quality

Cryopreservation of human semen has been associated with decreased acrosin activity (Schill 1975; Mack and Zaneveld 1987; Cross and Hanks 1991), impaired chromatin structure (Hammadeh et al. 2001b), reduced morphological quality of spermatozoa (Donnelly et al. 2001, Hammadeh et al. 2001b), increased acrosomal damage (Hammadeh et al. 2001a), post-freeze reduction of motility (Schill et al. 1986; McLaughlin et al. 1992), reduced DNA integrity (Donnelly et al. 2001; Chohan et al. 2004), reduced mitochondrial functions (O'Connell et al. 2002) and impaired ability of spermatozoa to penetrate cervical mucus. On the other hand, fresh and frozen-thawed human spermatozoa bind in a similar pattern to the zona pellucida in the hemizona assay (Gamzu et al. 1992). Nevertheless, swelling of the plasma membrane, acrosomal leakage and breakdown as well as lesions in the midpiece and the flagellum may lead to a substantial reduction of sperm function. Remarkably, programmed stage freezing using the cryopreservative glycerol is far superior to DMSO, yielding the best chances of penetrating zona-free hamster ova (Serafini et al. 1986).

There is no marker available to predict the freezability of individual semen samples (Centola et al. 1992). Delay of the freezing process for more than 1 h after semen production has a deleterious effect on the freezability of sperm (Yavetz et al. 1991). Seminal plasma and intracellular sperm Ca^{2+} concentrations were negatively correlated with post-thaw recovery of sperm motility (Meseguer et al. 2004). Studies using the hypoosmotic swelling test failed to show any correlation with the post-thaw motility or the survival rate of spermatozoa after cryopreservation (Chan et al. 1990). However, the hypoosmotic swelling test has been found suitable for assessing the viability of cryopreserved spermatozoa, which is of great importance for the identification of immotile, but still viable spermatozoa for successful ICSI (Esteves et al. 1996).

Clinical experience has demonstrated that the spermatozoa of some individuals have virtually no loss of motility and vitality, while others show such a tremendous cryoinjury that the application of cryopreservation in these cases was more than questionable before the ICSI era. In general, however, the survival rate 1 h after thawing of frozen semen is between 50 and 60 %; 4 h after thawing the survival rate decreases further to 35–40 %, whereas the motility loss of fresh semen within the same observation period is only 10–15 %.

II.4.17.6 Fertilization Rates with Cryopreserved Spermatozoa

Using cryopreserved donor spermatozoa within in vitro fertilization programmes, Trounson and Conti (1982) and Mahadevan et al. (1983) demonstrated that these spermatozoa yielded fertilization rates comparable to those achieved with fresh semen. The most predictive variable for pregnancy is the post-thaw motility (Mayaux et al. 1985). Using ICSI, only a few vital spermatozoa are needed after freezing and thawing for successful fertilization of oocytes. Thus, in contrast to the past, no minimal criteria for cryostorage of semen samples exist nowadays as long as at least some viable spermatozoa are present after thawing. Cryopreservation of ejaculated, epididymal and testicular spermatozoa does not affect ICSI results in terms of fertilization and pregnancy rates (Rubio et al. 1996; Ben Rhouma et al. 2003; Wood et al. 2003). However, the data about testicular spermatozoa are contradictory because single studies have reported a reduced fertilizing capacity of testicular spermatozoa with no decrease in pregnancy rates (Wood et al. 2002).

II.4.17.7 Cryobanking of Semen for Fertility Protection from Radiation or Cytotoxic Treatment

Testicular cancer is the most frequent cancer in men aged between 25 and 34 years. Other malignant diseases with high prevalence at a younger age are Hodgkin's disease and leukaemia. Most of these patients have not fathered children at the time of diagnosis (Köhn and Schill 1988).

Even though better surgical techniques and chemotherapeutic agents and regimens for the treatment of these diseases are available to maintain male fertility, it is not yet possible to predict accurately which of these men will regain spermatogenic function. Chemotherapeutic agents may cause azoospermia in up to 90–100% of adult men. Recovery of spermatogenesis depends on the regimen and dosage of chemotherapy with 15–30% of cancer patients having a complete loss of fertility. After completion of treatment for testicular cancer, recovery of spermatogenic function may take 2–3 years, sometimes more than 5–10 years. This is the reason why cryopreservation of semen from patients with malignant diseases before specific chemotherapy, radiation or surgical therapy is a realistic option to preserve fertility (Khalifa et al. 1992). In addition, for many young patients the availability of a sperm cryobank and the possibility of storing semen before chemotherapy is a great psychological relief. Interestingly, only a few patients (no more than 5–15%) will later call for their spermatozoa to be used for either IUI or in vitro fertilization (IVF) (Holland-Moritz and Krause 1990; Keck and Nieschlag 1993; Chung et al. 2004). For example, of 112 patients whose semen had been stored at the Munich sperm bank during 1974 and 1986, only 15 requested that for their spermatozoa be used for IUI or IVF (Köhn and Schill 1988). More than 55% of patients achieve pregnancies after assisted reproductive technologies (ART) with their frozen/thawed spermatozoa. The type of cancer has no effect on ART outcome (Agarwal et al. 2004). Hallak et al. (1998) reported why cancer patients stop storing their semen in a sperm bank programme. Only a minority of patients did not plan to have children. Most reasons included patient death or restored fertility.

A major problem of cancer patients is that 50% of them may have disease-intrinsic suppression of spermatogenesis (Lampe et al. 1997). There are no criteria available to predict the quality of cryopreserved spermatozoa from cancer patients (Krause and Brake 1994; Agarwal et al. 1996; Padron et al. 1997). However, deterioration in sperm function after cryopreservation of semen among patients with different malignancies and normal donors appears to be similar, indicating that the type of cancer is not related to the cryopreservation results. Sperm cryopreservation should also be recommended to oncological patients younger than 15 years, if they are able to produce a semen sample, because the freezability of these ejaculates is comparable to that of adult men ejaculates (Kamischke et al. 2004).

Through the introduction of ICSI, cryobanking of semen from cancer patients has to be completely reconsidered. In these cases, fertility should be protected and semen samples of any quality and even from testicular tissue have to be frozen and kept in liquid nitrogen (–196 °C) to be later available for ART.

In cases of non-obstructive azoospermia after chemotherapy testicular sperm extraction (TESE) is successful in more than 40% (Meseguer et al. 2003, Schrader et al. 2003). Cryopreservation of testicular tissue and TESE should also be considered in patients with bilateral testicular tumours and azoospermia, if frozen semen samples are not available (Köhn et al. 2001).

II.4.17.8 Autotransplantation of Germinal Epithelium

Prevention of fertility in childhood cancer patients by later autotransplantation of cryopreserved testicular stem cells will probably be a future option for this patient group. Although the clinical effectiveness of this procedure has not yet been proven in humans, it is already under discussion (Tournaye et al. 2004). Therefore, cryopreservation of testicular tissue from prepubertal boys with malignancies may be considered prior to radiation or chemotherapy.

Initiation of spermatogenesis was observed when testicular stem cells had been transplanted into the testes of mice with Sertoli cell only syndrome (Brinster and Avarbock 1994). The outcome of ICSI seems to be similar to that for controls in these mouse models (Goossens et al. 2003). Live births have also been reported after transplantation of spermatogonia from Long Evans rats to the seminiferous tubules of Sprague-Dawley rats after treatment with ciclosporin (Zhang et al. 2003).

However, the results of these experiments cannot simply be transferred to humans for a variety of aspects: influence of testicular damage after radiation or chemotherapy on autotransplantation; identification and isolation of human testicular stem cells; freezing protocols for testicular stem cells; transfer technique in humans; best age for autotransplantation in humans; safety aspects of autotransplantation (Brougham et al. 2003; Tournaye et al. 2004). Concerning the cryoprotectants and the optimal freezing protocol of testicular stem cells data are still contradictory (Tournaye et al. 2004). Frederickx et al. (2004) demonstrated reduced functional capacity in testicular stem cells after cryopreservation, whereas the survival rates were better.

The alternatives to autotransplantation of frozen/thawed testicular stem cells may be xenotransplantation into other species or in vitro maturation (Nordhoff and Schlatt 2003). However, the entry of germ cells into meiosis is one of the experimental problems that has to be addressed before clinical application of this method.

References

Agarwal A, Shekarriz M, Sidhu RK, Thomas AJ (1996) Value of clinical diagnosis in predicting the quality of cryopreserved sperm from cancer patients. J Urol 155:934–938

Agarwal A, Ranganathan P, Kattal N, Pasqualotto F, Hallak J, Khayal S, Mascha E (2004) Fertility after cancer: a prospective review of assisted reproductive outcome with banked semen specimens. Fertil Steril 81:342–348

Agca Y, Critser JK (2002) Cryopreservation of spermatozoa in assisted reproduction. Semin Reprod Med 20:15–23

Anger JT, Gilbert BR, Goldstein M (2003) Cryopreservation of sperm: indications, methods and results. J Urol 170:1079–1084
Bahadur G, Chatterjee R, Ralph D (2000) Testicular tissue cryopreservation in boys. Ethical and legal issues. Hum Reprod 15:1416–1420
Bell M, Wang R, Hellstrom WJG, Sikka SC (1993) Effect of cryoprotective additives and cryopreservation protocol on sperm membrane lipid peroxidation and recovery of motile human sperm. J Androl 14:472–478
Ben Rhouma K, Marrakchi H, Khouja H, Attalah K, Ben Miled E, Sakly M (2003) Outcome of intracytoplasmic injection of fresh and frozen-thawed testicular spermatozoa. A comparative study. J Reprod Med 48:349–354
Blackmore PF, Neulen J, Lattanzio F, Beebe SJ (1991) Cell surface-binding sites for progesterone mediated calcium uptake in human sperm. J Biol Chem 266:18655–18659
Bongso A, Jarina AK, Ho J, Ng SC, Ratnam SS (1993) Comparative evaluation of three sperm-washing methods to improve sperm concentration and motility in frozen-thawed oligozoospermic and normozoospermic samples. Arch Androl 31:223–230
Brennan AP, Holden CA (1995) Pentoxifylline-supplemented cryoprotectant improves human sperm motility after cryopreservation. Hum Reprod 10:2308–2312
Brinster RL, Avarbock MR (1994) Germline transmission of donor haplotype following spermatogonial transplantation. Proc Natl Acad Sci USA 91:11303–11307
British Andrology Society (1999) British Andrology Society guidelines for the screening of semen donors for donor insemination (1999). Hum Reprod 14:1823–1826
Brotherton J (1990) Cryopreservation of human semen. Arch Androl 25:181–195
Brougham MF, Kelnar CJ, Sharpe RM, Wallace WH (2003) Male fertility following childhood cancer: current concepts and future therapies. Asian J Androl 5:325–337
Centola GM, Raubertas RF, Mattox JH (1992) Cryopreservation of human semen. Comparison of cryopreservatives, sources of variability, and prediction of post-thaw survival. J Androl 13:283–288
Centola GM, Cartie RJ, Cox C (1995) Differential response of human sperm to varying concentrations of pentoxifylline with demonstration of toxicity. J Androl 16:136–142
Chan CC, Chen IC, Liu JY, Huang YC, Wu GJ (2004) Comparison of nitric oxide production motion characteristics of sperm after cryopreserved in three different preparations. Arch Androl 50:1–3
Chan SYW, Craft IL, Chan YM, Leong MKH, Leung CKM (1990) The hypoosmotic swelling test and cryosurvival of human spermatozoa. Hum Reprod 5:715–718
Chohan KR, Griffin JT, Carrell DT (2004) Evaluation of chromatin integrity in human sperm using acridine orange staining with different fixatives and after cryopreservation. Andrologia 36:321–326
Chung K, Irani J, Knee G, Efymow B, Blasco L, Patrizio P (2004) Sperm cryopreservation for male patients with cancer: an epidemiological analysis at the University of Pennsylvania. Eur J Obstet Gynecol Reprod Biol 113 (Suppl. 1):S7–S11
Clarke GN (1999) Sperm cryopreservation: is there a significant risk of cross-contamination? Hum Reprod 14:2941–2943
Critser JK, Huse-Benda AR, Aaker DV, Arneson BW, Ball GD (1988) Cryopreservation of human spermatozoa. III. The effect of cryoprotectants on motility. Fertil Steril 50:314–320
Cross NL, Hanks SE (1991) Effects of cryopreservation on human sperm acrosomes. Hum Reprod 6:1279–1283
De Jonge CJ, Han HL, Lawrie H, Mack SR, Zaneveld LJD (1991) Modulation of the human sperm acrosome reaction by effectors of the adenylate cyclase/cyclic AMP second-messenger pathway. J Exp Zool 258:113–125
Donnelly ET, Steele EK, McClure N, Lewis SE (2001) Assessment of DNA integrity and morphology of ejaculated spermatozoa from fertile and infertile men before and after cryopreservation. Hum Reprod 16:1191–1199
Esteves SC, Sharma RK, Thomas AJ, Agarwal A (1996) Suitability of the hypo-osmotic swelling test for assessing the viability of cryopreserved sperm. Fertil Steril 66:798–804
Esteves SC, Sharma RK, Thomas AJ Jr, Agarwal A (2000) Improvement in motion characteristics and acrosome status in cryopreserved human spermatozoa by swim-up processing before freezing. Hum Reprod 15:2173–2179
Fisch JD, Behr B, Conti M (1998) Enhancement of motility and acrosome reaction in human spermatozoa: differential activation by type-specific phosphodiesterase inhibitors. Hum Reprod 13:1248–1254
Frederickx V, Michiels A, Goossens E, De Block G, Van Steirteghem AC, Tournaye H (2004) Recovery, survival and functional evaluation by transplantation of frozen-thawed mouse germ cells. Hum Reprod 19:948–953
Gamzu R, Yogev L, Yavetz H, Homonnai ZT, Hiss Y, Paz G (1992) Fresh and frozen-thawed human sperm bind in a similar pattern to the zona pellucida in the hemizona assay. Fertil Steril 58:1254–1256
Gilmore JA, Liu J, Gao DY, Critser JK (1997) Determination of optimal cryoprotectants and procedures for their addition and removal from human spermatozoa. Hum Reprod 12:112–118
Goossens E, Frederickx V, De Block G, Van Steirteghem AC, Tournaye H (2003) Reproductive capacity of sperm obtained after germ cell transplantation in a mouse model. Hum Reprod 18:1874–1880
Hallak J, Sharma RK, Thomas AJ, Agarwal A (1998) Why cancer patients request disposal of cryopreserved semen specimens posttherapy: a retrospective study. Fertil Steril 69:889–893
Hammadeh ME, Georg T, Rosenbaum P, Schmidt W (2001a) Association between freezing agent and acrosome damage of human spermatozoa from subnormal and normal semen. Andrologia 33:331–336
Hammadeh ME, Greiner S, Rosenbaum P, Schmidt W (2001b) Comparison between human sperm preservation medium and TEST-yolk buffer on protecting chromatin and morphology integrity of human spermatozoa in fertile and subfertile men after freeze-thawing procedure. J Androl 22:1012–1018
Hammerstedt RH, Graham JK, Nolan JP (1990) Cryopreservation of mammalian sperm: what we ask them to survive. J Androl 11:73–88
Holland-Moritz H, Krause W (1990) Use of cryopreservation by tumor patients. Hautarzt 41:204–206
Hovatta O (2003) Cryobiology of ovarian and testicular tissue. Best Pract Res Clin Obstet Gynaecol 17:331–342
Hsieh YY, Tsai HD, Chang CC, Lo HY (2000) Cryopreservation of human spermatozoa within human or mouse empty zonae pellucidae. Fertil Steril 73:694–698
Kamischke A, Jurgens H, Hertle L, Berdel WE, Nieschlag E (2004) Cryopreservation of sperm from adolescents and adults with malignancies. J Androl 25:586–592
Kaneko S, Kobayashi T, Lee HK, Won WK, Oda T, Izumi Y, Ohono T, Iizuka R (1990) Cryogenic preservation of low-quality human semen. Arch Androl 24:81–86
Keck C, Nieschlag E (1993) Cryopreservation of spermatozoa and its importance in the management of malignant diseases. Fertilität 9:145–151
Khalifa E, Oehninger S, Acosta AA, Morshedi M, Veeck L, Bryzyski RG, Muasher SJ (1992) Successful fertilization and

pregnancy outcome in in-vitro fertilization uring cryopreserved/thawed spermatozoa from patients with malignant diseases. Hum Reprod 7:105 - 108

Köhn FM, Schill W-B (1988) The Munich cryopreserved sperm bank - intermediate 1974 - 1986 evaluation. Hautarzt 39: 91 - 96

Köhn FM, Volk R, Schill WB (1997) Cryopreservation of semen samples from severely oligozoospermic men. Hum Reprod 12 (Abstract Book 1):237

Köhn FM, Schroeder-Printzen I, Weidner W, Montag M, van der Ven H, Schill WB (2001) Testicular sperm extraction in a patient with metachronous bilateral testicular cancer. Hum Reprod 1:2343 - 2346

Krause W, Brake A (1994) Utilization of cryopreserved semen in tumor patients. Urol Int 52:65 - 68

Lacham-Kaplan O, Trounson A (1993) The effects of the sperm motility activators 2-deoxyadenosine and pentoxifylline used for sperm microinjection on mouse and human embryo development. Hum Reprod 6:945 - 952

Lampe H, Horwich A, Norman A, Nicholls J, Dearnaley DP (1997) Fertility after chemotherapy for testicular germ cell cancers. Clin Oncol 15:239 - 245

Linden JV, Centola G (1997) New American Association of Tissue Banks standards for semen banking. Fertil Steril 68:597 - 600

Mack SR, Zaneveld JD (1987) Acrosomal enzymes and ultrastructure of unfrozen and cryotreated human spermatozoa. Gamete Res 18:375 - 383

Mahadevan MM, Trounson AO, Leeton JF (1983) Successful use of human semen cryobanking for in vitro fertilization. Fertil Steril 40:340 - 343

Mayaux MJ, Schwartz E, Czyalik F, David G (1985) Conception rate according to semen characteristics in a series of 15,364 insemination cycles: results of a multivariate analysis. Andrologia 17:9 - 15

Mbizvo MT, Johnston RC, Baker GHW (1993) The effect of the motility stimulants, caffeine, pentoxifylline, and 2-deoxyadenosine on hyperactivation of cryopreserved human sperm. Fertil Steril 59:1112 - 1117

McLaughlin EA, Ford WCL, Hull MGR (1992) Motility characteristics and membrane integrity of cryopreserved human spermatozoa. J Reprod Fertil 95:527 - 534

Merino G, Martínez Chéquer JC, Barahona E, Bermúdez JA, Morán C, Carranza-Lira S (1997) Effects of pentoxifylline on sperm motility in normogonadotropic asthenozoospermic men. Arch Androl 39:65 - 69

Meseguer M, Garrido N, Remohi J, Pellicer A, Simon C, Martinez-Jabaloyas JM, Gil-Salom M (2003) Testicular sperm extraction (TESE) and ICSI in patients with permanent azoospermia after chemotherapy. Hum Reprod 18:1281 - 1285

Meseguer M, Garrido N, Martinez-Conejero JA, Simon C, Pellicer A, Remohi J (2004) Role of cholesterol, calcium, and mitochondrial activity in the susceptibility for cryodamage after a cycle of freezing and thawing. Fertil Steril 81:588 - 594

Nassar A, Mahony M, Blackmore P, Morshedi M, Ozgur K, Oehninger S (1998) Increase of intracellular calcium is not a cause of pentoxifylline-induced hyperactivated motility or acrosome reaction in human sperm. Fertil Steril 69:748 - 754

Nordhoff V, Schlatt S (2003) Present and future options for the preservation of testis tissue and function. Endocr Dev 5:136 - 155

O'Connell M, McClure N, Lewis SE (2002) The effects of cryopreservation on sperm morphology, motility and mitochondrial function. Hum Reprod 17:704 - 709

O'Donnell JM (2000) William Harvey Research Conference on PDE inhibitors: drugs with an expanding range of therapeutic uses. Expert Opin Investig Drugs 9:621 - 625

Padron OF, Sharma RK, Thomas AJ Jr, Agarwal A (1997) Effects of cancer on spermatozoa quality after cryopreservation: a 12-year experience. Fertil Steril 67:326 - 331

Paul M, Sumpter JP, Lindsay KS (1996) The paradoxical effects of pentoxifylline on the binding of spermatozoa to the human zona pellucida. Hum Reprod 11:814 - 819

Payne MA, Lamb EJ (2004) Use of frozen semen to avoid human immunodeficiency virus type 1 transmission by donor insemination: a cost-effectiveness analysis. Fertil Steril 81:80 - 92

Pérez-Sánchez E, Cooper TG, Yeung CH, Nieschlag E (1994) Improvement in quality of cryopreserved human spermatozuoa by swim-up before freezing. Int J Androl 17:115 - 120

Quinn P (1993) Cryopreservation. In: Marrs RP (ed) Assisted reproductive technologies. Blackwell, Oxford, pp 89

Rubio C, Minguez Y, Ruis A, Amorocho B, Romero J, De los Santos MJ (1996) Efficacy of sperm cryopreservation of ejaculated, testicular and epididymal spermatozoa for ICSI. Hum Reprod 11 (Abstract Book 1):89

Schill WB (1975) Acrosin activity of cryopreserved human spermatozoa. Fertil Steril 26:711 - 720

Schill WB (1986) Established and new approaches in medical treatment of male sterility. Fertilität 2:7 - 17

Schill WB, Bollmann W (1986) Semen preservation, insemination, in vitro fertilization. Urban and Schwarzenberg, Munich

Schill WB, Köhn FM (1997) Cryobanking of spermatozoa: is there a continuing need for semen cryopreservation? In: Waites GMH, Frick J, Baker GWH (eds) Current advances in andrology. Monduzzi Editore, Bologna, pp 371 - 382

Schill WB, Pritsch W, Preissler G (1979) Effect of caffeine and kallikrein on cryo-preserved human spermatozoa. Int J Fertil 24:27 - 32

Schill WB, Töpfer-Petersen E, Hoffmann R, Michalopoulos M, Rübekeil A (1986) Untersuchungen zur Schädigung von Kryosperma. In: Schill WB, Bollmann W (eds) Spermakonservierung, Insemination, In-vitro-fertilisation. Urban and Schwarzenberg, Munich, pp 35

Schrader M, Muller M, Sofikitis N, Straub B, Krause H, Miller K (2003) "Onco-tese": testicular sperm extraction in azoospermic cancer patients before chemotherapy-new guidelines? Urology 61:421 - 425

Schuster TG, Keller LM, Dunn RL, Ohl DA, Smith GD (2003) Ultra-rapid freezing of very low numbers of sperm using cryoloops. Hum Reprod 18:788 - 795

Serafini PC, Hauser D, Moyer D, Marrs RP (1986) Cryopreservation of human spermatozoa: correlations of ultrastructural sperm head configuration with sperm motility and ability to penetrate zona-free hamster ova. Fertil Steril 46:691 - 695

Sharma RK, Tolentino MV, Thomas AJ, Agarwal A (1996) Optimal dose and duration of exposure to artificial stimulants in cryopreserved human spermatozoa. J Urol 155:568 - 573

Sherman JK (1986) Current status of clinical cryobanking of human semen. In: Paulson JD, Negro-Vilar A, Lucena E, Martini L (eds) Andrology, male fertility and sterility. Academic Press, Orlando, pp 517

Stanic P, Sonicki Z, Suchanek E (2002) Effect of pentoxifylline on motility and membrane integity of cryopreserved human spermatozoa. Int J Androl 25:186 - 190

Stewart GJ, Tyler JP, Cunningham AL, Barr JA, Driscoll GL, Gold J, Lamont BJ (1985) Transmission of human T-cell lymphotropic virus type III (HTLV-III) by artificial insemination by donor. Lancet 2:581 - 585

Terriou P, Hans E, Giorgetti C, Spach JL, Salzmann J, Urrutia V, Roulier R (2000) Pentoxifylline initiates motility in spontaneously immotile epididymal and testicular spermatozoa and allows normal fertilization, pregnancy, and birth after intracytoplasmic sperm injection. J Assist Reprod Genet 17:194 - 199

Tesarik J, Mendoza C, Carreras A (1992) Effects of phosphodiesterase inhibitors caffeine and pentoxifylline on spontaneous and stimulus-induced acrosome reaction in human sperm. Fertil Steril 58:1185–1189
Tournaye H, Van der Linden M, Van den Abbeel E, Devroey P, Van Steirteghem A (1993a) Effects of pentoxifylline on in-vitro development of preimplantation mouse embryos. Hum Reprod 8:1475–1480
Tournaye H, Van der Linden M, Van den Abbeel E, Devroey P, Van Steirteghem A (1993b) Effects of pentoxifylline on implantation and post-implantation development of mouse embryos in vitro. Hum Reprod 8:1948–1954
Tournaye H, Devroey P, Camus M, Van der Linden M, Janssens R, Van Steirteghem A (1995) Use of pentoxifylline in assisted reproductive technology. Hum Reprod 10:72–79
Tournaye H, Goossens E, Verheyen G, Frederickx V, De Block G, Devroey P, Van Steirteghem A (2004) Preserving the reproductive potential of men and boys with cancer: current concepts and future prospects. Hum Reprod Update 10:525–532
Trounson AO, Conti A (1982) Research in human in vitro fertilization and embryo transfer. Br Med J (Clin Res Ed) 285: 244–248
Van der Elst J, Verheyen G, Van Steirteghem A (1997) Cryopreservation: sperms and oocytes. In: Rabe T, Diedrich K, Runnebaum B (eds) Manual on assisted reproduction. Springer, Berlin Heidelberg New York, pp 223
Wood S, Thomas K, Schnauffer K, Troup S, Kingsland C, Lewis-Jones I (2002) Reproductive potential of fresh and cryopreserved epididymal and testicular spermatozoa in consecutive intracytoplasmic sperm injection cycles in the same patients. Fertil Steril 77:1162–1166
Wood S, Sephton V, Searle T, Thomas K, Schnauffer K, Troup S, Kingsland C, Lewis-Jones I (2003) Effect on clinical outcome of the interval between collection of epididymal and testicular spermatozoa and intracytoplasmic sperm injection in obstructive azoospermia. J Androl 24:67–72
Yavetz H, Yogev L, Homonnai Z, Paz G (1991) Prerequisites for successful human sperm cryobanking: sperm quality and prefreezing holding time. Fertil Steril 55:812–816
Yogev L, Gamzu R, Botchan A, Homonnai ZT, Amit A, Lessing JB, Paz G, Yavetz H (1995) Pentoxifylline improves sperm binding to the zona pellucida in the hemizona assay. Fertil Steril 64:146–149
Yogev L, Gamzu R, Botchan A, Hauser R, Paz G, Yavetz H (2000) Zona pellucida binding improvement effect of different sperm preparation techniques is not related to changes in sperm motility characteristics. Fertil Steril 73:1120–1125
Zhang Z, Renfree MB, Short RV (2003) Successful intra- and interspecific male germ cell transplantation in the rat. Biol Reprod 68:961–967

II.4.18 Current Research and Future Prospects for Gene Therapy in Andrology

Y. Kojima, S. Sasaki, K. Kohri

Summary

- Clinical and basic research are in progress to develop gene-based interventions for the treatment of andrological disease including prostate cancer, male infertility and erectile dysfunction.
- Generally, gene transfer vectors can be roughly divided into two groups: viral and non-viral vectors.
- Prostate cancer is a particularly suitable target of research to study and use in gene therapy trials because the organ is expendable, the primary tumour is accessible and a circulating marker of response is readily available.
- Therapeutic strategies in prostate cancer can be subdivided into five categories: (1) induction of the immune response (immunotherapy), (2) correction of genetic alterations (corrective gene therapy), (3) enhancement of apoptosis, (4) suicide gene therapy and (5) viral-mediated oncolysis.
- Since testicular cells play a significant role in creating life and personality, safety precautions are very important and the expression of transferred genes must be well controlled.
- Adenoviral- and lentiviral-mediated gene transfer may be effective in transfecting testicular somatic cells, Sertoli and Leydig cells, and applicable to in vivo gene therapy for male infertility in the future.
- Molecules and enzymes that influence the signal-transduction pathway of corporeal smooth muscle relaxation represent potential targets for erectile dysfunction gene therapy.
- There are two problems with erectile dysfunction gene therapy: one is the relatively short duration of the physiological effect, and the other is the possibility of priapism through overexpression of the gene product.

II.4.18.1 Introduction

Gene transfer in vivo is a powerful tool for studying basic biological mechanisms and has many potential applications in medicine (Baum et al. 2003; Ratko et al. 2003). The use of gene transfer technology in developing novel therapies for disorders that currently lack effective treatment has markedly increased in the last decade. Clinical application of gene therapy was initially targeted to the treatment of inherited monogenetic disorders and cancers that were refractory to conventional treatment (Aguilar and Aguilar-Cordova 2003; Lundstrom and Boulikas 2003). Today, however, they are being developed for most tissues and for non-inherited multiple disorders. As of 2002, more than 400 clinical gene therapy protocols have been approved in the United States, about 75% of all protocols approved worldwide (Baum et al. 2003). Clinical and basic research are in progress to develop gene-based interventions for the treatment of andrological disease including prostate cancer, male infertility and erectile dysfunction (ED). This section summarizes the latest achievements and controversies in preclinical studies and clinical trials in this field of gene therapy.

II.4.18.2 Ethical Issues in Gene Therapy

There are several limitations, including ethical aspects, regarding research on genetic manipulation in human subjects. The ethical concept and principle for gene therapy vary from country to country. Basic common consensus throughout the world is to apply somatic gene therapy to a wide range of disorders, including inherited diseases and cancer (Smith 2003). Ethical issues on somatic gene therapy are primarily those concerned with the risk of this procedure, such as vector toxicity and oncogenesis. On the other hand, germline gene therapy is theoretically possible, but is rejected on the grounds that there is the possibility of disturbing the future generation without a precise understanding of the mechanism and control of gene expression (Spink 2004).

II.4.18.3 Gene Transfer Vectors

Of great importance in the gene therapy strategy is the vehicle used to carry and deliver the therapeutic gene. Many methods and techniques for in vivo gene transfer have been developed, and some of them have already been applied in clinical trials (Aguilar and Aguilar-Cordova 2003; Lundstrom and Boulikas 2003).

Generally, these can be roughly divided into two groups: viral and non-viral vectors (Table II.4.14). Viral vectors provide more efficient gene transfer and have a greater safety risk compared to use of non-viral vectors. They cover a wide range of viral species with different types of nucleic acid composition and characteristic features related to host cell specificity, expression pattern and duration as well as cytotoxicity. The introduction of viral vectors into several organs of various animals have been reported to elicit cytotoxicity, nonspecific inflammatory responses and antivector cellular immunity (Crystal 1995). For example, adenovirus-mediated gene transfer is the most widely used because of its high efficiency, but it is a high-risk biohazard. Obviously, application of viral vectors for clinical trials in humans requires serious consideration of safety aspects related to their use.

Table II.4.14. Properties of the main gene transfer vector systems

Viral vectors
ds DNA: adenovirus, adeno-associated virus, herpesvirus, baculovirus
ds RNA: retrovirus, lentivirus, poxvirus
ss RNA: alphavirus
Non-viral vectors
Naked DNA: injection, gene gun, electroporation, ultrasound, hydrodynamic pressure
Liposomes: cationic liposomes, neutral/zwitterionic
Polymers
Peptide–DNA complexes

By contrast, non-viral delivery of DNA in vivo has a much reduced biosafety risk by nature, but its weakness is the short-term and low level of expression. The simplest approach is the injection of naked DNA into the target organ. A more sophisticated approach is the use of physical techniques including electroporation, gene gun, ultrasound or hydrodynamic pressure to improve the efficiency of naked gene transfer. Electroporation is a well-established laboratory technique, and one of the most efficient non-viral methods of introducing exogenous molecules into cells by high-voltage electric pulses. Various chemical approaches such as the lipid-mediated system and polymer system have also been used to increase gene transfer efficiency and cell specificity.

It is essential to find a rational balance between feasibility, safety and efficacy when deciding on the clinical uses of these vectors, as well as when devising suitable regulations and guidelines. Gene transfer can take place in vivo or ex vivo. In vivo gene transfer is accomplished directly in the animal model or in the patient. For ex vivo gene transfer, cells from the experimental animal or patient are removed, gene transfer is accomplished in the laboratory and transduced cells are returned to the host (Baum et al. 2003).

II.4.18.4 Gene Therapy for Prostate Cancer

Radical prostatectomy and radiotherapy are the most common therapeutic modalities for localized prostate cancer. However, up to one-third of patients with prostate cancer with localized disease, who have undergone treatments with a curative intent, will experience disease recurrence and metastasis. Moreover, nearly 20% of newly diagnosed patients present with metastatic prostate cancer. Although androgen ablation therapy has been utilized in the treatment of advanced, recurrent or metastatic prostate cancer, the efficacy of this approach is limited by the development of hormone-refractory prostate cancer. Another novel treatment approach, such as gene therapy, for advanced and recurrent prostate cancer is needed to achieve long-term local control and particularly to develop effective systemic therapy for metastatic prostate cancer. Gene therapy is emerging as a promising adjuvant to conventional strategies, and several clinical trials have been performed (Steiner and Gingrich 2000; Mabjeesh et al. 2002; Collins et al. 2003; Foley et al. 2004; Mazhar and Waxman 2004).

Prostate cancer is a particularly suitable target of research to study and use in gene therapy trials because the organ is expendable, the primary tumour is accessible and a circulating marker of response is readily available. Many researchers around the world have tried gene therapy for prostate cancer by several methods. The adenoviral vector dominates as the vector of choice. The vast majority of trials employ intratumoural injection, while intravenous injection, which requires target bone metastases, is used only in a minor proportion (Maitland et al. 2004).

Therapeutic strategies in prostate cancer can be subdivided into five categories (Steiner and Gingrich 2000; Mabjeesh et al. 2002; Mazhar and Waxman 2004): (1) induction of the immune response (immunotherapy), (2) correction of genetic alterations (corrective gene therapy), (3) enhancement of apoptosis, (4) suicide gene therapy and (5) viral-mediated oncolysis.

II.4.18.4.1 Immunotherapy

The most popular clinical trial of prostate cancer gene therapy strategies is immunotherapy (Maitland et al. 2004). Application of immunotherapy may be most suitable for minimal residual disease settings rather than a large bulky tumour. Granulocyte-macrophage colony stimulating factor (GM-CSF), interleukin-2 (IL-2), IL-12, tumour necrosis factor-alpha (TNF-α) and interferon-gamma (IFN-γ) have emerged as cytokine genes with significant efficacy in inducing an anti-tumour immune response (Steiner and Gingrich 2000; Mabjeesh et al. 2002; Collins et al. 2003; Mazhar and Waxman 2004). Immunotherapy is divided into three approaches: direct intratumoural injection of cytokine genes, gene vaccine therapy and adoptive immunotherapy. Ex vivo treated tumour cells may be used for subcutaneous vaccination or treated effector cells may be infused intravenously as adoptive immunotherapy. There are a few promising results from immunotherapy in phase I trials with GM-CSF and IL-2 (Maitland et al. 2004). For example, the phase I trial of IL-2 gene therapy reported the safety of intraprostatic injection, with transient PSA-based responses seen in 16 of 24 patients with high-risk localized prostate cancer after therapy (Belldegrun et al. 2001).

II.4.18.4.2 Corrective Gene Therapy

Functional loss of tumour suppressor and cell cycle regulatory genes (*p53*, *nm23*, *PTEN*, *MMAC1*, retinoblastoma gene, *KAI1*, *p16*, *p27*) and overexpression of several oncogenes (c-*myc*, *bcl-2*, *ras* and *her2/neu*) have been implicated in prostate cancer oncogenesis or progression (Steiner and Gingrich 2000; Mabjeesh et al. 2002; Mazhar and Waxman 2004). Several gene-based approaches to replenish the genetic deficit or to suppress the activated oncogenic pathway have disrupted tumour growth in animal tumour models. Most corrective gene therapy strategies involve retroviral or adenoviral vectors administered by intratumoural injection.

II.4.18.4.3 Enhancing Apoptosis

The goal of this approach is to force the cancer cells irreversibly to programmed cell death by activating the apoptotic pathway (Garrison and Kyprianou 2004). Intratumoural injection of the adenoviral vector containing p53, fas ligand and caspase-7, which are critical modulators of apoptosis, significantly suppressed tumour growth due to enhanced programmed cell death. Adenoviral hammerhead ribozyme-mediated disruption of *bcl-2*, an oncogene with anti-apoptotic activity, has been reported to enhance apoptosis of prostate cancer cells. Other apoptosis-associated genes, including c-*cam*, TRAIL and *bax*, have been reported to induce apoptosis of prostate cancer by gene transfer (Maitland et al. 2004).

II.4.18.4.4 Suicide Gene Therapy

This approach relies on the conversion of an inactive prodrug into a toxic drug using an enzyme vectored only to target tumour cells. In this way, the active drug is limited to the transduced cells and adjacent surrounding cells, allowing higher drug concentrations with no increase in normal tissue toxicity. Two of the most widely utilized enzyme/prodrug systems are herpes simplex virus (HSV), thymidine kinase (tk), ganciclovir (GCV) and cytosine deaminase (CD)/5-fluorocytosine (5-FC). The tumour is destroyed by necrosis and apoptosis. Both systems are currently being evaluated in clinical trials for prostate cancer. In an extended phase I/II study, 36 prostate cancer patients with local recurrence after radiotherapy received adenoviral vector-mediated HSV-tk/GCV in situ gene therapy and showed a significant prolongation of the mean serum

PSA-doubling time (PSADT) from 15.9 to 42.5 months and in 28 of the injected patients (77.8%) there was a mean PSA reduction (PSAR) of 28% (Miles et al. 2001). Another group reported the results of a phase I trial of adenoviral vector mediated HSV-tk/CD in situ gene therapy, and 7 out of 16 (44%) patients demonstrated a more than 25% decrease in serum PSA, and 3 out of 16 (19%) patients demonstrated a more than 50% decrease in serum PSA (Freytag et al. 2002).

II.4.18.4.5 Virus-Mediated Oncolysis

Several viruses have, as part of their normal life cycle, a lytic phase that is lethal to the host cell, and are used as oncolytic viruses. The use of oncolytic herpes simplex virus and adenovirus for the treatment of prostate cancer cells has recently been developed (Nakamori et al. 2004). Replication of the adenovirus can be regulated by placing E1A and/or E1B under the control of a tissue-specific promoter, thereby restricting replication of the virus to those cells which make proteins that specifically bind promoter elements. The adenovirus vector with the E1A gene placed under control of a PSA minimal promoter enhancer, CG7060 (CN706), demonstrated potent PSA-selective cytotoxic activity in preclinical testing and a clinical trial (Nakamori et al. 2004). This strategy is still a relatively new development, although the PSA-controlled CG7060 was also well tolerated and achieved at least a 50% reduction in PSA levels in all treated patients (De Weese et al. 2001).

II.4.18.5 Gene Therapy for Male Infertility

There are two major problems concerning gene transfer to the testis for application in clinical trials. First, the possibility exists that gene transfer to the testis may affect not only the patient but also the patient's offspring, because the target cells are both somatic cells and germ cells. Second, there are still many points not yet clarified as to the mechanism of spermatogenesis, and the unambiguous identification of specific genetic defects has not been achieved (De Jonge and Barratt 2002). Male infertility may be related to genetic abnormalities or defects suspected to be the causes of male infertility in a substantial proportion of cases (Hargreave 2000; Cram et al. 2001). However, with few exceptions, the precise nature of the genetic lesions remains unclear. There are some problems that need to be solved before we can apply gene transfer to a clinical trial. The main purpose of gene transfer to testicular cells and sperm in animals has been to generate transgenic mice easily without microinjection, and to clarify the molecular mechanism of spermatogenesis. Clinically, however, testicular gene therapy may be useful for treatment of male infertility in the future. Since testicular cells play a significant role in creating life and personality, safety precautions are very important and the expression of transferred genes must be well controlled.

Some researchers reported gene transfer to animal testis by various methods (Table II.4.15, Fig. II.4.41). The liposome-mediated gene transfer results in transgene expression in sperm (Sato et al. 2002). Gene transfer by electroporation resulted in transfection of not only Sertoli cells and Leydig cells, but also spermatocytes (Umemoto et al. 2005). On the other hand, no evidence of spermatogenic cell transduction was observed with the adenoviral vector or lentiviral vector by either histological or mating experiments, and it was possible to transfect the Sertoli and Leydig cells (Ikawa et al. 2002; Kanatsu-Shinohara 2002; Kojima et al. 2003). In contrast, the retroviral vector could transduce male germ cells in vitro, and some of the offspring carried the transgene (Nagano et al. 2001). These results are particularly interesting from the viewpoint of gene therapy in the future. At present it is not possible to introduce a foreign gene accurately into a specific chromosomal locus. If a foreign gene is introduced into the spermatogenic cells, abnormal sperm would be formed. This would lower the fertilization rate and pregnancy rate, and increase the rate of anomalies. However, when the adenoviral vector and lentiviral vector are used, such problems can be avoided because of the biological characteristic that genes are not introduced into the spermatogenic cells. Although the slight

Table II.4.15. Characteristics of several vectors of the testicular gene transfer system

	Viral vector Adenovirus	Lentivirus	Non-viral vector Lipofection	Electroporation
Transgene expression cell				
Sertoli cell	+	+	–	+
Leydig cell	+	+	–	+
Germ cell	–	–	–	+
Sperm	–	–	+	+
Efficiency	++	++	+	+
Cytotoxicity	+	+	+	++
Inflammatory response	+	+	+	++
Cellular immunity	+	+	+	++
Expression periods	>2 months	>2 months	<1 week	<1 month

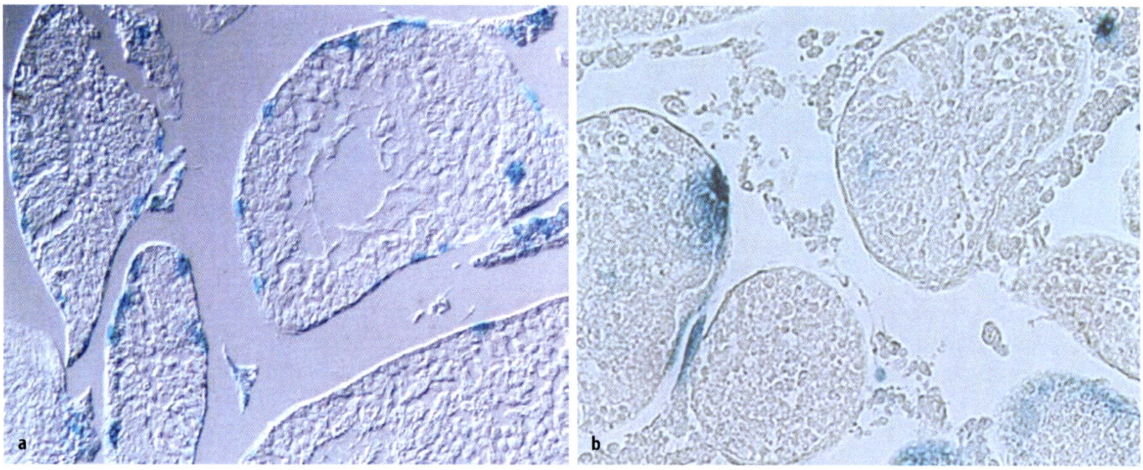

Fig. II.4.41. Light micrographs of testis after transfection by two methods. Transgene (β-galactosidase gene) expression showed blue staining. **a** Adenoviral vector, **b** Electroporation

spermatogenic damage and inflammatory response caused by these methods may present problems, adenoviral- and lentiviral-mediated gene transfer may be effective for transfecting testicular somatic cells, Sertoli and Leydig cells, and applicable to in vivo gene therapy for male infertility in the future.

There are a few reports about gene transfer to infertile mouse testis and restoration of spermatogenesis. Transfer of the Steel (*Sl*) gene into Sertoli cells by electroporation, adenoviral vector and lentiviral vector restored spermatogenesis in infertile *Sl/Sl* mutant mouse testes (Ikawa et al. 2002; Kanatsu-Shinohara 2002; Yomogida et al. 2002).

Several researchers have predicted that deletion and mutations in not only the Y chromosome (including azoospermia factors such as DAZ and RBM1), but also in both X-linked and autosomal testis-specific genes are significant causes of male infertility (Cram et al. 2001). Gene therapy to replenish these genetic deficits may be developed as a treatment for male infertility in the future. Based on the present ethical consensus, however, it would not be acceptable to let offspring be born in cases where paternity was obtained after genetic correction of a Y-chromosome microdeletion.

Compared with other organs, gene transfer into the testis requires careful consideration particularly for ethical reasons. We must clarify the mechanism of spermatogenesis, and develop a technique for safer and more efficient gene transfer.

II.4.18.6 Gene Transfer for Treatment of Erectile Dysfunction

To our knowledge, no gene therapy trials for patients with erectile dysfunction (ED) have been reported. Several researchers performed gene transfer to the penis using ED animal models including aged rats and diabetic rats (Schenk et al. 2001; Christ 2003; Gonzalez-Cadavid and Rajfer 2004). Most of the vectors used for gene transfer are viral vectors, such as adenovirus and adeno-associated virus.

Penile erection is induced by an increase in arterial inflow and a decrease in venous outflow from the penis, caused by relaxation of the penile corpus cavernosum. Therefore, molecules and enzymes that influence the signal-transduction pathway of corporeal smooth muscle relaxation represent potential targets for ED gene therapy (Table II.4.16).

The nitric oxide (NO)/guanylate cyclase/cGMP system plays a most critical role in the normal erectile process, and it seems a logical molecular target for gene

Table II.4.16. Gene therapy strategies for erectile dysfunction. (*BDNF* Brain-derived neurotrophic factor, *CGRP* calcitonin gene-related peptide, *eNOS* epithelial nitric oxide synthase, *iNOS* inducible NOS, *nNOS* neuronal NOS, *pNOS* probe NOS, *PDE* phosphodiesterase, *SOD* superoxide dismutase, *VEGF* vascular endothelial-derived growth factor)

In vivo gene therapy
1. NOS
iNOS, eNOS, nNOS (pNOS)
2. Other genes related to cavernosal relaxation
Maxi K^+ channels: hSlo
CGRP
VEGF
BDNF
SOD
Rho kinase
PDE V
Ex vivo gene therapy
Myoblast cell-mediated gene therapy

therapy. NO, the hydrolysis product of L-arginine by NO synthase (NOS), is the principal neurotransmitter mediating the relaxation of cavernous smooth muscle and penile erection. Therefore, several researchers tested NOS gene transfer in the animal ED model. There are three NOS isoforms: endothelial NOS (eNOS), neuronal NOS (nNOS) and inducible NOS (iNOS, specifically the PnNOS variant cloned from rat and human penis). Of the three isoforms, iNOS has often been selected for gene transfer to the penis, because it is not normally expressed in the penis, and is easily induced in penile smooth muscle cells. By injecting a plasmid containing iNOS cDNA in a liposomal preparation, the defective erectile response of the aged rat was corrected without side-effects (Garban 1997). Similar observations have been made utilizing an adenoviral construct of other isoforms of NOS, eNOS and nNOS, which is responsible for normal penile erection (Champion et al. 1999; Bivalacqua 2000; Magee et al. 2002; Bivalacqua et al. 2003). Also, the efficacy of gene therapy to ameliorate ED has been extended to other genes related to cavernosal relaxation (Christ et al. 1998; Champion et al. 1999; Bivalacqua et al. 2001; Christ 2002; Gholami et al. 2003; Seftel 2003). The ex vivo transfection of cell cultures with the desired gene construct, which are transplanted into the corpora cavernosa, have been recently established as more efficient methods. Myoblast cell-mediated gene therapy was suggested to be superior to plasmid or adenoviral injection, and forms the basis of future experiments to prepare for human trials (Tirney et al. 2001; Chancellor et al. 2003).

There are two problems with gene therapy: one is the relatively short duration of the physiological effect, another is the possibility of priapism by overexpression of the gene product. If these problems are solved, gene therapy shows promise as a potential cure for patients with ED.

II.4.18.7 Conclusions

Gene therapy is now evolving rapidly and gaining significant momentum as a therapeutic strategy for application in the near future. Many methods and techniques for gene transfer have been developed and some have already been applied in clinical trials. However, several problems and limitations have been pointed out. Additional clinical and basic research is needed to determine the future role of gene therapy.

References

Aguilar LK, Aguilar-Cordova E (2003) Evolution of a gene therapy clinical trial. From bench to bedside and back. J Neurooncol 65:307–315

Baum BJ et al (2003) Advances in vector-mediated gene transfer. Immunol Lett 90:145–149

Belldegrun A et al (2001) Interleukin 2 gene therapy for prostate cancer: phase I clinical trial and basic biology. Hum Gene Ther 12:883–892

Bivalacqua TJ (2000) Adenoviral gene transfer of endothelial nitric oxide synthase (eNOS) to the penis improves age-related erectile dysfunction in the rat. Int J Impot Res 12 [Suppl 3]:S8–S17

Bivalacqua TJ et al (2001) Gene transfer of prepro-calcitonin gene-related peptide restores erectile function in the aged rat. Biol Reprod 65:1371–1377

Bivalacqua TJ et al (2003) Gene transfer of endothelial nitric oxide synthase partially restores nitric oxide synthesis and erectile function in streptozotocin diabetic rats. J Urol 169:1911–1917

Champion HC et al (1999) Gene transfer of endothelial nitric oxide synthase to the penis augments erectile responses in the aged rat. Proc Natl Acad Sci USA 96:11648–11652

Chancellor MB et al (2003) Nitric oxide synthase gene transfer for erectile dysfunction in a rat model. BJU Int 91:691–696

Christ GJ (2002) K channels as molecular targets for the treatment of erectile dysfunction. J Androl 23:S10–S19

Christ GJ (2003) Frontiers in gene therapy for erectile dysfunction. Int J Impot Res Suppl 5:S33–S40

Christ GJ et al (1998) Intracorporal injection of hSlo cDNA in rats produces physiologically relevant alterations in penile function. Am J Physiol 275:H600–H608

Collins SJ et al (2003) Novel therapeutic strategies in prostate cancer management using gene therapy in combination with radiation therapy. World J Urol 2:275–289

Cram DS et al (2001) Male infertility genetics – the future. J Androl 22:738–746

Crystal RG (1995) Transfer of genes to humans: early lessons and obstacles to success. Science 270:404–410

De Jonge CJ, Barratt CL (2002) The future of reproductive cellular engineering in male infertility. Urol Clin North Am 29:809–815

DeWeese TL et al (2001) A phase I trial of CV706, a replication-competent, PSA selective oncolytic adenovirus, for the treatment of locally recurrent prostate cancer following radiation therapy. Cancer Res 61:7464–7472

Foley R et al (2004) Gene-based therapy in prostate cancer. Lancet Oncol 5:469–479

Freytag SO et al (2002) Phase I study of replication-competent adenovirus-mediated double suicide gene therapy for the treatment of locally recurrent prostate cancer. Cancer Res 62:4968–4976

Garban H (1997) Cloning of rat and human inducible penile nitric oxide synthase. Application for gene therapy of erectile dysfunction. Biol Reprod 56:954–963

Garrison JB, Kyprianou N (2004) Novel targeting of apoptosis pathways for prostate cancer therapy. Curr Cancer Drug Targets 4:85–95

Gholami SS et al (2003) The effect of vascular endothelial growth factor and adeno-associated virus mediated brain derived neurotrophic factor on neurogenic and vasculogenic erectile dysfunction induced by hyperlipidemia. J Urol 169:1577–1581

Gonzalez-Cadavid NF, Rajfer J (2004) Therapy of erectile dysfunction: potential future treatments. Endocrine 23:167–176

Hargreave TB (2000) Genetic basis of male infertility. Br Med Bull 56:650–671

Ikawa M et al (2002) Restoration of spermatogenesis by lentiviral gene transfer: offspring from infertile mice. Proc Natl Acad Sci USA 99:7524–7529

Kanatsu-Shinohara M (2002) Adenovirus-mediated gene delivery and in vitro microinsemination produce offspring from infertile male mice. Proc Natl Acad Sci USA 99: 1383–1388

Kojima Y et al (2003) Effects of adenovirus mediated gene transfer to mouse testis in vivo on spermatogenesis and next generation. J Urol 170:2109–2114
Lundstrom K, Boulikas T (2003) Viral and non-viral vectors in gene therapy: technology development and clinical trials. Technol Cancer Res Treat 2:471–486
Mabjeesh NJ et al (2002) Gene therapy of prostate cancer: current and future directions. Endocr Relat Cancer 9:115–139
Magee TR et al (2002) Gene therapy of erectile dysfunction in the rat with penile neuronal nitric oxide synthase. Biol Reprod 67:1033–1041
Maitland NJ et al (2004) Targeting gene therapy for prostate cancer. Curr Pharm Des 10:531–555
Mazhar D, Waxman J (2004) Gene therapy for prostate cancer. BJU Int 93:465–469
Miles BJ et al (2001) Prostate-specific antigen response and systemic T cell activation after in situ gene therapy in prostate cancer patients failing radiotherapy. Hum Gene Ther 12: 1955–1967
Nagano M et al (2001) Transgenic mice produced by retroviral transduction of male germ-line stem cells. Proc Natl Acad Sci USA 98:111–115
Nakamori M et al (2004) Potent antitumor activity after systemic delivery of a doubly fusogenic oncolytic herpes simplex virus against metastatic prostate cancer. Prostate 60: 53–60
Ratko TA et al (2003) Clinical gene therapy for nonmalignant disease. Am J Med 115:560–5699
Sato M et al (2002) Direct injection of foreign DNA into mouse testis as a possible in vivo gene transfer system via epididymal spermatozoa. Mol Reprod Dev 61:49–56
Schenk G et al (2001) Gene therapy: future therapy for erectile dysfunction. Curr Urol Rep 2:480–487
Seftel A (2003) Intracavernosal vascular endothelial growth factor (VEGF) injection and adeno-associated virus-mediated VEGF gene therapy and reverse venogenic erectile dysfunction in rats. J Urol 170:681
Smith KR (2003) Gene therapy: theoretical and bioethical concepts. Arch Med Res 34:247–268
Spink J (2004) Gene therapy progress and prospects: bringing gene therapy into medical practice: the evolution of international ethics and the regulatory environment. Gene Ther 11:1611–1616
Steiner MS, Gingrich JR (2000) Gene therapy for prostate cancer: where are we now? J Urol 164:1121–1136
Tirney S et al (2001) Nitric oxide synthase gene therapy for erectile dysfunction: comparison of plasmid, adenovirus, and adenovirus-transduced myoblast vectors. Mol Urol 5:37–43
Umemoto Y et al (2005) Gene transfer to mouse testes by electroporation and its influence on spermatogenesis. J Androl 26:264–271
Yomogida K et al (2002) Electroporated transgene-rescued spermatogenesis in infertile mutant mice with a Sertoli cell defect. Biol Reprod 67:712–717

II.4.19 Behavioural Therapy and Counselling

E.A. Jannini, A. Lenzi, G. Wagner

Summary

Some clinical aspects important for the diagnosis and therapy of andrological diseases have a deep behavioural impact, which are of particular practical interest to the clinical andrologist. It should be remembered that the diagnosis and therapy of andrological diseases interact with two biological functions – fertility and sexuality – that are more sensitive to psychological, educational, cultural, religious and social factors than any other body function. The clinical andrologist must take these aspects into account as an integral part of the pathophysiological mechanism and the entire process of diagnosis and therapy. Fertility, sexual, genetic and neoplastic andrological disorders require the clinician to give scientific information in the fundamental phase of counselling.

II.4.19.1 Fertility Problem Counselling

It is well known that infertility involves many psychological difficulties, both individual and marital. For this reason, andrological counselling is essential for infertile men. To provide methodologically correct counselling it is important to discriminate among the psychological factors involved in infertility: (1) psychosomatic factors as a cause of infertility; (2) the impact of infertility on psychological functioning (somatopsychic), both individual and marital; (3) strategies for coping with infertility conditions; and (4) the psychological impact of infertility diagnosis and treatments (De Gennaro et al. 2003).

The negative relationship between various stress conditions and female fertility has been amply described. In particular, psychological stress (high levels of depression or anxiety) is related to a lower pregnancy rate and in vitro fertilization (IVF) success rate. In fact, differences in stress conditions may significantly influence the outcome of IVF and intracytoplasmic sperm injection (ICSI) procedures.

The effect of stress on human semen quality is less clear. This phenomenon is especially important when counselling particular workers who, due to a physically or psychologically stressful job, may have a relatively great risk of infertility (Figà-Talamanca et al. 1996).When diagnosing and treating male infertility, such factors should be carefully considered as co-factors together with other (organic) pathologies or circumstances (Lenzi 1995).

The diagnosis of female infertility may have a large impact on men as they are becoming more involved in the diagnosis and treatment of infertility (Burns and

Covington 1999). However, their stress levels are greater in cases of male infertility, which may actually be more stressful for both partners than a diagnosis of female infertility. The male may feel completely excluded from the fertility decisional process: this should be avoided during counselling. The andrologist should appreciate the gender differences when counselling infertile couples and encourage them to share each other's feelings, which may help them to cope with any communication problems they experience. Also to be avoided is the situation in which the male patient feels himself an involuntary instrument of the reproductive process ("breeding bull" syndrome), or even a victim excluded from any participation. In these cases, both infertility itself and its evaluation and treatment are stressful experiences.

An ESHRE Guideline for Infertility Counselling emphasizes the importance of the psychological aspects of infertile couples, and especially of infertile men (Boivin and Kentenich 2002). Diagnosis and treatment of male infertility, together with the frequently extreme social pressure to become parents, can have a profound impact on psychological functioning and several male sexual dysfunctions often result. Reduced sexual activity, hypoactive sexual desire, erectile dysfunction and premature or retarded ejaculation can be encountered by clinical andrologists treating infertile patients (Lenzi et al. 2003). The requirement to produce a semen sample can itself cause difficulty or inability to ejaculate. These patients often state that they have no such problems under normal conditions.

Erectile dysfunctions are also common in both programmed intercourse during hormone-induced ovulation, and when semen collection is required for use in an assisted reproduction programme. In predisposed patients, the problem is caused by the necessity for an erection on demand. This can significantly interfere with the success of such therapies and should be discussed openly with the patient. To partially overcome these sexual symptoms, a type-V phosphodiesterase (PDE-5) inhibitor may be prescribed to patients collecting semen for artificial insemination and to male partners of couples before post-coital testing (Jannini et al. 2003a).

When fertility becomes the major issue for men with *impotentia ejaculationis* of any cause, ejaculation can be induced by penile vibratory stimulation for self- or intrauterine insemination or assisted conception (Jannini et al. 2002b). During the use of penile vibratory stimulation, contraction of abdominal muscles, spasticity below the level of spinal cord injury, knee and hip flexion and abduction of the thighs are common. This should be acknowledged during andrological counselling.

Another important role as counsellor regards the andrologist's explanation of the issue of timing. Couples must be informed of the duration of involuntary infertility they should undergo before seeking medical help, the adequate number of unprotected sexual acts per month and the correct timing of coitus during the female cycle. During infertility counselling the clinical andrologist must also address the psychological and sexual aspects for male infertile patients and, together with the other specialists (endocrinologist, gynaecologist, urologist, psychologist, etc.) responsible for the infertile couple's management, must decide whether and when to stop treatment of male infertility and opt for assisted reproduction techniques, taking care that they have fully explored all diagnostic and therapeutic andrological options, but not blindly continuing ineffective and stressful therapy (Lenzi 2003). However, in all cases, the andrologist should ensure not to take away hope from couples seeking fertility treatment.

II.4.19.2 Sexual Dysfunction

The availability of the first efficacious oral treatment for erectile dysfunction (see for review Jannini et al. 2003b) has led to a significant increase in numbers of men seeking andrological diagnosis and treatment. However, the apparently easy treatment approach has induced some clinicians to neglect counselling and the relational-interpersonal and psychological impact of sexual dysfunction and its diagnosis and treatment (McDowell et al. 2001).

II.4.19.2.1 Sexual Counselling

The objectives of counselling for male sexual dysfunction are summarized in Table II.4.17. Counselling effected in this way is an essential part of the therapeutic process, and in some patients is successful without any other intervention.

Male Counselling

A brief explanation of sexual physiology in dysfunctional men is no less essential than giving information on food intake to diabetic patients. Men's expectations of performance and genital size are frequently unrealistic and based on unscientific sources. This is dramatically evident in countries (such as Italy, Pinchera et al. 2003) where sexual education is still totally absent in all educational programmes. In addition, lack of counselling and explanations has been considered to be a principal cause of impotence in drug drop-outs (Jiann et al. 2004).

Table II.4.17. The clinical andrologist's sexual counselling decalogue

1. Giving time	Recent sexual anamnesis can be obtained using a simple questionnaire (Rosen et al. 1997) or a semi-structured interview (Petrone et al. 2003). Alternatively, it can be explored asking questions on the frequency of sex and on libido, erection (morning, masturbation, sexual), ejaculation and orgasm. The patient should also give his opinion of the couple's general life. Information (never sufficient for diagnosis) must be obtained on the timing and modalities of the sexual dysfunction. The simplest way to obtain critical information is to ask: "tell me about your last sexual experience" (Perelman 2003)
2. Explain sexual physiology	Many patients do not have a correct sexual culture. Some dysfunctions are due to ignorance or unrealistic expectations. In complicated cases, a professional cognitive restructuring technique is suggested (Rosen 2001)
3. Talk to the partner	The partner's point of view is fundamental in the assessment of a dysfunctional patient. In most cases, her information will be different to that obtained from the patient (onset and course of dysfunction, quality of couple's relationship, partner's role in the dysfunction). Ask the partner what would make her sex life better (Dunn 2004)
4. Avoid the psychogenic/organic dichotomy (Sachs 2000, 2003)	Patients should never feel their problem is "all in the mind". They are asking a medical doctor for a complete medical treatment
5. Medicalization	Medicalization is currently regarded as a bad term when applied to a function such as sex, commonly considered natural and instinctive. However, if a patient talks about sex with his physicians, he is consciously or unconsciously asking for the medicalization of his sexuality. The doctor should explain that sexual life is an essential part of quality of life (Wagner et al. 2000) and general health and that sexual dysfunction is a medical symptom with a medical therapy
6. Diagnosing	Never consider sexual dysfunction as a disease, but as a symptom of a disease that needs to be discovered. One of the major reasons for PDE5 inhibitor drop-out (up to 40–50%) is the lack of medical diagnostic efforts before its prescription. The first question (open or not) the patient has for the clinical andrologist is: "Doctor, why am I impotent/a premature ejaculator/do I have hypoactive desire?" In some patients, diagnosis is in itself therapeutic. Do not prescribe any medications before a check of blood chemistry, hormones and possibly vascular status
7. Identify risk factors	For a list of the numerous risk factors affecting male potency see Feldman et al. (1994). Prescription drug intake should be considered. Psycho-relational risk factors may also be identified (stress, fatigue, relationship problems, lack of stimulation)
8. Change lifestyle	After identification of risk factors, a change in lifestyle is prescribed (Derby et al. 2000). This should be considered by the patient as the price to be paid to obtain effective medical treatment
9. Personalize therapy	Using the information obtained, the therapy should be personalized. For example, a single, young impotent subject may benefit from a short-acting PDE5 inhibitor, while a middle-aged man in a stable relationship and with a history of smoking may be prescribed a long-acting inhibitor. Prescription information must be accurate to optimize therapeutic output (Jiann et al. 2004). Never use sentences like "let's try this drug" (a medical treatment is prescribed, not "tried"). Never use medication as a diagnostic probe (*ex juvantibus* criterion). In both cases the patient's mistrust will lower the pharmacological effect. When possible, dose vasoactive drugs to the vascular status
10. Follow-up	The patients must understand that pharmacological treatment for his sexual dysfunction is no different to other medical therapies. A scheduled follow-up, with frequent dose adjustments, and evaluation of the impact on the couple is needed

Marital Counselling

Counselling may uncover and resolve hidden conflicts (anger and grief). The clinician, who should try to facilitate communication between partners, may explore relationship issues. The physician's understanding strongly helps the couple seeking professional marital therapy in complicated cases. Clinical experience helps in recognizing couples (the majority, unfortunately, in many cultural environments) where sharing the proposal of an oral therapy for male sexual dysfunction could be harmful and dangerous, due to the widespread female opinion of the unnaturalness of pharmacological therapies. Only in some selected cases will counselling change this, allowing the ideal situation of the partner's participation in the therapy. The need of such a sharing in all couples, frequently stated as necessary in psycho-sexological literature, is unrealistic, perhaps hypocritical, and sometimes responsible for new marital problems, therapeutic failures and withdrawals.

II.4.19.2.2 Behavioural Therapy

Sex therapy is a collective term which indicates many behavioural models for short-term treatment of human sexual dysfunctions. The common aim of these therapies is to modify dysfunctional behaviour as directly as possible, taking into account the role of childhood conflicts, self-defeating attitudes and the quality of the partners' relationship. The groundbreaking work of Masters and Johnson (1970) is at the origin of behavioural therapies, which have been modernized with the so-called *new* sexual therapy of Kaplan (1974), who offered a psychodynamic, or transactional, account of the psychological causes of sexual dysfunction. While behavioural therapies were the first effective treatment of sexual symptoms (at least in some patients), they need further research and validation (Wagner and Green 1981).

The behavioural treatment of sexual disorders uses the theories of learning (Dengrove 1967). Sexological therapy starts from the approach that it is the couple, not the individual, who is dysfunctional. Involving the partner in this process can dispel misperceptions about the symptoms, decrease stress, enhance intimacy and the ability to talk about sex, and increase the chances of a successful outcome. Counselling sessions are also helpful in uncovering conflicts in the relationship, psychiatric problems and alcohol or drug misuse. For this reason, sexual homework assignments are often prescribed to the couple, such as the "sensate focus" in which partners take turns in giving and receiving stimulation in non-genital body areas. Basically, the method, developed as a therapy for impotence and then applied to other sexual disturbances, continues with non-demanding genital stimulation, which may proceed to erection. To specifically cure premature ejaculation, Masters and Johnson suggested the "squeeze" technique (squeeze the glans for about 20 s, immediately before ejaculation) and Kaplan the alternative stop-start method (when a man feels he is close to ejaculation, he stops and withdraws from the partner, and only restarts when he feels he has regained control) (see Jannini et al. 2002a, and references therein).

The major contribution of behavioural approaches to sexual dysfunction therapy has been the concept of patient non-liability. The therapist is responsible for the success of the treatment, so that the "spectator syndrome" and performance anxiety, very frequently present in sexual dysfunction, can be overcome. The clinical andrologist dealing with male sexual dysfunction should do the same, taking full responsibility for diagnosis and treatment.

In the last 30 years the only real novelty in the management of sexual diseases has been their medical treatment. In fact, behavioural therapies (Barnes 1999) are still used without substantial modification of the original definitions and format (Shover and Leiblum 1994). Although a success rate of 60–95% has been claimed for behavioural approaches to sexual dysfunction (Seftel and Althof 1997), the field of psycho-sexology has only later taken seriously the task of scientifically demonstrating the efficacy of sex therapies (Bancroft 1999). Following this path, talking therapies will continue to play a pivotal role in sexology, not as an alternative to but probably in conjunction with medical treatments in complicated cases. However, some points need to be addressed by a new research effort. The success rate of behavioural therapies has also been difficult to duplicate and verify in controlled studies (McCarthy 1989). This suggests three possible scenarios for the future: (1) the decline of sexual therapists without medical training, (2) the development of new roles for sex therapists and medical sexologists and (3) integration of the diagnostic and therapeutic roles of medical and non-medical practitioners. To obtain the last possibility, a renewed effort must be made to validate psychosexological therapies.

II.4.19.2.3 Finding the Clinical Andrologist's Therapeutic Path

After Master and Johnson's work (1970) the field of sexology was heavily dominated by psychologists. Impotence and ejaculatory dysfunctions were considered almost incurable diseases and physicians were not really interested in them. Later, when Helen Singer Kaplan and Gorm Wagner wrote the first book on sexual medicine (Wagner and Kaplan 1993), it was realized that most sexual problems were related to ordinary medical disorders or various surgical and pharmacological interventions and therefore should clearly be primarily diagnosed by, referred to and/or treated by a physician.

There are many men with sexual dysfunctions, and their number is expected to grow, as will awareness of the possibility of seeking help. It is clear that the best therapeutic results are obtained when the psycho-relational impact of diagnosis and therapy is taken into account (Leiblum and Rosen 2000). For this reason, an integrated model has been proposed, with responsibility for the management of dysfunctional patients shared between the doctor (exclusion of physical diseases and prescription of medicines) and the psychologist (taking care of the mind). There are several elements in favour of this model, but also several against, making it problematic. Any sexual dysfunction, even if caused by the most organic of causes, dramatically affects the couple's psychology, behaviour and relationship, with profound echoes in their life. Re-establishing erectile function or ejaculatory control and re-establishing satisfactory sexual interaction with the partner are totally different objectives, and when the latter is not achieved, men may re-present with treatment failure, or withdraw from treatment altogether. The risk with medical and surgical therapies is in fact their focus on the penis as the central dysfunctional element, failing to appreciate the couple as the real dysfunctional element. Furthermore, since sexology and sexual medicine are not taught in medical schools (Pinchera et al. 2003), physicians do not feel comfortable in the management of sexual health, and sentimental and sexual life appears as a dark room, complicated and time consuming. Psycho-sexology manuals try to demonstrate the difficulty of the setting of a patient with desire, erectile, or ejaculatory dysfunction. These are the main reasons why many specialists, such as diabetologists, cardiologists and neurologists, avoid tackling sexual health problems. Some urologists too consider their surgical culture inadequate to treat such symptoms. The help of a psycho-sexologist thus seems necessary.

Against the sometimes utopian integrated model are the problems of a lack of guarantee of its therapeutic outcome, the high cost of a talking therapy, and the fact that few psychologists are really able to achieve a good, effective relationship with their patients and a good partnership with the andrologists. The Global Study of Sexual Attitudes and Behaviours (GSSAB) survey demonstrated that, around the world, only 5.5% of men with a sexual dysfunction talked to a psychiatrist, psychologist or marriage counsellor about their sexual problems (Moreira et al. 2003). In addition, the distinction between body and mind is cultural and artificial, and frequently not appreciated by patients. Integrated medical and psycho-sexological sex therapy ["shared care" (Barnes 1999; Wagner et al. 2002)] requires mutual understanding and respect for the different disciplines involved in sexology (Jannini and Lenzi 2003). This is not always possible, due to both medical and psychological reductionisms.

For a practical use of behavioural therapies, the clinical andrologist must take diagnostic and therapeutic responsibility for all male patients with sexual problems, recognizing those who need more profound psychological help. Only in these selected cases, and only if very expert, skilful and honest therapists are available, should the patient and/or the couple be referred to a psycho-sexologist. In all other cases, the simple rules in Table II.4.17 should be followed. Marian Dunn, Director of the Center of Human Sexuality at the State University of NY, stated that "physicians must remember that they do not need to be expert sexologists, have perfect sexual relationship with their own partner, or share the values and attitudes of their patients to make them more comfortable discussing sexual matter; they need to be good interviewers, which requires a different skill set entirely" (Dunn 2004).

II.4.19.3 Genetic Counselling

According to the 1975 definition of the American Society of Genetics, genetic counselling is a complex process of communicating the medical aspects of a genetic disorder and their impact (Baker et al. 1998). It is a delicate matter, since many aspects are probabilistic, regarding risk (rarely certainty) or occurrence as disease recurrence in the family, thus involving the patient(s)' preventive options. The pivotal concept in genetic counselling is thus the estimation of the probability of occurrence of unbalanced progeny at birth and other unfavourable outcomes of pregnancy (miscarriages, stillbirths and early death).

There are various indications for genetic counselling (Table II.4.18). Some regard the clinical andrologist directly, but all may be a reason for andrological counsel-

Table II.4.18. Common indications for genetic counselling. Created with modifications from the text of Phadke (2004)

Directly involving the andrologist	Indirectly involving the andrologist
Genetic diseases (thalassaemia, Wilson's disease, haemophilia, mucopolysaccharidosis)	Management of Down's syndrome and other chromosomal disorders
Male chromosomal disorders (Robertsonian translocation, centrosomal inversion, Y chromosome microdeletion)	Presence of congenital malformations
Maternal age (risk of Down's syndrome and other chromosomal disorders)	Mental retardation, development delay, facial dysmorphism, neurological deficits
Exposure to known or suspected teratogens	Neurodegenerative diseases (focal neurological deficit, ataxia, spasticity, hypotonia, epilepsy)
Familial diseases and cancer (e.g. medullary thyroid carcinoma)	Acutely sick neonate
Consanguineous marriage	Ambiguous genitalia
Relatives of an individual with chromosome rearrangement	Short stature
Previous unexplained miscarriages and stillbirths	Childhood deafness
Abnormalities of sexual development	
DNA studies for paternity	

ling. The setting of genetic counselling is of paramount importance: a quiet and comfortable room is useful, as are allowing adequate time and fully respecting privacy. In the case of genetic counselling, possibly in contrast with other forms of counselling, both partners must be present. They usually pass from the initial phase of shock and denial, to a phase of anger and or/guilt. Before the final phase of acceptance and adjustment, many subjects experience anxiety and depression. The andrologist aware of these possibilities will understand overt and mute queries, minimizing the natural tension within the family (Michie et al. 1997).

The clinical andrologist may be involved in two kinds of genetic counselling: preventive counselling together with the gynaecologist, before pregnancy, and, with the geneticist and paediatrician, after the appearance of a genetic disease in a newborn child. In both cases, genetic counselling is an integral part of the management of genetic disorders, where clinicians can take over the responsibility of providing correct scientific information.

The role of the clinical andrologist in the psychoeducational process centred on genetic information is to facilitate the patient's ability to use counselling in a personal meaningful way. This is to minimize psychological distress and maximize personal control, allowing the couple to cope with the genetic disorder and reach an often dramatic reproductive decision (Phadke 2004). The andrologist's responsibility is to provide proper non-directive, non-coercive and non-judgemental counselling (Kessler 1997) to enable the couple to reach an informed decision. This is in fact the consultant's responsibility and right. For this reason, even if requested ("what would you do in similar situation?"), it is better not to give the client a personal opinion, although empathy and human participation should not be excluded.

After the decision, the consultant's follow-up is also important. Some andrologists believe that their duty is finished once the decision has been made. However, the couple should never be made to feel alone and their decision should be respected and supported, independently of the outcome and the counsellor's personal opinions.

There are some particular problems related to genetic counselling. Men with microdeletion of the Y chromosome, likely to be encountered in a fertility clinic, are requested with their partners to make a decision about their reproductive future. They need to understand that parental factors can be transferred to the male offspring. Similar problems may arise from cystic fibrosis transmembrane conductance regulator (CFTR) gene carriers (Dohle et al. 2002). The andrologist should explore the three possibilities: (1) ICSI, (2) insemination with donor semen and (3) no treatment. It has been demonstrated that most couples choose ICSI and that a minority prefer an alternative. Each andrologist should be aware of this and should try to counsel in an objective and optimal way, so that the couples can make well-informed choices about their reproductive future (Nap et al. 1999).

II.4.19.4 Cancer Counselling

Neoplastic diseases and their treatment alter the body image, leading to emotions that can profoundly disturb the patient and/or his partner. Sexual dysfunction is a common, sometimes enduring consequence of cancer treatment (Andersen 1990). A mental health professional can be presented to the patient as a functional and integral part of the oncology team. Patients may benefit from brief psychosexual interventions including education, counselling and support. However, since this coaching (Table II.4.19) is best performed in combination with symptom management, the andrologist should also be involved. It has been demonstrated that patients receiving careful counselling or behavioural therapy increase their compliance with chemotherapy treatments (Given et al. 2004).

Unfortunately, dealing with sexuality may disturb some andro-oncologists, despite the evidence that it is considered essential to the quality of life. Andrological cancers such as testicular, penile and prostatic neoplasia may have a particularly dramatic effect on sexuality. Anatomical mutilation of external genitalia (testicular and penile cancers), amputation of *nervi erigentes* (prostatic cancer), hormonal treatments affecting the libido directly and erection indirectly (prostatic cancer), together with radio- and chemotherapies (decreased libido, erectile and ejaculatory dysfunction, dyspareunia, infertility) frequently destroy the patient's idea that he is a sexually active subject (Stotts 2004). For this reason, to obtain both maximum therapeutic compliance and maximum life hope, cancer treatment has to include careful counselling. The clinician must know which cancers or therapies may cause sexual and reproductive dysfunctions.

In the counselling phase, the andrologist should be able to frankly discuss with the couple, if there is agreement, or with the patient alone, the possibility that the disease and its treatment may (not "will") cause serious damage to sexuality and fertility. A short explanation of the three phases of sexuality [desire, excitation (erection/lubrication), orgasm] is useful, as is an explanation of how cancer and its treatment may affect them. It is helpful to disclose the large individual variability. For example, only some chemically castrated men experience hypoactive sexual desire, and only some of them will have erectile dysfunction. Even more than other patients, the subject with cancer needs hope – at all ages. It is thus fundamental to discuss immediately

Table II.4.19. Coaching cancer patients about sexuality and fertility

1. Setting	Create privacy and confidentiality, be aware of cultural differences, be non-judgemental and respectful, avoid jargon (Sundquist 2003)
2. Education on the impact of serious systemic diseases on sexuality	The patient should be aware that any important disease might affect sexuality. This is an adaptive mechanism, but it is a good prognostic sign to resume sexual activity
3. Education on the impact of cancer on sexuality	The patient should be aware that the disease process (weight loss, muscle loss, anaemia, pain, fatigue, incontinence, neurological impairment, ascites, loss of sensation, depression) might affect sexual life, so that he can face it in the best way
4. Education on the impact of cancer treatments on sexuality	The patient must know a therapy's impact on sexual performance beforehand. However, he should also be informed that there is great variability in this
5. Education on the impact of cancer treatments on fertility	In patients with both good and bad prognosis, preservations of gametes before chemotherapy, radiotherapy and surgery should be discussed in counselling
6. Suggestions on improving intimate communication	Sex should be regarded as part of an intimate relationship, particularly important when facing cancer
7. Suggestions on resuming sex comfortably and how to mitigate sexual handicap	This is of particular importance in patients whose treatment has caused or will cause mutilation. In some cases, the importance of non-penetrative sex should be stressed
8. Self-help strategies to overcome specific sexual problems	A minority of patients may need specialized, intensive psychological treatment
9. Use of pro-sexual drugs as antidotes to anticancer therapy's side-effects	The use, when indicated, of hormones, PDE5 inhibitors, prostaglandins, even prostheses should be encouraged
10. Follow-up	For most patients, discussion of their quality of life and sexual issues after treatment is particularly important (Aass et al. 1993)

possible treatments for sexual dysfunction (hormones, oral treatment for impotence, prostheses). They must not be proposed as options, but as an important part of the treatment, alongside surgery or oncolytic drugs. Furthermore, the possibility of natural recovery should always be raised, as it has been demonstrated that sexual function has an excellent chance of rehabilitation (Von Eschembach and Schover 1984). In fact, while the highest incidence of sexual dysfunction in treated testicular cancer occurs within 6 months of therapy, most patients recover within the following 3 years and only 15% have long-term sexual dysfunction (Heidenreich and Hofmann 1999).

From a practical point of view, the clinical andrologist may introduce the evidence that many cancer patients experience some difficulties in their sexual life, asking if this has been the case for the patient. S/he can then ask if the patient feels any differences in himself or his body, and if the cancer (or its treatment) has changed his sexual functioning and the quality of his intimate relationship. His partner's reactions to the disease can also be explored (Sundquist 2003).

Andrological expertise should be involved in the management of male patients treated for any potentially curable cancer (Giwercman 2003). As chemotherapy and radiotherapy may lead to impairment of testicular function, cryopreservation of sperm must be considered as a part of the disease's treatment. While this is always true for potentially curable cancers, it is also important to consider sperm cryopreservation in diseases with a bad prognosis. In this case, the andrologist is considering the patient's desire to live on through his own semen.

There are particular issues regarding counselling in andrological cancers. Testicular cancer and Hodgkin's disease represent two of the most frequent pathologies in young adult males. Given that the incidence of these cancers is highest in the 20 to 35 age group, that prognosis has improved over recent years, and that antineoplastic treatment may induce minor or major alterations in spermatogenesis, including possible transitory or irreversible azoospermia, specific counselling followed by semen cryopreservation is essential (Gandini et al. 2003).

Prostatectomy is a frequent cause of impotence in the elderly. There are many treatment options, some well established (radical prostatectomy, external radiation therapy) and others experimental (cryosurgery, implant radiation or adjuvant hormonal therapy), with a multitude of opinions readily provided by the various physicians involved, friends, relatives and the media. The andrologist should give balanced information to allow the patient to participate in this often difficult decision (Montie 1994), but should also stress the possibility of sexual rehabilitation following traditional therapies with various medical and surgical approaches.

II.4.19.5 Gender Dysphoria

Macro and micro-anatomical differences in the bed nucleus of the stria terminalis (BSTc) and its sex reversal in the transsexual brain clearly support the paradigm that in transsexuals sexual differentiation of the brain and genitals may go into opposite directions and point to a neurobiological basis of gender identity disorder (Kruijver et al. 2000). This agrees with the evidence that gender dysphoria begins relatively early in life (around 5–6 years old).

The clinical andrologist plays a pivotal role in gender dysphoria disorder counselling. His sexological, medical and surgical expertise is essential for patients seeking help for this condition. After a tragic period of psycho-environmental reductionism, when psychoanalysis and psychotherapy were recommended in an attempt to induce the patient to accept his/her biological gender (Meyer 1979), the treatment of choice for true gender dysphoria is now hormonal, surgical and legal gender reassignment. However, differential diagnosis, although not easy, is essential before any treatment to distinguish between true ("primary") gender dysphoria (where the patient sexually and generally thinks of him/herself as a member of the opposite sex) and the "secondary" form, paraphilic behaviour (transvestic fetishism and autogynaephilia) where the subject is sexually aroused by cross-dressing and acting as a member of the opposite sex. Most of these cases require psychiatric aid, also for the reason that major psychiatric disturbances must be excluded before therapy. The andrologist may have a role as counsellor for male-to-female transsexuals undergoing female hormone treatment before final surgical gender reassignment (Table II.4.20). In this case, the clinicians should carefully anticipate the obstacles the patients may encounter. Many problems (drop-out, depression, suicide) can in fact be avoided when the patient's expectations are realistic (Carroll 2000).

Table II.4.20. The 10 tasks of the counsellor in gender dysphoria. (From Henry Benjamin International Gender Dysphoria Association 1998)

1. Diagnose gender dysphoria
2. Recognize co-morbid psychiatric disorders and seek professional help
3. Discuss the range of treatment options and their implications
4. Advise inclusion of psychotherapy, not to accept the biological gender, but to support the patient in his/her difficulties in gender reassignment
5. Ascertain eligibility and readiness for hormonal and surgical therapy
6. Make formal recommendations for medical and surgical therapy
7. Document the patient's relevant history in a letter of recommendation
8. Collaborate with a team of professionals with interest in gender identity disorders
9. Educate family members, employers and institutions about gender identity disorders
10. Follow-up medical and surgical therapies

Even if the large majority of adults with primary gender dysphoria cannot, or will not, accept their given biological gender through use of psychotherapy, supportive psychological help is almost always needed during the long journey to match the patient's body, social role and sexuality to his/her identity (Brown 1990).

Transsexuals often form support groups, magazines, newsletters, websites, forums and chat rooms: many of them are well informed and share information, but have a constant desire to be personally counselled and guided. The counsellor must be knowledgeable about the current DSM diagnosis of gender identity disorder (American Psychiatric Association 1996), and the most recent standards of care developed by the Harry Benjamin International Gender Dysphoria Association (1988). The andrologist should be able to counsel on dangerous behaviours (alcohol, drugs, prostitution) with a humanistic perspective, supporting the patient's empowerment of self-identification. Furthermore, the andrologist should educate family, relatives and friends about the patient's condition, also influencing public opinion where possible. Prejudices, homophobia and morbidness are still widely present even in the most civilized societies. The andrologist should fight against the common misconception that people who want to change sex are sexual deviants. Patients, who have often waited years before seeking medical help, are usually anxious for surgery as quickly as possible. The role of the andrologist as ounsellor is to give the patient an assessment period lasting between a year and 18 months, to give them experience ("real life" experience) of the sex they wish to become. Patients change their name, all their documentation and how they dress and conduct themselves with family and friends. During counselling, it should be made evident that the novelty of a relative's transsexualism may be a great shock for his/her family, but, with scientific, authoritative and empathic counselling, many adapt. The patient's children are also offered counselling and often accept the "new" parent.

References

Aass N, Grunfeld B, Kaalhus O, Fossa SD (1993) Pre- and post-treatment sexual life in testicular cancer patients: a descriptive investigation. Br J Cancer 67:1113–1117

American Psychiatric Association (1996) Diagnostic and statistical manual of mental disorders, III edn. American Psychiatric Association, Washington

Andersen BL (1990) How cancer affects sexual functioning. Oncology 4:81–94

Baker DI, Shutte JL, Unlamann WR (1998) A guide to genetic counselling. Wiley, New York

Bancroft J (1999) Sexual science in the 21st century: where are we going? A personal note. J Sex Res 36:226–229
Barnes T (1999) Integrated sex therapy: the interplay of behavioral, cognitive and medical approaches. In: Carson CC, Kirby ES, Goldstein I (eds) Textbook of erectile dysfunction. Isis Medical, Oxford, pp 465–484
Boivin J, Kentenich H (2002) Guidelines for counselling in infertility. ESHRE Monographs [Hum Reprod J Series]. Oxford University Press, Oxford
Brown GR (1990) A review of clinical approaches to gender dysphoria. J Clin Psychiatr 51:57–64
Burns LH, Covington SN (1999) Infertility counselling: a comprehensive handbook for clinicians. Parthenon, New York, pp 152
Carroll RA (2000) Assessment of gender dysphoria. In: Leiblum SR, Rosen RC (eds) Principles and practice of sex therapy, III edn. Guilford, New York, pp 368–397
De Gennaro L, Balistreri S, Lenzi A, Lombardo F, Ferrara M, Gandini L (2003) Psychosocial factors discriminate oligozoospermic from normozoospermic men. Fertil Steril 79:1571–1576
Dengrove E (1967) Behavior therapy for the sexual disorders. J Sex Res 3:49–61
Derby CA, Mohr BA, Goldstein I, Feldman HA, Johannes CB, McKinlay JB (2000) Modifiable risk factors and erectile dysfunction: can lifestyle changes modify risk? Urology 56: 302–306
Dohle GR, Halley DJ, Van Hemel JO, van den Ouwel AM, Pieters MH, Weber RF, Govaerts LC (2002) Genetic risk factors in infertile men with severe oligozoospermia and azoospermia. Hum Reprod 17:13–16
Dunn ME (2004) Restoration of couple's intimacy and relationship vital to re-establishing erectile function. J Am Osteopath Assoc 104 [3 Suppl 4]:S6–S10
Feldman HA, Goldstein I, Hatzichristou DG, Krane RJ, McKinlay JB (1994) Impotence and its medical and psychosocial correlates: results of the Massachusetts male Aging Study. J Urol 151:54–60
Figà-Talamanca I, Cini C, Varricchio GC, Dondero F, Gandini L, Lenzi A, Lombardo F, Angelucci L, Di Grezia R, Patacchioli FR (1996) Effects of prolonged autovehicle driving on male reproductive function: a study among taxi drivers. Am J Ind Med 30:750
Gandini L, Lombardo F, Salacone P, Paoli D, Anselmo AP, Culasso F, Dondero F, Lenzi A (2003) Testicular cancer and Hodgkin's disease: evaluation of semen quality. Hum Reprod 18:796–801
Given C, Given B, Rahbar M, Jeon S, McCorkle R, Cimprich B, Galecki A, Kozachik S, Brady A, Fisher-Malloy MJ, Courtney K, Bowie E (2004) Effect of behavioural intervention on reducing symptom severity during chemotherapy. J Clin Oncol 22:507–516
Giwercman A (2003) Gonadotoxic cancer treatment in males – a reason for andrological counselling? Radiother Oncol 68:213–215
Heidenreich A, Hofmann R (1999) Quality-of-life issues in the treatment of testicular cancer. World J Urol 17:230–238
Henry Benjamin International Gender Dysphoria Association (1998) The standards of care of gender identity disorders. Düsseldorf, Symposium, p 22
Jannini EA, Lenzi A (2003) Introduction to the integrated model: medical, surgical and psychological therapies for the couple. J Endocrinol Invest 26 [Suppl 3]:128–131
Jannini EA, Simonelli C, Lenzi A (2002a) Sexological approach to ejaculatory disorders. Int J Androl 25:317–323
Jannini EA, Simonelli C, Lenzi A (2002b) Disorders of ejaculation. J Endocrinol Invest 25:1006–1019
Jannini EA, Lenzi A, Wagner G (2003a) New perspectives in the pharmacotherapy of erectile dysfunction. IDrugs 6:1165–1172
Jannini EA, Lombardo F, Salacone P, Gandini L, Lenzi A (2003b) Treatment of sexual dysfunctions secondary to male infertility with sildenafil citrate. Fertil Steril 81:705–707
Jiann BP, Yu CC, Su CC, Huang JK (2004) Rechallenge prior sildenafil nonresponders. Int J Impot Res 16:64–68
Kaplan HS (1974) The new sex therapy: active treatment of sexual dysfunction. Brunner/Mazel, New York
Kessler S (1997) Psychological aspects of genetic counselling. Am J Med Gen 72:164–171
Kruijver FPM, Zhou J-N, Pool CW, Hofman MA, Gooren LJG, Swaab DF (2000) Male-to-female transsexuals have female neuron numbers in a limbic nucleus. J Clin Endocrinol Metab 85:2034–2041
Leiblum SR, Rosen RC (2000) Sex therapy in the age of Viagra. In: Leiblum SR, Rosen RC (eds) Principles and practice of sex therapy, III edn. Guilford, New York, pp 1–13
Lenzi A (1995) Male infertility: evaluation of human sperm function and its clinical application. J Endocrinol Invest 18:468–488
Lenzi A (2003) The role of the medical andrologist in the assisted reproduction era. J Endocrinol Invest 26:268–273
Lenzi A, Lombardo F, Salacone P, Gandini L, Jannini EA (2003) Stress, sexual dysfunctions, and male infertily. J Endocrinol Invest, 26 [Suppl 3]:72–76
Masters WH, Johnson VE (1970) Human sexual inadequacy. Little Brown, Boston, Mass.
McCarthy BW (1989) Cognitive-behavioral strategies and techniques in the treatment of early ejaculation. In: Leiblum SR, Rosen RC (eds) Principles and practice of sex therapy – update for the 1990s, 2nd edn. Guilford, New York, pp 141–167
McDowell AJ, Snellgrove CA, Bond MJ (2001) Beyond Viagra. Psychological issues in the assessment and treatment of erectile dysfunction. Aust Fam Physician 30:867–873
Meyer JM (1979) The theory of gender identity disorders. J Am Psychoanal Assoc 30:381–418
Michie S, Marteau TM, Bobrow M (1997) Genetic counseling. The psychological impact of meeting patient's expectations. J Med Gen 34:237–241
Montie JE (1994) Counseling the patient with localized prostate cancer. Urology 43 [Suppl 2]:36–40
Moreira E, Glasser DB, Laumann E, Nicolosi A, Brock G, Gingell C for the GSSAB Investigators' Group (2003) Help-seeking behavior for sexual problems according to gender: results from the global survey of sexual attitudes and behaviors. Proceeding of the VII Latin American Congress for the Study of Impotence and Sexuality, Cartagena, Colombia
Nap AW, Van Golde RJT, Tuerlings JHAM, De Sutter P, Pieters MHEC, Giltay JC, Kastrop PMM, Braat DDM, Kremer JAM (1999) Reproductive decisions of men with microdeletions of the Y chromosome: the role of genetic counselling. Hum Reprod 14:2166–2169
Perelman MA (2003) Sex coaching for physicians: combination treatment for patients and partner. Int J Impot Res 15 [Suppl 5]:S67–S74
Petrone L, Mannucci E, Corona G, Bartolini M, Forti G, Giommi G, Maggi M (2003) Structure interview on erectile dysfunction (SIEDY): a new, multidimensional instrument for quantification of pathogenetic issues on erectile dysfunction. Int J Impot Res 15:210–220
Phadke SR (2004) Genetic counselling. Indian J Pediatr 71: 151–156
Pinchera A, Jannini EA, Lenzi A (2003) Research and academic education in medical sexology. J Endocrinol Invest 26 [Suppl 3]:13–14
Rosen RC (2001) Psychogenic erectile dysfunction. Urol Clin North Am 28:269–278

Rosen RC, Riley A, Wagner G, Osterloh IH, Kirkpatrick J, Mishra A (1997) The international index of erectile function (IIEF): a multidimensional scale for assessment of erectile dysfunction. Urology 49:822–830

Sachs BD (2000) Contextual approaches to the physiology and classification of erectile function, erectile dysfunction, and sexual arousal. Neurosci Biobehav Rev 24:541–560

Sachs BD (2003) The false organic-psychogenic distinction and related problems in the classification of erectile dysfunction. Int J Impot Res 15:72–78

Seftel AD, Althof SE (1997) Premature ejaculation. In: Mulcahy JJ (ed) Diagnosis and management of male sexual dysfunction. Igaku-Shoin, New York, pp 196–203

Shover L, Leiblum S (1994) The stagnation of sex therapy. J Psychol Human Sexuality 6:5–10

Stotts RC (2004) Cancers of prostate, penis, and testicles: epidemiology, prevention, and treatment. Nurs Clin North Am 39:327–340

Sundquist K (2003) Sexuality and body image after cancer. Aust Fam Physician 32:19–22

Von Eschembach AC, Schover LR (1984) The role of sexual rehabilitation in the treatment of patients with cancer. Cancer 54:2662–2667

Wagner G, Green R (1981) Impotence – physiological, psychological, surgical diagnosis and treatment. Plenum, New York

Wagner G, Kaplan HS (1993) The new injection treatment for impotence. Medical and psychological aspects. Brunner and Mazel, New York

Wagner G, Fugl-Meyer KS, Fugl-Meyer AR (2000) Impact of erectile dysfunction on quality of life: patient and partner perspectives. Int J Impot Res 12 [Suppl 4]:S144–S146

Wagner G, Claes H, Costa P, Cricelli C, De Boer J, Debruyne FM, Dean J, Dinsmore WW, Fitzpatrick JM, Ralph DJ, Hakkett GI, Heaton JP, Hatzichristou DG, Mendive J, Meuleman EJ, Mirone V, Montorsi F, Raineri F, Schulman CC, Stief CG, Von Keitz AT, Wright PJ, Lygon Arms Group (2002) A shared care approach to the management of erectile dysfunction in the community. Int J Impot Res 14:189–194

II.4.20 Donor Insemination, Egg and Embryo Donation

G.T. Kovacs, A. Trounson, K. Dawson

Summary

- Donor insemination (DI) has been practised using fresh sperm for many decades.
- Before intracytoplasmic sperm injection (ICSI), donor insemination was the only option for men with severe oligospermia.
- The technique of cryobanking was adapted from experience with bovine artificial insemination.
- The development of sperm freezing and cryobanking enabled the separation of donation and treatment and improved donor screening, selection and matching.
- With the emergence of acquired immunodeficiency syndrome only cryostored, quarantined sperm from screened donors should be used.
- Screening for egg donors has a less logical basis.
- There is a steady move worldwide to "open donation" rather than "secretive".
- Using in vitro fertilization (IVF) technology, egg donation is equivalent to donor insemination in treating women with ovarian failure.
- Egg donation is widely accepted and practised worldwide.
- The use of embryo donation can be equated to "prenatal adoption".
- The use of embryo donation is a very resource-effective way of helping couples form families, especially if there is both a sperm and an oocyte problem.
- Counselling should be an integral part of all donor programmes.

II.4.20.1 Introduction

The use of donor sperm has provided a realistic option for "fathering" a family when a man lacks sufficient sperm to achieve fertilization, or is at risk of passing on a severe genetic condition to an offspring.

Egg donation is a similar solution for women with no fertile oocytes, or carrying a genetic risk.

Embryo donation is a new treatment that has become possible because of the availability of excess embryos that couples have in storage after in vitro fertilization (IVF) treatment, at a time when they have completed their family. Whilst many of these are destroyed, some couples do donate their embryos to other women.

This chapter provides an overview of the use of donor sperm, donor eggs and donor embryos (Fig. II.4.42). It concludes by considering the possibility of manufacturing gametes from embryonic stem cells, a process that could make gamete donation obsolete.

II.4.20.2 Donor Insemination

II.4.20.2.1 History of Sperm Donation

The first pregnancy from donor sperm in artificial insemination (DI) was reputed to occur during the battle of Waterloo, involving the sperm of a dead soldier (Jequier 2000). However, the use of DI did not start to be formalized until 1954 (Kleegman 1954), when the treatment of women using fresh donor semen was described

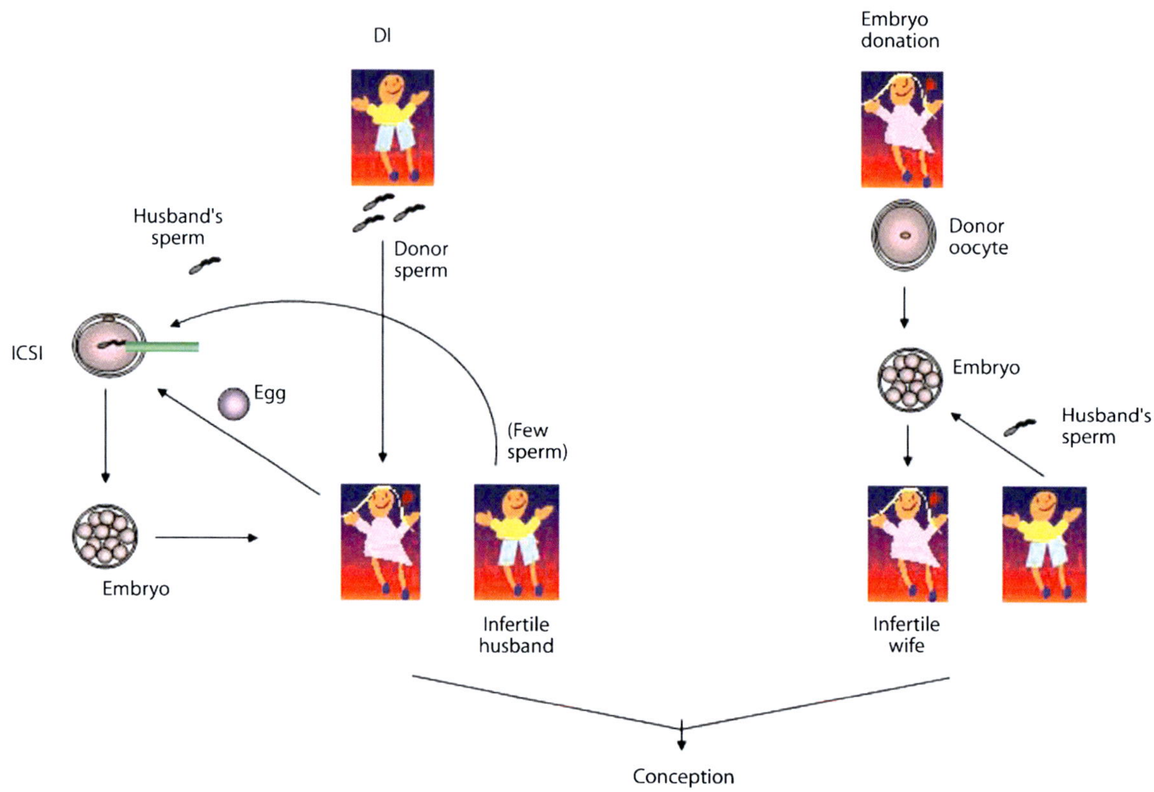

Fig. II.4.42. Donor insemination (*DI*), embryo donation and intracytoplasmic sperm injection (*ICSI*)

and the broad area of donor sperm use was considered, including indications for treatment, criteria for patient selection, choice of donor used, technique of insemination and relevant religious and legal considerations. Several series of DI were reported in the medical literature during the 1970s (Hill 1970; Warner 1974; Dixon and Buttram 1976; Leeton and Backwell 1976; Pennington and Naik 1977). The use of DI became more widespread with the development of sperm cryopreservation, or freezing, which allowed for both thorough screening of the donor sperm to be used and better matching of the donors and recipients (Bunge et al. 1954; Trounson et al. 1981).

II.4.20.2.2 Human Sperm Cryopreservation

A method of human sperm cryopreservation was originally described by Sherman (1962) as a "simple, efficient, reproducible combined freezing and storage method", where sperm were mixed with glycerol, frozen in nitrogen vapour at a rate of –16°C to –25°C per minute and then stored in liquid nitrogen.

Semen freezing was progressively improved (Mahadevan and Trounson 1980) and refined by optimization of the media used for dilution and freezing (Mahadevan and Trounson 1983) and more accurate determination of cooling and warming rates for freezing and thawing (Mahadevan and Trounson 1984). These methods, based on slow cooling in glycerol, were adopted widely for semen banking for IVF and for DI (Mahadevan et al. 1983). With minor modifications, these methods have been adopted for sperm cryopreservation around the world.

II.4.20.2.3 Screening of Semen Donors and Quarantine Period

With the reported spread of human immunodeficiency virus (HIV) through the use of donor sperm (Stewart et al. 1985; Wortley et al. 1998), it became apparent that semen needed to be frozen and quarantined to allow for the "window period" for antibody expression of the virus.

The guidelines operating in Australia (Reproductive Technology Accreditation Committee, Fertility Society of Australia) recommend a quarantine period of 6 months, in accordance with Britain (British Fertility Society) and the USA (American Society for Reproductive Medicine 2004).

The extent of screening for sexually transmitted diseases (STDs) varies internationally. All sperm donors are screened for HIV, hepatitis B and C, syphilis and gonorrhoea. Some centres also screen for chlamydia, ureaplasma, mycoplasma, trichomonas and cytomegalovirus (Olatunbosun et al. 1998). The potential recipients of donor sperm also undergo this screening.

II.4.20.2.4
Pre-Treatment Counselling of Recipient Couples

It is important that couples are properly informed about all aspects of DI before undergoing the procedure. The screening and selection of donors, the timing and technique of insemination, legal aspects of the treatment and psychosocial considerations for any child born need to be understood by the recipient couples. In some countries these aspects of DI are discussed between couples and the clinicians (Thompson and Boyle 1982). In other jurisdictions, such as the Australian State of Victoria, it is mandatory that this information be provided by a counsellor approved by the legislation that regulates Assisted Reproductive Technology (Infertility Treatment Act 1995).

II.4.20.2.5
Timing and Methods of Insemination

The initial timing of DI used simple biophysical characteristics such as mucus changes that correlate with sperm penetration capacity (Kremer 1965; Jequier 2000) and a temperature chart to confirm the occurrence of ovulation (Kovacs and Lording 1980). The use of mucus changes to predict ovulation had previously been used in family planning (Billings 1972). With the development of rapid serum and urinary luteinizing hormone (LH) assays (Stenman et al. 1985), the use of daily LH measurement was incorporated into DI to increase the efficiency of conception and to conserve semen supplies. With the availability of simple dipstick urinary LH assays that had been assessed as accurate for detecting ovulation (Elkind-Hirsch et al. 1986), the possibility of home monitoring became a reality, minimizing patient inconvenience. The woman would simply ring the clinic when the mid-cycle LH rise occurred, and insemination would be undertaken on the day of predicted ovulation, the day following the LH rise (Baker et al. 1986). Another option is to control the timing of ovulation by administering human chorionic gonadotrophin (hCG) when a pre-ovulatory follicle ($\geq$ 16 mm) is detected by ultrasound, thereby eliminating the need for monitoring for inseminating at the expected time of ovulation (Edwards and Steptoe 1975).

II.4.20.2.6
Method of Insemination

The primary requirement for insemination is that sufficient numbers of motile sperm reach the cervix and there are several methods for achieving this. The simplest way is to use a modified syringe to deposit sperm into the exocervix (Kovacs and Lording 1980). Other workers have reported the use of washed sperm resuspended in culture medium and intrauterine insemination, although this has not been shown to significantly improve results and is technically more demanding (Van Weert et al. 2004).

II.4.20.2.7
Results of Donor Insemination

Early reports of the outcome for DI were described as "overall success rates", the percentage of women who achieved a pregnancy. For example, in an initial series of 24 inseminated women, a mean success rate of 61% was reported (Behrman 1959). However, this makes no allowance for the number of cycles of insemination each woman has undergone to achieve pregnancy or to fail to become pregnant. More meaningful data are "per-cycle" pregnancy rates, but this measure again does not allow for the number of cycles of insemination that each woman may have had.

The best method of assessing success is by "life-table analysis". This type of analysis adjusts for patients who drop out, who may be resting, and takes into consideration what may have happened to these women if they had continued therapy. The first report of DI results using this method was in 1980 (Leeton et al. 1980) and a computer programme for constructing such a life table was also published (O'Connor and Trounson 1980). The life table pregnancy rates of two populations of patients can then be compared by the log rank test (Peto et al. 1977).

Pregnancy rates per cycle of between 10 and 20% have been reported for DI overall, with the most significant variable being the characteristics of the recipient (Hoy et al. 1999). It was shown by a large multicentre Australian study that the wives of azoospermic men had a higher pregnancy rate than the wives whose husbands had oligospermy, thereby proving the existence of a definite female infertility factor (Kovacs et al. 1982). It was also shown that women who had been pregnant once with DI had a higher pregnancy rate per cycle of treatment the second time around (Kovacs et al. 1983).

In a series of couples undergoing more than 1000 DI treatments in Victoria, Australia, it was found that about 75% of couples conceived within 24 DI treatments (Kovacs et al. 1988).

II.4.20.2.8
Treatment After Failed Donor Insemination

If several cycles of DI have not resulted in pregnancy, despite the woman having a laparoscopically diagnosed normal pelvis, the situation is similar to "unexplained subfertility". During the late 1980s Gamete IntraFallopian Transfer (GIFT) using donor sperm was a popular treatment for these patients, with a high rate of success (Kovacs and King 1994). GIFT is a treatment that involves laparoscopy and ultrasound guidance of a fine catheter to place both sperm and eggs into a woman's Fallopian tubes to allow fertilization to occur (Asch et al. 1986).

By analysis of the life table conception rates after DI treatment it was shown that it was probably cost-effective to change to treatment by IVF after six failed cycles of DI (Kovacs et al. 1988). With the improved outcomes of IVF and the relative invasiveness of GIFT, IVF with donor sperm is now the treatment of choice after failed DI (Kovacs et al. 1989).

II.4.20.2.9 Psychosocial Aspects of Donor Insemination

The technical aspects of DI are fairly simple (Kovacs et al. 1988), but when sperm banking and widespread insemination commenced in the late 1970s, there was concern about the psychosocial effects of DI for the couples treated. Studies at various stages of the treatment, however, provided reassurance that the use of DI had little effect on the recipient couples (Clayton and Kovacs 1980). The question that remained was whether children born from DI were detrimentally affected in any way. Studies of the DI children were needed.

The first of these studies involved the use of fresh and frozen sperm in Japan (Mochimaru et al. 1980). The study reported on the physical development of 133 children and the mental development of 40 children born following DI. They found no difference in physical development, but found that the mental development of DI children was superior to those conceived naturally. Studies of the children born from DI at 3 years of age found no difference in physical or mental development from children conceived naturally (Clayton and Kovacs 1982). Furthermore, the first controlled study of DI offspring compared with adoptees and naturally conceived children, using a quantitative Achenbach questionnaire to measure social adjustment, found that there was no difference between these three groups (Kovacs et al. 1993).

Golombok et al. (2002) reported a prospective study of the quality of parenting and psychological adjustment of DI children at the age of 12 years. They compared 37 DI families, 49 adoptive families, and 91 families with a naturally conceived child by standardized interview and questionnaire measures administered to mothers, fathers, children and teachers. The differences between DI families and the other family types reflected greater expressive warmth of DI mothers toward their children and less involvement in the discipline of their children by DI fathers. The DI children were well adjusted in terms of their social and emotional development. This study further confirmed the findings that DI children are no different from naturally conceived children with regard to psychosocial functioning. This well-adjusted characteristic of DI children was also found in children parented by either lesbian or heterosexual couples (Chan et al. 1998). We are currently surveying our families with children between 6 and 14 years on a family wellness study. Preliminary findings are that only 10 out of 114 couples have separated.

DI has been used widely to treat male subfertility and couples with unexplained subfertility (deKretser et al. 1986) before the availability of IVF and intracytoplasmic sperm injection (ICSI). These techniques have largely replaced DI for these indications.

II.4.20.2.10 Assisted Reproductive Technology (ART) and Male Factor Fertility

DI is still used today, but to a lesser extent. With the continued development of ART and the availability of ICSI (Palermo et al. 1992), together with the surgical recovery of sperm from the testicles of patients in cases of obstructive azoospermia and some cases of testicular malfunction (American Society for Reproductive Medicine 2004), the potential number of couples requiring DI has been significantly decreased. DI is now restricted to men where no sperm is available even by surgical retrieval, or for those couples who could attempt IVF but choose to use DI as an easier and cheaper option than ICSI (Fig. II.4.42).

II.4.20.3 Oocyte Donation

The concept is almost as simple as sperm donation: a woman undergoes controlled ovarian hyperstimulation, the oocytes are collected, but insemination is then undertaken using the recipient's partner's sperm. Once embryos are produced they can be transferred fresh or frozen. This requires that the endometrium of the recipient is synchronized to the donor.

To aid this, the endometrium of the recipient is prepared using hormone replacement therapy (HRT) with oestrogen and a progestogen.

II.4.20.3.1 History of Oocyte Donation

Whilst the concept of sperm donation has existed for a long time, egg donation only became possible with the development of IVF.

The first pregnancy from the donation of human oocytes was reported by the Monash group in 1983 (Trounson et al. 1983). In this case, a woman going through the Monash IVF programme donated one of her five eggs to a 38-year-old friend, with an 18-year history of subfertility and an infertile husband. Despite 15 attempts at donor insemination, and 4 tries at IVF she had failed to conceive. The donated egg was fertilized in vitro, and the embryo formed transferred into the recipient, resulting in a pregnancy, which then aborted at 9 weeks (Leeton 1992).

The first successful human birth was also reported from the Monash IVF team in 1984 (Lutjen et al. 1984).

Following this report oocyte donation was still a relative rare event, with only 90 pregnancies reported in Australia by 1989. In 1989 Serhal and Craft reported on 61 patients treated with donor eggs in the UK (Serhal and Craft 1989), and Rosenwaks et al. (1986), Navot et al. (1986) Asche et al. (1987) pioneered the technique in the USA, and Feichtinger and Kemeter (1985) in Europe.

A world survey in 1991 (King and Kovacs 1992) of 11 centres in Australia, Europe, USA, South America and Israel reported on 220 donor egg pregnancies. Fresh embryo transfers were twice as common as frozen transfers and the respective pregnancy rate per transfer was 26.7% compared to 14.7%.

II.4.20.3.2
Type of Oocyte Donors

The type of donor can broadly be classified as "anonymous" or "known". Anonymous donors are women who altruistically donate to an "oocyte bank" where the oocytes are used by someone not known to them, whereas "known donors" donate for someone they know – a friend or a relative. All types of known donations have been reported, sister:sister, mother:daughter, daughter:mother. It is of course important to exclude consanguinity by not using a relation of the male partner.

Another type of egg donation is what is now called "egg sharing", where a woman in an IVF treatment cycle shares her eggs with a recipient. This could be "obligatory" where the number of oocytes that can be inseminated is limited (in Monash in the 1980s) the reason being to restrict the number of embryos frozen, or "voluntary" where a woman decides to share with another. In some countries this "egg sharing" is financially compensated, so that a woman donating her eggs would be given a significant discount from her treatment cycle.

II.4.20.3.3
Screening of Oocyte Donors

Oocyte donation is completely different to sperm donation. The oocyte is collected, isolated from the follicular fluid, inseminated and cultured in vitro, with only the embryo produced being subsequently transferred. This is in contrast to DI where the ejaculate containing seminal plasma and white blood cells is injected into the recipient's body. Yet the routine of screening for oocyte donors has evolved to be virtually identical to that for sperm donors.

The reason for this is that oocyte donation was just evolving when the prospect of blood-borne infections became recognized, so it seemed reasonable to use the screening that evolved for sperm donors. This is not entirely logical, but has become accepted historically.

There have even been suggestions to freeze embryos from donated eggs, and not transfer them for at least 6 months, to allow for the "window period". However, as freezing and thawing would lose 30–40% of suitable embryos, and there is no evidence to show that HIV can be transmitted through egg donation, such suggestions have not been followed up.

II.4.20.3.4
Reasons for Oocyte Donation

The reason for the need for oocyte donation includes congenital absence of the ovaries (e.g. Turner's syndrome), premature ovarian failure (natural premature menopause or induced by chemotherapy and/or radiotherapy), surgical removal of the ovaries, or simply having ovaries that do not respond appropriately to stimulation for IVF. Women over 40 have a poor chance of conceiving with IVF with their own eggs, and for over a decade this has been increased to 30–50% with donor eggs (Serhal and Craft 1989). Another possible reason for egg donation is when the female carries an inherited condition.

II.4.20.3.5
Pre-treatment Counselling of Donors and Recipients

This was again modelled very much on pre donor insemination counselling. The counselling of oocyte donors of course is more involved, because, apart from discussion about social and legal factors, the risks of undergoing a stimulated IVF cycle, as well as the risks of oocyte collection and long-term medical considerations also have to be considered.

II.4.20.3.6
Timing and Methods of Transfer of Embryos Derived from Donated Oocytes

As most women receiving oocyte donation do not have ovarian function, the embryos produced are replaced in hormone replacement cycles. The endometrium is first stimulated by the administration of oral oestrogen, and the progesterone is administered to produce a secretory change. The embryos created are then transferred on the appropriate day after commencing progesterone, depending on their age.

In the rare situation where the recipient still has ovarian function, downregulation prior to using HRT is required.

II.4.20.3.7
Results of Oocyte Donation

The outcome of oocyte donation appears to relate to the age of the woman who donated the oocytes. Success rates approximate the best results obtained in IVF treatment. The age of the recipient does not seem to affect outcome, once the endometrium is prepared with HRT.

II.4.20.4
Embryo Donation

II.4.20.4.1
Historical/Source of Embryos

Following the successful cryopreservation of human embryos (Trounson and Mohr 1983), embryo freezing and the storage of frozen embryos by couples (cryobanking) became an integral part of IVF programmes. At the end of 2002, there were 92,541 frozen embryos in storage in Australia (Bryant et al. 2004). As a consequence, there are now many couples who have completed their families and still have embryos stored frozen. The options available to these couples include: discarding these embryos; donating the embryos for research; or donating the embryos to another couple. From a recipient couple's point of view, accepting these embryos is akin to "prenatal adoption". In the Australian State of Victoria, the Infertility Treatment Act 1995, which stipulates the provisions to be met by IVF clinics, clinicians, scientists and patients, specifies that frozen embryos must be discarded after 5 years in storage, if not used by the couple who produced them, or not donated to another couple. If a couple wishes to donate their frozen embryos for research, the IVF scientists and clinicians involved are required to obtain a licence for the proposed research from the National Health and Medical Research Council of Australia's Licensing Committee, a body established by federal and state legislation to monitor adherence to the relevant Acts.

The first report of embryo donation came from the Monash IVF Clinic in 1983 (Trounson et al. 1983). Reports from Brussels (Devroey et al. 1989) and Singapore (Chan et al. 1996) soon followed. There is, however, relatively little in the literature about embryo donation. A Pub Med search on embryo donation from 1983 to 2004 yielded 1023 references, with nearly 300 being editorial comments, nearly 100 being news columns, 229 discussing the ethics of embryo donation and 161 considering the international laws and other legal aspects.

Our initial experience with embryo donation was that only 10% of couples chose to donate embryos (Kovacs et al. 2003) and a survey in another clinic found that in their cohort of patients only 6% of couples chose embryo donation (Cattoli et al. 2004). A retrospective audit of 11.5 years of data (1991–2002), regarding the choices of couples relinquishing frozen embryos and the outcomes of embryo donation at Monash IVF in 2003 (at this time, the option of donating to research was not available in Victoria), found that of 1246 couples relinquishing frozen embryos, 1116 (89.5%) opted to discard rather than donate their embryos (Kovacs et al. 2003). Sixty-six percent of donated embryos survived thawing. From donated-embryo transfers to 50 women in 92 cycles, a 17.4% pregnancy rate per transfer cycle was achieved and 10 women delivered 11 healthy babies at term.

Lee and Yap (2003) reviewed the implications of embryo donation and the procedure used, from both the donor's and the recipient's viewpoint. They concluded that embryo donation might indeed be the answer to many infertile couples who would otherwise have as their only options childlessness or adoption. They reported that success rates of both fresh and freeze-thawed embryo transfers have been encouraging and there did not seem to be any long-term clinical implications for the offspring. There still remain, however, many legal and psychosocial issues associated with embryo donation that have yet to be fully analysed.

II.4.20.4.2
Techniques of Embryo Transfer

The technique of embryo transfer of thawed-frozen embryos is identical to frozen embryo transfers for couples using their own embryos.

Natural Cycles

For women with regular cycles, the use of natural cycles with monitoring of the spontaneous LH rise is the treatment of choice (Sathanandan et al. 1991).

- Embryos are thawed and transferred on the appropriate day.
- Ovulation is confirmed by a serum progesterone assay, and no hormonal supplements are necessary if progesterone is >0.31 ng/ ml, which indicates good follicular recruitment (Huang et al. 1996).

Hormone Replacement Cycles

For women with irregular cycles, HRT with or without downregulation, e.g. leuprolide acetate, should be used. Downregulation acts by suppressing gonadotrophin releasing hormone and hence gonadotrophin signals from the pituitary gland to the ovary, thereby allowing the cycle of oocyte development to be completely controlled by exogenous fertility drugs (Randall et al. 1996; Fabregues et al. 1998).

The methods used for frozen embryo transfers are identical to frozen embryo transfers of the couple's own embryos.

II.4.20.4.3
Success Rates

Published reports on the outcomes of embryo donation are limited, and most series have been small. For instance two US reports involved eight couples (Van Voorhis et al. 1999) and eight donated embryos (Lindheim and Sauer 1999). In one Finnish study involving 24 couples undertaking 54 treatment cycles, pregnancy rates ranged from 23 % to 57 % per cycle (Soderstrom-Anttila et al. 2001).

II.4.20.4.4
Psychosocial Aspects of Embryo Donation

There have been a number of publications about couples' attitudes to donating embryos. Newton et al. (2003) studied 51 couples who had embryos stored after IVF for longer than 3 years in Ontario, Canada. They found that patients were supportive of donor screening procedures, but less comfortable sharing non-identifying information. Comfort levels declined as information became increasingly personal. Willingness to donate was associated with greater comfort about disclosing personal information, a desire to know the outcome of donation and willingness to have future contact with a child, but not with current family size. They concluded that comfort in sharing information with a recipient couple is more important than acceptance of screening procedures, or attainment of family size.

Bangsboll et al. (2004) in Denmark, as well as Burton and Saunders (2004) in Perth, Australia, surveyed 235 couples who had embryos in storage that had been cryopreserved between 1 January 2000 and 30 June 2002. The response rate was 57 %, and 29 % of respondents (36/126) reported they would donate their embryos to research that would improve IVF techniques and 27 % (34/126) reported they would donate their embryos to stem-cell research, but only 15 % (19/126) would donate their embryos to another infertile couple.

Therefore, if the community wishes to make use of the valuable resource of stored embryos to help infertile couples, an education programme encouraging donation by those couples who have embryos in storage to complete their families is required. Such a programme has been implemented at Monash IVF, with a significant increase in the number of embryos available for donation.

II.4.20.5
Informing the Children of Their Origin

The use of DI, donor oocytes and donated embryos has been surrounded by two major issues since the 1990s: whether the donor involved should be anonymous or identified and whether the parents will tell the child about their origin.

The opinions of disclosure of their origin to the child born from the use of donor gametes range as follows: that it is a matter best left for the parents to decide (Patrizio et al. 2001; Shenfield and Steele 1997); that children born from the use of donor gametes should be told of their origin as soon as they can understand reproduction in general (McGee et al. 2001); that providing this information is in accord with international declarations on the rights of the child and is fundamental to the life-long well-being of that child (McWhinnie 1998, 2001); that imparting identifying information about the donor should only be considered when research provides proof that non-identifying information is insufficient for the well-being of donor children (Fortescue 2003).

In a random survey of the parents of DI children at Monash IVF, only 22 out of 74 couples had told their children of their origins, despite receiving counselling about the desirability of "openness". A study by Cook et al. (1995) also found that, in contrast to parents of adopted children and IVF children, no parents of DI children had disclosed information about their conception to the child. Problems inhibiting this disclosure were the father's infertility, how and when to tell the child and the lack of genetic information about the donor to provide to the child. A later study by Durna et al. (1997) found that most parents of DI children did not plan to tell their child of their origins. Unfortunately these parents had told others about the birth of their child from the use of donor gametes and may have set up the future possibility of accidental disclosure occurring. Some legislation, such as the Infertility Treatment Act 1995, aims to provide the storage of records that will enable a child born from the use of donor gametes or a donated embryo to trace their birth once they have reached maturity. The difficulty with this provision is that it only becomes useful when the parents are sufficiently informed to espouse complete openness with their child about its origins. To ensure such cooperation would require much education, understanding and rethinking of motivations in some cases. It is not something that will happen overnight or without responsible and responsive planning.

II.4.20.6 Looking to the Future

Gamete and embryo donation will probably remain options for patients with significant infertility and for perimenopausal and menopausal women who wish to have children. In the future, it may be possible to construct the equivalent of sperm and ova by the directed differentiation of embryonic stem cells into germ stem cells and gametes. In fact, this has already been reported in mice with the production of haploid spermatocyte-like cells (Geijsen et al. 2004), spermatozoa-like cells (Toyooka et al. 2003) and oocyte-like cells (Hubner et al. 2003). It is therefore feasible that similar pathways of differentiation will be found in the human and by using nuclear transfer techniques, it will be possible to produce embryonic stem cells from the patient's own somatic cells (Trounson 2001, 2005). These techniques have been established (Fig. II.4.43), although the normality of sperm- and oocyte-like cells has not been established as yet in mice. If these techniques are developed in the future, there may be little need for DI or embryo donation, although the additional costs of deriving the patient's own genetic gametes may be prohibitive for some patients. However, the desire to use one's own gametes for conception is extremely high and the stem cell technique will be sought by many patients.

References

Asch RH, Balmaceda JP, Ellsworth LR, Wong PC (1986) Preliminary experiences with gamete intrafallopian transfer (GIFT). Fertil Steril 45:366–371

Asche R, Balmaceda J, Ord T, Borrero C, Cefalu E, Gastaldi C, Rojas F (1987) Oocyte donation and gamete intrafallopian transfer as treatment for premature ovarian failure. Lancet i:687

Baker HW, Bangah ML, Burger HG, Kovacs GT, Summerbell D, Warnes GM (1986) Timing of ovulation by determination of the urinary luteinizing hormone surge with an enzyme-linked monoclonal antibody dipstick (OvuStick). Aust N Z J Obstet Gynaecol 26:79–83

Bangsboll S, Pinborg A, Yding Andersen C, Nyboe Andersen A (2004) Patients' attitudes towards donation of surplus cryopreserved embryos for treatment or research. Hum Reprod 19:2415–2419

Behrman SJ (1959) Artificial insemination. Fertil Steril 10:248–258

Billings JJ (1972) Ovulation method of family planning. Lancet 2:1193–1194

Borini A, Bonu MA, Coticchio G, Bianchi V, Cattoli M, Flamigni C (2004) Pregnancies and births after oocyte cryopreservation. Fertil Steril 82:601–605

Bryant J, Sullivan E, Dean J (2004) Assisted reproductive technology in Australia and New Zealand 2002. Assisted Reproductive Technology Series No. 8. Australian Institute of Health and Welfare National Perinatal Statistics Unit, Sydney

Bunge RG, Keettel WC, Sherman JK (1954) Clinical use of frozen semen: report of four cases. Fertil Steril 5:520–529

Burton PJ, Sanders K (2004) Patient attitudes to donation of embryos for research in Western Australia. Med J Aust 180:559–561

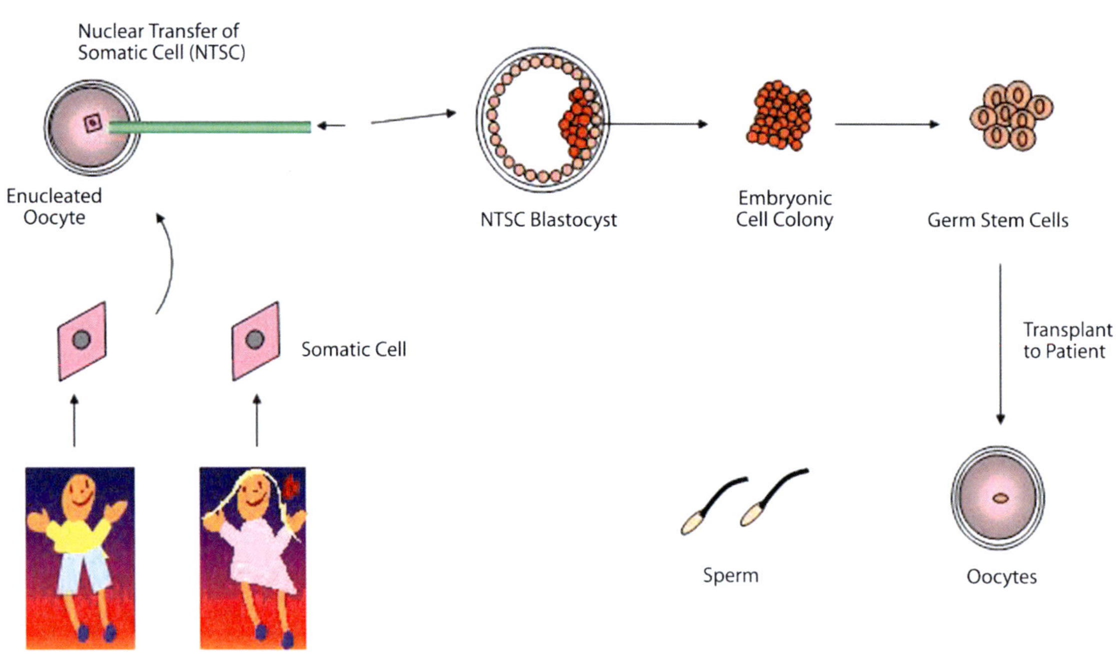

Fig. II.4.43. Future use of stem cells to re-establish gametes in sterile patients

Cattoli M, Borini A, Bonu MA (2004) Fate of stored embryos: our 10 years experience. Eur J Obstet Gynecol Reprod Biol 115 [Suppl 1]: S16–S18

Chan CL, Kumar J, Ong ML, Ng SC, Bongso TA, Ratnam SS (1996) The first frozen embryo donation pregnancy for hypergonadotrophic hypogonadism in Singapore – hormonal profile and obstetric outcome. Med J Malaysia 51:482–484

Chan R, Raboy B, Patterson C (1998) Psychosocial adjustment among children conceived via donor insemination by lesbian and heterosexual mothers. Child Dev 69:443–457

Clayton CE, Kovacs GT (1980) A.I.D. – a pretreatment social assessment. Aust N Z J Obstet Gynaecol 20:208–210

Clayton CE, Kovacs GT (1982) AID offspring: initial follow-up study of 50 couples. Med J Aust 1:338–339

Cook R, Golombok S, Bish A, Murray C (1995) Disclosure of donor insemination: parental attitudes. Am J Orthopsychiatry 65:549–559

deKretser D, Yates C, Kovacs G (1986) The use of in vitro fertilization in the management of male infertility. Clin Obstet Gynecol 12:767–773

Devroey P, Camus M, van den Abbeel E, van Waesberghe L, Wisanto A, van Steirteghem AC (1989) Establishment of 22 pregnancies after oocyte and embryo donation. Br J Obstet Gynaecol 96:900–906

Dixon RE, Buttram VC (1976) Artificial insemination using donor semen: a review of 171 cases. Fertil Steril 27:130–134

Durna EM, Bebe J, Steigrad SJ, Leader LR, Garrett DG (1997) Donor insemination: attitudes of parents towards disclosure. Med J Aust 167:256–259

Edwards RG, Steptoe PC (1975) Induction of follicular growth, ovulation and luteinization in the human ovary. J Reprod Fertil Suppl 22:121–163

Elkind-Hirsch K, Goldzieher JW, Gibbons WE, Besch PK (1986) Evaluation of the OvuSTICK urinary luteinizing hormone kit in normal and stimulated menstrual cycles. Obstet Gynecol 67:450–453

Fabregues F, Balasch J, Creus M, Civico S, Carmona F, Puerto B, Vanrell JA (1998) Long-term down-regulation does not improve pregnancy rates in an in vitro fertilization program. Fertil Steril 70:46–51

Feichtinger W, Kemeter P (1985) Pregnancy after total ovarioectomy achieved by ovum donation. Lancet ii:722–723

Fortescue E (2003) Gamete donation – where is the evidence that there are benefits in removing the anonymity of donors? A patient's viewpoint. Reprod Biomed Online 7:139–144

Geijsen N, Horoschak M, Kim K, Gribnau J, Eggan K, Daley GQ (2004) Derivation of embryonic germ cells and male gametes from embryonic stem cells. Nature 427:148–154

Golombok S, MacCallum F, Goodman E, Rutter M (2002) Families with children conceived by donor insemination: a follow-up at age twelve. Child Dev 73:952–968

Hill AM (1970) Experiences with artificial insemination. Aust N Z J Obstet Gynaecol 10:112–114

Hoy J, Venn A, Halliday J, Kovacs G, Waalwyk K (1999) Perinatal and obstetric outcomes of donor insemination using cryopreserved semen in Victoria, Australia. Hum Reprod 14:1760–1764

Huang JC, Jackson KV, Hornstein MD, Ginsburg ES (1996) The effect of elevated serum progesterone during ovulation induction in in vitro fertilization-embryo transfer. J Assist Reprod Genet 13:617–624

Hubner K, Fuhrmann G, Christenson LK, Kehler J, Reinbold R, De La Fuente R, Wood J, Strauss JF, 3rd, Boiani M, Scholer HR (2003) Derivation of oocytes from mouse embryonic stem cells. Science 300:1251–1256

Jequier A (2000) Male infertility: a guide for the clinician. Blackwell Science, Oxford

King C, Kovacs G (1992) Oocyte donation: review of results. In: Oocyte donation. Reprod Fertil Dev 4:60719–60724

Kleegman SJ (1954) Therapeutic donor insemination. Fertil Steril 5:7–31

Kovacs GT, King C (1994) The use of gamete intra-fallopian transfer with donor spermatozoa after failed donor insemination. Hum Reprod 9:859–860

Kovacs GT, Lording DW (1980) Artificial insemination with donor semen. Review of 252 patients. Med J Aust 2:609–612

Kovacs GT, Leeton JF, Matthews CD, Steigrad SJ, Saunders DM, Jones WR, Lyneham R, McMaster R (1982) The outcome of artificial donor insemination compared to the husband's fertility status. Clin Reprod Fertil 1:295–299

Kovacs GT, Baker HW, Vaux HA (1983) Outcome of AID in initial and subsequent courses of treatment. Clin Reprod Fertil 2:295–298

Kovacs G, Baker G, Burger H, De Kretser D, Lording D, Lee J (1988) Artificial insemination with cryopreserved donor semen: a decade of experience. Br J Obstet Gynaecol 95:354–360

Kovacs GT, King C, Rogers P, Wood C, Baker HW, Yates C (1989) In vitro fertilization, a practical option after failed artificial insemination with donor semen. Reprod Fertil Dev 1:383–386

Kovacs GT, Mushin D, Kane H, Baker HW (1993) A controlled study of the psycho-social development of children conceived following insemination with donor semen. Hum Reprod 8:788–790

Kovacs GT, Breheny SA, Dear MJ (2003) Embryo donation at an Australian university in-vitro fertilisation clinic: issues and outcomes. Med J Aust 178:127–129

Kremer J (1965) A simple sperm penetration test. Int J Fertil 10:209–215

Lee J, Yap C (2003) Embryo donation: a review. Acta Obstet Gynecol Scand 82:991–996

Leeton J (1992) Clinical oocyte donation. In: Oocyte donation. Reprod Fertil Dev 4:601–604

Leeton J, Backwell J (1976) Artificial donor insemination. Aust N Z J Obstet Gynaecol 16:45–47

Leeton J, Selwood T, Trounson A, Wood C (1980) Artificial donor insemination frozen versus fresh semen. Aust N Z J Obstet Gynaecol 20:205–207

Lindheim SR, Sauer MV (1999) Embryo donation: a programmed approach. Fertil Steril 72:940–941

Lutjen P, Trounson A, Leeton J, Findlay J, Wood C, Renou P (1984) The establishment and maintenance of pregnancy using in vitro fertilization and embryo donation in a patient with primary ovarian failure. Nature 307:174–175

Lutjen PJ, Findlay JK, Trounson AO, Leeton JF, Chan LK (1986) Effect on plasma gonadotropins of cyclic steroid replacement in women with premature ovarian failure. J Clin Endocrinol Metab 62:419–423

Mahadevan M, Trounson A (1980) Cryopreservation of human semen. In: Wood C, Leeton J, Kovacs G (eds) Artificial insemination by donor. Brown, Prior and Anderson, Melbourne, pp 19–32

Mahadevan M, Trounson AO (1983) Effect of cryoprotective media and dilution methods on the preservation of human spermatozoa. Andrologia 15:355–366

Mahadevan M, Trounson AO (1984) Effect of cooling, freezing and thawing rates and storage conditions on preservation of human spermatozoa. Andrologia 16:52–60

Mahadevan MM, Trounson AO, Leeton JF (1983) Successful use of human semen cryobanking for in vitro fertilization. Fertil Steril 40:340–343

McGee G, Brakman SV, Gurmankin AD (2001) Gamete donation and anonymity: disclosure to children conceived with donor gametes should not be optional. Hum Reprod 16:2033–2036

McWhinnie A (1998) Ethical dilemmas in the use of donor gametes. Med Law 17:311–317
McWhinnie A (2001) Gamete donation and anonymity: should offspring from donated gametes continue to be denied knowledge of their origins and antecedents? Hum Reprod 16:807–817
Mochimaru F, Sato H, Kobayashi T, Iizuka R (1980) Physical and mental development of children born through AID. In: David G, Price W (eds) Human artificial insemination and sperm cyropreservation. Plenum, London, pp 277–282
Navot D, Laufer N, Kopolovic J et al (1986) Artificially induced endometrial cycles and establishment of pregnancies in the absense of the ovaries. N Engl J Med314:806–811
Newton CR, McDermid A, Tekpetey F, Tummon IS (2003) Embryo donation: attitudes toward donation procedures and factors predicting willingness to donate. Hum Reprod 18:878–884
O'Connor A, Trounson A (1980) Assessment of artificial insemination success using life tables. In: Woog C, Leeton J, Kovacs G (eds) Artificial insemination by donor. Monash University Press, Melbourne, pp 33–37
Olatunbosun OA, Chizen DR, Pierson RA (1998) Screening of potential semen donors for sexual transmitted diseases. West Afr J Med 17:19–24
Palermo G, Joris H, Devroey P, Van Steirteghem AC (1992) Pregnancies after intracytoplasmic injection of single spermatozoon into an oocyte. Lancet 340:17–18
Patrizio P, Mastroianni AC, Mastroianni L (2001) Gamete donation and anonymity: disclosure to children conceived with donor gametes should be optional. Hum Reprod 16:2036–2038
Pennington GW, Naik S (1977) Donor insemination: report of a two-year study. Br Med J 1:1327–1330
Peto R, Pike MC, Armitage P, Breslow NE, Cox DR, Howard SV, Mantel N, McPherson K, Peto J, Smith PG (1977) Design and analysis of randomized clinical trials requiring prolonged observation of each patient. II. analysis and examples. Br J Cancer 35:1–39
Randall GW, Gantt PA, Gantt D, Kirk MJ, Romines N (1996) Elevated serum progesterone values at the time of ovulation induction in luteal leuprolide acetate-down-regulated GIFT cycles are associated with decreased clinical pregnancy rates. J Assist Reprod Genet 13:459–463
Rosenwaks Z, Veeck L, Hung-Ching L (1986) Pregnancy following transfer of in vitro fertilised donated oocytes. Fertil Steril 45:417–420
Salamonsen L, Healy D (eds) (1992) Oocyte donation. Reprod Fertil Dev 4:1–148
Sathanandan M, Macnamee MC, Rainsbury P, Wick K, Brinsden P, Edwards RG (1991) Replacement of frozen-thawed embryos in artificial and natural cycles: a prospective semi-randomized study. Hum Reprod 6:685–687
Serhal PF, Craft IL (1989) Oocyte donation in 61 patients. Lancet i:1185–1187
Shenfield F, Steele SJ (1997) What are the effects of anonymity and secrecy on the welfare of the child in gamete donation? Hum Reprod 12:392–395
Sherman J (1962) Preservation of bull and human spermatozoa by freezing in liquid nitrogen vapour. Nature 194:1291
Silber SJ, Devroey P, Tournaye H, Van Steirteghem AC (1995) Fertilizing capacity of epididymal and testicular sperm using intracytoplasmic sperm injection (ICSI). Reprod Fertil Dev 7:281–292; discussion 292–293
Soderstrom-Anttila V, Foudila T, Ripatti UR, Siegberg R (2001) Embryo donation: outcome and attitudes among embryo donors and recipients. Hum Reprod 16:1120–1128
Stenman UH, Alfthan H, Koskimies A, Seppala M, Pettersson K, Lovgren T (1985) Monitoring the LH surge by ultrarapid and highly sensitive immunofluorometric assay. Ann NY Acad Sci 442:544–550
Stewart GJ, Tyler JP, Cunningham AL, Barr JA, Driscoll GL, Gold J, Lamont BJ (1985) Transmission of human T-cell lymphotropic virus type III (HTLV-III) by artificial insemination by donor. Lancet 2:581–585
Thompson W, Boyle DD (1982) Counselling patients for artificial insemination and subsequent pregnancy. Clin Obstet Gynaecol 9:211–225
Toyooka Y, Tsunekawa N, Akasu R, Noce T (2003) Embryonic stem cells can form germ cells in vitro. Proc Natl Acad Sci USA 100:11457–11462
Trounson A (1992) The development of the technique of oocyte donation and hormonal replacement therapy: is oestrogen really necessary for the establishment and maintenance of pregnancy? Reprod Fertil Dev 4:671–679
Trounson AO (2001) The derivation and potential use of human embryonic stem cells. Reprod Fertil Dev 13:523–532
Trounson A (2005) Derivation characteristics and perspectives for mammalian pluripotential stem cells. Reprod Fertil Dev 17:135–41
Trounson A, Mohr L (1983) Human pregnancy following cryopreservation, thawing and transfer of an eight-cell embryo. Nature 305:707–709
Trounson AO, Matthews CD, Kovacs GT, Spiers A, Steigrad SJ, Saunders DM, Jones WR, Fuller S (1981) Artificial insemination by frozen donor semen: results of multicentre Australian experience. Int J Androl 4:227–234
Trounson A, Leeton J, Besanko M, Wood C, Conti A (1983) Pregnancy established in an infertile patient after transfer of a donated embryo fertilised in vitro. Br Med J (Clin Res Ed) 286:835–838
Van Voorhis BJ, Grinstead DM, Sparks AE, Gerard JL, Weir RF (1999) Establishment of a successful donor embryo program: medical, ethical, and policy issues. Fertil Steril 71:604–608
Van Weert JM, Repping S, Van Voorhis BJ, van der Veen F, Bossuyt PM, Mol BW (2004) Performance of the postwash total motile sperm count as a predictor of pregnancy at the time of intrauterine insemination: a meta-analysis. Fertil Steril 82:612–620
Warner MP (1974) Artificial insemination. Review after thirty-two years' experience. N Y State J Med 74:2358–2361
Wortley PM, Hammett TA, Fleming PL (1998) Donor insemination and human immunodeficiency virus transmission. Obstet Gynecol 91:515–518

II.4.21 Aesthetic Andrology: Surgical Interventions

R. Ponchietti

Summary

Surgery on the external male genitalia has developed for the management of congenital (hypospadias, epispadias) and acquired (Peyronie's disease, penile injuries and neoplasms) diseases of the penis; its main purpose is the achievement of functional and aesthetic results.

In the past 10 years penile lengthening and augmentation have been proposed as a cosmetic procedure for the normal penis and great interest in these procedures has been generated in the media.

- Penile size varies with ethnicity and this has to be remembered when evaluating a man with concerns about penile adequacy.
- Most men have a misconception about normal penile size and many patients interested in surgical penile augmentation have a penis within the normal size range.
- Surgical procedures aimed at increasing penile size are not standardized. Various complications have been reported. The most common procedures to lengthen the penis improve only its visual aspect because the length of penile structures remains unchanged.
- Men seeking penile augmentation surgery should be offered full counselling on the reliability and outcome of these procedures to avoid unrealistic expectations and post surgical disappointment.

Phalloplasty:

- Surgical reconstruction of the penis is a major challenge because of the functional and aesthetic targets that have to be addressed.
- Surgical procedures have to be tailored to the aetiology and entity of the mutilation.
- Flap transfer and subsequent penile prosthesis placement offer the best results in patients who have undergone partial or total penectomy for cancer.

Testicular prosthesis:

- The placement of a testicular prosthesis is not considered a merely aesthetic issue.
- The absence or the loss of a testis is a traumatic experience at any age and the restoration of the normal scrotal silhouette may prevent the psychological consequences of having an empty scrotum.
- Testicular prostheses have an excellent record of safety and efficacy and a low rate of post operative adverse effects.
- Because testicular cancer has become one of the most curable solid neoplasms, the placement of a testicular prosthesis represents an important step in counselling men undergoing surgery for testicular cancer.

Scrotal skin redundancy:

- The visual aspect of a normal penis may be affected by congenital or acquired abnormalities of the penile shaft and prepubic fat pad resulting in a hidden or concealed penis. This situation causes hygiene problems, predisposing to urinary infections and, in the adult, affecting vaginal penetration.
- Surgical correction of these situations has to be considered as a rehabilitative rather than a cosmetic procedure.

II.4.21.1 Normal Size Measurements of the Penis

Personal appearance and physical beauty are becoming very important in our societies and, as a consequence, both men and women are increasingly seeking cosmetic enhancement. Apart from purely aesthetic reasons, other motivations to have operations to achieve a more harmonious appearance or to treat the external signs of ageing include the desire to increase professional opportunities, to better adapt to the social environment and to improve affective relations.

The increasing interest in male genital aesthetics means that elective penile lengthening and girth enhancement have been proposed as a cosmetic procedure for the normal penis and an increasing number of men explore the possibility of this surgery.

Penile length is defined as the linear distance along the dorsal side of the penis extending from the pubo-penile skin junction to the tip of the glans. Indeed the true physiological length of the penis is the erect length, but it is not easy or feasible to make extensive observations, furthermore there are ethical problems associated with inducing erection especially in children and adolescents. The fully stretched, but still flaccid, penile length has been documented to provide reliable estimations of the potential maximal elongation in erection and may obviate the use of intracavernous drug injection, audiovisual aids or manual stimulation

Table II.4.21. Penile dimensions, according to ethnicity, in young adult males (n.a. not available)

Author	No. subjects	Age (years)	Ethnic group	Flaccid length (cm)	Stretched length (cm)	Erect length (cm)	Flaccid circumference (cm)
Schonfeld and Beebe (1942)	123	18 – 25	Caucasian	n.a	13.6	n.a	8.61
Ajamani et al. (1985)	320	17 – 23	Nigerian	8.2 ± 0.9	n.a.	n.a.	8.8 ± 0.02
Ponchietti et al. (2001)	3300	17 – 19	Caucasian	8.8 ± 1.88	12.6 ± 2.3	n.a.	9.8 ± 0.8
Schneider et al. (2001)	111	18 – 19	Caucasian	8.6	n.a.	14.4	n.a.
Son et al. (2003)	123	19 – 27	Korean	6.9 ± 0.8	9.6 ± 0.8	n.a.	8.5 ± 1.1

for estimating penile length during erection (Chen et al. 2000; Sengezer et al. 2002).

The development of male external genitalia is a phenomenon of pubescence and the adult stages are reached at the age 18 – 20 years in over 90 % of individuals; therefore, the data recorded from young males of this age group may be assumed to be the normal size of male genitalia (Table II.4.21).

These selected, homogeneous data on penile sizes in young adult males confirm that ethnic variations exist and have to be kept in mind when evaluating for short penis.

II.4.21.2 Indications and Contraindications for Penis Enlargement Surgery

In clinical practice we observe that concerns over penile size are not unusual in the male population; indeed most men have a misconception about the normal size of the penis and often misperceive their own normal penile size. As a matter of fact many patients with subjective feelings of penile inadequacy and who are interested in having surgical elongation procedures have a penis within the normal size range (Mondaini et al. 2002).

Penile augmentation surgery is not contraindicated in patients with a normal penile size, as it is a kind of aesthetic surgery; nevertheless, in some patients penile augmentation surgery may be motivated by a psychological difficulty rather than by a physical distress. Careful selection and proper counselling of candidates for penile augmentation surgery are strongly advised to avoid unrealistic expectations.

Penile elongation surgery has grown in popularity owing to the widespread advertising and media attention; however, it is claimed that these procedures are still experimental and many complications have been reported (Wessells et al.1996).

II.4.21.3 Preferred Techniques of Penis Enlargement Surgery

The widely used techniques are based on the advancement of the penis by releasing the suspensory ligament of the penis and advancing the infrapubic skin according to V-Y plasty or double Z plasty (Fig. II.4.44). Nevertheless these procedures to lengthen the penis improve only the visual aspect of the penis when flaccid, because the length of penile structures remains unchanged.

An aggressive approach has been described to enable genuine penile lengthening by means the inserting rib cartilage between the tip of the corpora cavernosa and glans cap (Perovic and Djordjevic 2000). Autologous fat injections into the tunica dartos have been used for penile thickening, but with poor results and a large number of aesthetic and functional deformities (Adler 1997). Alloderm grafts and saphenous grafts have been used with better results, but these techniques are still under evaluation (Austoni et al. 1999). Glans penis augmentation using injections of hyaluronic acid gel has been reported (Kim et al. 2003).

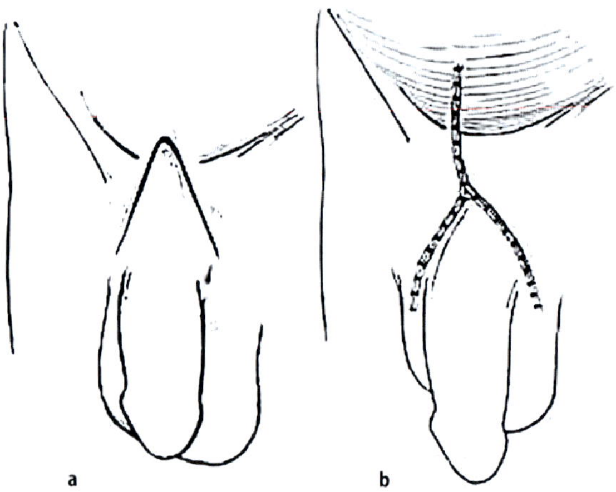

Fig. II.4.44. V-Y plasty for penile elongation

II.4.21.4 Phalloplasty

Penile amputation is an uncommon lesion resulting from accidental trauma, gunshot wounds, mutilation and surgery for penile cancer. The surgical reconstruction of the penis is a major challenge because of the functional and cosmetic targets that must be addressed, but at present there is no single gold standard technique for this procedure.

The development of techniques for phalloplasty has paralleled the evolution of flap transfer in reconstructive surgery. The improvement of these surgical procedures is mainly related to the increasing number of female transsexuals desiring the construction of a completely functional and aesthetically appealing penis at the time of female-to-male genital reassignment (Hage et al. 1993).

The aims of reconstructive surgery of the penis are:

- Creation of a competent neo-urethra to allow voiding while standing.
- Restoration of a phallus with both tactile and erogenous sensibility and enough bulk for implantation of a penile prosthesis.
- Aesthetic appearance of the neophallus.

In partial or total traumatic penile amputations the surgical replantation is the favoured approach; current replantation techniques rely on microsurgical approximation of the dorsal structures and cavernosal arteries with a high degree of success and restoration of sexual function. Tissue cold ischaemia times greater than 18 h are not unreasonable, allowing the patient to be transported to a centre where microvascular replantation can be performed (Lowe et al. 1991).

The reconstruction of a penile stump resulting from partial penectony for cancer can be managed by means of a (scrotal, abdominal or myocutaneous) flap transfer, the replacement of distal corpora cavernosa using a sleeve of Dacron or Gore-Tex and subsequent penile inflatable prosthesis placement (Mazza and Cheliz 2001).

For patients with severe penile injuries or penile cancer requiring total penectomy the type of phallic reconstruction should accommodate the patient's wish. Pedicle flaps still remain a valuable option if the patient desires a partial aspect of an aesthetic and functional penis. For total phallic reconstruction the microvascular forearm flap transfer, with its various modifications, and subsequent prosthetic placement offer the best aesthetic and functional results (Chang and Hwang 1984; Jordan 1999).

II.4.21.5 Testicular Prosthesis

Fantasies, beliefs, myths and cultural values emphasizing the importance of the testes are part of many cultures since Ancient times, so the emotional reactions related to the absence or loss of a testis deserve considerable attention at any age. The placement of a testicular prosthesis may be considered to restore the normal scrotal silhouette and prevent the potential psychological consequences of having an empty scrotum.

Boys with a solitary testis experience considerable ridicule and embarrassment about their genitalia and tend to avoid collective sport, public bathing and showering with mates, resulting in social isolation. Moreover for boys and adolescents, having two testes in the scrotum plays an important role in the development of sexual male identity.

The loss of a testis in an adult male represents a major traumatic experience: the patient's body image and self-esteem are impaired and he may feel genitally defective and develop serious behavioural disturbances.

Testicular cancer, although relatively rare, is the most common malignancy in men in the 15 to 35 age group. The dramatic improvement in survival resulting from the combination of effective diagnostic techniques, improved multidrug chemotherapeutic regimens and modification of surgical techniques has led to a decrease in patient mortality to less 5%. Orchiectomy is a curative treatment for testicular cancer, but these patients report more sexual dysfunction (erectile dysfunction, premature ejaculation) than do men in an age-matched group with other forms of neoplasm (Jonker-Pool et al. 1995). Because testicular cancer has become one of the most curable solid neoplasms, it is worth paying attention to the emotional distress caused by semicastration. Studies on patients receiving testicular prostheses after orchiectomy reported improved body image, less embarrassment at being naked with other men, a low frequency of sexual problems and a high rate of satisfaction (Lynch and Prior 1992; Incrocci et al. 1999).

The timing of performing a testicular implant is still under discussion, but indication for this procedure is not merely an aesthetic issue rather it represents an important step in counselling men undergoing surgery for testicular cancer (Adshead et al. 2001).

The main target in the management of patients with advanced prostate cancer is the suppression of circulating testosterone, and surgical castration has often been the gold standard of endocrine therapy. Although it is a curative treatment, bilateral orchiectomy is a severe assault to body image and sense of masculinity and may be unacceptable to some patients. In 1942 Riba introduced the subcapsular orchiectomy as a surgical procedure that is both effective at removing the testicular source of testosterone and also may overcome the cosmetic disadvantage of the empty scrotum. Surgical as well as medical castration produce the same effects in terms of lowering levels of plasma testosterone. Nevertheless, patients who underwent surgery reported more sexual dysfunction than those who did not have surgery, a difference that may be accounted for by psychological factors associated with the surgery. Medical hormone ablation is symbolically less drastic compared to surgical castration and therefore preferred by many patients with advanced prostate cancer (Fossa et al. 1994). If castration is planned, bilateral implantation of testicular prostheses might be considered to preserve the intact body image and concomitantly improve the quality of life of these patients.

Testicular prostheses are widely used to replace missing or removed testes with an excellent record of safety and efficacy and a low rate of postoperative adverse effects. Available gel-filled or silicone elastomer testicular implants approximate the shape, weight and softness of the normal testis. For patients with concerns about the safety of silicone prosthetics, the new saline-filled implants for testicular replacements may be used (Turek et al. 2004).

II.4.21.6 Scrotal Skin Redundancy

Several congenital or acquired deformities may cause an unpleasant appearance of the normal male external genitalia. This phenomenon, known as *hidden penis or concealed penis*, describes a spectrum of disorders from peno-scrotal webbing to a completely buried penis. The concealed penis occurs commonly in children and obese adolescents and in the most severe form the penis can disappear into the surrounding tissue, resulting in hygiene problems and predisposing to urinary tract infections.

Concealed penis in children is the result of a combination of factors affecting the visual aspect of a normal penis: occasionally the scrotal skin encroaches on the shaft of the penis producing a midline web extending often to the tip. The webbed penis can easily be corrected by a VY type of rearrangement of the scrotal skin with good aesthetic and functional results (Fig. II.4.45). The buried penis is often observed in obese infants or boys and refers to a penile shaft that is buried below the surface of the skin because of an abnormally prominent suprapubic fat pad and dense fibrous bands retracting and tethering the penis. Avoidance of circumcision is imperative in neonates and infants with a buried penis because it can worsen this condition resulting in a *trapped penis* which is cosmetically more devastating and more difficult to correct.

The pathophysiology of the buried penis in the adult differs from that in children and includes scar of the penile shaft, trauma, inguinal surgery, obesity and voluminous intrascrotal mass. The buried penis in adults is particularly debilitating, resulting in the inability to void while standing and affecting vaginal penetration.

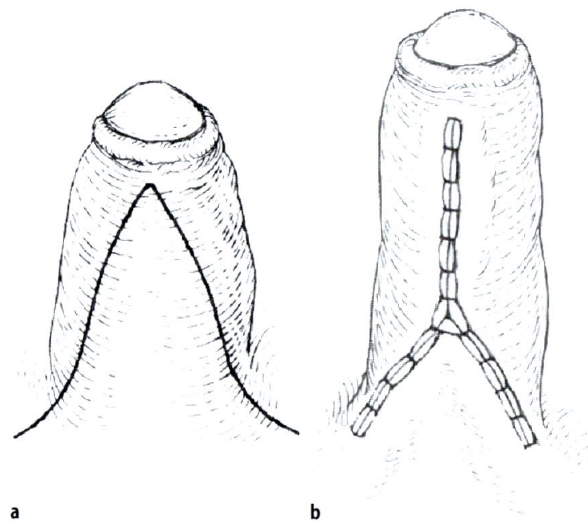

a b

Fig. II.4.45. V-Y plasty for webbed penis

Surgical correction of these situations is aimed at freeing the penis and restoring the normal aspect of external genitalia, and has to be tailored to their aetiology (Donatucci and Ritter 1998; Herndon et al. 2003). Such procedures have to be considered rehabilitative rather than purely cosmetic in nature.

References

Adler GJ (1997) Reconstruction of deformities resulting from penile enlargement surgery. J Urol158:2153–2157

Adshead J, Khouhene B, Wood J, Rustin G (2001) Testicular implants and patient satisfaction: a questionnaire-based study of men after orchiectomy for testicular cancer. BJU Int 88:559–562

Ajamani ML, Jain SP, Saxena SK (1985) Anthropometric study of male external genitalia of 320 healthy Nigerian adults. Anthropol Anz 43:179–186

Austoni E, Guarnieri A, Gatti G (1999) Penile elongation and thickening – a myth? Is there a cosmetic medical indication? Andrologia 31:45–51

Chang TS, Hwang WY (1984) Forearm flap in one-stage reconstruction of the penis. Plast Reconstr Surg 74:251–258

Chen J, Gefen A, Greenstein A, Matzkin H, Elad D (2000) Predicting penile size during erection. Int J Impot Res 12:328–333

Donatucci CF, Ritter EF (1998) Management of the buried penis in adults. J Urol 159:420–424

Elder JS, Keating MA, Duckett JW (1989) Infant testicular prostheses. J Urol 141:1413–1415

Fossa SD, Aass N, Opjordsmoen S (1994) Assessment of quality of life in patients with prostate cancer. Semin Oncol 5:657–661

Hage JJ, Bloem JJ, Suliman HM (1993) Review of the literature on techniques for phalloplasty with emphasis on the applicabilit in female-to-male transsexuals. J Urol 150:1093–1098

Herndon CD, Casale AJ, Cain MP, Rink RC (2003) Long term outcome of the surgical treatment of concealed penis. J Urol 170:1695–1697

Incrocci L, Bosch JL, Slob AK (1999) Testicular prostheses: body image and sexual functioning. BJU Int 84:1043–1045
Jonker-Pool G, Van Basten JP, Hoekstra HJ, Van Driel MF, Sleijfer DTH (1995) Testicular cancer and sexual dysfunction. Int J Impot Res 7:23–24
Jordan GH (1999) Penile reconstruction, phallic construction and urethral reconstruction. Urol Clin North Am 26:1–19
Kim JJ, Kwack TI, Jeon BG, Cheon J, Moon DG (2003) Human glans penis augmentation using injectable hyaluronic acid gel. Int J Impot Res 15:439–443
Lowe MA, Chapman W, Berger RE (1991) Repair of traumatically amputated penis with return of erectile function. J Urol 145:1267–1270
Lynch MJ, Prior JP (1992) Testicular prostheses: the patient's perception. Br J Urol 70:420–422
Mazza ON, Cheliz GMJ (2001) Glanuloplasty with scrotal flap for partial penectomy. J Urol 166:887–889
Mondaini N, Ponchietti R, Gontero P, Muir GH, Natali A, Di Loro F, Caldarera E, Biscioni S, Rizzo M (2002) Penile length is normal in most men seeking penile lengthening procedures. Int J Impot Res 14:283–286
Perovic SV, Djordjevic ML (2000) Penile lengthening. BJU Int 86:1028–1033
Ponchietti R, Mondaini N, Bonafè M, Di Loro F, Biscioni S, Masieri L (2001) Penile length and circumference: a study on 3,300 young Italian males. Eur Urol 39:183–186
Riba LW (1942) Subcapsular castration for carcinoma of prostate. J Urol 48:384–387
Schneider T, Sperling H, Lummen G, Syllwasschy J, Rubben H (2001) Does penile size in younger men cause problems in condom use? A prospective measurement of penile dimensions in 111 young and 32 older men. Urology 57:314–318
Schonfeld WA, Beebe GW (1942) Normal growth and variation in the male genitalia from birth to maturity. J Urol 48:759–777
Sengezer M, Ozturk S, Deveci M (2002) Accurate method for determining functional penile length in Turkish young men. Ann Plast Surg 48:381–385
Son H, Lee N, Huh JS, Kim SW, Paick JS (2003) Studies on self-esteem of penile size in young Korean military men. Asian J Androl 5:185–189
Turek PJ Master VA and The Testicular Prosthesis Group (2004) Safety and effectiveness of a new saline filled testicular prosthesis. J Urol 172:1427–1430
Wessells H, Lue TF, Mc Aninch JW (1996) Complications of penile lengthening and augmentation seen at 1 referral center. J Urol 155:1617–1620

II.4.22 Aesthetic Andrology: Skin Care for Men – Male Cosmetics and Cosmetic Dermatologic Procedures

C. Müller, W.-B. Schill

Summary

At present, there is a steady increase in medical-aesthetic procedures performed in men. The trend for well-groomed men will continue as men are interested in improving their outward appearance. Within the scope of **aesthetic andrology,** a variety of surgical, non-surgical and skin care techniques are used to achieve a vital, attractive and youthful appearance, resulting in increased self-confidence for professional, social and emotional competence. A self-confident appearance generally means more success in both one's job and private life.

II.4.22.1 Trends in Male Skin Care

As women have known for a long time, cosmetics constitute a weapon in the daily struggle for appreciation, esteem and success. It is now statistically proven that well-groomed men too have better career prospects and success with women. Long gone are the days when the use of toilet water and creams was regarded as unmanly. Inhibitions about buying special cosmetic products for men and going to a beauty parlour have recently diminished. Things that were coyly asked for some years ago are an expression of male emancipation today. According to a study commissioned by the Society for Rational Psychology in Munich, the "new man" is health conscious, pays attention to fitness, seeks a relationship based on partnership and regularly spends money on both scents and cosmetic care products.

The man of the new millennium is "metrosexual", giving way to his feminine side without being homosexual. He cares about his appearance to be different from people in the crowd or out of a self-confident attitude to his own body aesthetics.

The different composition of male skin and men's preference for tangy scents mean that special lines of cosmetic products are recommended. Men want easy-to-use products that are non-greasy, easy to spread and only lightly perfumed. As men are very practical, they like multi-functional products, e.g. a balm that can be used for both care after shaving and sun protection and additionally has an anti-ageing effect. Men also differ significantly from women in terms of personal hygiene. To men this means primarily body cleansing and shaving. Regular skin care with creams and lotions is generally not performed until concrete problems occur. However, there seems to be a gradual change in this purposeful behaviour, and the market has recognized the mood of the times.

II.4.22.2
Basic Concepts of Male Skin Science

II.4.22.2.1
Differences: Male – Female Skin

The distinction between male and female skin becomes apparent with the onset of puberty (Black et al. 1970; Shuster et al. 1970; Burton et al. 1972). Increased androgen production is responsible for a variety of differences. Testosterone, the main male hormone, is 95% produced by testicular Leydig cells and to a small extent in the adrenal cortex. It is converted to a biologically active form by the enzyme 5α-reductase. In the skin, hair follicles, prostate, liver and mammalian fat cells it is aromatized to 17β-oestradiol. Further metabolites are dihydrotestosterone and, to a lesser extent, oestradiol (Fritz 2003).

In the skin, testosterone can impair the epidermal barrier function. Intrauterinally, male fetuses demonstrated slower barrier development than did female fetuses. A greater epidermal barrier and faster barrier recovery were observed to occur during a testosterone-deficient state (Kao et al. 2001). In men, the surface of keratinocytes is statistically significantly lower than in premenopausal women, approximating that of postmenopausal women without hormonal substitution (Fluhr et al. 2001). However, there is no relationship between the keratinocyte surface and different functional skin parameters such as transepidermal water loss. Only skin resistance is affected by the surface.

Being approximately 25% thicker than female skin, male skin has a higher water binding capacity and is visually different, with greater roughness because of its thicker stratum corneum. The epidermis is better developed (by 12–24%) and strongly anchored in the corium. Epidermal thickness does not only depend on sex, but also on age. Based on radiographic measurements it was shown that the epidermis has a thickness of 1–1.7 mm in men under 65 years age, compared to 0.9–1.4 mm in women. This difference equalizes with advancing age: in men over 65 years it is still 0.7–1.2 mm, in women 0.6–1.2 mm. The corium of male skin contains a higher number of smooth muscle fibres compared to women, giving increased skin firmness. Likewise, the composition of the sebum is different. Throughout a man's life, sebum production (mainly stimulated by androgens) is significantly higher than that in women (Kavallunas et al. 1985). The increased lipid film on the skin surface of men delays cell desquamation. In contrast, women with advancing age are more prone to develop dry skin, as both ovarian and adrenal cortical androgen production gradually decrease after menopause.

Men perspire more rapidly and more strongly than women. The skin loses humidity, for which male skin requires increased hydration. These physiological differences are amplified by the lack of protection from weather influences through creams and make-up, and worsened by shaving and microtraumas.

Special Care for Male Skin?

The answer to this question is affirmative, as there are sex-specific variations. Comparing the skin of men with that of women, the following differences are found (Black et al. 1970; Shuster et al. 1975):

- Generally thicker skin
- Higher number of cell layers in the stratum corneum
- 15–24% stronger epidermis and better anchoring in the corium
- More smooth muscle fibres in the corium, resulting in greater firmness
- More hair follicles
- Increased sebaceous secretion with higher sebum production (androgen-dependent)
- Stable hydrolipid film with higher water binding capacity, moist skin
- Better circulation
- Skin pH ~ 5.4
- Higher initial collagen content, consecutively delayed skin ageing, but more marked wrinkle formation
- Less developed subcutaneous fatty tissue
- Lower sensitivity to external stimuli such as touch or temperature changes.

II.4.22.2.2
Male Skin Types

In men and women, skin types are generally distinguished as normal, oily (seborrhoeic), dry (sebostatic) and sensitive. The skin type may be subject to seasonal variations and depends on hormone levels, age and current state of health.

The predominant skin type in men is marked by increased sebum production. Men tend to have seborrhoeic skin with enlarged pores and blackheads and early onset of longer persisting and more severe acne.

Oily (seborrhoeic) Skin and Acne

Seborrhoea results from increased sebaceous secretion by excessive development of the lipophilic part of the hydrolipid film. Another pathophysiological cause of acne is androgen-dependent hyperkeratosis of the hair follicles and ducts of sebaceous glands as well as colonization by propionic bacteria. The stratum corneum of oily skin is relatively thick. Therefore, the skin appears poorly supplied with blood and pale. The shiny skin tends to large pores, blackheads and pustules. On the other hand, oily skin remains smooth, wrinkles develop later than in individuals with dry skin, and it is less sensitive to environmental influences.

Care comprises morning and evening cleansing with synthetic detergents (syndets) or lotions that mildly decrease the sebum output and prevent or delay new formation. Fat-free, non-irritating care products can be adjunctively applied. Suitable for acne are keratolytic agents (e.g. vitamin A acid derivatives, glycolic acid), antiseborrhoeic (benzoyl peroxide) and/or antibacterial additives. Supportively, glycolic acid peelings with astringent masks can be performed at regular intervals. Furthermore, regular manual acne treatment by a cosmetician will improve the skin appearance.

As seborrhoeic skin is the predominant male skin type, most care products for men on the market are designed for slightly oily skin.

Dry Skin

Dry skin is lipid-deficient. Loss of epidermal and sebaceous lipids leads to an altered composition of hydrolipid film and barrier lipids. There is a lack of natural humectants, particularly urea and essential fatty acids. The barrier function is weakened and transepidermal water loss increases. The skin appears dull and is tense, especially after washing. It is dry, rough and scaly and tends to premature wrinkle formation.

Care should be performed with moisturizing preparations that substitute the lacking skin lipids (e.g. ceramides) or stimulate their production. Only mild cleansers should be used and alcohol-containing facial tonics should be avoided.

Sensitive Skin

A survey in England in 2003 revealed that 30% of all men stated they had sensitive skin, and even more than 50% of women. The term "sensitive skin" is not clearly defined. It describes a skin condition that has a decreased stimulus threshold for irritative noxae which are influenced by both individual and environmental factors. The condition of the protective acid mantle and hydrolipid film as well as the barrier function are highly important for skin sensitivity. Increased transepidermal water loss is significant in the development of impaired barrier function. Typical signs of sensitive skin are redness, swelling, scaling, prickling, burning, itching and tension. Care of sensitive skin should be aimed at rehydration and restoration of a healthy skin barrier. Prevention of exogenous damage to the skin is decisive. Mild syndets instead of soaps should be used for cleansing. Suitable care products are well tolerated materials in base formulations. In addition, regular use of fragrance- and preservative-free creams is recommended, which contain natural humectants ("natural moisturizer") such as urea, lactic acid, ammonium lactate and alpha-hydroxy-acids at low concentrations. The number of different products used should be low because of the higher risk of irritation with varying ingredients and, thus, increased risk of allergic reactions (type IV hypersensitivity).

II.4.22.2.3 Ageing Skin – Extrinsic and Intrinsic Ageing

Ageing is a complex process. The skin is the organ that is most obviously affected by the ageing process. Closer examination reveals premature ageing in human skin areas that are exposed to external environmental influences, such as face and hands. Among the current theories of ageing, there is every reason to believe that accumulation of cell damage leads to what is perceived as ageing. During normal cell breathing, electrons are continuously lost, which results in the production of highly reactive molecules, reactive oxygen species (ROS). Skin ageing is a combination of intrinsic (genetically programmed, chronological) and extrinsic ageing determined by exogenous noxae. UV rays (photoageing), nicotine consumption, stress and unhealthy habits are responsible for premature skin ageing. The main mechanism of extrinsic skin ageing is the production of ROS, which cause the oxidation of DNA, proteins and membrane lipids (Beckmann and Ames 1997). For their protection the cells are equipped with a network of different repair systems and antioxidative mechanisms. However, overstrain of these protective systems can result in permanent cell damage and DNA impairment. Furthermore, UV radiation causes expression of metalloproteinases and, consequently, degradation of collagenous and elastic fibres. This results in loss of elasticity and consecutive formation of lines and wrinkles.

The processes of ageing differ in male and female skin. Visible skin ageing is observed earlier in women, but progresses more slowly. In men, the first signs of skin ageing occur around the age of 40 and are more vehement than in women. Initially fine lines rapidly develop to wrinkles and furrows. The skin gradually slackens because of increased elastosis. These clinical features of ageing are closely related to the total skin collagen content.

The higher initial skin collagen content is the reason why men seem to age later than women (Black et al. 1970; Shuster et al. 1970; Burton et al. 1972). Due to the influence of androgen, skin collagen fibres are more densely packed in men than in women. Likewise, the arrangement of dermal fibrils depends on age and sex. Thus, androgen production is primarily responsible for the sex-specific different skin collagen content (Shuster et al. 1975).

The development of innovative ingredients and optimized galenics have improved the therapeutic options in aesthetic dermatology for both the prevention and treatment of ageing. There is a steadily increasing demand for medical and sound cosmetic counselling for men with skin diseases, sensitive skin or who wish for purely prophylactic measures. Competent advice helps patients find their way in the vast market of different cosmetic products. This results in better compliance and endurance. Counselling should include a recommendation about especially well-tolerated cosmetics that are adapted to the individual skin to achieve optimization and maintenance of treatment results, particularly with regard to products that prevent ageing.

Apart from the simple prevention of harmful environmental influences on the skin, effective cosmetics can be used for additional prophylaxis against ageing. These enhance the skin's protective mechanisms and activate regenerative mechanisms. The therapy, or better prevention, of skin ageing thus represents an innovative concept of aesthetic dermatology. Particularly after minimally invasive methods such as chemical peeling and laser peeling it is most important to recommend a plan for behaviour and further treatment. Carefully selected products for follow-up therapy will contribute to an optimal, long-lasting result. Individualized light protection with skin-type-specific products is an absolute must which should be strongly advised to the patient.

II.4.22.2.4
Men's Beard

Male skin is significantly more hairy than female skin. In the lower third of the face, the beard area, there are between 5000 and 25,000 hairs. Because of the androgen influence, beard hair in men is markedly thicker and grows by 0.3–0.4 mm daily, i.e. almost 14 cm per year. A man spends about 3000 h or 140 days of his life shaving. This means stress to the skin. Daily shaving can be equated with intensive peeling, as outer skin particles with the protective hydrolipid film are also removed. Therefore, skin in this facial region is often irritated and particularly sensitive so that modern men use face care products after shaving. Especially in the case of dry skin electric shaving is better tolerated after pretreatment with shaving care products. A calming, alcohol-free lotion should be applied to skin with a tendency to erythema and irritations, to prevent further drying and irritation. Alcohol-containing aftershave products are suitable for very oily skin. Many men tend to develop folliculitis with inflammation and pustules in the beard area, caused by spreading of bacteria during shaving.

Dry shaving should be preferred to wet shaving in cases of acne and skin infections. A preshave tonic prior to shaving puts the hair into an upright position.

Wet shaving is generally more gentle and more thorough. It peels the skin, removing dead, dried skin particles. The face should first be washed with warm water and cleansing cream. Thereafter, shaving cream or foam is massaged into the skin and allowed to take effect for some minutes so that the stubble becomes soft and can be better cut. Foam remnants are first removed with warm, then with cold water. Aftershave tonic should only be used if the perfume ingredients are well tolerated by the skin. Otherwise, aftershave lotion, gel or balm are preferable as they are less irritative and give moisture to the skin.

II.4

II.4.22.3
Cosmetic Dermatologic Procedures

II.4.22.3.1
"Cosmeceuticals" – Anti-Ageing Products

For long-term treatment within the framework of skin ageing, various care products, so-called **anti-ageing products**, are available. Because of their high tolerability and specific adaptation to dermatologic needs, these stand out from common perfumery and drugstore cosmetics. "**Cosmeceuticals**" is a relatively new term from the USA (Gerny 2004). These products contain substances that lie between classic cosmetics and drugs. According to diagnosis, cosmeceuticals are applied on a skin-type-specific basis. The following agents should also be contained in anti-ageing creams for men: Anti-ageing preparations

- Vitamin A and derivatives
- Alpha-hydroxy acids (AHA)
- Antioxidants
  - Stabilized vitamin C (ascorbic acid)
  - Vitamin E (alpha-tocopherol)
  - Coenzyme Q 10
  - Polyphenols
- DNA repair enzymes
- UV protective filter (UV-A and UV-B spectrum)

Vitamin A and Derivatives

Apart from vitamin A (retinol), vitamin A acid (tretinoin) and the aldehyde retinal (retinaldehyde) have an effect on the nuclear receptor and thus on gene expression. Both dermal and epidermal effects have been demonstrated. The activity of collagen (type I and III) and elastin-degrading collagenases is inhibited. In addition, there is collagen neosynthesis and reorganization of damaged collagen and elastin fibres (Vahlquist et al. 1982; Griffith et al. 1993; Fisher et al. 1996).

Alpha-Hydroxy Acids (AHAs)

Some AHAs are natural agents, of which glycolic acid is the simplest one. Their spectrum extends from keratolysis to exfoliation, hydration and bleaching. Furthermore, they serve as vehicles for other agents. AHAs enhance cell proliferation, which results in thickening of the epidermis. By increased cell division the stratum granulosum becomes more prominent. This causes a reduction of transepidermal water loss, resulting in increased skin moisture. The collagen production is elevated by greater glycosaminoglycans (GAG) formation (Klein 2000).

Antioxidants

Antioxidants are agents that inhibit the harmful effects of ROS, thus protecting the skin from oxidative stress and resultant cell and tissue damage. Imbalance in the antioxidative and prooxidative systems causes damage to lipids, proteins and nucleic acids. The antioxidants include vitamins such as vitamin C and E, β-carotene and polyphenols (botanic antioxidants, "phytochemicals") such as flavonoids, green tea phenols, quercetin, resveratrol and silymarin (Elmets et al. 2001; Afaq and Mukthar 2002).

Stabilized Vitamin C (Ascorbic Acid)

The hydrophilic vitamin C influences skin differentiation and stimulates connective tissue metabolism by collagen-synthesizing enzymes and inhibition of collagenases (Nusgens et al. 2001). Furthermore, there is increased differentiation of epidermal ceramides (Galinski et al. 1985).

Vitamin E (Alpha-Tocopherol)

As a lipophilic antioxidant, vitamin E is able to quench free radicals. It also inhibits collagen- and elastin-degrading collagenases. It protects collagen biosynthesis and prevents GAG synthesis stimulated by ROS (Tanaka et al. 1993; Ricciarelli et al. 1999). Moreover, vitamin E influences cellular signal transduction by inhibiting protein kinase C activity. Oxidative stress and inhibition of collagenase activity are also reduced by other antioxidative agents, such as **coenzyme Q 10** and **flavonoids**, which have an additional photoprotective effect (Hoppe et al. 1999; Elmets et al. 2001; Krutmann and Hansen 2001).

DNA Repair Enzymes

Typical skin lesions are induced by UVB, i.e. DNA damage with the development of adverse photo products such as cyclobutane pyrimidine dimers. Dimerization can be stopped by photolyase-containing liposomes to enhance rapid repair of DNA damage. This process is called photoreactivation. Furthermore, the expression of matrix metalloproteinases is inhibited and immunosuppression is prevented (Krutmann and Hansen 2001).

Vitamin A acid and vitamin C preparations should be principally used in the evening. Other radical quenchers can also be applied every morning together with UV protective moisture care to attenuate light-induced skin ageing. Information on appropriate sun behaviour and use of adequate sun protection (UVA and UVB spectrum) should always take precedence over all care recommendations in terms of skin ageing.

Concluding Remarks

Fitness, freshness, naturalness and, to a certain extent, grooming are the key ideas in mediating the message "skin care for men". Traditionally, cosmetics for men and women are different with regard to their foundation and marketing strategy. Consequently, the response to these products varies: men strive for well-being and healthiness, while women attach importance to beauty and youthful appearance. The majority of men treat their skin in accordance with the necessity of shaving and body cleansing. However, the "modern man" is increasingly interested in presenting an attractive image to his environment, which fits in with his profession and lifestyle. This results in an increase of surgical and non-surgical aesthetic procedures on the one hand, and in the daily use of skin and body care products for well-being and delay of the ageing process on the other.

The products should be uncoloured, non-greasy, easy to apply and easy to spread. They should be rapidly absorbed, discreetly perfumed and have a fresh scent. Most popular with men are "easy-to-use" products, which are increasingly being marketed.

II.4.22.3.2 Minimally Invasive Aesthetic Procedures

In the twenty-first century world, men pay more and more attention to their appearance and health. In Germany, too, an increasing number of men decide to have medical-aesthetic treatments. About 15–20% of all men are interested in this subject. This follows a trend from the USA where no fewer than 30% of all beauty-aware patients are male. On the labour market the external appearance is also important for men, so that medical-aesthetic procedures are often requested for professional reasons. Well-groomed, good-looking men earn 25% more and find jobs more easily than their "untreated" colleagues.

According to statistics from the American Society for Aesthetic Plastic Surgery (ASAPS 2003), there was a 34% increase (2002–2003) in the total number of non-surgical procedures, such as injection of botulinum toxin or fillers like collagen, hyaluronic acid and polylactic acid, laser epilation, microdermabrasion and chemical peeling. Among these procedures, botulinum toxin treatment is the most popular. Therefore, the cosmetic uses of botulinum toxin are described in more detail in the following section.

Botulinum Toxin

To date, nearly all studies on the aesthetic use of botulinum toxin have been performed in women, as they are the main clientele. Recently, however, an increasing number of men have wanted treatment with botulinum toxin to reduce the signs of ageing. When applying botulinum toxin in practice, sex-specific differences in skin composition and musculature have to be considered. According to a pertinent study, at least twice the dose that is used in women is required for men to effectively treat glabellar lines (Carruthers, 61st Annual American Academy of Dermatology, San Francisco, 2003). This is explained by the fact that men have deeper wrinkles because of their thicker epidermis, lower amount of subcutaneous fatty tissue and, in particular, stronger muscle tone and larger muscle mass. Despite the higher doses, no additional side-effects or complications have been observed.

Basis and Effect of Botulinum Toxin A

Mimic wrinkles develop by contraction of the underlying musculature. With advancing age these wrinkles become increasingly visible because of elastosis and photoageing of the skin. Since 2000, the use of botulinum toxin A has gained increasing popularity, after a Canadian ophthalmologist discovered that the toxin, when used to treat muscular spasm, also had a "smoothing effect" on facial expression. The first publication about botulinum toxin A in cosmetic dermatology appeared in 1990. The American couple Carruthers, an ophthalmologist and a dermatologist, described how to correct glabellar lines by use of botulinum toxin A (Carruthers and Carruthers 1990).

Botulinum toxin induces chemical denervation of smooth muscles by cleaving proteins that inhibit the release of acetylcholine at the neuromuscular connection, consecutively causing temporary reversible paralysis of the injected muscles (Simpson 1981). Botulinum toxin A is an exotoxin produced by *Clostridium botulinum* in an anaerobic environment. It is a protein of 147 kDa with two subunits connected by disulphide bridges. The heavy chain (approx. 100 kDa) binds rapidly and irreversibly to presynaptically located receptors (sialoglycoproteins) at cholinergic nerve endings. This induces pinocytotic absorption of the whole molecule into the motor end-plate. The light chain is cleaved intracellularly, acting as a specific metalloprotease which specifically cleaves the synaptic target protein SNAP-25 (synaptosomal-associated protein of 25 kDa) (Binz et al. 1994). This protein activation is followed by irreversible blockage of acetylcholine release.

The clinical effect is observed after 24 – 72 h, reaching its maximum after 1 – 2 weeks and lasting for about 3 – 6 months. Thereafter, the muscles gradually regain their function by sprouting new nerve endings from the adjacent regions. Muscle biopsy samples from patients who had repeatedly received toxin injections did not show any signs of permanent degeneration in terms of atrophy.

There are seven serologically different, but structurally similar types of botulinum toxin (A to G), of which subtype A is the most effective and longest lasting (Hambleton 1992).

Three botulinum A products are currently available on the German market:

- Botox® (Allergan)
- Dysport® (Ipsen)
- Xeomin® (Merz)

which differ in their components, storability, shelf life and dosage. One unit of Botox®/Xeomin® corresponds to 3 – 4 units of Dysport®.

Conditions of Use

Thorough anatomic knowledge of the mimic musculature is a prerequisite for safe injection (Fig. II.4.46). Some special features of the facial musculature have to be considered. Most parts of the mimic musculature are not surrounded by a fascia. Depending on the region, it may be very difficult to distinguish between the individual muscle groups. Parts of the fibres merge into each other and run differently. Thus it is not possible to define particular injection points, but rather these should be considered as approximate points. Paresis of one muscle group may extend to an adjacent one. Depending on the dilution of the botulinum toxin A solution, the toxin diffuses to a varying degree, the effect gradually decreasing with a larger diffusion radius. Thus, it is the injected area rather than a specific point that is of prime importance for the effect of botulinum toxin A. A muscular agonist–antagonist system should be considered and observed while treatment is carried out.

Apart from the explanations mentioned before, the patient should be informed that use of botulinum toxin A for the indication of wrinkle treatment has not yet been approved and therefore must be declared as a healing trial. Thorough information should include a detailed listing of possible side-effects, alternative aesthetic methods and pretreatments. The patient should also be questioned for neurological and rheologic diseases, allergies and drug intake. Neuromuscular diseases, pregnancy and lactation period are considered contraindications; intake of anticoagulants is thought to be a relative contraindication. Asymmetries and

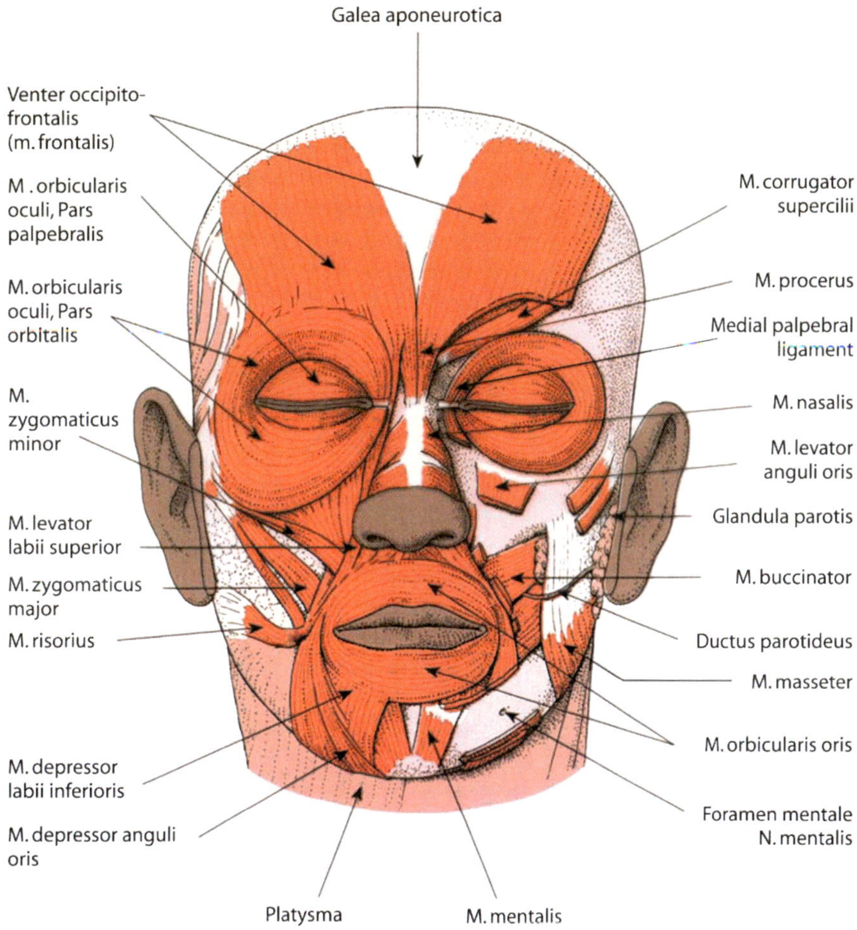

Fig. II.4.46. Muscles of facial expression – anterior view. Anatomic drawing of mimic musculature

neurological disturbances such as peripheral facial paresis should always be examined before treatment. Stigmatizing facial asymmetries can be equalized by targeted injections of side-adapted doses, higher doses per injection area being needed in male patients compared with female patients. Ideal candidates for botulinum toxin treatment are young and middle-aged men whose skin does not yet show severe sun damage (photoageing) and senile elastosis but who feel their facial wrinkles are disturbing.

Application of Botulinum Toxin A

Botulinum toxin A treatment is exemplarily demonstrated in four regions: glabella, forehead, periorbital area with chemical brow lift, corner of the mouth.

Selected locations of mimic wrinkles and suitability for botulinum toxin A:

- Glabellar region ("brow furrow")
- Forehead area
- Periorbital area ("crow's feet ","laugh wrinkles") with chemical brow lift
- Sagging of the corner of the mouth ("marionette lines")

Glabellar Wrinkles ("Brow Furrow")

Men often feel attractive and vital except for the deep furrow between their eyebrows. These vertical lines near the glabellar area indicate anger, trouble, stress and sometimes anxiety, i.e. negative emotions. Glabellar wrinkles are the main indication for botulinum toxin A injection in men.

Wrinkle development is caused by continuous traction of the mimic musculature, which in many cases becomes hypertrophic. This is because of frequent and strenuous activities that are required in modern civilized society.

Recently, many botulinum toxin A users have reported striking improvement of complaints such as tension headache and migraine. To date, there is no scientific reason for this phenomenon. It is noticeable that most injection points in the glabellar area correspond to acupuncture points (Sommer and Sattler 1999).

Glabellar wrinkles are caused by traction of several

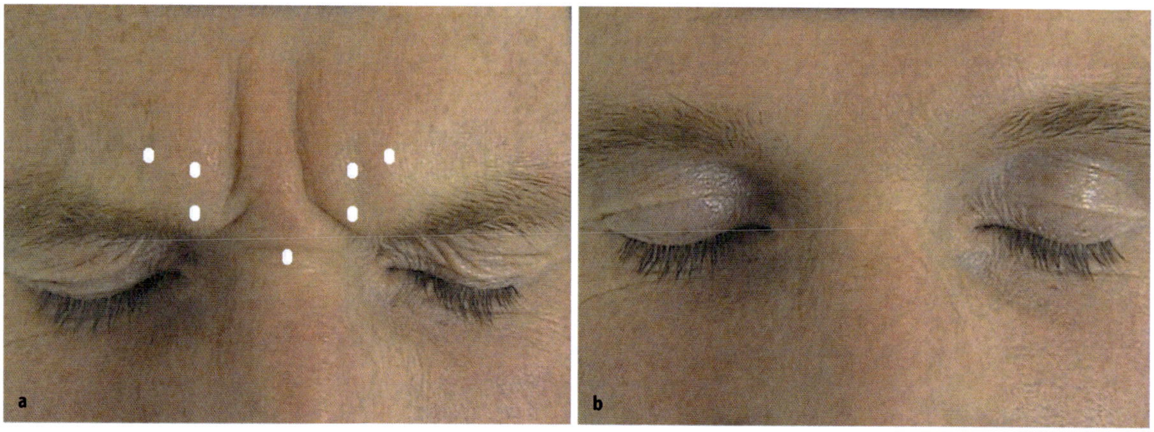

Fig. II.4.47a, b. Injection scheme for glabellar wrinkle. Glabellar wrinkle in tension 2 weeks before (**a**) and after injection (**b**)

muscles (Carruthers and Carruthers 1992, 1998a, b; Forster and Wulc 1998; Grablowitz 1999; Rzarny and Feller 2000). The corrugator muscle draws the eyebrow mediocaudally and the orbicularis oculi muscle medially. Caudally the eyebrow is drawn by the procerus muscle and the depressor supercilii muscle. As there are frequently variations in muscle anatomy, the individual eyebrow position should always be assessed prior to therapy. The dosage is determined by muscle mass; in men it is mostly twice or three times higher than in women. Various injection techniques have been reported in the literature. In general, the schemes describe two points of injection into the corrugator muscle. Another one or two points are placed into the procerus muscle. Further injection points are the lower part of the occipitofrontalis muscle, the lateral part of the corrugator muscle and the cranial of the orbicular muscle. The injection is made vertically (90%) to the skin surface (Fig. II.4.47).

A possible side-effect is lid ptosis, which has been reported to occur in between 0% and 15% of patients (Ascher et al. 1995; Garcia and Fulton 1996; Ahn et al. 2000).

Treatment of Glabellar Area

- Three to seven injection points
- Intramuscularly
- Bilaterally 0.5 – 1 cm above the cranial, medial orbital rim
- 1 cm laterally above the aforementioned point
- Never laterally to the mid-pupillary line
- Risk of lid ptosis increases with closer distance between lateral points and orbital cavity

Forehead Wrinkles

Transverse or longitudinal wrinkles across the forehead lead to a picture of "lofty brow", but may also express sorrow and scepticism. The younger the patient and the tighter the skin, the better is the treatment result. Older patients often use the lateral part of the occipitofrontalis muscle to even out an existing brow ptosis. Injection points and dosage are determined by eyebrow position and muscle thickness. The number of points depends on the forehead size. In general, 4 – 8 points are placed at a distance of 1 – 2 cm in 1 – 3 horizontal lines. Care should be taken above the orbit and laterally to the midpupil. Caution must be exercised in older patients who use their forehead muscle to lift the brow, and those whose eyebrows are located below or at the level of the orbital rim, as altered facial expression by deeper situated brows and possible lid ptosis may result for a period of at least 3 – 8 weeks (Carruthers et al. 1996; Sommer and Sattler 2000; Becker-Wegerich et al. 2001). Increased elevation of the lateral brows, which may occur because of hyperfunction of the lateral muscle and gives the patient a questioning facial expression ("Mephisto effect"), can be corrected at a later time by placement of one or two injection points along the forehead hair border or one injection point directly above the wrinkle.

Treatment of Forehead Wrinkles

- Four to eight injection points
- Individually dependent on brow position
- Distance of 1 – 2 cm in one to three lines
- **Caution** in the case of injections directly above the orbit or lateral to the midpupillary line because of lid ptosis

Chemical Brow Lift

The shape and curvature of the eyebrows are clearly different in men and women. Typically, masculine brows are strong and straight, while female brows are finer and curved upwards. In men, the distance between the lid and the brow is smaller. Brows that appear too straight or are sagging can be gently lifted by botulinum toxin A injections. This technique is called chemical brow lift (Huang et al. 2000). The toxin is injected into the lateral upper part of the orbicularis oculi muscle, the point being placed near the orbital rim and 1–2 cm above the lateral angle of the eye. Slight levation of the lateral brows occurs by counter-traction of the occipitofrontalis muscle. Ahn et al. (2000) observed an average brow elevation of 1.02 mm from the midpupil and of 4.83 mm from the lateral canthus. Brow lifting can also be achieved by widening of the eye. Tension of the orbicular muscle may lead to a mischievous or strained facial expression. This can be modified by botulinum toxin A injections into partial areas of the orbicular muscle so that the eye appears larger and wider and the patient's facial expression becomes open and beaming.

Periorbital Wrinkles, Lateral Canthal Rhytides ("Crow's Feet", "Laugh Wrinkles")

With increasing actinic elastosis over the course of the years, laugh wrinkles develop to crow's feet. The sphincter-like orbicularis oculi muscle, which runs circularly around the eye, is responsible for screwing up the eyes. The injection area is approximately 1 cm laterally to the orbital rim, with two to four points being placed at each side in a crescent-shaped manner. Injections are made at a 45° angle to the skin surface from the canthus outwards (Fig. II.4.48). Laterally to the orbital cavity there is a venous plexus consisting of branches of the superficial temporal vein. The patient should be informed that injury may result in the formation of haematoma.

In the case of marked lower lid wrinkles, a small amount of botulinum toxin A may be injected at one point each just below the lower lid in the midpupillary line and 0.5 cm laterally.

Treatment of Periorbital Wrinkles

- Two to four points
- Subcutaneously
- Crescent-shaped, approximately 1 cm laterally to the bony orbital rim
- Injection technique at 45° angle to skin surface
- Keep needle away from the eye!

Melomental Folds (Marionette Lines – Sagging of the Corner of the Mouth)

These vertical grooves at the lateral corners of the mouth give an impression of fixed disapproval or sadness. They appear in the early 40 s and may be more pronounced in those who have smoked. Men can disguise them with a beard. The depressor anguli oris muscle pulls the mouth corners down, opposing the elevation of the zygomaticus major and minor muscles. With selective chemodenervation of the depressor anguli oris, the zygomaticus becomes unopposed as an elevator of the corner of the mouth. The injection is made directly into the muscle, approximately 7 mm laterally and 8–10 mm caudally to the corner of the mouth (Grablowitz 1999; Sommer and Sattler 2000; Heckmann and Rzany 2002). If doses are too high or injections are placed too far medially, the depressor labii can be involved, which will cause flattening of the lower lip contour. Asymmetry may temporarily lead to severe functional loss, impairing eating, laughing and swallowing. In case of deep wrinkles, additional elevation can be achieved by augmentation with fillers 10–14 days later.

Treatment of Sagging Mouth Corners

- One point each per mouth corner
- Intramuscularly
- Always palpate depressor anguli oris muscle
- Approximately 7 mm laterally and 10 mm caudally to the mouth corner

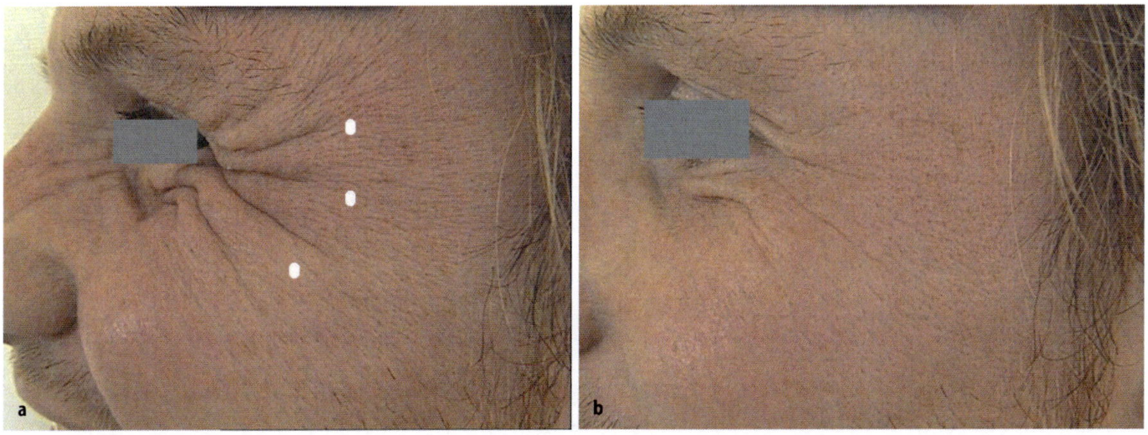

Fig. II.4.48a, b. Injection scheme for periorbital wrinkles. Periorbital wrinkles in tension 2 weeks before (**a**) and after injection (**b**)

Combination Procedures with Botulinum Toxin A

Botulinum toxin A as a monotherapy has been particularly successful in younger patients. As for mimic wrinkles in the upper facial third, the result in most cases corresponds to patient's and doctor's expectations. Concerning the glabellar area and crow's feet, further augmentation with fillers is generally not required after botulinum toxin A injection, except for glabellar wrinkles which cannot be completely eliminated. These cases can be treated with injectable fillers or solid implants. About 30 different injectables are currently on the market; most frequently used are resorbable fillers such as collagen and hyaluronic acid as well as autologous fat. After 3–8 months, these rapidly resorbable materials are no longer histologically demonstrable in the dermis (Alster 1998). Dislocation of the implanted substance does not occur because of diminished mimic muscle tension.

UV light and smoking (extrinsic ageing) or genetic factors (intrinsic ageing) intensify skin elastosis and accentuate mimic wrinkles so that the impression of skin ageing is even worse. To achieve an optimal result to the patient's satisfaction, botulinum A toxin should be combined with other methods of facial rejuvenation. Particularly in the lower facial third and perioral region as well as in cases of age-related skin changes and loss of substance in deeper tissue structures, the success of monotherapy is limited. Combination options include the filling substances mentioned before or other procedures for wrinkle treatment, such as skin resurfacing, lasering, chemical peel methods, dermabrasion and plastic surgery. The result of combined treatment can be markedly superior to that of monotherapy (Klein et al. 1997; Carruthers and Carruthers 1998a, b). Pretreatment with botulinum toxin A is a useful complement, which improves the long-term effect of filling materials or skin resurfacing methods. In general, it should be performed 10–14 days prior to the planned procedure. After this period, the maximal effect of botulinum toxin A on mimic musculature has been reached and the overlying skin has relaxed. Because of decreased mimic muscle traction, degradation of the filling materials is reduced and, thus, the long-term results are improved. In the case of resurfacing procedures, a positive effect by pretreatment with botulinum toxin A is gained in that collagen neosynthesis is unhindered. The new collagen bundles and elastic fibres do not follow the previous wrinkle pattern but can develop parallel to the skin surface. Thus, pretreatment with botulinum toxin A improves both the immediate and the long-term effect.

Chemical Peeling

In addition to improving the texture of the skin and reducing hyperpigmentation and mild wrinkling, peels are also useful in the treatment of acne and melasma. Chemical peels are categorized based on the depth of the procedure: superficial, medium or deep. Currently, superficial and medium-depth peels are the most frequently performed procedures. They do not significantly improve deep wrinkles or sagging skin, but can improve the colour and texture of the skin, thereby yielding a more youthful appearance. The deeper-depth peels that cause necrosis as far as the stratum reticulare are increasingly being supplanted by laser resurfacing, showing superior results with fewer complications.

Superficial peels induce necrosis of all parts of the epidermis, from the stratum granulosum to the basal cell layer (~0.06 mm). There is a wide variety of agents, including alpha hydroxy acids (AHAs), modified Jessners solution (resorcin, acid salicyl, acid lactic, ethanol 95 %) and trichloroacetic acid (TCA) 10–15 %. The ingredients are often used in combination. All of these solutions remove the superficial layer of the stratum corneum, yielding skin that is smoother in texture and more evenly pigmented.

The most commonly used AHA peeling is glycolic acid, known as "lunchtime peel", as the patients can return to work without any telltale signs after the procedure performed at lunch time. It has been reported that AHA-containing formulations exert profound influence on epidermal keratinization. Ditre et al. (1996) demonstrated that application of AHAs resulted in a 25 % increase of skin thickness, improved quality of the elastic fibres, increased density of collagen and increased mucopolysaccharides in the dermis, as shown by histology. Kim et al. (1998) found that glycolic acid treatments enhanced both fibroblast proliferation and collagen production in vitro. This results in two major effects: quickening of the cell cycle, which is slowed in aged skin, and smoothening of the stratum corneum.

Medium-depth peels (trichloroacetic acid at 35–40 % as standard solution) cause necrosis of the epidermis and part of the papillary dermis. Patients need to allow a recovery time of at least 10 days. On the first 2 days the skin appears slightly pink, and on the next 2 days it darkens. Peeling of the skin begins at day 5 and will be completed by day 10. The indications are the same as for superficial peelings, therefore severe acne scars, photoageing and wrinkles may respond better. Contraindications include patients with darker skin types, hyperpigmentation and scarring in the history and those who have been treated with isotretinoin or topical radiation.

For all peeling patients it is essential to avoid the sun and strictly use sun blockers because of postinflammatory hyperpigmentation. Furthermore, hydrochinone formulations should be used in patients with darker skin types after the peeling.

Soft Tissue Augmentation

There is a long history of soft tissue augmentation in cosmetic surgery. Fillers are natural or synthetic substances that are injected into the skin to correct depressed lesions or slight blemishes, such as wrinkles, scars, atrophic areas and small lips. The ideal fillers must have characteristics compatible with the tissues in which they are installed, they must not provoke rejection, reactions of inflammatory or immune types and finally they must yield an acceptable and persistent correction. It should be easy to obtain, implant and store, should be inexpensive, non-toxic, non-carcinogenic and long lasting. None of the available materials can yet meet all of these criteria. The panorama of the fillers is primarily composed of fillers of biological origin (autologous or heterologous) or of synthetic origin. As concerns the induced persistence and correction, these may be permanent or non-permanent. The fillers are injected under the skin to reduce irregularities such as wrinkles, pits and scars. The resorbable substances used for injection are primarily collagen, hyaluronic acid, polylactic acid, self-donated body fat and plasma gel.

Collagen

Injectable bovine collagen-containing products (e.g. Zyderm® I, II®, Zyplast® – Collagen Aesthetics) have been used for a long time and more frequently than any other material. There are differently concentrated collagens and are crosslinked, for example with glutaraldehyde, for deeper wrinkles and furrows. The application is to a superficial to medium dermal depth. The resulting correction is temporary because host collagenases displace collagen from the injection place in the dermis within 3–6 months after the procedure. Bovine collagen implants are expensive, must be refrigerated and pose the risk of allergy. Therefore, two allergy tests have to be performed 6 and 2 weeks prior to treatment. Indications include superficial wrinkles, horizontal forehead lines, glabellar lines, crow's feet, fine perioral lines and scars. Zyplast® is better suited for complete correction of deeper wrinkles and furrows, such as nasolabial folds, marionette grooves and deep scars. As an advantage, the collagen implants contain small amounts of lidocaine, which partially and temporarily numbs the treatment area.

Hyaluronic Acid

Hyaluronic acid is a glycosaminoglycan composed of repeating dimeric units of D-glucuronic acid and *N*-acetyl-glucosamine, for long-lasting effect the polymer is chemically modified. Hyaluronic acid products are injected into the dermis. There are different types of hyaluronic acid products, one type derived from animals (cockscomb, (Hylaform® – Medicis/Inamed), the others from bacterial cultures (Restylane® – Q-Med, Uppsala). Hyaluronic acid products are less expensive than collagen products, can be stored at room temperature, are easy to apply and no allergy tested is required. Adverse reactions include transient erythema, inflammation, bruising and tenderness at the treated area.

Poly-L-Lactic Acid (PLA)

Poly-L-lactic acid (PLA) Sculptra® (Sanofi Aventis) is one of the latest implants commercialized among bioresorbable fillers. This synthetic polymer is biocompatible, biodegradable, immunologically inert and free from toxicity. All these necessary properties provide theoretical safety. It is provided as freeze-dried material and can be stored at room temperature. After reconstitution with water Sculptra® has to be injected deeply into the dermis or into the subcutaneous tissue using a 26-gauge needle, stimulating the patient's own collagen synthesis. Therefore, the main indications of Sculptra® are the correction of significant wrinkles and furrows on the face. It has been used for the correction of nasolabial folds, marionette lines, mid and lower facial volume loss, jaw line laxity and other signs of facial ageing. Furthermore, Sculptra® is used especially for spread tissue augmentation for "face modelling", as for cheek lipoatrophies in HIV patients receiving antiprotease treatment. After two or three sessions, results are appreciable and equivalent to those achieved with other resorbable fillers, but seem to last longer (18–24 months). Sculptra® treatment provides a minimally invasive and effective facial enhancement correction with a low frequency of side-effects and no need for allergy testing. The clinical results using poly-L-lactic acid for soft tissue augmentation are comparable to autologous fat grafting (Woerle et al. 2004). Superficial injections should be avoided. They may increase the risk of persistent granulomas, which will be difficult to manage (Vochelle 2004).

Laser Epilation

Laser treatment for the removal of unwanted body hair is one of the hottest grooming trends, also for men. It has been proved to be effective and is commonplace throughout the world today. There are numerous lasers and light sources available for hair epilation. Compared to electrolysis as the only other proven method for permanent hair removal, laser epilation is expensive but much faster, with the result of permanent hair reduction up to 90–95% requiring multiple treatment sessions. It is much more comfortable especially for men, if used to remove hair from large areas such as the back or chest.

There are different types of laser systems for hair removal with different wavelengths. The optimal wavelength, pulse duration and fluence are essential to provide safe and permanent long-term hair removal.

Laser-assisted hair removal is based on the theory of selective photothermolysis. Thermal injury will be restricted to the hair follicle if the target chromophore – melanin – absorbs the laser energy in an amount of time (pulse width) that is equal to or less than the thermal relaxation time of melanin. The hair follicle is heated and destroyed while other structures are left unharmed. Light-skinned persons with dark hair are ideal for laser-assisted hair removal. Those with darker-skin types more often have negative side-effects from the procedure. Several treatments will be required for permanent hair reduction at certain time intervals. After the treatment consequent sun protection is necessary to prevent permanent pigment changes. Darker-skinned patients have the highest risk of developing pigmentation changes, besides crusting, blistering and scarring.

Outlook

At present, there is a steady increase in medical-aesthetic procedures performed in men. The trend for well-groomed men will continue as men are interested in improving their outward appearance. Within the scope of **aesthetic andrology**, a variety of surgical, non-surgical and skin care techniques are used to achieve a vital, attractive and youthful appearance, resulting in increased self-confidence for professional, social and emotional competence. A self-confident appearance generally means more success in both one's job and private life. Long gone are the years when men proudly presented their weather-beaten skin and furrows. Thus, men constitute about 10–15% botulinum toxin A users. Botulinum toxin seems to be an acceptable alternative to invasive cosmetic surgery. Injection of botulinum toxin A is a rapid, safe, effective and almost atraumatic method to correct mimic wrinkles for a period of 3–6 months.

References

Afaq F, Mukthar H (2002) Photochemoprevention by botanical antioxidants. Skin Pharmacol Appl Skin Physiol 15:297–306

Ahn MS, Catten M, Maas CS (2000) Temporal brow lift using botulinum toxin. A Plast Reconstr Surg 205:1129–1135

Alster AS (1998) Preoperative preparation for CO_2 laser resurfacing. In: Coleman WP, Lawrence N (eds) Skin resurfacing. Williams and Wilkins, Baltimore, Md., pp 171–179

Ascher B, Klap P, Marion MH, Chanteloub F (1995) Botulinum toxin in the treatment of fronto-glabellar and periorbital wrinkles. An initial study. Ann Chir Plast Esthet 40:76

Becker-Wegerich P, Rauch L, Ruzicka T (2001) Botulinum toxin A in the therapy of mimic facial lines. Clin Exp Dermatol 26:619–630

Beckmann KVB, Ames BN (1997) Oxidative delay of DNA. J Biol Chem 272:19633

Binz T, Blasi J, Yamasaki S et al (1994) Proteolysis of SNAP-25 by types E and A botulinal neurotoxins. J Biol Chem 269:1617

Black MM, Shuster S, Bottoms E (1970) Osteoporosis, skin collagen and androgen. Br Med J 4:773

Burton JL, Johnson C, Libman I (1972) Skin virilism in women with hirsutism. J Endocrinol 53:349

Carruthers JD, Carruthers JA (1992) Treatment of glabellar frown lines with C. botulinum-A exotoxin. J Dermatol Surg Oncol 18:17–21

Carruthers A, Carruthers J (1998a) Clinical indications and injection technique for the cosmetic use of botulinum A exotoxin. Dermatol Surg 24:1189–1194

Carruthers J, Carruthers A (1998b) The adjunctive usage of botulinum toxin. Dermatol Surg 24:1244–1247

Carruthers A, Carruthers J (1990) The treatment of glabellar furrows with botulinum A exotoxin. J Dermatol Surg Oncol 16:83

Carruthers A, Keine K, Carruthers J (1996) Cosmetic use of botulinum A exotoxin. J Am Acad Dermatol 34:788–797

Ditre CM, Griffin TD, Murphy GF, Sueki H, Telegan B, Johnson WC, Yu RJ, Van Scott EJ (1996) Effects of alpha-hydroxy acids on photoaged skin: a pilot clinical, histologic and ultrastructural study. J Am Acad Dermatol 34:187–195

Elmets CA, Singh D, Tubesing K, Matsui M, Kotiyar SK, Mukthar H (2001) Cutaneous photoprotection from ultraviolet injury by green tea polyphenols. J Am Acad Dermatol 44:425–432

Fisher GJ, Datta SC, Talwar HS (1996) Molecular basis of sun-induced premature skin ageing and retinoid antagonism. Nature 379:335–339

Fluhr JW, Pelosi A, Lazzerini S, Dikstein S, Berardesca E (2001) Differences in corneocyte surface area in pre- and post-menopausal women. Skin Pharmacol Appl Skin Physiol Suppl 14:10–16

Forster JA, Wulc AE (1998) Cosmetic use of botulinum toxin. Semin Ophthalmol 13:142–148

Fritz K (2003) In: Krutmann J, Diepgen T (eds) Hautalterung. Springer, Berlin Heidelberg New York, p 86

Galinski FA, Pfeiffer HP, Trüper HG (1985) 1,4,5,6-Tetrahydro-2-methyl-4-pyrimidincarboxylic acid, a novel cyclic amino acid from halophilic bacteria of the genus *Ectothiorhodospira*. Eur J Biochem 149:135–139

Garcia A, Fulton J (1996) Cosmetic denervation of the muscles of facial expression with botulinum toxin. A dose-response study. Dermatol Surg 22:39–43

Gerny H (2004) In: Worret WI, Gehring W (eds) Kosmetische Dermatologie. Springer, Berlin Heidelberg New York, pp 87–94

Grablowitz D (1999) Plastisch-ästhetische Indikationen im Gesichtsbereich. Urban and Vogel, Munich

Griffith CEM, Russman AN, Majmudar G, Singer RS, Hamilton TA, Voorhees JJ (1993) Restauration of collagen formation in photodamaged human skin by tretinoin (retinoic acid). N Engl J Med 329:530–535

Hambleton P (1992) Clostridium botulinum toxins: a general review of involvement in disease, structure, mode of action and preparation for clinical use. J Neurol 239:16

Harris B (1997) The aromatherapy database. Research into the physiological properties of essential oils and their components. St Helier, Jersey

Heckmann M, Rzany B (2002) Botulinumtoxin in der Dermatologie. Grundlagen und praktische Anwendung, Urban and Vogel, Munich

Hoppe U, Bergemann J, Diembeck W, Ennen J, Gohla S, Harris I, Jacob J, Kielholz J, Mei W, Pollet D, Schachtschabel D, Sauermann G, Schreiner V, Stab F, Steckel F (1999) Coenzyme

Q10, a cutaneous antioxidant and energizer. BioFactors 9: 371–378

Huang W, Rogachefsky AS, Foster JA (2000) Brow-lift with botulinum toxin. Dermatol Surg 26:55–60

Kao J, Garg A, Mao-Qiang M, Crumrine D, Ghadially R, Feingold KR, Elias PM (2001) Testosterone perturbs epidermal permeability barrier homeostasis. J Invest Dermatol 116:443–451

Kavallunas DR, Nacht S, Bogardus RE (1985) Men's skin care needs. Cosmetics Toiletries 100:29–32

Kim SJ, Park JH, Carruthers A, Carruthers J (1998) Increased in vivo collagen synthesis and in vitro cell proliferative effect of glycolic acid. Dermatol Surg 24:1054

Klein AW, Wexler P, Carruthers A, Carruthers J (1997) Treatment of facial furrows and rhytides. Analysis and treatment of the aging face. Dermatol Clin 15:595–607

Klein M (2000) AHA's provide novel approach to topical rejuvenation. Dermatology Times

Krutmann J, Hansen PM (2001) New developments in photoprotection of human skin. Skin Pharmacol Appl Skin Physiol 14:401–407

Nusgens BV, Humbert P, Rougier A, Colige AC, Haftek M, Lambert CA, Richard A, Creidi P, Laoiere CM (2001) Topically applied vitamin C enhances the mRNA level of collagen I and III, their processing enzymes and tissue inhibitors of matrix metalloproteinase 1 in the human dermis. J Invest Dermatol 116:853–859

Ricciarelli R, Maroni P, Ozer N, Zingg JM, Azzi A (1999) Age-dependent increase of collagenase expression can be reduced by alpha-tocopherol via protein kinase C inhibition. Free Radic Biol Med 27:729–737

Rzarny B, Feller G (2000) Korrektur mimischer Falten: Botulinumtoxin A. Kosmetische Medizin 3:136–142

Shuster S, Black MM, Bottoms E (1970) Skin collagen and thickness in women with hirsuties. Br Med J 4:772

Shuster S, Black MM, McVitie E (1975) The influence of age and sex on skin thickness, skin collagen and density. Br J Dermatol 93:639–643

Simpson LL (1981) The origin, structure and pharmacological activity of botulinum toxin. Pharmacol Rev 33:155

Sommer B, Sattler G (1999) Botulinum A exotoxin, headache and acupuncture. Presentation at the 20th Congress of the International Society for Dermatologic Surgery, Athens, Greece

Sommer B, Sattler G (2000) Botulinumtoxin in der ästhetischen Medizin. Blackwell, Berlin

Tanaka H, Okada T, Konishi H, Tsuji T (1993) The effect of reactive oxygen species on the biosynthesis of collagen and glycosaminoglycans in cultured human dermal fibroblasts. Arch Dermatol Res 185:351–355

Vahlquist A, Lee JB, Michaelsson G, Rollman O (1982) Vitamin A in human skin: II Concentrations of carotene, retinol and dehydroretinol in various components of normal skin. J Invest Dermatol 79:94–97

Vochelle D (2004) The use of poly-L-lactic acid in the management of soft-tissue augmentation: a five-year experience. Semin Cutan Med Surg 23:223–226

Woerle B, Hanke CW, Sattler G (2004) Poly-L-lactic acid: a temporary filler for soft tissue augmentation. Drugs Dermatol 3:385–389

Subject Index

MIX
Papier aus verantwortungsvollen Quellen
Paper from responsible sources
FSC® C105338

Printed by Books on Demand, Germany